Clinical Ocular Pharmacology

Second Edition

Clinical Ocular Pharmacology

Second Edition

Editor
Jimmy D. Bartlett, O.D., D.O.S.
Professor of Optometry, Department of Optometry, School of Optometry, University of Alabama at Birmingham, Birmingham, Alabama

Associate Editor
Siret D. Jaanus, Ph.D.
Professor of Pharmacology, Department of Basic and Visual Sciences, Southern California College of Optometry, Fullerton, California

Butterworth–Heinemann
Boston London Oxford Singapore Sydney Toronto Wellington

Every effort has been made to ensure the drug dosage schedules within this text are accurate and conform to standards accepted at time of publication. However, as treatment recommendations vary in the light of continuing research and clinical experience, the reader is advised to verify drug dosage schedules herein with information found on product information sheets. This is especially true in cases of new or infrequently used drugs.

Library of Congress Cataloging-in-Publication Data

Clinical ocular pharmacology.

Includes bibliographies and index.
1. Ocular pharmacology. I. Bartlett, Jimmy D. II. Jaanus, Siret D. [DNLM: 1. Eye—drug effects. 2. Eye Diseases—drug therapy. WW 166 C641]
RE994.C55 1989 617.7′061 88–7603
ISBN 0–7506–9322–3 (previously ISBN 0–409–90058–3)

British Library Cataloguing in Publication Data

Clinical ocular pharmacology—2nd ed.
1. Ophthalmology. Pharmacology
I. Bartlett, Jimmy D. II. Jaanus, Siret D. 617.7
ISBN 0–7506–9322–3 (previously ISBN 0–409–90058–3)

Butterworth–Heinemann
80 Montvale Avenue
Stoneham, MA 02180

10 9 8 7 6 5 4

Printed in the United States of America

To our families—
Cindy, Andrew, and Kenton,
and Jaak—
whose extreme sacrifice we have deeply felt.

Contents

Contributing Authors

Larry J. Alexander, O.D.
Professor of Optometry, Department of Optometry, School of Optometry, University of Alabama at Birmingham; Chief, Special Diagnostic Procedures Clinic, School of Optometry, University of Alabama at Birmingham, Birmingham, Alabama

David M. Amos, O.D.
Private Practice, Overland Park, Kansas; Consultant, Kansas City Veterans Administration Medical Center, Kansas City, Missouri; formerly, Associate Professor of Ophthalmology, Department of Ophthalmology, University of Kansas Medical Center, Kansas City, Kansas

Jimmy D. Bartlett, O.D., D.O.S.
Professor of Optometry, Department of Optometry, School of Optometry, University of Alabama at Birmingham, Birmingham, Alabama

Neal L. Burstein, Ph.D.
Associate Adjunct Professor, Department of Ophthalmology, University of California, Irvine, California

John G. Classé, O.D., J.D.
Associate Professor of Optometry, Department of Optometry, School of Optometry, University of Alabama at Birmingham, Birmingham, Alabama; Member of the Bar of Alabama

Richard J. Clompus, O.D.
Private Practice, West Chester, Pennsylvania; Adjunct Faculty, Pennsylvania College of Optometry, Philadelphia, Pennsylvania

Anthony P. Cullen, M.Sc., O.D., Ph.D., F.B.C.O.
Professor of Optometry, School of Optometry, University of Waterloo, Waterloo, Ontario, Canada; formerly, Associate Professor and Chief of Pathology Clinic, College of Optometry, University of Houston, Houston, Texas; formerly, Clinical Lecturer in Ophthalmology, College of Medicine, University of Saskatchewan, Saskatoon, Saskatchewan, Canada

J. Boyd Eskridge, O.D., M.Opt., M.Sc., Ph.D.
Professor of Optometry, Department of Optometry, School of Optometry, University of Alabama at Birmingham, Birmingham, Alabama

Murray Fingeret, O.D.
Chief, Optometry Section, St. Albans, New York Veterans Administration Extended Care Center, Brooklyn Veterans Administration Medical Center; Assistant Clinical Professor of Optometry, College of Optometry, State University of New York, New York, New York; Adjunct Assistant Professor of Optometry, Pennsylvania College of Optometry, Philadelphia, Pennsylvania

Eduardo Gaitan, M.D.
Professor of Medicine, School of Medicine, University of Mississippi, Jackson, Mississippi; Chief, Endocrinology Section, Jackson Veterans Administration Medical Center, Jackson, Mississippi; Attending Physician, University Hospital, University of Mississippi Medical Center, Jackson, Mississippi

Sally L. Hegeman, M.S., Ph.D.
Associate Professor of Pharmacology, Department of Visual Sciences, School of Optometry, Indiana University, Bloomington, Indiana; Adjunct Associate Professor of Pharmacology, Department of Pharmacology, School of Medicine, Indiana University

Jeffrey A. Hiett, O.D., M.S.
Chief, Optometry Program, American Lake Veterans

Administration Medical Center, Tacoma, Washington; Adjunct Assistant Clinical Professor of Optometry, College of Optometry, Pacific University, Forest Grove, Oregon

Siret D. Jaanus, Ph.D.
Professor of Pharmacology, Department of Basic and Visual Sciences, Southern California College of Optometry, Fullerton, California

William L. Jones, O.D.
Chief, Optometry Section, Veterans Administration Medical Center, Albuquerque, New Mexico; Clinical Instructor, Department of Surgery, School of Medicine, University of New Mexico; Adjunct Professor of Optometry, College of Optometry, University of Houston, Houston, Texas

Gerald E. Lowther, O.D., M.Sc., Ph.D.
Professor of Optometry, College of Optometry, Ferris State University, Big Rapids, Michigan; Chief, Contact Lens Service, College of Optometry, Ferris State University

Robert D. Newcomb, O.D., M.P.H.
Chief, Optometry Service, Veterans Administration Outpatient Clinic, Columbus, Ohio; Clinical Assistant Professor of Optometry, College of Optometry, The Ohio State University, Columbus, Ohio

Vincent T. Pagano, M.S., Ph.D.
Associate Professor of Pharmacology, Department of Biological Sciences, College of Optometry, State University of New York, New York, New York

John W. Potter, O.D.
Vice President and Clinical Director, VisionAmerica, Nashville, Tennessee; Adjunct Faculty, Southern College of Optometry, Memphis, Tennessee; Adjunct Faculty, Southern California College of Optometry, Fullerton, California; Distinguished Clinical Scholar, College of Optometry, State University of New York, New York, New York

Marlon L. Priest, M.D.
Associate Professor, Division of Emergency Services, Department of Surgery, School of Medicine,

University of Alabama at Birmingham, Birmingham, Alabama; Medical Director, Emergency Department, University Hospital, University of Alabama at Birmingham; Assistant Dean, University of Alabama School of Medicine

Leo Semes, O.D.
Associate Professor of Optometry, Department of Optometry, School of Optometry, University of Alabama at Birmingham, Birmingham, Alabama; Chief, Primary Care Vision Services, School of Optometry, University of Alabama at Birmingham; Director, Office of Continuing Education, School of Optometry, University of Alabama at Birmingham

Jack E. Terry, M.S., O.D.
Chief, Optometry Section, Surgical Service, Veterans Administration Medical Center, Huntington, West Virginia; Adjunct Assistant Professor of Pharmacology, School of Medicine, Marshall University, Huntington, West Virginia; Clinical Assistant Professor of Optometry, School of Optometry, Indiana University, Bloomington, Indiana; Adjunct Assistant Professor of Optometry, Pennsylvania College of Optometry, Philadelphia, Pennsylvania

William Wallace IV, O.D.
Vice President and Director of Professional Services, MediVision, Inc., Atlanta, Georgia; formerly, Director, Omni Eye Services of Atlanta, Atlanta, Georgia

David R. Whikehart, Ph.D.
Associate Professor of Physiological Optics, Department of Physiological Optics, School of Optometry, University of Alabama at Birmingham, Birmingham, Alabama; Associate Professor of Biochemistry, Department of Biochemistry, School of Medicine, University of Alabama at Birmingham

Diane P. Yolton, O.D., Ph.D.
Associate Professor, College of Optometry, Pacific University, Forest Grove, Oregon

Preface

The enthusiastic acceptance of *Clinical Ocular Pharmacology* has confirmed our belief that the approach to ocular pharmacology should be in the context of clinical practice, and that, as a distinct discipline, it should include strong emphasis in three fundamentally important areas—the actions of ocular drugs, drug use in clinical practice, and toxicology. The more basic concepts underlying the pharmacology of ocular drugs establish the foundation for their ultimate use in patient care. Moreover, since drugs are not used in isolation, it is important to stress adjunctive procedures that accompany the use of ocular pharmaceutical agents. To this end, we continue in this edition to emphasize both the diagnostic and therapeutic clinical procedures that have as their foundation the administration of drugs to the eye. Our purpose is to provide practical, clinically useful information based on currently accepted scientific principles and standards of practice.

For clarity of presentation the book has been expanded into five major parts. Substantial reorganization of the material in Part I should allow a better appreciation of ophthalmic drug formulations and routes of administration before considering the individual drug groups in Part II. We have attempted, throughout the text, to reduce redundancy and to make the discussions as concise as possible while still covering the salient features of each topic. Although difficult to accomplish in a multiauthored work, we have attempted to ensure consistency by adopting a standard format of presentation. Each of the chapters in Part II (Pharmacology of Ocular Drugs) discusses, where appropriate, the pharmacology, clinical uses, side effects, and contraindications of each drug. Each chapter in Part III (Ocular Drugs in Clinical Practice) considers, where appropriate, the etiology, diagnosis, and management of the clinical conditions for which ophthalmic drugs are indicated.

Every chapter has been extensively revised, with several being completely rewritten, to reflect the rapid development of the science of ocular pharmacology as well as the art of ocular drug use in clinical practice. New commercially available drugs and ocular devices are an important part of the text, and Part IV (Toxicology) has been greatly expanded to include virtually all major drug groups that are well documented to affect the eye and vision system. A section of color plates has been added to enhance both the quality and accuracy of represented clinical conditions and drug therapies. Part V (Legal Aspects of Drug Utilization) is new to this edition and attempts to set forth the relevant legal principles involving the use of drugs in patient care. A new feature of the Index is the inclusion of drug trade names typed in capital letters, which should allow easier recognition of commercially available products.

We are extremely delighted to welcome five new contributing authors, whose combination of exceptional talent and enthusiasm has culminated in chapters that are both timely and lucid. Our burden was made considerably lighter by the splendid cooperation shown by every contributor, for which we are most thankful.

The timely completion of this project would have been impossible without the strong support and encouragement from our families, friends, and colleagues. We are deeply grateful for the expert secretarial and word processing skills of Kim Humphreys, Pat Humpres, Affie Martin, Carolyn Rickels, and Glenda J. Sitland, who cheerfully and skillfully completed the arduous task of typing and preparing revisions for a manuscript exceeding 2000 pages. Patricia Carlson and Beth Laughlin were unfailing in their careful attention to exhaustive literature searches and other reference services. Cindy Bartlett, Ann Richardson, Beth Baker, and Dr. Brad Middaugh provided invaluable technical assistance, and Kim Washington contributed important clinical photographic support. We are especially indebted to Ken Norris, who helped to create and develop most of the new line drawings and graphics. Making significant contributions to the preparation of Chapter 6 (Anti-Infective Drugs) were Toni Chronister, Linda Coppedge, Alyson Harper, Carol Johnson, Laurel Gregory, Vickie Kelly, Douglas Melzer, Silvia Mende, Jan Merrell, Donna Rubrecht, and Alaina Softing.

We sincerely thank Barbara Murphy, whose motivating spirit confirmed the outstanding commitment of our publisher to this project. We were most fortunate to have the superb writing skills of our copy editor, Ann Calandro, whose contributions resulted in a considerably more readable text. And most of all we are particularly grateful for the insights and suggestions provided by our students and residents, and by practitioners and other users of this book, whose perspective has guided us in the preparation of this edition. It is to these individuals, and to their patients, that this book is directed.

JDB
SDJ

Preface to the First Edition

The evolution of health care is measured, in part, by the development of clinical knowledge and by the specific clinical procedures that become salient features of contemporary health care practice. Recent advances in eye care technology serve as valid testimony that this evolution does indeed occur. Just as health care practices in general have become more sophisticated and specialized, the diagnosis and management of ocular disorders in particular reflects this trend to specialization with the proliferation of numerous secondary and tertiary level procedures and services.

With this emphasis on specialization and sophisticated technology, the generalist who serves the eye has become increasingly more frustrated with his or her apparent abandonment and isolation. The generalist is being called upon to care for a greater variety of eye problems, yet has not had an appropriate literature available that addresses his or her needs as a sophisticated primary care practitioner.

Clinical Ocular Pharmacology has been written for optometry students and residents, practicing optometrists, family practice physicians, pediatricians, and other primary care practitioners who are in need of a text that can be used as a practical guide for the clinical utilization of ophthalmic drugs. Ophthalmology residents and practitioners of ophthalmology will find the book useful as an updated source of information regarding the contemporary use of ophthalmic drugs for ocular conditions commonly encountered in office practice.

Our goal has been to produce a book that emphasizes the clinical uses of ophthalmic drugs in the diagnosis and management of those ocular disorders most commonly encountered in primary care practice. To achieve this goal we have felt it first necessary to discuss in Section I the basic pharmacologic principles that govern the various classes of ophthalmic drugs. The reader will find here a discussion of those pharmacologic agents that have been demonstrated by their longevity to be useful in the diagnosis and treatment of ocular disease. Drugs that have only recently been introduced into contemporary practice are also considered, including pimaricin, timolol maleate, dipivalyl epinephrine, cytosine arabinoside, trifluorothymidine, and others. In addition to those drugs normally used in the diagnosis and treatment of ocular disease, Chapter 12 considers the preparations utilized in contact lens practice. Throughout Section I, lists of commercially available drugs have been prepared to represent agents commonly employed in clinical practice.

Section II considers the pharmacologic diagnosis and management of ocular disorders according to tissue site or clinical problem. This format and approach should be of greatest value to the student, resident, or practitioner who uses the text as a reference in the clinic, hospital, or office. Emphasis has been placed on both the diagnostic as well as the therapeutic uses of ophthalmic drugs in the context of total patient management and care. This approach allows the reader to better appreciate the utilization of ocular drugs as these drugs are used in clinical practice. Strong emphasis is therefore placed on etiology and differential diagnosis of those conditions discussed, for the effective and safe use of drugs for the treatment of ocular disease requires accurate and timely diagnostic skills as well as appreciation of the causes of those disorders. Where other, nonpharmacologic management modalities are employed, such as surgical or physical therapy, these have been mentioned so that the pharmacologic considerations are placed in proper perspective. The editors believe that this approach serves to better define and teach the relationship of ocular drug therapy to total patient care.

As more sophisticated methods are used in the clinical trials for ocular drugs, numerous side effects are being recognized. We consider in Section III important clinical aspects of drug toxicity. While Sections I and II discuss the important side effects of ocular drugs on the eye, Section III is designed to complement that discussion by considering adverse ocular effects of systemically administered drugs as well as the systemic side effects of drugs applied topically to the eye. The epidemiology and management of the latter group of side effects are considered in Chapter 30.

Throughout the text generic names of drugs are used, and these are occasionally followed in parentheses by proprietary names if a particular preparation is especially common or is the only preparation commercially available.

Because of the multiauthored nature of this text, some redundancy of material is inevitable. However, the editors have attempted to minimize redundancy by referring the reader, where appropriate, to other sections or chapters of the text. In this way completeness of individual discussions has been ensured while making the text as concise as possible.

The timely completion of this project would have been impossible without the able assistance, support, or encouragement from numerous individuals. We acknowledge the many hours of typing and preparation of the manuscript by Judy Badstuebner, Doris Caldwell, Hazel Davis, Dorinda Finke, Richard Hawkins, Debbie Hicks, Kim Humphreys, Pat Humpres, Margo Jeffrey, and Ann Simpson. This laborious task was accomplished speedily and with great skill.

The accuracy of many of the bibliographic citations and other reference services were provided by Patricia Carlson and Nancy Clemmons.

Ronald Amaker, John Carswell, Richard Morrison, and Danny Musick provided much of the clinical photography, and the editors express special gratitude to Ken Norris, whose artistic pen created many of the line drawings and graphics.

Dr. JoAnn Graffeo, Dr. Dennis Matthews, Allison Hendrick, and Ann Honeycutt contributed expert technical assistance.

The editors owe deep gratitude to Drs. Robert F. Furchgott, Alden N. Haffner, Richard L. Hopping, and Ronald P. Rubin for their unfailing faith and support. A special appreciation is due to Dr. John F. Amos, who provided continuous encouragement and direction.

Finally, the individuals who brought this book from an idea to a reality deserve special acknowledgment— the contributing authors, whose work constitutes the essence of the final product; the numerous optometrists, pharmacologists, and physicians who reviewed portions of the manuscript and offered helpful comments and suggestions; our students and faculty colleagues, whose encouragement and patience created a supportive environment in which to work; our spouses, whom we asked to endure the preparation of this book; and the publisher, whose interest in, and constant support of this project led to an exciting and satisfying publishing experience.

Jimmy D. Bartlett
Siret D. Jaanus

PART I

Fundamental Concepts in Ocular Pharmacology

There is no great danger in our mistaking the height of the sun, or the fraction of some astronomical computation; but here where our whole being is concerned, 'tis not wisdom to abandon ourselves to the mercy of the agitation of so many contrary winds.

—Hippocrates

CHAPTER 1

Basic Science of Ocular Pharmacology

Neal L. Burstein

Drugs affect ocular tissues based on the eye's special pharmacokinetic properties. Pharmacokinetics is the study of the time course of absorption, distribution, metabolism, and elimination of an administered drug.[1] Drug absorption depends on the drug's molecular properties, the viscosity of its vehicle, and the functional status of the tissue forming the barrier to penetration.[2] Drug distribution over time and bioavailability at the desired site of action can usually be predicted by the interrelationships of the eye's compartments and barriers.[3] Metabolism plays an important part in eliminating drugs and their sometimes toxic by-products from the eye and from the body.[4] Metabolic enzymes have recently been studied to assist in the design of prodrugs, molecules that are converted to an active form after tissue penetration has occurred.[5]

This chapter considers the unique structural aspects of ocular tissues as they relate to pharmacokinetics. Compartment models will be shown as an aid to understanding the path and time course followed by drugs in the eye. Receptor theory will be discussed, together with examples to illustrate how two drugs can compete for the same site of action. Examples of how ocular drugs are designed and formulated to enhance bioavailability will also be considered.

Physicochemical Factors Affecting Drug Bioavailability

Medicinal chemistry involves the study of existing drugs and the design and synthesis of molecules with im-proved activity, bioavailability, toxicity, and other characteristics. An understanding of any drug's action is based on analysis of its quantitative structure-activity relationships, which are unique to each molecular structure. Computer analysis of these relationships and of three-dimensional molecular conformations has contributed to rapid development in this field. Some of the quantifiable properties used in evaluating molecular drugs for therapeutic consideration are described below.

Solubility and Partition Coefficient

Molecular diffusion through cell membranes can occur by two major pathways.[6] The first is entry through the lipid portion of the membrane by lipophilic ("fat-loving") compounds. The second is diffusion through "water pores" in the membrane by hydrophilic ("water-loving") compounds. Since the cell membrane is largely composed of lipids, there are few restrictions on the penetration of lipophilic compounds, even considering molecular size. Hydrophilic compounds, in contrast, are more limited in diffusion except where an extracellular fluid pathway exists for transport.[7] The hydrophilic versus lipophilic migrational tendencies of a compound, as well as its absolute solubilities in each phase, greatly affect its pharmacokinetics.[8]

A useful expression for the relative lipophilic versus hydrophilic nature of a molecule is the octanol-water partition coefficient (OWPC). In a simple test, a molecular species is suspended and well stirred in a flask containing equal portions of buffered water and octanol. Organic solutes such as hexane are sometimes substituted for octanol as the lipid phase. The pH of the buffer is important, since it affects the partitioning of a weak acid or base. After equilibrium occurs, the two phases are each analyzed for concentration of the test species. The result is expressed as the log of concentration ratios between octanol and water. A wide range of solubilities in aqueous and lipid phases can be expressed by the coefficient derived from this method.[8,9]

Molecular Size and Shape

Molecular size is often less important than the molecular charge and partitioning characteristics in determining ocular drug penetration.[9] However, very large molecules are sterically hindered by their bulk, which impedes their diffusion through narrow spaces.[3] The size of a globular molecule increases as the cube root of the molecular weight, which is usually expressed in Daltons. The water of solvation surrounding a charged molecule must be considered in determining the total size for diffusion calculations. The diffusion coefficient decreases with increasing molecular size. The molecular configuration becomes important for proteins and other macromolecules, where the shape can vary from a folded globular form to an elongate helix.

In ophthalmic medications, the concentration of the active drug is usually expressed as a percentage. However, a high molecular weight compound will be present at a lower molarity than a smaller molecule when both are supplied at the same percentage. Some commercially available compounds that have similar active sites but have different groups substituted in the inactive portions of the molecule are supplied at concentrations that appear to be the same on a weight basis but vary considerably in molarity due to the difference in molecular size or in the size of the inactive ion.

Dissociation Constant

Any drug that is at least partially water soluble will ionize to a degree dependent on the molecule's ionizable groups and the solute's pH. Many ophthalmic drugs with charged groups act as weak bases. An example is pilocarpine hydrochloride, which undergoes hydrolysis to an equilibrium dependent on the hydrogen ion concentration, as follows:[10]

$$C_{11}H_{16}N_2O_2HCl \rightarrow C_{11}H_{16}N_2O_2H^+$$
Pilocarpine HCl   Pilocarpine ion

$$+ \quad Cl^-$$
Chloride ion   (1.1)

$$C_{11}H_{16}N_2O_2H^+ + HOH \rightarrow C_{11}H_{16}N_2O_2HOH$$
Pilocarpine ion   Pilocarpine base

$$+ \quad H^+$$
Hydrogen ion   (1.2)

The pK_b of a base is the pH at which 50% of the molecule is dissociated. Table 1.1 shows the pK_b for several ophthalmic drugs. At a pH lower than the pK_b, more than half the weak base is dissociated. Figure 1.1 shows the ion-base equilibrium of these drugs. Drugs such as pilocarpine that are present in both base and ionic forms at ocular pH penetrate most ocular barriers readily. When a drug is biologically active but has difficulty reaching its site of action, adjusting the dissociation constant by modifying ionizable groups can markedly alter drug penetration.[10] However, it is not practical to make the pH of formulations lower than 4 or higher than 10. The effects of pH on the storage properties and comfort of ophthalmic formulations are discussed later in this chapter.

TABLE 1.1
Percentage of Free Base in Equilibrium with Salts of Alkaloids

Drug	pK_b	pH 4.0	pH 7.4	pH 9.0
Atropine	4.35	0.0002	0.6	18.3
Ephedrine	4.64	0.0004	1.1	30.4
Procaine	5.15	0.001	3.4	58.5
Cocaine	5.59	0.004	8.9	79.6
Pilocarpine	7.15	0.141	78.1	99.3

From Hind HW, Goyan FM. A new concept of the role of hydrogen ion concentration and buffer systems in the preparation of ophthalmic solutions. J Am Pharm Assoc 1947;36:33–41.

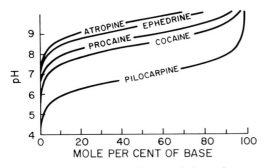

FIGURE 1.1 **The ion-base equilibrium of drugs that are weak bases is plotted as a function of pH. The pK$_b$ is the pH at which 50% of the drug is ionized (see Table 1.1 for numerical values). (Modified from Hind HW, Goyan FM. A new concept of the role of hydrogen ion concentration and buffer systems in the preparation of ophthalmic solutions. J Am Pharm Assoc 1947;36:33–41.)**

Ocular Tissue Structure and Pharmacokinetics

The eye is composed of numerous tissues, each of distinct developmental origin, and each with a specific role in the functioning visual system. These tissues include the smooth and striate musculature, a variety of simple and mucoid epithelia, connective tissues, sympathetic and parasympathetic nerves, and the retina. The retina itself is often considered a direct extension of the brain, since together with the optic nerve it is formed from an outfolding of the embryonic neural tube.

The organization of the eye must provide a path for light through the clear tissues that form the optical imaging system, while providing for the nutrition of those same tissues in the absence of a blood supply. This avascularity allows a direct route for ocular drug penetration without absorption by the systemic circulation.

In this section, some special properties of each of the eye's clear axial components will be discussed, together with their nutritional and metabolite exchange through the adjoining vascular tissues. A model will then be developed wherein the ocular tissues and fluids function as barriers and depots. Such a model can be useful in predicting ocular distribution of drugs over time.

Tear Structure and Chemical Properties

The tear film covering the cornea and defining the major optical surface of the eye is composed of three layers[11,12] (see Fig. 10.1). The outermost, oily layer is usually considered to be a lipid monolayer and is pro-

duced primarily by the meibomian glands located in the eyelids. The primary function of the oily layer is to stabilize the surface of the underlying aqueous fluid layer and retard evaporation. Tear surface lipids are readily washed away if the eye is flushed with saline or medication, resulting in a tear evaporation increase of more than tenfold.[13] Minor infections of the meibomian glands, particularly *Staphylococcus,* can also decrease tear film stability. This is due to an alteration of the chemical nature of meibum, the secretion product of the gland.

The aqueous phase of the tears comprises more than 95% of the total volume and covers the cornea with a layer that averages about 7 µm thick. This layer is inherently unstable, however, and begins to thin centrally at the end of each blink. The tear film in healthy subjects has a breakup time (BUT) that averages between 25 and 30 seconds.[14]

The inner, or basal, layer of the tears is composed of glycoproteins and is secreted by goblet cells in the conjunctiva. This mucinous layer is present both as a thin hydrophilic coating covering the cornea and conjunctiva and as thick rolls and strands that cleanse the tears of particulate debris at each blink (Fig. 1.2).[15] The pH of the tears is about 7.4,[16] and the tear layer contains small amounts of protein including lysozyme, lactoferrins, gammaglobulins, and other immune factors. The tears are primarily responsible for supplying the oxygen requirements of the corneal epithelium.

Tear Volume

The normal volume of the tear layer is 8 to 10 µl, including the fluid trapped in the folds of the conjunctiva.[17] A total volume of perhaps 30 µl can be held for a brief time if the eyelids are not squeezed after dosing. When a single drop of medication of 50 µl (1/20 ml) is applied, the nasolacrimal duct rapidly drains the excess. Increasing drop size, therefore, does not result in more medication penetrating the cornea.[18] However, the systemic load is increased linearly with drop size, since after drainage through the nasolacrimal duct the drug is usually absorbed through the nasal mucosa or swallowed. For drugs with major systemic side effects, such as β blockers, efforts have been made to limit drop size.[19] A metering dispenser delivering small drops (25 µl) has been introduced to decrease the ratio of systemic to ocular effect. Such a device, however, cannot take the place of careful supervision during initial dosing and monitoring of patient compliance.[20]

It is difficult to limit the volume of a drop dispensed by gravity from a dropper tip below about 25 µl, three times the normal tear reservoir. Chrai and associates[21] have proposed that the theoretical optimum volume of

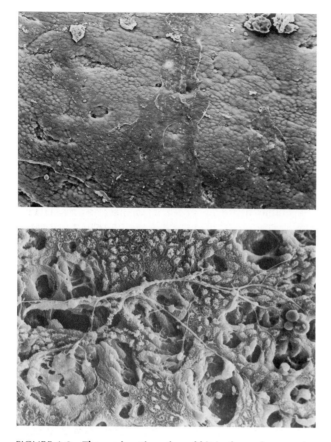

FIGURE 1.2 **The conjunctiva of a rabbit is shown by scanning electron microscopy with surface mucins intact. Note the sheets and folds that allow the mucins to entrap particles and remove them from the tears. The tears form a reservoir for drug compounds, including those that are delivered as particulate suspensions. (From Burstein NL. The effects of topical drugs and preservatives on the tears and corneal epithelium in dry eye. Trans Ophthalmol Soc UK 1985;104:402–409.)**

drug solution to deliver is zero volume, since increasing the instilled volume increases the volume lost and the percentage of drug lost. Although this theoretical extreme is impossible to achieve, it is practical to dispense accurately measured drops as small as 2 μl from a micrometer syringe by touching a flexible polyethylene tip to the conjunctiva (Color Plate I). For investigational purposes this allows instillation of drugs without greatly affecting size of the tear reservoir. The use of a mirror allows simple and convenient self-dosing using this means.

Tear Flow

The normal rate of basal (unstimulated) tear flow in humans is about 0.5 to 2.2 μl/min and decreases with age.[22] Tear flow rate is stimulated by the ocular irritation resulting from many topical medications. The concentration of drug available in the tears for transcorneal absorption is inversely proportional to the tear flow, due to the drug's dilution and removal by the nasolacrimal duct and by lid spillover. Therefore, both the flow rate and tear volume influence drug absorption by the anterior segment of the eye.[23]

When corneal absorption of a drug must be increased, a high tear film concentration can be prolonged by manually blocking the nasolacrimal ducts or by tilting the head back to reduce drainage.[24] Another effective technique to increase corneal penetration is to give a series of drops at intervals of about 10 minutes.[18] The size of the drops delivered has far less effect on ocular absorption than the repetition of doses. It has been determined that when several drops are given in rapid succession, the medications first applied are diluted and do not achieve full therapeutic potential.[21]

Patients with a flow rate near the lower limit of 0.5 μl/min, often due to aging or atrophy of the lacrimal ducts and glands, are usually considered to have dry eye (keratoconjunctivitis sicca).[25] This group includes many elderly patients, individuals with rheumatoid arthritis, some postmenopausal women, and persons with exposure keratitis associated with dry climate or dusty work conditions.[15] Several factors contribute to greatly increased drug absorption in these individuals. Their total tear volume is less than normal, so that a drop of medication is not diluted as much as usual. Because lacrimation is reduced, the drug is not rapidly diluted by tears and has a prolonged residence time next to the corneal surface, where the majority of absorption occurs. Since epithelial surface damage is usually present in patients with dry eye, the final result is greatly increased ocular absorption.

Drugs (e.g., pilocarpine) that cause rapid lacrimation by stinging or by stimulation of lacrimal glands in normal individuals, are formulated at high concentration to offset the dilution and washout that occur from tear flow. Patients with dry eyes, who do not lacrimate readily, can absorb greatly exaggerated doses of such medications. In children, who cry and lacrimate more easily than adults, rapid drug washout can prevent adequate absorption of topically applied medications.

Cornea and Sclera

The cornea is a five-layered, avascular structure[26] (Fig. 1.3). It comprises the major functional barrier to ocular penetration, and it is also the major site of absorption for topically applied drugs. The epithelium and stroma have a major influence on pharmacodynamics, since

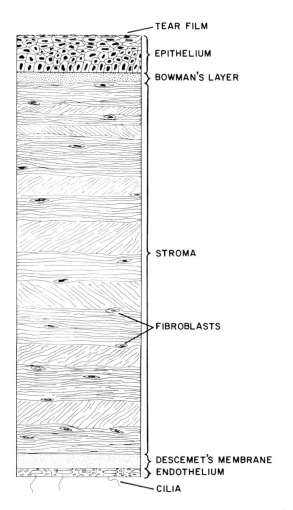

TEAR FILM

EPITHELIUM

BOWMAN'S LAYER

STROMA

FIBROBLASTS

DESCEMET'S MEMBRANE
ENDOTHELIUM

CILIA

FIGURE 1.3 **Cross-sectional diagram of the cornea. Note the epithelium is only about one-tenth the total corneal mass. Nevertheless, it can be considered a separate storage depot for certain lipophilic drugs.**

they constitute depots or reservoirs for lipophilic and hydrophilic drugs, respectively.

The sclera is an opaque, vascular structure continuous with the cornea at the limbus. The loose connective tissue overlying the sclera, the conjunctiva, is also vascularized. The conjunctiva and sclera, as routes of drug penetration, are responsible for less than one-fifth of all drug absorption to the iris and ciliary body. This is due to the extensive vascularization of these tissues, which results in removal of most drugs.[27,28] An elegant visualization of the route of scleral penetration was achieved by Bienfang,[29] who applied a piece of filter paper moistened with epinephrine to the white of the eye in a human subject. He was able to obtain mydriasis in an isolated sector of iris adjacent to the site of scleral application.

The conjunctival sac forms a large area, about 32 cm^2 for both eyes. Its surface functions as a major depot for some drugs that are superficially absorbed, then rereleased to the tears. Trapped particles from a suspension may allow active drug to dissolve slowly from the conjunctival sac and saturate tear drug levels.[30]

CORNEAL EPITHELIUM

The corneal epithelium is 5 to 6 cell-layers thick centrally, with 8 to 10 layers at the periphery. It is composed of a basal germinative layer, intermediate wing cells, and a surface squamous layer that possesses structures known as *zonula occludens,* or tight junctions. These junctions comprise a continuing border between epithelial cells formed by the fusion of the outer plasma membrane.[31] Mucopolysaccharides bound to the outer plasma membrane, shown in Figure 1.4A, stabilize the tears. The cornea relies on diffusion of nutrients from the aqueous humor to supply its metabolic needs.[16]

Over half the total corneal electrical resistance is contained in the uppermost squamous cell layer.[32] Since the epithelium in its healthy state presents a continuous layer of plasma membrane to the tear film, as shown in Figure 1.4B, it largely resists the penetration of hydrophilic drugs.[33] The anionic diagnostic agent, sodium fluorescein, is a good example. The amount of fluorescein penetrating the intact epithelium is small. If a slight break in the outer cellular layer occurs, then fluorescein can penetrate easily and is visible as a green stain for several minutes in the beam of a blue excitation filter. Epithelial erosion or the action of cationic preservatives can greatly increase the penetration of hydrophilic drugs in the same manner.

The interstices between the epithelial cell layers communicate directly by an aqueous pathway with the stroma and aqueous humor. This has been demonstrated by Tonjum,[34] who injected horseradish peroxidase, an enzyme used experimentally as a molecular tracer, into aqueous humor. It diffused readily across the entire cornea and accumulated adjacent to the epithelial tight junctional complex, where it was blocked from passage to the tear side. When applied to the tears, however, it did not penetrate the outer corneal layer.

Lipophilic drugs can readily enter the epithelium, since its barrier is composed of phospholipid membranes.[35] Since the epithelium contains more than two-thirds of the plasma membrane mass of the cornea, it is the most significant storage depot for agents that readily partition into lipid media. The release rate of drugs from the epithelium depends on their tendency to reenter an aqueous phase. Thus, agents that are very lipophilic have a very long half-life once in the

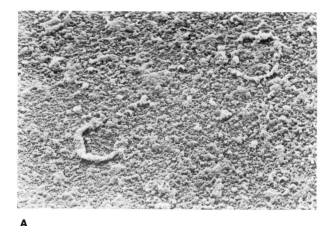

A

B

FIGURE 1.4   **Scanning electron micrographs of the corneal epithelium of a rabbit. *(A)* Mucins are fixed in place as they are normally, to stabilize the tear film. The pits seen in the photograph are normal for rabbits and are not present in humans. *(B)* The mucins are washed away by acetylcysteine to reveal the underlying pattern of microvilli and microplicae visible on the cell surface. (From Burstein NL. The effects of topical drugs and preservatives on the tears and corneal epithelium in dry eye. Trans Ophthalmol Soc UK 1985;104:402–409.)**

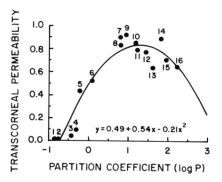

FIGURE 1.5   **Parabolic curve of corneal penetration versus octanol-water partition coefficient. As the drug becomes too lipophilic or too hydrophilic, penetration through the cornea is diminished. Reagent properties are given in Table 1.2. (Adapted from Kishida K, Otori T. Quantitative study on the relationship between transcorneal permeability of drugs and their hydrophobicity. Jpn J Ophthalmol 1980;24:251–259.)**

epithelium. Cyclosporins, for example, have a half-life of about 24 hours in epithelium and are effective when administered topically every 48 hours, since they have sufficient biologic activity to remain effective at the very low levels released from the cornea.[36]

To penetrate the cornea effectively, a drug must possess a balance of hydrophilic and lipophilic properties and must be able to partition between both media. This phenomenon is well known through the study of series of compounds of similar properties, such as β blockers.[37] A plot of partition coefficient versus corneal permeability usually results in the formation of a parabola.[8] An example is shown in Figure 1.5 (see also Table 1.2).[37] Molecular species with the appropriate partition coefficient at or near the peak are thus readily transferred through the cornea. Those with too low a coefficient do not penetrate well through the outer epithelial barrier. Those with too high a partition coefficient tend to remain in the epithelium and partition into the anterior chamber slowly, resulting in low but prolonged aqueous humor levels.[8]

CORNEAL STROMA

Bowman's layer is the modified outer border of stroma in humans. This layer is 8 to 14 μm thick and is composed of clear, randomly oriented collagen fibrils surrounded by mucoprotein ground substance.[26,38] Numerous pores in the inner structure allow the passage of terminal branches of corneal nerves from the stroma into epithelium. The surface of Bowman's layer adjoins the structurally distinct epithelial basal lamina. The drug penetration characteristics of Bowman's layer are probably similar to those of the stroma.

The stroma occupies 90% of the corneal thickness and contains about one-third of the cells of the cornea in the form of keratocytes, modified fibroblasts. The connective tissue of the stroma is composed of multiple layers of closely knit collagen bundles, or lamellae, arranged to distribute evenly the stress of the intraocular pressure to the limbus, the thickened zone that joins the cornea and sclera. The collagen bundles are hexagonally packed and more ordered in the cornea than in the sclera, and their organization, together with the interspersed proteoglycans, is largely responsible for the clarity of the cornea.[39] In the adult a small number of keratocytes is interspersed among the lamellae.

The collagen fibrils occupy space and also increase the path of diffusion, with the net effect of impeding

TABLE 1.2
Corneal Permeability and Properties of Some Reagents

No. Reagent (see Fig 1.5)	Molecular Weight (Daltons)	Partition Coefficient (Log P)	Transcorneal Permeability (μ mol)
1 Ethanolamine	61.1	−0.846	0.013
2 Sulfanilamide	172.2	−0.756	0.013
3 p-Aminobenzamide	136.2	−0.441	0.043
4 p-Aminoacetanilide	150.2	−0.308	0.094
5 p-Aminobenzylalcohol	123.1	−0.215	0.436
6 p-Aminophenylethanol	137.2	0.103	0.519
7 p-Methoxyaniline	123.2	0.807	0.909
8 p-Aminoacetophenone	135.2	0.829	0.838
9 Aniline	93.1	0.950	0.923
10 2,5-Dimethoxyaniline	153.2	1.198	0.859
11 p-Ethoxyaniline	137.2	1.240	0.792
12 p-Toluidine	107.2	1.445	0.775
13 Methylenedianiline	198.3	1.618	0.639
14 p-Chloroaniline	127.6	1.825	0.895

Adapted from Kishida K, Otori T. Quantitative study on the relationship between transcorneal permeability of drugs and their hydrophobicity. Jpn J Ophthalmol 1980;24:251–259.

diffusion by the equivalent of a fluid layer several times the actual stromal thickness. Nevertheless, the stroma is transparent to molecular species below about 500,000 Daltons.[3] The stroma serves as the major ocular depot for topically applied hydrophilic drugs, and the keratocytes presumably provide a reservoir for lipophilic compounds as well.

The inner border of the stroma is the endothelial basal lamina, termed Descemet's layer. Approximately 3 to 4 μm thick at birth, it becomes about 10 to 12 μm thick by 50 years of age. It is highly elastic and is formed of prenatal banded collagen and unbanded collagen secreted after birth by the endothelium. Descemet's layer stains distinctly periodic acid–Schiff (PAS) positive because of the presence of carbohydrate not found in stroma and has a structural pattern evident in cross-section that is not present in any other known tissue.[26,40] Descemet's layer appears to pass molecular species as readily as the stroma and is not known to act as a separate drug depot.

CORNEAL ENDOTHELIUM

The corneal endothelium, a monolayer of polygonal cells about 3 μm thick,[41] has a structure and properties unique in the body. It should not be confused with the blood vessel endothelium, which is of different developmental origin and has different characteristics. The nonregenerative property of the corneal endothelium requires that existing cells stretch to cover the space of any neighbors that are destroyed by physical damage or that senesce. The endothelial cell layer has the remarkable ability to pump its own weight in fluid in 5 minutes out from the stromal side into the anterior chamber. The intercellular borders form a junction that is open along its full length and that allows a rapid leakage of water and solutes in the reverse direction to the fluid pump.[40,42]

The fluid pump is probably a bicarbonate-based ion transport, which may be coupled to Na^+-K^+ ATPase by an unknown mechanism.[43,44] The leak is composed of a channel 12 μm long and 20 nm wide, narrowing to 5.0 nm at the edge facing the anterior chamber.[45] This space is large enough to conduct large molecules, such as 3.5 nm diameter colloidal gold and colloidal lanthanum particles as shown in Figure 1.6. The ultrastructure and ability to pass large molecules make the endothelial border a special type of leaky junction, rather than a tight junction (*zonula occludens*) as sometimes stated. Globular proteins above 1,000,000 Daltons cannot pass readily, but smaller molecules are not hindered. Pinocytosis does occur in the endothelium and allows the transport of high molecular weight proteins. Because of the thinness and small volume of the endothelial layer, it is not considered a major reservoir for drugs.[3]

The cornea can concentrate certain substances from the aqueous, allowing the corneal stroma to hold more drug than would be expected from its fluid mass. This may result from the constant inward leakage of whole aqueous from the anterior chamber to the stroma, offset by the return of osmotic water by the fluid pump. Fluorescein given by mouth or vein will thus accumulate rapidly in the corneal stroma from the aqueous.

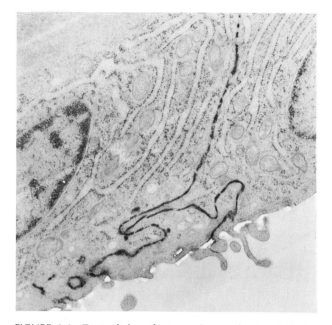

FIGURE 1.6 **Transmission electron micrograph of endothelial cells showing a border between two cells. The dense material is lanthanum, which was added 1 minute before the tissue was fixed by rapid freezing. The area of cytoplasm bordering cells at bottom center is probably an interdigitation from one of the two cells.**

An alternative explanation for this accumulation is the ionic binding of substances by negative charges in stroma, reducing the diffusible pool of solute. However, since fluorescein is itself an anion, this explanation is not fully satisfactory.[3]

Iris

The iris functions primarily to adjust the amount of light reaching the retina, simultaneously altering the visual depth of focus without changing the field of vision. It does this by controlling the total area of the visual pathway between the two major refractive components of the eye—the cornea and lens. It therefore contains pigment to absorb light. To accomplish this function two groups of muscles, the sphincter and the dilator, work in opposition. These are supplied by cholinergic and adrenergic innervation, respectively. Miosis (pupillary constriction) can be accomplished by endogenous or exogenous acetylcholine or by cholinergic stimulation. Mydriasis (dilation) can be accomplished by an adrenergic stimulant such as epinephrine, which acts on the dilator musculature, or by an antagonist to acetylcholine, which allows relaxation of the sphincter. The readily observed behavior of the iris has made its action an excellent model for the study of drug penetration in the human eye.[2]

The pigment granules of the iris epithelium absorb light and can also absorb lipophilic drugs. This type of binding is characteristically reversible, allowing release of drug over time. It is usually termed nonspecific or low-affinity binding, indicating that a specific high-affinity drug receptor is not involved. As a result, the iris can serve as a depot or reservoir for some drugs, concentrating and then releasing them for longer than otherwise expected.

Nonspecific binding can prevent or delay a single dose of a lipophilic drug from reaching an effective level within the eye. However, on multiple dosing, a saturation equilibrium is reached when the amount of drug being bound is the same as that being released from the reservoir. Once this occurs, effective dosing is achieved. Since individual iris pigmentation varies widely, some drugs show a far greater response after the first dose in blue-eyed individuals than in patients with dark irides. Shell[1] demonstrated constriction of the pupil (miosis) after a single dose of pilocarpine continuing for 4.7 hours in darkly pigmented subjects compared with 2 hours in subjects with blue eyes.

Aqueous Humor

Aqueous humor is formed by the ciliary body and occupies the posterior and anterior chambers, a compartment measuring about 0.2 ml, although the total volume decreases with age as the lens grows. The fluid is constantly generated by the pigmented and nonpigmented epithelium of the ciliary body, which is supplied by a rich bed of capillaries. It flows from the posterior chamber through the pupil and then slowly circles in the anterior chamber, circulated by the thermal differential between the cornea and the deeper ocular tissues.[46] The aqueous exits at the angle between the cornea and iris through the sieve-like trabecular meshwork. It then enters the canal of Schlemm, which leads directly into low-pressure episcleral veins and finally into the general circulation. Drugs absorbed through the cornea can leave the aqueous through this so-called conventional route or through the walls of the iris or other tissues comprising the margins of the anterior chamber, the "uveoscleral route" of aqueous humor outflow.

Ciliary Body

The ciliary body has the major function of aqueous humor production. Aqueous is composed of a clear ultrafiltrate of blood plasma devoid of large proteins, together with some substances actively transported across the blood-aqueous barrier. One example is ascorbate, essential for wound healing processes such as collagen synthesis, which is concentrated 100-fold from the blood.

The capillaries of the ciliary body are many and possess no tight junctions to limit the diffusion of drugs or proteins. However, drugs are usually limited by the apical tight junctions of the nonpigmented cells at the paired layers making up the ciliary epithelium.[47] Systemic drugs enter the anterior and posterior chambers largely by passing through the ciliary body vasculature and then diffusing into the iris where they can enter the aqueous humor.

The ciliary body is the major ocular source of drug-metabolizing enzymes, responsible for the two major phases of reactions that begin the process of drug detoxification and removal from the eye. The localization of these enzymes together in a single tissue is important, since the oxidative and reductive products from phase I reactions of the cytochrome P-450 system are highly reactive and potentially more toxic than the parent compounds.[4] Conjugation by glucuronidation, sulfonation, acetylation, methylation, or with amino acids or glutathione in phase II reactions can then be accomplished by detoxifying enzymes. The uveal circulation provides up to 88% of the total blood flow and can rapidly remove these conjugated products from the eye.[48] Melanin granules of the pigmented ciliary epithelium adsorb polycyclic compounds, such as chloroquine, storing them for metabolism and removal.[49]

Crystalline Lens

The normal human lens originates from a double layer of epithelium. Its thickened outer basal lamina (the capsule) is analogous to Descemet's layer. It grows to become a thick, flexible tissue composed of cells densely packed with clear proteins known as crystallins. The flexibility is reduced by 50 years, diminishing accommodation.[50] The capsule reaches a thickness of several microns anteriorly and is 10 times thinner posteriorly. The anterior lens epithelium is the most active region metabolically, conducting cation transport and cell division. This region is also the most prone to damage from drugs or toxic substances.[51]

Hydrophilic drugs of high molecular weight cannot be absorbed by the lens from the aqueous humor, since the lens epithelium provides a major barrier to entry.[52] The capsule prevents the entry of large proteins. Lipid-soluble drugs, however, can pass slowly into and through the lens cortex.[51] Fluorescein, a hydrophilic molecule, can penetrate the capsule and reach the nucleus in a few weeks.[46] The lens can be viewed primarily as a barrier to rapid penetration of drugs from aqueous to vitreous humor.

The lens grows with age, and colorations or opacities may develop and interfere with vision. Cataract formation is hastened by some miotics, steroids, and phenothiazines.[51] Aldose reductase inhibitors, which prevent the conversion of sugars to polyols, have been shown to prevent or delay diabetic cataract.[53] Levels of glutathione and other compounds drop during the formation of some kinds of cataract.[54] There is currently great interest in the pharmacokinetics of delivery and penetration of such compounds into the crystalline lens.

When cataracts require lens removal to restore vision, the kinetics between aqueous and vitreous humor change. A major barrier to molecular transport is removed, and more rapid exchange of aqueous and vitreous contents occurs. In one experimental study,[55] the concentration of a topically applied anti-inflammatory agent, flurbiprofen, was increased in retinal tissues, vitreous humor, and choroid after lens removal.

Vitreous Humor

The vitreous humor is a viscoelastic connective tissue composed of small amounts of glycosaminoglycans including hyaluronic acid, and proteins such as collagen. The collagen fibrils are anchored directly to the basal lamina, which forms the boundaries of the lens, the ciliary body epithelium, and the neuroglial cells of the retina.[56] Although the anterior vitreous is cell-free, the posterior vitreous contains a few phagocytic cells called hyalocytes and is sometimes termed the cortical tissue layer.[57]

At birth, the material of the vitreous is gel-like in humans and primates. A central remnant of the hyaloid artery, Cloquet's canal, which is free of collagen fibrils, runs from the posterior lens capsule to the optic disc. Since the total volume of the vitreous expands with age while the amount of hyaluronate remains constant, the gel-like material develops a central viscous fluid lake, completely surrounded by the gel vitreous. These events can cause condensation and tearing of the sheath of Cloquet's canal, forming structures termed floaters, which can interfere with vision.[58,59]

The vitreous comprises approximately 80% of the ocular mass and for small molecules may be considered an unstirred fluid with free diffusion.[60] Some molecular species can diffuse between the posterior chamber and the vitreous. However, very high molecular weight substances, such as hyaluronate, are held in place by the zonules and lens capsule and diffuse out of the vitreous only after intracapsular lens extraction.[61-64]

From this discussion it is apparent that the vitreous can serve as a major reservoir for drugs as well as a temporary storage depot for metabolites. For low molecular weight substances, there exists a free path of diffusion from the ciliary body and hence the posterior aqueous humor.

Hydrophilic drugs such as gentamicin, which do not cross the blood-retinal barrier readily, have a prolonged half-life of 24 hours or more in the vitreous humor.[3] Their major route of exit is across the lens zonules and into the aqueous humor, then through the aqueous outflow pathways. For the vitreous to act as a depot for these drugs, they must be injected or introduced by iontophoresis.[63,65]

Retina and Optic Nerve

Tight junctional complexes, *zonula occludens,* in the retinal pigment epithelium (RPE) prevent the ready movement of antibiotics and other drugs from the blood to the retina and vitreous. Since the retina is a developmental derivative of the neural tube wall and can be viewed as a direct extension of the brain, it is not surprising that the blood-retinal barrier somewhat resembles the blood-brain barrier in form and function. Experimental evidence for this similarity comes from the work of Cunha-Vaz,[66,67] who showed that histamine does not alter the vascular permeability of the retina but does alter that of all other ocular tissues. In this trait the retina closely resembles the brain.

The capillaries of the retina are lined by continuous, close-walled endothelial cells, which are the primary determinant of the molecular selectivity that is the blood-retinal barrier's major function.[68,69] Bruch's membrane is a prominent structure associated with the retinal-vitreous barrier, yet it contributes relatively little to the barrier's filtration properties.

The barrier protects against the entry of a wide variety of metabolites and toxins and is effective against most hydrophilic drugs, which do not cross the plasma membrane. Glucose, however, can cross much more easily than would be expected from its molecular structure, an example of diffusion probably facilitated by an active transport system such as a transmembrane carrier molecule. Lipophilic drugs cross the barrier easily in either direction due to their membrane fluidity. A number of agents can cause retinal toxicity, including topical epinephrine, systemic digitalis, phenothiazines, quinine, quinoline derivatives, and methyl alcohol.[70,71] A growing number of substances have been shown to be transported from the vitreous and retina into the blood plasma, including ions, drugs, and the prostaglandins associated with ocular inflammation.[72–74]

The optic nerve is of interest here since some drugs are toxic to this tissue.[71,75] The antibiotics chloramphenicol, ethambutol, streptomycin, and sulfonamides can cause optic neuritis. Vitamin A, especially in large doses, can cause papilledema. Digitalis can cause retrobulbar neuritis.

Blood Supply and Removal of Drugs and Metabolites

The parenteral route of administration is effective only for drugs of low systemic toxicity that can be introduced into the eye at therapeutic concentrations. An important example of systemic dosing is the case of internal ocular infections, such as endophthalmitis, where a high concentration of antibiotic must be maintained. The systemic dose is sometimes augmented by topical drug applications to the eye.[76]

Some drugs are especially useful for topical ocular dosing due to their unacceptability as systemic medications. Drugs that are highly effective may be toxic to liver or kidney, preventing systemic use. They are often well suited for topical use in the eye or for injection, since they are rapidly diluted by the bloodstream to levels that are nontoxic.

The bloodstream is responsible for removing drugs and drug metabolites from ocular tissues. The two circulatory pathways in the eye, the retinal vessels and the uveal vessels, are quite different. The retinal vessels can remove many drugs, metabolites, and such agents as prostaglandins from the vitreous humor and retina, apparently by active transport.[69] The uveal vessels remove drugs by bulk transport from the iris and ciliary body. The direct outflow pathway from aqueous humor through trabecular meshwork and canal of Schlemm into the episcleral vessels is another major source of drug removal from the eye.

Compartment Theory and Drug Kinetics

The eye is a unique structure, since several of its fluids and tissues—the tear film, cornea, aqueous humor, lens, and vitreous humor—are almost completely transparent. These components of the optical system have no direct blood supply in the healthy state. Each can be considered a separate chamber or compartment. A compartment is defined here as a region of tissue or fluid through which a drug can diffuse and equilibrate with relative freedom. Each compartment is generally separated by a barrier from other compartments so that flow between adjacent compartments takes more time than diffusion within each compartment.

The tears are an example of a compartment with constant turnover, since the inflow of lacrimal fluid is constant and equal to the outflow through the puncta. Consider the fate of sodium fluorescein, a diagnostic tracer representative of a highly hydrophilic drug. Once instilled, it mixes rapidly with the tears, and the tear flow carries away a portion per unit time dependent on the drug concentration present. This can be expressed by the first derivative expression:

$$\frac{dC_d}{dt} = k_0 C_d t \qquad (1.3)$$

where C_d = the concentration of drug in tears at time t;

dC_d/dt = the change in concentration C_d during an interval of time;

and k_0 = a proportionality constant of drug loss to the nasolacrimal duct dependent on the flow rate and volume of the tear compartment.

On integration, equation 1.3 becomes:

$$C_d t = C_{d_o} k_0 t \qquad (1.4)$$

where $C_d t$ = the concentration of drug at any time, t;

C_{d_o} = the initial concentration of drug;

e = the base of natural logarithms;

and k_0 = the rate constant already defined.[77]

Approximately 99% of fluorescein will exit the tears by lacrimal drainage, yet a very small amount will penetrate the corneal epithelial barrier and enter the stroma. A barrier is a region of lower permeability or restricted diffusion that exists between compartments. If we consider the epithelium as a barrier to drug penetration from the tears, and the bulk of the cornea as a compartment, we now have a two-compartment model. In the absence of an active transport mechanism, drugs diffuse across barriers according to the laws of thermodynamics, from a region of higher to one of lower concentration. Fick's first law of diffusion states that the rate of diffusion across a barrier is proportional to the concentration gradient between the compartments on either side of the barrier:

$$\frac{dC_d}{dt} = k_{dc} A (C_d - C_c) \qquad (1.5)$$

where dC_d/dt = the net drug moving from tears to cornea per unit of time;

A = the area of the tear-corneal interface;

C_d = concentration of drug in tears;

C_c = concentration of drug in cornea; and

k_{dc} = the permeability constant from tears to cornea. The permeability constant in the reverse direction would be k_{cd}.[3]

The permeability constant, k_{dc}, is specific to a given drug and represents the net number of moles that cross a unit area of the membrane in unit time under unit concentration difference.[6] It is subject to modification by many factors, including other drugs, preservatives, infection, inflammation, or nervous control. Such modifications can greatly affect drug bioavailability at the desired site of action.

From Fick's law, the rate of diffusion of a drug across a barrier is linearly dependent on the concentration difference between the compartments on either side of the barrier. As soon as the concentration of drug in the cornea equals that in the tears, drug no longer penetrates inward. Therefore, corneal absorption depends on the integral, or "area under the curve," of tear film concentration over the first 10 to 20 minutes after instillation of a drug, as indicated by the shaded area in Figure 1.7.

The diffusion of drug from the cornea to the aqueous humor is similar to that for tears to cornea, except that

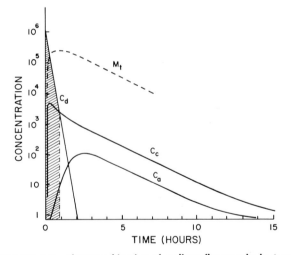

FIGURE 1.7 **Pharmacokinetics of sodium fluorescein in tears, cornea, and aqueous humor after instillation. The concentration of fluorescein in each compartment is plotted as a function of time. The tear concentration (C_d) falls rapidly, and significant drug is transferred to the cornea only while the tear concentration remains higher than the corneal concentration (C_c). The cornea then functions as a storage depot for the aqueous humor, whose concentration (C_a) parallels that of the cornea for many hours. The dotted line M_t represents the total mass of the drug in all tissues. This curve can be experimentally verified in the living human eye by fluorophotometry. (Modified from Maurice DM, Mishima S. Ocular pharmacokinetics. In: Sears ML, ed. Pharmacology of the eye. Handbook of experimental pharmacology. Berlin: Springer-Verlag, 1984;69:19–116.)**

for the corneal depot, the aqueous humor will receive the major proportion of drug. Both lateral diffusion across the limbus and diffusion back across the epithelium contribute relatively little to the total diffusion. The rate is:

$$\frac{dC_c}{dt} = k_{ca}A\,(C_c - C_a) \qquad (1.6)$$

where dC_c/dt = the amount of drug penetrating the barrier during a unit of time;
   A = the area of the tear-corneal interface;
   C_c = concentration of drug in cornea;
   C_a = concentration of drug in aqueous; and
   k_{ca} = the permeability constant from cornea to aqueous.

Since the majority of the corneal drug depot eventually enters the aqueous humor, the aqueous level rises over about 3 hours to a maximum. After this time, the concentration in the cornea, C_c, and in the aqueous humor, C_a, drop in parallel as the aqueous humor level decays logarithmically, as shown in Figure 1.7.

To complete the model, the elimination transfer coefficient from the aqueous to the blood plasma, k_{ap}, is defined by:

$$\frac{dC_a}{dt} = k_{ap}\,(C_p r_{ap} - C_a) \qquad (1.7)$$

where C_a and C_p are the drug concentrations in aqueous and plasma, respectively; and r_{ap} is the value of the ratio of C_a/C_p at steady state.[3] The plasma is usually considered an infinite sink for the drug, unless a systemic dose has been given.

The compartment model just described can estimate the concentrations of drugs within various ocular tissues. A more complex compartment model, which includes drug movement through the posterior aqueous, vitreous, and retina, is shown in Figure 1.8. This model becomes useful when a drug is introduced directly into the vitreous or systemic circulation, or when the very slight amount of a topically applied drug reaching the lens, vitreous, or retina must be considered.

The molecular properties of drugs influence which tissues will act as reservoirs for them, and which will act as barriers. The modeling parameters may vary considerably for drugs with different penetration and partitioning properties. The distribution and elimination of a lipophilic drug that is also water-soluble and penetrates the corneal epithelium readily will occur more rapidly than the example of fluorescein illustrated in Figure 1.7.

Active Transport and Diffusion Kinetics

Drug distribution usually depends on the rate of passive diffusion within and between compartments and is governed by the barrier resistance between any two compartments where the distribution is unequal at a given time. In some cases, however, molecules accumulate against a concentration gradient on one side of a barrier.[6] Either of two phenomena is responsible for such an observation. First, biochemical reactions or coupled pumping mechanisms in the cell may provide the energy necessary for active transport.[7] Second, a high degree of nonspecific binding due to ionic or other forces may cause an apparent accumulation of molecules against a concentration gradient.[3]

The properties of passive drug release from a tissue or from an artificial device can vary under certain circumstances. One example is zero-order kinetics, a term used when the release of a drug is constant over time. Zero-order kinetic conditions are satisfied when the concentration of a drug released over time is independent of concentration. Drugs usually obey zero-order kinetics when there is a rate-limiting barrier, as when a carrier system is saturated by an excess of drug. An example of drug dosing by zero-order kinetics is the Ocusert, which is a small membrane-bound delivery system designed for insertion in the conjunctival sac (see Fig. 2.19). A reservoir of medication is released at a nearly constant rate over a 1-week period.[1]

First-order kinetics is most commonly encountered in ocular drug movement (Fig. 1.9). Here, the rate of movement is directly proportional to the concentration difference across the barrier, $C_o - C_i$, and changes with time as the concentration differential across the barrier changes. The passive diffusion of molecules across a nonsaturated barrier generally adheres to first-order kinetics.[6]

Second-order and higher kinetics depend on the variable concentrations of two or more molecular species, as, for example, when a drug is converted by an enzyme to or from an active form. This type of kinetics is more often encountered with enzymes and their cofactors acting on substrates than in transport.

Properties of Receptors

Endogenous hormones and neurotransmitters are internally secreted substances that change tissue responses by binding at sites of action known as receptors. Exogenous drugs, with some notable exceptions, are administered compounds that mimic, block, or change the response of tissue receptors to endogenous molecules. The response of each tissue to a given drug

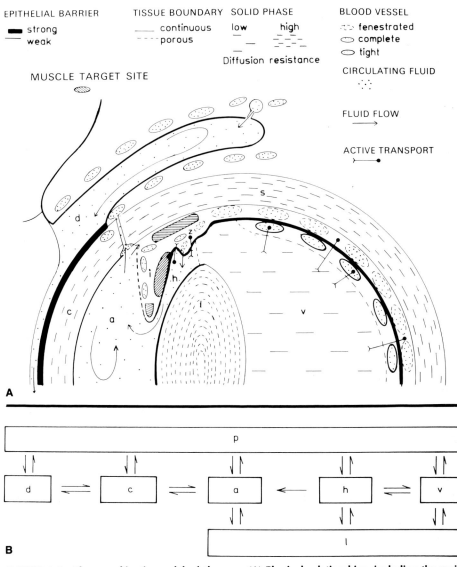

FIGURE 1.8 **Pharmacokinetic model of the eye.** *(A)* **Physical relationships, including the major barriers and active pumping mechanisms.** *(B)* **Compartment model. p, plasma; d, tear reservoir; c, cornea; a, anterior chamber aqueous; h, posterior chamber aqueous; l, lens; i, iris; z, ciliary body; s, sclera; v, vitreous humor. (From Maurice DM, Mishima S. Ocular pharmacokinetics. In: Sears ML, ed. Pharmacology of the eye. Handbook of experimental pharmacology, Berlin: Springer-Verlag, 1984;69:19–116.)**

depends on the type and number of receptors it contains, as well as the recent history of stimulation, which in part determines their current status.

Tissue Receptor Site

The drug receptor initially represented an abstract mathematical concept designed to fit experimental data. In recent years the isolation of well-defined membrane molecules, some of which have been successfully isolated, purified, and reconstituted by modern techniques, has led to new knowledge of receptor function.[78]

A receptor is viewed as a molecule or molecular complex residing in the membrane of a cell that binds a ligand and initiates or redirects cellular activity. A ligand is an endogenous hormone, neurotransmitter, or exogenous drug or substance with high affinity and high specificity for receptor binding. The ligand binding to the receptor may be by weak van der Waals

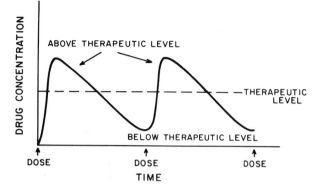

FIGURE 1.9   First-order kinetics of ocular drugs in solution or ointment. This results in periods of overdosage and underdosage. (Modified with permission from Place V, Benson H. Local effects of topically applied steroids. J Steroid Biochem 1975;6:717–722, copyright 1975, Pergamon Press, Ltd.)

forces, by attraction of oppositely charged ionic pairs, by covalent bonding, or by a combination of these.[79] The specific effect of a ligand is presumed to be caused by the interaction with its receptor, which is viewed as a reversible, biomolecular interaction.[80] The mammalian receptor model, as represented here, cannot be applied directly to the effects of membrane-active anesthetic agents nor to the actions of antimicrobial compounds.

Second Messengers

Once bound, certain hormones or agonist drugs are internalized and metabolized. During this process, they can produce an effect within the cell or tissue, mediated by the production of an internal signal molecule. In the case of β-adrenergic receptors, Sutherland and associates[81,82] were the first to demonstrate that ligand binding causes activation of adenylate cyclase. This results in the internal production of cyclic adenosine monophosphate (cAMP), a so-called second messenger that serves to transmit and amplify the effects of the ligand. By comparison, the epidermal growth factor (EGF) receptor is a 170 kDalton transmembrane polypeptide that becomes phosphorylated at an internal tyrosine residue on activation and stimulates ornithine decarboxylase activity.[83] The net result of this action is to stimulate cell division.

Agonists, Partial Agonists, and Antagonists

More than one ligand is often required to bind to a cell in order to elicit a detectable threshold response,

and the response may increase in proportion to increasing concentration of the ligand. A dose-response curve can thus be generated to show the effects of increasing drug levels. Usually this reaches a plateau beyond which no further increase in cell activity can be elicited by increasing the drug level.

A theoretical concentration-effect curve is shown in Figure 1.10. The proportion of maximal activity, $E_A/E_{A\ max}$, is a function of the molar concentration of the agonist, A. Note that at both very low and very high concentrations of agonist, asymptotic changes in activity occur. Over the central range of the drug-receptor interaction, a nearly linear dose-response function is generated. The concentration of drug that yields half-maximal effect is used to calculate the drug's intrinsic affinity for the receptor and is often expressed as the negative logarithm of molar concentration, pD_2.[80]

A partial agonist is defined as a ligand that binds to a receptor without producing the maximal response possible, even at high concentration. There is no direct relationship between a ligand's binding affinity and intrinsic activity; these two independent properties together determine drug activity. As an example, a drug that binds strongly yet does not cause maximal response can act simultaneously as a partial agonist and as an antagonist, because it blocks other ligands from binding and eliciting the maximal or normal response.

An antagonist can block stimulation of a drug receptor by binding at a site interfering with the ligand

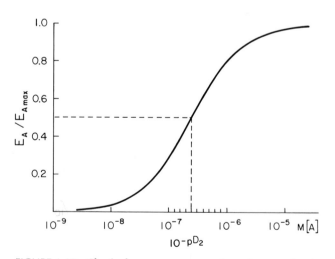

FIGURE 1.10   Classic dose-response curve for a drug agonist, A. The sigmoid curve defines the theoretical effect on a specific receptor for varying concentrations of the agonist. The value labelled pD_2 is the negative log of the molar concentration of agonist producing 50% of maximal receptor effect, the ED_{50}. (From Van Den Brink FG. General theory of drug-receptor interactions. In: Van Rossem JM, ed. Kinetics of drug action. Handbook of experimental pharmacology, Berlin: Springer-Verlag, 1977;47.)

binding site of the receptor. It may also alter the molecular conformation of the binding site to prevent binding. Antagonists can be classified as competitive or noncompetitive inhibitors, depending on whether they compete for the same molecular binding site as the ligand. Depending on the type of antagonist interacting with the receptor, differences occur in the agonist dose-response curve. Since antagonists often bind strongly, remaining in position on the receptor without internalization or destruction, they can exert their effects at very low concentration and act as powerful drug substances.

Competitive Inhibition

Drug molecules that bind to the same receptor site as the endogenous ligand, or agonist, can physically block the latter's access to the receptor. These drugs are termed competitive inhibitors. A competitive inhibitor blocks the action of a hormone or neurotransmitter at a receptor site. The degree of inhibition depends on the concentration of antagonist and its properties relative to the agonist.

A sufficiently high concentration of ligand will overcome the action of a competitive inhibitor, as shown in Figure 1.11. The competitive inhibitor is administered at 5 different concentrations. Each increase in concentration of antagonist causes a shift of the agonist function, requiring an increased concentration of agonist to elicit a given response.

A competitive inhibitor may reduce or block the action of an endogenous hormone. Competitive inhibitors, however, often have an intrinsic partial agonist activity of their own. Graded transitions between agonist and antagonist activity are a common feature of molecular structure-activity relationships.[84]

Noncompetitive Inhibition

A noncompetitive inhibitor blocks the action of a drug on its receptor independent of ligand concentration, often with powerful and long-lasting effects. One reason for this is that antagonists often have extremely high or irreversible affinity for the receptor site. Another is that, unlike agonists, antagonists often do not allow the receptor to complete its cycle of internalization and activation, which would restore the receptor to its active state. This may occur in several ways. The antagonist may interact with a different type of receptor in the same cell, thus changing the affinity between the ligand and its receptor. This is termed a metactoid interaction.[80] An example is shown in Figure 1.12. Here, an increasing concentration of antagonist causes a lessened maximal response by any concentration of agonist.

Regulation of Receptors

The body can adjust the sensitivity of a tissue to naturally released transmitter substances in both health and disease. For instance, following nerve damage, less total transmitter is released than normally occurs. To compensate, a greater number of receptor molecules are produced at the effector site. This response, referred to as up regulation, allows fine adjustment of the receptor sensitivity to the range of ligand activity present at the synapse.

The reverse can also occur. If an endogenous neurotransmitter is present at abnormally high levels, the number of receptors present for that drug may be reduced proportionately to compensate and allow normal physiologic function. This can also occur when a drug substance is administered at frequent intervals; it is termed down regulation.[85]

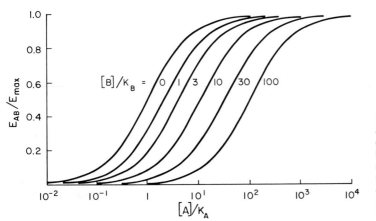

FIGURE 1.11 **Theoretical shift of dose-response curve for agonist A in the presence of increasing concentrations of competitive antagonist B. Characteristically, although a higher concentration of A is required to elicit a given response in the presence of B, there is no change in curve shape or height. (From Van Den Brink FG. General theory of drug-receptor interactions. In: Van Rossem JM, ed. Kinetics of drug action. Handbook of experimental pharmacology, Berlin: Springer-Verlag, 1977;47.)**

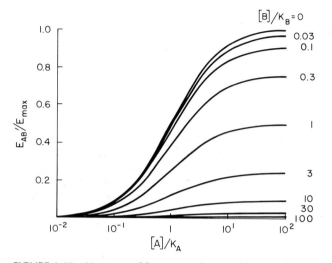

FIGURE 1.12   Noncompetitive antagonism. In this example, increasing concentration of B causes decreasing receptor response to A. The concentration-effect curves are all in the same position in relation to the concentration axis, but their maximum heights differ. (From Van Den Brink FG. General theory of drug-receptor interactions. In: Van Rossem JM, ed. Kinetics of drug action. Handbook of experimental pharmacology, Berlin: Springer-Verlag, 1977; 47.)

Adrenergic agonists typically produce a strong response on initial application, then have reduced effect when dosing is continued at frequent intervals. Adrenergic receptors have been shown to be regulated experimentally in corneal tissue in response to epinephrine.[86] When drug use is discontinued, normal sensitivity returns in a few days. Antagonist drugs generally cause less down regulation than agonists, or none at all, since they do not stimulate maximal receptor response.

Properties of Drug Formulations Affecting Bioavailability

Biopharmaceutics involves the development of optimum dosage forms for the delivery of a given drug.[1] In this section some of the properties of ocular formulations will be considered for their effects on drug bioavailability. Side effects of drugs and preservatives will also be discussed.

Bioavailability

Bioavailability describes the amount of drug present at the desired receptor site. The dose level producing a response that is 50% of maximum is termed the ED_{50}

(see Fig. 1.10). An effective dose level must be present for a time sufficient to produce the desired action. The requirements for concentration and time to achieve ED_{50} differ widely depending on the drug's mechanism of action and the desired response. The following are two challenging examples of drug bioavailability problems selected to illustrate markedly different requirements for effective therapeutic dosing.

A bicarbonate pump located in the membrane of the ciliary body is important in the production of aqueous humor. Inhibition of the enzyme carbonic anhydrase (CA) reduces the ciliary body fluid output by as much as one-third.[87] Such inhibition is desirable in treating glaucoma, since it lowers intraocular pressure. The CA enzyme must be almost completely inhibited to produce the desired reduction of fluid transport. This can easily be achieved in a tissue bath where a sufficiently high concentration of a competitive inhibitor such as acetazolamide can be maintained. However, orally administered carbonic anhydrase inhibitors of sufficient dosage to allow therapeutic ocular effects can also cause acidosis and gastric upset. Topical application of carbonic anhydrase inhibitors has not yet achieved clinical success due to the problem of insufficient corneal penetration and bioavailability. A variety of carbonic anhydrase inhibitors with fluorine and other substitutions have been screened in recent years in attempts to find a suitable topical agent.

Epidermal growth factors (EGF), derived originally from mouse salivary glands, are of interest in corneal epithelial wound healing and potentially in stimulating endothelial cell division as well. They are medium-length peptides that can stimulate DNA synthesis and reproduction in epithelial and certain other cells. A single dose of EGF, internalized through the cell receptors, can cause events leading to mitosis. Great success has been achieved in obtaining cell growth in culture. However, prolonged contact for at least 20 minutes with the cell membrane is required to stimulate binding and internalization. A complicating factor is that in high concentration, EGF actually inhibits cell reproduction. Moreover, it is not easy to demonstrate efficacy using topically applied EGF due to the rapidly changing concentration in the tear film, which is initially so high that it is inhibitory, and becomes so low that it is ineffectual in minutes.[83] Research is now directed at methods of altering cells at secondary receptor sites to render them more receptive to rapid binding and incorporation of EGF. Such methods use the same property of interaction of receptors already described for metactoid receptor antagonism.

These two examples illustrate the bioavailability considerations that must be taken into account in the practical design of drugs that are to be therapeutically useful in humans once a mechanism of action is characterized.

Active Ingredients

Therapeutic and diagnostic drugs given topically or systemically can have major effects on uptake of other drugs, due to their own actions on tissue permeability, blood flow, and fluid secretion. Preservatives, buffers, and vehicles also can have significant effects on drug absorption.[88] Table 1.3 categorizes some topical medications and preservatives and their effects on the corneal epithelium, evaluated by scanning electron microscopy.[89]

Many drugs used to treat glaucoma decrease aqueous humor formation and thereby slow their own kinetics of removal and removal of other drugs by the aqueous route. In a like manner, anti-inflammatory agents compensate for the increased permeability of the blood-aqueous barrier and help to bring it back within normal limits, thus altering the kinetics of drugs within the

eye. Many similar examples of drug modification of pharmacokinetics can be found (e.g., the inhibition of tear flow by systemically administered anticholinergic agents).

Stability, Buffering, and Osmolarity

No complex drug molecule is indefinitely stable in solution. The determination of drug stability is of major concern to the pharmaceutical industry. In the United States, a manufacturer must demonstrate that at least 90% of the labelled concentration of a drug is present in the active form after storage at room temperature for the shelf life requested. In many cases, a manufactured drug may contain 110% of the labelled amount of medication, so that 18% of the drug can degrade before the minimum acceptable level is

TABLE 1.3
Effects of Topical Ocular Drugs, Vehicles, and Preservatives on the Corneal Epithelium of the Rabbit Eye

Topical Preparation			*SEM[a] Evaluation of Effects on Corneal Epithelium*
Preparations causing no epithelial damage		%	
Drugs	Atropine	1.0	Surface epithelial microvilli normal in size, shape, and
	Chloromycetin	0.5	distribution
	Epinephryl borate	1.0	No denuded cells
	Gentamicin	0.3	Cell junctions intact
	Proparacaine	0.5	Plasma membranes not wrinkled
	Tetracaine	0.5	Usual number of epithelial "holes"
Vehicles	Boric acid in petrolatum-mineral oil	5.0	
	Methylcellulose	0.5	
	Polyvinyl alcohol	1.6	
	Saline	0.9	
Preservatives	Chlorobutanol	0.5	
	Disodium edetate	0.1	
	Thimerosal	0.01	
Preparations causing moderate epithelial damage		%	
Drugs	Echothiophate iodide	0.25	Most cells normal
	Pilocarpine	2.0	Some cells showed loss of microvilli and wrinkling of plasma
	Fluorescein	2.0	membranes
	Fluor-I-Strip (wet with 1 drop 0.9% saline)		A small number of cells showed disruption of plasma membrane with premature cellular desquamation
Preparations causing important epithelial damage		%	
Drugs	Cocaine	4.0	Complete loss of microvilli
	Neopolycin	(no BAK)	Wrinkling of plasma membranes
			Premature desquamation of top layer of cells
Preservatives	Benzalkonium chloride	0.01	Severe epithelial microvillous loss
Drug + preservative	Pilocarpine	2.0	Severe membrane disruption
	Gentamicin	0.3	Death and desquamation of two superficial layers of cells over
	Benzalkonium chloride	0.01	3-hour period

[a]Scanning electron microscope.
Adapted from Pfister RR, Burstein NL. The effects of ophthalmic drugs, vehicles, and preservatives on corneal epithelium: A scanning electron microscope study. Invest Ophthalmol 1976;15:246–259.

reached. A shelf life of less than 18 months usually makes warehousing and distribution of a drug economically impractical, unless the drug is in very high demand.

Once a sealed bottle is opened, the contents are subject to the risk of excessive oxidation and microbial contamination. The bottle may be subject to heating if left on a table, in a car, or in a pocket. These conditions all contribute to accelerated drug degradation. Diagnostic agents must be replaced on a routine basis to prevent their use too long after opening. This is particularly true for topical anesthetics, which can rapidly deteriorate once opened. Any drug that has a brownish discoloration or that stings more than usual should be suspect, even if still apparently in date.

Drugs formulated in an acid solution are sometimes more stable than those at neutral or alkaline pH, particularly when the drug is a weak base.[10] Often such a drug must be stored at an acid pH to increase protonation and prevent rapid degradation. Polypeptides such as growth factors, which are now of interest in ophthalmic formulations, may require alkaline storage. In the eye, the normal pH is approximately 7.4.[16] Tear pH can remain altered for over 30 minutes after addition of a strongly buffered solution. A change of tear pH can cause such irritation and stimulation of lacrimation that drug penetration is decreased. The use of a low concentration of buffer in the drug vehicle can allow the natural ocular buffering system to reestablish normal tear film pH rapidly after drug instillation.

Occasionally, an important drug is not stable in solution. As an example, an antioxidant such as sodium metabisulfite must be added to the formulation of adrenergic drugs such as epinephrine to prevent the rapid formation of a brownish degradation product that is irritating. An extreme stability problem is posed by acetylcholine, a very useful drug in rapidly and reversibly constricting the pupil in some surgical procedures such as cataract extraction. This agent degrades within minutes in solution. Therefore, a system for packaging has been developed using a sterile aqueous solution in one compartment and lyophilized (freeze-dried) drug in the other. A plunger displaces a stopper between chambers, allowing mixing just before use.

Osmolarity is influenced by all molecules in a formulation with colligative properties, including drug, buffer salts, vehicle, and preservative. An osmolarity of 290 milliOsmoles (mOsm) is equivalent to 0.9% saline, and this is the value sought for most ophthalmic as well as intravenous medications. The ocular tear film has a wide tolerance for variation in osmotic pressure. However, increasing tonicity above that of the tears causes immediate dilution by osmotic water movement from the lids and eye.[90] Hypotonic solutions are sometimes used to treat dry eye conditions and reduce tear osmolarity from abnormally high values.[91]

Preservatives

The formulation of ocular medications has included antimicrobial preservatives since the historic problem of fluorescein contamination in the 1940s. *Pseudomonas,* a soil bacterium that can cause corneal ulceration, uses the fluorescein molecule as an energy source for metabolism, and many years ago it caused serious consequences for the practitioner who kept an unpreserved solution in the office to assist in the the diagnosis of corneal abrasions. As a result of several tragic infections, two actions have been taken by manufacturers. First, fluorescein is now most commonly supplied as a dried preparation on filter paper, preventing the growth of pathogens.[88] Second, as a precautionary measure, all ophthalmic solutions designed for nonsurgical, multiple use after opening now contain preservatives. However, as noted by Lemp,[92] preservatives employed at high concentrations can irritate and damage the ocular surface.

Preservatives currently available for commercial use are of two distinct types. One group, the surfactants, are ionically charged molecules that disrupt the plasma membrane and are usually bactericidal. The other group of chemical toxins includes the metals mercury and iodine and their derivatives as well as alcohols. These compounds block the normal metabolic processes of the cell. They are considered bacteriostatic if they only inhibit growth, or bactericidal if they destroy the ability of bacteria to reproduce. In contrast to antibiotics, which selectively destroy or immobilize a specific group of organisms, the preservatives act nonselectively against all cells.

The quaternary surfactants benzalkonium chloride and benzethonium chloride are preferred by many manufacturers because of their stability, excellent antimicrobial properties in acid formulation, and long shelf life. They have long been known to increase drug penetration. However, they exhibit toxic effects on both the tear film and the corneal epithelium.[93,94] This toxicity is increased by acidity of the formulation.[95]

A single drop of 0.01% benzalkonium chloride can break the superficial lipid layer of the tear film into numerous oil droplets.[12] This is because benzalkonium chloride can insert into the lipid monolayer of the tear surface and disrupt it by detergent action. Benzalkonium chloride thus reduces by one-half the tear film breakup time.[96] Repeated blinking does not restore the lipid layer for some time. The inclusion of benzalkonium chloride in artificial tear formulations is questionable, since its characteristics do not include protection of corneal epithelium or promotion of a stable oily tear surface.

Surfactants' ability to disrupt membranes or to alter their permeability is related to their charge and to the size of their hydrophobic (lipophilic) group. These agents are usually cationic. Marsh and Maurice[97] studied the ability of cationic surfactants to alter corneal permeability. They observed a significant increase in permeability that, however, was coupled with objectionable irritation. Cadwallader[98] studied the effects of benzalkonium chloride of varying molecular chain lengths and found that the C_{14} length was the most toxic. This length would most easily fit into the bilaminar model of the plasma membrane first proposed by Davson and Danielli[6,99] (Fig. 1.13).

Chlorhexidine is a diguanide that contains two charges arranged so that it does not intercalate readily into the phospholipid membrane. It is useful as an antimicrobial agent in the same range of concentrations as is benzalkonium chloride, yet it is used at lower concentrations in marketed formulations. It does not alter corneal permeability to the same degree as does benzalkonium chloride.[99] There may be two major reasons for this. First, its structure is such that it has two positive charges that are separated by a long carbon backbone, and it cannot intercalate into a lipid layer in the same manner as does benzalkonium chloride. Second, Green[100] has shown that proteins neutralize the toxicity of chlorhexidine, and this may occur in the tear film.

Of the mercurial preservatives, thimerosal is less subject to degradation into toxic mercury than either phenylmercuric acetate or phenylmercuric nitrate. Thimerosal is most effective in weakly acidic solutions. Some patients develop a contact sensitivity and must discontinue use after a few weeks of exposure.[101] Since thimerosal affects internal cell respiration and must be present at high continuous concentrations to have biologic effects, its dilution by the tear film prevents short-term epithelial toxicity on single application.[102] It has no known effects on tear film stability. A concentration of 1% thimerosal is required to equal the effects on corneal oxygen consumption of 0.025% benzalkonium chloride.[103]

Chlorobutanol is less effective than benzalkonium chloride as an antimicrobial and tends to disappear from bottles during prolonged storage.[104] There appears to be no allergic reaction associated with prolonged use. However, chlorobutanol is not a highly effective preservative when used alone.[88,105]

Methylparaben and propylparaben have been introduced into some medications in recent years, especially artificial tears and nonmedicated ointments. They can cause allergic reactions and are unstable at high pH.[105]

Disodium ethylene diamine tetra-acetic acid (EDTA)

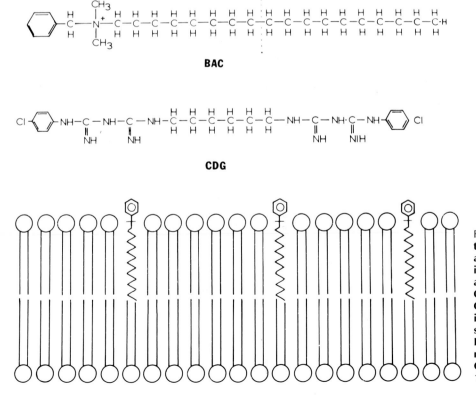

BAC

CDG

FIGURE 1.13 **Comparison of the structures of benzalkonium chloride (BAC) and chlorhexidine (CDG). Benzalkonium chloride can intercalate readily into a plasma membrane, as seen below. Chain length affects binding ability. Chlorhexidine cannot bind effectively into the membrane and causes far less surface disruption. (From Burstein NL. Preservative alteration of corneal permeability in humans and rabbits. Invest Ophthalmol Vis Sci 1984;25:1453–1457.)**

is a special type of molecule known as a chelating agent that can preferentially bind and sequester divalent cations in the increasing order: Ca^{++}, Mg^{++}, Zn^{++}, Pb^{++}. Its role in preservation is to assist the action of thimerosal, benzalkonium chloride, and other agents. Contact dermatitis is known to occur from EDTA.[105]

When instilled topically in the eye, mercurial and alcoholic preservatives are rapidly diluted below the toxic threshold by tears. However, surfactant preservatives rapidly bind by intercalating into the plasma membrane and can increase corneal permeability before dilution can occur. The changed barrier property of the cornea can allow large hydrophilic molecules to penetrate the cornea far more readily.

Vehicles

An ophthalmic vehicle is an agent other than a drug or preservative added to a formulation to provide proper tonicity, buffering, and viscosity to complement drug action.[104,106] The use of one or more high molecular weight polymers increases the viscosity of the formulation, delaying washout from the tear film and increasing bioavailability of drugs. Polyionic molecules can bind at the corneal surface and increase drug retention as well as stabilize the tear film. Petrolatum or oil-based ointments provide even longer retention of drugs at the corneal surface and provide a temporary lipid depot.

The monomer unit structure of the vehicle is the most important property in controlling the behavior of the material, followed by the molecular weight and viscosity. In the manufacture and purification of polymers, a range of molecular sizes is usually present in the final product.[107]

Molecular viscosity, M_v, the most important property in controlling residence time in the tear fluid, is measured in centistokes. It is a nonlinear function of molecular weight and of concentration. Thus, a 2% solution of polymer in water usually will not give a viscosity twice that of a 1% solution. Each batch of a commercial polymer must therefore be measured for viscosity at the appropriate concentration. The addition of salts can affect the final viscosity of some polymers. Divalent anions and cations can have a major effect on the conformation of polymers in solution, occasionally causing incompatibilities when formulations are mixed together in the eye.

POLYVINYLPYRROLIDONE

Polyvinylpyrrolidone (PVP) (U.S. Pharmacopeia name: povidone) is the homopolymer of N-vinyl-2-pyrrolidone (Fig. 1.14), which was used as a blood plasma substitute during World War II. Although considered to be a nonionic polymer, it has specific binding and detoxification properties that are of great interest in health care. As an example, it complexes iodine, reducing its toxicity 10-fold, while still allowing bactericidal action to occur. This occurs through the formation of iodide ions by reducing agents in the polymer, which then complex with molecular iodine to give tri-iodide ions.[107] Povidone can also complex with mercury, nicotine, cyanide, and other toxic materials to reduce their damaging effects.[108]

The pharmacokinetics of povidone are well understood as a result of its experimental use to determine the properties of pores in biological membranes. Povidone molecules can readily penetrate hydrophilic pores in membranes if they are small enough, and they are also taken up by pinocytotic vesicles. Apparently pov-

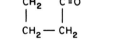

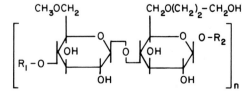

FIGURE 1.14 **Comparison of the structure of three viscosity-enhancing vehicles. These can all be modified by chain length change or by substitution of functional groups.**

idone is not detectably bound to membrane surfaces and hence does not provide long-lasting viscosity enhancement beyond the normal residence time in the tears.

Povidone has very low systemic toxicity, shows no immune rejection characteristics, and is easily excreted by the kidneys at molecular weights up to 100,000 Daltons.[109] The pK_a of the conjugate acid (PVP ·H^+) is between 0 and 1, and the viscosity of povidone does not change until near pH 1, when it doubles. Therefore, there should not be any appreciable ionic character to the PVP chain at pharmaceutical or physiologic pH values. However, with ionic cosolutes, anions are bound much more readily than cations by povidone. Cosolute binding can cause a change in the size of the polymer coil, influencing the viscosity and other properties of the solution.

POLYVINYL ALCOHOL

Introduced into ophthalmic practice in 1942, polyvinyl alcohol (PVA) is a water-soluble viscosity enhancer with both hydrophilic and hydrophobic sites[106] (see Fig. 1.14). A common concentration used in ophthalmic preparations is 1.4%.[104] It has been found useful in the treatment of corneal epithelial erosion and dry eye syndromes, since it is nonirritating to the eye and actually appears to facilitate healing of abraded epithelium.[110] It is also used to increase the residence time of drugs in the tears, aiding ocular absorption.[111]

HYDROXYPROPYL METHYLCELLULOSE

Like polyvinyl alcohol, the viscosity enhancer hydroxypropyl methylcellulose (HPMC) is available in a variety of molecular weights and in formulations with different group substitutions. The basic structure is shown in Figure 1.14. It has been shown to prolong tear film wetting time and to increase the ability of fluorescein and dexamethasone to penetrate the cornea. HPMC 0.5% has been shown to exhibit twice the ocular retention time of 1.4% PVA.[112,113]

POLYIONIC VEHICLES

Recent advances in chemical synthesis and in an understanding of the tear film of the eye have resulted in the development of compounds that have two or more regions, which vary in their lipophilic nature and in their binding. The first of these to be tested in the eye was poloxamer 407, a polyionic vehicle with a hydrophobic nucleus of polyoxypropylene, and hydrophilic end groups of polyoxyethylene.[114] The conceptual function of this vehicle in the tear film is shown in Figure 1.15.

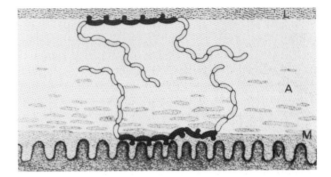

FIGURE 1.15 **Poloxamer 407, represented schematically in the tear film. The lipophilic center of the molecule tends to bind at the corneal surface, while the hydrophilic end chains stabilize the tears. Such polyionic vehicles may provide improved drug delivery in the future. L, lipid layer; A, aqueous layer; M, mucin layer. (From Waring GO, Harris RR. Double-masked evaluation of a poloxamer artificial tear in keratoconjunctivitis sicca. In: Leopold IH, Burns RP, eds. Symposium on ocular therapy. New York: John Wiley & Sons, 1979;11:127–139. Reprinted by permission of John Wiley & Sons, Inc.)**

One advantage of poloxamers is their ability to produce an artificial microenvironment in the tear film, which can greatly enhance the bioavailability of lipophilic drugs such as steroids. In one series of experiments in rabbits[a], a 10-fold increase in penetration of progesterone was achieved with a poloxamer vehicle.

Future advances in polymer chemistry are likely to provide polyionic vehicles that greatly assist therapeutic drugs in molecular partitioning and membrane penetration into the eye.

OINTMENTS

Ointments are commonly used for topical application of drugs to the eye. These vehicles are primarily mixtures of white petrolatum and liquid mineral oil with or without a water-miscible agent such as lanolin.[115] The mineral oil is added to the petrolatum to allow the vehicle to melt at body temperature, while the lanolin is added to the nonemulsive ointment base to absorb water. This allows for water and water-soluble drugs to be retained in the delivery system. Commercial ophthalmic ointments are derivatives of a hydrocarbon mixture of 60% petrolatum USP and 40% mineral oil USP, forming a molecular complex that is semisolid but that melts at body temperature.[116] In general, ointments are well tolerated by the ocular tissues, and when antibiotics are incorporated, they are usually more stable in ointment than in solution.[117]

---

[a]Krezanoski JZ, Weinreb R, Polanski J, Burstein NL, unpublished data, 1981.

The primary clinical purpose for an ointment vehicle is to increase the ocular contact time of the applied drugs. The ocular contact time is about twice as long in the blinking eye and 4 times longer in the nonblinking (patched) eye compared with a saline vehicle.[115] Ointments are retained longer in the conjunctival sac because the large molecules of the ointment are not easily removed into the lacrimal drainage system by blinking. Another factor in the prolonged retention is that a component of tears is a nonpolar oil. Because ointments are also nonpolar oil bases, they are readily absorbed by the precorneal and conjunctival tear films.[118] Because they markedly increase contact time, ointments are used to increase drug absorption for nighttime therapy or for conditions in which antibiotics are delivered to a patched eye, such as corneal abrasions. They are also useful in children, since they do not wash out readily with tearing.

A disadvantage of ointments is the difficulty of self-administration, particularly by the partially sighted patient who may occasionally traumatize the ocular surface with the applicator tip. In addition, dosing is imprecise. Furthermore, many patients report transient blurred vision with the use of ophthalmic ointments. Since they cause blurred vision, ointments are not often used for daytime therapy except where necessitated by postsurgical, infectious, or other special circumstances. Some patients will incur contact dermatitis from ophthalmic ointments, especially atropine ointment and formulations containing neomycin.

IONIC COUPLING AGENTS

From the preceding discussion of membrane permeability, it is obvious that a drug that can temporarily assume lipophilic properties can permeate the cornea readily. One of the strategies that has been attempted experimentally is the coupling of an anion and a cation to form a complex with the charges masked, so that membrane crossing is more easily accomplished. Although this approach has not yet resulted in a commercial formulation, it is noteworthy that a combination of cationic and anionic drugs in the tear film may complex and facilitate the penetration of both.

DRUG RELEASE SYSTEMS

Soft contact lenses absorb drugs from solution and then slowly release them when placed on the eye.[119] This form of drug therapy can be valuable when continuous treatment is desired.[120]

Advanced drug release systems have been designed based on the insertion of a solid device in the eye. There are two major types. The first is a device of low permeability filled with drug. The second is a polymer that is completely soluble in lacrimal fluid, formulated with drug in its matrix (Table 1.4).[120] Both of these systems can be made to approach zero-order kinetics.[1] The advantages of these systems are significant for the treatment of certain conditions, including glaucoma, and for those drugs that do not produce toxic effects when delivered in this manner. To date, the expense of the slow-release inserts compared with the economy of eye drops has hindered their acceptance. However, both theory and clinical experience support the rationality of this approach to ocular dosing. Future improvements in technology and reduced cost would allow increased use of this dosage form.

Prodrugs

When the metabolite of a molecule is more active at the receptor site than is the parent form, the compound is often termed a prodrug. To be therapeutically useful, a prodrug must metabolize predictably to the effective drug form before it reaches the receptor site. The greatest advantage of prodrugs is the potential to add groups that mask features of the drug molecule that prevent penetration or have other undesirable effects.

TABLE 1.4
Polymers Used for Making Inserts

Natural products
  Gelatin
  Alginates
  Pectins
  Tragacanth
  Karaya gum
  Carrageenan
  Agar
  Arabic gum
Starch derivatives
  Starch acetate
  Hydroxyl starch ethers
  Hydroxypropyl starch
Cellulose derivatives
  Methylcellulose
  Carboxymethylcellulose
  Hydroxyethylcellulose
Acrylates
  Polyacrylic acid salts
  Ethyl acrylates
  Polyacrylamides
Polyvinyl derivatives
  Polyvinyl alcohol
  Polyvinylpyrrolidone
  Polyvinyl methyl ether
Miscellaneous
  Polyethylene oxide
  Xanthan gum

From Chiou GCY, Watanabe K. Drug delivery to the eye. Pharmacol Ther 1982;17:269–278.

Prodrug design can be a useful way of increasing a therapeutic agent's penetration through corneal or other barriers.

Dipivalyl epinephrine is the first successful example of the ophthalmic prodrug concept. A pair of pivalyl groups can be attached to the two charged groups on epinephrine. This diesterification increases epithelial penetration 10-fold due to the lipophilic nature of the modified prodrug.[1] The pivalyl groups are removed by esterases in the cornea, leaving epinephrine to act at the receptor site. This special delivery mechanism allows a topically applied concentration of the dipivalyl derivative only one-tenth that of epinephrine to achieve bioavailability equivalent to epinephrine.[5] Systemic absorption of the drug is thereby greatly reduced. This drug has achieved wide acceptance for the treatment of glaucoma since its introduction.

A prodrug that by virtue of lipophilicity can cross the blood-vitreous barrier into the vitreous humor might then be metabolized into a drug that has a greater ionic charge and that therefore cannot recross the barrier readily. An anti-inflammatory drug or antibiotic of low systemic toxicity could thus be introduced by the systemic route into the eye at relatively infrequent intervals, becoming trapped by metabolic alteration, then supplying the aqueous and corneal tissues with a near-zero-order supply of drug over a prolonged period. The vitreous could thus become a drug reservoir of major consequence.

The future design and use of prodrugs holds much promise in ocular drug delivery, particularly where lipophilic prodrugs can be induced to penetrate the blood-vitreous barrier readily, then be metabolized to a form that is trapped in the vitreous compartment. Such drugs, because of selective permeability, could reach an effective concentration in the eye by entrapment within the vitreous compartment. A major problem with this approach is that the brain might sequester drug in the same manner as the vitreous humor. This could potentially be avoided by identifying a suitable enzyme that is present in vitreous humor and not in the brain.

Ocular Drug Development and the Patient

Many steps are involved in the successful design of an ocular drug formulation. The first is selection of an appropriate drug molecule that maximizes therapeutic benefit and bioavailability while minimizing toxicity. A formulation must then be developed to include a vehicle, a preservative, and a buffer. Stability, toxicity, and efficacy must then be evaluated for the complete formulation. An effective dosing regimen must also be developed before beginning clinical trials on a wide scale. The Food and Drug Administration (FDA) is involved in evaluating these steps to provide formulations that are efficacious and safe.

Of the numerous factors that influence ocular drug distribution, the most important remains that of patient compliance. Determining the proper dosage regimen and getting the patient to administer the medication is a primary responsibility of the practitioner. These factors are considered in Chapter 2.

References

1. Shell JW. Pharmacokinetics of topically applied ophthalmic drugs. Surv Ophthalmol 1982;26:207–218.
2. Burstein NL, Anderson JA. Review: Corneal penetration and ocular bioavailability of drugs. J Ocular Pharm 1985; 1:309–326.
3. Maurice DM, Mishima S. Ocular pharmacokinetics. In: Sears ML, ed. Pharmacology of the eye, Handbook of experimental pharmacology. Berlin: Springer-Verlag, 1984; 69:19–116.
4. Shichi H. Biotransformation and drug metabolism. In: Sears ML, ed. Pharmacology of the eye, Handbook of experimental pharmacology. Berlin: Springer-Verlag, 1984;69:117–148.
5. Anderson JA, Davis WL, Wei CP. Site of ocular hydrolysis of a prodrug, dipivifrin, and a comparison of its ocular metabolism with that of the parent compound, epinephrine. Invest Ophthalmol Vis Sci 1980;19:817–823.
6. Davson H, Danielli JF. The permeability of natural membranes. Cambridge: University Press, 1943.
7. Ussing HH. Transport of electrolytes and water across epithelia. Harvey Lectures, Series 59, 1965.
8. Hansch C, Clayton JM. Lipophilic character and biological activity of drugs. II. The parabolic case. J Pharm Sci 1973; 62:1–21.
9. Kishida K, Otori T. Quantitative study on the relationship between transcorneal permeability of drugs and their hydrophobicity. Jpn J Ophthalmol 1980; 24:251–259.
10. Hind HW, Goyan FM. A new concept of the role of hydrogen ion concentration and buffer system in the preparation of ophthalmic solution. J Am Pharm Assoc 1947; 36:33–41.
11. Holly FJ. Formation and stability of the tear film. Int Ophthalmol Clin 1973;13:73–96.
12. Holly FJ. Tear film formation and rupture. In: Holly FJ, ed. The precorneal tear film. Dry Eye Institute, 1986.
13. Mishima S, Maurice DM. Oily layer of tear film and evaporation from corneal surface. Exp Eye Res 1961;1:39–45.
14. Norn MS. Desiccation of the precorneal tear film. I. Corneal wetting-time. Acta Ophthalmol 1969;47:865–880.
15. Burstein NL. The effects of topical drugs and preservatives on the tears and corneal epithelium in dry eye. Trans Ophthalmol Soc UK 1985;104:402–409.
16. Hind HW, Goyan FM. The hydrogen ion concentration and osmotic properties of lacrimal fluid. J Am Pharm Assoc 1949;38:477–479.

17. Mishima S, Gasset A, Klyce SD Jr, Baum JL. Determination of tear volume and tear flow. Invest Ophthalmol 1966;5:264–276.

18. Chrai SS, Makoid MC, Eriksen SP, Robinson JR. Drop size and initial dosing frequency problems of topically applied ophthalmic drugs. J Pharm Sci 1974;63:333–338.

19. Patton TF, Francoeur M. Ocular bioavailability and systemic loss of topically applied ophthalmic drugs. Am J Ophthalmol 1978;85:225–229.

20. Kaila T, Salminen L, Huupponen R. Systemic absorption of topically applied ocular timolol. J Ocular Pharm 1985;1:79–83.

21. Chrai SS, Patton TF, Mehta A, Robinson JR. Lacrimal and instilled fluid dynamics in rabbit eyes. J Pharm Sci 1973;62:1112–1121.

22. Lamberts DW. Dry eye and tear deficiency. Int Ophthalmol Clin 1981;22:123–130.

23. Mishima S. Clinical pharmacokinetics of the eye. Invest Ophthalmol Vis Sci 1981;21:504–541.

24. Fraunfelder FT. Extraocular fluid dynamics: How best to apply topical ocular medications. Trans Am Ophthalmol Soc 1976;74:457–487.

25. Roen JL, Stasior OG, Jakobiec FA. Aging changes in the human lacrimal gland: Role of the ducts. CLAO J 1985;11:237–242.

26. Spencer WH, ed. Ophthalmic pathology: An atlas and textbook, 3 vols., ed. 3. Philadelphia: W.B. Saunders Co, 1985.

27. Ahmed I, Patton TF. Importance of the noncorneal absorption route in topical ophthalmic drug delivery. Invest Ophthalmol Vis Sci 1985;26:584–587.

28. Doane MG, Jensen AD, Dohlman CH. Penetration routes of topically applied eye medications. Am J Ophthalmol 1978;85:383–386.

29. Bienfang DC. Sector pupillary dilatation with an epinephrine strip. Am J Ophthalmol 1973;75:883–884.

30. Ehlers N. On the size of the conjunctival sac. Acta Ophthalmol 1965;43:205–210.

31. Porter KR, Bonneville MA. Fine structure of cells and tissues, ed. 3. Philadelphia: Lea & Febiger, 1968.

32. Klyce SD. Electrical profiles in the corneal epithelium. J Physiol 1972;226:407–429.

33. Maurice DM. Review: The permeability of the cornea. Ophthal Lit 1953;7:1–26.

34. Tonjum AM. Permeability of rabbit corneal epithelium to horseradish peroxidase after the influence of benzalkonium chloride. Acta Ophthalmol 1975;53:335–347.

35. Swan KC, White NG. Corneal permeability. I. Factors affecting penetration of drugs into the cornea. Am J Ophthalmol 1942;25:1043–1057.

36. Wiederholt M, Kössendrup D, Schulz W, Hoffmann F. Pharmacokinetics of topical cyclosporin A in the rabbit eye. Invest Ophthalmol Vis Sci 1986;27:519–524.

37. Huang HS, Schoenwald RD, Lach JL. Corneal penetration behavior of beta blocking agents. II. Assessment of barrier contributions. J Pharm Sci 1983;72:1272–1279.

38. Hogan MJ, Alvarado JA, Weddell JE. Histology of the human eye. Philadelphia: W.B. Saunders Co, 1971.

39. Maurice DM. The chemical and physical basis of corneal transparency. Biochemistry of the eye, Symp. Tutzing Castle, August 1966; 51–61.

40. Davson H. Physiology of the eye. New York: Academic Press, 1980.

41. Johnston MC, Noden DM, Hazelton RD, et al. Origins of avian ocular and periocular tissues. Exp Eye Res 1979;29:27–43.

42. Maurice DM. The cornea and sclera. In: Davson H, ed. The eye. New York: Academic Press, 1984;1b.

43. Hodson S, Miller F. The bicarbonate ion pump in the endothelium which regulates the hydration of rabbit cornea. J Physiol 1976;263:563–577.

44. Whigham C, Hodson S. The movement of sodium across short-circuited rabbit corneal endothelium. Curr Eye Res 1985;4:1241–1245.

45. Burstein NL, Maurice DM. Cryofixation of tissue surfaces by a propane jet for electron microscopy. Micron 1978;9:191–198.

46. Maurice DM. The use of fluorescein in ophthalmological research. The Friedenwald Memorial Lecture. Invest Ophthalmol 1967;6:464–477.

47. Burstein NL, Fischbarg J, Liebovitch L. Electrical potential, resistance, and fluid secretion across isolated ciliary body. Exp Eye Res 1984;39:771–779.

48. Friedman E, Kopald HH, Smith TR, Mimura S. Retinal and choroidal blood flow determined with krypton-85 anesthetized animals. Invest Ophthalmol 1964;3:539–547.

49. Yamashita H, Uyama M, Sears ML. Comparative study by electron microscopy of response to urea between ciliary epithelia of albino and pigmented rabbits. A function of the ciliary pigmented epithelium. Jpn J Ophthalmol 1981;25:313–320.

50. Fisher RF, Hayes BP. Thickness and volume constants and ultrastructural organization of basement membrane (lens capsule). J Physiol 1979;293:229–245.

51. Paterson CA. Effects of drugs on the lens. In: Ellis PP, ed. Side effects of drugs in ophthalmology. Int Ophthalmol Clin 1971;11:63–98.

52. Kaiser RJ, Maurice DM. The diffusion of fluorescein in the lens. Exp Eye Res 1964;3:156–165.

53. Kinoshita JH. Mechanisms of cataract formation. Invest Ophthalmol 1974;13:713–724.

54. Reddy VN. Metabolism of glutathione in the lens. Exp Eye Res 1971;11:310–328.

55. Anderson JA, Chen CC, Vita JB, Shackleton M. Disposition of topical flurbiprofen in normal and aphakic rabbit eyes. Arch Ophthalmol 1982;100:642–645.

56. Balazs EA. Physiology of the vitreous body in retinal surgery with special emphasis on reoperations. In: Schepens CL, ed. Proceedings of the II Conference of the Retina Foundation, Ipswich, May 30–31, 1958. St. Louis: C.V. Mosby Co, 1960.

57. Balazs EA. Molecular morphology of the vitreous body. In: Smelser GK, ed. The structure of the eye. New York: Academic Press, 1961; 293–310.

58. Balazs EA, Flood MT. Age-related changes in the physical and chemical structure of human vitreous (abstr.). Third International Congress for Eye Research, Osdaka, Japan, 1978.

59. Balazs EA, Denlinger JL. The vitreous. In: Davson H, ed. The eye, ed. 3. New York: Academic Press, 1984;1a:533–589.

60. Maurice DM. The exchange of sodium between the vitreous body and the blood and aqueous humour. J Physiol 1957; 137:110–125.

61. Osterlin S. On the molecular biology of the vitreous in the aphakic eye. Acta Ophthalmol 1977;55:353–361.

62. Osterlin S. Vitreous changes after cataract extraction. In: Freeman HM, Hirose T, Schepens CL, eds. Vitreous surgery and fundus diagnosis and treatment. New York: Appleton-Century-Crofts, 1977.

63. Maurice DM. Injection of drugs into the vitreous body. In: Leopold IH, Burns RP, eds. Symposium on ocular therapy. New York: John Wiley & Sons, 1976;9:59–71.

64. Balazs EA, Denlinger JL. The pharmacology of the vitreous. In: Dikstein S, ed. Drugs and ocular tissues. Basel: S. Karger, 1977; 524–538.

65. Burstein NL, Bernacchi D, Leopold IH. Gentamicin iontophoresis into vitreous humor. J Ocular Pharm 1985;1:363–368.

66. Cunha-Vaz J. The blood-ocular barriers. Surv Ophthalmol 1979;23:279–296.

67. Henkind P. Ocular circulation. In: Records RE, ed. Physiology of the eye and visual system, Hagerstown, MD: Harper & Row, 1975;5:98–155.

68. Bill A. The blood-aqueous barrier. Trans Ophthalmol Soc UK 1986;105:149–155.

69. Alm A, Bill A. Ocular circulation. In: Moses R, ed. Adler's physiology of the eye: Clinical applications, ed. 8. St. Louis: C. V. Mosby Co, 1987.

70. Cerasoli JR. Effects of drugs on the retina. In: Ellis PP, ed. Side effects of drugs in ophthalmology. Int Ophthalmol Clin 1971;11:121–136.

71. Leopold IH. Ocular complications of drugs: Visual changes. JAMA 1968;205:631.

72. Bito LZ, Davson H, Levin E, et al. The relationship between the concentration of amino acids in the ocular fluids and the blood plasma of dogs. Exp Eye Res 1965;4:374–380.

73. Bito LZ. Absorptive transport of prostaglandins from intraocular fluids to blood: A review of recent findings. Exp Eye Res 1973;16:299–306.

74. Bito LZ, DeRousseau CJ. Transport functions of the blood-retinal barrier system of the micro environment of the retina. In: Cunha-Vaz J, ed. Blood-retinal barriers. 1980; 133–163.

75. Leibold JE. Drugs having a toxic effect on the optic nerve. In: Ellis PP, ed. Side effects of drugs in ophthalmology. Int Ophthalmol Clin 1971;11:137–158.

76. Leopold IH. Anti-infective agents. In: Sears ML, ed. Pharmacology of the eye, Handbook of experimental pharmacology. Berlin: Springer-Verlag, 1984;69:385–458.

77. Riggs DS. The mathematical approach to physiological problems. A critical primer. Cambridge, MA: The M.I.T. Press, 1963.

78. Levitzki A. Reconstitution of membrane receptor systems. Biochim Biophys Acta 1985;822:127–153.

79. Goldstein A, Aronow L, Kalman SM. Principles of drug action. New York: Harper & Row, 1974.

80. Van den Brink FG. General theory of drug-receptor interactions. In: Van Rossum JM, ed. Kinetics of drug action. Berlin: Springer-Verlag, 1977.

81. Caron MC, Mukherjee C, Lefkowitz RJ. β-Adrenergic receptors. In: Smythies JR, ed. Receptors in pharmacology. New York: Marcel Dekker, 1978;97–122.

82. Sutherland EW, Rall TW. The relation of adenosine-3', 5'-phosphate and phosphorylase to the actions of catecholamines and other hormones. Pharmacol Rev 1960;12:265–299.

83. Burstein NL. Review: Growth factor effects on corneal wound healing. J Ocular Pharm 1987;3:263–277.

84. Triggle DJ. Receptor theory. In: Smythies JR. Receptors in pharmacology. New York: Marcel Dekker, 1978;1–66.

85. Gavin JR, Roth J, Neville DM, et al. Insulin-dependent regulation of insulin receptor concentrations: A direct demonstration in cell culture. Proc Natl Acad Sci USA 1974;71:84–88.

86. Candia OA, Neufeld AH. Topical epinephrine causes a decrease in density of beta-adrenergic receptors and catecholamine-stimulated chloride transport in the rabbit cornea. Biochim Biophys Acta 1978;543:403–408.

87. Becker B. Decrease in intraocular pressure in man by a carbonic anhydrase inhibitor, Diamox. Am J Ophthalmol 1954;37:13–15.

88. Burstein NL. Corneal cytotoxicity of topically applied drugs, vehicles, and preservatives. Surv Ophthalmol 1980;25:15–30.

89. Pfister RR, Burstein NL. The effects of ophthalmic drugs, vehicles, and preservatives on corneal epithelium: A scanning electron microscope study. Invest Ophthalmol 1976; 15:246–259.

90. Maurice DM. The tonicity of an eye drop and its dilution by tears. Exp Eye Res 1971;11:30–33.

91. Gilbard JP, Kenyon KR. Tear diluents in the treatment of keratoconjunctivitis sicca. Ophthalmology 1985;92:646–650.

92. Lemp MA, Goldberg M, Roddy MR. The effect of tear substitutes on tear film breakup time. Invest Ophthalmol 1975;14:255–258.

93. Burstein NL. Preservative cytotoxic threshold for benzalkonium chloride and chlorhexidine digluconate in cat and rabbit corneas. Invest Ophthalmol Vis Sci 1980;19:308–313.

94. Leopold IH. Local toxic effect of detergents on ocular structures. Arch Ophthalmol 1945;34:99–102.

95. Keller N, Moore D, Carper D, Longwell A. Increased corneal permeability by the dual effects of transient tear film acidification and exposure to benzalkonium chloride. Exp Eye Res 1980;30:203–210.

96. Wilson WS, Duncan AJ, Jay JL. Effect of benzalkonium chloride on the stability of the precorneal tear film in rabbit and man. Br J Ophthalmol 1975;59:667–669.

97. Marsh RJ, Maurice DM. The influence of non-ionic detergents and other surfactants on human corneal permeability. Exp Eye Res 1971;11:43–48.

98. Cadwallader DE, Ansel HC. Hemolysis of erythrocytes by antibacterial preservatives. II. Quaternary ammonium salts. J Pharm Sci 1965;54:1010–1012.

99. Burstein NL. Preservative alteration of corneal permeability in humans and rabbits. Invest Ophthalmol Vis Sci 1984; 25:1453–1457.

100. Green K, Livingston V, Bowman K. Chlorhexidine effects on corneal epithelium and endothelium. Arch Ophthalmol 1980;98:1273–1278.

101. Abrams JD, Davies TG, Klein M. Mercurial preservatives in eye-drops. Br J Ophthalmol 1965;49:146–147.

102. Burstein NL, Klyce SD. Electrophysiologic and morphologic effects of ophthalmic preparations on rabbit cornea epithelium. Invest Ophthalmol Vis Sci 1977;16:899–911.

103. Burton GD, Hill RM. Aerobic responses of the cornea to ophthalmic preservatives, measured in vivo. Invest Ophthalmol Vis Sci 1981;21:842–845.

104. Mullen W, Shepherd W, Leibowitz J. Ophthalmic preservatives and vehicles. Surv Ophthalmol 1973;17:469–483.

105. Mondino BJ, Salamon SM, Zaidman GW. Allergic and toxic reactions in soft contact lens wearers. Surv Ophthalmol 1982;26:337–344.

106. Hind HW. Aspects of contact lens solutions. The Optician, May 2, 1975.

107. Molyneux P. The physical chemistry and pharmaceutical applications of polyvinylpyrrolidone. In: Digenis GA, Ansell J, eds. Proceedings of the International Symposium on Povidone. Louisville: University of Kentucky College of Pharmacy, 1983.

108. Shelanski HA, Shelanski MV, Cantor A. Polyvinyl pyrrolidone (PVP)—a useful adjunct in cosmetics. J Soc Cos Chem 1954;5:129–132.

109. Schwartz FL. Evaluation of the safety of povidone and crospovidone. Yakuzaigaku 1981;41:205–217.

110. Sabiston DW. The dry eye. Trans Ophthalmol Soc NZ 1969;21:96–100.

111. Krishna N, Mitchell B. Polyvinyl alcohol as an ophthalmic vehicle: Effect on ocular structures. Am J Ophthalmol 1965;59:860–864.

112. Linn ML, Jones LT. Rate of lacrimal excretion of ophthalmic vehicles. Am J Ophthalmol 1968;65:76–78.

113. Trueblood JH, Rossomondo RM, Carlton WH, Wilson LA. Corneal contact times of ophthalmic vehicles. Arch Ophthalmol 1975;93:127–130.

114. Waring GO, Harris RR. Double-masked evaluation of a poloxamer artificial tear in keratoconjunctivitis sicca. In: Leopold IH, Burns RP, eds. Symposium on ocular therapy. New York: John Wiley & Sons 1979;11:127–139.

115. Fraunfelder FT, Hanna C. Ophthalmic drug delivery systems. Surv Ophthalmol 1974;18:292–298.

116. Scruggs J, Wallace T, Hanna C. Route of absorption of drug and ointment after application to the eye. Ann Ophthalmol 1978;10:267–271.

117. Mackeen DL. Aqueous formulations and ointments. Int Ophthalmol Clin 1980;20:79–92.

118. Hardberger R, Hanna C, Boyd CM. Effects of drug vehicles on ocular contact time. Arch Ophthalmol 1975;93:42–45.

119. Kaufman HE, Uotila MH, Gasset AR, et al. The medical uses of soft contact lenses. Trans Am Acad Ophthalmol Otolaryngol 1971;75:361–373.

120. Chiou GCY, Watanabe K. Drug delivery to the eye. Pharmacol Ther 1982;17:269–278.

CHAPTER 2

Clinical Administration of Ocular Drugs

Jimmy D. Bartlett
Anthony P. Cullen

The successful diagnosis and management of ocular disease requires that appropriate routes of drug administration be used to obtain the desired beneficial therapeutic effect. Furthermore, drugs that are misused or inappropriately administered may contribute to iatrogenic ocular or systemic disease. An understanding of the basic principles of pharmacokinetics and bioavailability as applied to the eye, which are considered in Chapter 1, serves as the basis for a rational clinical approach to the ocular delivery of drugs through various routes.

This chapter considers guidelines for drug administration in clinical practice, the various methods employed to deliver drugs to the eye, ophthalmic prescription writing, patient compliance, and some legal aspects associated with drug administration.

Principles of Drug Administration

Patient History

A systematic case history is essential before any drug is administered. Not only does a careful history alert the practitioner to possible adverse drug reactions, but it also helps him or her choose the best preparation for the patient. The practitioner should consider the following areas of historical information before administering or prescribing any drug.

CONCOMITANT MEDICATIONS

Drug interactions can play a significant role in potentiating drug effects and may exacerbate any potential adverse reaction. For example, topically administered epinephrine or phenylephrine may potentiate the adrenergic effects of systemically administered tricyclic antidepressants,[1] and topically administered β blockers may potentiate the effects of systemic β-adrenergic blocking drugs. In this regard it is important for the clinician to be aware of any over-the-counter (OTC) preparations that the patient may not consider "drugs"—especially those for hay fever, colds, anxiety, and gastrointestinal disorders—that are likely to affect the autonomic nervous system. Because of individual idiosyncrasies, rules for drug interactions are far from established.

ALLERGIES

Although the risk of anaphylactic reactions associated with topically administered drugs is extremely remote, inquiry regarding a history of drug allergies is essential. Hypersensitivity to thimerosal and other mercury compounds is not uncommon among contact lens patients, and knowledge of allergy to systemically administered antibiotics will be helpful in the administration of topical antibiotics. Cross-sensitivity of proparacaine with other local anesthetics is quite rare and is usually not an important clinical consideration (see Chapter 4), but a history of hypersensitivity to specific local anesthetics should nevertheless be noted.

CARDIOVASCULAR DISEASE

Patients with systemic hypertension, arteriosclerosis, and other cardiovascular diseases may be at risk with high concentrations of topically administered adrenergic agonists such as phenylephrine. Repeated topical doses or soaked cotton pledgets placed in the conjunctival sac have been associated with significant adverse cardiovascular effects.[1]

THYROID DISEASE

Because of increased catecholamine activity in patients with hyperthyroidism, elevated blood pressure or other adverse cardiovascular effects can occur when patients with Graves' disease are administered adrenergic agonists.

DIABETES MELLITUS

Slower drug detoxification and excretion in patients with diabetes may result in prolonged drug activity. Systemic administration of hyperosmotic agents such as glycerin can cause clinically significant hyperglycemia. Administration of corticosteroids may also represent a significant risk because of drug-induced hyperglycemia. Furthermore, it is often more difficult to achieve a widely dilated pupil with topically administered mydriatics, thus tempting the practitioner to exceed the minimum dosage with the attendant risk of adverse systemic side effects.

SEIZURE DISORDERS

The practitioner should be cautious in the use of central nervous system (CNS) stimulants such as cyclopentolate. High concentrations of such drugs in normal children have resulted in transient CNS effects, and the risk is somewhat greater in untreated patients with documented seizure disorders.[2,3]

EMOTIONAL DISTURBANCES

Anxiety and emotional instability can be associated with psychogenic reactions that may appear to be drug related. Such reactions include vasovagal syncope. Attention to the patient's systemic medications and various innuendos made during the initial patient interview may alert the clinician to such a possibility.

PREGNANCY

Systemic drugs should not be administered to pregnant patients unless absolutely essential for their well-being or that of the fetus. Most topically administered drugs, however, are permissible if given in relatively low concentrations for brief periods.[4]

RESPIRATORY DISORDERS

Because topically applied β blockers can induce asthma or dyspnea in patients with preexisting chronic obstructive pulmonary disease (COPD),[5–7] the practitioner should inquire about a history of pulmonary disorders before initiating glaucoma treatment with β-adrenergic blocking agents.

OTHER SYSTEMIC DISEASES

Occasionally other systemic disorders can be affected by topically applied medications. Examples include myasthenia gravis, which can be worsened with topical timolol,[8] and erythema multiforme (Stevens-Johnson syndrome), which can be caused or exacerbated by topical ocular sulfonamides.[9,10] Chapter 31 discusses in further detail the relationship between topical ocular therapy and systemic disease.

Clinical Procedures that May Be Influenced by Drugs

Since various clinical procedures can be influenced by previously administered drugs, these procedures should be performed before drug application. This practice not only protects the clinician legally, but also provides valuable information regarding contraindications to the intended drugs as well as certain baseline clinical information that may be unobtainable following drug administration. Such procedures include the following.

VISUAL ACUITY

Corrected visual acuity should be the initial clinical test performed at each and every patient visit. This "entrance" visual acuity measurement protects the clinician legally and provides baseline information when patients are monitored on successive visits. Topically applied ointments, for example, can reduce vision, since these preparations often have a transient detrimental effect on visual acuity.

PUPIL EXAMINATION

Since a meaningful evaluation of pupils following drug-induced mydriasis or miosis is impossible, pupillary examination, including pupil size and responsiveness, should be recorded before instilling mydriatics or miotics. The presence and nature of the direct reflexes should be recorded, as well as the presence or absence of a Marcus Gunn sign.

MANIFEST REFRACTION

Since topically applied cycloplegics will often affect the manifest (subjective) refractive error, refraction influenced by drugs is undesirable. When indicated, cycloplegic refraction may be performed following the initial manifest refraction (see Chapter 17).

AMPLITUDE OF ACCOMMODATION

Because of the obvious effects of anticholinergic agents on accommodation, amplitude of accommodation should be measured before administering cycloplegics.

TESTS OF BINOCULARITY

Evaluation of binocular vision, including accommodation-convergence relationships, should be performed before administering cycloplegics. In many cases these drugs will produce dramatic alterations in the observed heterophoria or heterotropia measurements. An esotropia associated with uncorrected latent or manifest hyperopia will often worsen under cycloplegia.

BIOMICROSCOPY

The possibility of compromising the corneal epithelium with topically applied drugs (particularly anesthetics) or with procedures such as applanation tonometry and gonioscopy emphasizes the importance of evaluating the cornea and other anterior segment structures before instilling any drug, including dyes. The indiscrete application of a sodium fluorescein–impregnated filter paper strip may result in corneal-staining patterns associated with the iatrogenic foreign body abrasion. Since the application of certain mydriatics such as phenylephrine can produce nonpathologic cells in the anterior chamber, it is of diagnostic importance to know whether such cells are iatrogenic. Thus, careful evaluation of the aqueous, using a conical slit lamp beam, before pupillary dilation with such drugs is essential. Furthermore, examination of the anterior chamber angle will be of value before administering mydriatics for pupillary dilation (see Chapter 16). In other instances, certain drugs should precede others so that the corneal epithelium and precorneal tear film are not disturbed. For example, sodium fluorescein should be instilled for determining the tear breakup time (BUT) prior to administering a topical anesthetic for tonometry, since the latter agent can adversely affect the BUT measurement.

TONOMETRY

In eyes with narrow anterior chamber angles, it is important to record the intraocular pressure before dilating the pupil with mydriatics. Although cycloplegics can cause minor elevation of pressure even in eyes with open angles,[11,12] acute and dangerous pressure elevation is common in eyes undergoing attacks of angle-closure glaucoma induced by mydriatics. Thus,

baseline tonometry is essential before dilating pupils in eyes with narrow angles.

TESTS OF CARDIOVASCULAR STATUS

Since some topically administered drugs affecting the autonomic nervous system (e.g., atropine, timolol, epinephrine) can affect systemic blood pressure and cardiac activity, it is of value to note pulse strength, regularity, and rate during routine sphygmomanometry.

Adverse Drug Reactions

Adverse reactions to ocular drugs are not uncommon, but serious reactions are extremely rare. In most instances these adverse reactions are manifestations of drug hypersensitivity (allergy) or toxicity.

With judicious use, the possibility of anaphylactic shock associated with topically administered ocular drugs is considerably remote. The long-term topical application of drugs is more likely to result in less serious hypersensitivity reactions. Most drugs are nonproteins and are not themselves antigenic. However, metabolic by-products can combine with body proteins to form antigens. These, in turn, combine with antibodies, which may initiate the characteristic allergic inflammatory response. Hypersensitivity responses are generally unpredictable reactions; they include conditions such as blepharoconjunctivitis associated with topically administered neomycin (see Color Plate II), itching and hyperemia associated with thimerosal or chlorhexidine in contact lens preparations, or the stringy discharge accompanying the topical administration of cyclopentolate.

In determining sensitivity to a medication, a number of procedures can help but are not always reliable. These include applying some of the agent to the skin and patching, scratching, or pricking the area. Alternatively, the medication may be injected intradermally or applied in a weak concentration to the conjunctiva. It is also essential to consider the patient's history of previous reactions to topically administered drugs. If a patient is found, by testing or history, to be allergic to a particular preparation, this fact should be recorded in the patient's chart and an alternative drug selected. Management of the mild hypersensitivity reactions that occasionally occur from topical application of ocular drugs is considered in subsequent chapters.

Drug toxicities are responses that can frequently be anticipated or at least explained pharmacologically. For example, topically administered proparacaine is known to loosen the corneal epithelium. Desquamation of epithelium following the administration of proparacaine is an undesirable response occurring as a manifestation of this drug's toxicity. Toxic signs associated with drugs affecting the autonomic nervous system are particularly easy to predict. Topically administered atropine, for example, may be associated with tachycardia, xerostomia, and other manifestations of anticholinergic activity. Bronchospasm, bradycardia, and systemic hypotension associated with the topical administration of timolol and other β blockers are also predictable systemic toxicities easily explained on the basis of these drugs' pharmacologic activity.

OCULAR EFFECTS OF LOCALLY ADMINISTERED DRUGS

Numerous adverse ocular effects from topically administered drugs have been observed[13] (Table 2.1). Topically administered ophthalmic medications can produce adverse ocular effects through a variety of mechanisms, including immunologic, photoimmunologic or phototoxic, irritative, or toxic cumulative deposition, alteration of melanotic pigmentation, and microbial imbalance.[14] The ocular or adnexal tissues respond by manifesting cutaneous changes; papillary, follicular, keratinizing, or cicatrizing conjunctivitis; epithelial, ulcerative, vascularizing, or cicatrizing keratitis; hyperpigmentation or hypopigmentation; or infectious complications.[15] The clinician administering or prescribing ocular drugs must be aware of these potential iatrogenic complications.

In general, any topically applied drug can elicit a hypersensitivity reaction. As previously mentioned, such local allergic reactions are particularly common with neomycin and with thimerosal and chlorhexidine employed as preservatives in various contact lens preparations. The practitioner should diminish the risk of allergic responses by carefully questioning the patient about any previous drug reactions.

Iatrogenic infection is possible with locally applied drugs, but it can usually be avoided by handling medications with care and by using single-dose containers when available. Since airborne contamination is normally of little significance,[16] the principal source of pathogens is the dropper tip that has been allowed to come in contact with the nonsterile surface of the patient's lids, lashes, or face or of the practitioner's fingers.[17,18] Care must therefore be exercised during instillation of topical medications. In addition, labeled expiration dates should be respected, and old or contaminated solutions should be discarded.

Mydriatics should be used with caution in patients with extremely narrow anterior chamber angles. Such drugs may precipitate an attack of acute angle-closure glaucoma.

The degradation products of topically applied solutions (e.g., epinephrine) can be irritating and can compromise corneal and other ocular tissues. Drugs

TABLE 2.1
Adverse Ocular Effects from Topically Administered Drugs

Eyelids
  Urticaria and angioedema
  Allergic contact dermatoconjunctivitis
  Allergic contact dermatitis
  Photoallergic contact dermatitis
  Irritative or toxic contact dermatitis
  Phototoxic dermatitis
  Cumulative deposition
  Melanotic hyperpigmentation or hypopigmentation
  Microbial imbalance

Conjunctiva
  Anaphylactoid conjunctivitis
  Allergic contact (dermato)conjunctivitis
  Cicatrizing allergic conjunctivitis
  Nonspecific (papillary) irritative or toxic conjunctivitis
  Follicular irritative or toxic conjunctivitis
  Cicatrizing and keratinizing irritative or toxic conjunctivitis (including pseudotrachoma)
  Cumulative deposition
  Microbial imbalance

Cornea
  Anaphylactoid keratitis
  Allergic contact keratitis
  Irritative or toxic keratitis
  Phototoxic keratitis
  Toxic calcific band keratopathy
  Pseudotrachoma
  Cumulative deposition
  Microbial imbalance

Intraocular pressure
  Elevation (glaucoma)
  Reduction (hypotony)

Uvea
  Hypertrophy of pupillary frill (iris "cyst")
  Iridocyclitis
  Iris sphincter atrophy

Crystalline lens
  Anterior subcapsular opacification
  Posterior subcapsular opacification

Retina
  Detachment
  Cystic or hemorrhagic toxic maculopathy

Modified from Wilson FM. Adverse external ocular effects of topical ophthalmic medications. Surv Ophthalmol 1979;24(2):57–88.

should preferably be stored away from sunlight and in a cool location to prevent rapid deterioration.

Drug interactions can play an important role in precipitating adverse ocular side effects. Adverse interactions with systemically administered medications, such as the depression of hydroxyamphetamine mydriasis in patients taking methyldopa,[16] should be anticipated and avoided.

Various pathologic conditions of the eye may affect its response to topically administered drugs. Particularly important are the denervation syndromes such as Horner's, Riley-Day, and Adie's, in which low concentrations of topically applied drugs affecting the autonomic nervous system can produce ocular responses normally encountered only with higher concentrations. In addition, patients with Down's syndrome may demonstrate hyperreactivity to topically administered atropine.[19]

Any clinical procedure that compromises the integrity of the corneal epithelium can enhance the penetration of topically administered drugs. The prior application of a topical anesthetic may facilitate absorption of subsequently applied drugs.[20] Phenylephrine 0.125%, which normally does not dilate the pupil, can produce mydriasis after applanation tonometry or after instillation of a topical anesthetic.[16]

The abuse of topically administered drugs, either by practitioner or patient, can cause significant ocular toxicity. Infiltrative keratitis has occurred from the chronic use of anesthetic drops by patients for relief of pain associated with corneal abrasions.[21] Bilateral posterior subcapsular cataracts developed in a 24-year-old patient following the topical administration of prednisolone acetate 0.12% twice daily for 4 years.[22] Practitioners should carefully monitor patients treated with drugs known to have significant ocular or systemic toxicities.

Topically administered drugs most often associated with significant adverse ocular reactions are summarized in Table 2.2.

SYSTEMIC EFFECTS OF LOCALLY ADMINISTERED DRUGS

Topically applied ocular drugs may in some cases cause significant systemic effects. After instillation into the conjunctival sac, drugs are absorbed into the systemic circulation through the conjunctival capillaries; the nasal mucosa after passage through the lacrimal drainage system; or through the oral pharynx or the gastrointestinal tract after swallowing.[23] Since topically applied drugs avoid the metabolic transformation and detoxification normally occurring in the gut wall and liver, these drugs can exert a substantial pharmacologic effect as great as a similar oral or parenteral dose. Table 2.3 lists the quantities of topically applied drugs according to solution concentration. Note that topically applied doses often exceed the minimum toxic systemic dose.

Significant effects on the cardiovascular system can be exerted by topically administered adrenergic agonists such as epinephrine and phenylephrine. Anticholinergic drugs can have significant effects on the CNS—toxic disorders such as cortical disturbances, cerebellar dysfunction, and confusional psychosis may occur. CNS toxicity is particularly common with high doses of topically administered cyclopentolate.[23] Toxic effects on the autonomic nervous system may be produced by direct-acting cholinergic or anticholinesterase agents. Evidence of muscarinic toxicity such as nausea, vomiting, sweating, abdominal cramps, diarrhea, and salivation may predominate. Respiratory distress due to bronchiolar spasm may be associated with β blockers. There have been reports of bone marrow depression and death attributable to the chronic topical

TABLE 2.2
Topically Administered Drugs Commonly Associated with Adverse Ocular Reactions

Drug	CDC	PK	PC	FC	EIOP	HPF	ISA	ASC	PSC	RD	TM	CA	EOI	DCE
					Adverse Ocular Reactions									
Neomycin	X	X	X											
Gentamicin	X	X	X											
Tetracycline		X	X											
Idoxuridine	X	X	X	X										
Miotics			X	X			X			X				
Atropine	X													
Mydriatics					X									
Preservatives		X	X											
Corticosteroids					X				X				X	
Anticholinesterases						X		X	X					
Epinephrine	X										X			
Timolol		X										X		
Anesthetics														X

CDC, contact dermatoconjunctivitis; PK, punctate keratopathy; PC, papillary conjunctivitis; FC, follicular conjunctivitis; EIOP, elevated intraocular pressure; HPF, hypertrophy of pupillary frill; ISA, iris sphincter atrophy; ASC, anterior subcapsular cataract; PSC, posterior subcapsular cataract; RD, retinal detachment; TM, toxic maculopathy; CA, corneal anesthesia; EOI, extraocular infection; DCE, desquamation of corneal epithelium. Adapted from Wilson FM. Adverse external ocular effects of topical ophthalmic medications. Surv Ophthalmol 1979;24(2):57–88.

TABLE 2.3
Quantities (mg) of Topically Applied Drugs according to Solution Concentration

Drops	Approximate Milliliters	Concentration (%)												
		0.03	0.06	0.12	0.25	0.50	1.0	2.0	3.0	4.0	5.0	6.0	8.0	10.0
1	0.05	0.02	0.03	0.06	0.125	0.25	0.50	1.0	1.5	2.0	2.5	3.0	4.0	5.0
2	1.10	0.03	0.06	0.12	0.250	0.50	1.00	2.0	3.0	4.0	5.0	6.0	8.0	10.0
4	0.20	0.06	0.12	0.24	0.500	1.00	2.00	4.0	6.0	8.0	10.0	12.0	16.0	20.0
6	0.30	0.09	0.18	0.36	0.750	1.50	3.00	6.0	9.0	12.0	15.0	18.0	24.0	30.0
8	0.40	0.12	0.24	0.48	1.00	2.00	4.00	8.0	12.0	16.0	20.0	24.0	32.0	40.0
10	0.50	0.15	0.30	0.60	1.25	2.50	5.00	10.0	15.0	20.0	25.0	30.0	40.0	50.0
12	0.60	0.18	0.36	0.72	1.50	3.00	6.00	12.0	18.0	24.0	30.0	36.0	48.0	60.0

Based on 20 drops/ml.

administration of chloramphenicol.[24] Topically administered corticosteroids can also produce toxic systemic effects, notably Cushing's syndrome. The epidemiology, diagnosis, and management of adverse systemic effects of topically applied ocular drugs are discussed in Chapter 31.

The prevention of toxic systemic effects associated with topically applied ocular drugs is largely a matter of a very careful patient interview and examination before administering or prescribing any medication. The patient history is vital, since it serves to identify the patient with drug allergies, the patient taking systemic medications likely to interact adversely with the locally applied drug, and the patient who is otherwise at risk for adverse systemic side effects. Adherence to the following general guidelines will usually reduce the risk of adverse reactions.[25,26]

- Store all medications out of children's reach. As few as 20 drops of 1% atropine can be fatal if swallowed.[27]
- Wipe excessive solution or ointment from the lids and lashes after instillation.
- Use the lowest concentration and least dosage frequency consistent with a drug's clinical purpose. Avoid overdosage. Drug dosages should generally be reduced in neonates because of differences in relative volumes of the body fluid compartments, reduced binding of drugs to plasma proteins, immaturity of the enzymatic mechanisms for drug inactivation, and incomplete development of the blood-brain barrier.
- Drug application should be conservative in patients with hyperemic conjunctivae. The existence of hyperemia increases the rate of systemic drug absorption through the conjunctival capillaries.
- Before any drug is administered or prescribed, consider its potential adverse effects relative to its potential diagnostic or therapeutic benefit to the patient.
- Caution patients, or their parents, to use prescribed medication only as directed. Contrary to what some patients or parents may expect, there is no additional benefit from receiving more than the prescribed amount of drug.
- Recognize adverse drug reactions. Often the practitioner fails to recognize the clinical signs of drug toxicity or allergy, which can occur as quickly as a few seconds or minutes following drug administration, or after months or years.
- Environmental temperature and humidity may play a role in the toxicity of cycloplegic agents. Heat and humidity place greater demands on the body's thermoregulatory centers. Toxicity may thus occur more readily because of inhibition of perspiration and its decreased evaporation. This reduces body heat dissipation. It seems advisable, therefore, to use conservative dosages when administering cycloplegics in hot and humid environments.
- Manual depression of the puncta (see Fig. 2.5) can reduce systemic drug absorption by inhibiting initial nasolacrimal drainage. It is prudent to use this procedure in the office or recommend it for home use in patients who are at high risk for systemic complications associated with certain topically applied drugs, such as β-adrenergic blocking agents.

OCULAR EFFECTS OF SYSTEMICALLY ADMINISTERED DRUGS

The mechanisms contributing to the adverse ocular effects of systemically administered drugs are complex. These mechanisms, as well as a description of the ocular toxicities themselves, are discussed in Chapter 30.

The most frequently used methods of drug administration are described in the following sections.

Topical Administration

Topical application, the most common route of administration for ophthalmic drugs, is convenient, simple, and noninvasive, and the patient can self-administer the medication. On the other hand, the need to rely on the patient to carry out proper treatment is one of the most significant factors in noncompliance.

The two primary sources of drug loss in topical administration are diffusion into the circulating blood and escape into the canal of Schlemm through the aqueous.[28] Diffusion into the circulating blood takes place through the blood vessels of the conjunctiva, episclera, intraocular vessels, and vessels of the nasal mucosa and oral pharynx after drainage through the nasolacrimal system. Because of these blood and aqueous losses of drug, topically administered medications do not typically penetrate in useful concentrations to the posterior ocular structures and therefore are of no therapeutic benefit for diseases of the posterior segment. The occurrence of systemic side effects sometimes associated with the topical application of ocular drugs has created much interest in devising various drug delivery systems to minimize the risk of systemic toxicity. The following discussion considers these and other forms of topical drug delivery systems.

Solutions and Suspensions

Solutions are the most commonly used mode of delivery for topical ocular medications. Solutions or suspensions are usually preferred over ointments, since the former are more easily instilled, interfere less with vision, and have fewer potential complications.[29] Dis-

advantages of topically applied solutions, however, include short ocular contact time,[29] imprecise and inconsistent delivery of drug, frequent contamination,[30] and the possibility of ocular injury with the dropper tip.[31,32] Furthermore, aqueous suspensions have the problem of precipitation. Suspensions must be resuspended by shaking to provide an accurate dosage of drug, and the degree of resuspension varies considerably among preparations and among patients. The best corticosteroid formulations, for example, are not always adequately resuspended even by the most compliant and carefully instructed patient.[33]

STORAGE

Solutions of drugs should be stored in the examination room in a manner allowing easy identification of labels (Fig. 2.1). Since containers of solutions often differ little in size, shape, or labelling, numerous cases have been reported of bottle confusion between drugs with similar packaging.[34–36] The drug name should be confirmed by inspection each and every time a medication is used.

To help reduce confusion in labelling and identification among various topical ocular medications, drug-packaging standards have been proposed.[37] When fully implemented by the ophthalmic drug industry, the standard colors for drug labelling and bottle caps will include yellow, blue, or both for β blockers, red for mydriatics and cycloplegics, green for miotics, gray for nonsteroidal anti-inflammatory drugs, and brown or tan for anti-infective agents.

Many practitioners have been annoyed by the bubbles contained in even the more viscous gonioscopic or fundus contact lens solutions. These troublesome

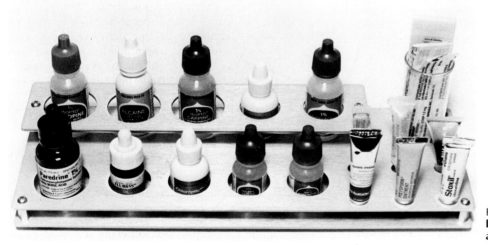

FIGURE 2.1 **Drug storage tray allows easy identification of packaging labels.**

bubbles can be minimized or eliminated by simply storing the solution inverted in the plastic vial in which many topical ophthalmic preparations are commercially packaged (Fig. 2.2). In this way the bubbles float to the top of the solution during storage and do not subsequently interfere with the diagnostic procedure.

As stated previously, expiration dates of solutions should be respected. The practitioner should periodically survey the ophthalmic preparations in the office and discard solutions that have reached the expiration date. The use of old solutions can increase the practitioner's liability as well as introduce the risk of potential drug toxicity or iatrogenic infection. Some commonly employed ophthalmic solutions, such as proparacaine, may change color, indicating deterioration (Fig. 2.3). Others, however, will show no visible signs of deterioration.

TECHNIQUES OF INSTILLATION

Traditionally, two methods have been commonly used to instill topical ocular solutions.

1. With the patient looking down and the upper lid retracted, apply 1 or 2 drops of solution to the superiorly exposed bulbar conjunctiva.
2. With the patient's head inclined backward so that the optical axis is as nearly vertical as possible, retract the lower lid and stabilize the upper lid. Instruct the

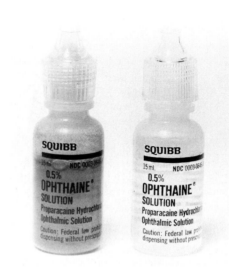

FIGURE 2.3   **Change in color of proparacaine solution (left) indicates deterioration of the preparation.**

patient to elevate the globe to move the cornea away from the instillation site to minimize the blink reflex. Instill the solution, keeping the dropper tip at least 2 cm from the globe to avoid contact contamination (Fig. 2.4). After the lids are gently closed, caution the patient to avoid lid squeezing, and rotate the globe downward to bring the cornea into maximum contact with the instilled drug. Apply pressure with the fingertips over the lower puncta and canaliculi to minimize nasolacrimal drainage[38] (Fig. 2.5), maintaining this position for approximately 1 minute.[39]

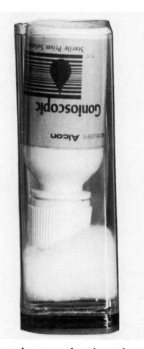

FIGURE 2.2   **Inverted storage of gonioscopic solution minimizes interference by bubbles.**

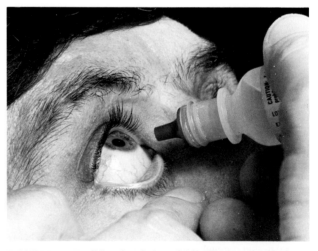

FIGURE 2.4   **Traditional technique for instillation of topical ocular solutions. Patient's head is inclined backward, lower lid is retracted, globe is elevated, and the dropper tip is maintained at least 2 cm from the globe.**

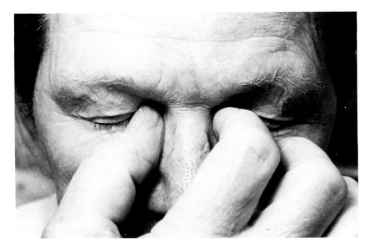

FIGURE 2.5 **Nasolacrimal drainage of solutions may be minimized by applying pressure over the lower puncta and canaliculi.**

Various modifications of the latter technique have resulted in increased ocular contact time for the applied solution.[25,26] Fraunfelder[40] modified the procedure by gently pulling the lid away from the globe at right angles to the plane of the head, placing the drop in the inferior conjunctival sac without touching ocular tissues or lashes, and after waiting to allow gravity to deliver the drop to the most dependent area of the fornix, moving the lid parallel to the plane of the head until it comes in contact with the globe (Figs. 2.6 and

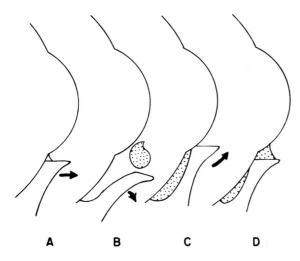

A   B   C   D

FIGURE 2.6 **Schematic representation of technique described by Fraunfelder[40] to administer topical solutions to the eye. *(A)* The lid is gently pulled away at right angles to the plane of the head. *(B)* The drop is placed in the inferior conjunctival sac without touching ocular tissues or lashes. *(C)* After waiting a moment to allow gravity to deliver the drop to the most dependent area of the fornix, the lid is then moved parallel to the plane of the head until it comes in contact with the globe. *(D)* A portion of the drop is entrapped under the eyelid. (From Fraunfelder FT. Extraocular fluid dynamics: How best to apply topical ocular medication. Trans Am Ophthalmol Soc 1976;74:457–487, with permission of the author and publisher.)**

2.7). This "pouch" method thus allows the topically applied solution to act as a "depot" deposit. Even with the patient's head vertical and with a normal blink rate, or with the lids closed, 80% or 96% of the drop, respectively, remains in the ocular area for 5 minutes.[40] This method increases the ocular retention rate of a 13 μl drop twice as much over simply applying drops to the superior bulbar conjunctiva, and the effect is even more striking with the more flaccid lids commonly encountered in older age groups.[40] Regardless of the method of initial drop instillation, closure of the lids following drop instillation markedly increases the contact time of the drug with the ocular tissues.[40] Tables 2.4 and 2.5 summarize the recommended procedures for drop instillation.

McGraw and Rollins[41] have further modified the procedure described by Fraunfelder.[40] Since gravity

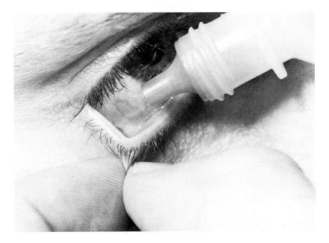

FIGURE 2.7 **Technique described by Fraunfelder[40] to administer topical solutions to the eye. The drop is placed in a "pouch" created by gently pulling the lower lid away at right angles to the plane of the head.**

TABLE 2.4
**Recommended Procedure for Instilling Topical
Ocular Solutions**

1. Tilt patient's head backward
2. Instruct patient to direct gaze toward ceiling
3. Gently grasp lower outer eyelid below lashes and pull eyelid away from globe
4. Without touching lashes or eyelids, instill 1 drop of solution into conjunctival sac
5. Continue to hold eyelid in this position for a few seconds to allow solution to gravitate into deepest portion of lower fornix
6. Instruct patient to gaze downward while lifting the eyelid upward until it contacts the globe
7. Instruct patient to gently close eyes
8. Patient should keep eyes closed for 1 to 2 minutes

TABLE 2.5
**Instructions to Patients for Self-Administration
of Medication**

1. Tilt head backward
2. With clean hands, gently grasp lower outer eyelid below lashes and pull eyelid away from the eye
3. Place dropper over eye by looking directly at it
4. Just before applying a drop, look upward
5. After applying the drop, look downward for a few seconds
6. Lift eyelid upward until it contacts the eye
7. Gently close eyes for 1 to 2 minutes

plays an important role in tear flow dynamics, following drop instillation and lid closure the patient is instructed to direct the head and eyes toward the feet for 3 minutes. This procedure also increases the bioavailability of topically administered drugs compared with the conventional techniques of instillation.

Administering topical solutions to children is often disconcerting. Several techniques may be used to facilitate drug administration to these patients.[26] The child's hand can be placed on his or her forehead, which proprioceptively reinforces upward gaze. The child's palpebral aperture can be widened for drop instillation by instructing the child to open the mouth. A spread of the neural impulse from the mesencephalic root of the fifth cranial nerve to the nucleus of the levator may explain the effectiveness of this maneuver.[26] Another useful method of administering drops to the uncooperative pediatric patient is to instruct the child to close the eyes. The child usually will not resist

and will be unable to see the approach of the dropper bottle. By gently retracting the lower lid, a small opening through the lashes into the conjunctival sac is created, and the drop can be subsequently instilled.[26]

The self-administration of topical solutions by the elderly patient can sometimes be difficult because of arthritis, tremors, or other physically debilitating diseases. The instillation of ocular drugs may be facilitated in these patients by using a pair of spectacle lenses into which a hole has been drilled through the center of each lens.[42,43] The patient inserts the dropper tip into the hole, gazes superiorly, and squeezes the bottle (Fig. 2.8). Only polycarbonate lenses should be used, since there is considerable risk associated with drilling into a conventional glass or plastic lens. Various commercial devices are also available.[44]

Solutions characterized by significant local toxicity or staining potential (e.g., silver nitrate and rose bengal) can be instilled using a cotton swab as applicator. This technique serves essentially to minimize drop size and subsequent overflow onto the patient's cheek or clothing.

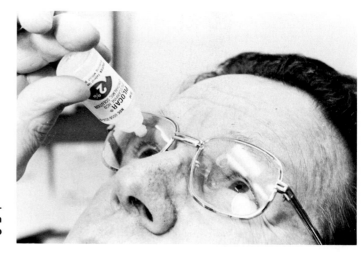

FIGURE 2.8 **Modification of polycarbonate spectacle lenses to facilitate drop instillation. After a hole is drilled through the center of each lens, the patient inserts the dropper tip into the hole, gazes superiorly, and squeezes the bottle.**

Sprays

Since ophthalmic solutions contain not only active drugs but also preservatives, buffers, and stabilizing agents, the topical administration of solutions to the eye is often an unpleasant procedure associated with significant burning, stinging, lacrimation, and emotional ambivalence on the patient's part. Topical sprays represent an alternative method of administering ophthalmic solutions that may be less irritating and less objectionable. Pilocarpine, epinephrine, and other agents were once commercially available in mist-dispensing bottles, but these are no longer manufactured. Combinations of mydriatics and cycloplegics such as phenylephrine-tropicamide or phenylephrine-tropicamide-cyclopentolate can be used as sprays for routine mydriasis in adults or for cycloplegia in children.[45]

The spray can be produced by using a refillable perfume atomizer (Fig. 2.9) that has first been sterilized with ethylene oxide gas before filling with the appropriate mydriatic or cycloplegic combination (see Chapter 16). The unit is held 5 to 10 cm from the eye before activating the spray. The volume of a single spray emanating from such a system is often comparable to the volume of a drop obtained from a standard eyedropper.

One advantage of a spray is that the drug can be applied to closed eyelids. Following drug application, the patient should be instructed to blink. If the medication reaches the precorneal tear film, mild stinging is expected. After blinking several times, the patient should wipe off the excess solution. Subjectively, spray directed to closed eyelids is much less irritating than the irritation experienced with topical drops. Furthermore, the reaction may be delayed until several mo-

ments after the patient blinks. If there is no mild burning or stinging after the eye has been sprayed, it is likely that none of the drug reached the precorneal tear film from the lid margin,[45] and another application is necessary. This may occur in patients who have tightly closed lids in which redundancy of the skin shields the lid margins from the spray.

The use of sprays is a rapid, effective, and often a less irritating method for drug delivery. There is less resistance from the patient when the spray is directed to the closed eye. The clinical use of mydriatic and cycloplegic sprays has been well tolerated by patients and is particularly well received by children because the patient does not need to assume an awkward position to receive the spray.

The use of mydriatic sprays often allows satisfactory pupillary dilation for fundus examination. No significant difference has been noted between the dilation produced by drugs administered as topical drops and as a spray[45] (Figs. 2.10 and 2.11).

Ointments

Solutions are the most commonly used vehicles for topical ocular medications, but ointments are also commonly used for application to the eye.

When applied to the inferior conjunctival sac, ophthalmic ointments melt quickly, and the excess spreads out onto the lid margins, lashes, and skin of the lids depending on the amount instilled and on the extent of lacrimation induced by any irritation. The

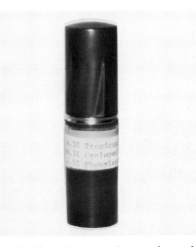

FIGURE 2.9 **Refillable perfume atomizer can be used to deliver solutions in the form of a spray.**

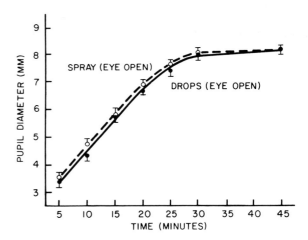

FIGURE 2.10 **Comparison of mean pupil sizes of eyes that received mydriatic drops while open, compared with fellow eyes that received the same mydriatic drugs as a spray while open. Brackets represent the standard error. (From Sharp J, Hanna C. Use of a spray to deliver drugs to the eye. J Arkansas Med Soc 1977;73:462–463, with permission of the authors and publisher.)**

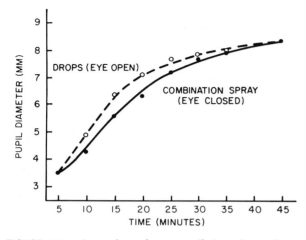

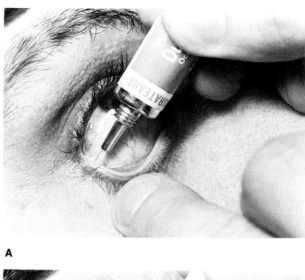

A

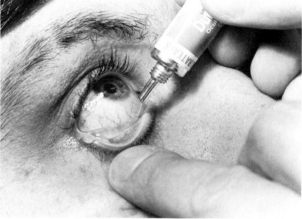

B

FIGURE 2.11 **Comparison of mean pupil sizes of eyes that received a combination mydriatic spray while closed, compared with fellow eyes that received the same mydriatic drugs as a drop while open. (From Sharp J, Hanna C. Use of a spray to deliver drugs to the eye. J Arkansas Med Soc 1977;73:462–463, with permission of the authors and publisher.)**

FIGURE 2.12 **Technique of ointment instillation. With the globe elevated and the lower lid retracted, ointment is instilled into the inferior conjunctival sac in a sweeping fashion from lateral canthus (A) to medial canthus (B).**

ointment at the lid margins acts as a reservoir and enhances drug contact time.[46]

TECHNIQUES OF APPLICATION

Ointments are instilled by instructing the patient to elevate the gaze, and, with the lower lid retracted, the ointment is instilled into the inferior conjunctival sac in a sweeping fashion from canthus to canthus (Fig. 2.12). For daytime use at least 1 cm of ointment is generally applied. Volumes of 0.1 ml or more are often instilled, which frequently leads to complaints of blurred vision. Therefore, if the ointment is not to be applied at bedtime or used under a pressure patch, smaller volumes of ointment should be instilled, since the maximum volume of the conjunctival sac is only about 0.025 ml.[33]

An alternative method of application is to place the ointment on a cotton-tipped applicator and apply it to the upper lid margin and lashes as well as the medial and lateral canthi.[47] In this way the ointment causes minimal blurring of vision, and drug irritation is minimized. In addition, the ointment acts as a drug reservoir and will have a therapeutic effect for approximately 6 hours. This method of application may be of practical value in the treatment of ocular infections in all patients, but especially those in the pediatric and geriatric age groups.

Once the ointment has been instilled, the bioavailability of subsequently instilled solutions may be altered, since the solution is blocked from contact with the ocular surface.[48] Thus, whenever both solution and

ointment formulations are used in therapy, the solution should be instilled before ointment application.

COMPLICATIONS

Since ointments are characterized by prolonged ocular contact time, contact dermatitis of the lids sometimes occurs during use of ointments containing sensitizing agents such as atropine or neomycin. Hypersensitivity to the incorporated preservatives may also occur.

As mentioned previously, one of the most frequent adverse effects from ophthalmic ointments is the report of blurred vision. This problem can often be alleviated or minimized by simply reducing the volume of ointment instilled.

The effect of ophthalmic ointments on the healing of corneal wounds has received considerable attention. Early formulations of ophthalmic ointments contained waxy grades of petrolatum or unwashed lanolin, which interfered with corneal wound healing.[49,50] Contemporary ophthalmic ointments, however, are nonemulsive and do not contain the coarse grade of white petrolatum.[49] Ophthalmic ointments contain the less viscous petrolatum or are made even less viscous by the addition of liquid mineral oil. Since highly purified lanolin has little or no inhibitory effect on the healing of epithelial wounds,[50] occasionally purified lanolin is added to the white petrolatum–mineral oil nonemulsive base, allowing water and many water-soluble drugs to be retained in the nonemulsive ointment preparation. These ointments cause no significant inhibition of corneal wound healing, even when maximum dosage frequencies of every 30 minutes are employed.[49]

It is rare for ointment to become entrapped within the cornea.[48,51,52] The inability to trap ophthalmic ointments during corneal wound healing appears to be related to the rapid melting of these preparations. Almost all commercial ophthalmic ointments melt below body temperature and become an oil within minutes. This rapid melting allows the ointment to float above the precorneal tear film and permits migration and mitosis of the underlying epithelial cells without interference. Entrapment of ointment occurs only after direct injection into the stroma or, rarely, in corneal wounds in which stroma-to-stroma contact occurs anterior to the ointment. However, "pseudoentrapment" of ointment in the cornea sometimes occurs in corneal lesions that have been administered ointments and pressure patched, and that have stromal loss or distortion of the normal stromal architecture. This allows ointment globules to lie below the corneal surface.[51] Although the clinical picture is that of a cluster of large ointment globules lodged within the corneal defect, the ointment is actually entrapped only within the wound exudates below the plane of the corneal surface (Fig. 2.13). No treatment is necessary, since the ointment usually extrudes spontaneously within 24 to 48 hours even if the pressure dressing is continued. No complications are associated with this condition.

Although it has been generally assumed that ointments are not eliminated through the nasolacrimal drainage system,[46,53] Scruggs and associates[46] have shown that topically applied ophthalmic ointments do travel through the lacrimal drainage system, although more slowly than do solutions. These investigators demonstrated that the total amount of drug absorbed systemically is similar regardless of whether solution or ointment is used. However, the slower drainage of ointments through the nasolacrimal system and therefore slower systemic absorption may explain why sys-

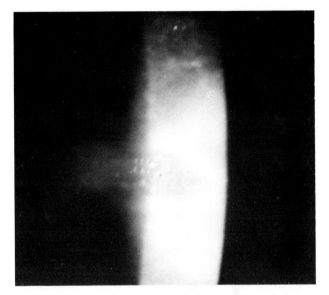

FIGURE 2.13 **Pseudoentrapment of ointment in cornea in case of recurrent corneal erosion. Photograph was taken 3 hours after removal of firm pressure dressing. (From Fraunfelder FT, Hanna C, Woods AH. Pseudoentrapment of ointment in the cornea. Arch Ophthalmol 1975;93:331–334. Copyright 1975, American Medical Association.)**

temic drug toxicity is much less common with topical ointments than with solutions. Another important factor contributing to the reduced systemic toxicity of ointment preparations is that a much smaller total amount of drug is delivered by an ointment compared to the "bolus" effect of drop therapy.[48] On the other hand, serious side effects can indeed occur with ointment therapy. Death has occurred following the administration of topical atropine ointment.[54,55]

Considering the characteristics and complications inherent in the use of ophthalmic ointments, the following guidelines are suggested for their clinical utilization.[56]

- Ointments may be used immediately after intraocular surgery under a conjunctival flap or in corneal incisions with excellent wound approximation, since the risk of entrapment of ointment is minimal. Do not use ointments, however, in any surgical wound in which there is a question of wound integrity, such as when difficulty is experienced maintaining the anterior chamber at surgery. In such cases, delay ointment medication until several days after the first dressing change.
- Use ointments with caution in jagged or flaplike corneal lacerations, in eyes with impending corneal perforation, and in open conjunctival lacerations.

- Ointments can be used routinely for superficial corneal abrasions. However, any abrasion involving corneal tissues deeper than the epithelium should be managed on an individual basis depending on the configuration of the wound edges.
- Ointments may be applied to corneal ulcers with little risk of entrapment or inhibition of wound healing. However, use them with caution in ulcers with an impending perforation or in ulcers with large overhanging margins, since there is a risk of ointment entrapment under a flap.

Lid Scrubs

Application of solutions or ointments directly to the lid margin is especially helpful in treating seborrheic or infectious blepharitis. This direct application is probably more effective therapeutically than is the simple instillation of topical solutions or ointments into the conjunctival sac. After applying several drops of the antibiotic solution or detergent, such as baby shampoo, to the end of a cotton-tipped applicator, the solution is applied to the lash line of the lid margin with the eyelids either opened or closed (Fig. 2.14). Antibiotic ointments are applied in the same way.

Gels

Pilocarpine is commercially available as a gel.[57,58] The ocular hypotensive and miotic effects of this formulation have been compared with traditional drop instillation. The 4% pilocarpine gel is packaged in a tube

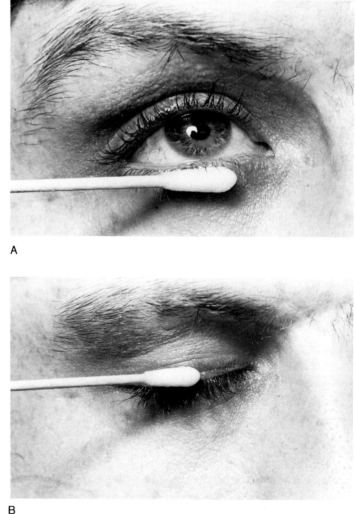

A

B

FIGURE 2.14 **Technique of lid scrub. Drug application to the lid margin is accomplished with a cotton-tipped applicator applied to the opened** *(A)* **or closed** *(B)* **eyelids.**

similar to that in which ophthalmic ointments are packaged. A practical advantage of this sustained pulse delivery system is the once-daily dosage regimen, usually administered at bedtime. Other advantages include improved patient compliance as well as a reduction in ocular or systemic toxicity because of the lower total dose of pilocarpine administered. The major disadvantage of pilocarpine gel is its significant loss of ocular hypotensive effect during the hours before the next bedtime dose.[59] A minor side effect is superficial corneal haze, which may occur after long-term (>8 weeks) use.[57]

Solid Delivery Devices

One of the significant problems with the delivery of drugs in solution is that the drug administration is pulsed, with an initial period of overdosage followed by a period of relative underdosage (see Fig. 1.9). With only a few exceptions, the development of solid drug delivery devices has been an attempt to overcome this disadvantage.

HYDROGEL CONTACT LENSES

The effect of topically applied ophthalmic drugs can be enhanced by several methods. "Lamellae," described as early as 1948, were atropine-containing gelatin wafers intended for placement in the conjunctival sac. A Russian study in 1966[60] reported use of pilocarpine-impregnated discs of polyvinyl alcohol that were designed to provide sustained miosis and reduce intraocular pressure. The use of soft contact lenses as a vehicle for the delivery of pilocarpine was first suggested by Sedlacek, a Czechoslovakian ophthalmologist, in 1965.[61] In the United States the use of hydrogel contact lenses for drug delivery was initially proposed by Waltman and Kaufman in 1970.[62] The use of hydrogel lenses to prolong drug contact with the eye and to promote drug penetration into the eye seems to be effective at least for some of the medications studied.

Drugs penetrate hydrogel contact lenses at a rate depending on the pore size between the cross-linkages of the three-dimensional lattice structure of the lens, on the concentration of drug in the soaking solution, soaking time, water content of the lens, and the molecular size of the drug. Lenses with higher water contents absorb more water-soluble drug for later release into the precorneal tear film.[29,63–65] For example, the Poly HEMA lens, consisting of 42% water, releases approximately 62% of impregnated pilocarpine after 30 minutes of wear, whereas the Sauflon lens, consisting of 85% water, releases about 95% of impregnated pilocarpine (Fig. 2.15).[56] However, it may not be prac-

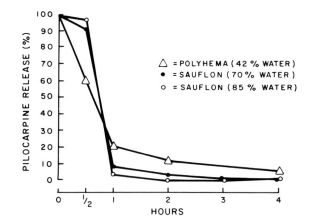

FIGURE 2.15 **Pilocarpine release (%) from hydrogel lenses with 3 different water contents. (From Ruben M, Watkins R. Pilocarpine dispensation for the soft hydrophilic contact lens. Br J Ophthalmol 1975;59:455–458, with permission of the authors and publisher.)**

tical to equate the percentage of pilocarpine released in vivo with the concentration actually available in the precorneal tear film because of variables such as amount of water lost from the lens by evaporation and temperature, and the rate of tear flow or water flow into the lens from the cornea. The rates of drug entry into the polymer and the subsequent passage of drug into the cornea depend on the specific physical properties of the drug as well as those of the polymer used.[65] Although no specific pore structure exists in hydrogel lens materials, drugs with molecular weights over 500 generally have difficulty entering the substance of the polymer.[65]

The degree of permeability is also related to lens thickness. A thinner lens allows a greater amount of topically applied drug to pass into the lens-cornea interface, whereas a thicker lens stores a greater amount of the drug without releasing it to the cornea.[65]

Maximum drug delivery is obtained by presoaking the lens.[62,66–69] This produces a more sustained high yield of drug.[66] In addition, a prolonged soaking to a state of equilibrium before clinical use produces a more standardized form of presoaked lens.

In addition to pilocarpine,[64,66,67,70–73] many other drugs have been used in hydrogel contact lens delivery systems. The release rates of antibiotics, including chloramphenicol, tetracycline, bacitracin, gentamicin and polymyxin B, have been studied.[74] Bacitracin is released from the lens somewhat more rapidly than is polymyxin B, but after 5 hours the content of both antibiotics in the contact lens is about the same, approximately 40% of the original amount. Chloramphenicol and tetracycline are both easily released from hydrogel contact lenses, chloramphenicol more rapidly than tetracycline. About 50% of the tetracycline and 75% of the chloramphenicol is released during the first 3 hours.

Other drugs have been delivered with these lenses, including ethylenediaminetetraacetic acid (EDTA) for alkali burns.[74] In some cases 48 hours of intensive treatment with these agents using hydrogel contact lenses may be more effective than more traditional methods of treatment of severe chemical burns. Other drugs used in conjunction with soft contact lenses have included cystein hydrochloride,[74] acetylcysteine,[75] lubricating solutions,[76] normal saline solution,[71] IDU,[71] corticosteroids,[71] and hypertonic solutions.[29]

Early in the use of hydrogel contact lenses as a drug delivery system it was suggested never to soak lenses in solutions containing preservatives, since the prolonged delivery of relatively high concentrations of preservatives might be toxic to the eye, producing ocular irritation as well as superficial punctate erosions of the cornea.[73] More recently, however, Lemp[76] found no evidence of benzalkonium chloride in hydrogel contact lenses used as drug delivery devices. He also failed to find clinical evidence of corneal toxicity associated with the preservative. Thus, the use of ophthalmic medications containing benzalkonium chloride as a preservative in conjunction with hydrogel contact lenses is probably a clinically acceptable procedure. Further studies, however, are needed to clarify the safety of other preservatives used in conjunction with this drug delivery system.

Currently, therapeutic soft contact lenses for drug delivery appear to be of greatest clinical value in the treatment of bullous keratopathy, dry eye syndromes, and corneal conditions requiring protection.[29] The most significant disadvantage of this mode of therapy, however, is the rapid loss of most drugs from the lens.

Since drug-impregnated hydrogel lenses are characterized by first-order kinetics,[69] they only occasionally offer any significant advantage over topically applied solutions or ointments. Hence, this method of drug administration has not become popular. In addition, since the most advantageous way to use soft contact lenses as drug delivery devices is to soak them with medication before fitting, this poses some potential logistic problems for the patient as well as for the practitioner.[77]

FILTER PAPER STRIPS

Two staining agents, sodium fluorescein and rose bengal, are commercially available as drug-impregnated filter paper strips (Fig. 2.16). This form of drug delivery allows these agents to be more easily administered to the eye in dosage amounts adequate for their intended clinical purpose. Administration of excessive drug is eliminated, thus avoiding unintentional staining of lid tissues or the patient's clothing. Furthermore, the availability of fluorescein-impregnated paper strips eliminates the risk of solution contamination with *Pseudomonas aeruginosa*. For administration, the drug-impregnated paper strip is moistened with a drop of tap water, normal saline, or irrigating solution, and the applicator is gently touched to the superior or inferior bulbar conjunctiva or to the inferior conjunctival sac. Some practitioners prefer to moisten the fluorescein-impregnated strip with a drop of rose bengal solution before application, allowing for the simultaneous administration of both the sodium fluorescein and the rose bengal. To avoid the risk of cross-contamination between eyes, the practitioner should use separate applicators for drug delivery to eyes with suspected infection.

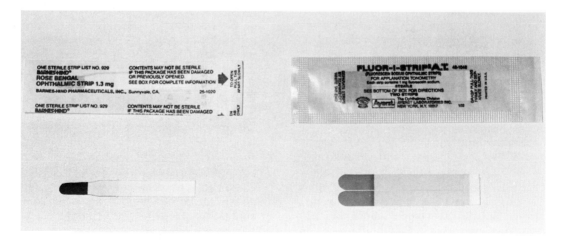

FIGURE 2.16   **Drug-impregnated filter paper strips. Rose bengal (left) and sodium fluorescein (right).**

OPHTHALMIC RODS

Ophthalmic rods (Basotherm Ophthalmica, Biberack, West Germany) are plastic rods 5 cm long with a single dose of a diagnostic or therapeutic drug coating the flat tip. Although not commercially available in the United States, they may be used by the practitioner or patient, and they provide an alternative delivery method that may improve compliance in patients who experience difficulty in using eyedrops.[78]

COTTON PLEDGETS

Cotton pledgets saturated with ophthalmic solutions are of value in several clinical situations. These devices allow prolonged ocular contact time with solutions that are normally topically instilled into the eye. A pledget is constructed by simply teasing the cotton tip of an applicator to form a small (approximately 5 mm), elongated body of cotton. After placing 1 or 2 drops of the ophthalmic solution on the pledget, the device is placed into the inferior conjunctival fornix (Fig. 2.17). The clinical use of pledgets is usually reserved for administration of mydriatic solutions such as cocaine, phenylephrine, or hydroxyamphetamine. This method of drug delivery allows maximum mydriasis in attempts to break posterior synechiae, to dilate sluggish pupils, or mydriasis of the inferior pupillary quadrant for intentional sector dilation of the pupil (see Chapter 16).

ARTIFICIAL TEAR INSERT

Katz and Blackman[79] first described in 1977 a soluble ophthalmic drug delivery insert developed in the United States. This device has been studied as a means for treating dry eye syndromes and is now commercially available (Lacrisert, Merck Sharp & Dohme). The Lacrisert consists of a rod-shaped pellet of hydroxypropyl cellulose without preservative. In its dehydrated state, each dosage unit measures approximately 1 mm in diameter and 4 mm in length and contains 5 mg of the unmedicated synthetic polymer. It is supplied to the patient in hermetically sealed blister packs and is inserted into the inferior conjunctival fornix with a specially designed applicator (Fig. 2.18). Following placement into the conjunctival sac, its hypertonicity causes it to absorb fluid from the capillaries of the conjunctiva, and it consequently swells, becoming a gelatinous mass. During the following several hours the insert dissolves and releases the polymer into the tear film.

This device is useful for patients with moderate to severe dry eye syndromes for whom conventional therapies have failed or are inconvenient. Although the device is reasonably well tolerated and generally does not migrate or become displaced, the most annoying side effect, associated with the intense release of polymer, is blurring of vision after 4 to 6 hours.[80,81] Many patients are able to minimize or eliminate the blurred vision by removing the insert after 3 to 4 hours and inserting a second device several hours later, or by inserting the device at bedtime. Since transient blurring of vision is common, patients should be instructed to be cautious when operating hazardous machinery or driving a motor vehicle.[82]

The continuous delivery of a tearlike substance may be more similar to the natural physiologic condition than is the intermittent instillation of artificial tears and lubricants, and in patients with chronic severe dry

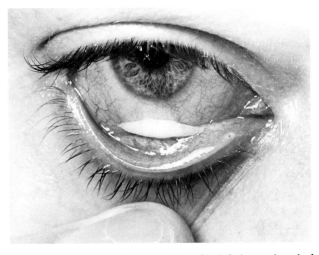

FIGURE 2.17   **Cotton pledget positioned in inferior conjunctival fornix.**

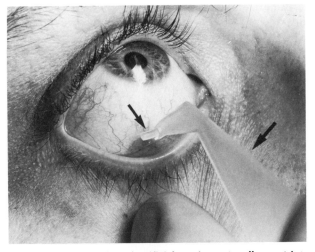

FIGURE 2.18   **Insertion of artificial tear insert (small arrow) into inferior conjunctival fornix with specially designed applicator (large arrow).**

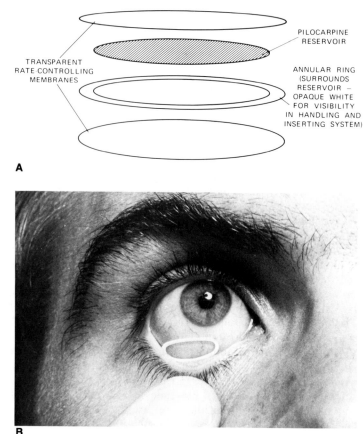

FIGURE 2.19   *(A)* **Schematic diagram of pilocarpine Ocusert.** *(B)* **Ocusert in situ.**

eye syndromes may more satisfactorily alleviate both objective corneal findings as well as subjective symptoms.[80] Since the duration of action of the insert is about 24 hours in most patients, once-daily application is usually sufficient to relieve symptoms associated with severe dry eye syndromes. Some patients, however, may require twice-daily application.

MEMBRANE-BOUND INSERTS

Thin, multilayered, drug-impregnated, copolymeric plastic devices placed into the conjunctival sac have been designed to release a specified amount of drug over an extended period. The first such device marketed in the United States became commercially available in 1974 (Ocusert, Alza). The device consists of a two-membrane sandwich of ethylene vinylacetate with a pilocarpine reservoir in the center. A white titanium dioxide ring incorporated between the copolymeric membranes aids in visualizing and handling the insert (Fig. 2.19). This elliptical device contains one of two commercially available quantities of pilocarpine. The pilocarpine is bound to alginic acid and is present as a free base, partly in an ionized (water-soluble) and

partly in an un-ionized (lipid-soluble) form.[69] The device is sterile and contains no preservatives. The physical and drug release characteristics of the Ocusert are listed in Table 2.6.[31,83]

Membrane-controlled drug devices such as the Ocusert are characterized by zero-order drug delivery, in which the drug is released into the tear film at a

TABLE 2.6
Characteristics of the Pilocarpine Ocusert

Characteristics	*Pilo-20*	*Pilo-40*
Long axis (mm)	13.4	13.0
Short axis (mm)	5.7	5.5
Thickness (mm)	0.3	0.5
Weight of device (mg)	19.0	29.0
Weight of drug (mg)	5.0	11.0
Pilocarpine release rate (μg/hr)	20	40
Therapeutic lifetime (days)	7	7
Total pilocarpine released (mg)	3.4	6.7

Modified from Novak S, Stewart RH. The Ocusert system in the management of glaucoma. Tex Med 1975;71(12):63–65, with permission of the authors and publisher.

constant rate over almost the entire lifetime of the device.[69,80,84] Drug release terminates when the reservoir is exhausted. The controlled rate of drug delivery is provided by interaction between the polymeric membrane molecules and the molecules of the drug contained in the reservoir. A major factor in the rate of drug release is the driving force of the concentration gradient that is maintained by the saturated concentration of drug within the reservoir. As long as this gradient exists, there is zero-order drug delivery through the membrane.[80] Another factor in the rate of drug release is the concentration of drug outside the membrane. Released drug must be removed, or the driving force (gradient) will be diminished. The eye provides an excellent environment for such a drug delivery system because tear flow prevents the buildup of a stagnant layer of drug around the device. The pilocarpine contained within the central reservoir is in equilibrium between the ionized, water-soluble form and the unionized, lipid-soluble form. In the aqueous tear layer, the lipid form of the drug is released.[80] During the initial 6 to 8 hours following insertion of the device, there is a higher pulse release of pilocarpine from the device due to the amount of drug previously equilibrated into the barrier membranes.[80,84–87] During this period, the Ocusert releases 3 to 4 times the amount of pilocarpine it does at later times.[86] Following this initial period, the pilocarpine is released at a constant rate of 20 μg/hr (Ocusert Pilo-20) or 40 μg/hr (Ocusert Pilo-40) for approximately 7 days. Figure 2.20 illustrates the time course of pilocarpine release from the Ocusert Pilo-20 system.

Because of individual differences, direct comparisons between the Ocusert systems and various concentrations of pilocarpine drops cannot be made. However, a majority of patients controlled with pilocarpine 0.5%

and 1% drops can usually be controlled with the Ocusert Pilo-20.[86] Most patients who require 2% or 4% solutions of pilocarpine will require the Ocusert Pilo-40 (Fig. 2.21).

The clinical advantages of the pilocarpine Ocusert over pilocarpine drops are numerous. One of the distinct advantages of the Ocusert is the substantially less total drug delivered to the eye for adequate control of intraocular pressure. Such reservoir membrane delivery systems are capable of only a very low drug release rate, but since these systems are characterized by zero-order drug delivery, the therapeutic effect can be achieved with much smaller amounts of drug. The Ocusert Pilo-20 unit releases 3.4 mg of drug over a 7-day period, while the Ocusert Pilo-40 unit contains twice the amount of pilocarpine and releases it at twice the rate. By comparison, administration of 1 drop (0.05 ml) of 2% pilocarpine solution 4 times daily delivers 28 mg of drug per eye over a 7-day period, 4 or 8 times the amount released from an Ocusert over the same period.[88] Since the total dose of pilocarpine delivered by the Ocusert is considerably less than that delivered by pilocarpine drop instillation, the risk of ocular or systemic pilocarpine toxicity is reduced. In patients with open but narrow anterior chamber angles, pilocarpine can precipitate angle closure by inducing pupillary block and forward movement of the lens-iris diaphragm.[89] Although both the Pilo-20 and Pilo-40 Ocusert systems produce shallowing of the anterior chamber, the shallowing produced by the Ocusert (0.08 mm with Pilo-20) is less than that produced by 2% pilocarpine drops (0.265 mm).[89,90]

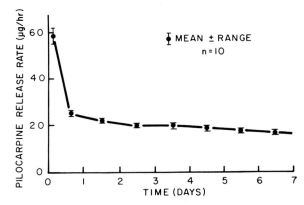

FIGURE 2.20 **Time course of pilocarpine release from the Ocusert Pilo-20 system. (Modified from Shell JW, Baker RW. Diffusional systems for controlled release of drugs to the eye. Ann Ophthalmol 1974;6:1037–1045.)**

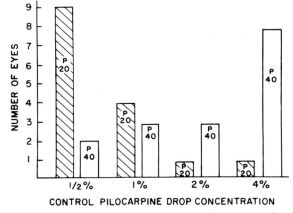

FIGURE 2.21 **Comparison of concentration of Ocuserts Pilo-20 and Pilo-40 with concentration of pilocarpine drops administered 4 times daily. (Modified from Quigley HA, Pollack IP, Harbin TS. Pilocarpine Ocuserts. Long-term clinical trials and selected pharmacodynamics. Arch Ophthalmol 1975;93:771–775. Copyright 1975, American Medical Association.)**

In addition, visual disturbances associated with drug-induced miosis or myopia do not occur to the same extent with the Ocusert systems as they do with pilocarpine solutions (Fig. 2.22). In one study,[90] average pupil size after the instillation of 2% pilocarpine solution was 1.35 mm; after insertion of the Ocusert Pilo-20 it was 3.0 mm. There was a mean increase of crystalline lens thickness of 0.24 mm in the pilocarpine solution–treated group, whereas the increase was only 0.03 mm in the group treated with the Ocusert Pilo-20. The mean accommodative myopia was significant for the solution-treated group (3.10 D) but was negligible for the Ocusert-treated group (0.45 D). In the younger age group, the changes were more pronounced. There was a mean accommodative myopia of 5.84 D in the solution-treated group between the ages of 20 and 40 years, and the maximum accommodative myopia was 11.0 D. In the age group between 40 and 60, the maximum accommodative myopia was 5 D after instillation of 1 drop of 2% pilocarpine. After age 60 years, however, accommodative myopia was usually insignificant, reaching a maximum of only 1.25 D in the Ocusert-treated group.

Since the device is inserted only once per week, drug application is convenient and results in good patient compliance. The Ocusert enjoys a distinct advantage for patients who must rely on others for treatment, such as children and the elderly. Since the Ocusert offers continuous drug release, diurnal variations of intraocular pressure may be stabilized in patients who might otherwise require the longer-acting anticholinesterase agents. In addition, the constant release of pilocarpine is a safeguard against dangerously high intraocular pressures caused by the irregular instillation of drops. This is especially important for the elderly patient whose ability to instill pilocarpine regularly is questionable. The Ocusert is ideal for treating young adults who require better control of intraocular pressure than is obtainable with topical epinephrine, but who have contraindications to β blockers and are intolerant of the accommodative myopia induced by pilocarpine solutions.

Despite the numerous advantages inherent in the pilocarpine Ocusert, this membrane-bound insert has not achieved widespread popularity in clinical practice. The major problems preventing satisfactory use of the Ocusert in practice are foreign body sensation, especially when it becomes folded, and difficulty with retention of the device.[83] When the Ocusert becomes folded, it must be replaced with a fresh one because it usually cannot be straightened to its original smooth shape. Retention problems may be solved in some cases by instructing the patient to wear the device in the superior fornix, especially while sleeping. Other significant disadvantages associated with the device include the need for detailed instruction and encouragement of patients and significantly higher cost compared with pilocarpine drops. The cost of a monthly supply of the Ocusert can range from 7 to 10 times the cost of pilocarpine drops. In addition, many patients who are accustomed to eyedrop therapy simply prefer their eyedrops and are reluctant to use any new therapeutic modality. Table 2.7 summarizes the clinical advantages and disadvantages of the pilocarpine Ocusert.

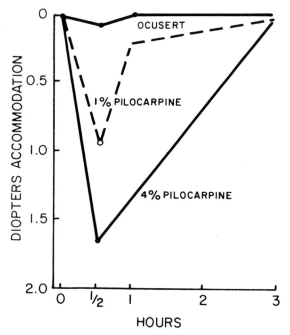

FIGURE 2.22 **Accommodative spasm resulting from 1 drop of 4% pilocarpine, 1 drop of 1% pilocarpine, or pilocarpine Ocusert. (Modified from Brown HS, Meltzer G, Merrill RC, et al. Visual effects of pilocarpine in glaucoma. Arch Ophthalmol 1976; 94:1716–1719. Copyright 1976, American Medical Association.)**

Liposomes

Liposomes are spherical vesicles composed of synthetic phospholipid bilayers that may be used to encapsulate a particular drug. Because of their size (0.01 to 10 μm diameter), liposomes tend not to cross capillary walls; thus, when topically instilled into the conjunctival sac, they are lost through the nasolacrimal system unless they bind to the superficial cells of the cornea or conjunctiva.[91] Barza and associates[92] have suggested that amphotericin B incorporated into liposomes produces less toxic response than commercial amphotericin B when injected intravitreally in Rhesus monkeys. Assil and Weinrob[93] have demonstrated in rabbits that liposomal-entrapped cytarabine injected subconjuncti-

TABLE 2.7
Clinical Advantages and Disadvantages of the Pilocarpine Ocusert

Advantages	Disadvantages
• Constant, continuous drug delivery	• Requires detailed patient instruction
• Less ocular and systemic drug toxicity	• Retention difficulties and loss
• Less frequent application	• Foreign body sensation
• Less miosis	• High cost
• Less accommodative myopia	
• Less reduction in visual acuity	
• Better patient compliance	
• Treatment reliability in children and elderly	
• Better control of diurnal variations in IOP	

IOP, intraocular pressure.

vally allows sustained delivery of the drug to the eye. However, much clinical and technical development appears to remain before liposomes become viable as a clinical method of topical ocular drug delivery.[94]

Continuous Flow Devices

When relatively small amounts of drug are required for delivery to the eye, the use of solutions, ointments, or inserts is usually satisfactory. However, when large volumes of fluids are required, such as in the treatment of acute chemical burns, severe ocular infections, or the application of enzyme inhibitors to retard corneal ulceration, other drug delivery systems are necessary. Various methods for delivering large volumes of fluids continuously to the eye have been developed.

CONVENTIONAL IRRIGATING SYSTEMS

Extraocular irrigation is often employed in the initial treatment of ocular foreign bodies or chemical burns in an effort to dislodge the foreign material. It is also used to remove excessive drug from the eye following fluorescein or rose bengal staining or following gonioscopic or fundus contact lens procedures in which viscous lens-bonding solutions have been used. The conventional delivery system for irrigation fluids consists simply of the container of irrigating solution and a means—usually a tissue, towel, or emesis basin—with which to collect the fluid after bathing the eye. The patient should be in a supine position with head tilted toward the side to be irrigated (Fig. 2.23). The irrigating solution should be at room temperature to minimize patient discomfort during the procedure. With the patient's upper and lower lids retracted, the clinician gently bathes the extraocular surfaces with the solution, taking care to collect the fluid in the tissue, towel, or emesis basin and to avoid staining the pa-

tient's clothing. In most cases no topical anesthesia is required, except if the patient, because of severe pain or ocular involvement, is unable to open the eye.

A simple, inexpensive, yet effective ocular irrigation unit can be assembled by using a standard 1000 ml bottle or bag of sterile normal saline commonly em-

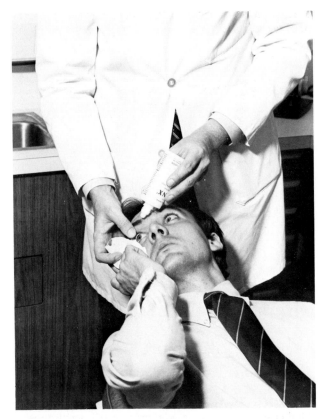

FIGURE 2.23 **Conventional irrigation system. Patient's head is tilted toward the side to be irrigated, and the irrigation solution is collected in a tissue after it has bathed the extraocular tissues.**

ployed for intravenous infusion, intravenous tubing with stopcock (needle removed), and a hanger made from a metal bracket and threaded ring (Fig. 2.24).[95] The bag and tubing can be hung from a wall or, alternatively, from a mobile stand. A mobile stand allows the unit to be moved to any treatment room. Such a unit permits irrigation at rates varying from the standard intravenous drip to a maximum of 200 ml/min. Excess irrigating solution is collected in an emesis basin.

The obvious limitation of these conventional irrigating systems is the need to have an attendant administer the fluid, but the advantage is the ease and simplicity with which the solution can be administered. In addition, conventional irrigating systems represent the most cost-effective means of administering fluids continuously to the eye.

CONTINUOUS IRRIGATING SYSTEMS

To circumvent the need for an attendant to administer the irrigating fluid or drug, various methods have been developed that enable the continuous delivery of fluid on a long-term basis. Most methods that have been devised for continuous ocular irrigation are suitable for relatively short periods in nonambulatory patients. Polyethylene tubing is sometimes simply passed with a minor surgical procedure through the lid and into the

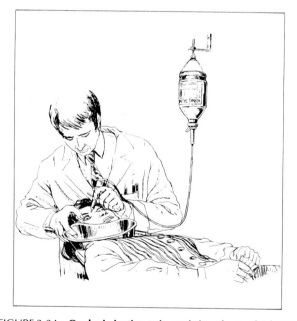

FIGURE 2.24 **Ocular irrigation unit consisting of a standard 1000 ml bottle of sterile normal saline, intravenous tubing with stopcock (needle removed), and a hanger. (From Flora MR. How to make a simple ocular irrigation unit. Rev Optom 1980;117:59, with permission of the author and publisher.)**

conjunctival fornix, and the fluid or drug to be perfused is supplied from an overhead infusion bottle. The tubing is anchored to the skin with sutures at the zygoma and forehead and may also be secured by tape. An adaptor may be attached to the tubing and to the intravenous infusion apparatus, allowing the system to be disconnected for ambulation. In many patients this apparatus is tolerated well with no apparent discomfort. Continuous irrigation of the extraocular tissues by this method may be superior to other modes of drug administration because of its constantly high drug titers and its gentle debridement.

In cases in which it is undesirable to penetrate the lids surgically, various configurations of tubing, loops, rings, and haptic contact lens shells have been successfully employed. Corneoscleral contact lenses, however, have the disadvantage of pressure on the cornea, poor permeability to oxygen, and frequent complaints of pain or discomfort.

Regardless of the method employed for continuous irrigation, certain precautions should be observed when administering antibiotics as constant lavage to the ocular surface.[96] Careful attention must be paid to the possibility of systemic toxicity resulting from absorption of drug. In addition, when antibiotics are maintained in solution for many hours, there is always risk of a significant deterioration of the drug before the drug reaches the patient. This is particularly true of ampicillin, which can lose 10% of its activity per hour at room temperature.[96] Some drugs are unstable in acid media, while other drugs lose their activity in alkaline solution. Some drugs may be adversely affected by the presence of calcium in solution. Furthermore, vitamin B complex and vitamin C inhibit the activity of chloramphenicol, penicillin G, and erythromycin. These observations suggest that the administration of antibiotics by continuous perfusion may carry a significant risk of drug degradation or incompatibility. When continuous irrigation with antibiotics is warranted, the administration of mixtures of antibiotics should be avoided, and solutions should be freshly prepared every 4 to 6 hours.[96]

MOBILE SYSTEMS

The long-term continuous perfusion of the ocular surface offers a therapeutic advantage in many ambulatory patients, such as those with severe keratoconjunctivitis sicca, Sjögren's syndrome, or the severe corneal involvement associated with Stevens-Johnson syndrome. In some patients the inconvenience of frequent topical instillation of solutions necessitates a more satisfactory mode of drug delivery. Insert devices are usually not capable of containing the volume of fluid required, typically 2 to 5 ml/day. The advent of mobile, self-contained fluid pumping devices has offered a distinct advantage in the treatment of such patients. Most of these units consist of a power source, a fluid reservoir, a mechanism to drive the fluid, and a means of delivering the fluid to the eye.[97] Although most of the readily available fluid pumps were originally designed for anticancer chemotherapy, several of these devices have been adapted for ocular use[97–99] (Fig. 2.25).

Although satisfaction with these pumping systems is largely based on the increased convenience and ocular comfort afforded patients with severe dry eye syndromes, many patients express concern about the cosmetic appearance of the apparatus. Some patients, in an effort to minimize the effect of the bulk and weight of the device, have constructed varieties of halters and bags that are carried under their clothing or in a shirt pocket, or that are held by a belt around the waist. Depending on the system and on the drugs perfused, complications have included infection, crystallization and sludging of the drug within the tubing, and slippage of the tubing.[99]

Animal experiments suggest that implantable pumping devices may have practical application in the delivery of drugs to the eye. In some systems the implanted fluid reservoir can be refilled by a percutaneous injection through a self-sealing rubber septum, thus circumventing the inconvenience of carrying an exposed pump.[97] Implantable pumps have not yet been approved for fluid delivery to the human eye.

Periocular Administration

When higher concentrations of drugs, particularly corticosteroids and antibiotics, are required than can be delivered to the eye by topical, oral, or parenteral administration, local injections into the periocular tissues can be considered. Periocular drug administration includes the routes of subconjunctival, anterior sub-Tenon's, posterior sub-Tenon's, and retrobulbar administration.

Subconjunctival Injection

Although repeated topical applications of most ocular drugs will achieve intraocular drug levels comparable to those achieved with subconjunctival injections, subconjunctival injections offer an advantage in the administration of drugs, such as antibiotics, with poor intraocular penetration. Although the value of subconjunctival injections as a useful route of drug administration is still somewhat questionable, this mode of drug delivery appears to offer the following advantages.[29]

- High local concentrations of drug can be obtained with the use of small quantities of medication, thereby avoiding adverse systemic effects.
- High tissue concentrations can be obtained with drugs that poorly penetrate the epithelial layer of the cornea or conjunctiva.
- This method is useful in patients who will not reliably use topical medication.
- Drugs can be injected at the conclusion of surgery to avoid the necessity of topical or systemic drug therapy.

Subconjunctival injection involves passing the needle between the anterior conjunctiva and Tenon's capsule (Fig. 2.26). This can be performed through the lid, as illustrated in Figure 2.26, or directly into the subconjunctival space. Although the injection can be placed in any quadrant, the superotemporal quadrant is preferred, since this is the only quadrant between two rectus muscles that is not traversed by a portion of an oblique muscle or a tendon. In some cases, however, an injection site adjacent to the intraocular inflammation may be desirable. Since Tenon's capsule lies between the injected drug and the globe, the amount of drug absorbed across the sclera is minimized. In fact, the mechanism of drug absorption following subconjunctival injection may relate to simple leakage of drug through the needle puncture site with subsequent absorption through the cornea.[100] McCartney and associates,[101] however, have shown that, at least for corticosteroids, a subconjunctivally administered drug does penetrate the underlying sclera, suggesting a rationale for placing the drug directly adjacent to the site of inflammation rather than injecting it randomly.

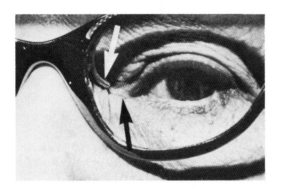

FIGURE 2.25 **Sigmamotor battery-driven pump. Fluid is delivered to the eye from the pump by a thin tubing that is led along a spectacle frame and enters the inferior conjunctival sac from the nasal side (arrows). (From Dohlman CH, Doane MG, Reshmi CS. Mobile infusion pumps for continuous delivery of fluid and therapeutic agents to the eye. Ann Ophthalmol 1971;3:126–128, with permission of the authors and publisher.)**

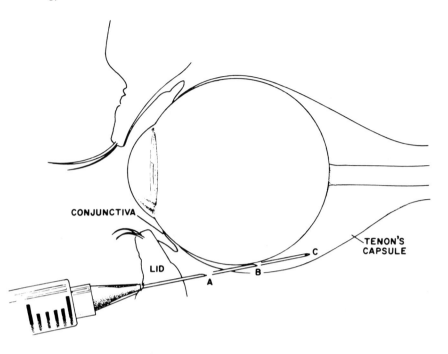

FIGURE 2.26 **Relative positions of peri-ocular injections.** *(A)* **Subconjunctival.** *(B)* **Sub-Tenon's.** *(C)* **Retrobulbar.**

The specific technique of drug administration used by most practitioners is relatively simple.[102] After the eye is anesthetized with a drop of local anesthetic such as proparacaine instilled 5 times at 1 minute intervals, the patient is instructed to look down while the upper eyelid is retracted. The conjunctiva is grasped with fine-toothed forceps between the superior and lateral rectus muscles and midway between the limbus and equator of the eye, and the drug is injected with a 25- or 27-gauge hypodermic needle. Following injection, the puncture site is firmly grasped with forceps for a few minutes to prevent leakage of drug after the needle has been withdrawn. An eye pad is applied for several hours. Although most patients often feel minor discomfort for 24 to 36 hours, they are usually able to continue with their daily activities.

Probably the greatest clinical benefit associated with the subconjunctival route of drug administration is in the treatment of severe corneal disease such as bacterial ulcers. Much higher concentrations of antibiotics can be achieved in the affected corneal tissues with subconjunctival injection than can be obtained by systemic drug administration.[96] Subconjunctival antibiotic administration is also useful as an initial supplement to the systemic antibiotic treatment of bacterial endophthalmitis. A variety of ocular diseases are treated with subconjunctival corticosteroids. Mydriatrics, however, are seldom injected subconjunctivally, since pledget application offers comparable intraocular drug levels.

When contemplating subconjunctival antibiotic

therapy, the practitioner should keep in mind the compatibility of the various antibiotics. Some broad-spectrum antibiotics inactivate or are antagonistic to each other, such as chloramphenicol and gentamicin. As a precaution against interaction of antagonistic drugs, it is advisable to avoid the subconjunctival injection of different antibiotics at the same injection site. If more than one antibiotic is required, the second drug should be injected at a separate site with a second syringe. In addition, the practitioner should judiciously select for administration only those drugs causing relatively little local inflammation (e.g., gentamicin and oxacillin). Certain drugs, such as methicillin and cephalothin, may cause moderate degrees of local inflammation when injected subconjunctivally.[96]

Anterior Sub-Tenon's Injection

Although the terms *subconjunctival* and *anterior sub-Tenon's* are often used interchangeably, they are technically different forms of drug administration. Either one of two techniques may be used.[103]

1. Prepare the skin of the lower lid with an alcohol pad. With the patient looking superiorly and nasally, puncture the skin at the junction of the outer and middle third of the lower lid just above the orbital rim using a 15 mm ($\frac{5}{8}$ inch), 25- or 27-gauge needle attached

to a disposable tuberculin syringe. Pass the needle inward until its hub noticeably indents the skin of the lower lid (see Fig. 2.26). To test whether the needle is resting within a vessel, attempt to aspirate blood. If no blood is withdrawn, inject the drug at a slow to moderate rate. The patient usually feels little discomfort.

2. After instilling a topical anesthetic such as proparacaine, instruct the patient to look away from the desired site of injection. Grasp the bulbar conjunctiva and Tenon's capsule with toothed forceps, and pass a 15 mm ($\frac{5}{8}$ inch), 25- or 27-gauge needle attached to a disposable tuberculin syringe under the forceps in the desired quadrant of injection. The conjunctiva and Tenon's capsule are easily perforated, and the injection is directed posteriorly in a plane that is parallel to the optic nerve. After attempting to aspirate blood, inject the drug at a slow to moderate rate into the space beneath Tenon's capsule.

Sub-Tenon's injection offers no significant advantages over subconjunctival drug administration. In fact, sub-Tenon's injection delivers lower quantities of drug to the eye and is associated with a greater risk of perforating the globe.[96] Despite these disadvantages, however, sub-Tenon's injections are occasionally used in the treatment of severe iritis or iridocyclitis.

Posterior Sub-Tenon's Injection

As with the subconjunctival and anterior sub-Tenon's routes of administration, posterior sub-Tenon's injections can be administered through two routes, conjunctival or skin. In the conjunctival route, the conjunctiva is anesthetized with a topical anesthetic such as proparacaine, or with an anesthetic-moistened applicator applied to any of the 4 quadrants deep into the fornix. With the patient looking away from the quadrant of injection, a 15 mm ($\frac{5}{8}$ inch), 25-gauge needle attached to a tuberculin syringe is passed into the fornix through the conjunctiva without grasping it. To minimize the risk of perforating the globe, the tip of the needle may be moved from side to side as it is passed posteriorly following the curvature of the globe. Since neither the injected drug nor the tip of the needle is visible during the injection procedure, the precise location of the inoculation site is unknown. However, the posterior portion of Tenon's space is the desired target. The technique for drug administration through the skin is precisely the same as that used for a standard retrobulbar injection in the inferior temporal orbit. It may be performed through a small bleb of lidocaine infiltrated into the skin of the lid. Since a 15 mm ($\frac{5}{8}$

inch) needle is used for the procedure, the injection is not considered a retrobulbar technique.[104]

Posterior sub-Tenon's injection of corticosteroids is most often used in the treatment of equatorial and midzone posterior uveitis, including inflammation of the macular region. In the treatment of macular disease, however, there may be little difference in clinical effectiveness between a posterior sub-Tenon's injection and retrobulbar injection, because these tissue spaces freely intercommunicate.[28] Because of the curvature of the eye, the tip of the needle in a retrobulbar procedure is unlikely to be any closer to the macula than the needle tip in the posterior sub-Tenon's technique. Consequently, a sub-Tenon's injection is often preferred in such instances, since it is usually somewhat more comfortable than the retrobulbar injection and somewhat safer, with fewer complications, than the retrobulbar procedure.[28]

Retrobulbar Injection

Drugs have been administered by retrobulbar injection for at least 75 years.[105,106] The procedure was originally developed to anesthetize the globe, and this remains its principal clinical use. However, antibiotics, vasodilators, corticosteroids, and alcohol have also been administered through this route. Currently, retrobulbar anesthetics are used routinely, retrobulbar corticosteroids are used occasionally (although their clinical value remains controversial and unproved), and retrobulbar alcohol is rarely administered.

The specific technique usually involves injection through the skin of the lower lid with a 23- or 25-gauge needle inserted immediately above the inferotemporal orbital rim and directed toward the orbital apex[105,107] (see Fig. 2.26). Retrobulbar injections may also be administered inside the lower eyelid through the conjunctival fornix. In general, 35 mm ($1\frac{3}{8}$ inch) needles are usually adequate to deliver the drug within the muscle cone, although 50 mm (2 inch) needles can be used to produce a deeper anesthetic injection to ensure a more complete motor block. Blunted needles may reduce the likelihood of hemorrhage.

The volume of the retrobulbar injection varies greatly depending on the drug injected.[105] Anesthetic solutions are usually employed in volumes of 1.5 to 6.0 ml. Steroids are usually administered in volumes of 0.5 to 1.0 ml. When retrobulbar alcohol is administered, a 1.0 or 2.0 ml injection of an anesthetic is usually given a few minutes before the injection of a similar amount of absolute alcohol to reduce the initial pain associated with the alcohol. Regardless of the drug to be injected, however, it is advisable to attempt aspiration of blood before injecting any significant amount of medication, to ensure that the tip of the needle is not within a blood vessel. It has also been suggested that injecting small amounts of the drug as the needle is gently inserted may tend to push away tissues from the needle tip. Supplemental measures following injection include massage after anesthetic injections to increase diffusion of the drug; also, following alcohol injection, ice compresses are often applied to reduce lid and conjunctival swelling.[108]

Retrobulbar injections have been used for a variety of ocular diseases. Dramatic relief of pain has often been achieved with retrobulbar injection of alcohol. In most cases, this therapy has been reserved for patients with blind eyes, such as in absolute glaucoma, but it has also been used in the partially sighted. Duration of relief of pain may be for several months or as long as a year or more. Although intraocular pressure is lowered in many patients, this does not often occur in patients with absolute glaucoma. Although retrobulbar injections of alcohol may offer an alternative to enucleation of blind and painful eyes, they should not be used if the internal structures of the eye cannot be examined. The incidence of unsuspected melanomas in such eyes is alarmingly high, and misdiagnosis or mismanagement could result if retrobulbar alcohol therapy were used.[105]

Although the use of retrobulbar steroids is controversial, this therapeutic modality has been advocated and continues to be used in the treatment of optic neuritis, Graves' ophthalmopathy, and inflammatory diseases of the posterior segment, including the macula. In some instances retrobulbar steroid therapy has been successful when high doses of oral steroids have failed to produce a satisfactory clinical response. The singular advantage of retrobulbar steroid therapy is that higher local drug concentrations can be obtained with less systemic toxicity than is possible with high doses of systemic steroids.[109]

Complications of Periocular Injection

Because of the disadvantages and complications associated with periocular drug administration, this form of drug delivery should generally be reserved for ocular disorders that fail to respond adequately to topical drug therapy. A major disadvantage of subconjunctival injections is the very low tissue drug concentrations during the intervals between injections.[96] In addition, local side effects include massive subconjunctival hemorrhage, markedly irritated eyes, dellen formation, chemosis, pain, and retained subconjunctival drug deposits.[29] Since periocular drug administration involves injection directly into the ocular tissues, patient apprehension is also a significant limiting factor.

Although serious complications with retrobulbar injections are uncommon, numerous complications have been reported[28,104,105,110] (Table 2.8). These include retrobulbar hemorrhage, which occurs in 1% to 2% of patients receiving anesthetic injections. The incidence is higher when longer needles are used. Some eye surgeons believe that the incidence of retrobulbar hemorrhage is lower with larger (lower gauge) needles and with blunted tips. Most retrobulbar hemorrhages, however, are of little consequence because they resolve spontaneously without sequelae. Conjunctival and eyelid ecchymoses are common but usually subside without treatment. In addition, proptosis, corneal exposure, and elevated intraocular pressure can occur. Bradycardia associated with the oculocardiac reflex has been observed. Occlusion of the central retinal artery as well as optic atrophy have followed retrobulbar injections.[115,116] The latter complication may occur from direct injury to the nerve itself or from secondary hemorrhage, resulting in compression of nutrient vessels to the nerve. A transient reduction in visual acuity almost always occurs following retrobulbar injection of anesthetics. Extraocular muscle palsies, ptosis, and pupillary abnormalities frequently occur as well, but recovery is usually complete within hours. However, following retrobulbar alcohol injections, extraocular muscle palsies and ptosis may persist for weeks or months.[117,118] Chemosis, lid swelling, and pain may be pronounced following these injections. Cardiovascular and CNS toxicity can occur if the medication is inadvertently injected into the vascular system or subarachnoid space.[119,120]

Numerous complications have been associated with the periocular administration of corticosteroids. Glau-

---

TABLE 2.8
Complications of Retrobulbar Injections

- Retrobulbar hemorrhage
- Conjunctival and eyelid ecchymosis
- Proptosis
- Exposure keratopathy
- Elevated intraocular pressure
- Respiratory arrest
- Bradycardia
- Central retinal artery/vein occlusion
- Optic atrophy
- Transient reduction in visual acuity
- Extraocular muscle palsies
- Ptosis
- Pupillary abnormalities
- Chemosis
- Eyelid swelling
- Pain
- Cardiovascular or CNS drug toxicity
- Accidental perforation of the globe

coma has resulted from the periocular injection of such drugs. Surgical excision is the only means of removing this material once it is deposited.[28,121] Diplopia and limited elevation of the involved eye have followed the periocular injection of steroids into the region of the superior fornix.[110] Cataract has also been reported as a complication of periocular steroids.[104] One patient developed numerous complications following a series of 20 retrobulbar injections of steroid administered weekly for the treatment of presumptive toxoplasmic retinitis.[104] Complications included pseudoptosis, proptosis, Cushing's syndrome, systemic hypertension, increased susceptibility to bruises, and weight loss. Intralesional periocular injection of steroids has resulted in both retinal and choroidal vascular occlusion.[122,123]

One of the most significant and serious complications associated with periocular injections is accidental perforation of the globe.[103,114,124–126] Steroid preparations have been accidentally injected into the choroidal vasculature, retina, and the intraocular compartment.[127] The globe can be perforated so easily, and without noticeable resistance, that the practitioner may not know when the globe has been penetrated.[125] In some cases perforation may go undetected for several weeks. The immediate effects associated with perforation of the globe during periocular steroid administration may include pain, reduced vision, ocular hypertension, ocular hypotony, an obvious white mass in the vitreous cavity, visible subretinal material, or intraocular hemorrhage. Delayed effects have included pseudohypopyon in aphakia from prolapse of drug from the vitreous cavity, vitreoretinal traction bands, preretinal membrane formation, retinal detachment, toxic pigmentary atrophy, and ascending optic atrophy.[114,125,126] The injected intraocular steroid material may require 6 to 8 weeks to disappear, which is followed by either complete recovery of vision or permanent vision loss of varying degrees.

The use of periocular injections less than 6 weeks following cataract extraction is contraindicated.[103] The tendency for the patient receiving a periocular injection to squint or squeeze the lids during the procedure mandates that the procedure be delayed until the surgical wound has adequately healed.

Intracameral Administration

Intracameral administration involves injecting a drug directly into the anterior chamber of the eye. The most common clinical application is the injection of viscoelastic substances into the anterior chamber during cataract extraction to protect the corneal endothelium.

When antibiotics are used, however, this procedure is associated with a significant risk of operative complications as well as drug toxicity but has the advantage of rapidly achieving high intraocular concentrations of drug. Intracameral antibiotic administration may be particularly valuable in the treatment of nonsterile conditions requiring surgery, such as closure of a ruptured operative wound or repair of a laceration.[128] Only very minute quantities of antibiotics are tolerated in the anterior chamber (Table 2.9). Irrigation of the anterior chamber with excessive amounts of antibiotics often causes destruction of the corneal endothelium, dense corneal opacification, iritis with neovascularization, or cataract.

Intravitreal Administration

The risks inherent in intravitreal injection are as significant as those associated with intracameral administration and probably outweigh any possible benefit in almost all circumstances. In general, the intraocular injection of drugs is primarily reserved as an heroic effort to rescue eyes with severe acute intraocular inflammation or eyes that have failed to respond to other, more conservative methods of therapy. In these instances, since the vitreal penetration of antibiotics in therapeutic concentrations following systemic or subconjunctival administration is usually inadequate (except for systemically administered chloramphenicol and subconjunctivally administered penicillin G), intravitreal injection seems to be superior to subconjunctival or intracameral injection as the preferred route of drug administration.[129] Consequently, intravitreal antibiotics may be the treatment of choice for endophthalmitis in which the organism, or at least its morphology or

TABLE 2.9
Antibiotics Tolerated by Intracameral Injection

Antibiotic	Dosage
Bacitracin	500–1000 units
Chloramphenicol	1–2 mg
Colistin	0.1 mg
Erythromycin	1–2 mg
Neomycin	2.5 mg
Penicillin G	1000–4000 units
Methicillin	1 mg
Polymyxin B	0.1 mg
Streptomycin	0.5–5 mg
Tetracycline	2.5–5 mg

Modified from Leopold IH. Antibiotics and antifungal agents. Problems and management of ocular infections. Invest Ophthalmol 1964;3:504–511, with permission of the author and publisher.

staining characteristics, is known. Table 2.10 lists antibiotics that have been tolerated by intravitreal injection. In addition, intravitreal liquid silicone has been used for several decades in the treatment of complicated retinal detachment.[130,131]

A technique for intravitreal injection has been described by Peyman and Sanders.[132] This technique involves an operating room procedure in which, following a retrobulbar block and topical anesthesia, an anterior chamber paracentesis is performed, and sclera is exposed in the superotemporal or inferotemporal quadrant approximately 5 to 6 mm posterior to the limbus. Following an incision into the vitreous, 0.2 ml of vitreous is aspirated with a 22-gauge needle. The antibiotic is then injected through a 27-gauge needle.

Iontophoresis

In the early part of this century iontophoresis was commonly used in the treatment of ocular infections, but this procedure is almost never used today.[96,133] The technique involved applying to the patient's eye a cup containing a solution of antibiotic. An electrode was attached to the bottom of the cup, and another electrode was usually held by the patient to complete the circuit. Current was passed through this circuit in a direction appropriate to the net charge of the active portion of the antibiotic molecule. This technique was used to enhance the corneal penetration of water-soluble antibiotics to achieve adequate therapeutic intraocular drug levels. More recently, iontophoresis has been used to achieve deep conjunctival anesthesia to permit the surgical removal of chalazions and conjunctival concretions. The procedure has also been employed in the administration of 6-hydroxydopamine to produce a chemical sympathectomy in the treatment of glaucoma and of cisplatin (Platinol) for the chemotherapy of basal cell and squamous cell carcinomas.[134] It may also be useful as an adjunct to deliver topical aminoglycosides to the eye in patients with severe bacterial keratitis.[135]

Oral Administration

Although topical administration is the easiest and most convenient form of drug delivery to the eye, some forms of ocular disease require systemic drug administration to achieve adequate therapeutic levels of drug in specific ocular tissues. In addition, some drugs are commercially available in formulations suitable only

TABLE 2.10
Antibiotics Tolerated by Intravitreal Injection

Antibiotic	Intravitreal Dosage (mg)	Duration of Vitreous Therapeutic Level (hr)	Duration of Aqueous Therapeutic Level (hr)
Aminoglycosides			
Gentamicin	0.4	72–96	—
Tobramycin	0.5	96	96
Kanamycin	0.5	24–72	—
Penicillins			
Methicillin	2.0	40	—
Ampicillin	5.0	48	24
Carbenicillin	2.0	16–24	—
Antifungal			
Amphotericin B	5–10 μg	—	—
Miscellaneous			
Cephaloridine	0.25	—	—
Erythromycin	0.5	24	—
Clindamycin	1.0	16–24	—
Chloramphenicol	2.0	24	24

Modified from Peyman G, Sanders D. Advances in uveal surgery, vitreous surgery, and the treatment of endophthalmitis. New York: Appleton-Century-Crofts, 1975.

for systemic use, while other drugs are clinically effective only when systemically administered. Examples of such drugs include the carbonic anhydrase inhibitors for the treatment of glaucoma, steroids and diuretics for the treatment of Graves' ophthalmopathy, and analgesics for the management of pain associated with severe corneal abrasions. In some instances oral administration may be the most effective route of drug delivery. For example, the oral antibiotic therapy of preseptal cellulitis, and the oral antihistaminic therapy of acute allergic dermatoblepharitis, will result in a more rapid clinical response than the respective topical antibiotic or antihistaminic therapies. On the other hand, oral antibiotic therapy may be less effective in the treatment of bacterial corneal ulcers, endophthalmitis, and other disorders that respond more favorably to topical or periocular drug administration.

Some oral preparations for ocular use are available as sustained-release formulations, notably acetazolamide. Although a single dose of acetazolamide will reduce intraocular pressure up to 12 hours, a single dose of sustained-release acetazolamide will produce a comparable effect lasting 20 hours.[28] Advantages of sustained-release medication include more constant delivery of drug without the exaggerated "pulses" associated with uncoated medication release and better patient compliance, since the drug is administered at less frequent intervals.

Oral fluorescein, described by Burke in 1910 as a stain for active fundus lesions, was reintroduced in the United Kingdom in the 1970s for fundus fluorography.[136] The risk of an anaphylactic reaction is much less than when the fluorescein is administered intravenously for angiographic purposes. Although no toxic reactions have been reported, oral administration of sodium fluorescein has not yet been approved by the Food and Drug Administration (FDA).[137]

Since the risk of systemic drug toxicity and allergy is greater with systemically administered drugs, the practitioner should carefully question the patient regarding drug allergies or previous drug toxicities before administering or prescribing oral medication. In addition, more careful monitoring of patients is required to ascertain side effects that may be associated with the prescribed drug. Complications associated with drug interactions may also be encountered, and the practitioner should be alert to anticipate these interactions before prescribing oral medications. Unlike most dosage schedules for topically applied drugs, dosage schedules for orally administered drugs usually differ greatly in their recommendations for adults and children. The clinician should generally adhere to those pediatric and adult dosage recommendations contained in the commercially available package inserts.

Parenteral Administration

Subcutaneous Injection

The ophthalmic use of subcutaneous injections is normally limited to infiltration anesthesia for minor surgical procedures of the eyelids, and to the emergency management of anaphylaxis with subcutaneous epinephrine. The inner aspect of the forearm is an easily accessible and convenient location for the subcutaneous injection of epinephrine. The use of subcutaneous epinephrine in the management of anaphylactoid reactions is discussed in Chapter 31.

Intramuscular Injection

Hydroxycobalamin (vitamin B_{12}) and some antibiotics (e.g., penicillin) are often most appropriately administered through the intramuscular route. If intramuscular injections are required in infants, these should be administered anteriorly in the mid-portion of the quadriceps, since the sciatic nerve lies near the surface and can be damaged by the traditional upper-outer quadrant injection.[28]

Intravenous Injection

In the treatment of endophthalmitis and other severe ocular infections, the continuous intravenous infusion of various antibiotics may be required. Such continuous infusion can be accomplished with the traditional intravenous apparatus or, more recently, using the AR/MED (Alza Corporation) infusor, which is worn on the arm and permits outpatient treatment even when continuous drug infusion is required. This infusor consists of a disposable cartridge containing a pressurized drug reservoir that holds 25 ml of drug, and a control unit with an adjustable, precalibrated valve and a bacterial filter.[138] A flow line attached to a catheter carries the drug solution, and continuous parenteral administration of medication is possible at rates of 0.4 to 2.0 ml/hr. Patients are able to change the cartridges safely and easily.

Acute infectious retinitis of presumed viral origin has been successfully managed with intravenous acyclovir.[139] Certain antibacterial agents such as ampicillin, chloramphenicol, and erythromycin penetrate into the eye at higher initial concentrations and maintain comparable intraocular levels when administered as a single intravenous "pulse" compared with administration by continuous infusion.[28] Thus, a single intravenous injection may be superior to continuous intravenous infusion to achieve a high initial intraocular drug concentration that will be maintained for at least 4 hours. However, although effective serum levels of antibiotics may be achieved by this route, tear levels may be subtherapeutic for corneal infections.[140]

Ophthalmic Prescription Writing

Ophthalmic drug prescriptions do not differ significantly from those for other pharmaceutical agents.[141] The trend toward the use of commercially prepared combinations of drugs formulated in suitable vehicles has greatly simplified the writing of ophthalmic prescriptions. As with other prescriptions, the basic elements of the ophthalmic prescription include the patient demographic data, the inscription, the subscription, and the signatura.

The inscription consists of the name of the prescribed drug and may be in either generic or proprietary form. If the drug is formulated in varying concentrations, the desired concentration should be specified. Many commercially prepared combination drugs, such as antibiotic-corticosteroid preparations, are available in only one fixed-ratio formulation such that specific concentrations of the component drugs need not be specified. The specific dosage form (e.g., solution, ointment) should be included in the inscription.

The subscription consists of the quantity of drug to be dispensed by the pharmacist. The specific number of dosage units (volume of solution, number of tablets, etc.) should be clearly specified. Only the quantity sufficient for the clinical condition for which the medication is being prescribed should be ordered, since excess drug may be stored by the patient for later use in ocular conditions that may be totally unrelated to the initial disease episode.

The signatura includes the instructions to the patient for use of the prescribed medication. Inadequate and incomplete prescription instructions to the patient may be the single most important factor contributing to noncompliance.[142] Incomplete, inadequate, or vague instructions occur in a substantial number of prescriptions. Vague directions serve only to confuse the patient and motivate him or her not to comply with the intended therapy. For this reason, instructions should be clear, concise, and unambiguous. The practitioner should reread the prescription for clarity and accuracy before issuing it to the patient.

Use of phrases such as "as directed" and "p.r.n." (as needed) should be avoided, since these serve only to increase the frequency of dosaging errors by the patient.[142] The frequency of use of "as directed" and "p.r.n." in ophthalmic prescriptions compared with other pharmaceutical prescriptions is shown in Table 2.11. Because of such ambiguous prescription labeling, patients have been known to drink eyedrops intended for glaucoma or for conjunctivitis.[143] It therefore appears totally inappropriate to assume that patients will always be able to recall what was intended by the phrase "as directed." Furthermore, use of "p.r.n." is discouraged, since this instruction encourages self-assessment, self-diagnosis, and drug abuse potential. Few patients can accurately and objectively assess their clinical condition and therapeutic needs. Many patients will often resume taking the medication at a later date for a disorder totally unrelated to the initial disease.

Figure 2.27 illustrates properly completed ophthalmic

TABLE 2.11
Frequency of Use of "as directed" and "p.r.n." on Ophthalmic and Other Randomly Selected Prescriptions

Dosage Form	Number of Prescriptions	Percentage of Total	Number of Times "as directed" Utilized		Number of Times "PRN" Utilized	
Oral solids	14,104	70.62	921	(6.53%)	2,046	(14.51%)
Oral liquids	2,389	11.96	151	(6.32%)	382	(15.99%)
Dermatologicals	1,095	5.48	157	(14.30%)	128	(11.69%)
Vaginal preparations	660	3.31	94	(14.24%)	44	(6.67%)
Ophthalmics	486	2.43	61	(12.6 %)	70	(14.40%)
Suppositories	385	1.93	41	(10.6 %)	83	(21.56%)
Otics	312	1.56	21	(6.7 %)	53	(16.99%)
Miscellaneous	541	2.71	102	(18.8 %)	133	(24.58%)
Total	19,972	100.00	1548	(7.75%)[a]	2,939	(14.72%)[a]

[a]Average percentage.
Reprinted with permission from *Patient Counseling and Health Education,* Winter/Spring 1979, Excerpta Medica, Princeton, N.J.

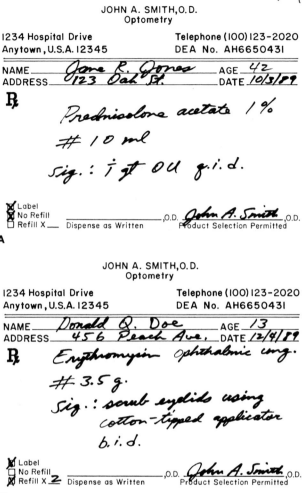

4th generation fluoroquinolones gatifloxacin (Zymar) moxifloxacin (Vigamox)

FIGURE 2.27 **Properly completed ophthalmic drug prescriptions. *(A)* Ophthalmic suspension. *(B)* Ophthalmic ointment.**

drug prescriptions. To enhance patient compliance, the prescription label should reflect as many of the following points as are applicable.[142]

- Amount of drug to be taken in a single dose
- Total number of doses to be taken daily
- Timing or frequency of administration of the medication
- Route of administration
- Purpose of the medication, if appropriate
- Name of the medication
- Maximum amount of the drug that can be used in one day (as with "p.r.n." medications)
- Length of time for which the medication should be used
- Number of refills permitted
- Other drugs, foods, or concomitant activities that should be avoided
- Proper storage technique
- Any other information that may be pertinent to the patient's condition or drug therapy regimen

It is axiomatic that the handwritten prescription should be legible. The chances of error on the pharmacist's part are compounded by poorly written or illegible prescriptions. In fact, several cases of accidental substitution of acetohexamide (Dymelor), an oral hypoglycemic agent, for acetazolamide (Diamox), a carbonic anhydrase inhibitor, have been reported.[144] A number of similar features exists between the two drugs, including the fact that both medications are formulated as 250 mg white tablets and have similar generic and proprietary names. Hence, the importance of legible handwriting is emphasized.

Another potential factor in prescription writing errors involves the use of incorrect Latin abbreviations. Although the trend in contemporary prescription writing is to use English rather than the traditional Latin phrases, numerous Latin abbreviations remain in common use. The abbreviations most often used in ophthalmic prescription writing are listed in Table 2.12.

TABLE 2.12
Latin Abbreviations Used in Prescription Writing

Abbreviation	*Latin*	*English Meaning*
a.c.	ante cibum	before meals
b.i.d.	bis in die	twice a day
c̄	cum	with
caps.	capsula	capsule
d.	dies	day
gt(t).	gutta(e)	drop(s)
h.	hora	hour
h.s.	hora somni	at bedtime
o.d.	oculus dexter	right eye
o.h.	omni hora	every hour
o.s.	oculus sinister	left eye
o.u.	oculus uterque	each eye
p.c.	post cibum	after meals
p.o.	per os	by mouth
p.r.n.	pro re nata	as needed
q.	quaque	each, every
q.h.	quaque hora	every hour
q.i.d.	quater in die	four times a day
s̄	sine	without
sig.	signa	label
sol.	solutio	solution
tab.	tabella	tablet
t.i.d.	ter in die	three times a day
ung.	unguentum	ointment
ut dict.	ut dictum	as directed

Patient Compliance

The term *noncompliance* implies that the patient is responsible for self-administration of the prescribed medication and is at fault when it is not administered. The term *drug defaulting,* on the other hand, implies that the medication is administered but in an inappropriate fashion. Wide variation exists in the degree to which drugs are misused, ranging from 4% to 87% for drug defaulting and from 25% to 50% for noncompliance in the ambulatory population.[142,145] Patients exhibit noncompliance or drug defaulting in a variety of ways.

- Patients fail to take medication. Of drug prescriptions, 3% to 7% are never filled, and as many as 40% of defaulting patients never have any intention of following the practitioner's instructions.[146] Failure to take medication is the most common and most serious form of noncompliance.
- Patients may take medication for the wrong purpose. This often occurs when the patient receiving multiple medications becomes confused regarding the purpose for each drug, or the patient might use outdated medication for a purpose other than that for which it was originally prescribed.
- Patients may unintentionally skip dosages, intentionally administer inadequate dosages, or prematurely discontinue therapy.
- Patients sometimes take medication excessively in hopes of increasing the benefit derived from the drug. This is probably the least common form of defaulting.[145]
- Improper timing of medication dosages may occur[147] when patients do not comprehend the importance of adequate intervals between drug administrations. Patients receiving medication on a three times a day (t.i.d.) or four times a day (q.i.d.) schedule may separate successive dosages by 0 to 24 hours.[145] The greater the number of drugs to be taken and the more complex the schedule of administration, the more likely that improper dosaging intervals will occur.
- Patients may employ an improper technique of drug administration that might diminish the beneficial therapeutic effect derived from the drug. In addition, as many as 33% of patients over age 60 years have been reported to have difficulty using child-resistant containers and may be too embarrassed to admit this to the practitioner.[146]

In general medical practice, the rate of patient noncompliance is greatest in the less serious conditions, when the consequences are often relatively insignificant compared with acute symptomatic illnesses. Unfortunately, noncompliance with glaucoma therapy may be relatively high, since this disease is rarely associated with pain or immediate disability. Many reasons exist for noncompliance,[142,145] as noted in Table 2.13. Noncompliance does not correlate reliably with patient age, sex, race, education, occupation, diagnosis, or severity of disease as perceived by the practitioner.[145] Contrary to popular opinion, noncompliance is not restricted to the lower socioeconomic groups or to less educated patients. Furthermore, many cases of noncompliance can be predicted,[145] including the patient who returns with a 6-month-old bottle of timolol prescribed for his glaucoma, the patient who "just ran out of drops yesterday," the patient who misses multiple appointments, and the patient who is receiving pilocarpine therapy but who has normal-sized, reactive pupils.

The most important contribution to compliance with drug therapy appears to be the patient's understanding of his or her illness, the importance of therapy, and the instructions for use of the prescribed drug(s).[142] The clinician's willingness to consider the possibility of poor compliance is essential for a successful solution to the problem. Nonjudgmental questions should be asked, such as "You are not doing quite as well as I had anticipated; is there something about the treatment that I did not explain?" Since possibly two-thirds of compliance problems arise from faulty comprehension on the patient's part, the clinician should ascertain the patient's understanding of techniques such as drop instillation, lid scrubs, insertion of ocular inserts, and meibomian gland expression before the patient leaves the office. The patient might be asked, "Do you have any questions I have not answered today?" Patient comprehension may be improved by using nontechnical language. Since many patients express anxiety or fear during the initial interview with the practitioner, it is

TABLE 2.13
Reasons for Noncompliance

- Advancing age
- Duration of drug therapy
- Number of drugs in the treatment regimen
- Frequency of drug administration
- Drug-induced adverse effects
- Relief of symptoms
- Fear of drug dependency
- Unpalatable dosage form
- Inadequate patient-doctor relationship
- Excessive waiting time in the office
- Cost of medication
- Carelessness
- Complexity of the therapeutic regimen
- Family instability
- Lack of symptoms

not surprising that numerous patients fail to remember the detailed instructions given during the office visit. Most patients fear the possibility of physical illness, and this fear is compounded if their condition is serious enough to require medication. The only certain way to ensure that the patient fully understands the practitioner's instructions is to ask, before the office visit ends, "Repeat for me what you have heard me ask you to do." More general and less specific questions such as, "Do you understand?" are only likely to elicit a socially acceptable affirmative response. Repetition can also improve comprehension. Written instructions for reading at home are beneficial, as is positive reinforcement from spouse, friend, or various family members. Instructions for the proper use of prescribed medication should not necessarily be restricted to fit the dimensions of the prescription label. If necessary, supplemental labelling should be attached to the drug container.[148] The combination of a complete prescription label and appropriate verbal counseling appears to be effective in improving compliance.[142]

Since less complicated tasks are easier to learn, especially for the elderly, the use of simplified treatment programs also improves compliance. Once-daily or twice-daily therapeutic programs are easier to understand, are often less costly, and fit more readily into the patient's daily lifestyle. If possible, the total number of medications prescribed should be limited, since considerable confusion may arise in the taking of multiple daily medications. Of utmost importance is the forewarning regarding expected or potential drug-induced side effects. Patient compliance can often be improved substantially if the patient is cautioned to anticipate side effects rather than allowing the patient to encounter them unexpectedly.

Legal Aspects of Drug Administration

Documentation of Administered Drugs

In a litigation-conscious society, the practitioner should seize every opportunity to diminish the risk of liability. The recording of administered, dispensed, or prescribed drugs is an easy and practical means of reducing such liability. The practitioner should record the specific name of the drug (either generic or proprietary), the concentration or dosage unit, the quantity administered or prescribed, and the time of day if administered in the office. This practice not only ensures proper documentation of administered or prescribed drugs for future clinical reference, but also serves to reduce the practitioner's liability should an adverse reaction occur that is allegedly associated with the drug. The practi-

tioner may devise a shorthand nomenclature for the documentation of drugs that are administered on a routine basis. For example, for routine dilation of the pupil, "1 gt M_1 + P_1 OU × 1" might represent "1 drop of 1% Mydriacyl and 1 drop of 1% Paredrine in both eyes for one application." Use of shorthand abbreviations is also convenient in the long-term management of glaucoma patients (see Table 29.21). This nomenclature allows rapid recording of routinely administered or prescribed drugs, which saves time in the busy office while maintaining desired legal standards. Of course, copies of written or verbal drug prescriptions should be maintained as part of the patient's clinical chart.

Unlabelled Uses

The legal implications of the drug package insert have been challenged. In some cases, however, various courts have recognized that drugs may be used for clinical indications other than those specified in the package insert.[149] Dosage schedules different from those specified in the package insert may be prescribed for the patient's benefit if consistent with sound scientific rationale and medical practice.[150,151] However, it has not been clearly established whether an approved drug may be used for an unapproved purpose without first obtaining an application for an Investigative New Drug (IND). For example, sodium fluorescein has been approved in the United States for administration intravenously and topically but not orally. At the very least, patients should be informed of the nature of the intended therapy, and the practitioner should obtain the patient's written permission (informed consent) before beginning such treatment. Since drug-related side effects are a significant cause of malpractice litigations, it is essential that patients understand the risks of potential side effects.

It has been recognized that the package insert may not contain the most recent information about a drug and that the clinician should be free to use the drug for an indication not in the package insert when such use is part of the rational practice of medicine intended for the patient's benefit.[149] It appears that if there is documented use for a drug in the medical literature or at a medical meeting, an IND is not necessary. However, if the drug has not been demonstrated to be useful for a nonapproved purpose, then it is considered experimental, and an IND should be obtained.[a]

In determining what constitutes sound medical practice in malpractice litigations, the package insert is

---

[a]Personal Communication, Joel S. Mindel, M.D., Ph.D.

admissible into evidence, but it does not establish conclusively the standards of acceptable practice or that departure from the directions contained in the package insert is negligence. One of the best protections against unfavorable malpractice verdicts is to prescribe medications in the patient's best interest according to rational standards of medical practice.

The Drug Enforcement Administration

In the United States the regulation of the distribution and dispensing of CNS drugs with significant potential for abuse was completely revised by the Comprehensive Drug Abuse Prevention and Control Act of 1970, more commonly known as the Controlled Substances Act.[152] This law is regulated by the Drug Enforcement Administration (DEA) of the U.S. Department of Justice. In addition, various state and city laws usually exist to regulate drugs with serious abuse potential. On May 1, 1971, the Controlled Substances Act of 1970 became fully effective and, except for the Durham-Humphrey Amendment, which delineated whether certain drugs may be sold over the counter (without prescription) or dispensed only on prescription, superseded all previously enacted narcotic laws controlling prescription drugs.[152] Because of the legal implications in the use of narcotic and other drugs of abuse, it is worthwhile to summarize the practitioner's responsibilities in the clinical use of these drugs.

The DEA defines an individual practitioner as a physician, dentist, veterinarian, or other individual licensed, registered, or otherwise permitted by the United States or the jurisdiction in which he or she practices to dispense a controlled substance in the course of professional practice.[153] Conversely, the practitioner who wishes to employ any drug regulated by the Controlled Substances Act must be registered with the DEA. Note, however, that federal DEA registration is predicated on individual state law requirements. Optometrists and other health care providers practicing in states that do not authorize those practitioners to use controlled substances are not eligible for DEA registration.[152]

Drugs included within the jurisdiction of the Controlled Substances Act are divided into 5 "schedules," each designated by a Roman numeral (Table 2.14). Schedule I drugs are those that have no accepted medical use in the United States and that have a high abuse potential, including LSD, heroin, marijuana, and peyote, and may include investigational controlled substances.

Schedule II drugs have a high abuse potential with severe psychologic or physical dependence liability but have a currently accepted medical use with strict lim-

TABLE 2.14
Controlled Substances Commonly Used in Outpatient Ophthalmic Practice

Schedule	Drug
I	Not commercially available
II	Cocaine
	Oxycodone
III	Aspirin with codeine
	Acetaminophen with codeine
	Acetaminophen with hydrocodone
IV	Chloral hydrate
V	None commonly used

itations. Drugs in this schedule include certain narcotics, stimulants, and depressants such as codeine, meperidine, morphine, amphetamines, phenobarbital, and cocaine. Prescriptions for drugs in schedule II must be typewritten or be in ink or indelible pencil, must be personally signed by the prescribing practitioner, and are not refillable.

Drugs included in schedule III have an abuse potential less than those in schedules I and II. Abuse of these drugs may lead to low or moderate physical dependence or to high psychologic dependence. Schedule III drugs may contain limited quantities of certain narcotic drugs and nonnarcotic drugs such as chlorhexadol, nalorphine, and paregoric.

Drugs in schedule IV have lower abuse potential than do those in schedule III, and abuse of these drugs may lead to limited physical or psychologic dependence. Chloral hydrate, chlordiazepoxide (Librium), diazepam (Valium), meprobamate (Equanil), and propoxyphene (Darvon) are representative drugs in this schedule. Prescriptions for schedules III and IV drugs may be oral or written and may be refilled up to 5 times within 6 months if authorized by the prescribing practitioner.

Drugs included in schedule V have limited abuse potential and consist primarily of preparations containing limited quantities of drugs generally used for antitussive and antidiarrheal purposes. Prescriptions for drugs in schedule V may be refilled as authorized by the prescribing practitioner, and some preparations in this category are available over the counter.

The practitioner has numerous responsibilities in conforming to the Controlled Substances Act. This act requires separate registration of each principal place of professional practice and periodic renewal of DEA registration. The practitioner must record his or her registration number on all prescription orders for controlled substances and must maintain an inventory of stocked controlled substances. However, inventory records of schedule II drugs are not required if these substances are either administered to a patient during professional practice or if a prescription order is written. The practitioner must also file a revised registration form if his or her practice location changes and must keep a record of controlled substances in schedules II to V that he or she dispenses. Complete and accurate inventory records are also required for nonnarcotic controlled substances in schedules II to V if the patient is charged for these drugs in addition to the regular professional fee. Because of these and other technical details, DEA-registered practitioners have been known to innocently violate the law in their use of controlled substances. Strict observation of the regulations is required. Note also that most state and local jurisdictions have their own rules and regulations for the professional use of narcotics. Federal DEA laws may be superseded by a stricter local narcotic regulation.

Issues of informed consent, negligence, product liability, and other legal aspects of drug use are discussed in detail in Part V of this book.

References

1. Fraunfelder FT, Scafidi AF. Possible adverse effects from topical ocular 10% phenylephrine. Am J Ophthalmol 1978;85(4):447–453.
2. Kennerdell JS, Wucher FP. Cyclopentolate associated with two cases of grand mal seizure. Arch Ophthalmol 1972;87:634–635.
3. Awan KJ. Adverse systemic reactions of topical cyclopentolate hydrochloride. Ann Ophthalmol 1976;8:695–698.
4. Fraunfelder FT, Samples JR. Ophthalmic medications during pregnancy. JAMA 1988;259:2021–2022.
5. Van Buskirk EM. Adverse reactions from timolol administration. Ophthalmology 1980;87(5):447–450.
6. Fraunfelder FT. Ocular β-blockers and systemic effects. Arch Intern Med 1986;146(6):1073–1074.
7. Roholt PC. Betaxolol and restrictive airway disease. Arch Ophthalmol 1987;105(9):1172.
8. Verkijik A. Worsening of myasthenia gravis with timolol maleate eyedrops. Ann Neurol 1985;99(2):211–212.
9. Gottschalk HR, Stone OJ. Stevens-Johnson syndrome from ophthalmic sulfonamide. Arch Dermatol 1976;112(4):513–514.
10. Genvert GI, Cohen EJ, Donnenfeld ED, et al. Erythema multiforme after use of topical sulfacetamide. Am J Ophthalmol 1985;99(4):465–468.
11. Harris LS. Cycloplegic-induced intraocular pressure elevations. A study of normal and open-angle glaucomatous eyes. Arch Ophthalmol 1968;79:242–246.
12. Portney GL, Purcell TW. The influence of tropicamide on intraocular pressure. Ann Ophthalmol 1975;7:31–34.
13. Wilson FM. Adverse external ocular effects of topical ophthalmic therapy. An epidemiologic, laboratory, and clinical study. Trans Am Ophthalmol Soc 1983;81:854.
14. Wilson FM. Adverse external ocular effects of topical ophthalmic medications. Surv Ophthalmol 1979;24(2):57–88.
15. Fiore PM, Jacobs IH, Goldberg DB. Drug-induced pemphigoid. A spectrum of diseases. Arch Ophthalmol 1987;105:1660–1663.
16. Lyle WM, Hopkins GA. The unwanted ocular effects from topical ophthalmic drugs. Their occurrence, avoidance and reversal. J Am Optom Assoc 1977;48(12):1519–1523.
17. Coad CT, Osato MS, Wilhelmus KR. Bacterial contamination of eyedrop dispensers. Am J Ophthalmol 1984;98:548.
18. Schein OD, Wasson PJ, Boruchoff SA, et al. Microbial keratitis associated with contaminated ocular medications. Am J Ophthalmol 1988;105:361–365.
19. Priest JH. Atropine response of the eyes in mongolism. J Dis Child 1960;100(6)869–872.
20. Lyle WM, Bobier WR. Effects of topical anesthetics on phenylephrine-induced mydriasis. Am J Optom Physiol Opt 1977;54(5):276–281.
21. Michaels RH, Wilson FM, Grayson M. Infiltrative keratitis from abuse of anesthetic eyedrops. J Indiana State Med Assoc 1979;72(1):51–54.
22. Gasset AR, Bellows RT. Posterior subcapsular cataracts after topical corticosteroid therapy. Ann Ophthalmol 1974;6(12):1263–1265.
23. Davidson SI. Systemic effects of eye drops. Trans Ophthalmol Soc UK 1974;94:487–495.
24. Fraunfelder FT, Bagby GC, Kelly DJ. Fatal aplastic anemia following topical administration of ophthalmic chloramphenicol. Am J Ophthalmol 1982;93(3):356–360.
25. Bartlett JD. Administration of and adverse reactions to cycloplegic agents. Am J Optom Physiol Opt 1978;55(4):227–233.
26. Gray LG. Avoiding adverse effects of cycloplegics in infants and children. J Am Optom Assoc 1979;50(4):465–470.
27. Havener WH. Ocular pharmacology. St. Louis: C.V. Mosby Co, 1978;4:248.
28. Havener WH. Ocular pharmacology. St. Louis: C.V. Mosby Co, 1978;4:19–38.
29. Fraunfelder FT, Hanna C. Ophthalmic drug delivery systems. Surv Ophthalmol 1974;18(4):292–298.
30. Templeton WC, Eiferman RA, Snyder JW, et al. *Serratia* keratitis by contaminated eyedroppers. Am J Ophthalmol 1982;93:723–726.
31. Halberg GP, Kelly SE, Morrone M. Drug delivery systems for topical ophthalmic medication. Ann Ophthalmol 1975;7(9):1199–1209.
32. Nelson JD. Corneal abrasion resulting from a unit dose artificial tear dispenser. Am J Ophthalmol 1987;103(3):333–334.
33. MacKeen DL. Aqueous formulations and ointments. Int Ophthalmol Clin 1980;20(3):79–92.
34. Katz NNK, Foer EG. Ophthalmic drugs with similar packaging (letter). Am J Ophthalmol 1982;93(2):253–254.
35. Ling RTK, Villalobos R, Latina M. Inadvertent instillation of Hemoccult Developer in the eye. Arch Ophthalmol 1988;106:1033–1034.
36. Mauger T. Sodium hydroxide masquerading as a contact lens solution. Arch Ophthalmol 1988;106:1037.
37. Fraunfelder FT. Drug-packaging standards for eye drop medications. Arch Ophthalmol 1988;106:1029.

38. Zimmerman TJ, Kooner KS, Kandarakis AS, et al. Improving the therapeutic index of topically applied ocular drugs. Arch Ophthalmol 1984;102(4):551–552.

39. Levine L. Effective degree of mydriasis with phenylephrine and tropicamide. J Am Optom Physiol Opt 1976;53(12):774–785.

40. Fraunfelder FT. Extraocular fluid dynamics: How best to apply topical ocular medication. Trans Am Ophthalmol Soc 1976;74:457–487.

41. McGraw BF, Rollins CL. Method for increasing bioavailability of cycloplegics. J Am Optom Physiol Opt 1978;55(12):795–800.

42. Freeman MI. A method for delivery of ocular medication. Bull Mason Clin 1975;29:114.

43. Tennant JS. Instillation of eye drops (letter). Am J Ophthalmol 1979;87(1):104–105.

44. Sheldon GM. Self-administration of eyedrops. Ophthal Surg 1987;18:393–394.

45. Sharp J, Hanna C. Use of a spray to deliver drugs to the eye. J Arkansas Med Soc 1977;73(11):462–463.

46. Scruggs J, Wallace T, Hanna C. Route of absorption of drug and ointment after application to the eye. Ann Ophthalmol 1978;10(3):267–271.

47. Wallace T, Hanna C, Boozman F, et al. New application of ophthalmic ointments (letter). JAMA 1975;233(5):418.

48. Robin JS, Ellis PP. Ophthalmic ointments. Surv Ophthalmol 1978;22(5):335–340.

49. Hanna C, Fraunfelder FT, Cable M, et al. The effect of ophthalmic ointments on corneal wound healing. Am J Ophthalmol 1973;76(2):193–200.

50. Heerema JC, Friedenwald JS. Retardation of wound healing in the corneal epithelium by lanolin. Am J Ophthalmol 1950;33(9):1421–1427.

51. Fraunfelder FT, Hanna C, Woods AH. Pseudoentrapment of ointment in the cornea. Arch Ophthalmol 1975;93(5):331–334.

52. Fraunfelder FT, Hanna C, Cable M, et al. Entrapment of ophthalmic ointment in the cornea. Am J Ophthalmol 1973;76(4):475–484.

53. Norn MS. Role of the vehicle in local treatment of the eye. Acta Ophthalmol 1964;42(4):727–734.

54. Heath WE. Death from atropine poisoning. Br Med J 1950;2:608.

55. Hughes CA. Poisoning from use of atropine ointment 1 percent. Trans Ophthalmol Soc UK 1938;58:444–446.

56. Fraunfelder FT, Hanna C. Ophthalmic ointment. Trans Am Acad Ophthalmol Otolaryngol 1973;77:467–475.

57. Johnson DH, Kenyon KR, Epstein DL, et al. Corneal changes during pilocarpine gel therapy. Am J Ophthalmol 1986;101(1):13–15.

58. Johnson DH, Epstein DL, Allen RC, et al. A one-year multicenter clinical trial of pilocarpine gel. Am J Ophthalmol 1984;97(6):723–729.

59. Goldberg I, Ashburn FS, Kass MA, et al. Efficacy and patient acceptance of pilocarpine gel. Am J Ophthalmol 1979;88(5):843–846.

60. Yakovlev AA, Lenkevich MM. Use of pilocarpine impregnated alcohol films in the treatment of glaucomatous patients. Vestn Oftal 1966;79(6):40–42.

61. Sedlacek J. Possibility of the application of ophthalmic drugs with the use of gel contact lenses. Cesk Oftal 1965;21:509–512.

62. Waltman SR, Kaufman HE. Use of hydrophilic contact lenses to increase ocular penetration of topical drugs. Invest Ophthalmol Vis Sci 1970;9(4):250–255.

63. Scullica L, Squeri CA, Ferreri G. "Minor" applications of soft contact lenses. Trans Ophthalmol Soc UK 1977;97(1):159–161.

64. Ruben M, Watkins R. Pilocarpine dispensation for the soft hydrophilic contact lens. Br J Ophthalmol 1975;59(8):455–458.

65. Aquavella JV. New aspects of contact lenses in ophthalmology. Adv Ophthalmol 1976;32:2–34.

66. Hillman JS. Management of acute glaucoma with pilocarpine-soaked hydrophilic lens. Br J Ophthalmol 1974;58(7):674–679.

67. Podos SM, Becker B, Asseff C, et al. Pilocarpine therapy with soft contact lenses. Am J Ophthalmol 1972;73(3):336–341.

68. Maddox YT, Bernstein HN. An evaluation of the Bionite hydrophilic contact lens for use in a drug delivery system. Ann Ophthalmol 1972;4(9):789–802.

69. Lamberts DW. Solid delivery devices. Int Ophthalmol Clin 1980;20(3):63–77.

70. Hillman JS, Marsters JB, Broad A. Pilocarpine delivery by hydrophilic lens in the management of acute glaucoma. Trans Ophthalmol Soc UK 1975;95(1):79–84.

71. Wilson M, Leigh E. Therapeutic use of soft contact lenses. Proc R Soc Med 1975;68(1):55–56.

72. Marmion VJ, Jain MR. Role of soft contact lenses and delivery of drugs. Trans Ophthalmol Soc UK 1976;96(2):319–321.

73. Kaufman HE, Uotila MH, Gasset AR, et al. The medical uses of soft contact lenses. Trans Am Acad Ophthalmol Otolaryngol 1971;75:361–373.

74. Krejci L, Brettschneider I, Praus R. Hydrophilic gel contact lenses as a new drug delivery system in ophthalmology and as a therapeutic bandage lenses. Acta Univ Carol (Med) (Praha) 1975;21(5/6):387–396.

75. Shaw EL, Gasset AR. Management of an unusual case of keratitis mucosa with hydrophilic contact lenses and N-acetylcysteine. Ann Ophthalmol 1974;6(10):1054–1056.

76. Lemp MA. Bandage lenses and the use of topical solutions containing preservatives. Ann Ophthalmol 1978;10(10):1319–1321.

77. Busin M, Spitznas M. Sustained gentamicin release by presoaked medicated bandage contact lenses. Ophthalmology 1988;95:796–798.

78. Gwon A, Borrmann LR, Duzman E, et al. Ophthalmic rods. New ocular drug delivery devices. Ophthalmology 1986;93:82–85.

79. Katz IM, Blackman WM. A soluble sustained-release ophthalmic delivery unit. Am J Ophthalmol 1977;83:728–734.

80. Zimmerman TJ, Leader B, Kaufman HE. Advances in ocular pharmacology. Ann Rev Pharmacol Toxicol 1980;20:415–428.

81. LaMotte J, Grossman E, Hersch J. The efficacy of cellulosic ophthalmic inserts for treatment of dry eye. J Am Optom Assoc 1985;56(4):298–302.

82. Lacrisert Product Information, Merck and Co. Inc., West Point, Pennsylvania, 1981.

83. Novak S, Stewart RH. The Ocusert system in the management of glaucoma. Tex Med 1975;71(12):63–65.

84. Shell JW, Baker RW. Diffusional systems for controlled release of drugs to the eye. Ann Ophthalmol 1974;6(10): 1037–1045.

85. Pollack IP, Quigley HA, Harbin TS. The Ocusert pilocarpine system: Advantages and disadvantages. South Med J 1976;69(10):1296–1298.

86. Quigley HA, Pollack IP, Harbin TS. Pilocarpine Ocuserts. Long-term clinical trials and selected pharmacodynamics. Arch Ophthalmol 1975;93(9):771–775.

87. Ros R, Greve E, Dake C, et al. Ocusert (proceedings). Ophthalmologica 1977;175(1):38–39.

88. Hitchings RA, Smith RJH. Experience with pilocarpine Ocuserts. Trans Ophthalmol Soc UK 1977;97(1):202–205.

89. Drance SM, Mitchell DWA, Schulzer M. The effects of Ocusert pilocarpine on anterior chamber depth, visual acuity, and intraocular pressure in man. Can J Ophthalmol 1977;12(1):24–28.

90. Francois J, Goes F, Zagorski Z. Comparative ultrasonographic study of the effect of pilocarpine 2% and Ocusert P 20 on the eye components. Am J Ophthalmol 1978; 86(2):233–238.

91. Lee VHL, Urrea PT, Smith RE, et al. Ocular drug bioavailability from topically applied liposomes. Surv Ophthalmol 1985;29(5):335–348.

92. Barza M, Baum J, Tremblay C, et al. Ocular toxicity of intravitreally injected liposomal amphotericin B in Rhesus monkeys. Am J Ophthalmol 1985;100(8):259–263.

93. Assil KK, Weinreb RN. Multivesicular liposomes. Sustained release of the antimetabolite cytarabine in the eye. Arch Ophthalmol 1987;105(3):400–403.

94. Khoobehi B, Peyman GA, McTurnan WG, et al. Externally triggered release of dye and drugs from liposomes into the eye. An in vitro and in vivo study. Ophthalmology 1988;95:950–955.

95. Flora MR. How to make a simple ocular irrigation unit. Rev Optom 1980;117(1):59.

96. Baum JL, Barza M, Weinstein L. Preferred routes of antibiotic administration in treatment of bacterial ulcers of the cornea. Int Ophthalmol Clin 1973;13(4):31–37.

97. Doane MG. Methods of ophthalmic fluid delivery. Int Ophthalmol Clin 1980;20(3):93–101.

98. Dohlman CH, Doane MG, Reshmi CS. Mobile infusion pumps for continuous delivery of fluid and therapeutic agents to the eye. Ann Ophthalmol 1971;3(2):126–128.

99. Ralph RA, Doane MG, Dohlman CH. Clinial experience with a mobile ocular perfusion pump. Arch Ophthalmol 1975;93(10):1039–1043.

100. Wine NA, Gornall AG, Basu PK. The ocular uptake of subconjunctivally injected C^{14} hydrocortisone. I. Time and major route of penetration in a normal eye. Am J Ophthalmol 1964;58(3):362–366.

101. McCartney HJ, Drysdale IO, Gornall AG, et al. An autoradiographic study of the penetration of subconjunctivally injected hydrocortisone into the normal and inflamed rabbit eye. Invest Ophthalmol 1965;4(3):297–302.

102. Garber MI. Methylprednisolone in the treatment of exophthalmos. Lancet 1966;1(7444):958–960.

103. Giles CL. Bulbar perforation during periocular injection of corticosteroids. Am J Ophthalmol 1974;77(4):438–441.

104. Nozik RA. Periocular injection of steroids. Trans Am Acad Ophthalmol Otolaryngol 1972;76(3):695–705.

105. Ellis PP. Retrobulbar injections. Surv Ophthalmol 1974;18(6):425–430.

106. Feibel RM. Current concepts in retrobulbar anesthesia. Surv Ophthalmol 1985;30(2):102–110.

107. Lichter PR. Avoiding complications from local anesthesia. Ophthalmology 1988;95:565–566.

108. May DR, May WN. Decreasing discomfort caused by retrobulbar alcohol injection. Am J Ophthalmol 1981;95(2):262–263.

109. Freeman WR, Green RL, Smith RE. Echographic localization of corticosteroids after periocular injection. Am J Ophthalmol 1987;104(3):281–288.

110. Raab EL. Limitation of motility after periocular corticosteroid injection. Am J Ophthalmol 1974;78(6):996–998.

111. Wittpenn JR, Rapoza P, Sternberg P, et al. Respiratory arrest following retrobulbar anesthesia. Ophthalmology 1986;93(6):867–870.

112. Brookshire GL, Gleitsmann KY, Schenk EC. Life-threatening complication of retrobulbar block. A hypothesis. Ophthalmology 1986;93(11);1476–1478.

113. Javitt JC, Addiego R, Friedberg HL, et al. Brain stem anesthesia after retrobulbar block. Ophthalmology 1987;94(6):718–724.

114. Morgan CM, Schatz H, Vine AK, et al. Ocular complications associated with retrobulbar injections. Ophthalmology 1988;95:660–665.

115. Sullivan KL, Brown GC, Forman AR, et al. Retrobulbar anesthesia and retinal vascular obstruction. Ophthalmology 1983;90(4):373–377.

116. Pautler SE, Grizzard WS, Thompson LN, et al. Blindness from retrobulbar injection into the optic nerve. Ophthal Surg 1986;17(6):334–337.

117. Antoszyk AN, Buckley EG. Contralateral decreased visual acuity and extraocular muscle palsies following retrobulbar anesthesia. Ophthalmology 1986;93:462–465.

118. Martin SR, Baker SS, Muenzler WS. Retrobulbar anesthesia and orbicularis akinesia. Ophthal Surg 1986;17(4):232–233.

119. Ahn JC, Stanley JA. Subarachnoid injection as a complication of retrobulbar anesthesia. Am J Ophthalmol 1987;103(2):225–230.

120. Friedberg HL, Kline OR. Contralateral amaurosis after retrobulbar injection. Am J Ophthalmol 1986;101(6):688–690.

121. Mills DW, Siebert LF, Climehaga DB. Depot triamcinolone-induced glaucoma. Can J Ophthalmol 1986;21(4):150–152.

122. Shorr N, Seiff S. Central retinal artery occlusion associated with periocular corticosteroid injection for juvenile hemangioma. Ophthal Surg 1986;17(4):229–231.

123. Thomas EL, Laborde RP. Retinal and choroidal vascular occlusion following intralesional corticosteroid injection of a chalazion. Ophthalmology 1986;93(3):405–407.

124. Perry HT, Cohn BT, Nauheim JS. Accidental intraocular

injection with Dermojet syringe (letter). Arch Dermatol 1977;113(8):1131.

125. Schlaegel TF, Wilson FM. Accidental intraocular injection of depot corticosteroids. Trans Am Acad Ophthalmol Otolaryngol 1974;78(6):847–855.

126. Schneider ME, Milstein DE, Oyakawa RT, et al. Ocular perforation from a retrobulbar injection. Am J Ophthalmol 1988;106:35–40.

127. Andrew NC, Zdenek GJ. Intraocular injection of Depomedrone. Br J Ophthalmol 1986;70:298–300.

128. Havener WH. Ocular pharmacology. St. Louis: C. V. Mosby Co, 1978;4:118–119.

129. Goldman HB. Peri- and intra-ocular drug therapy in the treatment of endophthalmitis. Ophthalmol Semin 1977; 2(2);167–201.

130. Chan C, Okun E. The question of ocular tolerance to intravitreal liquid silicone. A long-term analysis. Ophthalmology 1986;93(5):651–660.

131. Grisolano J, Peyman GA. Special short needles to inject and aspirate high-viscosity silicone oil. Arch Ophthalmol 1986;104(4):608.

132. Peyman GA, Sanders D. Advances in uveal surgery, vitreous surgery, and the treatment of endophthalmitis. New York: Appleton-Century-Crofts, 1975.

133. Hughes L, Maurice DM. A fresh look at iontophoresis. Arch Ophthalmol 1984;102(12):1825-1829.

134. Luxenberg MN, Guthrie TR. Chemotherapy of basal cell and squamous cell carcinoma of the eyelids and periorbital tissues. Ophthalmology 1986;93:504–510.

135. Rootman DS, Hobden JA, Jantzen JA, et al. Iontophoresis of tobramycin for the treatment of experimental *pseudomones* keratitis in the rabbit. Arch Ophthalmol 1988;106:262–265.

136. Cullen AP. Fluorescein angiography of the ocular fundus. Am J Optom Physiol Opt 1979;56(9):592–596.

137. Balogh VJ. The use of oral fluorescein angiography in idiopathic central serous choroidopathy. J Am Optom Assoc 1986;57(12):909–913.

138. Kent S. Continuous drug delivery methods reflect progress in therapy for chronic diseases. Geriatrics 1977;32(9):146–149.

139. Blumendranz MS, Culbertson WW, Clarkson JG, et al. Treatment of the acute retinal necrosis syndrome with intravenous acyclovir. Ophthalmology 1986;93(3):296–300.

140. Woo WL, Johnson AP, Insler MS, et al. Gentamicin, tobramycin, amikacin and netilmicin levels in tears following intravenous administration. Arch Ophthalmol 1985; 103(2):216–218.

141. Potter JW, Christensen BJ, Goldstein TJ. Optometric prescription writing. J Am Optom Assoc 1985;56(5):383–385.

142. Covington TR, Porter ME, See K. Improper prescription instructions: A factor in patient compliance. Patient Couns Health Educ 1979;1(3):97–100.

143. Fritz MH. Eye drops. J Med Assoc State Ala 1977;47(4):32–33.

144. Hargett NA, Ritch R, Mardirossian J, et al. Inadvertent substitution of acetohexamide for acetazolamide. Am J Ophthalmol 1977;84(4):580–583.

145. Ashburn FS, Goldberg I, Kass MA. Compliance with ocular therapy. Surv Ophthalmol 1980;24(4):237–248.

146. Davidson SI. Noncompliance in ophthalmology. International symposium on drug-induced ocular side effects and ocular toxicology. Portland, Oregon, March 13–15, 1980.

147. Kass MA, Meltzer DW, Gordon M. A miniature compliance monitor for eyedrop medication. Arch Ophthalmol 1984;102(10):1550–1554.

148. Ullman S, Pflugfelder SP. A supplemental labeling system for topical medication. Am J Ophthalmol 1987;103(3):335.

149. Mindel JS, Goldstein JI. Non-approved use of Food and Drug Administration approved drugs (editorial). Am J Ophthalmol 1979;88(3 Pt 2):626–628.

150. Johnson DW. Adverse drug reaction reporting—critical but easy. International symposium on drug-induced ocular side effects and ocular toxicology. Portland, Oregon, March 13–15, 1980.

151. Roth SH. Drug use, the package insert, and the practice of medicine. Arch Intern Med 1982;142(5):871–872.

152. Bartlett JD, Wood JW. Optometry and the Drug Enforcement Administration. J Am Optom Assoc 1981;52(6):495–498.

153. 21 CFR, Section 1304.02. Washington, DC: U.S. Government Printing Office, 1987.

PART II

Pharmacology of Ocular Drugs

Drug therapy must be based upon correlation of effects of drugs with physiologic, biochemical and microbiologic kinetic aspects of diseases. Only through basic knowledge can we understand toxicology and limitations of drugs and how these can be overcome.

—I.H. Leopold

CHAPTER 3

Drugs Affecting the Autonomic Nervous System

Siret D. Jaanus
Vincent T. Pagano
Jimmy D. Bartlett

Drugs that affect the autonomic nervous system (ANS) are an extremely important group of agents used for ophthalmic diagnostic and therapeutic purposes. Included in this group are drugs that influence pupil size, accommodation, and intraocular pressure.

A brief overview of the ANS will be presented to aid in understanding the pharmacologic actions of drugs discussed in this chapter.[1] Individual drugs will then be considered in terms of their pharmacology, clinical uses, side effects, and contraindications.

Functional Concepts

Anatomic Characteristics

The ANS is widely distributed throughout the body and acts primarily on an involuntary or unconscious basis. Anatomically, it consists essentially of two major divisions: (1) the adrenergic or sympathetic outflow, and (2) the cholinergic or parasympathetic outflow (Fig. 3.1). Each division consists of 2 sets of neurons. The cell bodies of both divisions originate in the central nervous system (CNS), and their axonal fibers extend into the periphery, where they terminate on collections of cells in clusters called ganglia. These fibers are referred to as the preganglionic portion of each division. Axons arising from the ganglia then extend to the target organs, commonly referred to as the effector sites. These neuronal fibers are termed postganglionic fibers.

Cells that give rise to neurons of the adrenergic division are located primarily in the intermediolateral columns of the spinal cord, from C8 to L2 or L3. Preganglionic adrenergic neurons generally extend their axons only a short distance to reach ganglia close to the CNS. The postganglionic neurons, however, travel varying distances to reach their respective target organs.

The preganglionic neurons of the cholinergic division arise from 3 different outflow regions of the CNS—the midbrain, the medulla oblongata, and the sacral portion of the spinal cord. The midbrain outflow consists of fibers arising from the Edinger-Westphal nucleus of the third cranial nerve, and these fibers synapse within the ciliary ganglion in the orbit. The medullary outflow comprises the cholinergic components of the seventh, ninth, and tenth cranial nerves. The sacral portion consists of fibers that arise in the second, third, and fourth segments of the spinal cord.

The anatomic location of the preganglionic neurons of each division has given rise to such additional terminology as *thoracolumbar* for the adrenergic and *craniosacral* for the cholinergic outflow.

Certain functional differences exist between the two

Parasympathetic nerves   Sympathetic nerves

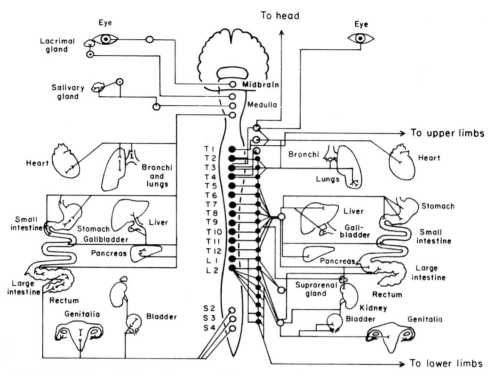

FIGURE 3.1 **Autonomic innervation to various organs. (Redrawn from a Sandoz Pharmaceuticals publication.)**

divisions of the ANS. Adrenergic neurons are widely distributed throughout the body. Although the adrenergic system generally has short preganglionic fibers, a preganglionic adrenergic fiber may travel considerable distances and pass through several ganglia before synapsing with a postganglionic neuron. In addition, one preganglionic neuron may synapse with many postganglionic neurons. This anatomic relationship results in diffuse adrenergic discharges on stimulation of the division.

In contrast, the cholinergic system has long preganglionic and short postganglionic fibers. The terminal ganglia are very near or on the organ of innervation. Responses on stimulation are therefore more discrete and limited. In addition, the relationship between preganglionic and postganglionic neurons appears to be 1:1 in many instances.

The adrenergic and cholinergic divisions are also often viewed as physiologic antagonists. If one system stimulates an effector site, the other usually inhibits that particular function. However, their actions on certain organs can also be independent.

The term *catecholamine* is used synonymously for adrenergic agents that contain the catechol nucleus[1].

This term, therefore, includes norepinephrine and epinephrine as well as dopamine and the synthetic adrenergic-stimulating agent isoproterenol (Fig. 3.2).

Transmitter Substances

There is now ample evidence that chemical substances are liberated from nerve terminals during stimulation. These agents act to pass the nerve impulse across the neuron-neuron or neuron-effector site junctions (Fig. 3.3).

The chemical transmitter at preganglionic sites in both divisions of the ANS is acetylcholine (ACh). In the cholinergic division, ACh is also the transmitter at all postganglionic nerve terminals to effector sites. In addition, ACh is also the transmitter at sympathetic nerve endings supplying the sweat glands in humans as well as those supplying the adrenal medulla.

Norepinephrine, also referred to as noradrenaline, is the transmitter at the nerve terminal of postganglionic adrenergic fibers. In addition, norepinephrine and its methylated derivative, epinephrine, are present in the adrenal medulla, which is considered part of the adrenergic division. Epinephrine does not participate

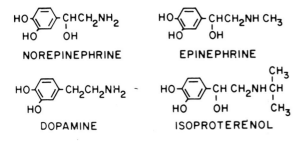

FIGURE 3.2   **Molecular structures of the catecholamines.**

as a transmitter substance in the ANS, but on adrenergic stimulation it is released from the adrenal medulla directly into the circulating blood. Epinephrine constitutes 80% of the active substance released by the medulla, with norepinephrine contributing the other 20%.

Because of their respective transmitters released from postganglionic neurons, the parasympathetic division is more commonly referred to as the cholinergic system, while the sympathetic division is referred to as the adrenergic system.

Divisions of the Autonomic Nervous System

The Cholinergic System

ACh is synthesized inside the cholinergic nerve fiber by combination of choline with the acetyl group from acetylcoenzyme A. The reaction is catalyzed by the enzyme choline acetyltransferase. Following its synthesis, ACh is stored in the nerve terminal in membrane-bound structures called *vesicles.* On arrival of the nerve impulse, ACh is released from nerve endings in quantal amounts. Following its release into the synaptic space, ACh diffuses to the postsynaptic site, where it performs its designated physiologic function (Fig. 3.4).

The action of neurotransmitters at postsynaptic sites involves interaction with structures or sites called *receptors,* which are thought to be unique and specific for a particular neurotransmitter. In both the cholinergic and adrenergic divisions, the receptors on autonomic ganglia are referred to as *nicotinic.* Receptor sites responding to postganglionic cholinergic stimulation are classified as *muscarinic* or *nicotinic.*

Following its release, the action of ACh is terminated by at least two enzymes called *cholinesterases,* which rapidly hydrolyze the ACh to choline and acetic acid (see Fig. 3.4). Acetylcholinesterase (AChE), also known as true or specific cholinesterase (ChE), is responsible for the hydrolysis of ACh in the process of cholinergic transmission. Butyrocholinesterase (BuChE), also known as serum esterase or pseudo-ChE, is present mainly in plasma, liver, and other organs but only to a limited extent in neuronal elements of the CNS and peripheral nervous system. Its physiologic function is less well defined than that of AChE. The activity of the cholinesterase enzymes can be inhibited by drugs, as discussed in this chapter.

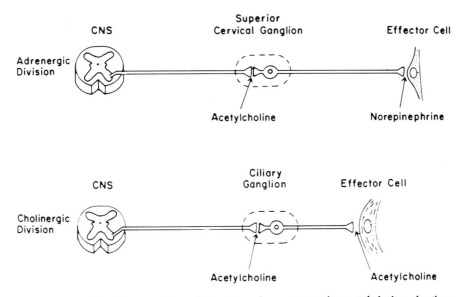

FIGURE 3.3   **Schematic presentation of the autonomic neurotransmitters at their sites of action.**

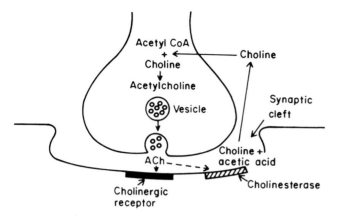

FIGURE 3.4 **Cholinergic nerve terminal depicting synthesis, storage, release, and termination of action of acetylcholine (ACh).**

The Adrenergic System

Norepinephrine is synthesized by a series of steps from the amino acid, tyrosine (Fig. 3.5). Epinephrine is formed in the adrenal medulla by methylation of norepinephrine.

As with ACh, the catecholamines also appear to be stored in membrane-bound structures called vesicles in both adrenergic nerve terminals and the adrenal medulla. In the adrenal medulla, methylation of norepinephrine takes place in the cytoplasm. Norepinephrine leaves the vesicle, is methylated, and then reenters a different set of intracellular vesicles, where it is stored until released.

Following their release, the catecholamines, like ACh, are thought to interact with specific receptors at their respective target sites. On the basis of experimental evidence, the terms α and β receptors were proposed by Ahlquist. The two receptor types have been further subdivided into α_1, α_2 and β_1, β_2 on the basis of the relative effects observed with various excitatory and inhibitory adrenergic agents.

The α_1-adrenergic receptors generally mediate excitory responses, except in the intestine, where response to α_1 stimulation is inhibitory. The α_2 receptors are thought to be located, at least in part, on presynaptic nerve terminals, since activation of these receptors with certain exogenous agents has been shown to inhibit norepinephrine release.

The β receptors mediate inhibitory responses, except in the heart, where the response to adrenergic stimulation is increased heart rate and contractility. The cardioreceptor sites have been designated as β_1, with all other sites in the adrenergic division thus far designated as β_2 (Table 3.1).

The actions of norepinephrine and of epinephrine are terminated by several mechanisms (see Fig. 3.5). These include reuptake into the nerve terminals, diffusion away from the junctional sites, and metabolic transformation by the enzymes monoamine oxidase (MAO) and catechol-O-methyltransferase (COMT).

In contrast to the cholinergic division, metabolic transformation plays a minor role in the inactivation process of endogenous as well as administered catecholamines. The major mechanism for terminating the actions of the adrenergic transmitters is reuptake into the nerve terminals. Drugs that inhibit reuptake, such as cocaine, potentiate the effects of endogenous norepinephrine as well as exogenously administered adrenergic stimulating agents.

Norepinephrine that is not found in vesicles within the nerve terminals is metabolized by MAO present in adrenergic nerve terminals. Endogenous circulating as well as administered catecholamines are inactivated primarily by COMT present in the liver.

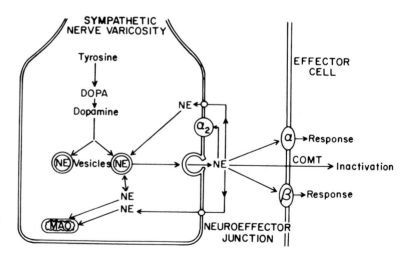

FIGURE 3.5 **Adrenergic nerve terminal (varicosity) depicting synthesis, storage, release, and termination of action of norepinephrine.**

TABLE 3.1
Effector Site Responses to Adrenergic Stimulation

Site	Receptor Types	Response
Eye		
Iris dilator	α_1	Contraction (mydriasis)
Ciliary muscle	β	Relaxation
Aqueous humor	β_2	Increased outflow; increased formation
	α	Slight decrease in formation
Conjunctival blood vessels	α	Vasoconstriction
	β_2	Vasodilation
Mueller's muscle	α	Contraction (lid retraction)
Heart		
S-A node	β_1	Increased heart rate
Atria	β_1	Increased contractility and conduction velocity
A-V node	β_1	Increased automaticity and conduction velocity
Ventricles	β_1	Increased contractility, conduction velocity, and automaticity
Smooth Muscle		
Arteries		
Coronary	α, β_2	Dilation; constriction
Abdominal viscera	α, β_2	Constriction
Pulmonary	α, β_2	Dilation
Intestine	α_1, β_1, β_2	Decreased motility
Stomach	α_2, β_2	Decreased motility
Bronchial	β_2	Relaxation
Bladder	β	Relaxation (usually)
Sphincters	α	Contraction
Spleen	α, β_2	Contraction (usually)
Ureter	α	Increased motility and tone (usually)
Glands		
Bronchial	α_1, β_2	Secretion increased or decreased
Pancreas		
Acini	α	Decreased secretion
Islets	α_2, β_2	Decreased secretion
	β_2	Increased secretion
Salivary	α_1	Potassium and water secretion
	β	Amylase secretion
Sweat	α	Localized secretion (e.g., palms)
Liver	α, β_2	Glycogenolysis, gluconeogenesis

Adapted from Mayer SE. Neurohumoral transmission and the autonomic nervous sytem. In: Gilman AG, Goodman LS, Rall TW, et al., eds. The pharmacological basis of therapeutics. New York: Macmillan Co, 1985; Chap. 4.

Adrenergic Agents

Adrenergic Innervation to the Eye

The sympathetic innervation to the eye originates from the posterior and lateral nuclei of the hypothalamus. Fibers descend through the lateral aspects of the brainstem to the intermediolateral columns in the cervical cord. Myelinated preganglionic neurons emerge from the thoracic section (C_8–T_2) of the spinal cord through the anterior roots and ascend over the apex of the lung through the stellate ganglion and the cervical sympathetic chain to synapse in the superior cervical ganglion (Fig. 3.6). This part of the pathway comprises the preganglionic portion.[2]

Unmyelinated fibers emerge from the superior cervical ganglion and course toward the cavernous sinus by following the carotid plexus adjacent to the carotid artery. There the fibers cross over the sixth cranial nerve and join the ophthalmic division of the fifth nerve. The fibers then bypass the ciliary ganglion and accompany the long ciliary nerves to the iris dilator

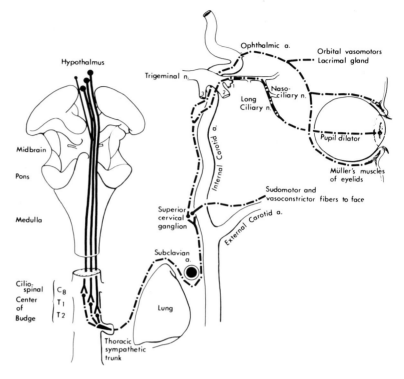

FIGURE 3.6 **The oculosympathetic pathway. Note its origin in the hypothalamus and its course through the brainstem and cervical spinal cord (central or first-order neuron), the upper thorax and lower neck (preganglionic or second-order neuron), and upper neck, middle cranial fossa, cavernous sinus, and orbit as it finally reaches Mueller's muscle of the lid and the iris dilator muscle (postganglionic or third-order neuron). (From Glaser JS. The pupils and accommodation. In: Duane TD, Jaeger EA, eds. Clinical ophthalmology. Hagerstown, MD: Harper & Row, Publishers, 1987, with permission of the author and publisher.)**

muscle and Mueller's muscle of the eyelid, thus completing the postganglionic portion of the oculosympathetic pathway (see Fig. 3.6).[2]

Sympathetic neuronal control of human ciliary muscle activity is less well established. Sympathetic nerves reach the ciliary muscle through the uveal blood vessels in close association with arteries and terminal arterioles. The distribution of the adrenergic fibers in the ciliary muscle appears to vary in different species. In primates, sympathetic nerve terminals can generally be found in the anterior portion of the ciliary muscle. The posterior half of the trabecular meshwork and the inner wall of Schlemm's canal also contain adrenergic nerve terminals.[3] Adrenergic nerve stimulation induces relaxation of the ciliary muscle.

Certain orbital muscles also receive adrenergic innervation. The tonic contraction of the tarsal smooth muscle of the upper lid (Mueller's muscle) is under adrenergic control. The convergence mechanism through the lateral rectus muscle is also at least partially controlled by adrenergic innervation.[4]

In addition to the control exerted on intraocular and orbital muscles, receptors for adrenergic agents are also present in the cornea, lens, and retina.

Cornea

Although the cornea possesses adrenergic nerve endings in both epithelium and stroma during the embry-

onic and neonatal phase of development, epithelial terminals appear to be lacking in adult tissue.[5] However, studies using radiolabeled compounds with specific affinity for β-receptor groups indicate that adult corneal epithelium is densely packed with β receptors.[6]

The cornea responds to adrenergic agonists in several ways. Mitosis is inhibited, and collagenase production decreases.[7,8] Chloride transport is enhanced.[9] Adenylate cyclase and cyclic adenosine monophosphate (AMP)-dependent protein kinase activities are stimulated.[10] The presence of the latter enzymes suggests that cyclic AMP may help regulate corneal physiology.

Lens

The lens, surrounded by the aqueous humor containing varying amounts of norepinephrine and epinephrine, responds to adrenergic stimulation with enhanced production of cyclic AMP.[11] During growth of the lens, catecholamines appear to interact synergistically with chalones, proteins that specifically inhibit mitosis of the lens epithelium.[12]

Retina

In the retina, cells containing catecholamines have been found in the inner plexiform layer corresponding to amacrine cells, the anterior border of the inner nuclear layer, and the ganglion cell layer. The only catecholamine demonstrated thus far in the retina has been dopamine. Since adrenergic activity has been demonstrated only in layers conveying evoked visual excitations, it has been proposed that adrenergic mechanisms are involved in cross-retinal transfer of visual excitations.[13]

Adrenergic Receptors

The localization of adrenergic receptor types in ocular tissue has been investigated in several species including humans, using primarily isolated ocular muscle strips.[14-21] The distribution of receptor types exhibits certain species specificity (Table 3.2).

The human dilator muscle has predominantly α-adrenergic receptors and very few β. Pharmacologically it responds to α-receptor stimulators as well as mixed α- and β-receptor agonists. Mydriasis, however, is inhibited by pharmacologic agents classified as α-receptor antagonists.

The sphincter muscle appears to contain both α and β receptors in equal amounts. In vitro, sphincter muscle strips respond poorly to catecholamines, but both contraction and relaxation can be elicited. It has been proposed that adrenergic stimulation produces an α activation of the dilator, resulting in dilator contraction, and β activation of the sphincter, relaxing the latter muscle fibers.

In the epithelium and core of the ciliary processes, β-receptor types appear to dominate, although evidence exists for the presence of few α receptors. Stimulation with adrenergic agonists results in ciliary muscle relaxation and reduction of intraocular pressure.

Evidence has accumulated indicating that each of the two types of adrenergic receptors may exist in more than one subtype.[19] Although both α_1, α_2 and β_1, β_2 receptor sites have been postulated in the eye, the receptor subtypes are not well defined in ocular tissue. Studies on human ciliary processes from donor eyes indicate a predominance of β_2-adrenergic receptors.[18] However, there is evidence that both β_1 and β_2 types of receptors are involved in control of intraocular pressure. Repeated β_1-receptor stimulation appears to increase intraocular pressure, whereas β_2-receptor stimulation rapidly reduces intraocular pressure.[22] Little data are presently available that clarify the distribution of α-receptor subtypes in ocular tissue. However, there is now some evidence that α_2 receptors may possibly exist in the vertebrate retina. Using bovine eyes, Bittiger and associates[23] and Osborne[24] showed that radioactive α_2-receptor agonists show greater affinity for [^{3}H] ligand-binding sites than compounds known to have α_1-receptor affinity. If these findings are true, then it is possible that norepinephrine may play a transmitter role in the retina.

Adrenergic Agonists

Adrenergic agonists are useful for a variety of clinical conditions related to the eye, including mydriasis for fundus evaluation, reduction of intraocular pressure in glaucoma, vasoconstriction of the conjunctiva, and relief of minor allergic reactions.

Norepinephrine

Stimulation of the adrenergic nerve fibers to the iris or intraocular injection of norepinephrine causes pupillary dilation and reduces intraocular pressure.[25-27] The observed effects with topical norepinephrine are dose dependent and reach a maximum at certain dose levels[27] (Fig. 3.7).

The effect of topical norepinephrine on intraocular pressure was first described by Hofmann in 1954.[25] Following topical application to the eye, norepinephrine's ability to lower intraocular pressure varies. Pretreatment with an anesthetic enhances its pressure-lowering effects.

The greater efficacy of norepinephrine following ocular injection or prior use of a topical anesthetic indicates difficulty in corneal penetration following topical application to the eye. Norepinephrine is a

TABLE 3.2
Distribution of Adrenergic Receptors in Humans and Other Species

	Iris Dilator	Iris Sphincter	Ciliary Muscle
Cat	Mainly α, some β	Mainly β, some α	Mainly β, some α
Rabbit	Mainly α, few β	Mainly β, few α	Mainly α, few β
Monkey	Mainly α, very few β	Mainly α, perhaps β	Exclusively β, no α
Man	Mainly α, very few β	α and β in equal amounts	Mainly β, very few or no α

Adapted from van Alphen GWHM. The adrenergic receptors of the intraocular muscles of the human eye. Invest Ophthalmol 1976; 15:502–505.

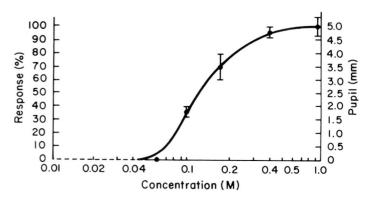

FIGURE 3.7   **Dose-response curve of normal adult subjects to topical application of 50 µl l-norepinephrine bitartrate. Responses represent mean maximal dilation of all eyes. (From Langham ME, Kitazawa RL, Hart RW. Adrenergic responses in the human eye. J Pharmacol Exp Ther 1971;179:47–55.)**

highly water-soluble compound. Pretreatment with an anesthetic induces changes in corneal epithelial permeability (see Chapter 15), which allows for greater penetration of the polar norepinephrine molecules across the lipoidal corneal barrier.

Experimental observations indicate a possible physiologic role for norepinephrine on aqueous outflow mechanisms, possibly by acting on the trabecular meshwork. It has little if any effect on aqueous humor production.[25]

Epinephrine

PHARMACOLOGY

Epinephrine, the major hormone secreted by the adrenal medulla, reaches the eye through the systemic circulation. Chemically it resembles norepinephrine, with the addition of a methyl group on the side chain nitrogen (see Fig. 3.2). Epinephrine is a direct-acting sympathomimetic amine with combined α and β receptor-stimulating capability. In solution it exhibits both lipid and water solubility, and corneal penetration occurs following topical application to the eye.

Use of a 1% to 2% topical solution results in a typical triple response of conjunctival decongestion, slight mydriasis, and reduction of intraocular pressure.[28] The effect on ocular pressure outlasts the vasoconstrictor and mydriatic effects. The pupillary dilation is maximum approximately 2 hours following instillation and gradually diminishes over 12 hours. At lower concentrations, epinephrine is a relatively poor mydriatic in the normal eye. The drug's mixed α and β actions, its rapid destruction, and the corneal epithelial barrier at least in part explain the clinical effects. The mydriatic effect of epinephrine is enhanced when the cornea is traumatized or when the drug is applied by prolonged contact by employing a cotton pledget.[28,29]

Since the major clinical usefulness of epinephrine lies in its ability to lower intraocular pressure in both primary and secondary open-angle glaucoma, it is this aspect that has been most actively investigated. Despite abundant research, however, controversy still remains on the mechanism whereby epinephrine produces its pressure-lowering effects. Species differences among experimental animals and inability to use certain techniques in humans restrict experimental comparison.[30]

Both a decrease in aqueous formation and an increase in outflow facility have been demonstrated in normal subjects and in patients with glaucoma.[31–34] Harris and associates[34] studied the effects of varying concentrations of epinephrine on aqueous humor inflow and facility of outflow. Concentrations as low as 0.06% reduced intraocular pressure, but no change in outflow facility was measured until 1.0% epinephrine was used. These investigators suggested that the observed effects were due to epinephrine's action on two different types of receptors. With lower concentrations of epinephrine, aqueous formation is reduced. Concentrations of 1.0% or greater increase the facility of outflow.

The effects of epinephrine on intraocular pressure have been studied with fluorophotometric techniques combined with tonography and tonometry.[35–37] These studies show that epinephrine produces an increase in the rate of aqueous production 2 to 5 hours after treatment. Moreover, tonographic results indicate a significant mean increase in outflow facility following epinephrine therapy.[37] In addition to enhancement of pressure-dependent facility of outflow as measured by tonography, a pressure-independent uveoscleral pathway for aqueous outflow has been demonstrated by Bill[38] in monkeys and confirmed in humans.[36] Thus, it appears possible that the effect of epinephrine in lowering intraocular pressure may be primarily to enhance outflow facility.

Experimental observations have further suggested that the effects of epinephrine on intraocular pressure may be mediated by a cyclic AMP–dependent mechanism.[39] A significant elevation of aqueous cyclic AMP levels has been observed in rabbits 30 minutes following epinephrine treatment, with peak levels at 1 to 4 hours. A rise in cyclic AMP levels thus appears to precede the maximal ocular hypotensive effect of epinephrine treatment.[40] These observations, as well as the effect of epinephrine on aqueous formation, need further elucidation.

Becker and associates[41] found that treatment with topical epinephrine hydrochloride decreased intraocular pressure more than 5mm Hg in 88% of patients with primary open-angle glaucoma but in only 31% of patients with secondary glaucoma. In the same study, premature ventricular contractions were demonstrated in 69% of patients with primary open-angle glaucoma but in only 19% of patients with secondary glaucoma. This suggests that epinephrine has a greater ocular as well as cardiac responsiveness in patients with primary open-angle glaucoma compared with those with secondary glaucoma.

CLINICAL USES

Glaucoma Therapy.   Epinephrine is one of the oldest ocular hypotensive agents currently used in clinical practice. It is commercially available as an ophthalmic solution and is prepared as the hydrochloride, borate, or bitartrate salt (Table 3.3). Although these preparations are therapeutically equal when administered in equivalent doses of epinephrine base, a 2% solution of epinephrine bitartrate is equivalent to approximately 1% solution of the hydrochloride or borate.

Epinephrine is available in concentrations from 0.25% to 2%, and the usual dosage schedule involves instillation twice daily. When using epinephrine compounds, the concentration of the base (see Table 3.3) should be taken into consideration. Most practitioners prefer the hydrochloride or borate salt rather than the bitartrate because of the higher concentrations of the free epinephrine base in the first two. Some epinephrine compounds are commercially packaged in combination with pilocarpine. All such preparations contain epinephrine bitartrate and thus contain only about half the free epinephrine base of the labeled concentration. However, these preparations may simplify use of the combined medications when such combination is warranted.

Epinephrine may be considered for some patients an initial drug of choice in the therapy of both primary open-angle glaucoma and, when treated, ocular hypertension.[42] The absence of associated miosis and accommodative spasm makes epinephrine a useful drug in the treatment of glaucoma in prepresbyopic patients who have critical vision requirements, since epinephrine allows adequate control of intraocular pressure in many patients without impairing visual acuity or inducing refractive changes.[43] It is particularly useful in patients who would sustain significant adverse visual effects from pilocarpine solutions or other miotics.

Epinephrine solutions are unstable when exposed to light or to the open atmosphere. Since oxidation products of epinephrine can cause adverse ocular effects, the patient should be advised regarding proper storage and the need for replacing solutions that become discolored or that contain a precipitate.

Vasoconstriction.   The vasoconstrictor effect of epinephrine contributes to its clinical usefulness as a topical decongestant to prevent hemorrhages from small ocular vessels during surgery, and it reduces systemic absorption of local anesthetics.[29]

Epinephrine in a 1:1000 concentration will constrict the superficial conjunctival vessels. With repeated ap-

TABLE 3.3
Ophthalmic Adrenergic Agonists

Generic Name	Trade Name	Manufacturer	Labeled Concentration (%)
Epinephrine bitartrate	Epitrate	Ayerst	2
Epinephrine borate	Epinal	Alcon	0.5, 1
	Eppy/N	Barnes-Hind	0.5, 1, 2
Epinephrine hydrochloride	Epifrin	Allergan	0.25, 0.5, 1, 2
	Glaucon	Alcon	1, 2
Dipivefrin	Propine	Allergan	0.1
Phenylephrine hydrochloride	Neo-Synephrine	Winthrop	2.5, 10
	AK-Dilate	Akorn	2.5, 10
	Mydfrin	Alcon	2.5
	Ocu-Phrin	Ocumed	2.5, 10
Hydroxyamphetamine hydrobromide	Paredrine	SKF	1

plication it will also constrict the episcleral vessels. Thus, if applied to a red eye, prompt blanching suggests a diagnosis of conjunctivitis rather than of episcleritis. Although this epinephrine test may be useful in the differential diagnosis of the red eye, it is considered less reliable than other ocular signs.[29]

The vasoconstrictor effect of epinephrine usually lasts for less than 1 hour. Moreover, the blanching is usually followed by reactive hyperemia. Its short action and the frequent rebound effect preclude the use of topical epinephrine as a decongestant for nonspecific chronic irritations or allergy.[29].

Epinephrine is useful clinically in a 1:50,000 concentration as a vasoconstrictor in anesthetic solutions for local injection. The vasoconstriction caused by epinephrine delays absorption of the anesthetic. The anesthetic effect is thus prolonged at the site of injection, and possible systemic toxicity is reduced.[29]

The vasoconstrictor effect of epinephrine can reduce or arrest hemorrhages from small arterioles and capillaries during ocular surgical procedures. Solutions of 1:1000 applied to the wound surface can prevent oozing from vessels and thus facilitate manipulation of the eye.

SIDE EFFECTS

Following topical application to the eye, epinephrine is taken up and stored in various ocular tissues. The primary sites are the iris, the ciliary body, and, to a lesser extent, the choroid. Far less is found in the retina and optic nerve. If the treated eye is aphakic, significantly more epinephrine appears in the choroid, and uptake into the retina and optic nerve is also enhanced.[44] Following topical administration significant amounts are also found in nonocular tissues, particularly those of the heart and the spleen.[44]

The topical use of epinephrine in glaucoma therapy can be accompanied by a number of adverse effects (Table 3.4). However, unlike pilocarpine and other

TABLE 3.4
Side Effects of Topical Epinephrine

Ocular Effects	Systemic Effects
Irritation and lacrimation	Severe headache
Conjunctival hyperemia	Palpitations
Allergic blepharoconjunctivitis	Tachycardia
Adrenochrome pigmentation	Premature ventricular
Adrenochrome staining of soft contact lenses	contractions
Pupillary dilation	Hypertensive crisis
Elevation of intraocular pressure	Anxiety
Cystoid macular edema	

miotics, epinephrine does not impair visual acuity, since it has no effect on refractive error and produces little or no mydriasis. Local ocular reactions, such as burning, conjunctival hyperemia, allergy, and irritation, occur in about 25% of patients.[45] Although changing to another salt form of epinephrine will often reduce these effects, the associated side effects cause discontinuation of the drug in about 20% to 50% of cases.[46]

Epinephrine may cause true allergic reactions, characterized by lid dermatitis, irritation, lacrimation, and diffuse conjunctival hyperemia. The prevalence of drug-induced allergic blepharoconjunctivitis is as high as 15%. Experimental observations have indicated that the allergic reactions are most likely due to the epinephrine or its oxidation products rather than to the vehicle. Patients who demonstrate hypersensitivity reactions have not been sensitive when the vehicle was applied alone.[47] If the continued use of epinephrine is required, these reactions may be treated with the concomitant administration of corticosteroids such as fluorometholone (FML). The lid dermatitis can often be prevented by applying a bland ophthalmic ointment to the eyelids before instilling epinephrine.

Injection of epinephrine solution into the anterior chamber can cause increased corneal thickness and loss of corneal endothelial cells.[48] The toxicity appears to be due to the low pH of the vehicle formulation, caused by the presence of the antioxidant, sodium bisulfite.

Prolonged use of topical epinephrine can result in localized pigment (adrenochrome) deposits. These occur most frequently in the palpebral conjunctiva (Fig. 3.8), but lid margin pigmentation and, on rare occasions, corneal pigmentation can occur. The black to brown pigment is most likely oxidation products of epinephrine.[29] Although adrenochrome deposits within the palpebral conjunctiva are not uncommon, they rarely, if ever, produce irritation and thus are of no consequence. Diffuse adrenochrome staining of hydrophilic contact lenses (Fig. 3.9) may also occur.[49,50] Such staining of soft contact lenses with epinephrine can occur within 2 to 6 weeks of initial topical epinephrine therapy.

Epinephrine will produce pupillary dilation in some patients. This effect is especially pronounced when epinephrine is used in combination with timolol or other β blockers.[42] Thus, epinephrine may precipitate acute angle-closure glaucoma in patients with narrow angles.

Occasionally, the use of epinephrine may be associated with a significant and prolonged rise of intraocular pressure in patients with primary open-angle glaucoma.[51] This occurs in the absence of any gonioscopically visible changes in the angle, but tonographic findings show the pressure rise to be associated with impaired outflow facility. Although the mechanism of

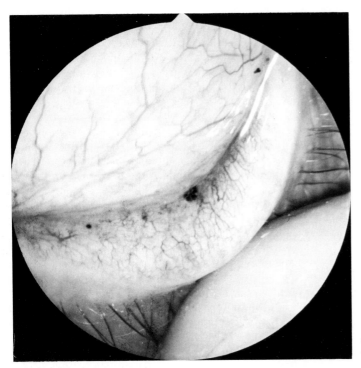

FIGURE 3.8   **Adrenochrome deposits in palpebral conjunctiva of patient using topical epinephrine for treatment of primary open-angle glaucoma. (Courtesy Lyman C. Norden, O.D.)**

this phenomenon is unknown, it calls for caution in the use of epinephrine in uniocular patients or in those with advanced glaucoma. This hazard appears to be less significant if miotics are simultaneously employed.[51]

Epinephrine maculopathy can occur in aphakic patients.[52] This macular toxicity occurs in 20% to 30% of aphakic eyes undergoing treatment with epinephrine. Experimental evidence indicates that topical epinephrine reaches the retina in significantly higher concentrations in aphakic than in phakic eyes.[44] Epinephrine applied topically to one eye reaches the retina, choroid, and optic nerve of both eyes. If the treated eye is aphakic, the amount reaching the posterior pole of the eye is much greater on that side.[53] The maculopathy is characterized by edema, usually cystic, with or without small flame-shaped hemorrhages.[54] The mechanism by which epinephrine produces cystoid macular edema is unknown, but both the clinical and fluorescein angiographic features of the maculopathy often cannot be distinguished from those observed in other conditions of cystoid macular edema, including the Irvine-Gass syndrome.[54] Clinically, visual acuity may be a poor indicator of epinephrine maculopathy, since only small acuity changes are present in some patients despite prominent leakage of dye on fluorescein angiography.[55] Thus, if treatment with epinephrine is required in some aphakic patients, periodic angiography may be advisable.

Topical administration of epinephrine can also result in systemic side effects[56] including severe headache, palpitations, tachycardia, premature ventricular contractions, and hypertensive crisis (up to 230 mm Hg systolic).[41,46] The β-receptor stimulatory effects on the cardiovascular system are responsible for most of these reactions. These systemic effects may at times be reduced or eliminated by instructing the patient to depress the puncta manually (see Fig. 2.5) following instillation of the drug.

The amount of epinephrine absorbed systemically from topical glaucoma therapy can be comparable to amounts used parenterally for various conditions. One drop of 2% epinephrine contains about 1.0 mg of drug. The usual systemic dose is about 0.1 to 0.5 mg.[57] Because of the possible cardiac effects following sys-

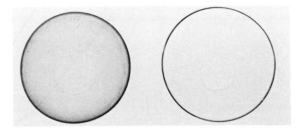

FIGURE 3.9   **Diffuse adrenochrome staining of hydrophilic contact lens (left) compared with normal lens (right).**

temic absorption of topically applied epinephrine, this agent must be used with caution in patients with cardiovascular disease, as discussed in the following section.

CONTRAINDICATIONS (TABLE 3.5)

Because epinephrine may cause pupillary dilation, it should be avoided in patients with narrow angles. Epinephrine should generally be avoided in aphakic or pseudophakic patients because of the risk of cystoid macular edema. In addition, adrenochrome staining of soft contact lenses precludes the simultaneous use of topical epinephrine in patients who wear such lenses.

Epinephrine should be used with caution in patients with cardiovascular disease, including ischemic heart disease; in patients with marked systemic hypertension; and in patients with hyperthyroidism, who may be sensitized to catecholamines.[58] This is particularly true if such patients are being treated for primary open-angle glaucoma rather than for one of the secondary glaucomas. Epinephrine must be used cautiously in patients treated with MAO inhibitors or tricyclic antidepressants because these drugs increase the sensitivity of adrenergic receptors, possibly resulting in exaggerated pressor responses such as hypertension or cardiac arrhythmia.[46] The use of epinephrine should be interrupted before general anesthesia with anesthetics (e.g., cyclopropane or halothane) that sensitize the myocardium to catecholamines.[59]

Dipivalyl Epinephrine

PHARMACOLOGY

Dipivalyl epinephrine (DPE, dipivefrin) is an analog of epinephrine formed by the addition of two pivalic acid groups to the hydroxyls of epinephrine (Fig. 3.10). This alteration of the epinephrine molecule creates a prodrug that is more lipophilic and better absorbed into the eye than is epinephrine. Subsequent to its corneal penetration, DPE is converted to epinephrine within the eye.[63]

Comparison of the partition coefficients of DPE and of epinephrine indicates that DPE is 100 to 600 times as lipophilic as epinephrine. Further studies using radioactively labeled compounds have revealed that 10 times as much DPE as epinephrine is absorbed by the rabbit eye.[64] In human eyes, however, the corneal penetration is 17 times greater than that of epinephrine.[65]

DPE is rapidly hydrolyzed to epinephrine by tissue esterases in the cornea and anterior chamber. Human plasma also catalyzes DPE to epinephrine, with a half-life of 18 minutes.[65]

Following topical application to the eye, DPE lowers intraocular pressure when used in concentrations of 0.025, 0.1, and 0.5%.[66] The ocular hypotensive response reaches a maximum in 4 to 8 hours and is sustained for about 12 hours. DPE 0.1% produces an effect approximately equipotent to 2% epinephrine or 2% pilocarpine. Ocular pressure reductions of 24% have been reported with 0.1% DPE as compared to 27% with 2% epinephrine.[67] With long-term use the ocular hypotensive effect appears to be maintained.[65]

The mechanism of action of DPE in lowering intraocular pressure appears to be similar to that of epinephrine. Both a reduction of aqueous formation and enhanced aqueous outflow have been demonstrated.[66] Moreover, as observed with epinephrine, DPE also causes a biphasic response on intraocular pressure.[67] An initial hypertensive phase, lasting less than 2 hours, is followed by a prolonged hypotensive phase. However, the initial hypertensive response is eliminated if an α-adrenergic blocker is also used. An initial reduction in outflow facility following administration of DPE has been linked with the ocular hypertensive effect. In the rabbit eye, the hypotensive effect of DPE is accompanied by a corresponding increase in cyclic AMP levels of the aqueous humor.[66]

Several investigators[68–71] have studied the effect of combined therapy with DPE and other drugs. In contrast to the effect observed with the combination of epinephrine and timolol (see below), combined ther-

TABLE 3.5
Contraindications to Epinephrine

- Narrow angles
- Aphakia/pseudophakia
- Hydrophilic contact lens wear
- Cardiovascular disease
- Hyperthyroidism
- Concomitant therapy with MAO inhibitors or tricyclic antidepressants
- General anesthesia with anesthetics that sensitize the myocardium to catecholamines

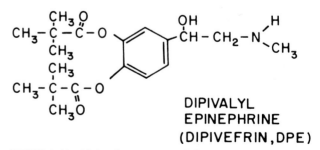

FIGURE 3.10 **Molecular structure of dipivalyl epinephrine.**

apy with DPE and timolol produces a consistent and additive ocular hypotensive response. Moreover, Mindel and associates[71] have shown that the combined use of DPE and echothiophate reduces intraocular pressure further than does the combined use of epinephrine and echothiophate.

DPE also produces a dose-dependent mydriasis.[66] Dilation of the pupil has been observed with 0.1% and 0.5% concentrations but not with lower DPE concentrations. In one study[72] the mydriatic effect of 0.1% DPE averaged 0.65 mm as compared to 0.55 mm with 2% epinephrine. Although these increases in pupil size were statistically significant, there was no significant difference in pupillary dilation between the two drugs. However, there is little, if any, correlation between the mydriatic and ocular hypotensive effects of DPE. The 0.025% concentration reduces intraocular pressure without apparent effects on pupil size.[66] Although DPE is a more potent mydriatic at the 0.25% concentration than at 0.1%, these concentrations appear to be equipotent in reducing intraocular pressure.[63]

CLINICAL USES

DPE is the first prodrug to become commercially available for use in ophthalmic practice. Its use is limited to the treatment of glaucoma.

Presently DPE is available as a 0.1% ophthalmic solution (see Table 3.3). When employed in its usual dosage schedule of twice daily, it appears to be an effective and safe alternative to epinephrine. It is especially useful for patients who are intolerant of epinephrine preparations, and for those patients predisposed to adverse systemic side effects from epinephrine. DPE has become the adrenergic agonist of choice because it can be used concomitantly with topical β-blocker therapy without loss of additivity. Many patients unable to tolerate epinephrine preparations are able to satisfactorily tolerate DPE, but the converse is not true.[42]

In contrast to epinephrine preparations, DPE may be used in patients wearing soft contact lenses without significant risk of adrenochrome staining.[49] The addition of 2 pivalyl groups to form the dipivalyl epinephrine molecule may render the drug less subject to oxidation and therefore may prevent the formation of breakdown products that stain the contact lens. Thus, this epinephrine analog is useful in the treatment of glaucoma patients who must also wear soft contact lenses.

SIDE EFFECTS

Because of the reduced concentration of DPE, there is a significant reduction of dose-related side effects,

both extraocular and systemic, compared with epinephrine preparations. Thus, certain ocular side effects with topical epinephrine are minimized with DPE, especially early in therapy.[65,66,72,73] Patients usually experience minimal ocular discomfort. Tearing, conjunctival hyperemia, corneal edema, and blurred vision are rare. There are also fewer allergic reactions. As a consequence, the vast majority of patients who are unable to tolerate epinephrine may be placed on DPE without significant ocular side effects.[74,75] Adrenochrome deposits in the conjunctiva occur less frequently than with epinephrine. The lower incidence of adverse reactions, particularly extraocular side effects, could be due to the reduced availability of active drug when applied topically. This can also explain the lack of hydrophilic lens discoloration in patients using DPE for glaucoma.[76] No staining of lenses occurred in 5 patients monitored up to 84 weeks.

Systemic effects are also significantly reduced.[65,66,72,73] Cardiac arrhythmias and elevated systemic blood pressure are less likely to occur with DPE, since these reactions are related to the total amount of epinephrine administered. With DPE, the concentration of epinephrine in the systemic circulation at any given time is much less.

With long-term use of DPE the incidence of ocular toxicity may increase. In 1 study,[76] 3 of 27 patients developed follicular conjunctivitis after 18 to 22 months of therapy.

Liesegang[77] observed large bulbar conjunctival follicles in 12 patients after 3 to 31 months of therapy. Associated symptoms were generally mild and included gradual onset of heaviness of the eyes, mild itching, or irritation. Most patients experienced mild to moderate conjunctival injection. When DPE was discontinued, the follicles resolved within 1 to 3 months. This reaction is believed to be toxic rather than allergic because conjunctival smears showed the presence of a few neutrophils, as commonly seen in drug reactions.[78] Eosinophils were not present in the conjunctival smears of these patients.[78]

In a 3-year follow-up of 14 patients receiving topical 0.1% DPE, 4 developed severe blepharoconjunctivitis, which resolved on withdrawal of the drug. Two of the 4 patients had a previous history of epinephrine intolerance. Three patients had asymptomatic conjunctival hyperemia after 30 months of DPE exposure. None of the 14 patients had conjunctival pigment deposits or cardiovascular effects.[79]

Although the extraocular effects are generally less with DPE than with epinephrine, intraocular complications would still be expected because the active drug in the eye is epinephrine. In aphakic patients, maculopathy remains a distinct possibility.[80]

CONTRAINDICATIONS

Contraindications to the use of DPE are the same as those for epinephrine. However, since the risk of adverse systemic side effects with DPE is considerably less than with epinephrine, the systemic contraindications are considered relative rather than absolute.

Phenylephrine

PHARMACOLOGY

Phenylephrine is a synthetic sympathomimetic amine structurally similar to epinephrine. It differs chemically from the natural amine only in lacking 1 hydroxyl group in position 4 on the benzene ring. It acts directly on α receptors and has little or no effect on β receptors. A minor part of its pharmacologic effects may be attributed to release of norepinephrine from adrenergic nerve terminals.

Ophthalmic preparations of phenylephrine range in concentration from 0.12% to 10% (Tables 3.3, 3.6).[28] In solution phenylephrine is clear and is colorless to slightly yellow. Like all adrenergic agonists, it is subject to oxidation on exposure to air, light, or heat. Phenylephrine solutions may darken with time and should not be used if the solution turns brown or if a precipitate forms. To prolong its shelf life, an antioxidant, sodium bisulfite, is frequently added to the vehicle. Since commercially available phenylephrine preparations vary in stability, the manufacturer's instructions should be followed concerning expiration date and proper storage. Loss of activity may occur without visible color change.

Following topical application, phenylephrine contracts the iris dilator muscle and smooth muscle of the conjunctival arterioles, causing pupillary dilation and blanching of the conjunctiva, respectively.[81] Mueller's muscle of the upper lid is stimulated, which may widen the palpebral fissure. Intraocular pressure may decrease in normal eyes and in eyes with open-angle glaucoma.[82] The ocular hypotensive effect of phenylephrine is usually less pronounced and more variable than that of epinephrine.

CLINICAL USES

For mydriasis, concentrations of 2.5% or 10% are available. Maximum dilation occurs in 45 to 60 minutes depending on the concentration instilled (Fig. 3.11). Recovery from mydriasis occurs in about 6 hours.[83–85,436] The virtual absence of an effect on the ciliary muscle produces mydriasis with little or no effect on accommodation. However, the 10% concentration can occasionally produce a brief cycloplegic effect. In 1 group of young adults, 10% phenylephrine produced an av-

TABLE 3.6
Ophthalmic Decongestant Preparations

Generic Name	Trade Name	Manufacturer	Concentration (%)
Phenylephrine hydrochloride	Relief	Allergan	0.12
	Prefrin Liquifilm	Allergan	0.12
	Prefrin—A[a]	Allergan	0.12
	AK-Nefrin	Akorn	0.12
	Isopto Frin	Alcon	0.12
	Zincfrin	Alcon	0.12
Naphazoline hydrochloride	Albalon Liquifilm	Allergan	0.1
	Albalon–A[a] Liquifilm	Allergan	0.05
	Clear Eyes	Ross	0.012
	Degest 2	Barnes Hind	0.012
	Naphcon–A[a]	Alcon	0.025
	Naphcon	Alcon	0.012
	Allerest Eye Drops	Pharmacraft	0.012
	Vasoclear	Iolab	0.02
	Vasocon–A[a]	Iolab	0.05
	AK-Con Ophthalmic	Akorn	0.1
Oxymetazoline	OcuClear	Schering	0.025
Tetrahydrozoline hydrochloride	Murine Plus	Ross	0.05
	Optigene 3	Pfeiffer	0.05
	Soothe Eye Drops	Alcon	0.05
	Visine	Leeming	0.05

[a]Decongestant/antihistamine combination.

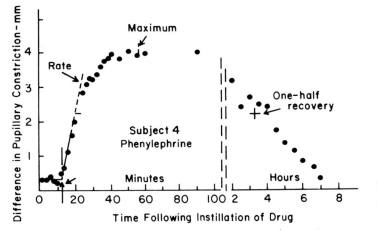

FIGURE 3.11   **Time course of mydriasis with 10% phenylephrine hydrochloride. (From Gambill HD, Ogle KN, Kearns TP. Mydriatic effect of four drugs determined by pupillograph. Arch Ophthalmol 1967;77:740–746. Copyright 1967, American Medical Association.)**

erage reduction of 0.66 D in amplitude of accommodation at 30 minutes following drug instillation. The effect disappeared within 2 hours.[86] Other studies have shown that, routinely, the instillation of 1 drop of 10% phenylephrine does not result in significant refractive changes.[87]

Dose-response curves for phenylephrine indicate an increasing mydriatic effect with concentrations up to 5%.[85] Between 5% and 10% the curve begins to plateau, and little additional effect is observed by increasing the concentration of the solution to 10% (Fig. 3.12). Since the study was performed with fresh solutions of phenylephrine hydrochloride, differences in vehicle content and instability during storage of the commercial solutions may in part explain the observed effects.

Dilation of the pupil with 2.5% and 10% commercial preparations has been studied in patients selected at random and not controlled for age or color of irides.[88,89] The results indicate that the higher concentration does not necessarily produce a significantly greater mydriasis. The data also appear to indicate that the 10% concentration may be a more effective mydriatic in blue irides than is the 2.5% concentration, although

no statistically significant difference was observed.[89] Other investigators have reported that dark irides dilate more poorly than do light irides with adrenergic mydriatics.[83,85]

In certain instances phenylephrine may also dilate the pupil at concentrations much lower than 2.5%. The mydriatic effect of 0.125% phenylephrine has been compared in unabraded and posttonography eyes.[90] Three of 10 patients with unabraded corneas showed significant pupillary dilation of 1.0 to 1.5 mm following instillation of 2 drops of 0.125% phenylephrine as compared with the saline control eye. In posttonography patients the test eye was dilated in all instances as compared with the control eye.

Procedures that alter corneal epithelial integrity can affect the response to certain ophthalmic drugs such as phenylephrine.[91] Use of a topical anesthetic or corneal trauma from procedures such as tonometry, gonioscopy, or tonography can compromise corneal epithelial integrity and facilitate the pharmacologic effects.

The mydriatic response of phenylephrine can be affected by the prior instillation of a topical anesthetic.[92–94] Using commercially available solutions of phenylephrine, Jauregui and Polse[92] found that prior

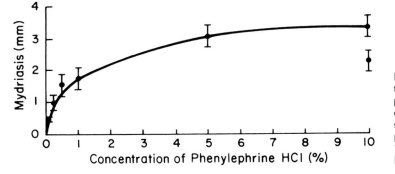

FIGURE 3.12   **Dose-response curve of mydriasis obtained with varying concentrations of freshly prepared phenylephrine hydrochloride. The lower point at 10% concentration represents response to a 10% commercial solution of phenylephrine hydrochloride. (Published with permission from the American Journal of Ophthalmology 70:729–733, 1970. Copyright by the Ophthalmic Publishing Company.)**

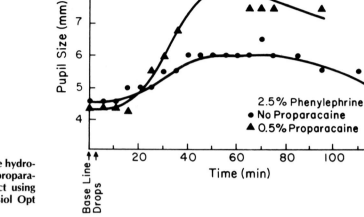

FIGURE 3.13   **Mydriatic effect of 2.5% phenylephrine hydrochloride with and without prior instillation of 0.5% proparacaine. (From Jauregui MJ, Polse KA. Mydriatic effect using phenylephrine and proparacaine. Am J Optom Physiol Opt 1974;51:545–549.)**

instillation of proparacaine 0.5% enhanced the mydriatic effect of 2.5% phenylephrine by 2 mm (Fig. 3.13). The time to produce 1 mm of dilation was reduced by 10 to 15 minutes, and the duration of mydriasis was increased by 1 hour. Kubo and associates[87]

studied the effects of 0.125, 0.5, 1.0, and 2.0% phenylephrine with and without prior instillation of proparacaine 0.5% in four subjects (Fig. 3.14). The anesthetic enhanced the mydriatic effects of 0.5, 1.0, and 2.0% concentrations. The 0.125% concentration produced

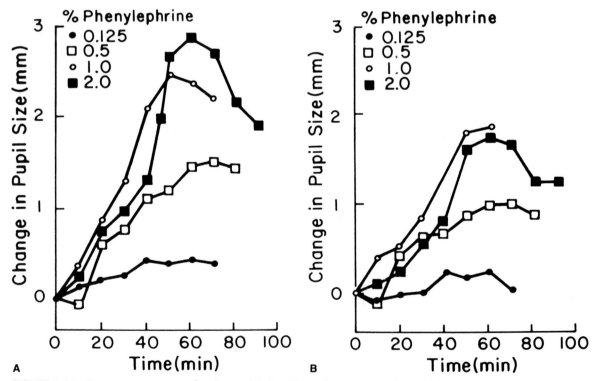

FIGURE 3.14   **Dose-response curves showing mydriasis with varying concentrations of phenylephrine with and without prior instillation of 0.5% proparacaine.** *(A)* **Phenylephrine and proparacaine.** *(B)* **Phenylephrine alone. (From Kubo DJ, Wing TW, Polse KA, et al. Mydriatic effects using low concentrations of phenylephrine hydrochloride. J Am Optom Assoc 1975; 46:817–822.)**

little or no dilation with or without the prior instillation of the anesthetic. The limited sample size in both these studies, however, makes it difficult to draw conclusions applicable to a general patient population.

Lyle and Bobier[94] compared the effects of anesthetics on mydriasis with phenylephrine 1.0% and 10%. Applying a topical anesthetic to one eye before applying phenylephrine 1.0% to both eyes caused more dilation in the eye that received the anesthetic (Table 3.7). The magnitude of the response appeared to vary with iris color. Light irides were generally more responsive in both the presence and the absence of the anesthetic. Prior application of 1 drop of proparacaine 0.5%, benoxinate 0.4%, or tetracaine 0.5% followed by 1 drop of phenylephrine 10% resulted in somewhat less mydriasis (1.22 mm average increase with proparacaine) than was produced by the 1% concentration and anesthetic (2.5 mm more dilation in eyes receiving both drugs). No significant differences were observed between the effects of the three different anesthetics.

In addition to its usual mydriatic effect, phenylephrine has several other clinical uses. The drug can be a valuable aid in breaking posterior synechiae. Application of the 10% solution to the cornea preceded by a topical anesthetic is usually recommended to help break the adhesion.[81]

The drug is also used concomitantly with echothiophate to prevent the formation of miotic cysts during treatment of open-angle glaucoma or accommodative esotropia. Addition of the 2.5% concentration to the echothiophate regimen is recommended.[95] The mechanism whereby phenylephrine prevents cyst formation is not known; however, inhibition of the intense miosis may account, at least in part, for the beneficial effect.

Ptosis resulting from sympathetic denervation such as in Horner's or Raeder's syndromes may respond to topical phenylephrine.[29] Dramatic effects on the uneven palpebral apertures are sometimes observed (see Fig. 19.13).

Individuals with poor vision due to lens opacities may sometimes benefit from topical phenylephrine. In patients who are unable or unwilling to undergo surgery, phenylephrine-induced pupillary dilation may improve vision.

Phenylephrine can also be used as a diagnostic test for Horner's syndrome.[96] Phenylephrine in the 1% concentration can markedly dilate the pupil with postganglionic sympathetic denervation. It will cause minimal or no dilation in the normal eye. If the lesion is central or preganglionic, the affected pupil will respond in a manner similar to the normal eye, since denervation hypersensitivity is minimal or absent.

Phenylephrine 0.12% or 0.125% is contained in several over-the-counter (OTC) collyria designed to cause vasoconstriction and thereby "whiten the eye"[90] (see Table 3.6). It is also added to other ophthalmic medications such as ocular antihistamines, corticosteroids, and antibiotics. These agents, particularly the OTC preparations, may be administered indiscriminately by the user. Since phenylephrine can induce

TABLE 3.7
Comparative Mydriatic Effect of 1% Phenylephrine with and without Previous Instillation of a Topical Anesthetic

Subject	Iris Color	Anesthetic and 1% Phenylephrine			Phenylephrine	Difference in Pupil Sizes at Time of Maximum Dilation (mm)
		Time to Reach 1 mm Dilation (min)	Maximum Dilation (mm)	Time of Maximum Dilation (min)	Change in Pupil Size (mm)	
1	Blue	15.5	4.0	40	+0.2	3.8
2	Blue	20.0	4.4	45	+0.6	3.8
3	Blue	23.0	3.1	50	+0.1	3.0
4	Gray	32.0	2.7	60	−0.1	2.8
5	Gray	25.0	3.0	60	0.0	3.0
6	Gray	32.0	2.2	60	0.0	2.2
7	Brown	29.0	3.9	60	+0.5	3.4
8	Brown	—	0.8	55	0.0	0.8
9	Brown	34.4	1.7	55	+0.7	1.0
10	Brown	46.0	1.1	75	+0.3	0.8
Mean		28.5	2.7	56	+0.2	2.5
						(More dilation in the eye that received 2 drugs)

Adapted from Lyle W, Bobier W. Effects of topical anesthetics on phenylephrine-induced mydriasis. Am J Optom Physiol Opt 1977; 54:276–281.

pupillary dilation at low concentrations, the use of these agents requires caution in eyes predisposed to angle-closure glaucoma, especially if the cornea is damaged or diseased.

SIDE EFFECTS

Topical instillation of phenylephrine can be accompanied by clinically significant local and systemic reactions.

Ocular Effects (Table 3.8). Local adverse reactions can include transient pain, lacrimation, and keratitis.[97] The effect of commercial 2.5% and 10% phenylephrine has been studied in intact and denuded rabbit and cat corneas.[98,99] Topical application to denuded corneas caused a significant increase in corneal thickness and ultrastructural changes in the endothelium. With the epithelium intact, corneal thickness did not change, but the epithelium and anterior stroma demonstrated some structural changes. Although the corneal edema and cytotoxic effect of phenylephrine was more pronounced in corneas with the epithelium removed, these results are obscured by the fact that in both instances a topical anesthetic was used before application of phenylephrine.

Phenylephrine eyedrops have been reported to cause an allergic dermatoconjunctivitis.[100,437] The reaction consists of a "scalded" appearance around the eye.

Phenylephrine can cause the release of pigmented granules from the iris.[101,102] The pigment appears in the aqueous (aqueous floaters) 30 to 40 minutes following instillation of the 5% or 10% concentration. These floaters usually disappear within 12 to 24 hours. The release of pigment is related to age and color of the iris, occurring more frequently in older individuals with brown irides. Further investigation has revealed that the pigmented granules have the same characteristics as melanin derived from the pigmented epithelium of the iris. It has been postulated that phenylephrine may cause rupture of the pigmented epithelial cells of the iris, and since this phenomenon has been observed primarily in older patients, it may be due to aging changes in the neuroepithelium.[101]

In patients over age 50 years, phenylephrine also appears to cause a rebound miosis the day after drug administration.[102] Moreover, instillation of phenylephrine at that time causes a diminished mydriatic response.[85] Similarly, with chronic use of the drug reduced dilation frequently occurs, making long-term, frequent use clinically unsatisfactory. Chronic use of phenylephrine at low concentrations for ocular vasoconstriction can result in rebound congestion of the conjunctiva.[97]

Phenylephrine has also been shown to decrease conjunctival PO_2.[103] Following instillation of 1 drop of 2.5% phenylephrine into the inferior conjunctival fornix, a 46% reduction in PO_2 was observed for about 80 minutes. This observation suggests that conjunctival hypoxia could occur with long-term use of this agent in clinical situations such as prevention of miotic-induced iris cysts and sustained pupillary dilation during and following intraocular surgery.

Systemic Effects (see Table 3.8). Systemic hypertension following administration of topical ocular phenylephrine was first observed in animals by Heath in 1936.[104] Since then numerous case reports have described acute hypertensive episodes and associated complications with the 10% ophthalmic preparation.[81,105–111]

McReynolds and associates[105] reported an increase in blood pressure in 6 of 100 patients administered topical 10% phenylephrine. In each of the 6 subjects the increase in pressure was less than 10 mm Hg. Samantary and Thomas[110] studied 60 patients following 3 applications of the 10% solution in each eye at 10-minute intervals. Thirty minutes following the last drop, systolic elevations of 10 to 40 mm Hg and diastolic elevations of 10 to 30 mm Hg occurred in all subjects. In each case pulse rate decreased 10 to 20 beats per minute.

In contrast to these observations, other investigators have reported a lack of systemic vasopressor response with the 10% concentration.[88,112] In 1 study,[88] a group of subjects ranging in age from 21 to 53 years received 2 drops of 10% phenylephrine in one eye every 15 minutes for 90 minutes. No rise in blood pressure occurred 90 minutes after the last drop. Brown and associates[104] conducted a double-blind study comparing the systemic hypertensive effects of topical 10% phenylephrine with 1% tropicamide, a drug with no known vasopressor effect, in patients of both sexes with an age range of 13 to 89 years. A total of 6 drops of each drug was administered over a 4-minute period to each

TABLE 3.8
Side Effects of Topical Phenylephrine

Ocular Effects	Systemic Effects
Transient pain	Systemic hypertension
Lacrimation	Occipital headache
Keratitis	Subarachnoid hemorrhage
Pigmented aqueous floaters	Ventricular arrhythmia
Rebound miosis	Tachycardia
Rebound conjunctival congestion	Reflex bradycardia
	Blanching of skin

eye of all subjects. No statistically significant differences between the 2 groups with respect to drug effects on blood pressure or pulse rate were observed. The percentage of individual blood pressure elevations greater than 15 mm Hg at 5, 15, and 30 minutes following drug instillation in both the phenylephrine and tropicamide groups is shown in Figure 3.15.

Data collected by the National Registry of Drug-Induced Ocular Side Effects suggest that in the general population, there may be a group of patients with certain risk factors for side effects from topical ocular 10% phenylephrine.[103] Of 15 patients with myocardial infarcts, 11 died following topical application of 10% phenylephrine. The average age of these patients was 71 years, and 9 had a history of cardiovascular disease. The epidemiologic significance of these data is discussed in Chapter 31.

The effects of 2.5% phenylephrine on systemic blood pressure and pulse have also been investigated.[113–115] Jennings and Sullivan[115] observed no significant change in systolic and diastolic blood pressures in a group of 252 patients ranging in age from 3 to 92 years. Kumar and Packer[114] reported 2 cases of acute systemic hypertension following instillation of 2.5% phenylephrine. Both patients, 69 and 71 years of age, were scheduled for surgery, and each received multiple drops of the phenylephrine. The medical history of one patient included diabetes and cardiac disease.

It is likely that age as well as physical status determines the patient's response to topical ocular phenylephrine. Neonates respond to 10% phenylephrine with significant increases in blood pressure.[108] Patients who are insulin-dependent diabetics may demonstrate increased systolic and diastolic blood pressure in response to topical 10% phenylephrine.[116] Similarly, individuals with idiopathic orthostatic hypotension respond to low concentrations of phenylephrine with marked blood pressure elevations. In 1 group of patients, a significant increase in blood pressure occurred following instillation of 1 drop of 2.5% phenylephrine solution in each eye. Heart rate was unaffected.[117]

Other systemic reactions reported with topical ocular phenylephrine include severe occipital headache, subarachnoid hemorrhage,[105] ventricular arrhythmias,[111] tachycardia,[110] reflex bradycardia,[118] ruptured aneurysm, and blanching of the skin.[98]

Patients taking certain systemic medications are also more sensitive to the pressor effects of phenylephrine. In individuals taking atropine, the pressor effect of phenylephrine is augmented and tachycardia can occur.[118] Tricyclic antidepressants and MAO inhibitors also potentiate the cardiovascular effects of topical phenylephrine.[119] The concomitant use of phenylephrine is contraindicated with these agents, even up to 21 days following cessation of MAO inhibitor therapy.[120] Similarly, patients taking reserpine, guanethidine, or methyldopa are at increased risk for adverse pressor effects from topical phenylephrine[116] because of denervation hypersensitivity accompanying the chemical sympathectomy.

Systemic reactions to 2.5% phenylephrine following topical ocular application to an intact eye have rarely been reported in adults.[111] However, an acute rise in systolic blood pressure has occurred in a 1-year-old child following the instillation of 0.5 ml of 2.5% phenylephrine during nasolacrimal duct probing.[121] A few seconds following application of the drug to the conjunctiva to clear the surgical field, systolic blood pressure increased to 200 mm Hg. The pressure returned to normal within 20 minutes with no adverse sequelae. In this situation a relatively high dose of drug was applied to an eye already hyperemic and irritated due to probing. This most likely enhanced systemic absorption of the drug. Since the patient weighed only 10 kg, the dose relative to body size was also large.

The threshold dosage of phenylephrine in the average adult has been estimated to be 0.4 mg intravenously, 2 mg subcutaneously, and 50 mg orally.[118] The upper limit for safe dosage in normal adults is about 1.5 mg intravenously and 300 mg subcutaneously. Since 1 drop of 10% phenylephrine contains 5 mg of drug, multiple applications can result in overdosage, especially if absorption from the site of administration is enhanced or if the patient is compromised by age, body size, concomitant medications, or trauma.

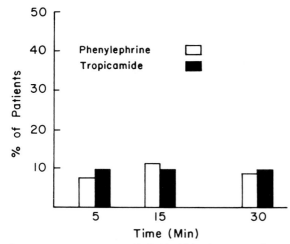

FIGURE 3.15 **Percentage of individual blood pressure elevations greater than 15 mm Hg at 5, 15, and 30 minutes in subjects receiving 10% phenylephrine or 1% tropicamide. (From Brown MM, Brown GC, Spaeth GL. Lack of side effects from topically administered 10% phenylephrine eye drops. Arch Ophthalmol 1980;98:487–489. Copyright 1980, American Medical Association.)**

It is not known to what extent topical ocular phenylephrine is absorbed into the vascular system. However, since the drug causes local vasoconstriction, this can possibly diminish flow to receptor sites for the drug.

CONTRAINDICATIONS

Based on data submitted to the National Registry of Drug-Induced Ocular Side Effects and those acquired by previous investigators, the following guidelines for the clinical use of 10% phenylephrine are suggested.[111,116,117]

- Use phenylephrine 10% with caution in patients with cardiac disease, idiopathic orthostatic hypotension, hypertension, aneurysms, insulin-dependent diabetes, and advanced arteriosclerosis.
- Give only one application of the 10% concentration per hour to each eye.
- The drug is contraindicated in patients taking MAO inhibitors, tricyclic antidepressants, reserpine, guanethidine, or methyldopa.
- Concomitant use of topical phenylephrine is discouraged in atropinized patients, since tachycardia and hypertension can occur.
- Prolonged irrigation, application with a conjunctival pledget, or subconjunctival injection of the 10% solution is not recommended.
- Only the 2.5% solution is recommended for infants and the elderly.

Since the 10% concentration appears to be associated with an increased risk of significant adverse ocular and systemic reactions, the 2.5% solution, with appropriate precautions, is recommended for routine use.[111]

Hydroxyamphetamine

PHARMACOLOGY

Hydroxyamphetamine (β-4-hydroxyphenylisopropylamine) is similar in chemical structure to epinephrine. Its primary pharmacologic action is thought to be due to release of norepinephrine from adrenergic nerve terminals, since guanethidine, an agent known to deplete norepinephrine, abolishes its adrenergic stimulatory effects.[122] In addition, hydroxyamphetamine has been shown to inhibit monoamine oxidase as well as the reuptake of norepinephrine into the nerve terminal.[123,124] It may also directly stimulate α- and possibly β-receptor sites, although this effect has been considered minimal and probably clinically insignificant.[125]

Hydroxyamphetamine has little if any effect on accommodation or the refractive state.[87,126] It also does not raise intraocular pressure in eyes with open anterior chamber angles.[126]

CLINICAL USES

Topical instillation of a 1% solution in eyes with normal adrenergic innervation causes mydriasis and vasoconstriction.[83,84,126] However, hydroxyamphetamine is used only as a mydriatic agent. Maximum dilation occurs within 60 minutes, and the total duration of mydriasis is about 6 hours (Fig. 3.16).

Several investigators have compared the mydriatic effects of phenylephrine and hydroxyamphetamine. Gambill and associates[84] compared 10% phenylephrine with several drugs including 1% hydroxyamphetamine. The time to maximum dilation was similar (70.2 minutes for phenylephrine and 64.8 minutes for hydroxyamphetamine). The amount of mydriasis produced was somewhat greater with 10% phenylephrine, 2.42 mm as compared to 1.93 mm with hydroxyamphetamine. Barbee and Smith[83] also found similar mydriatic effects for 10% phenylephrine and 1% hydroxyamphetamine in normal subjects ranging in age from 16 to 60 years.

Semes and Bartlett[127] compared the mydriatic effect of 2.5% phenylephrine to 1% hydroxyamphetamine in a group of 28 young adult subjects without ocular disease. The two agents produced a nearly equal pupillary dilation (Fig. 3.17). The maximum effect with both drugs occurred at about 45 minutes.

Hydroxyamphetamine is clinically useful for differentiating between preganglionic and postganglionic sympathetic denervation.[96,125] Since the drug stimulates release of endogenous norepinephrine from its stores in adrenergic nerve terminals, it will, depending on the extent of damage, fail to dilate a pupil with postganglionic sympathetic denervation. However, if the lesion causing a Horner's syndrome is central or preganglionic, hydroxyamphetamine should cause normal mydriasis, since the nerve endings of the postganglionic fibers should contain normal amounts of norepinephrine and thus respond normally.[96]

SIDE EFFECTS

The clinical use of hydroxyamphetamine for routine mydriasis has been much less frequent than that of phenylephrine, although hydroxyamphetamine appears to be effective while causing little if any ocular irritation. It has been suggested that this drug may be a safe mydriatic to use in eyes with shallow anterior chambers, since because of its indirect action, it may be more readily counteracted with miotics.[128] In patients with open-angle glaucoma hydroxyamphetamine elevates intraocular pressure minimally if at all. Reductions of intraocular pressure have also been reported.[129]

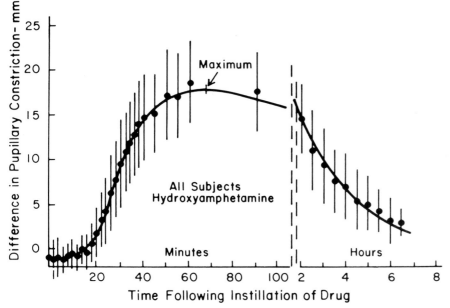

FIGURE 3.16 **Time course of mydriasis following instillation of 1% hydroxyamphetamine. (From Gambill HD, Ogle KN, Kearns P. Mydriatic effect of four drugs determined by pupillograph. Arch Ophthalmol 1967;77:740–746. Copyright 1967, American Medical Association.)**

The actions of hydroxyamphetamine on the cardiovascular system differ in certain respects from those of phenylephrine. The drug can raise blood pressure,[115] but unlike phenylephrine the pressor response is characterized by tachyphylaxis.[130] The drug can also produce sinoauricular tachycardia and ventricular arrhythmia following systemic administration.[131]

Other adverse reactions observed with subcutaneous or oral doses of hydroxyamphetamine include head-

ache, sweating, nausea, and vomiting. In all instances relatively large doses were administered.[126]

Adverse systemic reactions to topical ocular hydroxyamphetamine have not been reported in the literature. However, this might be explained by its lower frequency of use compared with other mydriatic agents.

CONTRAINDICATIONS

Contraindications to the topical use of hydroxyamphetamine for routine mydriasis are similar to those of phenylephrine. However, because of its tachyphylaxis and ineffectiveness in postganglionic denervation, hydroxyamphetamine may be a safer mydriatic for use in patients with insulin-dependent diabetes, idiopathic orthostatic hypotension, or chemical sympathectomy produced by therapy with systemic guanethidine, reserpine, or methyldopa. Thus, hydroxyamphetamine seems to be less strongly contraindicated than phenylephrine in certain high-risk patients.

Cocaine

PHARMACOLOGY

Cocaine is a naturally occurring alkaloid present in the leaves of the shrub *Erythroxylon coca* and other species of trees indigenous to Peru and Bolivia. Chemically it is an ester of benzoic acid with a nitrogen-containing base.

Cocaine exhibits several pharmacologic effects. Following local application it acts as an anesthetic by blocking the initiation and conduction of nerve impul-

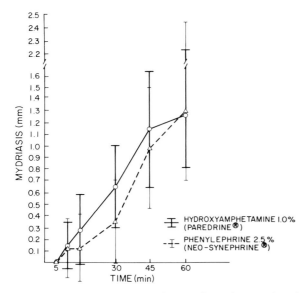

FIGURE 3.17 **Comparison of mydriatic effect of 2.5% phenylephrine and 1% hydroxyamphetamine in young adult subjects. (From Semes LP, Bartlett JD. Mydriatic effectiveness of hydroxyamphetamine. J Am Optom Assoc 1982;53:899–904.)**

ses. It also blocks neuronal reuptake of norepinephrine, thus potentiating adrenergic activity. Moderate doses increase heart rate and cause vasoconstriction. The most striking systemic effect of cocaine is CNS stimulation.[60]

The ocular effects of cocaine include anesthesia, mydriasis, and vasoconstriction. Topical application of a 1% to 4% solution produces anesthesia within 1 minute. Depending on the concentration used, the effect can last up to 20 minutes or longer.[61] The mydriatic effect of cocaine depends on the presence of a functioning adrenergic innervation. Following topical application to the eye, the pupil begins to dilate within 15 to 20 minutes.[62] The maximum effect, which is typically less than 2 mm of dilation, occurs within 40 to 60 minutes, and the pupil may remain dilated for 6 or more hours. The mydriasis is accompanied by a vasoconstriction that causes blanching of the conjunctiva.[61]

Topical application of cocaine can result in serious corneal epithelial damage. Repetitive use results in grossly visible gray corneal pits and irregularities. Cocaine is also readily absorbed through the mucous membranes into systemic circulation.[62]

CLINICAL USES

Because of its deleterious effects on the corneal epithelium, cocaine's clinical uses are limited. Although it is no longer used for such routine ophthalmic procedures as tonometry, the drug can be helpful in the diagnosis of Horner's syndrome (see Chapter 18). Additionally, due to its ability to loosen the corneal epithelium, it can be helpful in the debridement of dendritic ulcers.[61]

SIDE EFFECTS

The most striking effect of systemic absorption of cocaine is CNS stimulation. This effect is responsible for cocaine's addictive property. Moderate doses of cocaine can also increase heart rate and raise body temperature.[61]

Topical use on the eye can result in severe ocular tissue damage (see Chapter 4). Systemic absorption through mucous membranes is rapid and has been compared to that of intravenous administration.[61]

Ephedrine

PHARMACOLOGY

Ephedrine, a naturally occurring alkaloid, was used in China for over 5000 years before it was introduced to Western medicine in 1924. Synthesized in 1927, it resembles both epinephrine and amphetamine in its actions. Ephedrine stimulates both α and β receptors and, in addition, owes part of its action to release of norepinephrine from the adrenergic nerve terminal. It also exhibits tachyphylaxis, and doses given in rapid succession become less effective. Oral administration of therapeutic doses causes peripheral vasoconstriction, elevation of blood pressure, bronchiolar relaxation, stimulation of respiration, and dilation of the pupil.[132]

Instillation of ephedrine into the eye produces both mydriasis and vasoconstriction of extraocular vessels.[133] One drop of a 4% or 5% solution causes maximum dilation in 30 minutes. The mydriatic effect depends on iris color. Individuals with blue irides respond with greater dilation than do those with brown irides.[134] Ephedrine appears to be ineffective as a mydriatic agent in blacks.[83,133,134]

Although ephedrine usually has no effect on intraocular pressure in the normal eye, pressure may occasionally be reduced.[135] Accommodation is usually not affected or is slightly reduced.[133]

Topical administration can also cause a widening of the palpebral aperture. This is due to a stimulatory effect on Mueller's muscle of the upper lid.

CLINICAL USES

The primary ophthalmic use of ephedrine is as a topical vasoconstrictor for ocular decongestion (see Table 3.6). It can blanch the conjunctiva at relatively low concentrations, such as 0.1%.[29]

SIDE EFFECTS

Topical instillation of ephedrine in concentrations sufficient for mydriasis can be quite irritating. A transient hyperemia usually occurs because of the stinging effect of the preparation. As with other adrenergic agonists, acute angle-closure glaucoma can occur if the anterior chamber is abnormally shallow and the angle is narrow.[128] When ephedrine is used repeatedly as a decongestant, loss of its vasoconstrictor effect can occur, and rebound conjunctival hyperemia may force discontinuation of the drug.

The cardiovascular actions of ephedrine are similar to those of epinephrine but last about 10 times as long.[132] The drug can elevate systolic blood pressure, and the pulse pressure usually increases. The pressor effects are due primarily to cardiac stimulation.[130] CNS effects are similar to those of the amphetamines but are much less marked.

CONTRAINDICATIONS

Contraindications to the topical use of ephedrine are similar to those of epinephrine and phenylephrine.

Imidazole Derivatives

PHARMACOLOGY

Three agents, naphazoline, tetrahydrozoline, and oxymetazoline, are commercially available for ocular vasoconstriction. They differ structurally from other adrenergic agonists by replacement of the benzene ring with an unsaturated ring. In general, the imidazole derivatives exhibit greater α- than β-adrenergic receptor activity. Following systemic administration a pressor response is observed.[132] Unlike other adrenergic amines, they depress rather than stimulate the CNS.[130]

CLINICAL USES

Following topical application to the eye, naphazoline, tetrahydrozoline, and oxymetazoline will constrict the conjunctival vessels, and thus these agents are employed clinically as topical ocular decongestants.[136–139] Hurwitz and Thompson[137] studied the effects of 0.1% naphazoline hydrochloride in over 100 patients with normal and congested eyes from various causes. Slit-lamp evaluation revealed constriction of conjunctival vessels, with no effect on the deep vessels. Patients with scleritis and episcleritis also exhibited no noticeable constriction of these vessels. An increase in pupil size of 1 to 3 mm occurred in 68 of 120 eyes. Subjects with lightly pigmented irides appeared to be more sensitive to the mydriatic effects of naphazoline. Pupils that dilated with the 0.1% solution showed only a slight reduction in the pupillary light response. Twenty eyes demonstrated an increase in intraocular pressure of 3 to 7 mm Hg. No relationship was noted between preinstillation pressures and pressure increases following drug application.

No effect on the amplitude of accommodation has been observed with 0.1% naphazoline.[137,138] Miller and Wolf[140] compared with a placebo the effects of 0.05% naphazoline hydrochloride, 0.5% antazoline phosphate, and a combination of both components in a double-blind study of 51 patients with the clinical diagnosis of allergic conjunctivitis. Naphazoline performed better than the placebo on all parameters tested and was more effective than antazoline except for pruritis. Naphazoline alone reduced lacrimation and pain better than antazoline alone or the two agents combined. The combination provided greater relief of pruritis and photophobia, but for relief of conjunctival inflammation naphazoline alone performed equally as well as the combination product.

Tetrahydrozoline has also been evaluated in patients with conjunctival hyperemia due to a variety of ophthalmic conditions.[138,139] A solution of 0.1% was tested in a group of 94 patients with degrees of hyperemia ranging from mild injection to severe congestion and inflammation.[138] Most eyes blanched within 45 seconds following instillation, and the effect lasted for up to 4 hours in the majority of cases. Use of a weaker solution of 0.05% gave similar results.

Menger[139] evaluated the effects of 0.05% tetrahydrozoline in 1156 patients with allergic or chronic conjunctivitis. Of 348 patients with allergic conjunctivitis good results were obtained in 67% and fair results in 30% of the cases. Similar observations were reported in patients with chronic conjunctivitis and nonspecific conjunctivitis with hyperemia. The duration of the beneficial effect varied from 1 to 4 hours.

Tetrahydrozoline does not appear to alter pupil size or raise intraocular pressure.[139] Certain patients experience a mild, transient stinging sensation immediately following instillation of the drops.[139]

Tetrahydrozoline also appears to be safe for use in cataract patients. Menger[139] reported more than 100 patients with various stages of lens opacities who exhibited no significant changes in the course of development of cataracts or intraocular pressure while using this agent.

Oxymetazoline became available for ocular use in 1987 as a 0.025% eyedrop in a boric acid solution. Previously it was used to treat congestion of the nasal mucosa, where it exhibited a rapid onset and long duration of action without producing significant rebound congestion or systemic effects.[141]

The effectiveness of oxymetazoline as an ocular decongestant has been demonstrated in several double-blind clinical trials in which allergic, noninfectious, and chlorine conjunctivitis were treated with the 0.025% concentration.[141–144] Breaky and associates[142] reported results with the 0.025% concentration in a double-blind multicenter trial of 158 patients with allergic and noninfectious conjunctivitis. Two drops of oxymetazoline or placebo were placed into each eye four times daily for 1 week. Overall, 84% of the allergic and 94% of the noninfectious conjunctivitis group were improved, compared with 58% and 51%, respectively, in the placebo group. Duzman and associates[144] studied the effects of twice-daily instillation of oxymetazoline or placebo in patients with bilateral allergic or environmental conjunctivitis, classified as moderate to severe conjunctival hyperemia. Symptoms of burning, itching, tearing, and foreign body sensation were significantly improved in the oxymetazoline-treated group as compared with a control group.

The onset of action of oxymetazoline can be apparent 5 minutes following instillation, with the peak effect at 60 minutes. The effect can last up to 6 hours.

Oxymetazoline 0.025% appears to be relatively free of ocular and systemic side effects. Samson and associates[141] compared the effects of oxymetazoline 0.025% with phenylephrine 0.12% (Prefrin) and placebo on pupil size and accommodation using infrared electronic pupillography. Clinically significant changes in pupil diameter or near-point recession were not observed. Intraocular pressure, pupillary response to light, and visual acuity also appeared not to be altered.[141-144] One case of lid retraction has been associated with use of oxymetazoline.[142] No significant systemic side effects, such as changes in heart rate or blood pressure, have been observed with ocular administration of this agent.[143]

Few studies have been reported comparing the commercially available ocular decongestants (see Table 3.6). Butler and associates[145] compared 3 OTC vasoconstrictor agents, tetrahydrozoline 0.05%, naphazoline 0.012%, and phenylephrine 0.12%, in 40 adult subjects with no ocular disease. No significant changes in pupil size or anterior chamber angle ratios were observed. However, the effect of these three agents on intraocular pressure varied. Tetrahydrozoline significantly lowered intraocular pressure at 30 minutes, whereas naphazoline produced a higher average intraocular pressure than the control at all measured times (Fig. 3.18).

Abelson and associates[146] have compared the ability of certain ocular decongestants to counteract histamine-induced erythema. Naphazoline ranging in concentration from 0.012 to 0.1%, tetrahydrozoline 0.05%, and phenylephrine 0.12% were studied in a double-masked fashion in 6 human volunteers with no ocular disease. All the preparations tested produced blanching of the histamine-induced conjunctival hyperemia. However, naphazoline 0.02% produced a statistically greater blanching of the conjunctiva when compared with other nonprescription decongestants containing 0.05% tetrahydrozoline or 0.12% phenylephrine. Moreover, no significant differences were observed

with preparations containing 0.02%, 0.05%, or 0.1% naphazoline. The effect of naphazoline 0.02% was also comparable to a preparation containing 0.05% naphazoline combined with 0.5% antazoline phosphate.

Abelson and associates[147] have also compared the tolerance and rebound vasodilation effects of naphazoline and tetrahydrozoline in 11 normal subjects. Naphazoline caused a significantly greater reduction in redness at 1, 3, and 5 hours after instillation. After repeated 10-day use, tetrahydrozoline tended to lose its whitening ability when compared with naphazoline. Neither of the two agents produced rebound vasodilation.

Clinical studies have also been carried out to compare oxymetazoline (OcuClear) with naphazoline (Vasocon) and tetrahydrozoline (Visine) using the chlorine conjunctivitis model.[148] Subjects' eyes were experimentally irritated with a 1-minute rinse of chlorinated water. Comparing OcuClear to Vasocon and Visine, OcuClear showed a somewhat faster onset, longer duration of action, and better decongestant effect.

SIDE EFFECTS

Because of the relatively low concentrations required for ocular decongestion, the imidazole derivatives generally do not cause systemic side effects when used in the manufacturer's recommended dosage range. Patients should be cautioned, however, that liberal use can lead to excessive systemic absorption with the possibility of cardiac irregularities and hypertension.

Ocular side effects, including pupillary dilation and elevation of intraocular pressure, can occur and have been observed with naphazoline 0.1%.[126] In addition,

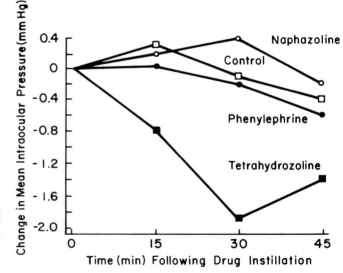

FIGURE 3.18 **Mean intraocular pressure changes following instillation of commercially available OTC decongestants containing naphazoline 0.012%, tetrahydrozoline 0.05%, or phenylephrine 0.12%. A commercial artificial tear preparation was used as the control. (From Butler K, Thompson JP, Yolton DP. Effects of nonprescription ocular decongestants. Rev Optom 1978;11:49-52.)**

prolonged ophthalmic use of vasoconstrictor agents may lead to epithelial xerosis in certain patients with ocular disease, particularly in the caruncle and surrounding eyelid margin.[149]

Rebound congestion has not been reported following ophthalmic use of naphazoline[126] or tetrahydrozoline.[138,139] Topical ocular use of these agents reduces conjunctival sac temperature.[150] Their vasoconstrictor action has been suggested as a possible mechanism for this effect.

CONTRAINDICATIONS

Contraindications to the imidazole derivatives as topical ocular decongestants are similar to those of epinephrine and phenylephrine. However, the low concentrations employed do not appear to subject the patient to significant risk for adverse ocular or systemic reactions.

Adrenergic Antagonists: β-Adrenergic Blocking Agents

Propranolol

PHARMACOLOGY

Drugs that block β receptors (Table 3.9) have proved useful in the management of cardiovascular disorders such as hypertension, arrhythmias, and angina pectoris. Of the available preparations, propranolol remains the most widely used systemic agent. It is a nonselective β-receptor antagonist, blocking both β_1 and β_2 receptors competitively. Propranolol also appears to be free of any intrinsic β-agonist properties.[151]

CLINICAL USES

In 1967 Philips and associates[152] observed that patients treated with propranolol for cardiovascular disorders had lowered intraocular pressures. Subsequent trials

TABLE 3.9
Ocular β-Adrenergic Blocking Agents

Drug	Receptor Blocked	Concentration (%)
Befunolol	$\beta_1 + \beta_2$	0.25, 0.5
Betaxolol	β_1	0.5
Bupranolol	$\beta_1 + \beta_2$	0.05, 0.1, 0.25, 0.5
Carteolol	$\beta_1 + \beta_2$	1, 2
Levobunolol	$\beta_1 + \beta_2$	0.5
Metipranolol	$\beta_1 + \beta_2$	0.1, 0.3, 0.6
Timolol	$\beta_1 + \beta_2$	0.25, 0.5

with oral propranolol in glaucoma patients revealed that the intraocular pressure-lowering effect was not maintained in all patients with long-term therapy. In addition, the oral use of propranolol is accompanied by a lowered systemic blood pressure and sometimes cardiac difficulties.[153]

Subsequent to the observations on systemic use, several investigators evaluated the effects of topical propranolol in glaucomatous eyes.[154,155] In one study 7 of 10 patients exhibited reduced intraocular pressure with 1.0% propranolol eyedrops. The mean maximum reduction of pressure was 4.35 mm Hg.[155]

Propranolol has also been used in conjunction with other glaucoma medications such as epinephrine.[156] The effects of the two agents in reducing intraocular pressure appear to be additive.

SIDE EFFECTS

Although topical propranolol does not affect pupil size, it has several other undesirable side effects. Stinging and irritation are common following topical instillation. Allergic reactions have been observed. In addition, the known local anesthetic properties of propranolol have been reported to affect corneal sensitivity.[155]

Topical propranolol also causes systemic side effects. Decreased heart rate and cardiac difficulties are not uncommon.[155]

Lack of a significant effect on intraocular pressure and the high incidence of adverse effects limit the usefulness of propranolol for control of intraocular pressure.

Timolol

PHARMACOLOGY

In 1978 timolol maleate became the first β-adrenergic blocking agent in the United States to receive Food and Drug Administration (FDA) approval as an ophthalmic preparation for the treatment of open-angle glaucoma, aphakic glaucoma, and the secondary glaucomas. Like propranolol, it is a nonselective β antagonist. However, timolol is 5 to 10 times more potent than propranolol as a blocking agent for β receptors.[156] It appears to lack the demonstrable local anesthetic properties of propranolol and exhibits minimal β-agonist activity.[151] Oral administration of timolol has been shown to be effective for treatment of certain cardiovascular conditions such as hypertension.[151,157]

Timolol maleate (Timoptic) is supplied as the levoisomer in dosage strengths of 0.25% and 0.5%. The solution is buffered to a pH of 6.5 to 7.5 and is preserved with 0.01% benzalkonium chloride. It is heat stable at room temperature but must be protected from light.[158] The expiration date is 2 years. For patients who are sensitive to benzalkonium chloride, a preservative-free formulation of timolol (Ocudose) is available. This formulation is supplied in a unit-dose package, designed to be used once and discarded. It differs from Timoptic only in the absence of the preservative.

The fate of topically instilled timolol has been studied in animals and humans. In rabbits radioactively labeled timolol has been shown to be present in the aqueous humor, whereas timolol and its metabolites are present in the serum, lung, kidney, and liver.[159] One to 7 hours following instillation of 2 drops of 0.5% timolol into eyes of patients about to undergo cataract surgery, aspirated aqueous has revealed concentrations of timolol ranging from 150 ng/100 mg during the first 2 hours to 10 ng/100 mg at 7 hours.[160]

Plasma levels of timolol following topical application to the eye have been analyzed in children and adults. Peak plasma levels occur 1 to 2 hours following administration (Fig. 3.19).[161–163] Passo and associates[162] found the mean plasma timolol concentration to be 0.34 ng/ml 12 hours after the previous night's administration in 10 patients over age 60 who received chronic timolol therapy for open-angle glaucoma. One hour after receiving drops the levels rose to 1.34 ng/ml. When punctal occlusion was applied, the mean 1 hour plasma timolol level diminished to 0.9 ng/ml, approximately 40% less than that observed without punctal occlusion (Fig. 3.20). Plasma levels were higher in children and ranged from 3.5 ng/ml in a 5-year-old child to 34 ng/ml in a 3-week-old infant (Fig. 3.21). It is likely that some patients using topical timolol attain therapeutic plasma levels of timolol.[163] Systemic side effects observed with topical timolol are similar to

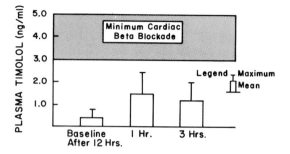

FIGURE 3.19   **Histogram showing mean and maximum plasma levels of timolol just before and 1 and 3 hours after instilling 1 drop of 0.5% timolol maleate into each eye. Baseline level was taken 12 hours after the previous night's dosage. (From Passo MS, Palmer EA, Van Buskirk EM. Plasma timolol in glaucoma patients. Ophthalmology 1984;91:1361–1363.)**

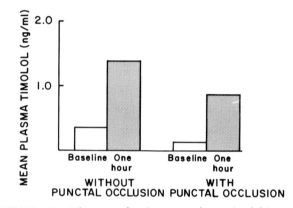

FIGURE 3.20   **Histogram showing mean plasma timolol in 9 patients immediately before (baseline) and 1 hour after instilling 1 drop of 0.5% timolol maleate into each eye, with and without punctal occlusion. (From Passo MS, Palmer EA, Van Buskirk EM. Plasma timolol in glaucoma patients. Ophthalmology 1984; 91:1361–1363.)**

FIGURE 3.21   **Histogram showing mean plasma timolol measured on 9 separate occasions under general anesthesia in 5 children (ages 3 weeks to 5 years) receiving topical timolol for glaucoma. Time elapsed from drop instillation is noted below each bar. The mean 1 hour adult level is included for comparison. (From Passo MS, Palmer EA, Van Buskirk EM. Plasma timolol in glaucoma patients. Ophthalmology 1984;91:1361–1363.)**

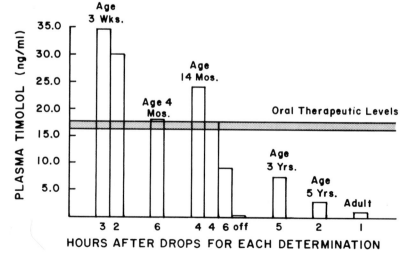

those observed with oral β-blocking agents. High plasma levels following topical ocular use most likely explain the systemic effects encountered with ocular timolol.[164]

Katz and associates[165] first studied the actions of single-dose administration of 0.5%, 1.0%, and 1.5% timolol in volunteers with no obvious ocular disease. Their results indicated that all the tested concentrations reduced intraocular pressure with no significant differences among the three concentrations. Subsequent studies[166,167] in patients with primary open-angle glaucoma have demonstrated a significant reduction in intraocular pressure when one eye of each patient was treated with timolol 0.5% and 1.5% as compared with a placebo. An interesting and unexplained result is the observation that the nonmedicated eyes of the timolol-treated groups also showed a pressure decrease over the same period (Figs. 3.22 A, B). This effect may suggest that systemically absorbed drug is active in the fellow eye or, alternatively, that timolol may be active through some central mechanism. Often there is no significant difference in the hypotensive response between the treated and the untreated eye in individual patients.[168]

Furthermore, dose-response curves following a single administration of timolol using concentrations of 0.1%, 0.25%, 0.5%, and 1.0% have demonstrated that 0.5% gives the maximal ocular hypotensive effect.[169] Further studies have confirmed the efficacy of timolol when administered to glaucomatous eyes for prolonged periods.[170,171]

When used alone as a topical ocular hypotensive agent, timolol is effective in reducing intraocular pressure by approximately 20% to 30% compared with pretreatment values.[172] The duration of the ocular hypotensive response following the instillation of 1 drop is about 24 hours.[173]

When the ocular hypotensive effectiveness of timolol is compared with that of pilocarpine, timolol is at least as, and often more, effective than pilocarpine in reducing intraocular pressure.[168,172,174] In addition, timolol produces less variation in the diurnal curves than does pilocarpine.[174] Thus, timolol appears to reduce intraocular pressure around the clock more effectively than does pilocarpine. When the ocular hypotensive effectiveness of timolol is compared with that of epinephrine, timolol clearly decreases intraocular pressure more effectively than does epinephrine.[175,438] Furthermore, timolol decreases intraocular pressure at least as effectively as acetazolamide.[176]

Boger and associates[170] showed that when timolol is administered to untreated glaucoma patients, the drug is maximally effective in the first few days after beginning therapy, but after the first several days the intraocular pressure rises slightly ("escapes") to a somewhat higher intraocular pressure that is still lower than the

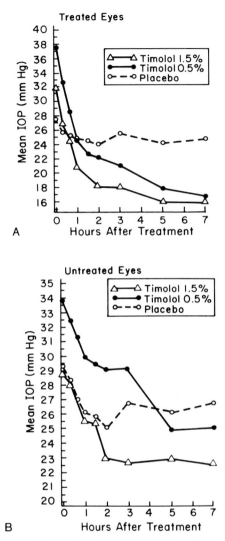

FIGURE 3.22 **Comparison of time-course of effect on treated (A) and untreated (B) eyes following instillation of 0.5 and 1.5% timolol. (From Zimmerman TJ, Kaufman HE. Timolol: A β-adrenergic agent for the treatment of glaucoma. Arch Ophthalmol 1977;95:601–604. Copyright 1977, American Medical Association.)**

untreated value. Neufeld and associates[6] have shown that the number of β receptors in ocular tissue increases with continued timolol therapy. This makes the cells more sensitive to adrenergic stimulation and thus may lessen the effect of β-blockade. This effect is transient, since it occurs only during the first few days of treatment. Thus, certain patients may have an initial dramatic response to timolol, followed by a rise in intraocular pressure.

Most studies[177–180,439] have confirmed the long-term efficacy of timolol in patients responsive to it. Patients will typically reach a plateau that remains level, with little dissipation of the pressure-lowering effect. Katz and associates[180] studied the effect of timolol 0.5% in over 2200 patients for periods up to 3 years. Mean intraocular pressure was 27.7 mm Hg before treatment and decreased to 19.7 mm Hg after 6 months of therapy. Thereafter the mean pressure remained relatively constant (between 19.7 and 18.8 mm Hg) for up to 3 years (Fig. 3.23).

An additive effect on intraocular pressure can occur when timolol is used in combination with other glaucoma medications such as miotics, epinephrine, and carbonic anhydrase inhibitors.[169,176,181–185] Radius and associates[169] first demonstrated an additional ocular hypotensive effect in rabbit eyes when norepinephrine and epinephrine were used in conjunction with timolol. Subsequent studies in patients with open-angle glaucoma have supported the clinical usefulness of concurrent administration of acetazolamide[176,183] and epinephrine[181,182,184–185] with timolol in the control of intraocular pressure.

However, because of the opposing pharmacologic actions of epinephrine and timolol, several investigators[186–189] have studied the effectiveness of glaucoma therapy with concomitant epinephrine and timolol. These results indicate that the combined administration of epinephrine and timolol, unlike epinephrine combined with other antiglaucoma agents, produces little if any additive effect, suggesting that their coadministration is essentially nonproductive. Although an initial additive ocular hypotensive effect is observed when epinephrine is added to the drug regimen of patients already receiving timolol, a complete loss of this additive effect occurs when patients are maintained on both drugs.[189] To minimize this loss of drug additivity, the epinephrine may be administered 3 to 4 hours following the timolol dose,[186] or such patients may be

treated with epinephrine, followed by the intermittent addition of timolol in "pulses."[189] Such pulsed administration of timolol for 2 to 3 weeks to patients on epinephrine may provide better control of intraocular pressure than would the simultaneous administration of both drugs.

When topical timolol is administered to patients receiving oral β-blocking agents for the treatment of systemic hypertension, there is a significant further reduction of intraocular pressure.[190] Although patients undergoing such systemic β-blocking therapy can benefit in some cases from additive topical timolol treatment, topical timolol therapy alone appears to give maximum reduction of intraocular pressure.[190] This appears to suggest, however, that the use of topical timolol is not contraindicated in patients undergoing oral β-blocking therapy for systemic hypertension, since a further reduction of intraocular pressure may occur.

The mechanisms of action associated with the combined actions of timolol and various other ocular hypotensive agents remain a matter of speculation. Since both acetazolamide and timolol reduce aqueous humor formation,[191,192] their effect on intraocular pressure could well be additive. The observation that both β-adrenergic antagonists and β-adrenergic agonists lower intraocular pressure is of clinical as well as theoretical significance.

Treatment of open-angle glaucoma with epinephrine alone significantly increases aqueous outflow facility 2 weeks following initiation of therapy.[32,33,185,193,194] When timolol is added to epinephrine, 2 weeks following initiation of the combined therapy outflow decreases significantly. In the reverse sequence, when epinephrine is added to patients already receiving timolol, there is a further reduction of intraocular pressure after 2 weeks of combined therapy. However, the additive effect of epinephrine diminishes during further therapy and becomes insignificant after an additional 6 weeks.[185,195] Thus, the effects of epinephrine and timolol on intraocular pressure appear to be additive only for a 2-week period.

From the above clinical observations and the findings of other investigators that timolol reduces intraocular pressure by inhibiting aqueous formation without affecting the facility of outflow,[166,196] it has been postulated that timolol blocks the effects of epinephrine on outflow—the proposed mechanism whereby epinephrine increases outflow is by stimulation of β receptors in the outflow tract.[185] Experimental data from studies in monkey eyes lend support to this theory of the action of epinephrine. Injection into the anterior chamber of isoproterenol, a β-receptor agonist, results in increased facility of outflow.[197] In contrast, stimulation of α receptors produces only a minor change in facility of outflow.[198]

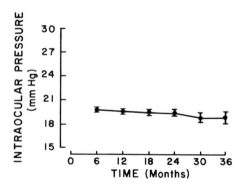

FIGURE 3.23 **Mean intraocular pressure and 95% confidence intervals across time for patients treated with timolol ophthalmic solution.** (From Katz IM, Kulaga SF, Gould LA, et al. Long-term tolerability and efficacy of timolol ophthalmic solution. Glaucoma 1987;9:84–88.)

Based on their clinical observations and the experimental data in primate eyes, Thomas and Epstein[185] have proposed a model of ocular adrenergic receptor action that may explain, at least partially, the pharmacologic effects of the β agonist, epinephrine, and β antagonists such as timolol in human eyes with glaucoma (Fig. 3.24). According to this model, β receptors play a role in both aqueous inflow and outflow. β receptors involved in outflow could be located in the trabecular meshwork, and stimulation with a β agonist, like epinephrine, produces an increase in facility of outflow. Receptors mediating inflow are possibly located in the ciliary processes, and stimulation with epinephrine produces an increase in aqueous production. Blocking the inflow receptor sites with a β antagonist, such as timolol, decreases aqueous production.

From this model it is postulated that the initial stimulation of β receptors in the outflow tract by epinephrine alone enhances facility of outflow and simultaneously increases aqueous production by stimulation of β receptors involved with aqueous inflow. Fluorophotometric studies in normal human eyes support the hypothesis that topical epinephrine increases aqueous production and enhances facility of outflow.[36] The addition of timolol blocks the effects of epinephrine on aqueous outflow and reduces the rate of aqueous production by blocking β receptors involved in inflow. Since timolol has a greater affinity for β receptors than does epinephrine,[19] its addition to epinephrine therapy can thus gradually lessen the additive effect on intraocular pressure by interfering with the β effects of epinephrine on outflow.

This model also provides a role for α receptors in control of intraocular pressure. It is postulated that α receptors located in walls of blood vessels supplying the ciliary processes will be stimulated through the α-agonist effects of epinephrine. The resulting constriction of these vessels will decrease blood flow and consequently decrease aqueous production.

Although further clinical and experimental data are needed to substantiate it, this model is an interesting hypothesis of the current state of knowledge. Perhaps as additional data become available on ocular receptor subtypes, the effects on β_1 and β_2 as well as α_1 and α_2 receptors will further clarify the actions of adrenergic agonists and antagonists in the control of intraocular pressure.

CLINICAL USES

Following its introduction into clinical practice in 1978, timolol quickly became a drug of first choice for the treatment of glaucoma. This popularity was largely due to its ocular hypotensive effectiveness in most types of glaucoma.

Timolol is commercially available as an ophthalmic solution in concentrations of 0.25% and 0.50%. Although timolol has a 24-hour duration of intraocular pressure reduction, it is usually administered twice daily to minimize diurnal pressure variations. However, some authors[199] recommend initiating therapy with once-daily administration and, if the response is inadequate, increasing the administration to twice daily. This practice minimizes ocular and systemic side effects and the possible development of drug tolerance.

One of the significant advantages of timolol compared with pilocarpine solutions is its less frequent instillation, which improves patient compliance.

Kass and associates[200] assessed compliance with timolol treatment in 110 patients with an eyedrop monitor that recorded electronically the date and time of drug administration over a 4- to 6-week period. The overall rate of compliance was 82.7%, with great variation among patients. This rate is higher than the 76% compliance observed with pilocarpine.

Except for combined timolol-epinephrine therapy, timolol appears to cause a significant reduction of intraocular pressure in long-term therapy when used together with most other glaucoma medications, including pilocarpine, carbachol, and acetazolamide.[201] Although pilocarpine and epinephrine are less effective in black patients than white, timolol appears to be equally effective in both.[172]

Because of the wide variety of timolol-induced ocular and systemic side effects, some of which are quite serious, conservatism is indicated in selecting patients to whom timolol is administered. Timolol is effective in the treatment of primary open-angle glaucoma, aphakic glaucoma, and ocular hypertension. It is also effective in the treatment of angle-closure glaucoma and many secondary glaucomas, including uveitic, neo-

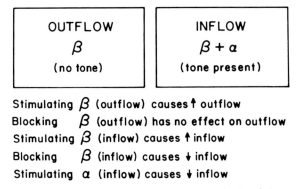

FIGURE 3.24   **Proposed model for the actions of epinephrine and timolol at their respective receptor sites and effects on aqueous dynamics. (From Thomas JV, Epstein DL. Study on the additive effects of timolol and epinephrine in lowering intraocular pressure. Br J Ophthalmol 1981;65:596–602.)**

vascular, and pseudophakic.[172] Timolol is also effective in the treatment of congenital glaucoma.[202] However, it is recommended that the lowest effective dosage be used and the pediatric patient carefully monitored for possible ocular or systemic complications.

One of the most useful indications for timolol is in the treatment of secondary glaucoma, in which timolol usually reduces intraocular pressure as effectively as does the combination of epinephrine and acetazolamide.[172] Timolol is also indicated in glaucomas that are extremely difficult to control with more traditional drug therapy. In such cases the use of timolol may eliminate or delay the need for laser or filtering surgery.

Patients under 40 years of age are likely to benefit from timolol therapy because it eliminates the pupillary constriction and accommodative spasm associated with the use of miotics. Timolol is particularly useful for patients with cataract because of the lack of pupillary constriction. In addition, the drug provides a useful alternative for patients who are uncontrolled with DPE and for those who do not tolerate or are uncontrolled with pilocarpine.

SIDE EFFECTS

Although topical timolol therapy results in ocular hypotensive effects with a relatively high therapeutic index, its frequent and long-term use has revealed both ocular and systemic side effects. Timolol is well tolerated by patients for whom there is no specific contraindication to its use, but therapy must be discontinued in about 10% of patients because of side effects.[203]

Ocular Effects (Table 3.10).   The most frequently observed adverse ocular reactions include ocular irritation, corneal complications, and visual or refractive disturbances.[180,203–209] However, one of the factors responsible for the clinical acceptance of timolol is the fact that the incidence of ocular side effects is less than that of pilocarpine (Fig. 3.25).

Burning and tearing following instillation, as well as foreign body sensation, stinging, and itching, have been reported with increasing frequency. Although these effects are generally tolerable, in some patients therapy with timolol must be discontinued.[204]

Transient dry eye syndromes following long-term treatment have been reported in several patients.[205,206] A reduction in tear film stability can occur with timolol therapy.[210] Rose bengal staining may reveal simultaneous diffuse punctate staining of the cornea. In one study[205] the symptoms were relieved by withdrawing the drug, but in another study[206] the symptoms lasted only 3 to 13 days despite continuation of drug therapy. Treatment with 0.5% timolol twice daily does not ap-

TABLE 3.10
Ocular Side Effects of Topical Timolol

- Irritation and itching
- Tearing
- Dry eye
- Superficial punctate keratitis
- Corneal hypoesthesia
- Allergic blepharoconjunctivitis
- Blurred vision
- Photophobia
- Persistent hypotony

pear to reduce tear flow or lysozyme concentration 12 months after initiation of therapy.[207]

Superficial punctate keratitis, possibly associated with corneal anesthesia in some patients, has been reported. Following discontinuation of timolol therapy, the keratitis disappears and normal corneal sensitivity returns within several weeks.[208] It has not been determined with certainty if timolol, like propranolol, exhibits some anesthetic properties.

Allergic blepharoconjunctivitis with lid edema, conjunctival injection, and chemosis has also been observed.[209]

Although burning or pain on instillation of timolol often completely resolves during the first week of therapy, blurred vision is a more persistent problem and is one of the more frequent reasons for discontinuing timolol therapy.[172] In presbyopic patients, substitution of timolol for miotic therapy can result in hyperopia.[203] Other complaints include nonspecific blurring of central vision for both distance and near. No change in

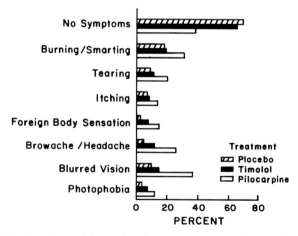

FIGURE 3.25   **Incidence of ocular symptoms with placebo (N = 82), timolol (N = 1,796–1,896), and pilocarpine (N = 317). (From Katz IM, Kulaga SF, Gould LA, et al. Long-term tolerability and efficacy of timolol ophthalmic solution. Glaucoma 1987;9:84–88.)**

the refractive status has been observed in some of these patients, while in others myopia of 1.5 to 3.0 D is present that resolves following cessation of timolol therapy.[209]

Dilated, almost fixed pupils have been observed in several patients undergoing concomitant therapy with timolol and epinephrine.[172] There appears to be a slightly greater dilation in eyes treated with both epinephrine and timolol than when epinephrine alone is administered.[187] Persistent hypotony secondary to timolol may rarely occur but can force termination of treatment.[172]

Less frequently reported adverse ocular reactions include macular edema in aphakics, macular hemorrhage, retinal detachment, uveitis, and progressive cataracts.[203,209]

Systemic Effects (Table 3.11). More than half the side effects reported in association with topical timolol therapy involve systemic reactions.[211] These side effects are essentially the same as those observed from systemically administered β-blocking agents. Although most patients tolerate topical timolol well, there is an increased potential for adverse systemic side effects in

TABLE 3.11
Systemic Side Effects of Topical Timolol

Central Nervous System
  Headache
  Lethargy
  Lightheadedness
  Weakness
  Fatigue
  Mental depression
  Dissociative behavior
  Memory loss

Cardiovascular
  Bradycardia
  Palpitations
  Systemic hypotension
  Syncope
  Cardiac arrhythmia
  Congestive heart failure

Respiratory
  Bronchospasm
  Dyspnea
  Pulmonary edema
  Exacerbation of asthma

Dermatologic
  Skin rash

Gastrointestinal
  Nausea
  Vomiting
  Diarrhea
  Abdominal pain

Orthopaedic
  Joint pain

elderly patients because these patients often have flaccid lids that permit greater volumes of drug to be retained in the conjunctival fornices, allowing for increased systemic drug absorption following drainage through the nasolacrimal system.[212]

The most frequent systemic side effects involve the CNS. Complaints of lethargy, lightheadedness, weakness, fatigue, mental depression, dissociative behavior, and memory loss are most common.[203,211] The onset of symptoms varies from a few days to months following initiation of therapy. In most cases these symptoms are mild and transient. However, in certain patients timolol must be discontinued because of these CNS effects.[203]

The second most frequently observed side effects involve the cardiovascular system. These reactions appear to be characteristic of β blockade and include bradycardia, palpitations, systemic hypotension, and syncope.[203] Katz and associates[180] measured a pulse rate decrease of 3.8 to 8.2 beats/min over a 27-month period. The mean pulse rate did not fall below 68 beats/min at any evaluation point. Cardiac arrhythmias consisting of heart block or atrial fibrillation usually subside following discontinuation of timolol therapy.[182] A reflex tachycardia (10 beats/min) following cessation of timolol therapy has also been reported.[213]

Respiratory symptoms following initiation of timolol therapy have been reported with increasing frequency. Even when used in the recommended dosages, timolol may cause a significant decrease in airflow in patients with chronic airflow obstruction. Wheezing and dyspnea are the most frequently observed respiratory effects. Pulmonary edema and exacerbation of asthma have occurred with 0.5% timolol.[209,214] Acute bronchospasm has occurred in previously asymptomatic asthmatic patients following the topical use of timolol.[215]

Other systemic problems occurring with topical timolol include dermatologic complications and gastrointestinal distress.[203,209] Diffuse pruritic skin rashes have occurred, occasionally associated with scalp alopecia and increased skin pigmentation. These reactions resolve when drug therapy is discontinued. Symptoms of gastrointestinal problems include nausea, vomiting, diarrhea, and abdominal pain. These symptoms are usually transient and do not necessitate termination of drug administration.

CONTRAINDICATIONS

Although timolol is well tolerated by the majority of patients for whom it seems indicated, this drug should be used with caution in certain patients (Table 3.12).

Timolol should be used with caution in infants and young children with congenital glaucoma.[216]

TABLE 3.12
Contraindications to Timolol

- Congenital glaucoma
- Narrow angles
- Labile diabetes
- Chronic obstructive pulmonary disease
- Heart block

Eyes with potential angle-closure glaucoma may require a miotic and should therefore not be treated with timolol alone.[203] Because of the increased risk of pupillary dilation, the concomitant use of timolol and epinephrine is hazardous in such patients and should be avoided.

Since nonselective β-blocking agents such as timolol can increase the tendency to hypoglycemia and prolong its duration, the use of topical timolol is contraindicated in patients with labile diabetes.[217]

Timolol should be used with caution in patients with chronic obstructive pulmonary disease, including asthma, chronic bronchitis, and emphysema. Since it is possible for β-blocking drugs, such as timolol, to aggravate or induce bronchospasm in such patients, it is advisable to perform baseline respiratory function studies before initiating therapy.[218] Spirometric evaluation following institution of timolol therapy may be useful to identify patients in whom bronchospasm develops following commencement of therapy.[219] In general, however, it is best to avoid timolol in patients with asthma and other obstructive pulmonary diseases.

Although patients with decompensated congestive heart failure should not be treated with β-blocking drugs in any form, patients with well-compensated heart failure who are receiving medical treatment may be administered topical timolol as long as the cardiac status is closely monitored.[218] Timolol, however, should be avoided in patients with first-degree heart block with a PR-segment interval greater than 0.24 seconds, in patients with second- or third-degree heart block, or in patients with sinus bradycardia with a pulse rate less than 55 beats/min.[218] Concomitant therapy with oral β-blocking agents is not a contraindication to topical timolol, since patients who are already tolerating a β blocker are not likely to encounter difficulty with the additional topical timolol.[218] However, it is advisable to obtain an electrocardiogram (ECG) in patients who are to be administered timolol if they have cardiac disease. This will identify patients who may be more likely to sustain adverse cardiac complications. When the advisability of topical timolol therapy is in question, the patient should probably be evaluated by an internist or cardiologist before initiating therapy. As a general rule, however, patients who would encounter

adverse effects from systemic β blockade are probably poor candidates for timolol therapy.

Levobunolol

PHARMACOLOGY

Levobunolol, like timolol, is a β_1- and β_2-receptor antagonist. It is equipotent on both types of receptors and exhibits little intrinsic sympathomimetic or local anesthetic effect.[220] Initially developed to treat systemic hypertension and ischemic heart disease, levobunolol can be as effective as timolol in decreasing intraocular pressure in glaucomatous eyes.[221] Duzman and associates[221] have shown that twice-daily instillation of 0.5% timolol as compared with 0.5% or 1% levobunolol produces similar changes in intraocular pressure.

Partamian and associates[222] studied the pressure-lowering effects of levobunolol at concentrations of 0.03%, 0.3%, 0.6%, 1%, and 2% in a double-masked study in patients with ocular hypertension. Intraocular pressure was decreased significantly from baseline levels at all concentrations tested. Subsequent clinical trials[223–227] have compared the effects of 0.5% and 1% levobunolol on intraocular pressure. Twice-daily instillation reduces intraocular pressure between 6.1 and 9.6 mm Hg, and the 0.5% and 1% concentrations demonstrate similar long-term efficacy.

Once-daily administration of levobunolol has also been shown to be effective in controlling intraocular pressure in primary open-angle glaucoma and in patients with ocular hypertension.[224–229,440,441] In a 3-month, double-masked clinical trial, 92 patients with open-angle glaucoma or ocular hypertension received levobunolol 0.5% or 1% or timolol 0.5% daily in both eyes. The overall mean decrease in intraocular pressure was 7.0 mm Hg, 6.5 mm Hg and 4.5 mm Hg, respectively.[228] A reason for the greater effectiveness of levobunolol could be that its major metabolite, dihydrolevobunolol, is equipotent to levobunolol and has a plasma half-life of 7 hours, compared with 6 hours for levobunolol and 2 hours for timolol. Since a once-daily instillation of topical antiglaucoma medication may decrease the incidence and severity of systemic side effects and be a regimen with which patients can more easily comply, further long-term studies are needed to compare the sustained efficacy of once-daily 0.5% levobunolol instillation.

The effects of levobunolol 0.5% on aqueous humor dynamics appear to be similar to those of timolol.[230] Like timolol, levobunolol lowers intraocular pressure primarily by decreasing aqueous production. No effects on uveoscleral flow, outflow facility, or episcleral venous pressure have been observed with this agent.

Levobunolol can also lower intraocular pressure in the healthy eye.[220] In addition, uniocular administration results in a contralateral pressure-lowering effect in the untreated eye.[221]

CLINICAL USES

Levobunolol (Betagan) is commercially available at 0.5% concentration with polyvinyl alcohol 1.4% and with benzalkonium chloride 0.004% as the preservative.[231] It is usually administered twice daily, although some patients may be controlled initially with only one instillation per day. In clinical practice the reduction in intraocular pressure levobunolol produces is similar to the effects observed with timolol.[220] In addition, levobunolol can be used in combination with dipivefrin without loss of additivity.[442] Continued use of this nonselective β-blocking agent will demonstrate whether its ocular hypotensive efficacy is maintained with long-term treatment.

SIDE EFFECTS

Instillation of levobunolol is associated with relatively few side effects.[224–227] Transient ocular stinging and burning may occur following instillation (Fig. 3.26). Occasionally patients experience a reduction of two or more lines of visual acuity when measured on the standard Snellen chart. Changes in pupil size, corneal sensitivity, or Schirmer tear test values occur infrequently.[220] An apparent drug-related blepharitis has been reported with levobunolol.[226] Two of 50 patients in a double-masked, randomized study developed this condition after 7 months of treatment.

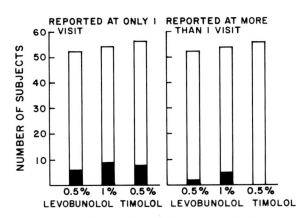

FIGURE 3.26 **Incidence of ocular burning and stinging with levobunolol and timolol. (Published with permission from the American Journal of Ophthalmology 99:11–17, 1985. Copyright by the Ophthalmic Publishing Company.)**

Systemic effects following topical ocular use of levobunolol are similar to those observed with timolol. This is not surprising, since both drugs are nonselective β blockers and thus affect both β_1- and β_2-receptor sites. Changes in mean heart rate and blood pressure have been observed with 0.5% levobunolol.[224–227] Although Novack and associates[232] found no significant decrease in heart rate with the 0.5% concentration, a decrease in heart rate of 4 to 5 beats/min for both 0.5% timolol and 0.5% levobunolol has been reported in 1 controlled study.[227] Overall mean decreases in systolic blood pressure were 12 to 14 mm Hg for levobunolol 0.5% and 19 mm Hg for timolol 0.5%. For diastolic blood pressure, a mean decrease of 4 to 6 mm Hg was observed for levobunolol and 11 mm Hg for timolol. Other investigators have reported similar values.[224,225,227,228] In general, the observed effects on heart rate and blood pressure are of limited clinical significance.[224,227]

Plasma levels of levobunolol following topical administration of 0.5% and 1% concentrations have been analyzed by Novack and associates.[232] On day 7 following initiation of levobunolol administration, plasma levels ranged from 0 to 1.1 ng/ml and from 0 to 1.2 ng/ml for the 0.5% and 1% concentrations, respectively. These levels are significantly lower than those reported with oral doses. One hour following a 3 mg oral dose, plasma levels rose to 19 ng/ml.

Auscultatory findings of the heart and lungs are usually normal, and blood chemistry and hematologic values appear to be unaltered by long-term use of topical levobunolol.[224,226]

CONTRAINDICATIONS

Contraindications to the use of topical levobunolol are the same as for timolol.

Betaxolol

PHARMACOLOGY

Introduced in 1985, betaxolol is the first cardioselective, β_1-adrenergic antagonist available in the United States for topical ocular use. Oral and intravenous administration lower blood pressure substantially in patients with systemic hypertension. Its relative lack of effect on β_2 receptors has made it useful in patients with chronic obstructive airway disease.[220]

Its mechanism of action in lowering intraocular pressure appears to be similar to that of timolol and levobunolol. Using the technique of fluorophotometry to measure aqueous production, and tonography to determine outflow resistance, Reiss and associates[233] observed a suppression in aqueous production but no consistent effect on outflow resistance.

Berrospi and Leibowitz[234] tested for a 12-month period the effects of 0.25% betaxolol in 12 patients with primary open-angle glaucoma or ocular hypertension. A 30% to 35% decrease in intraocular pressure was observed in all patients, and the effect was maintained during the 1-year observation period. Similar results with betaxolol have been reported by other investigators.[235,236]

The ocular hypotensive effect of betaxolol has been compared in several studies with that of timolol.[237–239] The results suggest that betaxolol and timolol at the 0.25% and 0.5% concentrations are about equally effective in lowering intraocular pressure. However, in one double-masked, randomized, 6-month trial,[240] the median intraocular pressure was consistently lower with timolol 0.5% than with betaxolol 0.5%. Adjunctive glaucoma therapy was required in 8 patients in the betaxolol group, compared with only 1 patient in the timolol group. A similar study comparing levobunolol with betaxolol indicated that, although both agents were effective, levobunolol provided a greater reduction of intraocular pressure than did betaxolol.[448]

CLINICAL USES

Betaxolol (Betoptic) is commercially available at 0.5% concentration with benzalkonium chloride 0.01%, edetate disodium, sodium chloride, hydrochloric acid, or sodium hydroxide to adjust pH.[231] It is usually administered twice daily to control intraocular pressure. About 2 weeks of therapy is required for the maximal observed effect on intraocular pressure to occur.[220]

SIDE EFFECTS

The most frequently observed ocular side effect with betaxolol is mild to moderate burning or stinging following instillation.[235,236,240,443] In one study,[237] 30% of patients receiving betaxolol 0.5% complained of ocular discomfort compared with only 9% of patients receiving timolol 0.5%. These symptoms are usually not severe enough to warrant discontinuation of treatment.[235]

Betaxolol appears to be relatively free of adverse structural or functional ocular effects. Pupil size, corneal sensitivity, and basal tear production are not altered by this agent.[235–240] Visual acuity as measured on the Snellen chart also does not seem to be affected.[235]

Since betaxolol is a selective, β_1-adrenergic blocking agent, it should theoretically not affect pulmonary function. Since glaucoma is often present in older patient populations where obstructive airway disease may coexist, a cardioselective β-blocking agent may be a better choice than a nonselective β blocker, which can both decrease heart rate and increase respiratory resistance.[444] Several investigators[234,235—240] have studied the effects of betaxolol 0.25%, 0.5%, and 1% on cardiopulmonary function in patients without obvious airway disease. No significant differences in pulse rate, blood pressure, respiratory rate, or spirometric measurements have been observed during rest or exercise when betaxolol is compared with timolol 0.5% or placebo in healthy subjects.

Although several controlled studies[241–243] have indicated that the use of betaxolol in patients with pulmonary disease does not result in significant effects on respiratory function, others have observed adverse effects in clinical use.[244,245] Schoene and associates[241] evaluated the effects of betaxolol 1% in 9 patients with pulmonary disease who had demonstrated bronchoconstriction to timolol 0.5%. Spirometric measurements, respiratory rate, blood pressure, and pulse rate were monitored for 4 hours following instillation of the drug. Although timolol elicited a 25% decrease in forced expiratory volume (FEV), betaxolol had no significant effect on airflow. Van Buskirk and associates[243] evaluated betaxolol 0.5% in 11 patients with reactive airway disease. Eight of these patients had previous timolol therapy discontinued after pulmonary symptoms or complications developed. After 2 weeks of twice-daily betaxolol administration, mean FEVs were measured and compared with pretherapy baseline values. Pulmonary function was not altered by betaxolol.

Dunn and associates[244] evaluated betaxolol in patients with documented adverse pulmonary effects to timolol. In the 8 patients tested, there was little decrease in the average FEV. However, 5 of the 8 had a decrease in FEV of 15% or greater at 1 or more times following betaxolol administration. Harris and associates[245] reported 5 patients who experienced symptoms of pulmonary distress with betaxolol 0.5% administered twice daily. Three of the patients were known asthmatics, while 2 had no history of respiratory disease. In each case the respiratory symptoms resolved when betaxolol was discontinued.

Pulmonary function tests can prove valuable in identifying patients at possible risk of systemic β_2 blockade when ophthalmic β blockers are used to control intraocular pressure. Other systemic side effects less commonly associated with betaxolol include severe depression, disorientation, vertigo, rhinitis, dysuria, and prolonged prothrombin time.[246,247] Bradycardia and sinus arrest have also been reported.[247,248]

CONTRAINDICATIONS

Contraindications to the use of topical betaxolol are the same as for timolol and levobunolol. Betaxolol, however, can be used more safely in patients with chronic obstructive pulmonary disease.

Miscellaneous β Blockers

Other β blockers that have been evaluated topically on the eye for possible ocular hypotensive effects include metipranolol, metoprolol, carteolol, pindolol, atenolol, and nadolol (see Table 3.9).[249–252,445] None has shown clinical advantages over timolol, levobunolol, or betaxolol.

Metipranolol, a nonselective β-blocking agent, has been available in Europe for control of intraocular pressure. Metipranolol 0.6% has been compared with levobunolol 0.5% in a 3-month clinical trial for efficacy, safety, and comfort in patients with glaucoma and ocular hypertension.[249] Both drugs lowered intraocular pressure to the same degree, but metipranolol caused more burning and stinging. Both agents caused a slight decrease in heart rate and blood pressure. Long-term use of metipranolol and other topical β blockers will determine the comparative efficacy and advantages of this class of drugs.

Oral use of β blockers can also affect intraocular pressure (see Chapter 7). Oral administration of propranolol has been shown to decrease pressure in eyes with normal and elevated intraocular pressure. When oral propranolol is added to the therapeutic regimen in individuals whose intraocular pressure is controlled with timolol, pressure is further reduced.[250] Other oral β blockers that have been investigated include pindolol, atenolol, timolol, bupranolol, and nadolol.[251] Patients who are receiving oral β blockers for other conditions can also be given topical β blockers, which enhances the intraocular pressure-lowering effect of topical β blockers.

"Soft" β Blockers

More recently, attempts have been made to develop β blockers with fewer systemic side effects. The acidic metabolite of metoprolol, a β-blocking agent, has been converted into various lipophilic esters referred to as "soft" β blockers. Tests in rabbits show that these compounds exhibit a long-lasting effect on intraocular pressure and are rapidly hydrolyzed in the blood to inactive acidic metabolites. Their rapid systemic hydrolysis could thus potentially eliminate the undesirable systemic side effects associated with ocular use of the presently available β-blocking agents.[253]

α-Adrenergic Blocking Agents

With only a few exceptions the clinical usefulness of these agents in ophthalmic practice is limited. They have been used in the therapy of glaucoma and to reverse the mydriasis induced by adrenergic agonists.

Thymoxamine

PHARMACOLOGY

Thymoxamine hydrochloride is a competitive antagonist of α-adrenergic receptors. When given intravenously, it antagonizes the hypertensive effects of norepinephrine and epinephrine.[254,255] It dilates human arteries in vitro[256] and therefore has been used in various vasospastic conditions such as Raynaud's disease, femoral artery occlusion, and chilblain.[257]

Pau[258] first reported the topical ocular use of thymoxamine in 1955. He applied a 5% solution topically to the eye and reported pupillary constriction and extreme ocular discomfort. Thirteen years later, Turner and Sneddon[259] observed that pretreatment with 0.1% thymoxamine prevented the mydriatic response to 10% phenylephrine and 2% ephedrine. Thymoxamine also rapidly reversed the pupillary dilation caused by 1% hydroxyamphetamine.

Thymoxamine does not reverse the mydriasis produced by the cholinergic blocking agent tropicamide, nor does it reverse the reduction in amplitude of accommodation produced by tropicamide. Thymoxamine does, however, reverse any effects on accommodation produced by adrenergic agonists such as ephedrine.[260]

The pupillary constriction produced by thymoxamine, unlike the cholinergic miotics, is not accompanied by a shallowing of the anterior chamber[261,262] (Fig. 3.27). Since thymoxamine has no apparent effect on the ciliary body, it should not alter the size or position of the lens.

CLINICAL USES

Mapstone[263] has presented theoretical evidence that the use of a cholinergic stimulatory agent such as pilocarpine to induce miosis, following the use of an adrenergic mydriatic such as phenylephrine, increases the risk of angle-closure glaucoma. Not only does spasm of accommodation occur with pilocarpine, but, in addition, stimulation of the dilator and sphincter muscles simultaneously is most likely to produce shallowing of the anterior chamber and to result in pupillary block.

Unlike pilocarpine, thymoxamine appears to be an effective and safe miotic for reversing phenylephrine-induced mydriasis.[447] Moreover, the miosis is maintained long after the phenylephrine effect has dissipated.[264] In addition, thymoxamine acts almost as rapidly as pilocarpine in reversing phenylephrine-induced mydriasis. One drop of 0.5% thymoxamine reverses the mydriasis of 10% phenylephrine to the premydriatic

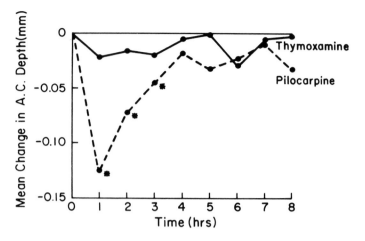

FIGURE 3.27 **Mean change in anterior chamber depth in 11 patients following instillation of 0.5% thymoxamine or 2% pilocarpine. Asterisks indicate values that are significant at P < 0.05. (From Saheb NE, Lorenzetti D, Salpeter CS. Effect of thymoxamine and pilocarpine on the depth of the anterior chamber. Can J Ophthalmol 1980;15:170–171.)**

pupillary diameter within 30 minutes.[207] In comparison, the mean time for reversal of phenylephrine mydriasis with 1.0% pilocarpine is 22 minutes.[265]

Since the miotic effect of thymoxamine appears to occur without an accompanying shallowing of the anterior chamber, it may prove useful for treatment of acute angle-closure glaucoma. Ten patients with angle-closure glaucoma were treated with 0.5% thymoxamine every minute for 5 minutes and then every 15 minutes for up to 3 hours. Of the 10 patients, 8 were successfully treated with thymoxamine alone.[266]

Thymoxamine has also been evaluated and appears to be of value as a diagnostic agent for differentiating angle-closure glaucoma from open-angle glaucoma with narrow angles.[257] Since thymoxamine produces miosis without affecting intraocular pressure, facility of outflow, rate of aqueous formation, or permeability of the blood-aqueous barrier,[267,268] the angle can be opened for a sufficient time without affecting the ciliary muscle.[257] Thus, if elevated intraocular pressure is reduced to normal following instillation of thymoxamine, the diagnosis is angle closure. If the intraocular pressure is only partially reduced, the diagnosis is combined mechanism glaucoma (combination of angle-closure and open-angle glaucoma). If the intraocular pressure remains elevated, the diagnosis is open-angle glaucoma with narrow angles, where the narrow angles do not contribute to the elevated pressure.

Thymoxamine has been suggested as a potential treatment in pigmentary glaucoma and pigmentary dispersion syndrome. Campbell[269] has postulated that mechanical rubbing between the anterior ciliary zonules and the peripheral iris in predisposed eyes is the cause of the loss of iris pigment. A drug such as thymoxamine, which can cause a flat and taut iris without affecting accommodation, may reduce or prevent the mechanical contact between the iris and the zonules and may be useful for long-term treatment of the glaucoma.

The effect of thymoxamine on intraocular pressure has also been investigated in healthy eyes and in patients with open-angle glaucoma. Marmion[270] reported that 1.0% thymoxamine reduced intraocular pressure in nonglaucomatous eyes. Subsequently 1.0% thymoxamine was tested in patients with open-angle glaucoma,[271,272] but no significant reduction in intraocular pressure occurred. Moreover, there was a slight reduction in the facility of outflow,[271] making thymoxamine an ineffective drug for the treatment of glaucoma.

Thymoxamine may be useful for reversal of eyelid retraction in patients with Graves' ophthalmopathy. Dixon and associates[273] observed substantial narrowing in 75% of palpebral fissures in patients with various types of lid retraction after topical application of 0.5% thymoxamine. The nonresponders included 1 patient with an orbital pseudotumor and patients with longstanding and stable euthyroid eye disease. The effect lasted for 5 hours following thymoxamine administration.

Another potential use for thymoxamine may be the treatment of persistent mydriasis after penetrating keratoplasty for keratoconus. This mydriasis is usually nonresponsive to direct and indirectly acting cholinergic agonists. Wand and Grant[257] have reported success with topical 0.5% thymoxamine in 1 case of persistent mydriasis in which both pilocarpine and echothiophate failed to constrict the pupil.

More recently, thymoxamine 0.1% in a buffered solution has been administered intracamerally during extracapsular cataract extraction.[274] Thymoxamine 0.1%, when administered with ACh, produces a more profound and prolonged miosis than does ACh alone.

SIDE EFFECTS

The topical ocular use of thymoxamine is accompanied by a transient stinging sensation.[264,266] The burning sensation is less intense with the 0.5% solution compared with the 1.0% solution. Conjunctival hyperemia may last several hours following application of the 0.5% solution,[266] and chemosis may result with higher concentrations.[254]

Ptosis has been observed with topical thymoxamine in concentrations exceeding 1.0%. Two cases of drug-induced Horner's syndrome have been reported,[254,264] but this has not occurred with use of the 0.5% solution.[266]

Thymoxamine appears to be relatively free of side effects when administered by the oral, intravenous, or subcutaneous routes. Reported effects have included facial flushing, vertigo, headaches, nausea, and diarrhea.[257]

Tolazoline and Phentolamine

Although classified as α-receptor blocking agents, these two drugs have a wide range of pharmacologic actions including antihistaminic, cholinergic, and adrenergic stimulation as well as antagonism of adrenergic activity. When given intravenously, they produce both vasodilation and cardiac stimulation.[151]

The ocular use of these two agents is limited. Tolazoline has been used both orally and by retrobulbar injection to treat central retinal artery occlusion.[275] Although tolazoline can dilate retinal vessels, successful treatment of this disorder is rare due to the disease process itself. Tolazoline therapy has also been unsuccessfully attempted for arrest of degenerative macular disease.[276]

Although both these drugs have been suggested for control of ocular hypertension, their clinical usefulness in glaucoma therapy has not been substantiated.

Dapiprazole

PHARMACOLOGY

A more recently developed α-adrenergic antagonist, dapiprazole, produces miosis and reduces intraocular pressure following topical instillation on the eye.[277-280] Concentrations ranging from 0.12% to 1.5% significantly reduce pupil size and intraocular pressure in both normal and glaucomatous eyes.[277,278] The miotic effect is concentration-dependent and can last up to 6 hours following instillation. Intraocular pressure can be reduced significantly for up to 6 hours.[277]

CLINICAL USES

Dapiprazole has been most extensively studied in Europe to treat both angle-closure and open-angle glaucoma, and also to reverse mydriasis due to tropicamide. Dapiprazole 0.25% and 0.5% is effective in cases of angle-closure glaucoma,[277-279] and in patients with gonioscopically narrow angles, the drug has been effective in preventing angle closure.[279]

The miosis produced by dapiprazole 0.5% begins 10 minutes following instillation and results in a significant reduction in pupil size, compared with the contralateral eye treated with 1% tropicamide alone.[280,281] Since the miosis is due to α-receptor blockade in the iris dilator muscle, there is no shifting of the iris-lens diaphragm with subsequent shallowing of the anterior chamber.

SIDE EFFECTS

The topical use of dapiprazole can be accompanied by a burning sensation and conjunctival hyperemia.[277] No significant changes in visual acuity, accommodation, or slit-lamp findings have been reported,[277,279] and systemic changes, such as in pulse rate or blood pressure, have also not been observed.[277]

Adrenergic Neuronal Blocking Agents

These drugs interfere with the release of norepinephrine at the postganglionic adrenergic nerve ending. The resultant effect on the effector sites allows these agents to be clinically useful for ocular conditions such as glaucoma, ptosis, and lid retraction.

Guanethidine

PHARMACOLOGY

Guanethidine exerts its blocking effect on the adrenergic system through a complex mechanism. Initially it causes release of norepinephrine from the nerve ending. This is followed by inhibition of both transmitter release and reuptake of catecholamine into the neuronal stores. A hypersensitivity to adrenergic agonists ensues, evident by their intensified action on the end organs.[151]

The actions of guanethidine on the eye have been demonstrated by continuous recording of pupillary responses following the instillation of a 10% solution[282] (Fig. 3.28). At 30 minutes following instillation of the drug the pupil is widely dilated. This mydriasis is presumed to be due to the release of neurotransmitter from the nerve endings of the dilator muscle. The palpebral fissure also widens. The mydriatic effect gradually attenuates, and at 5 hours following administration of guanethidine the pupil is smaller than is the opposite control. At 24 hours the characteristic features of Horner's syndrome become evident, including miosis, ptosis, and conjunctival congestion. This effect lasts for several days.

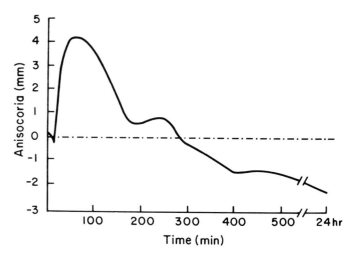

FIGURE 3.28   Continuous recording of pupillary responses following instillation of 10% solution of guanethidine. (From Falter RT, Thompson HS. Mechanism of guanethidine's sympatholytic action: A pupillographic demonstration. In: Blodi FC, ed. Curr Con Ophthalmol, St. Louis: C.V. Mosby Co, 1974;4:65–71.)

CLINICAL USES

Keates and associates[283] first reported the potential usefulness of guanethidine in primary open-angle glaucoma in 1960. Topical administration of 2%, 5%, and 10% solutions reduced intraocular pressure slightly. The ocular hypotensive effect occurs within 1 hour and usually lasts for 3 to 4 hours. Similar effects on intraocular pressure have been observed by Paterson and Paterson[271] with concentrations ranging from 1% to 5%. Patients with primary open-angle glaucoma were instructed to apply the drug twice daily. The results demonstrated an initial effective reduction in intraocular pressure that lasted for about 1 month, at which time little ocular hypotensive effect remained. The reduction in intraocular pressure is believed to be due to an increase in facility of outflow, followed at approximately 12 hours by inhibition of aqueous formation.

Since tissues treated with guanethidine become sensitized to adrenergic stimulation, the ocular effects of combining adrenergic agonists with guanethidine have been studied. Jablonski[284] demonstrated that 5% guanethidine potentiated the mydriatic effects of both topical 10% phenylephrine and subconjunctival injections of epinephrine.

The combined effects of guanethidine and epinephrine for control of primary open-angle glaucoma have also been investigated.[271,285–288] Paterson and Paterson[271] observed a greater reduction of intraocular pressure when 5% guanethidine was combined with 1.0% epinephrine (Fig. 3.29). Moreover, the reduction in pressure was still maintained after 12 months. However, side effects occurred frequently with these concentrations. Lower concentrations of guanethidine and epinephrine appear to reduce the incidence of these adverse effects. Concentrations of guanethidine ranging from

0.25% to 1.0% have been combined with 0.25% to 1.0% epinephrine and compared with 1% epinephrine alone.[286–288] The ocular hypotensive effect of 1.0% guanethidine with 0.5% epinephrine was greater than with 1.0% epinephrine alone.

Guanethidine is also of value in the treatment of lid retraction.[289] Topical 10% guanethidine produces both cosmetic and symptomatic improvement in patients with lid retraction associated with Graves' ophthalmopathy.

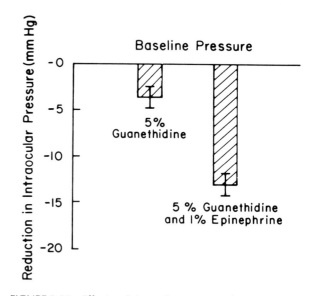

FIGURE 3.29   Effect on intraocular pressure of 5% guanethidine alone and combined with 1% epinephrine. (From Paterson HD, Paterson G. Drug therapy of glaucoma. Br J Ophthalmol 1972; 56:288–294.)

SIDE EFFECTS

Adverse effects with combined use of epinephrine and guanethidine are somewhat greater than with use of 1% epinephrine alone.[286] Persistent hyperemia and slight ocular pain occur more frequently with combined use.

6-Hydroxydopamine (6-OHDA)

PHARMACOLOGY

This agent is structurally similar to norepinephrine. It differs in the position of one hydroxyl group that, in the case of 6-OHDA, is on the benzene ring, while in norepinephrine it is on the β carbon of the side chain.[132]

Administration of 6-OHDA results in selective destruction of peripheral and central adrenergic nerve terminals.[290] The initial effect, however, is adrenergic stimulation and appears to be due to the endogenous release of norepinephrine. This is followed by a response comparable to adrenergic nerve section or the administration of guanethidine. The end result is a reversible chemical sympathectomy. Adrenergic hypersensitization occurs to exogenously administered catecholamines.[291]

The mechanism of action of 6-OHDA is not well understood. The amine is thought to accumulate in the adrenergic neuron. Uptake by the neuronal amine pump seems to be a prerequisite for its destructive effect on the nerve terminals.[290]

The ocular effects of 6-OHDA were first investigated by Holland and Mims in 1971.[291] Studies in experimental animals revealed that topical application of 6-OHDA by a special corneoscleral contact lens or by subconjunctival injection lowers intraocular pressure and produces a hypersensitization to both α- and β-adrenergic agonists. Subsequently it was shown that 6-OHDA can also induce ocular hypersensitization to epinephrine in patients with open-angle glaucoma[292,293] (Fig. 3.30). The intraocular pressure reduction begins within a few hours following administration of 6-OHDA, with a maximum effect occurring at about 3 days and returns to baseline levels within 2 to 3 weeks. Between the second and third weeks a hypersensitivity reaction to topical epinephrine occurs.[293]

When used in conjunction with topical epinephrine, a single subconjunctival injection of 6-OHDA may significantly decrease the intraocular pressure for about 12 weeks in over half the patients in whom it is used.[293,294] Following administration of 6-OHDA alone, the mean decrease in intraocular pressure may be 50% during the first 14 days, and following topical administration of 1% epinephrine, the mean reduction in intraocular pressure may be as much as 40%, which lasts for as long as 3 months.[293] Because of the short-lived effect

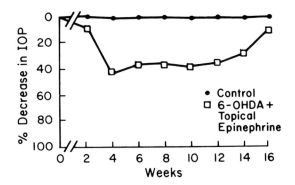

FIGURE 3.30 **Effect on intraocular pressure of 6-hydroxydopamine followed by topical epinephrine 1% compared with the control eye receiving usual glaucoma medication. (From Diamond JG. 6-hydroxydopamine in the treatment of open-angle glaucoma. Arch Ophthalmol 1976;94:41–47. Copyright 1976, American Medical Association.)**

of 6-OHDA, chemical sympathectomy with this agent is of little practical value when it is used alone for glaucoma therapy, and therefore must be used in conjunction with topical epinephrine.

Mydriasis appears as early as 1 hour following instillation of 6-OHDA. The pupil returns toward a miotic state within 24 hours. During the hypersensitivity phase to epinephrine, instillation of 0.125% to 2.0% epinephrine produces mydriasis.[294]

CLINICAL USES

Chemical sympathectomy with 6-OHDA followed by topical therapy with epinephrine has demonstrated considerable potential in the medical management of patients with primary open-angle glaucoma. Following chemical sympathectomy, the previously innervated tissue becomes hypersensitive to adrenergic agonists, and the subsequent use of topical epinephrine may be employed to reduce intraocular pressure more effectively. Although still an experimental procedure and therefore not used in clinical practice, the use of 6-OHDA with epinephrine offers promise for its clinical effectiveness in reducing intraocular pressure.

In the treatment of glaucoma, 6-OHDA has been used in concentrations of 1% and 2% and has been administered by subconjunctival injection or by iontophoresis. In one study[294] a second application of 6-OHDA was required after 12 weeks in 37% of patients and after 20 weeks in 67%. Thus, since most patients will require further administration of 6-OHDA within 5 months of initial therapy, iontophoresis appears to be a much more practical method of drug delivery; repeated administration of 6-OHDA by subconjunctival injection may cause subconjunctival scarring.[295,296]

Cholinergic Agents

Cholinergic Innervation to the Eye

The cholinergic innervation to the eye originates in the Edinger-Westphal nucleus (EWN) located within the mesencephalon. Preganglionic parasympathetic fibers emerge from the EWN, exit the CNS through the third cranial nerve (oculomotor), and proceed to the ciliary ganglion, where they synapse with postganglionic fibers and enter the globe through the short ciliary nerves and pass to and terminate on the iris sphincter muscle and ciliary body[2] (Fig. 3.31). The neurotransmitter at the ciliary ganglion synapse is ACh. The neurotransmitter at the effector cell junction, i.e., the sphincter and ciliary muscle, is also ACh.

Because of its variable size, the pupil controls the amount of light reaching the retina. Pupil size is determined predominantly by varying degrees of parasympathetic innervation to the sphincter muscle, which contracts accordingly, resulting in a corresponding degree of pupillary constriction. Sympathetic innervation, which is secondary, maintains a persistent tone in the dilator muscle, aiding relaxation of the sphincter and resulting in dilation. The degree of parasympathetic innervation to the sphincter muscle is governed by two important pupillary reflexes: the light reflex and the near reflex. The near reflex consists of the accommodation and convergence reflexes. Afferent pathways of both light and near reflexes terminate in the EWN. The efferent pathway from the EWN is the same for both the light reflex and the near reflex (see Fig. 3.31).

The lacrimal gland also receives parasympathetic innervation. Preganglionic fibers originate near the superior salivary nucleus in the pons. They travel with the seventh nerve until they join and synapse with the sphenopalatine ganglion. The postganglionic fibers become part of the fifth nerve and pass to the lacrimal gland through the lacrimal nerve (see Fig. 3.31).[297] Although the mechanism of neural control over normal tear secretion is poorly understood, it is clear that parasympathetic innervation is responsible for tear production in weeping.[297]

Other targets of cholinergic stimulation or blockade by drugs include the cornea, lens, and retina.

Cornea

The mammalian corneal epithelium contains very high levels of ACh and correspondingly high activities of choline acetylase and acetylcholinesterase. There is a certain amount of data suggesting that corneal epithelial nerves that mediate corneal sensation are cholinergic. It appears, however, that the cholinergic system may have additional roles, one possibility being the regulation of corneal hydration and epithelial ionic transport.[298]

Lens

The lens capsule epithelium contains cholinesterase (ChE).[299,300] Anticholinesterases such as demecarium and echothiophate have produced lens opacities, but this effect is not attributed to cholinesterase inhibition.[301] There is speculation that anticholinesterase-induced lenticular opacities result from proliferation of epithelial cells due to wrinkling of the lens capsule brought about by prolonged decreased tension on the zonules.

Retina

Several studies performed on mammalian retinas, including those of humans, have demonstrated the presence of significant activity of choline acetyltrans-

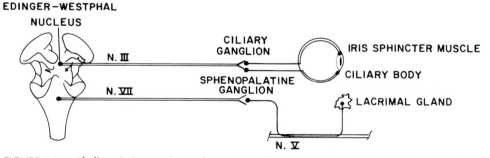

FIGURE 3.31   **Cholinergic innervation to the eye (iris sphincter muscle and ciliary body) and lacrimal gland.**

ferase,[302–304] ACh,[305,306] and acetylcholinesterase,[304,307–309] most of which occurs in the amacrine cells of the inner plexiform layer. These results provide considerable evidence suggesting the existence of a cholinergic amacrine system in the retina.

Cholinergic Receptors

Cholinergic receptors have been identified in ocular tissue as well as in other peripheral autonomic effectors by the use of pharmacologic and biochemical procedures. In both human and nonhuman mammalian iris sphincter tissue[310–314] and ciliary body,[315–319] these receptors have been shown to be of the muscarinic type. Muscarinic agonist action at these receptor sites constricts the pupil, contracts the ciliary muscle, and, in general, lowers intraocular pressure.

In the human retina, evidence has been offered for a population of both muscarinic and nicotinic receptors in the inner plexiform layer,[320] which suggests that cholinergic neurotransmission occurs in the retina. One related clinical implication is that cholinergic agonists and antagonists may have the potential to affect human vision.

Cholinergic Agonists

Cholinergic agonists are drugs that produce biologic responses similar to those of acetylcholine. They are also known as *parasympathomimetics, cholinomimetics,* or *miotics.* Certain ones have been employed clinically for their ocular therapeutic effects and for some diagnostic purposes. Therapeutic uses include the management of glaucoma (see Chapter 29) and the treatment of accommodative esotropia (see Chapter 28). As diagnostic agents, they have been useful in tests for pupillary abnormalities (see Chapter 18). They have also been employed to reverse the effects of topical ophthalmic diagnostic agents such as cycloplegics and mydriatics. In addition, they can be administered intraocularly to induce miosis during intraocular surgery.

Cholinergic agonists have been referred to as *parasympathomimetics* because they mimic the actions of the parasympathetic nervous system. In the case of certain cholinergic drugs such as physostigmine and echothiophate, the term is inadequate, since some of these agents have somatic effects in addition to cholinergic action. Cholinergic agonists are usually classified according to their mechanism of action, i.e., direct-acting or indirect-acting (Table 3.13). The direct-acting drugs activate cholinergic receptors directly at receptor

TABLE 3.13
Classification of Cholinergic Agonists

Direct-acting
  Acetylcholine
  Methacholine
  Pilocarpine
  Carbachol

Indirect-acting (anticholinesterases)
  Reversible
    Physostigmine
    Neostigmine
    Edrophonium
    Demecarium
  Irreversible
    Echothiophate
    Diisopropylfluorophosphate (DFP)

sites on the postsynaptic membranes of the nerves and postjunctional membranes of effector cells or at the neuroeffector junction. The indirect-acting drugs exert their cholinergic effects primarily by inhibiting cholinesterase enzymes, thereby making increased amounts of ACh available at cholinergic receptors.

The cholinesterase inhibitors are subclassified as reversible and irreversible (see Table 3.13). Physostigmine, a reversible ChE inhibitor, is a tertiary amine with a carbamyl ester linkage (Fig. 3.32). In cationic form it associates with the active center of the enzyme, serving as an alternate substrate. This interaction cleaves the alcoholic portion of physostigmine and produces the carbamylated enzyme that is stable for 2 to 4 hours.[321] Subsequently the inhibited enzyme is hydrolyzed and regenerated (Fig. 3.33). Because the enzyme is regenerated, the enzyme inhibitory action of physostigmine is considered to be reversible. Neostigmine, a quaternary amine (see Fig. 3.32), has the same mechanism. Edrophonium, a simple analog of neostigmine that lacks a carbamyl group (see Fig. 3.32), imparts a less potent and shorter inhibition of enzyme action.

The irreversible cholinesterase inhibitors (Fig. 3.34) are exemplified by the organophosphate compound, echothiophate iodide. This agent inhibits cholinesterases by forming a covalent bond on the esteratic site of the enzyme (Fig. 3.35). The consequence of this action is the long-term inactivation of cholinesterases, thus referred to as being *irreversible.* Agents of this type are indicated for use in conditions that require a relatively long duration of action, such as accommodative esotropia and advanced primary open-angle glaucoma. Another organophosphate with similar indications and effects is diisopropylfluorophosphate (DFP).

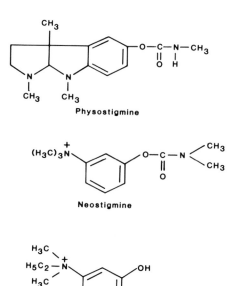

FIGURE 3.32 **Reversible cholinesterase inhibitors.**

Direct-Acting Agents

ACETYLCHOLINE

As mentioned previously, ACh is the neurotransmitter released from presynaptic nerve endings at the following peripheral sites.

- All autonomic ganglia, i.e., sympathetic as well as parasympathetic

- Adrenal medulla
- Postganglionic cholinergic nerve endings, i.e., all parasympathetic postganglionic nerves, and postganglionic sympathetic nerves that innervate generalized sweat glands and blood vessels of skeletal muscles
- Somatic nerves at the skeletal neuromuscular junction.

The biologic activity elicited by the release of ACh at these sites is controlled and terminated primarily by

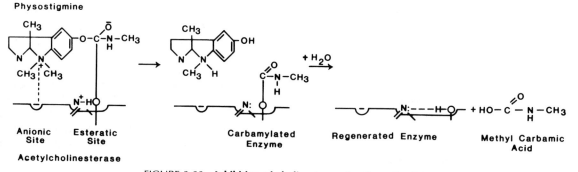

FIGURE 3.33 **Inhibition of cholinesterase by physostigmine.**

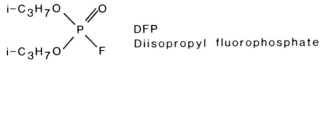

DFP
Diisopropyl fluorophosphate

Echothiophate Iodide
Phospholine Iodide

FIGURE 3.34   **Irreversible cholinesterase inhibitors.**

enzymatically mediated hydrolysis of ACh. Other influences are diffusion away from the receptors and protein binding. The enzymes involved in the cleavage (hydrolysis) of acetylcholine into choline and acetic acid are acetylcholinesterase (AChE, specific or true cholinesterase) and butyrocholinesterase (BuChE, nonspecific or pseudocholinesterase).

Certain anticholinesterases are employed clinically as ophthalmic therapeutic agents. Note also that certain insecticides contain organophosphate compounds that have anticholinesterase activity. Undue exposure to these chemicals can result in adverse effects commensurate with parasympathetic predominance—gastrointestinal disturbances, bradycardia, increased salivation, lacrimation, mucous secretions, wheezing, miosis, and ciliary spasm. Since ACh is a neurotransmitter at certain CNS sites, excessive cholinergic stimulation resulting from significant amounts of cholinergic drug passage into the CNS can produce toxic effects ranging from mental confusion to generalized convulsions.[321]

ACh is commercially available as an ophthalmic preparation (acetylcholine chloride solution 1:100) (Table 3.14) and is indicated for rapid and complete miosis during surgical procedures such as cataract extraction, penetrating keratoplasty, and iridectomy. Since it is ineffective when applied topically to the cornea, it must be placed directly onto the exposed iris during the surgical procedure. However, acetylcholine ophthalmic solution appears to be safe and effective for intraocular use. As indicated previously, ACh exerts its cholinergic-stimulating effects by interacting directly with cholinergic receptors. Its effects are brief due to its susceptibility to cholinesterases. Prolonged miosis may be achieved by applying a longer-acting miotic (e.g., pilocarpine) topically on the cornea before applying a surgical dressing; however, the disadvantages associated with longer-acting agents include increased postoperative pain and inflammation. ACh is not practical in the management of glaucoma and for other therapeutic and diagnostic uses because of its short duration of action and relative ineffectiveness when applied topically to the eye.

METHACHOLINE (MECHOLYL)

Pharmacology.   Methacholine chloride, a choline ester, is a direct-acting cholinergic agonist. Since it is hydrolyzed by AChE at a slower rate than ACh and is resistant to hydrolysis by pseudocholinesterase, its action is more prolonged, and therefore it is potentially useful as a medicinal agent. Its peripheral site of action is predominantly at muscarinic receptors; it lacks significant nicotinic action. Accordingly, systemically administered methacholine produces cholinergic effects with relative selectivity for the cardiovascular system. These effects vary with the dose and route of administration. A moderate vasodilatation and transient reduction in blood pressure with compensatory tachycardia or serious cardiac arrhythmias may occur following systemic administration.

Echothiophate Iodide

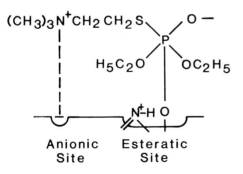

Anionic
Site

Esteratic
Site

Acetylcholinesterase

FIGURE 3.35   **Inhibition of cholinesterase by echothiophate.**

TABLE 3.14
Commercially Available Direct-Acting Miotics

Generic Name	Trade Name	Manufacturer	Concentration
Acetylcholine chloride	Miochol	Iolab	Powder, 20 mg, for reconstitution to 1:100 solution
Carbachol, intraocular	Miostat	Alcon	0.01%
Carbachol, topical	Isopto Carbachol	Alcon	0.75, 1.5, 2.25, 3%
Pilocarpine HCL solution	Pilocarpine HCl	(Various)	0.5, 1, 2, 4, 6%
	Isopto Carpine	Alcon	0.25, 0.5, 1, 2, 3, 4, 5, 6, 8, 10%
	Pilocar	Iolab	0.5, 1, 2, 4, 6%
	Adsorbocarpine	Alcon	1, 2, 4%
	Akarpine	Akorn	1, 2, 4%
	Almocarpine	Ayerst	1, 2, 4%
Pilocarpine nitrate solution	P.V. Carpine Liquifilm	Allergan	1, 2, 4%
Pilocarpine insert	Ocusert Pilo-20	Alza	20 µg/hr
	Ocusert Pilo-40		40 µg/hr
Pilocarpine gel	Pilopine H.S.	Alcon	4%

Clinical Uses. From an ophthalmic standpoint methacholine is important only from a historical perspective, since it is no longer commercially available. Methacholine was rarely administered systemically, probably because of its potential adverse cardiovascular effects. However, its structural characteristics rendered it useful as a topically applied ophthalmic drug in the diagnosis of Adie's pupil. It is a quaternary amine and is highly polar, and therefore is poorly soluble in lipids. When several drops of a 2.5% solution (without wetting agent) are applied topically to eyes that have normally innervated pupils and intact corneal epithelial cells, no significant pupillary response occurs because inadequate amounts of drug penetrate the cornea into the aqueous. However, when the same solution is applied to an eye with Adie's pupil, an intense miosis results due to supersensitivity to methacholine.[322]

In Adie's pupil the parasympathetic sensitization has been attributed to a lesion in the ciliary ganglion or in its postganglionic fibers. A positive reaction to the methacholine test has also been reported in patients with familial dysautonomia,[323] hereditary amyloidosis,[324] and diabetes mellitus.[325] In addition, positive reactions can occur in the normally innervated iris of eyes with damaged corneal epithelium. This may occur in eyes to which wetting agents or topical anesthetics have been applied immediately before the test, in patients with dry eye syndrome, or after tonometry.[326]

PILOCARPINE

Pharmacology. An alkaloid of natural plant origin, pilocarpine is a direct-acting cholinergic agonist used primarily to treat glaucoma. Pilocarpine is a tertiary amine (Fig. 3.36) with a dominant action at muscarinic sites both peripherally and centrally. Like other choline esters, it affects the cardiovascular system, exocrine glands, and smooth muscle.

The effects of pilocarpine on the cardiovascular system are complex. Small doses injected intravenously briefly reduce blood pressure, as would be anticipated because the response to muscarinic receptor stimulation in the vasculature is vasodilatation with a subsequent fall in blood pressure. However, some evidence suggests that there are postsynaptic muscarinic receptors in autonomic ganglia that may mediate a vasopressor action.[327] Therefore, under certain circumstances pilocarpine can increase blood pressure.

Exocrine glands are particularly sensitive to pilocarpine. Pilocarpine, 5 to 15 mg administered subcutaneously, has been used both to increase salivation and as a diaphoretic. Increased salivation, sweating, and mucous membrane and gastric secretions have been reported as side effects of pilocarpine administration.[327]

The action of pilocarpine on smooth muscle (effectors containing muscarinic receptors) generally results in contraction. Pilocarpine enhances the tone and motility in the gastrointestinal tract, ureters, urinary bladder, gallbladder, and ciliary ducts. Since bronchiolar musculature contracts, asthmatic attacks may be precipitated. The response of intraocular smooth muscle to pilocarpine is pupillary constriction, spasm of accommodation, and reduction of intraocular pressure.[327]

Although the precise mechanism by which pilocarpine reduces intraocular pressure has not been established, the most widely accepted explanation involves direct stimulation of the longitudinal muscle of the

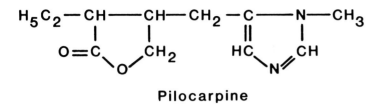

Pilocarpine

FIGURE 3.36 **Molecular structure of pilocarpine.**

ciliary body, which, in turn, affects the scleral spur, widening the trabecular spaces and allowing for increased aqueous outflow.[328] On long-term administration, there is evidence that pilocarpine may also decrease aqueous formation. There appears to be no significant difference between healthy and glaucomatous eyes, including those with ocular hypertension, in the degree to which pilocarpine reduces intraocular pressure. In each case pilocarpine reduces intraocular pressure about 10% to 40%.[328] On long-term administration pilocarpine has increasing hypotensive effects in concentrations up to 4%, but when used in higher concentrations it appears to have little additional effect.[329] This ocular hypotensive response is influenced by the ocular pigmentation. Blue eyes demonstrate maximal ocular hypotensive responses, while darkly pigmented eyes demonstrate a relative resistance to intraocular pressure reduction (Table 3.15).[330] This dose-response effect should be considered when treating black patients with glaucoma. Such patients may require pilocarpine solutions in concentrations exceeding 4%.

Pilocarpine also exerts a substantial influence on the diurnal variation of intraocular pressure. The drug significantly reduces the diurnal intraocular pressure variation in patients with glaucoma (Fig. 3.37).[331]

Because of its activity at cholinergic receptor sites (muscarinic) on the iris sphincter and ciliary muscles, pilocarpine causes pupillary constriction and varying degrees of accommodative spasm, depending on the patient's age.

In addition, most eyes with primary open-angle glaucoma that are treated with pilocarpine will demonstrate narrowing of the anterior chamber angle and thickening of the crystalline lens following each instillation of the drug (Figs. 3.38 and 3.39).[332] These effects are measurable within 15 minutes, maximum in 1 hour, and usually dissipate after 2 hours.[332] However, in about 15% of eyes with primary open-angle glaucoma undergoing long-term pilocarpine therapy, the drug induces a deepening of the anterior chamber and flattening of the lens, an effect that is not apparently observed in healthy eyes.[332] The reasons for this paradoxical cycloplegia are unknown.

Clinical Uses

Glaucoma Therapy.   Since its introduction into clinical practice in 1876, pilocarpine has remained the most useful miotic for management of primary open-angle glaucoma, acute angle-closure glaucoma, and many secondary glaucomas. Pilocarpine is commercially available as an ophthalmic solution in concentrations from 0.25% to 10% (see Table 3.14). It is commercially available in concentrations from 1% to 6% in combination with 1% epinephrine bitartrate (0.5% free epinephrine base). The 2% concentration is available in combination with physostigmine. These preparations are designed to simplify drug usage when the combination of agents is warranted. In addition, a sustained release, membrane-bound drug delivery system (Ocu-

TABLE 3.15
Mean Applanation Intraocular Pressures after Topical Pilocarpine in Open-Angle Glaucoma Patients with Differing Iris Color (± SEM)

Group	Baseline R	Baseline L	1% Solution R	1% Solution L	4% Solution R	4% Solution L	8% Solution R	8% Solution L
Blue[a] (N = 8)	29.28 ±2.23	29.28 ±1.84	21.63 ±1.25	30.63 ±2.48	19.00 ±0.91	29.37 ±2.98	18.80 ±1.41	29.48 ±2.73
Brown[a] (N = 7)	28.55 ±1.93	29.05 ±2.15	24.58 ±2.24	29.00 ±2.52	20.10 ±2.10	27.28 ±2.78	20.14 ±2.43	28.00 ±2.46
Black[a] (N = 9)	28.15 ±2.03	28.29 ±1.94	24.22 ±1.41	28.10 ±1.30	22.10 ±1.60	27.11 ±1.27	21.11 ±1.61	27.10 ±1.38

[a]Blue, blue-eyed white patients; Brown, brown-eyed white patients; Black, black patients.
Modified from Harris LS, Galin MA. Effect of ocular pigmentation on hypotensive response to pilocarpine. Am J Ophthalmol 1971; 72:923–925.

DIURNAL INTRAOCULAR PRESSURES IN PATIENTS (14 EYES) WITH GLAUCOMA

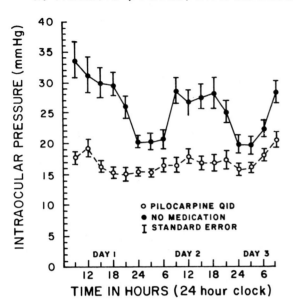

FIGURE 3.37   **Effect of pilocarpine on diurnal variation of intraocular pressure. (From Worthen DM. Effect of pilocarpine drops on the diurnal intraocular pressure variation in patients with glaucoma. Invest Ophthalmol 1976;15:784–787.)**

sert) is available that delivers pilocarpine at carefully controlled rates of 20 or 40 μg/hr. More recently, pilocarpine has become commercially available as a 4% ophthalmic gel that is supplied in 5 g tubes.[28]

The dosage frequency for pilocarpine solutions is usually 4 times daily. Twice-daily dosage usually results

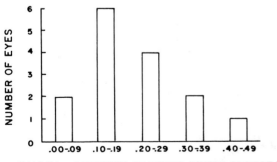

FIGURE 3.38   **Frequency distribution of maximal changes in anterior chamber depth found in 85% of cases following instillation of 1% to 4% pilocarpine. (From Abramson DH, Chang S, Coleman J. Pilocarpine therapy in glaucoma. Effects on anterior chamber depth and lens thickness in patients receiving long-term therapy. Arch Ophthalmol 1976;94:914–918. Copyright 1976, American Medical Association.)**

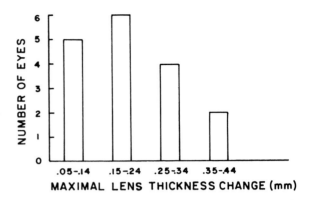

FIGURE 3.39   **Frequency distribution of maximal changes in lens thickness found in 85% of cases following instillation of 1% to 4% pilocarpine. (From Abramson DH, Chang S, Coleman J. Pilocarpine therapy in glaucoma. Effects on anterior chamber depth and lens thickness in patients receiving long-term therapy. Arch Ophthalmol 1976;94:914–918. Copyright 1976, American Medical Association.)**

in inadequate control of intraocular pressure.[333] Moreover, because patients instructed to use drops 4 times daily frequently will use them only 2 or 3 times per day, it is often unwise to recommend the use of pilocarpine solutions in dosage frequencies less than 4 times daily. Although pilocarpine is available in concentrations exceeding 4%, there is usually no advantage in using such concentrations except in black patients and in patients with very darkly pigmented irides.[332,333]

Pilocarpine remains one of the most useful drugs in the management of glaucoma. Compared with other ocular hypotensive agents, pilocarpine significantly reduces intraocular pressure in most patients while causing relatively few side effects. It is particularly useful for reducing intraocular pressure in patients with primary open-angle glaucoma and for relieving acute angle-closure attacks. The use of pilocarpine for hastening the resolution of hyphema has been advocated, although such use is of unproved benefit.[332,333]

The maximum ocular hypotensive effect achieved with the Ocusert system occurs about 2 hours after insertion of the device and lasts about 7 days (see Fig. 2.20). Thus, this device facilitates patient compliance because it requires less frequent application compared with the instillation of pilocarpine drops 4 times daily. The Ocusert Pilo-20 delivers about 20 μg of pilocarpine per hour and has a hypotensive effect approximately equivalent to 1% to 2% pilocarpine solution instilled every 6 hours.[334] The Ocusert Pilo-40 delivers about 40 μg of pilocarpine per hour and has a hypotensive effect approximately equivalent to 2% to 4% pilocarpine solution instilled every 6 hours. The Ocusert is supplied in packages containing 8 individual sterile units. The advantages of the Ocusert compared with pilocarpine solutions can include improved patient compliance, convenience, and continuous control of intraocular pressure. In addition, disturbances of vision are less pronounced than with the topical drug.[335] Miosis with the Ocusert is nearly always less intense and less variable than with pilocarpine solutions. In general, the Ocusert provides less frequent, less intense, and fewer fluctuations of vision (refraction, distance vision, near vision, and miosis) compared with pilocarpine solutions.[336]

The visual effects from the Ocusert Pilo-20 system do not differ substantially from those of the Ocusert Pilo-40 system, except for some additional miosis with the latter. Although drug-induced myopic changes may occur with the Ocusert, these are generally low and are more easily corrected with spectacles than are the more highly variable refractive changes associated with pilocarpine drops.[336] Since the Ocusert is sterile and is packaged without preservatives, allergic reactions attributable to a preservative are eliminated. Because of its low but constant rate of drug release, the Ocusert system delivers only one-fourth to one-eighth the total pilocarpine dosage administered by topical drops during 7 days. Thus, the risk of systemic as well as ocular side effects is decreased.

Major disadvantages associated with the Ocusert include difficulty with retention and unnoticed loss of the unit from the eye, rupture of the membrane resulting in excessive medication delivery, and high cost compared with pilocarpine solutions. Several studies[336,337] have shown that only about 50% of patients are successful in wearing the device after 3 months. The major reasons for discontinuing the device usually relate to discomfort, difficulty in retaining the device, and difficulty with insertion and removal. The most critical period of adjustment appears to be the first 2 weeks. Novak and Stewart[336] found that 71% of the unsuccessful patients discontinued the unit by the end of the first week. Age may also be a significant factor in success. Novak and Stewart[336] found that 74% of the unsuccessful patients were age 60 years or older. Because of the problems of retention, foreign body sensation, difficulty with insertion and removal, and high cost, the Ocusert has not achieved widespread popularity as a drug delivery system for pilocarpine.

The importance of proper patient selection for the Ocusert cannot be overemphasized. Since patients must be motivated to learn the proper insertion, removal, and use of the device, it is helpful to point out, before the patient uses the unit, the potential minor problems associated with the device, including foreign body sensation and difficulty with retention. The Ocusert is of particular benefit for the young glaucoma patient (under 40 years of age) who requires pilocarpine but who cannot tolerate the drug-induced accommodative spasm

and refractive changes associated with pilocarpine solutions or gel. The fact that the Ocusert provides continuous control of intraocular pressure may be a significant advantage for elderly patients whose ability to regularly instill pilocarpine solutions may be questionable. On the other hand, since some degree of manual dexterity is required to insert, position, and remove the device correctly, the Ocusert is a poor choice for patients with severe arthritis, tremors, or other fine motor problems unless the patient has some assistance from a spouse, family member, or attendant. Unfortunately, these patients represent a substantial proportion of the glaucoma population. Older patients who are content with their present therapy and who appear to be reluctant to consider the Ocusert are unlikely to be successful with the device. Likewise, patients who express anxiety regarding foreign objects in the eye are also unlikely to tolerate the device.

The Ocusert can be used concomitantly with various other antiglaucoma medications. The release rate of pilocarpine from the device is not influenced by oral carbonic anhydrase inhibitors or topical solutions of β blockers or epinephrine. In addition, concomitant therapy with topical antibiotics or corticosteroid preparations may be employed, and topical anesthetics and sodium fluorescein can be used for tonometry without removing the device.[28]

The patient should receive detailed instructions in the office on the use of the Ocusert and should demonstrate to the practitioner his or her ability to insert, adjust, and remove the unit. Retention problems can often be solved by instructing the patient to wear the device in the upper fornix, especially while sleeping. If other pilocarpine preparations have been used, these should be discontinued when Ocusert therapy is initiated. However, other concomitant medications may initially be continued but then subsequently discontinued according to how the intraocular pressure responds to the Ocusert. On follow-up, the patient should be questioned about comfort, retention, difficulty with insertion or removal, and convenience. The effect of the device on vision should also be ascertained. If the intraocular pressure is higher than desirable, other antiglaucoma medications may be prescribed. On the other hand, if the intraocular pressure is lower than necessary and the patient is using other medications, the concentrations of these medications can be adjusted accordingly.

The usual dosage of pilocarpine gel is a one-half-inch ribbon applied in the lower conjunctival sac of the affected eye(s) once a day at bedtime. Adverse effects associated with the once-daily dosage of the 4% gel are not significantly different qualitatively or quantitatively from those reported with the 4-times-daily instillation of the 4% drops.[446] Krause and associates,[338] however, have demonstrated that the drops tend to amplify myopia and impair nocturnal visual acuity more than does the gel. Moreover, there was no significant difference between the two dosage forms regarding other parameters such as pupillary diameter, intraocular pressure, visual acuity, and range of accommodation.

Pilocarpine is also indicated, along with other agents, to treat acute angle-closure glaucoma. During an acute angle-closure attack, intraocular pressure is often in excess of 60 mm Hg. At those high pressures the iris sphincter is unresponsive to pilocarpine. Topical β blockers or systemic hyperosmotic agents such as oral glycerin are indicated initially to bring the pressure down to below 50 to 60 mm Hg. In addition, carbonic anhydrase inhibitors such as oral or intravenous acetazolamide are also used. The reduction in vitreous volume by the hyperosmotics helps prevent the forward movement of the lens caused by pilocarpine.[29]

Accommodative Esotropia.   Although pilocarpine has been used therapeutically in the treatment of accommodative esotropia, it is not considered the best drug for this purpose. The anticholinesterase agents are preferred.

Counteracting Effects of Mydriatics.   Pilocarpine 1% is sometimes used to counteract the effects of mydriatics after ocular examination. However, the use of miotics after mydriatics and cycloplegics should be dis-couraged. The clinician should be aware of the ocular effects of pilocarpine when applied after drug-induced mydriasis or cycloplegia. Pilocarpine has a more rapid effect in reversing the dilatation produced by adrenergic mydriatics (e.g., phenylephrine, hydroxyamphetamine) than it does with anticholinergic mydriatics (e.g., cyclopentolate, tropicamide). It has been shown that 1 drop of 1% pilocarpine completely reverses the maximal mydriasis produced by 1 drop of 10% phenylephrine in about 22 minutes.[265] However, a prolonged miosis (4 to 6 hours) follows (Figs. 3.40 and 3.41). An additional disadvantage is a prolonged, annoying accommodative spasm.

As mentioned previously, pilocarpine is not as prompt in reversing anticholinergic-induced maximal mydriasis. Anastasi and associates[265] have shown that 1 drop of 1% pilocarpine takes 3.5 hours to fully reverse the pupil maximally dilated by 1 drop of 0.5% tropicamide and 28 hours to restore to normal the pupil maximally dilated by 1 drop of 2% homatropine. Thus, it appears that 1% pilocarpine is of little value in reversing anticholinergic-induced pupil dilatation.

O'Connor Davies[339] suggests that 0.25% physostigmine (a cholinesterase inhibitor) would be more effective in counteracting the mydriasis induced by anticholinergics because it is more powerful and longer acting than is pilocarpine. However, one should be aware of the disadvantages of strong miotics such as the anticholinesterases and concentrations of pilocar-

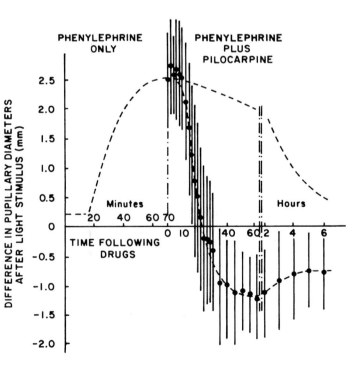

FIGURE 3.40   **Mean mydriasis-miosis time curve for 10% phenylephrine. The upper line shows the mean mydriasis curve, while the lower line shows the mean pupillary diameter following instillation of 1% pilocarpine at the time of maximal mydriasis. The vertical lines represent 1 standard deviation from the mean. (From Anastasi LM, Ogle KN, Kearns TP. Effect of pilocarpine in counteracting mydriasis. Arch Ophthalmol 1968;79:710–715. Copyright 1968, American Medical Association.)**

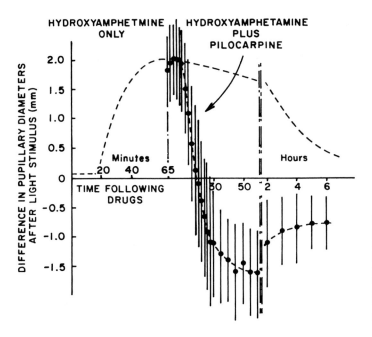

FIGURE 3.41 **Mean mydriasis-miosis time curve for 1% hydroxyamphetamine. The upper line shows the mean mydriasis curve, while the lower line shows the mean pupillary diameter following instillation of 1% pilocarpine at the time of maximal mydriasis. The vertical lines represent 1 standard deviation from the mean. (From Anastasi LM, Ogle KN, Kearns TP. Effect of pilocarpine in counteracting mydriasis. Arch Ophthalmol 1968;79:710–715. Copyright 1968, American Medical Association.)**

pine exceeding 2%. These agents produce strong contractions of the ciliary muscle, causing zonular relaxation with subsequent thickening and forward movement of the lens. These events significantly increase the chances of producing pupillary block, thereby impeding the passage of aqueous from the posterior chamber to the anterior chamber (see Fig. 16.8). In certain patients acute angle-closure glaucoma has been attributed to the use of miotics.[340]

As an alternative to the use of pilocarpine or anticholinesterase agents for constricting dilated pupils following fundus examination, thymoxamine, an α-adrenergic blocker, may be employed. This sympatholytic agent has been recommended by Mapstone[264] for producing effective miosis without the undesirable side effects of cholinergic miotics.

Differential Diagnosis of the Fixed, Dilated Pupil

Pilocarpine is used in the differential diagnosis of the fixed, dilated pupil. Mydriasis of neurologic origin (third-nerve palsy) responds readily to normal concentrations (0.5% to 1%) of pilocarpine, whereas there is no response when the etiology is due to anticholinergic causes. For example, a pupil dilated by inadvertently rubbing atropine or antimuscarinic alkaloids from wild plants such as jimson weed into the eye will not constrict in response to the topical application of pilocarpine 1%. On the other hand, a pupil dilated from third-nerve palsy would promptly constrict in response to instillation of pilocarpine. Thus, the instillation of pilocarpine enables one to differentiate a benign disorder (anticholinergic mydriasis) from a condition with

potentially grave consequences (third-nerve palsy). Specific clinical procedures are discussed in detail in Chapter 18.

The use of pilocarpine 0.125% or 0.1% has replaced the earlier test employing methacholine 2.5% in the diagnosis of Adie's pupil. One drop of the pilocarpine solution applied to each eye will constrict the Adie's pupil, with little or no response observed in the healthy eye. False-positive results may occur in eyes that have abraded corneal epithelium from trauma, contact lens wear or prior application of ophthalmic solutions containing wetting agents. Infrequently, false-negative results may also occur.

Side Effects.   Although pilocarpine is still an important agent for the medical management of many patients with glaucoma, numerous side effects, both ocular and systemic, may be associated with its use in long-term therapy (Tables 3.16 and 3.17). Systemic side effects are rare, but ocular reactions are relatively common and necessitate discontinuation of the drug in a substantial number of patients. One of the most annoying side effects is accommodative spasm, which can last for 2 to 3 hours following instillation of the topical solution. For this reason patients under 40 years of age generally find pilocarpine intolerable.[341] This effect can be minimized by using the lower concentrations, by changing to the gel or Ocusert system, or by treating the symptoms by prescribing a clip-on minus spectacle prescription during the period of blurred vision.[342] Because the accommodative spasm and resulting drug-induced myopia is variable with pilocarpine

TABLE 3.16
Systemic Side Effects of Cholinergic-Anticholinesterase Drugs

- Headache
- Browache
- Marked salivation
- Profuse perspiration
- Nausea
- Vomiting
- Bronchospasm
- Pulmonary edema
- Systemic hypotension
- Bradycardia
- Generalized muscular weakness
- Increased tone and motility of gastrointestinal tract (abdominal pain, diarrhea)
- Respiratory paralysis[a]

[a]May occur when anticholinesterase agents are not discontinued before use of succinylcholine during elective surgery.

drops, permanent spectacle prescriptions usually cannot be prescribed to overcome this problem. Fortunately, these visual disturbances are less frequent and less pronounced in older patients.

In addition to accommodative spasm, a significant ocular problem associated with the use of pilocarpine is miosis. The drug-induced pupillary constriction can visually incapacitate patients with nuclear sclerotic and posterior subcapsular cataracts. Moreover, with long-term use, pilocarpine has been shown to hasten the development of cataract.[343] The reduction in visual acuity or difficulty in dim illumination associated with the miotic pupil can be overcome by the concomitant use of topical phenylephrine.[344,345] In eyes with open angles, dilation of the pupil with phenylephrine does not adversely affect control of intraocular pressure but may

TABLE 3.17
Ocular Side Effects of Cholinergic-Anticholinesterase Drugs

- Accommodative spasm
- Miosis
- Follicular conjunctivitis
- Pupillary block with secondary angle-closure glaucoma
- Band keratopathy[a]
- Allergic blepharoconjunctivitis
- Retinal detachment
- Conjunctival injection[b]
- Lid myokymia[b]
- Anterior subcapsular cataract[c]
- Iris cyst formation[c]

[a]Associated with pilocarpine solutions containing phenylmercuric nitrate as preservative.
[b]Usually subsides within several days or weeks as treatment continues.
[c]Associated with anticholinesterase agents.

provide sufficient improvement in visual acuity to permit the patient to tolerate miotic therapy, which might otherwise prove functionally incapacitating.[344] All topical antiglaucoma medications can be continued while the patient uses 2.5% or 10% phenylephrine in the morning on awakening and then throughout the day and evening as required.[344] The practitioner must be cautious to use only adrenergic mydriatics for this purpose, since anticholinergic mydriatics are well known to elevate intraocular pressure. In addition, such use of phenylephrine is contraindicated in eyes with narrow angles. The pilocarpine should be regularly discontinued for several days at least twice a year so that the pupils may be pharmacologically dilated for careful stereoscopic examination of the optic disc and retina. Not only does this facilitate evaluation of the glaucomatous damage to the optic nerve, but it also serves to prevent permanent miosis, which can result from loss of tone in the iris dilator muscle and fibrosis of the iris sphincter muscle.[343]

Except for accommodative spasm and drug-induced myopia in young patients, the most common side effect of pilocarpine is follicular conjunctivitis.[346] This is usually alleviated by changing the drug therapy to carbachol.

Another side effect of pilocarpine therapy, as mentioned previously, is pupillary block with subsequent angle closure, which almost always occurs in patients with narrow angles who have advancing cataracts.[59] With forward displacement of the lens-iris diaphragm associated with the advancing cataract, and the physiologic action of the pilocarpine, angle closure becomes progressively superimposed on the underlying component of open-angle glaucoma, but often in a subacute or chronic manner.[59]

Band keratopathy is rare in patients receiving long-term pilocarpine therapy. It has been associated with pilocarpine solutions containing phenylmercuric nitrate (PMN) as a preservative.[347] There have been no cases of such band keratopathy developing in patients using pilocarpine without PMN. The calcium deposition is treated with topical applications of ethylenediaminetetraacetic acid (EDTA).

Occasionally allergic conjunctivitis and dermatitis develop after prolonged therapy.[348] In these instances, the preservative, particularly benzalkonium chloride, is usually implicated. Changing to a formulation with a different preservative often alleviates the problem.[348]

The association of miotic therapy and retinal detachment has been a subject of controversy. Although there is no factual evidence linking miotic therapy with retinal detachment, there is circumstantial evidence—time interval between institution of miotic therapy and retinal detachment, and type of detachment—that strong miotics such as the anticholinesterase drugs may precipitate retinal detachment.[349] Since myopic patients and patients with preexisting peripheral retinal disease have a higher incidence of retinal detachment than do those with healthy eyes, it seems possible that such patients might have a greater risk of developing retinal detachment following miotic therapy than do those with normal eyes. Because of the risk of retinal detachment, especially in myopic patients and patients with preexisting peripheral retinal disease, occasional retinal examinations are an important part of the follow-up of patients receiving pilocarpine therapy.

Other ocular side effects include ciliary and conjunctival congestion, lid myokymia, frontal headache, and ocular or periorbital pain.[343] Most of these signs and symptoms tend to disappear within several days or weeks as treatment continues.

Adverse systemic reactions associated with the cholinergic activity of pilocarpine are rare but occasionally observed in patients who misuse their medication or who are given frequent instillations of the drug in the treatment of acute angle-closure glaucoma. The systemic toxicity of pilocarpine can be significant and, occasionally, even life threatening (see Table 3.16).[350] Although the symptoms of nausea, diaphoresis, and weakness frequently experienced by patients undergoing attacks of acute angle closure are often attributed to the glaucoma attack itself, these symptoms are often caused by the high doses of pilocarpine. Other systemic manifestations may include salivation, lacrimation, vomiting, and diarrhea. Bronchiolar spasm and pulmonary edema can occur, causing patients with asthma to sustain a frank asthmatic attack.[348]

When pilocarpine therapy is initiated, the patient should be advised of potential ocular or systemic side effects, with the suggestion that, after 7 to 10 days of continued use, these reactions will either disappear or become tolerable. Providing this information usually improves patient compliance with the medication and improves the patient's confidence in the prescribing practitioner.

Contraindications (Table 3.18).   Pilocarpine is contraindicated in patients with cataract, especially nuclear sclerotic and posterior subcapsular, because it can affect vision and may accelerate the formation of lens opacities.[348] It is generally contraindicated in patients under 40 years of age because of the intolerable accommodative spasm and refractive changes. Since breakdown of the blood-aqueous barrier occurs with the use of pilocarpine and other miotics, particularly in the presence of neovascular and uveitic glaucoma, pilocarpine should be avoided in such patients.[341]

To prevent retinal detachment, miotic therapy should be instituted gradually in patients with high myopia, peripheral retinal disease predisposing to retinal de-

TABLE 3.18
Contraindications to Cholinergic-Anticholinesterase Drugs

- Presence of cataract
- Patients under 40 years of age
- Neovascular and uveitic glaucoma
- History of retinal detachment
- Asthma or history of asthma
- Phakic eyes[a]
- Surgical procedures employing succinylcholine[a]

[a]Anticholinesterase agents

tachment, and in aphakic patients. This can be accomplished by using low concentrations of pilocarpine and increasing as necessary. Likewise, pilocarpine should be avoided in patients with a history of retinal detachment. Ideally, every patient should have a thorough peripheral retinal examination with the binocular indirect ophthalmoscope through widely dilated pupils before initiating pilocarpine therapy.[349] If lattice degeneration or other peripheral retinal disease is found that predisposes to retinal detachment, the area should be prophylactically treated before miotic therapy.[349] During the course of treatment every patient should be instructed to report any flashes, spots, or floaters. These will necessitate prompt reexamination of the peripheral retina with the pupil dilated.

Pilocarpine should generally be avoided in patients with asthma or a history of asthma. As previously mentioned, pilocarpine in concentrations exceeding 2% is contraindicated in acute angle-closure glaucoma because these concentrations can lead to further shallowing of the anterior chamber as well as permanent peripheral anterior synechiae and angle closure.[343] Furthermore, pilocarpine in concentrations of 4% or more should be used with caution in patients with narrow angles, since these concentrations may lead to attacks of acute angle closure.[343]

The necessity of administering pilocarpine solutions 4 times daily makes this form of therapy a poor choice in patients who are likely to demonstrate poor compliance with medication schedules. In these instances the practitioner should select an alternative drug, such as a β blocker or dipivefrin, that requires less frequent instillation.

CARBACHOL

Pharmacology.   Carbachol, another choline ester, is also a direct-acting cholinergic agonist. It is completely resistant to hydrolysis by cholinesterases (AChE or BuChE). Consequently, its tenure in the body is prolonged enough so that it is adequately distributed to low blood-flow areas and has sustained local effects.

Its peripheral actions are both muscarinic and nicotinic (autonomic ganglia in particular), exhibiting a certain degree of selectivity for urinary bladder and gastrointestinal tract. In addition to the drug's direct action, it is believed that carbachol acts partly through an indirect mechanism involving the displacement of ACh from cholinergic nerve terminals.[327]

Carbachol is considerably more potent in its pupillary effects than ACh, methacholine, and pilocarpine in vitro.[327] However, when topically applied to the eye, carbachol exerts less miotic action than do pilocarpine and physostigmine.[351] A plausible explanation is that because carbachol is poorly lipid soluble, its intraocular bioavailability is considerably less than the more lipid-soluble pilocarpine and physostigmine.[29] Corneal penetration of carbachol has been enhanced by the addition of 0.03% benzalkonium chloride (BAK). The clinical implication is that carbachol should be used with caution in eyes with abraded corneas to avoid considerably increased penetration, which can lead to corneal cytotoxic effects, excessive miosis, ciliary spasm, and systemic toxicity.

Clinical Uses.   Carbachol is commercially available as the chloride salt for topical ocular application in concentrations of 0.75%, 1.5%, 2.25%, and 3.0% (see Table 3.14). Although it has been generally stated that carbachol ophthalmic solutions should contain 0.03% BAK to be clinically effective, certain frequently used commercial preparations presently available contain only 0.005% BAK as a preservative. However, these solutions contain 1% hydroxypropyl methylcellulose as a vehicle that promotes more prolonged contact of the active ingredient to the ocular surface, thereby enhancing intraocular penetration. It appears that the latter formulations are clinically effective and less irritating than are those containing 0.03% BAK.[29]

In addition to topical preparations, carbachol is available for intraocular use to produce miosis during surgery. Since carbachol is a potent miotic, this preparation is considerably less concentrated than are the topical solutions. It is available as a 0.01% sterile balanced salt solution with no preservatives and is supplied in 1.5 ml sterile glass disposable vials. The dose is 0.5 ml applied by gentle irrigation. An effective, prolonged miosis ensues 2 to 5 minutes after application.

The topical solutions are indicated for lowering elevated intraocular pressure in primary and some secondary open-angle glaucomas. Carbachol is extremely effective in controlling intraocular pressure in glaucoma, more so than other miotics such as pilocarpine.[352] Since its action is prolonged, carbachol is instilled less frequently than are shorter-acting miotics. It is usually instilled 2 or 3 times daily, but because of

poor ocular penetrability, more frequent applications may be necessary. However, since carbachol has the disadvantage of having relatively more severe local side effects than does pilocarpine, its use is limited to patients who have become allergic or refractory to pilocarpine.

Side Effects.   Systemic absorption from recommended dosages of carbachol used in the treatment of glaucoma appears to be insignificant, since systemic toxicity is not common. However, inadvertent increased systemic absorption of carbachol can produce a variety of effects (see Table 3.16). Ocular effects (see Table 3.17) include miosis, transient conjunctival and ciliary injection, and ciliary spasm with a resultant temporary decrease in visual acuity. Allergy has been rare and retinal detachment has been reported.

Contraindications.   Conditions precluding the use of carbachol include corneal abrasions and known allergies to any of its ingredients (see Table 3.18). The drug should be avoided in anterior uveitis and neovascular glaucoma because its vasodilatory effects cause increased inflammation. Caution should be observed when administering the drug to patients with bronchial asthma, gastrointestinal spasms, peptic ulcers, urinary tract obstructions, acute cardiac failure, and Parkinson's disease. Carbachol should be applied conservatively after procedures that reduce or disrupt the corneal epithelial barrier and conjunctiva such as in gonioscopy or tonometry or after topical anesthesia. As previously mentioned, these procedures promote excessive intraocular and systemic absorption of the drug with resultant increased local side effects and increased probability of systemic effects. If extreme miosis occurs, the patient should be advised to be cautious when driving at night or when engaging in hazardous activities in poor illumination.[28,29]

Anticholinesterase Agents

PHYSOSTIGMINE

Pharmacology.   Physostigmine, an alkaloid originally isolated from the Calabar bean, is a tertiary amine with a carbamyl ester linkage (see Fig. 3.32). It is an indirect-acting cholinergic agonist that exerts its cholinergic action by inhibiting cholinesterases, thus enhancing the effects of endogenous ACh. After a few hours, the inhibited enzyme is regenerated. Because the enzyme inhibition is not permanent, physostigmine is classified as a reversible cholinesterase inhibitor.[321]

Unlike the previously mentioned quaternary compounds, the choline esters, this alkaloid has a high degree of lipid solubility and therefore is readily distributed to central as well as to peripheral tissue. Because of its indirect action, physostigmine acts at those sites where ACh is released by nerve impulses. Because of the diverse locations of cholinergic synapses, both peripheral and central, the pharmacologic responses to physostigmine are potentially complex. Effector organ responses are due to the stimulation of both muscarinic receptors (central and peripheral) and nicotinic receptors (ganglionic and at the skeletal neuromuscular junction).[321]

The net pharmacologic effects, however, are largely influenced by dose and route of administration. Since physostigmine is not usually indicated for systemic administration, systemic side effects occur primarily from overdose of the topical ophthalmic preparation.

The iris sphincter and ciliary muscles continuously receive parasympathetic impulses; therefore, when a solution of physostigmine (0.25% or 0.5%) is applied topically to the eye, it exerts a sustained stimulation of intraocular muscle by inhibiting cholinesterase enzymes, resulting in miosis and spasm of accommodation. Pupillary constriction begins in about 5 to 10 minutes and is maximal in about 30 minutes, remaining so for 3 to 4 hours. Miosis diminishes gradually up to about 12 hours but may be evident for 3 to 4 days, particularly if the ointment is used.[29] Pupillographic studies have shown that physostigmine enhances the pupillary responses to light.[353] The spasm of accommodation begins in about 20 minutes and subsides after 2 to 3 hours if near work (reading, etc.) is not attempted during that period. However, a certain degree of irritability in the ciliary muscle remains, and it is possible that spasm may be elicited at any time. This undesirable effect of physostigmine is a distinct disadvantage compared with pilocarpine. The extent of spasm and associated ocular discomfort is dose related; that is, it occurs minimally with the lower concentration (0.25%).

The enhancement of ciliary muscle contraction by this drug has been shown to increase the accommodation induced per given amount of convergence.[354]

Therefore, accommodative blur in young patients being treated with topical physostigmine would not be an unexpected complaint.

The local and intraocular vascular responses to physostigmine are significant. Marked conjunctival vasodilatation occurs after instillation. Capillary permeability increases. The increased vasodilatation in the anterior uveal region is opposed by the contracted ciliary muscle, diminishing blood supply to that area. Simultaneously the dilated choroidal veins become more patent and facilitate blood flow away from the uveal tract. As a result, the overall intraocular content of fluid decreases, and there is a certain degree of intraocular pressure reduction.[355] In addition to its vascular ocular hypotensive effects, physostigmine lowers intraocular pressure by stimulating the longitudinal muscle of the ciliary body, opening up the trabecular meshwork and increasing aqueous outflow.

Clinical Uses.   Physostigmine ophthalmic preparations are available in sterile aqueous solutions, 0.25% and 0.5%, as the salicylate and in ointment form, 0.25%, as the sulfate (Table 3.19). A commercially prepared physostigmine-pilocarpine combination is also available. This contains physostigmine 0.25% and pilocarpine HCl 2%. Aqueous solutions that have been sterilized and that incorporate adequate antioxidant (e.g., sodium bisulfite) and are buffered at pH 3.6 to 3.8 should be stable for about 1 year if stored at 25°C. Solutions that have turned pink due to oxidation of the alkaloid are likely to have lost potency and are usually irritating. These should be discarded.[28]

Physostigmine is indicated primarily for lowering intraocular pressure in primary and some secondary open-angle glaucomas. Although effective as an ocular hypotensive agent, it is not the drug of first choice because of the undesirable ocular effects it produces. However, the ophthalmic ointment, because of its prolonged effect, is sometimes prescribed for bedtime use.

Although not currently advocated, physostigmine has been used to counteract the effects of anticholinergic mydriatics after ocular examination. It appears that a 0.25% solution of physostigmine is more effec-

TABLE 3.19
Commercially Available Anticholinesterase Miotics

Generic Name	Trade Name	Manufacturer	Concentration (%)
Echothiophate	Phospholine Iodide	Ayerst	Powder for reconstitution to 0.03, 0.06, 0.125, 0.25
Physostigmine	Eserine Sulfate	(Various)	Ointment, 0.25
	Isopto Eserine	Alcon	Solution, 0.25, 0.5
Demecarium	Humorsol	MSD	Solution, 0.125, 0.25
Isofluorphate	Floropryl	MSD	Ointment, 0.025

tive than 2% pilocarpine in restoring normal pupil size 40 minutes after dilation with cyclopentolate 0.1%.[339] An additional advantage of physostigmine is that its miotic effect is significantly more prolonged than is that of pilocarpine. This feature is necessary when counteracting mydriasis. It must be recognized, however, that a certain degree of lid twitching and ciliary spasm may persist when physostigmine is used in this way. As discussed previously, the likelihood of pupillary block is also increased, especially in eyes with narrow angles.

Physostigmine may be used in the treatment of phthiriasis palpebrarum. The anticholinesterase action has a lethal effect on the *Phthirus pubis* organism. The drug is applied as a lid scrub several times daily.

As an antidote for anticholinergic toxicity (atropine, scopolamine, cyclopentolate, and various phenothiazines and tricyclic antidepressants), physostigmine salicylate 1 to 4 mg administered subcutaneously or intravenously is effective within minutes in reversing the life-threatening central and peripheral toxic effects of these drugs.[356,357] Note that when physostigmine is administered systemically as an antidote, it is destroyed within 2 hours; therefore, repeated doses may be necessary.[321]

Side Effects.   Physostigmine produces one or more of the following undesirable local effects in and around the eye: stinging, conjunctival hyperemia, accommodative spasm, induced myopia, browache, and headache. Another common local effect of physostigmine observed after ocular instillation is lid twitching due to the prolonged action of ACh on the nicotinic receptors in the striated lid muscle (palpebral portion of the orbicularis). In addition, allergic irritation may develop, usually in the form of follicular conjunctivitis associated with epithelial keratitis.[355] Prolonged drug contact in the presence of this condition may lead to a pseudotrachoma.[355] Prolonged use may cause the formation of cysts (hypertrophy) of the pigmented epithelium at the pupillary margin (Fig. 3.42). Because of its ability to increase capillary permeability, this agent may activate latent iritis or uveitis. Pupillary block may follow physostigmine instillation, particularly with the higher concentrations, leading to a paradoxical increase in intraocular pressure. Long-term use may produce lens opacities, retinal detachment, conjunctival thickening, and stenosis of the puncta. In addition, posterior synechiae may develop; this can be averted by dilating the pupil once or twice a year.

Undesirable systemic effects (see Table 3.16) can occur from topical ocular administration, particularly if the patient does not apply pressure over the lacrimal canaliculi (see Fig. 2.5) after instilling the drug. In addition to the usual peripheral muscarinic side effects

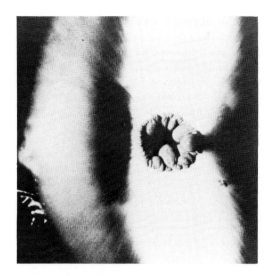

FIGURE 3.42   **Iris cysts associated with topical anticholinesterase therapy. (From Sugar HS. Pitfalls in the medical treatment of simple glaucoma. Ann Ophthalmol 1979;11:1041–1050.)**

produced by cholinergic agents, a certain degree of central muscarinic effects, such as respiratory depression, is possible, particularly in overdose. Nicotinic effects are also possible. These include muscular twitching, leading to convulsions.[321]

Accidental ingestion of physostigmine (approximate minimum lethal dose [MLD] is 0.06 g) is treated by immediately evacuating the stomach by gastric lavage or use of an emetic. The specific antidote is atropine sulfate (1 to 2 mg every 15 to 30 minutes) as long as symptoms persist.[358] Management of systemic toxicity associated with topical anticholinesterase therapy is discussed further in Chapter 31.

NEOSTIGMINE

Pharmacology.   Neostigmine, like physostigmine, is a phenyl ester of an alkyl carbamic acid (see Fig. 3.32). Unlike physostigmine, it is a quaternary amine and is therefore highly ionic and less lipid soluble. It is an indirect-acting cholinergic agonist, exerting its effect by inhibiting AChE reversibly, as does physostigmine. Its sites of action parallel those of physostigmine, having both muscarinic and nicotinic actions. In therapeutic doses, however, its distribution to the CNS is much less. On skeletal muscle, it has a direct stimulating action in addition to its anti-ChE effect,[359] a property that renders it useful in the diagnosis and treatment of myasthenia gravis.[360]

Clinical Uses.   Because of its poor lipid solubility, the efficacy of neostigmine as a topically applied miotic in the treatment of glaucoma has been less than desirable.

Although it has been used as an alternative to certain other miotics (e.g., physostigmine, pilocarpine), commercially prepared ophthalmic solutions of neostigmine are not currently available.

The main indications for use of neostigmine currently are the treatment of myasthenia gravis, for stimulating evacuation of the urinary bladder, screening for pregnancy, and as an antidote for tubocurarine. Neostigmine is available for oral use (neostigmine bromide) and parenteral administration (neostigmine methylsulfate).[321]

Side Effects.   Adverse effects of neostigmine are similar to those of physostigmine.

DEMECARIUM

Pharmacology.   Demecarium, structurally, is the result of linking two molecules of neostigmine (see Fig. 3.32). The connection is at their carbamate nitrogens through a series of 10 methylene groups. The pharmacologic consequences of this synthesis are increased potency and longer duration of action. Demecarium inhibits cholinesterases (AChE and BuChE), as does neostigmine. The sites of pharmacologic action are the same as those of physostigmine.[321]

Clinical Uses.   Because of its potency and sustained action, demecarium is not intended for systemic use. It is employed solely for topical use in the eye. The onset of miosis after 1 drop of the 0.125% or 0.25% ophthalmic solution is within 1 hour; miosis reaches a maximum in 2 to 4 hours and lasts for 3 to 10 days or longer. Intraocular pressure decreases within a few hours, is lowest at 24 hours, and may last for several days.[29]

Since it is a powerful anticholinesterase agent, demecarium produces undesirable local ocular effects similar to those produced by physostigmine. Of particular importance is the possibility of a transient paradoxical increase in intraocular pressure following initial use. Therefore, tonometer readings have been recommended hourly for 3 to 4 hours after the first instillation.[28]

Aqueous ophthalmic solutions of demecarium are available in two concentrations as the bromide salt (0.125% and 0.25%) (see Table 3.19). They are supplied in ophthalmic dispensers with a controlled dropper tip.[28]

Demecarium is indicated for the treatment of primary and some secondary open-angle glaucomas, preferably only when shorter-acting miotics such as pilocarpine and carbachol become inadequate.[29] Maximal efficacy can be obtained by individualized dosage. The adult dosage for glaucoma is 1 to 2 drops topically twice a day. Systemic side effects may be minimized by compressing the lacrimal canaliculi for at least 1 minute following application. Hands should be washed immediately thereafter, since absorption through the skin is likely as well as inadvertent oral ingestion. Satisfactory pressure reductions with the use of demecarium have been reported in patients with primary open-angle glaucoma not controlled adequately by certain other miotics.[361]

Side Effects.   Adverse effects and precautions for demecarium are similar to those for physostigmine.

EDROPHONIUM (TENSILON)

Pharmacology.   Edrophonium is a simple analog of neostigmine that lacks a carbamyl group (see Fig. 3.32). Classified as a reversible ChE inhibitor, its action is mainly on the skeletal neuromuscular junction and is brief. Part of its stimulating effects at the skeletal neuromuscular junction has been attributed to a direct action.[321]

Clinical Uses.   Because of its short duration and minimal muscarinic effects, edrophonium is considered to be the drug of choice for the diagnosis of myasthenia gravis. In the myasthenic patient, 2 to 10 mg of edrophonium administered intravenously will briefly improve muscular strength. This response constitutes the basis of the Tensilon test for diagnosing myasthenia and titrating the effectiveness of medications with which the patient is being treated.[362] Edrophonium chloride (Tensilon) is commercially available for this test as a parenteral injection in ampules and vials containing 10 mg/ml.[28] Tonography has been employed in the detection of a positive response to edrophonium in the myasthenic patient.[363] An immediate increase in intraocular pressure of 2 to 5 mm Hg constitutes a positive response in the tonography test.

Side Effects.   Side effects from edrophonium testing are uncommon; however, pretreatment with atropine reduces the incidence of undesirable effects such as hypotension, bradycardia, and syncope as well as involuntary defecation and cardiac arrest.[364]

DIISOPROPYLFLUOROPHOSPHATE (ISOFLUOROPHATE, DFP)

Pharmacology.   DFP belongs to a class of compounds known as organophosphorous anticholinesterase agents. Its structure (see Fig. 3.34) implies high lipid solubility and potential for producing alkylphosphorylation of cholinesterase. This drug produces an irreversible inactivation of both AChE and BuChE, with a preferential affinity for the latter enzyme. The mechanism by which it inhibits ChE involves the formation of a covalent bond with the esteratic site of the active center of the enzyme. The resultant phosphorylated enzyme is very stable. With time (minutes to hours) stability is enhanced. Simultaneously, spontaneous hydrolysis occurs at an insignificantly slow rate, resulting in an inconsequential amount of regenerated enzyme.[321] Accordingly, increased amounts of neurotransmitter (ACh) at the receptors in effector organs mediate prolonged increased cholinergic activity.

The pharmacologic effects of DFP are qualitatively similar to those of physostigmine. The primary differences are intensity and duration of action; in the case of DFP, AChE activity returns only when new enzyme is synthesized. An important characteristic of DFP relating to its potential systemic pharmacologic or toxic effects is its lipid solubility, which gives rise to its widespread distribution throughout the body. It readily penetrates the blood-brain barrier. Consequently, if sufficient amounts enter the CNS, reactions ranging from anxiety to tremors, convulsions, coma, and respiratory arrest can occur.[321]

Peripheral effects are muscarinic and nicotinic. As expected, the anticholinesterase action of DFP gives rise to activation of exocrine glands innervated by cholinergic nerves (lacrimation, salivation, sweating, bronchiolar and gastrointestinal secretions). The net effects of DFP on the heart are due to ganglionic (predominantly parasympathetic) and postganglionic parasympathetic stimulation; i.e., bradycardia, slowed AV conduction, and heart block.[321]

Blood pressure changes produced by this drug are variable, since it can exert its effects in the CNS, autonomic ganglia, adrenal medulla, the heart, and cholinergically innervated blood vessels.[321]

A single topical application of a 0.1% oily solution of DFP to the eye produces miosis that begins within 5 to 10 minutes, becomes maximal (pinpoint size) in 15 to 20 minutes, and lasts for 1 to 4 weeks. It causes a decrease in intraocular pressure that is maximal in 24 hours and returns to normal within 1 week. There is a marked and persistent ciliary spasm that induces myopia that may last for several days; accompanying pain may be exacerbated by attempts to accommodate. In addition, there is a marked vasodilatation, which results in an increased protein content in the aqueous and edema of the ciliary processes. This precludes the use of DFP in narrow angle glaucoma and in conditions with intraocular inflammation such as uveitic glaucoma. DFP may precipitate pupillary block.[29]

DFP is unstable in aqueous solutions. Commercially produced 0.1% solutions having a vehicle of peanut oil have been discontinued; however, a 0.025% ophthalmic ointment is currently available (see Table 3.19).[28]

Clinical Uses.   Oily solutions of DFP have been used in the management of primary open-angle glaucoma that is unresponsive to the shorter-acting miotics; however, only the 0.025% ointment is currently available. A small amount (¼ inch strip) of ointment is initially applied every 8 to 72 hours. Intraocular pressure should be reduced within a few hours. During this period, the patient should be supervised and tonometry performed hourly for 3 to 4 hours to detect possible paradoxical increases in intraocular pressure.[29]

Currently, DFP ointment is being employed satisfactorily in the diagnosis and management of accommodative esotropia. An apparent advantage is fewer systemic side effects than with another widely used organophosphate agent, echothiophate.[365]

DFP can be used as a diagnostic aid in patients with equal visual acuity in both eyes to determine if an accommodative component plays a role in the esotropia of young children with normal hyperopic refractive errors. The ointment (¼ inch strip) is applied to the conjunctival sac every night for 2 weeks. If the esotropia is relieved or reduced, an accommodative component is demonstrated.

In the therapy of accommodative esotropia in which there is no amblyopia or anisometropia, a ¼ inch strip of ointment is applied nightly for 2 weeks; reductions in frequency of dosage thereafter depend on the length of time the eyes remain straight without ointment; however, if good results cannot be maintained with dosage intervals of at least 48 hours, the therapy should be discontinued. Reevaluation of the patient's status after 2 months usually indicates that continued therapy is necessary. On occasion, therapy may be discontinued after a few months.[29]

Another clinical indication for DFP ointment is treatment of phthiriasis palpebrarum. A single application as a lid scrub seems to be effective. Since this compound is absorbed through the skin, it should be used sparingly.

Side Effects.   Prolonged systemic absorption of adequate amounts of DFP can produce local and systemic cholinergic side effects previously described. However, systemic side effects arising from the application of DFP ointment every other night or less are usually minimal.[365] On rare occasions, patients complain of cough or nasal congestion; these symptoms cease when the medication is discontinued.[366] Infrequently, patients complain about blurred vision, photophobia, and browache, but these effects are transient.[366]

An important potential side effect is the development of iris cysts, particularly in children; however, the incidence is minimal when DFP is applied every other night or less frequently. These cysts appear on the pupillary margin as multiple nodules (see Fig. 3.42). It has been reported that daily use of DFP in young children has produced a significant number of iris cysts. The average time of appearance was 10 weeks. In some cases visual acuity may be reduced to 20/200 (6/60) by the cysts. Fortunately, these lesions spontaneously disappear after discontinuation of the drug with no serious sequelae.[367] Histopathologically, iris cysts are not true cysts but rather represent hypertrophy of the pigmented cells of the pupillary frill. The development of iris cysts can be prevented by the concurrent administration of topical phenylephrine,[95] which probably acts to minimize the initial intense miosis produced by the anticholinesterase agent and thus reduces the stimulation of hypertrophy.

Some important potential drug interactions should be kept in mind when using DFP. The prior topical administration of reversible cholinesterase inhibitors such as neostigmine or physostigmine will antagonize the effects of irreversible ChE inhibitors including DFP. This occurs because AChE will have been inhibited by the relatively short-acting physostigmine or neostigmine first. Since DFP cannot inhibit the already inhibited enzyme, it becomes metabolized and excreted before AChE is freed of the shorter-acting drug.[321]

Because of possible respiratory collapse, the depolarizing muscle relaxant succinylcholine, which is employed during certain surgical procedures along with general anesthesia, should be administered with extreme caution to patients receiving cholinesterase inhibitors. Normal dosages of succinylcholine under these conditions can act as overdoses because its rate of metabolism (by cholinesterase) and resulting detoxification is reduced. As a result of the excessive action of succinylcholine, the diaphragm and intercostal muscles become paralyzed.[321]

Other potential drug-drug interactions include possible undesirable additive effects when DFP is administered to patients being treated systemically with other anticholinesterase agents or direct-acting cholinergic drugs. Anticholinesterase insecticides and pesticides may add to the effects of DFP or other organophosphates such as echothiophate.

Before using DFP or other organophosphates, it is important to be aware of the usual contraindications, warnings, and precautions associated with cholinesterase inhibitors (see Physostigmine).

Accidental ingestion of sufficient amounts of DFP or other organophosphate anticholinesterases can be fatal. The cause of death is respiratory failure due to a combination of obstructed airway (increased tracheobronchial and salivary secretions, laryngospasm, bronchoconstriction), central respiratory depression and weakness or paralysis of muscles of respiration (diaphragm, intercostal, and accessory muscles), and cardiovascular collapse (bradycardia and decreased cardiac output).

Severe acute toxicity is managed initially by maintenance of a patent airway and gastric lavage. A sufficient amount of atropine (2 to 4 mg intravenously or intramuscularly) should be administered initially. An additional 2 mg should be administered every 3 to 10 minutes until muscarinic symptoms abate.[321] Atropine reverses the muscarinic symptoms; however, it does not antagonize the peripheral nicotinic effects (initial stimulation and subsequent depolarizing blockade of skeletal muscle). A cholinesterase reactivator such as pralidoxime (Protopam) is necessary to reverse the nicotinic effects. Pralidoxime is given by intravenous infusion 20 to 40 mg/kg body weight up to 1 g slowly over one-half hour. The dosage is repeated in 1 hour if effective.[368] Pralidoxime is effective only if it is given before the organophosphate-cholinesterase compound becomes stable (minutes to hours). Additional supportive measures such as artificial respiration and oxygen administration may be necessary.[321]

ECHOTHIOPHATE

Pharmacology. Echothiophate, like isoflurophate (DFP), is an organophosphorous compound, specifically a phosphorylthiocholine (see Fig. 3.34). It is a cholinergic agonist because it inhibits cholinesterases (AChE and BuChE, with a propensity to inhibit the former), thereby enhancing the effects of endogenously released acetylcholine. Its mechanism of enzyme inhibition is similar to that of DFP. Like DFP, it interacts with the esteratic subsite in the active center of ChE; however, the quaternary ammonium radical within the echothiophate molecule is responsible for additional bonding at the anionic subsite. The result is a stable complex that is responsible for the drug's potent and prolonged irreversible activity. Significant spontaneous regeneration of active enzyme requires several hours; however, it occurs at a more rapid rate than with DFP. As with DFP, there is an enhanced stability of the phosphorylated enzyme over time.

The quaternary nitrogen of echothiophate imparts the property of low lipid solubility. Consequently, echothiophate's penetration of the blood-brain barrier is theoretically limited. This expectation is corroborated by studies that have shown that none of the symptoms of toxic doses of echothiophate in animals is attributable to cholinesterase inhibition in the CNS; death was caused by peripheral toxic effects, including paralysis of muscles of respiration and excessive bronchial constriction.[369] As expected, the pharmacologic effects of echothiophate are very similar to the peripheral effects of DFP.

A solution of echothiophate applied topically to the eye results in miosis that begins within 10 to 45 minutes and may last for 1 to 4 weeks. Accompanying reduction of intraocular pressure is maximal after 24 hours, lasting for as long as 4 days.[370] Its pressure-reducing effect has been attributed to an increase in facility of aqueous outflow.

Echothiophate ophthalmic solutions are commercially available as the iodide salt in concentrations of 0.03, 0.06, 0.125, and 0.25% (see Table 3.19). Because it has a relatively short shelf life, echothiophate iodide must be prepared fresh on dispensing; therefore it is supplied as a powder in the appropriate amount for reconstitution. A diluent containing a buffer and preservatives is added. After reconstituting, the refrigerated solution will be useful for up to 6 months. Solutions stored at room temperature will maintain stability for only 1 month.[28] Thus, it is wise to recommend refrigeration.

Clinical Uses. The main indications for echothiophate are in the treatment of advanced primary and some secondary open-angle glaucomas not controlled by shorter-acting miotics, epinephrine, β blockers, carbonic anhydrase inhibitors, or combinations thereof and in the diagnosis or treatment of accommodative esotropia.

In the treatment of glaucoma the therapeutic objective is to achieve optimal control of intraocular pressure on a diurnal basis, since significant diurnal variations in intraocular pressure can cause progressive visual field loss in patients who are inadequately controlled. Echothiophate is advantageous in this respect and is the most widely used anticholinesterase agent for this purpose. It has been demonstrated that 0.06% echothiophate solution administered once or twice a day and supplemented by acetazolamide and epinephrine has greater effectiveness than pilocarpine and supplements in maintaining pressure at 20 mm Hg or below.[371]

Certain precautions should be observed before initiating echothiophate therapy. Gonioscopy should be performed to rule out narrow angles or shallow anterior chambers. Anticholinesterases should be avoided in patients with active or quiescent uveitis or if uveitis is precipitated. The patient should be advised to compress the canaliculus for at least 1 minute following instillation to minimize systemic absorption. Temporary discontinuation of the medication is indicated if systemic side effects appear. Patients exposed to carbamate or organophosphate insecticides should be warned of their additive effects with anticholinesterases. Preventive measures such as wearing respiratory masks and frequent washing and clothing changes should be recommended.

Anticholinesterases should be used with caution or avoided in patients with illnesses that would be exacerbated by increased cholinergic stimulation; for example, asthma, gastrointestinal disturbances, bradycardia, heart block, recent myocardial infarct, epilepsy, parkinsonism, and history of or predisposition toward retinal detachment.[321]

With initial dosing, tonometric measurements should be performed if possible each hour for 3 to 4 hours because of the possibility of a paradoxical increase in intraocular pressure. Periodic pressure determinations thereafter at different times in the day are suggested to determine continued effectiveness.

In the treatment of primary open-angle glaucoma, the instillation of 0.03% echothiophate on retiring and in the morning is recommended for obtaining as smooth a diurnal pressure curve as possible; however, a single dose per day (at bedtime) or every other day is satisfactory in some patients. The daily dose should always be instilled at bedtime to avoid the inconvenience of drug-induced miosis and accommodative spasm. If results are inadequate, the higher concentrations of echothiophate may be necessary. When used in its highest concentrations, echothiophate has an ocular hypotensive effect that is considerably more pronounced than that of pilocarpine or carbachol. These latter drugs must be discontinued before instituting echothiophate therapy because the simultaneous use of these drugs provides no additional benefit yet increases the risk of systemic toxicity.

Because of their pharmacologic mechanism, the anticholinesterases cause an accumulation of ACh at the neuroeffector junction. Accordingly, a decrease in the nerve impulse is required for accommodation. This reduction in accommodative effort results in a concomitant reduction in accommodative convergence. Echothiophate is therefore useful in the diagnosis of accommodative esotropia. If 1 drop of a 0.125% solution applied to each eye at bedtime for 2 to 3 weeks brings about a favorable response (straightening of eyes), an accommodative component to the esotropia is revealed.

In the treatment of accommodative esotropia, the lowest concentration and frequency that give satisfactory results are recommended. Therefore, after the initial diagnostic regimen, dosage is reduced to 0.125% applied every other day or 0.06% every day. Dosages may be further reduced if the favorable response is maintained. After 1 to 2 years, the drug should be gradually withdrawn. If the deviation recurs after this period, alternate forms of therapy are suggested.

Side Effects.   The side effects and complications associated with echothiophate are essentially the same as are those associated with the other anticholinesterase agents. The major ocular complication of echothiophate is the development of cataract, usually characterized by anterior subcapsular vacuoles (Fig. 3.43).[346] However, evidence suggests that echothiophate and the other anticholinesterase agents accelerate nuclear sclerosis and posterior subcapsular changes.[346,372] Thus, echothiophate and the other anticholinesterases are more useful in aphakic than in phakic patients. There is a greater risk of retinal detachment with the use of echothiophate than with pilocarpine or carbachol. Reversible iris cysts are a well-known complication of all the anticholinesterase agents, including echothiophate. The iris cysts at the pupillary margin occur primarily in young patients and can decrease vision and produce visual field changes that mimic those of glaucoma. The development of such cysts can be minimized by the concomitant use of 2.5% or 10% phenylephrine. Patients treated with echothiophate may develop constant tearing associated with stenosis of the puncta, but this usually disappears following discontinuation of the drug.[346]

Systemic absorption of echothiophate may lead to significant side effects, characterized by intense gastrointestinal symptoms including diarrhea, nausea, and vomiting.[346] These have been attributed to inhibition of cholinesterase. Determination of cholinesterase content in red blood cells usually reveals low values in symptomatic patients. Normal values range between 0.6 and 1.1 units. Values less than 0.4 units are usually found in persons exposed to significant amounts of anticholinesterases. Although low values are not conclusive regarding a drug-induced effect, normal values rule out a drug-related etiology.

Since patients using echothiophate and other anticholinesterase agents have markedly lower plasma and red blood cell cholinesterase, the action of succinylcholine used in general anesthesia may be prolonged, leading to prolonged postoperative respiratory paralysis.[348] The dangers of using echothiophate in patients exposed to organophosphate insecticides or fertilizers and in patients undergoing treatment with anticholinesterase drugs for myasthenia gravis must be emphasized. Under these conditions echothiophate can cause intense intestinal cramps, CNS symptoms, cardiac arrest, hypotension, or respiratory failure. Manual depression of the lacrimal canaliculi should be mandatory following instillation of the drug to prevent or minimize these systemic side effects.

Contraindications.   Echothiophate is contraindicated in phakic glaucoma patients because of the greater risk for the development of cataract compared with the use of the shorter-acting miotics. Echothiophate is also contraindicated in patients with peripheral retinal disease that would predispose to retinal detachment.[345]

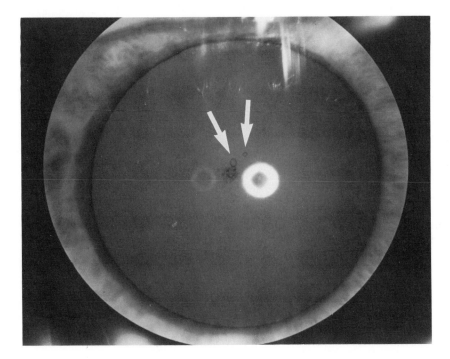

FIGURE 3.43 **Anterior subcapsular cataract (arrows) in a patient treated with anticholinesterase miotics. Pupil has been dilated for photography. White annular ring is photographic artifact. (Courtesy David M. Amos, O.D.)**

This drug should be discontinued several weeks before surgical procedures employing succinylcholine. It should be discontinued 4 to 6 weeks before intraocular surgery to minimize its inflammatory effects and to diminish conjunctival and episcleral bleeding during conjunctival dissection.[373] As with all miotics, it should be avoided in uveitic glaucoma because of the vasodilatation and aggravation of the uveitis.

Comparative Therapeutic Effectiveness of Cholinergic Drugs

Cholinergic agonists may be classified into three major groups according to their effectiveness in reducing intraocular pressure (Table 3.20). All the drugs in each group have approximately equal pressure-lowering effects. Changing from one drug within a group to another drug within the same group offers no additional ocular hypotensive potential. The practitioner must change from a drug within group I to a drug within group II, or from group II to group III, to achieve a more intense cholinergic (and thus ocular hypotensive) effect. It should be emphasized, however, that these groupings represent generalizations only, and that in clinical practice exceptions do exist. These categorizations serve to lend perspective in the use of miotics in the treatment of glaucoma and to allow the practitioner to more rationally anticipate therapeutic results.

Cholinergic Antagonists

Drugs that block the effects of ACh at muscarinic receptor sites in the iris sphincter and ciliary muscles have proved clinically useful, particularly for pupillary dilation, cycloplegic refraction, and management of iridocyclitis. The anticholinergic agents in current clinical use are atropine, homatropine, scopolamine, cyclopentolate, and tropicamide.

Atropine

PHARMACOLOGY

Atropine, a naturally occurring alkaloid, was first isolated from the belladonna plant, *Atropa belladonna*, in its pure form in 1831.[374] The stability of atropine is both pH and temperature dependent. At 20°C, the half-life of atropine is 2.7 years in a pH 7 solution, and 27.0 years at pH 6. At 30°C its stability is reduced to 0.61 years at pH 7 and 6.1 years at pH 6.[375] At the physiologic pH, atropine with a pK_a of 9.8 is partially in an un-ionized state.[376] This enhances intraocular absorption of the drug following its topical application to the eye. Atropine is the most potent mydriatic and cycloplegic agent presently available. Depending on the concentration used, mydriasis may last up to 10 days and cycloplegia, 7 to 12 days (Table 3.21). Atropine is available commercially as a sulfate derivative in 0.5% and 1% concentration in ointment form, and in 1%, 2%, and 3% solution[28] (Table 3.22).

The intraocular distribution of atropine has been studied following subconjunctival injection of the radioactive drug in rabbits.[377] At 90 minutes significant radioactivity is exhibited by the cornea, aqueous, and vitreous. Lower concentrations are present in the iris, ciliary body, and retina. By 5 hours, 95% of the radioactivity has left the ocular tissues as the atropine is excreted in the urine.

Lussana,[378] in 1852, was the first to study the effect of atropine on the eyes as part of a general study of its systemic actions. Following oral ingestion of atropine, the pupil dilated, vision became blurred, and the ability to do near work was lost.

Feddersen[379] is credited with the first extended study of the ocular effects of atropine sulfate following top-

---

TABLE 3.20
Comparative Therapeutic Effectiveness of Cholinergic Agonists

Group I	*Group II*	*Group III*

Pilocarpine
  1%–6% q.i.d.
	Carbachol
	  3.0% t.i.d.
		Echothiophate
		  0.125%–0.25% b.i.d.

Pilocarpine Ocusert
  20–40 μg/h
	Echothiophate
	  0.06% b.i.d.	

Carbachol 0.75%–1.5% q.i.d.		
Echothiophate 0.03% b.i.d.		

Adapted from Richardson KT. Pharmacology. In: Duane TD, ed. Clinical ophthalmology. Hagerstown, MD: Harper & Row, 1981; 3, Chap. 56:1–10.

TABLE 3.21
Mydriatic and Cycloplegic Properties of Anticholinergic Agents

Drug	Strength of Solution[a] (%)	Mydriasis		Paralysis of Accommodation	
		Maximal (minutes)	Recovery[b] (days)	Maximal (minutes)	Recovery[c] (days)
Atropine sulfate	1.0	30–40	7–10	60–180	7–12
Homatropine hydrobromide	1.0[d]	40–60	1–3	30–60	1–3
Scopolamine hydrobromide	0.5	20–30	3–7	30–60	5–7
Cyclopentolate hydrochloride	0.5–1.0	30–60	1	30–60	1
Tropicamide	0.5–1.0	20–35	0.25	30–45	0.25

[a]One instillation of 1 drop of solution.
[b]To within 1 mm of original pupillary diameter.
[c]To within 2 diopters of original amplitude of accommodation; ability to read fine print is possible by the third day after atropine and scopolamine and by 6 hours after homatropine instillation.
[d]Full mydriasis and loss of accommodation require instillation of a 5% solution.
Adapted from Weiner N. Atropine, scopolamine, and related antimuscarinic drugs. In: Gilman AG, Goodman LS, Rall TW, et al., eds. The pharmacological basis of therapeutics. New York: Macmillan Co, 1985;7:130–144.

ical application of a 1% solution. Following the instillation of 1 drop, the mydriatic effect began at 12 minutes and reached a maximum in 26 minutes. The pupil began to return to normal in 2 days and reached preinstillation size by the tenth day. The cycloplegic effect began in 12 to 18 minutes and reached maximum by 160 minutes. Accommodation began to return in 42 hours, and full accommodative ability was usually attained within 8 days.

Wolf and Hodge[380] observed a similar time course of action for 1% atropine sulfate in a series of 46 eyes (Fig. 3.44). In addition, these authors reported wide variations in individual responses to topical ocular atropine. Pigment binding has been suggested to explain, at least in part, this effect. When applied to heavily pigmented eyes, atropine exhibits a relatively slow onset and prolonged duration of cycloplegic effect. Moreover, the degree of mydriasis obtained is less, particularly in eyes of black patients.[29] Salazar and associates[381] reported that pigmented rabbit and human irides accumulate greater amounts of radioactive ^{3}H-atropine than nonpigmented irides in vitro. On repeated washing, the atropine blockade of nonpigmented iris could be easily removed, while that in the pigmented iris was retained. Thus, the smaller magnitude of the mydriatic effect with atropine in humans may be explained, at least in part, by the initial loss of administered drug to pigment cells. The prolonged

TABLE 3.22
Mydriatic-Cycloplegic Preparations

Generic Name	Trade Name	Manufacturer	Concentration (%)
Atropine sulfate	Atropine Sulfate Ophthalmic	(Various)	Ointment 1
	Isopto Atropine Ophthalmic	Alcon	Solution 0.5, 1, 3
	Atropisol Ophthalmic	Iolab	Solution 0.5, 1, 2
	Atropine Sulfate S.O.P.	Allergan	Ointment 0.5, 1
	Atropine-Care Ophthalmic	Akorn	Solution 1
Homatropine HBr	AK-Homatropine	Akorn	Solution 5
	Homatropine Ophthalmic	(Various)	Solution 5
	Isopto Homatropine	Alcon	Solution 2, 5
Scopolamine HBr	Isopto Hyoscine	Alcon	Solution 0.25
Cyclopentolate	Cyclogyl	Alcon	Solution 0.5, 1, 2
	AK-Pentolate	Akorn	Solution 0.5, 1
Tropicamide	Mydriacyl Ophthalmic	Alcon	Solution 0.5, 1
	Tropicacyl	Akorn	Solution 0.5, 1

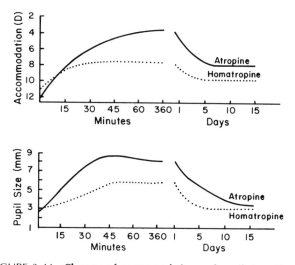

FIGURE 3.44 **Changes of accommodation and pupil size after administration of 1% solution of atropine sulfate and 1% solution of homatropine hydrobromide. (Modified from Wolf AV, Hodge HC. Effects of atropine sulfate, methylatropine nitrate (Metropine) and homatropine hydrobromide on adult human eyes. Arch Ophthalmol 1946; 36:293–301.)**

effect in the more heavily pigmented eye is attributed to the subsequent release of accumulated drug over time onto the muscarinic receptors of the iris and ciliary body.

In addition to pigment binding, the actions of atropine can be affected by the enzyme atropinase (atropinesterase) present in certain species of rabbits, which hydrolyzes the drug and thereby limits its duration of action.[382] Rabbits with and without the enzyme present in the serum exhibit an average half-life for recovery of atropine mydriasis of 12.4 and 96 hours, respectively. Atropinase-negative rabbits show a prolonged effect with atropine, similar to the time course in humans, who lack the enzyme.

CLINICAL USES

Refraction.   Atropine is useful for cycloplegic refraction, particularly for the younger, actively accommodating child with suspected accommodative esotropia (see Chapter 17). It should never be used for cycloplegic refraction of adults because the prolonged paralysis of accommodation renders the patient visually handicapped.

For purposes of cycloplegic refraction atropine solution is usually administered 3 times per day for 2 to 3 days before refraction. There is no particular justification for this dosage regimen, which may lead to overdosage in some cases. The drug is usually administered at home by an individual who has been instructed in the proper method of drug instillation. To prevent excessive systemic absorption of atropine by

the nasal mucosa, it is advised that pressure be placed over the lacrimal canaliculi immediately following drug instillation in the lower cul de sac (see Fig. 2.5).

Iridocyclitis.   Atropine is extremely useful in the treatment of anterior uveal inflammation. It relieves the pain associated with the inflammatory process by relaxing the ciliary muscle spasm and helps prevent posterior synechiae by dilating the pupil. With the pupil dilated, the area of posterior iris surface in contact with the anterior lens capsule decreases. Moreover, the cycloplegia produced by atropine is of additional value in reducing both the thickness and the convexity of the lens. If posterior synechiae should develop even when the pupil is dilated, there is less chance of iris bombé.[383]

Atropine may also help to restore toward normal the excessive permeability of the inflamed vessels and thereby reduce cells and protein in the anterior chamber (aqueous flare).[383]

Treatment of Myopia.   It has been suggested that topical ocular use of atropine may prevent the progression of myopia.[384] By placing the ciliary muscle at rest, accommodation is relaxed, and the tension that produces elongation of the eye may be reduced. However, clinical trials using atropine for myopia control are difficult to interpret due to variations in patient selection and differences in mode and duration of treatment. With administration of 1% atropine for 1 to 8 years, the decrease in myopia in treated eyes of children has usually been less than 0.5 D.[385,386] Although Sampson[387] reported that instillation of 1% atropine for 20 months to children aged 7 to 14 years seemed to prevent the progression of myopia, on discontinuation of the drops only 12% maintained improvement for more than 6 months. Additional studies with better control are needed to evaluate the efficacy of atropine and other cholinergic antagonists in myopia control.

Amblyopia.   Use of atropine can be an alternative to patching of the normal eye in the treatment of suppression amblyopia. The resultant cycloplegic blur in the eye with normal vision may force fixation with the amblyopic eye.

Since therapy with anticholinergics will be successful only if the reduction in visual acuity of the normal eye exceeds that of the amblyopic eye, multiple daily instillations may be required.[388] Although pharmacologic occlusion can improve visual acuity in amblyopic eyes, care is needed, since penalization can result in amblyopia in eyes with normal acuity.[389]

Provocative Testing for Glaucoma.   Atropine and other cholinergic antagonists can be useful in inducing acute angle-closure glaucoma in eyes with suspected narrow angles. Since mydriasis can lead to pupillary block, a narrow angle may be occluded. However, not all eyes with suspected narrow angles or a history of angle-closure attacks respond positively to the cholinergic blocking agents[390] (see Chapter 16).

SIDE EFFECTS

Toxic reactions can occur following topical use of atropine, particularly in children (Table 3.23).

Ocular Effects.   Ocular reactions include direct irritation from the drug preparation itself, possibly due to the presence of the preservative chlorobutanol; allergic contact dermatitis; risk of angle-closure glaucoma; and elevation of intraocular pressure in patients with open angles.[29,391]

The allergic reaction to atropine generally involves the eyelids and manifests itself as an erythema, with pruritus and edema. Allergic papillary conjunctivitis and keratitis have also occurred.[392]

In general, topical atropine as well as other cholinergic antagonists increase the patient's risk for angle-closure glaucoma. However, the risk of inducing angle closure in eyes without previous history of attacks is very remote. Keller[393] reviewed the literature on this subject and concluded that with proper precautions, the risk of precipitating an angle-closure attack is, at most, 1 in 183,000 in the general population and 1 in 45,000 in the population over age 30 years. It has also been argued that a pharmacologically provoked attack of angle closure may be in the patient's best interest, since a diagnosis can be made immediately and appropriate treatment provided before a spontaneous attack occurs.

Patients with open-angle glaucoma may experience an elevation of intraocular pressure. The effect is unpredictable, since not all patients respond to cholinergic antagonists with intraocular pressure elevations. The mechanisms involved in the pressure rise are not completely understood. The pressure elevation appears to be related not to the degree of mydriasis attained, but, rather, to a decrease in facility of aqueous outflow.[29]

TABLE 3.23
Toxic Reactions to Atropine in Children

- Diffuse cutaneous flush
- Thirst
- Fever
- Urinary retention
- Tachycardia
- Somnolence – sleepy
- Excitement and hallucinations

Systemically administered atropine may also cause mydriasis and raise intraocular pressure in normotensive patients with open-angle glaucoma. Following intramuscular injection of 0.6 to 0.8 mg of atropine, 3 of 8 patients developed 0.5 to 1.5 mm mydriasis.[394] A mean increase of 8 cm in the near point of accommodation following atropine administration was also reported. In another study 100 normotensive patients, ranging in age from 16 to 40 years, were given atropine intramuscularly, 0.016 mg/kg body weight. Thirteen of the subjects developed pupillary dilation of 2 mm or less, and 9 developed ocular pressure elevations of 3 mm Hg or less.[395]

Eyes with open-angle glaucoma respond variably to systemic atropine. In one study 34 eyes with open-angle glaucoma were maintained on glaucoma therapy while atropine 0.01 mg/kg body weight was injected intramuscularly. In 12 eyes the intraocular pressure increased from 2 to 5 mm Hg. However, the overall differences observed in both pupil size and intraocular pressure were not statistically significant.[396]

Systemic Effects.   Systemic reactions from the topical administration of atropine have also occurred. Following its application to the eye, systemic absorption of drug occurs primarily from the conjunctival vessels and the nasal mucosa.

The adverse systemic reactions appear to be dosage dependent, although patients vary in susceptibility.[374] Systemic peripheral effects occur with low doses, which generally do not produce central symptomatology. Depression of salivation and drying of the mouth are usually the first signs of toxicity. Slightly higher dosages produce facial flushing and inhibit sweating. At 20 times the minimum dose where adverse systemic symptoms begin to appear, CNS manifestations can occur.[397]

Deaths have been attributed to topical ocular atropine. Six reported cases in the literature have occurred in children 3 years of age and under. The dosages applied ranged from 1.6 mg to 18 mg, but the cases are rather poorly documented. All the children appeared to be either sickly or to have motor and mental retardation.[398-400] However, what these cases imply is that care must be taken not to overdose small children. Caution must be exercised particularly with lightly pigmented individuals, Down's syndrome children, and children with spastic paralysis or brain damage.[397]

The treatment of atropine overdosage is largely symptomatic, with prevention of hyperpyrexia and dehydration. Sedation with diazepam has been advocated. The specific antidote for CNS toxicity is physostigmine (Antilirium) in a subcutaneous dose of 0.25 mg in children and 1 to 2 mg in adults. The initial dose can be supplemented as needed every 15 minutes by doses of similar magnitude.[383]

Homatropine

PHARMACOLOGY

Homatropine is about one-tenth as potent as atropine and has a shorter duration of mydriatic and cycloplegic action (see Table 3.21). It is partly synthetic and partly, like atropine, from the plants of the Solanaceae family.[401] It is quite stable in solution. At physiologic pH, homatropine with a pK_a of 9.9 is about 0.32% un-ionized.[402] Homatropine is commercially available as the bromide salt in concentrations ranging from 2% to 5% (see Table 3.22).

Following topical instillation of a 1% solution, maximum mydriasis occurs in 40 minutes. Recovery requires about 1 to 3 days.[380] The amount and duration of cycloplegia produced by homatropine are significantly less than that produced by a comparable dose of atropine (see Fig. 3.44).

CLINICAL USES

Due to its prolonged mydriatic effect and relatively weak cycloplegic action, particularly in darkly pigmented irides, homatropine is not a drug of choice for fundus examination or cycloplegic refraction. Its primary clinical usefulness is in the treatment of iridocyclitis, where its effects are similar to those of atropine. It also serves as a substitute for atropine in patients with known sensitivities to that drug.

SIDE EFFECTS

The toxic effects of homatropine are indistinguishable from those of atropine, and the treatment is the same.[403]

Scopolamine (Hyoscine)

PHARMACOLOGY

The antimuscarinic potency of scopolamine on a weight basis is greater than that of atropine. Except for a shorter duration of mydriatic and cycloplegic action at the dosage levels used clinically, its effects are similar to those of atropine (see Table 3.21). Although previously available in both ointment and solution, scopolamine is currently available as the bromide salt in solution at 0.25% concentration (see Table 3.22).

Marron[404] studied the mydriatic and cycloplegic effects of 0.5% solution of scopolamine in subjects ranging from 15 to 37 years of age. Maximum pupillary dilation occurred at 20 minutes. This effect lasted for 90 minutes, and the pupil returned to its preinstillation size by the eighth day. The maximum cycloplegic effect occurred at 40 minutes, with amplitude of accommodation at 1.6 D. This accommodative effect lasted for at least 90 minutes and gradually returned by the third day to a level where the average patient could read.

CLINICAL USES

Since patients tend to exhibit a higher incidence of toxic reactions to scopolamine[383] than to other anticholinergic agents, it is not a drug of first choice for cycloplegic refraction or treatment of anterior uveal inflammations. Its use is reserved primarily for patients who exhibit sensitivity to atropine.

SIDE EFFECTS

Although adverse reactions from scopolamine are quite similar to those from atropine, CNS toxicity appears to be more common with scopolamine. In a series of several hundred patients whose pupils were dilated with 1% scopolamine, 7 cases of confusional psychosis were observed. The reactions included restlessness, confusion, hallucinations, incoherence, violence, amnesia, unconsciousness, spastic extremities, and vomiting and urinary incontinence.[405] However, no deaths have been reported from topical ocular use of scopolamine. Treatment of toxic reactions is the same as that for atropine toxicity.

Cyclopentolate

PHARMACOLOGY

Cyclopentolate was introduced into clinical practice in 1951.[406] A stable, water-soluble ester with a pK_a of 8.4, cyclopentolate is primarily in an ionized state at physiologic pH.[378] It is commercially available in 0.5, 1, and 2% solutions (see Table 3.22).

The mydriatic and cycloplegic properties of cyclopentolate have been studied and compared with other available anticholinergic agents by several groups of investigators.[407-410] Essentially the same techniques have been used in these studies for determining onset, intensity, and duration of action. Usually the 0.5% or 1% concentrations were used, and the subjects were classified according to age and race.

In whites, 2 drops of 0.5% cyclopentolate instilled 5 minutes apart, or 1 drop of 1% solution, produces maximum mydriasis within 20 to 30 minutes. The average pupil size is usually 7.0 to 7.5 mm. In black patients, two instillations of 0.5% produce a 6.0 mm pupil in 30 minutes and a 7.0 mm pupil at 60 minutes following instillation of the first drop.[406,409] Cyclopentolate is also a less effective mydriatic in whites with dark irides. The pupil size in these patients is an average of 6.5 mm at 30 minutes and 7.0 mm at 60 minutes. Full recovery from mydriasis occurs within 24 hours.

Maximum cycloplegia in whites occurs within 30 to 60 minutes following instillation of 2 drops of 0.5% or 1 drop of 1% solution. The residual accommodation ranges between 1.00 D and 1.75 D, with an average of 1.25 D.[406] The cycloplegic effect usually dissipates within 24 hours.

In groups of black patients ranging in age from 9 to 40 years, 1% cyclopentolate has been reported to produce satisfactory cycloplegia in 98% of patients. The 0.5% concentration was effective in only 66% of the same individuals. The average residual accommodation was 1.75 D following use of 1% cyclopentolate.[408]

Cyclopentolate does not alter intraocular pressure in normal eyes. Tonometry performed in a series of patients ranging from age 4 to 93 years before and after instillation of 0.5% and 1% cyclopentolate revealed no statistically significant differences in the readings.[406,409]

CLINICAL USES

Cyclopentolate is a useful cycloplegic agent for routine cycloplegic refractive procedures in nearly all age groups, especially infants and young children. Its cycloplegic effect is superior to that of homatropine[406,408] and closely parallels that of atropine in older children and adults, but with a relatively faster onset and shorter duration (see Table 3.21). Pupils dilated with cyclopentolate do not constrict when exposed to intense light such as that of the binocular indirect ophthalmoscope or during fundus photography.

Although full recovery from mydriasis and cycloplegia generally occurs within 24 hours, most patients have sufficient recovery of accommodative amplitude to permit reading in 6 to 12 hours. Moreover, unlike with atropine and homatropine, onset of maximum cycloplegia generally approximates the onset of maximum mydriasis.[406,411]

Cyclopentolate is also useful in the treatment of iridocyclitis, particularly in patients sensitive to atropine. If the inflammation is severe, more frequent instillations may be necessary, since its duration of action is less than that of atropine.

SIDE EFFECTS

Ocular Effects.   The most common ocular side effect is transient stinging on initial instillation.[392] The degree of irritation appears to be concentration dependent, with the 0.5% solution causing the least amount of burning and tearing.

Allergic reactions to cyclopentolate are quite rare and may go unrecognized by the practitioner. However, Havener[29] has observed several cases of redness and discomfort in eyes of patients following in-office use of cyclopentolate. The symptoms consist of irri-tated, diffusely red eyes that develop within minutes of drug instillation. Lacrimation, stringy white mucus discharge, and blurred vision are prominent, but itching is not a significant complaint. Similar symptoms occur at each office visit if cyclopentolate is used. A diffuse superficial punctate keratitis typically accompanies the reaction.

Topically applied cyclopentolate can increase intraocular pressure in patients with primary open-angle glaucoma, and it may precipitate an attack of acute glaucoma in patients with narrow angles.[412,413] Harris[413] reported that 1 of 4 eyes with open-angle glaucoma will respond to topical 1% cyclopentolate with a significant elevation of intraocular pressure, whereas only 1 out of 50 normal eyes would respond in a similar manner. The intraocular pressure rise usually begins within 1 hour, reaches a maximum at 2 hours, and returns to preinstillation levels by 4 hours.

Systemic Effects.   Systemic cyclopentolate toxicity is dose related and evolves in a manner similar to that of atropine.[414] However, unlike atropine, cyclopentolate causes more CNS effects.[414-418]

The CNS disturbances are characterized by signs and symptoms of cerebellar dysfunction and visual as well as tactile hallucinations. These can include drowsiness, ataxia, disorientation, incoherent speech, restlessness, and emotional disturbances (Table 3.24). The CNS effects are particularly common in children with use of the 2% concentration,[413,414] but multiple instillations of the 1% solution may also cause the same symptoms.[414,415] Binkhorst and associates[415] evaluated 40 children before and after use of the 2% solution. Of these children, 5 exhibited transient psychotic reactions within 30 to 45 minutes following instillation of the drops. The symptoms included restlessness with aimless wandering, irrelevant talking, visual hallucinations, memory loss, and faulty orientation as to time and place. Psychotic reactions have been reported with the 1% concentration following instillation of 2 drops in each eye in children and adults.[414,417,418] In addition, adults have also complained of drowsiness, nausea, or

TABLE 3.24
Side Effects of Cyclopentolate

Ocular Effects	*Systemic Effects*
Irritation and lacrimation	Drowsiness
Conjunctival hyperemia	Incoherent speech
Allergic blepharoconjunctivitis	Ataxia
Elevated intraocular pressure	Disorientation
	Restlessness
	Visual hallucinations

weakness. All reactions subside usually within 2 hours in adults and 4 to 6 hours in children, without permanent sequelae. However, cyclopentolate is not without possible serious toxic effects. Two cases of grand mal seizure have been reported with use of the 2% solution.[419]

Peripheral effects typical of atropine, such as flushing or dryness of the skin or mucous membranes, have not been observed with cyclopentolate in children or in adults. Moreover, temperature, pulse, blood pressure, and respiration are generally not affected.[414–418]

Treatment of cyclopentolate toxicity is the same as that for atropine toxicity. Since toxic reactions occur more commonly with the 2% solution or with multiple instillations of 1%, the smallest possible dose should be used and care should be taken with very young children and with those persons at special risk, such as debilitated or aged patients.

Tropicamide

PHARMACOLOGY

A synthetic derivative of tropic acid, tropicamide became available for ocular use in 1959. With a pK_a of 5.37, it is only about 2.3% ionized at physiologic pH. The un-ionized molecules can readily diffuse the lipid portion of the corneal epithelium, and thus a greater concentration of drug can reach the receptor sites than is the case with atropine, homatropine, and cyclopentolate, with pK_a values of 9.8, 9.9, and 8.4, respectively.[376] The relatively greater diffusibility of tropicamide may also account for its faster onset and shorter duration of action compared with those of other anticholinergic agents. Tropicamide is commercially available as 0.5% and 1% solutions (see Table 3.22)

Merrill and associates[411] were first to report the effects of 0.5% and 1% solution of tropicamide in human eyes. Maximum mydriasis occurred in 25 to 30 minutes following instillation of either the 0.5% or the 1% concentration. The 1% produced an average increase of 4.0 mm in pupil size at 30 minutes. Thereafter, the pupil diameter began to decrease, reaching preinstillation size at 6 hours. The effect of the 0.5% solution on mydriasis was only slightly less than that of the 1% concentration.

Tropicamide has been reported to provide sufficient mydriasis for routine ophthalmoscopy at concentrations as low as 0.25%. Gettes[420] reported that 1 drop of 0.25% tropicamide provided a 5 mm or greater dilation in most subjects except for blacks, whose eyes dilated to a lesser degree. Pollack and associates[421] observed no significant differences in pupil size under normal or bright illumination in 8 male whites, aged 22 to 32 years, following instillation of 1 drop of tropicamide 0.25%, 0.5%, 0.75%, or 1% (Fig. 3.45).

Since, in general, the pupils of diabetic patients are resistant to dilation with anticholinergic agents, adequate mydriasis with tropicamide alone is usually not achieved in these patients. A combination of tropicamide and phenylephrine produces adequate dilation in most cases, particularly since the pupil of diabetic patients shows supersensitivity to adrenergic agonists.[422]

The maximum cycloplegic effect also occurs at 30 minutes following instillation. Unlike the mydriatic effects, there may be a difference on accommodation between the two commercially available concentrations of tropicamide, the 1% producing a somewhat greater loss of accommodation.[411] The average residual accommodation with 1% tropicamide was 1.60 D at 30 minutes and 2.40 D at 40 minutes. Gettes[420] studied the cycloplegic effect of 1% tropicamide and found it to be clinically effective in 90% of the eyes tested, provided that a second drop was instilled 5 to 25 minutes after the first, and provided also that the examination was performed 20 to 35 minutes following instillation. Accommodation returns to preinstillation values within 6 hours.

Pollack and associates[421] studied the cycloplegic effects of 0.25%, 0.5%, 0.75%, and 1% tropicamide. Some inhibition of accommodation occurred with each concentration of tropicamide, and the effects were dose related. The maximum residual accommodation ranged from 3.17 D for the 0.25% concentration to 1.30 D for the 1% concentration. The maximum cycloplegic ef-

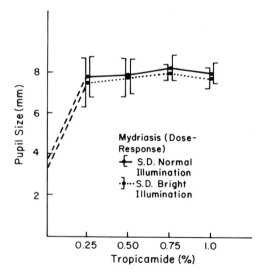

FIGURE 3.45 **Mean mydriatic dose-response curves for tropicamide 0.25, 0.5, 0.75, and 1% under normal and bright illuminance. (From Pollack SL, Hunt JS, Polse KA. Dose-response effects of tropicamide HCl. Am J Optom Physiol Opt 1981;58:361–366.)**

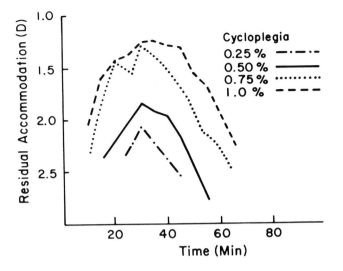

FIGURE 3.46 **Mean residual accommodation for tropicamide over the period of maximum cycloplegia. (From Pollack SL, Hunt JS, Polse KA. Dose-response effects of tropicamide HCl. Am J Optom Physiol Opt 1981;58:361–366.)**

fects for all subjects occurred 30 to 35 minutes following instillation. Significant differences in cycloplegic effects were found between the 0.25% and 1% solutions but not among 0.5%, 0.75%, or 1% concentrations. Figure 3.46 illustrates the residual accommodation during the period of maximum cycloplegia for all concentrations of tropicamide tested. Two diopters or less of residual accommodation were present for at least 40 minutes with the 0.75% and 1% concentrations and for about 15 minutes with the 0.5% concentration. A mean residual accommodation of 2.2 D was present following the application of 0.25% tropicamide. This

effect was sufficient to incapacitate the subjects for most near vision tasks for 40 to 60 minutes.

The mydriatic effect of tropicamide has been compared to that of homatropine and of cyclopentolate.[411,425] Merrill and associates[411] reported that whereas tropicamide 0.5% or 1% produced maximum mydriasis within 30 minutes, cyclopentolate 1%, homatropine 5%, or phenylephrine 10% did so in 60 to 90 minutes. Moreover, the degree of mydriasis at 30 minutes was greater with tropicamide than with the other drugs tested.[411] Gambill and associates[84] compared the mydriatic effects of tropicamide 0.5%, homatropine 2%, phenylephrine 10%, and hydroxyamphetamine 1%. Tropicamide had the fastest onset and greatest intensity of mydriatic action (Fig. 3.47).

The cycloplegic effectiveness of tropicamide has been compared to that of cyclopentolate and homatropine.[411,423-425] Merrill and associates[411] observed that the maximum cycloplegic effect of 1% tropicamide at 30 minutes was greater than that obtained from 1% cyclopentolate or 5% homatropine but was much shorter, with clinically effective cycloplegia maintained only up to 35 minutes following instillation of a single drop. Gettes and Belmont[423] compared the effects of tropicamide 1%, cyclopentolate 1%, and homatropine 4% combined with hydroxyamphetamine 1%. Two instillations of each drug were given 5 minutes apart, and measurement of accommodation was performed 20 to 40 minutes after the second drop. Figure 3.48 summarizes the results. Although the initial intensity of the cycloplegic effect of tropicamide was nearly equal to that of cyclopentolate, accommodation rapidly returned after 35 minutes. Cyclopentolate remained consistently effective after 25 minutes for the duration of the measurement. The homatropine-hydroxyamphe-

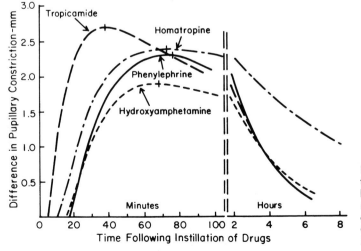

FIGURE 3.47 **Onset, intensity, and duration of mydriasis for tropicamide 0.5%, homatropine 2%, phenylephrine 10%, and hydroxyamphetamine 1% measured by electronic pupillography. (From Gambill HD, Ogle KN, Kearns TP. Mydriatic effect of four drugs determined by pupillograph. Arch Ophthalmol 1967;77:740–746. Copyright 1967, American Medical Association.)**

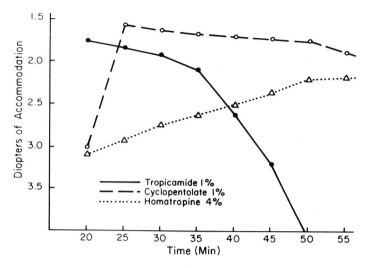

FIGURE 3.48 **Average residual accommodation with tropicamide 1%, cyclopentolate 1%, and homatropine 4% in adult patients. (From Gettes BC, Belmont O. Tropicamide: Comparative cycloplegic effects. Arch Ophthalmol 1961;66:336–340. Copyright 1961, American Medical Association.)**

tamine combination exhibited a slower onset, reaching clinically effective levels of cycloplegia for refraction at 45 to 55 minutes. In similar studies using tropicamide 1%, cyclopentolate 1%, or homatropine 5%, 2 drops to each eye, Milder[424] observed that cyclopentolate and homatropine were superior to tropicamide in 92% and 80% of patients, respectively. Moreover, the magnitude of residual accommodation was inversely related to age, being greater than 2.5 D with tropicamide in patients under 40 years of age (Table 3.25).

Prior application of a topical anesthetic appears to prolong tropicamide's mydriatic and cycloplegic actions.[426] Mordi and associates[426] reported that prior instillation of proparacaine 0.5% in blue-green eyes prolonged both the time required for 50% recovery to normal pupil size and the time during which mydriasis is maintained within 90% of maximum. In brown-hazel eyes the time for recovery to 50% was lengthened by 30 minutes, but the time during which mydriasis re-

mained 90% of maximum was not lengthened by prior application of the anesthetic. The time during which cycloplegia was maintained within 90% of maximum was extended by 3 to 4 minutes in all eyes, regardless of degree of pigmentation.

CLINICAL USES

Due to its relatively fast onset, short duration, and sufficient intensity of action, tropicamide is considered the drug of choice for ophthalmoscopy and other procedures where mydriasis is desirable. Moreover, unlike with atropine, homatropine, or cyclopentolate, pupillary dilation with tropicamide appears to be independent of iris pigmentation. Dillon and associates[427] achieved a minimum of 6 mm pupil size with 0.5% tropicamide in subjects with light and dark irides. No significant differences in amplitude of dilation occurred

TABLE 3.25
Residual Accommodation Following Instillation of Tropicamide 1%, Homatropine 5%, or Cyclopentolate 1%

Age (yr)	Number of Subjects	Tropicamide (30 min)	Homatropine or Cyclopentolate (60 min)
0–9	6	6.25 D	2.50 D
10–14	20	3.65	2.40
15–19	7	3.20	1.40
20–29	7	3.10	1.40
30–39	7	2.60	2.00
40+	3	1.70	1.10

From Milder B. Tropicamide as a cycloplegic agent. Arch Ophthalmol 1961;66:60. Copyright 1961, American Medical Association.

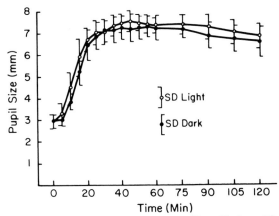

FIGURE 3.49   **Comparison of mean pupillary dilation with 0.5% tropicamide in subjects with light and dark irides. (From Dillon JR, Tyhurst CW, Yolton RL. The mydriatic effect of tropicamide on light and dark irides. J Am Optom Assoc 1977;48:653–658.)**

that a combination of 0.1% tropicamide and 1% hydroxyamphetamine was effective for routine ophthalmoscopic examinations. Brown and Hanna[430] compared 0.1% tropicamide and 1% phenylephrine suspended in 1% methylcellulose to 1% tropicamide and 10% phenylephrine administered as drops. Both combinations produced nearly equal dilation at 30 minutes. The average residual accommodation measured 1.8 D at 45 minutes with the methylcellulose mixture. The mydriatic effect of a mixture of 0.75% tropicamide and 2.5% phenylephrine has been compared to that of the separate instillation of 1% tropicamide and 10% phenylephrine in 100 white patients ranging in age from 14 to 85 years.[431] Both direct and indirect ophthalmoscopy were performed on each patient. The low-concentration mixture produced average pupil sizes of 7.4 mm and 7.5 mm in blue and brown irides, respectively, compared with an average dilation of 7.6 mm in all subjects with the separate instillation of 10% phenylephrine and 1% tropicamide (Fig. 3.50). Cycloplegic effects were not evaluated, but one could presume, based on the data of Pollack and associates,[421] that accommodation was reduced equally with both drug regimens.

The advantage of tropicamide as compared to other mydriatic-cycloplegic agents is its fast onset and relatively short duration of action. Clinically, it is important to remember that tropicamide has a greater mydriatic than cycloplegic effect, and thus, unlike with cyclopentolate and other anticholinergics, mydriasis does not necessarily indicate adequate cycloplegia for refraction.

with respect to iris pigmentation or race of subjects (Fig. 3.49).

For clinical situations where only mydriasis is necessary, it is desirable to obtain pupillary dilation with minimum paralysis of accommodation so as not to interfere with near vision tasks. To achieve clinically useful mydriasis with minimal accommodative paralysis, various combinations of drugs have been investigated. Priestly and associates[428] evaluated a combination of cyclopentolate 0.2% and phenylephrine 1% (Cyclomydril). This combination produced satisfactory mydriasis 30 minutes following instillation. However, the effect on accommodation with Cyclomydril is equal to or greater than with tropicamide 1%.[429,430] Other investigators have tested various concentrations of tropicamide with adrenergic agonists. Gettes[425] reported

SIDE EFFECTS

Tropicamide, especially at the 1% concentration, can produce transient stinging on instillation. As with the

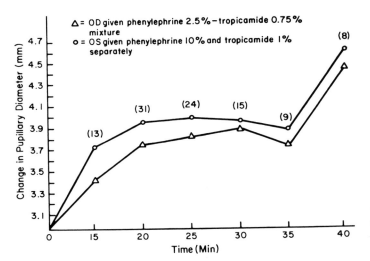

FIGURE 3.50   **Changes in pupil diameter with 1 drop of phenylephrine 2.5% and tropicamide 0.75% in right eye, and 1 drop of phenylephrine 10% and tropicamide 1% in left eye. (From Forman AR. A new low-concentration preparation for mydriasis and cycloplegia. Ophthalmology 1980;87:213–215.)**

other mydriatic-cycloplegics, it can raise intraocular pressure in eyes with open-angle glaucoma. The pressure elevation is usually less than 5 mm Hg and can be considered insignificant in most patients, since it will subside in several hours without damaging the optic nerve.[432]

Adverse systemic reactions to tropicamide are quite rare. Wahl[433] has reported one such reaction in a 10-year-old white male. Immediately following instillation of 1 drop of 0.5% tropicamide into each eye, the patient fell from the chair to the floor unconscious. This was followed by generalized muscular rigidity, pallor, and cyanosis. Within a few minutes the patient became flaccid and regained consciousness, but he remained in a state of generalized weakness and drowsiness. About 1 hour after the onset of the episode, his vital signs were normal and he was fully recovered. Wahl classified this reaction as acute hypersensitivity manifested by anaphylactic shock. The spontaneous recovery, however, argues against an anaphylactic mechanism. Others have suggested the possibility that psychomotor factors may play a role in such reactions. Yolton and associates[434] and Applebaum and Jaanus[435] have observed no adverse reactions associated with the use of tropicamide in over 12,000 drug applications in patients undergoing ophthalmoscopy.

Since tropicamide is devoid of vasopressor effect,[112] it is probably one of the safest mydriatic agents for use in patients with systemic hypertension, angina, or other cardiovascular disease.

REFERENCES

1. Weiner N, Taylor P. Neuro-humoral transmission: The autonomic and somatic nervous systems. In: Gilman AG, Goodman LS, Rall TW, Murad F, eds. The pharmacological basis of therapeutics. New York: Macmillan Co, 1985;Chap. 4.
2. Zinn KM. The pupil. Springfield, IL: Charles C Thomas, 1972; Chap. 2.
3. Ehinger B. A comparative study of the adrenergic nerves to the anterior eye segment of some primates. Z Zellforsch 1971;116:157–177.
4. Lowenfeld IE. Mechanisms of reflex dilation of the pupil; historical review and experimental analysis. Doc Ophthalmol (Den Haag) 1958;12:185–448.
5. Laties A, Jacobowitz D. A histochemical study of the adrenergic and cholinergic innervation of the anterior segment of the rabbit eye. Invest Ophthalmol 1964;3:592–600.
6. Neufeld AH, Zawistowski KA, Page ED, Bromberg BB. Influences on the density of beta adrenergic receptors in the cornea and iris-ciliary body of the rabbit. Invest Ophthalmol 1978;17:1069–1075.
7. Butterfield LC, Neufeld AH. Cyclic nucleotides and mitosis

8. Waltman SR, Yarian D, Hart W, Becker B. Corneal endothelial changes with long-term topical epinephrine therapy. Arch Ophthalmol 1977;95:1357–1358.
9. Zadunaisky JA, Lande MA, Chalfie M, Neufeld AH. Ion pumps in the cornea and its stimulation by epinephrine and cAMP. Exp Eye Res 1973;15:577–584.
10. Walkenback RJ, Le Grand RD. Adenylate cyclase activity in bovine and human corneal endothelium. Invest Ophthalmol Vis Sci 1982;22:120–124.
11. Kahan A. Effects of adrenergic activators and inhibitors on the eye. In: Szekeres L, ed. Adrenergic activators and inhibitors. Handbuch Pharm 1981;8:319–344.
12. Voaden MS. A chalone in the rabbit lens. Exp Eye Res 1968;7:326–331.
13. Kramer SG. Dopamine: A retinal neurotransmitter. I. Retinal uptake, storage, and light-stimulated release of H3-dopamine in vivo. Invest Ophthalmol 1971;10:438–452.
14. Van Halpern GWHN, Kern R, Robinette SL. Adrenergic receptors of the intraocular muscles. Arch Ophthalmol 1965;74:253–259.
15. Laties A, Jacobowitz D. A comparative study of the autonomic innervation of the eye in monkey, cat and rabbit. Anat Rec 1966;156:383–389.
16. Kern R. Die adrenergischen receptoren der intraocularen muskelin des menschen. Graef Arch Klin Exp Ophthal 1970;180:321–348.
17. Langham ME, Diggs E. β-adrenergic responses in the eyes of rabbits, primates and man. Exp Eye Res 1974;19:281–295.
18. Nathanson JA. Human ciliary process adrenergic receptor: pharmacological characterization. Invest Ophthalmol Vis Sci 1981;21:798–804.
19. Lahar M, Melamed E, Dafna Z, Alas D. Localization of beta-receptors in the anterior segment of the rat eye by a fluorescent analogue of propranolol. Invest Ophthalmol 1978;17:645–651.
20. Neufeld AH, Page Ed. In vitro determination of the ability of drugs to bind to adrenergic receptors. Invest Ophthalmol Vis Sci 1977;16:1118–1124.
21. Bhargava G, Mahman MH, Katzman R. Distribution of β-adrenergic receptors and isoproterenol-stimulated cyclic AMP formation in monkey iris and ciliary body. Exp Eye Res 1980;31:471–477.
22. Langham ME, Krieglstein GK. The biphasic intraocular pressure response of rabbits to epinephrine. Invest Ophthalmol Vis Sci 1976;15:119–127.
23. Bittiger H, Heid J, Wigger N. Are only 2 adrenergic receptors present in the bovine retina? Nature 1980;287:645–647.
24. Osborne NN. Binding of (-) ³H noradrenaline to bovine membrane retina. Evidence for the existence of 2- receptors. Vis Res 1982;22:1401–1407.
25. Hofmann H. Noradrenaline in der augenheilkunde. Klin Monatsbl Augenheil Kd 1954;124:63–76.
26. Owe-Larsson A. The local effect on the eye of noradrenaline. Acta Ophthalmol 1956;34:27–34.
27. Langham ME, Diggs EM. Adrenergic responses in the human eye. J Pharmacol Exp Ther 1971;179:47–55.
28. Henkind P, Walsh JB, Berger AW, eds. Physicians' desk

reference for ophthalmology. Oradell, NJ:Medical Economics, 1988.

29. Havener WH. Ocular pharmacology. St. Louis: C.V. Mosby, 1983;Chap. 12.

30. Holland MG. Autonomic drugs in ophthalmology: some problems and promises. III. Sympathomimetic drugs. Ann Ophthalmol 1974;6:875–888.

31. Weekers R, Delmarcelle Y, Gustin J. Treatment of ocular hypertension by adrenaline and diverse sympathomimetic amines. Am J Ophthalmol 1955;40:666–672.

32. Ballintine EJ, Garner L. Improvement of the coefficient of outflow in glaucomatous eyes. Arch Ophthalmol 1961; 66:314–317.

33. Becker B, Pettit TH, Gay AS. Topical epinephrine therapy of open angle glaucoma. Arch Ophthalmol 1961;66:219–225.

34. Harris LS, Galin MA, Lerner R. The influence of low dose L-epinephrine on intraocular pressure. Ann Ophthalmol 1970;2:253–257.

35. Jones RF, Maurice DM. New methods of measuring the rate of aqueous flow in man with fluorescein. Exp Eye Res 1966;5:208–220.

36. Townsend DJ, Brubaker RF. Immediate effect of epinephrine on aqueous formation in the normal human eye as measured by fluorophotometry. Invest Ophthalmol 1980; 19:256–266.

37. Schenker HI, Yablonski ME, Podos SM, Linder L. Fluorophotometric study of epinephrine and timolol in human subjects. Arch Ophthalmol 1981;99:1212–1216.

38. Bill A. Early effect of epinephrine on aqueous humor dynamics in Verret monkeys. Exp Eye Res 1969;8:35–43.

39. Neufeld AH, Jampol LM, Sears ML. Cyclic AMP in the aqueous humor. The effects of adrenergic action. Exp Eye Res 1972;14:242–250.

40. Boas RS, Messenger MJ, Mittag TW, Podos SM. The effects of topically applied epinephrine and timolol on intraocular pressure and aqueous humor cyclic-AMP in the rabbit. Exp Eye Res 1981;32:681–690.

41. Becker B, Montgomery SW, Kass MA, Shin DH. Increased ocular and systemic responsiveness to epinephrine in primary open-angle glaucoma. Arch Ophthalmol 1977;95:789–790.

42. Podos SM, Ritch R. Epinephrine as the initial therapy in selected cases of ocular hypertension. Surv Ophthalmol 1980;25:188–194.

43. Tredici TJ. Screening and management of glaucoma in flying personnel. Aerospace Med 1980;50:34–41.

44. Kramer SG. Epinephrine distribution after topical administration to phakic and aphakic eyes. Trans Am Ophthalmol Soc 1980;78:947–981.

45. Durkee D, Bryant BG. Drug therapy in glaucoma. Am J Hosp Pharm 1979;35:682–690.

46. Sugar SH. Pitfalls in the medical treatment of simple glaucoma. Ann Ophthalmol 1979;11:1041–1050.

47. Aronson SB, Yamamoto EA. Ocular hypersensitivity to epinephrine. Invest Ophthalmol 1966;5:75–80.

48. Edelhauser HF, Hyndiuck RA, Zeeb A, Schultz RO. Corneal edema and the intraocular use of epinephrine. Am J Ophthalmol 1982;93:327–333.

49. Sugar J. Adenochrome pigmentation of hydrophilic lenses. Arch Ophthalmol 1974;91:11–12.

50. Mahmood MA, Pillai S. Epinephrine staining of soft contact lens. Arch Ophthalmol 1987;105:1021–1022.

51. Lee PF. The influence of epinephrine and phenylephrine on intraocular pressure. Arch Ophthalmol 1958;60:863–867.

52. Kolker AE, Becker B. Epinephrine maculopathy. Arch Ophthalmol 1968;79:552–562.

53. Becker B, Morton WF. Topical epinephrine in glaucoma suspects. Am J Ophthalmol 1966;62:272–277.

54. Michels RG, Maumenee AE. Cystoid macular edema associated with topically applied epinephrine in aphakic eyes. Am J Ophthalmol 1975;80:379–388.

55. Mackool RJ, Muldoon T, Fortier A, Nelson D. Epinephrine induced cystoid macular edema in aphakic eyes. Arch Ophthalmol 1977;95:791–793.

56. Ballin N, Becker B, Goldman ML. Systemic effects of epinephrine applied topically to the eye. Invest Ophthalmol 1966;5:125–129.

57. Davidson SI. Systemic effects of eye drops. Trans Ophthalmol Soc UK 1974;94:487–495.

58. Schwartz B. Primary open-angle glaucoma. In: Duane TD, ed. Clinical ophthalmology. Hagerstown, MD: Harper & Row, 1981;3:52.

59. Van Buskirk EM. Hazards of medical glaucoma therapy in the cataract patient. Ophthalmology 1982;89:238–241.

60. Ritchie JM, Greene NM. Local anesthetics. In: Gilman AG, Goodman LS, Rall TW, Murad F, eds. The pharmacological basis of therapeutics. New York: Macmillan Co, 1985; Chap. 15.

61. Altman AJ, Albert DM, Fournier GA. Cocaine's use in ophthalmology: Our 100-year heritage. Surv Ophthalmol 1985;29:300–306.

62. Friedman JR, Whiting DW, Kosmorsky GS, Burde RM. The cocaine test in normal patients. Am J Ophthalmol 1984;98:808–810.

63. Mandell AI, Podos SM. Dipivalyl epinephrine (DPE): A new prodrug in the treatment of glaucoma. In: Leopold IH, Burns RP, eds. Symposium on ocular therapy. New York: John Wiley & Sons, 1977;10:109–117.

64. Wei C, Anderson JA, Leopold IH. Ocular absorption and metabolism of topically applied epinephrine and a dipivalyl ester of epinephrine. Invest Ophthalmol 1978;17:315.

65. Mandell AI, Stentz F, Kitabicki AE. Dipivalyl epinephrine: a new prodrug in the treatment of glaucoma. Trans Am Acad Ophthalmol Otolaryngol 1978;85:268–274.

66. Kaback MB, Podos SM, Harbin TS, et al. The effects of dipivalyl epinephrine on the eye. Am J Ophthalmol 1976;81:768–772.

67. Mindel JS, Koenigsberg AM, Kharlamb AP, et al. The effect of echothiophate on the biphasic response of rabbit ocular pressure to dipivefrin. Arch Ophthalmol 1982;100:147–151.

68. Thorson JC. Concomitant glaucoma therapy with dipivefrin and timolol maleate. Trans Ophthalmol Soc NZ 1981;33:24–26.

69. Frumar KD, McGuinness R. A study of the intraocular pressure lowering effect of timolol and dipivalyl epinephrine. Trans Ophthalmol Soc NZ 1981;33:27–29.

70. Keates EV, Stone RA. Safety and effectiveness of concom-

itant administration of dipivefrin and timolol maleate. Am J Ophthalmol 1981;91:243–248.

71. Mindel JS, Yablonski ME, Tavitian HO, et al. Dipivefrin and echothiophate. Arch Ophthalmol 1981;99:1583–1586.

72. Kohn AN, Moss AP, Hargett NA, et al. Clinical comparison of dipivalyl epinephrine and epinephrine in the treatment of glaucoma. Am J Ophthalmol 1979;87:196–201.

73. Kerr CR, Hass I, Drance SM, et al. Cardiovascular effects of epinephrine and dipivalyl epinephrine applied topically to the eye in patients with glaucoma. Br J Ophthalmol 1982;66:109–114.

74. Yablonski ME, Shin DH, Kolker AE. Dipivefrin use in patients with intolerance to topically applied epinephrine. Arch Ophthalmol 1977;95:2157–2158.

75. Theodore J, Leibowitz HM. External ocular toxicity of dipivalyl epinephrine. Am J Ophthalmol 1979;88:1013–1016.

76. Newton MJ, Nesburn AB. Lack of hydrophilic lens discoloration in patients using dipivalyl epinephrine for glaucoma. Am J Ophthalmol 1979;87:193–195.

77. Liesegang TJ. Bulbar conjunctival follicles associated with dipivefrin therapy. Ophthalmology 1985;92:228–233.

78. Wilson FM. Adverse external ocular effects of topical ophthalmic medications. Surv Ophthalmol 1979/80;24:57–88.

79. Wandel T, Spinak M. Toxicity of dipivalyl epinephrine. Ophthalmology 1981;88:259–260.

80. Bigger JF. Dipivefrin and glaucoma. Perspect Ophthalmol 1980;4:87–90.

81. Heath P, Geiter CW. Use of phenylephrine hydrochloride (Neosynephrine) in ophthalmology. Arch Ophthalmol 1949;41:172–177.

82. Lee PF. The influence of epinephrine and phenylephrine on intraocular pressure. Arch Ophthalmol 1958;60:863–867.

83. Barbee R, Smith WA. A comparative study of mydriatic and cycloplegic agents. Am J Ophthalmol 1957;44:617–622.

84. Gambill HD, Ogle KN, Kearns TP. Mydriatic effect of four drugs determined by pupillograph. Arch Ophthalmol 1967;77:740–746.

85. Haddad NJ, Moyer NJ, Riley FC. Mydriatic effect of phenylephrine hydrochloride. Am J Ophthalmol 1970;70:729–733.

86. Briggs RA, Alpern M, Bennett DR. The effect of sympathomimetic drugs upon amplitude of accommodation. Am J Ophthalmol 1959;48:169–172.

87. Roth N. Refractive state after instillation of paredrine and neosynephrine. Br J Ophthalmol 1968;52:763–767.

88. Smith RB, Read S, Oczypik PM. Mydriatic effect of phenylephrine. Eye Ear Nose Throat Monthly 1976;55:133–134.

89. Neuhaus RW, Hepler RS. Mydriatic effect of phenylephrine 10% vs phenylephrine 2.5% (aq). Ann Ophthalmol 1980;12:1159–1160.

90. Weiss DI, Shaffer RN. Mydriatic effects of one-eighth percent phenylephrine. Arch Ophthalmol 1962;68:727–729.

91. Marr WG, Wood R, Senterfit L, Sigelman S. Effect of topical anesthetics on regeneration of corneal epithelium. Am J Ophthalmol 1957;606–610.

92. Jauregui MJ, Polse KA. Mydriatic effect using phenylephrine and proparacaine. Am J Optom Physiol Opt 1974;51:545–549.

93. Kubo DJ, Wing TW, Polse KA, Jauregui M. Mydriatic effects using low concentrations of phenylephrine hydrochloride. J Am Optom Assoc 1975;46:817–822.

94. Lyle WM, Bobier WR. Effects of topical anesthetics on phenylephrine-induced mydriasis. Am J Optom Physiol Opt 1977;54:276–281.

95. Chiri NB, Gold AA, Breinin G. Iris cysts and miotics. Arch Ophthalmol 1964;71:611–616.

96. Thompson HS, Menscher JH. Adrenergic mydriasis in Horner's syndrome; hydroxyamphetamine test for diagnosis of postganglionic defects. Am J Ophthalmol 1971;72:472–480.

97. Meyer SM, Fraunfelder FT. Phenylephrine hydrochloride. Ophthalmology 1980;87:1177–1180.

98. Edelhauser HF, Hine JE, Pederson H, Van Horn D, Schultz RO. The effect of phenylephrine on the cornea. Arch Ophthalmol 1979;97:937–947.

99. Cohen KL, Van Horn DL, Edelhauser HF, Schultz RO. Effect of phenylephrine on normal and regenerated endothelial cells in cat cornea. Invest Ophthalmol Vis Sci 1979;18:242–249.

100. Hanna C, Brainard J, Augsburger KD, Roy RH, et al. Allergic dermatoconjunctivitis caused by phenylephrine. Am J Ophthalmol 1983;95:703–704.

101. Mitsui Y, Takagi Y. Nature of aqueous floaters due to sympathomimetic mydriatics. Arch Ophthalmol 1961;65:626–631.

102. Haddad NJ, Moyer NJ, Riley FC. Mydriatic effect of phenylephrine hydrochloride. Am J Ophthalmol 1970;70:729–733.

103. Isenberg SJ, Green BF. Effect of phenylephrine hydrochloride on conjunctival PO_2. Arch Ophthalmol 1984;102:1185–1186.

104. Heath P. Neosynephrine hydrochloride. Some uses and effects in ophthalmology. Arch Ophthalmol 1936;16:839–846.

105. McReynolds W, Havener W. Henderson J. Hazards of the use of sympathomimetic drugs in ophthalmology. Arch Ophthalmol 1956;56:176–179.

106. Lanche R. Systemic reactions to topical epinephrine and phenylephrine. Am J Ophthalmol 1966;61:95–98.

107. Solosko D, Smith R. Hypertension following 10% phenylephrine ophthalmic. Anesthesiol 1972;36:187–189.

108. Borromeo-McGrail V, Borduik J, Keitel H. Systemic hypertension following ocular administration of 10% phenylephrine in the neonate. J Pediatr 1973;51:1032–1036.

109. Wilensky J, Woodward H. Acute systemic hypertension after conjunctival instillation of phenylephrine hydrochloride. Am J Ophthalmol 1973;76:156–157.

110. Samantary S, Thomas A. Systemic effects of topical phenylephrine. Ind J Ophthalmol 1975;23:16–17.

111. Fraunfelder FT, Scafidi AF. Possible adverse effects from topical ocular 10% phenylephrine. Am J Ophthalmol 1978;85:862–868.

112. Brown MM, Brown GC, Spaeth GL. Lack of side effects from topically administered 10% phenylephrine eyedrops. Arch Ophthalmol 1980;98:487–488.

113. Fraunfelder FT, Meyer SM. Possible cardiovascular effects secondary to topical ophthalmic 2.5% phenylephrine. Am J Ophthalmol 1985;99:362–363.

114. Kumar V, Packer AJ, Choi WW. Hypertension following 2.5% phenylephrine ophthalmic drops. Glaucoma 1985; 7:131–132.

115. Jennings BJ, Sullivan DE. The effect of topical 2.5% phenylephrine and 1% tropicamide on systemic blood pressure and pulse. J Am Optom Assoc 1986;57:382–389.

116. Kim JM, Stevenson CE, Mathewson HS. Hypertensive reactions to phenylephrine eyedrops in patients with sympathetic denervation. Am J Ophthalmol 1978;85:862–868.

117. Robertson D. Contraindication to the use of ocular phenylephrine in idiopathic orthostatic hypotension. Am J Ophthalmol 1979;87:819–822.

118. Keys A, Violante A. The cardiocirculatory effects in man of Neo-Synephrine. J Clin Invest 1942;21:1–21.

119. Stack DDC. Effects of giving vasopressors to patients on monoamine oxidase inhibitors. Lancet 1962;1:1405–1406.

120. Neo-Synephrine Hydrochloride package insert. Winthrop Laboratories, NW-147 U. Revised, November, 1976;1–8.

121. Wellwood M, Goresky GV. Systemic hypertension associated with topical administration of 2.5 percent phenylephrine HCL. Am J Ophthalmol 1982;93:369–374.

122. Sneddon JM, Turner P. The interaction of local guanethidine and sympathomimetic amines in the human eye. Arch Ophthalmol 1969;81:622–627.

123. Rutledge CO. The mechanism by which amphetamine inhibits oxidative elimination of norepinephrine in man. J Pharmacol Exp Ther 1970;171:188–196.

124. Caldwell J, Sever PS. The biochemical pharmacology of abused drugs. I. Amphetamines, cocaine and LSD. Clin Pharmacol Ther 1974;16:625–638.

125. Thompson HS, Mensher JH. Reply: hydroxyamphetamine test in Horner's syndrome. Am J Ophthalmol 1975;79:525–526.

126. Abbott WO, Henry CM. Paredrine (β-4-hydroxyphenyli-sopropylamine): A clinical investigation of a sympathomimetic drug. Am J Med Sci 1937;193:661–673.

127. Semes LP, Bartlett JD. Mydriatic effectiveness of hydroxyamphetamine. J Am Optom Assoc 1982;53:899–904.

128. Gartner S, Billet E. Mydriatic glaucoma. Am J Ophthalmol 1957;43:975–976.

129. Kronfeld PC, McGarry HI, Smith HE. The effect of mydriatics upon the intraocular pressure in so called primary wide-angle glaucoma. Am J Ophthalmol 1943;26:245–252.

130. Hanna C. Tachyphylaxis. Some cardiovascular actions of hydroxyamphetamine and related compounds. Arch Int Pharmacodyn 1960;128:469–480.

131. Aviado DM. Cardiovascular effects of some commonly used pressor amines. Anesthesiol 1959;20:71–97.

132. Weiner N. Norepinephrine, epinephrine and the sympathomimetic amines. In: Gilman AG, Goodman LS, Rall TW, et al., eds. The pharmacological basis of therapeutics. New York: Macmillan Co., 1986; Chap. 8.

133. Chen KK, Poth EJ. Ephedrine as a mydriatic in Caucasians. Am J Med Sci 1929;178:203–209.

134. Obianww HO, Rand MJ. The relationship between the mydriatic action of ephedrine and the color of the iris. Br J Ophthalmol 1965;49:264–270.

135. Mitchell DWA. The effect of ephedrine instillation on intraocular pressure. Br J Physiol Opt 1957;14:38–42.

136. Babel J. Action of 2-(1-naphthylmethyl) imidazoline hydrochloride on the eye. Schweiz Med Wochschr 1941;71:561–575.

137. Hurwitz P, Thompson JM. Use of naphazoline (Privine) in ophthalmology. Arch Ophthalmol 1950;43:712–717.

138. Grossmann EE, Lehman RH. Ophthalmic use of tyzine. Am J Ophthalmol 1956;42:121–123.

139. Menger HC. New ophthalmic decongestant, tetrahydrozoline hydrochloride. JAMA 1958;170:178–179.

140. Miller J, Wolf EM. Antazoline phosphate and naphazoline hydrochloride, singly and in combination for the treatment of allergic conjunctivitis—a controlled double-blind clinical trial. Ann Allergy 1975;35:81–86.

141. Samson CR, Danzig MR, Sasovetz D, Thompson HS. Safety and toleration of oxymetazoline ophthalmic solution. Pharmatherapeutica 1980;2:347–352.

142. Breaky AS, Cinotti AA, Hirshman M, Skowron RA, et al. A double-blind, multi-centre controlled trial of 0.025% oxymetazoline ophthalmic solution in patients with allergic and non-infectious conjunctivitis. Pharmatherapeutica 1980;2:353–356.

143. Duzman E, Anderson J, Vita JB, Lue JC, et al. Topically applied oxymetazoline. Arch Ophthalmol 1983;101:1122–1126.

144. Duzman E, Warman A, Warman R. Efficacy and safety of topical oxymetazoline in treating allergic and environmental conjunctivitis. Ann Ophthalmol 1986;18:28–31.

145. Butler K, Thompson JP, Yolton DP. Effects of non-prescription ocular decongestants. Rev Optom 1978;115:49–52.

146. Abelson MB, Yamamoto GK, Allansmith MR. Effects of ocular decongestants. Arch Ophthalmol 1980;98:856–858.

147. Abelson MB, Butrus SI, Weston JH, Rosner B. Tolerance and absence of rebound vasodilation following topical ocular decongestant usage. Ophthalmology 1984;91:1364–1367.

148. Schering Laboratories, July 1987.

149. Lisch K. Bindehautalterationen durch sympathomimetika. Klin MBl Augenheilk 1978;173:404–406.

150. Salem H, Dunn BJ, Loux JJ. Conjunctival temperature: a measure of ocular decongestant and antiinflammatory activity. Ann Ophthalmol 1975;7:819–824.

151. Weiner N. Drugs that inhibit adrenergic nerves and block adrenergic receptors. In: Gilman AG, Goodman LS, Rall TW, et al., eds. The pharmacological basis of therapeutics. New York: Macmillan 1985;9:176–210.

152. Philips CI, Howitt G, Rowlands DJ. Propranolol, an ocular hypotensive agent. Br J Ophthalmol 1967;51:222–226.

153. Cote G, Drance SM. The effect of propranolol on human intraocular pressure. Can J Ophthalmol 1968;3:207–212.

154. Bucci MG, Giraldi JP, Missiroli A, Virno N. La Somministrazione locale del propranololo rella terpia del glaucoma. Bol Ocul 1968;47:51–60.

155. Vale J, Gibbs ACC, Phillips CI. Topical propranolol and ocular tension in the human. Br J Ophthalmol 1972;56:770–775.

156. Weinstein P. Receptor paralyzing agents applied in the treatment of glaucoma simplex. Intern Zeitschrift für Klin Pharmak Ther Toxikol 1969;2:374–375.

157. Hall RA, Robson RD, Share NN. Timolol maleate: a new

beta-adrenergic receptor blocking agent. Arch Int Pharmacodyn Ther 1975;213:251–263.

158. Merck Sharp and Dohme. Product information summary. Merck and Co., West Point, PA, 1978.

159. Schmitt C, Lotti US, Le Douarec JC. Penetration of timolol into the rabbit eye after ocular instillation and intravenous injection. Arch Ophthalmol 1980;98:547–551.

160. Phillips CI, Bartholomew RS, Kazi G, et al. Penetration of timolol eye drops into human aqueous humor. Br J Ophthalmol 1981;65:593–595.

161. Affrime MB, Lowenthal DT, Tobert JA, et al. Dynamics and kinetics of ophthalmic timolol. Clin Pharmacol Ther 1980;27:471–477.

162. Passo MS, Palmer EA, Van Buskirk EM. Plasma timolol in glaucoma patients. Ophthalmology 1984;91:1361–1363.

163. Fraunfelder FT, Meyer SH. Systemic side effects from ophthalmic timolol and their prevention. J Ocul Pharmacol 1987;3:177–184.

164. Scriabine A, Torchiana ML, Stavorski JM, et al. Some cardiovascular effects of timolol, a new beta adrenergic blocking agent. Arch Int Pharmacodyn Ther 1973;205:76–93.

165. Katz IM, Hubbard WA, Getson AJ, Gould AL. Intraocular pressure decrease in normal volunteers following timolol ophthalmic solution. Invest Ophthalmol 1976;15:489–492.

166. Zimmerman TJ, Kaufman HE. Timolol: A β-adrenergic blocking agent for the treatment of glaucoma. Arch Ophthalmol 1977;95:601–604.

167. Zimmerman TJ, Kaufman HE. Timolol dose response and duration of action. Arch Ophthalmol 1977;95:605–607.

168. Kwitko GM, Shin DH, Ahn BH, et al. Bilateral effects of long-term monocular timolol therapy. Am J Ophthalmol 1987;104:591–594.

169. Radius RL, Diamond GR, Pollack IP, Langham ME. Timolol: A new drug for management of chronic simple glaucoma. Arch Ophthalmol 1978;96:1603–1608.

170. Boger WP III, Puliafito CA, Steinert RF, Langston D. Long-term experience with timolol ophthalmic solution in patients with open-angle glaucoma. Ophthalmology 1978;85:259–267.

171. Willcockson J, Willcockson T. Long-term timolol use in patients with chronic open-angle glaucoma: Results of a 40-month study. Glaucoma 1982;4:155–158.

172. Wilson CP, Spaeth GL, Poryzees E. The place of timolol in the practice of ophthalmology. Ophthalmology 1980;87:451–454.

173. Zimmerman TJ, Kaufman HE. Timolol—dose response and duration of action. Arch Ophthalmol 1977;95:605–607.

174. Hass I, Drance SM. Comparison between pilocarpine and timolol on diurnal pressure in open-angle glaucoma. Arch Ophthalmol 1980;98:480–481.

175. Secter RA, Elenbaas JK, Hamburger S. Update on drug therapy. II. Timolol maleate ophthalmic solution. JAMA 1980;35:31–33.

176. Berson FG, Epstein DL. Separate and combined effects of timolol maleate and acetazolamide in open-angle glaucoma. Am J Ophthalmol 1981;92:788–791.

177. Steinert RF, Thomas JV, Boger WP. Long-term drift and continued efficacy after multiyear timolol therapy. Arch Ophthalmol 1981;99:100–103..

178. Maclure GM. Chronic open angle glaucoma treated with timolol. A four year study. Trans Ophthalmol Soc UK 1983;103:78–83.

179. Blumenthal M, Yalon M, Rothkoff L, et al. Effectiveness study of longterm timolol therapy. Glaucoma 1984;6:28–30.

180. Katz IM, Kulaga SF, Gould AL, et al. Long-term tolerability and efficacy of timolol ophthalmic solution. Glaucoma 1987;9:84–88.

181. Keates EU. Evaluation of timolol maleate combination therapy in chronic open-angle glaucoma. Am J Ophthalmol 1979;88:565–571.

182. Nielsen NV. Timolol: Hypotensive effect used alone and in combination for treatment of increased intraocular pressure. Acta Ophthalmol 1978;56:504–509.

183. Kass M, Korey M, Gordon M, Becker B. Timolol and acetazolamide. Arch Ophthalmol 1982;100:941–942.

184. Obstbaum SA, Galin MA, Katz IM. Timolol: effect on intraocular pressure in chronic open-angle glaucoma. Ann Ophthalmol 1978;10:1347–1351.

185. Thomas JV, Epstein DL. Timolol and epinephrine in primary open-angle glaucoma. Transient additive effect. Arch Ophthalmol 1981;99:91–95.

186. Cyrlin MN, Thomas JV, Epstein DL. Additive effect of epinephrine to timolol therapy in primary open-angle glaucoma. Arch Ophthalmol 1982;100:414–417.

187. Korey MS, Hodapp E, Kass MA, et al. Timolol and epinephrine. Long-term evaluation of concurrent administration. Arch Ophthalmol 1982;100:742–746.

188. Schenker HI, Yablonski ME, Podos SM, Linder L. Fluorophotometric study of epinephrine and timolol in human subjects. Arch Ophthalmol 1981;99:1212–1214.

189. Thomas JV, Epstein DL. Study of the additive effect of timolol and epinephrine in lowering intraocular pressure. Br J Ophthalmol 1981;65:596–602.

190. Mare N, Alvan G, Calissendorff BM, et al. Additive intraocular pressure reducing effect of topical timolol during systemic β-blockade. Acta Ophthalmol 1982;60:16–23.

191. Becker B. Decrease in intraocular pressure by a carbonic anhydrase inhibitor, Diamox. Am J Ophthalmol 1954;37:13–15.

192. Coakes RL, Brubaker RF. The mechanism of timolol in lowering pressure in the normal eye. Arch Ophthalmol 1978;96:2045–2048.

193. Krill AE, Newell FW, Novak M. Early and long-term effects of levo-epinephrine. Am J Ophthalmol 1965;59:833–839.

194. Richards JSF, Drance SM. The effect of 2% epinephrine on aqueous humor dynamics in the human eye. Can J Ophthalmol 1967;2:259–263.

195. Goldberg I, Ashburn FS, Palmberg PF, et al. Timolol and epinephrine: A clinical study of ocular interactions. Arch Ophthalmol 1980;98:484–486.

196. Sonntag JR, Brindley GO, Shields MB. Effect of timolol therapy on outflow facility. Invest Ophthalmol Vis Sci 1978;17:293–296.

197. Neufeld AH. Influence of cyclic nucleotides on outflow facility in the vervet monkey. Exp Eye Res 1978;27:387–397.

198. Bill A, Heilmann K. Ocular effects of clonidine in cats and monkeys. Exp Eye Res 1975;21:481–488.

199. Valon M, Urinowsky E, Rothkoff L, et al. Frequency of timolol administration. Am J Ophthalmol 1981;92:526–529.

200. Kass MA, Gordon M, Morley RE, et al. Compliance with

topical timolol treatment. Am J Ophthalmol 1987;103:188–193.

201. Keates EU. Evaluation of timolol maleate combination therapy in chronic open-angle glaucoma. Am J Ophthalmol 1979;88:565–571.

202. Hoskins HD, Hetherington J, Magee SD, et al. Clinical experience with timolol in childhood glaucoma. Arch Ophthalmol 1985;103:1163–1165.

203. McMahon CD, Shaffer RN, Hoskins HD, Hetherington J. Adverse effects experienced by patients taking timolol. Am J Ophthalmol 1979;88:736–738.

204. Katz IM, Kasdin SL. Safety and tolerability of timolol maleate ophthalmic solution in perspective. J Ocul Therap Surg 1981;Nov-Dec: 76–80.

205. Frais MA, Bayley TJ. Ocular reaction to timolol maleate. Post Grad Med J 1979;55:884–885.

206. Nielsen NE, Eriksen JS. Timolol: Transitory manifestations of dry eyes in long-term treatment. Acta Ophthalmol 1979;57:418–424.

207. Coakes RL, Mackie IA, Seal DV. Effects of long-term treatment with timolol on lacrimal gland function. Br J Ophthalmol 1981;65:603–605.

208. Van Buskirk EM. Corneal anesthesia after timolol maleate therapy. Am J Ophthalmol 1979;88:739–743.

209. Van Buskirk EM. Adverse reactions from timolol administration. Ophthalmology 1980;87:447–450.

210. Strempel I. The influence of topical β-blockers on the breakup time. Ophthalmologica 1984;189:110–115.

211. Wilson RP, Spaeth GL. Use of timolol. JAMA 1979;242:1849.

212. Van Buskirk EM, Fraunfelder FT. Timolol and glaucoma. Arch Ophthalmol 1981;99:696.

213. Ros FE, Drake CL. Timolol eye drops. Bradycardia or tachycardia. Doc Ophthalmol 1979;48:283–289.

214. Jones FL, Ekberg NL. Exacerbation of asthma by timolol. N Engl J Med 1979;301:270.

215. Charan NB, Lakshimarayan S. Pulmonary effects of topical timolol. Arch Intern Med 1980;140:843–844.

216. Olson RJ, Bromberg BB, Zimmerman TJ. Apneic spells associated with timolol therapy in a neonate. Am J Ophthalmol 1979;88:120–122.

217. Nielsen AK. Timolol topically and diabetes mellitus. JAMA 1980;244:2263.

218. Burggraf GW, Munt PW. Topical timolol therapy and cardiopulmonary function. Can J Ophthalmol 1980;15:159–160.

219. Schoene RB, Martin TR, Charan NB, French CL. Timolol-induced bronchospasm in asthmatic bronchitis. JAMA 1981;245:1460–1461.

220. Novack GD. Ophthalmic beta blockers since timolol. Surv Ophthalmol 1987;31:307–327.

221. Duzman E, Ober M, Scharrer A, Leopold IH. A clinical evaluation of the effects of topically applied levobunolol and timolol on increased intraocular pressure. Am J Ophthalmol 1982;94:318–327.

222. Partamian LG, Kass MA, Gordon M. A dose-response study of the effects of levobunolol on ocular hypertension. Am J Ophthalmol 1983;95:229–232.

223. Bensinger RE, Keates EU, Gofman JD, et al. Levobunolol: A three month efficacy study in the treatment of glaucoma and ocular hypertension. Arch Ophthalmol 1985;103:375–378.

224. Cinotti A, Cinotti D, Grant W, et al. Levobunolol vs timolol in open angle glaucoma and ocular hypertension. Am J Ophthalmol 1985;99:11–17.

225. Ober M, Scharrer A, David E, et al. Long-term ocular hypotensive effect of levobunolol: Result of a one-year study. Br J Ophthalmol 1985;69:593–599.

226. Berson FG, Cohen HB, Foerster RJ, et al. Levobunolol compared with timolol for the long-term control of elevated intraocular pressure. Arch Ophthalmol 1985;103:379–382.

227. Greyer O, Lazar M, Novack GD, et al. Levobunolol compared with timolol for the control of elevated intraocular pressure. Ann Ophthalmol 1986;18:289–292.

228. Wandel T, Charap AD, Lewis RA, et al. Glaucoma treatment with once-daily levobunolol. Am J Ophthalmol 1986;101:298–304.

229. Wandel T, Fishman D, Novack GD, et al. Ocular hypotensive efficacy of 0.25% levobunolol instilled once daily. Ophthalmology 1988;95:252–255.

230. Yablonski ME, Novack GD, Burke PJ, et al. The effect of levobunolol on aqueous humor dynamics. Exp Eye Res 1987;44:49–54.

231. Physicians Desk Reference. Oradell, NJ: Medical Economics, 1987.

232. Novack GD, Liu DS, Kelley EP, et al. Plasma levobunolol levels following topical administration with reference to systemic side effects. Ophthalmologica 1987;194:194–200.

233. Reiss GR, Brubaker RF. The mechanism of betaxolol, a new ocular hypotensive agent. Ophthalmology 1983;90:1369–1372.

234. Berrospi AR, Leibowitz HM. Betaxolol. A new β-adrenergic blocking agent for treatment of glaucoma. Arch Ophthalmol 1982;100:943–946.

235. Radius RL. Use of betaxolol in reduction of elevated intraocular pressure. Arch Ophthalmol 1983;100:898–901.

236. Feghali JG, Kaufman PL. Decreased intraocular pressure in the hypertensive human eye with betaxolol, a β-adrenergic antagonist. Ophthalmology 1985;100:777–782.

237. Berry DP, Van Buskirk EM, Shields MB. Betaxolol and timolol. A comparison of efficacy and side effects. Arch Ophthalmol 1984;102:42–45.

238. Levy NS, Boone L, Ellis E. A controlled comparison of betaxolol and timolol with long-term evaluation of safety and efficacy. Glaucoma 1985;7:54–62.

239. Stewart RH, Kimbrough RL, Ward RL. Betaxolol vs timolol. A six month double-blind comparison. Arch Ophthalmol 1986;104:46–48.

240. Allen RC, Hertzmark E, Walker AM, et al. A double-masked comparison of betaxolol vs timolol in treatment of open-angle glaucoma. Am J Ophthalmol 1986;101:535–541.

241. Schoene RB, Abuan T, Ward RL, Beasley CH. Effects of topical betaxolol, timolol and placebo on pulmonary function in asthmatic bronchitis. Am J Ophthalmol 1984;97:86–92.

242. Ofner S, Smith TJ. Betaxolol in chronic obstructive pulmonary disease. J Ocul Pharmacol 1987;3:171–173.

243. Van Buskirk EM, Weinreb RN, Berry DP, et al. Betaxolol in patients with glaucoma and asthma. Am J Ophthalmol 1986;101:531–534.

244. Dunn TL, Gerber MJ, Shen AS, et al. The effect of topical

ophthalmic instillation of timolol and betaxolol on lung function in asthmatic subjects. Ann Rev Respir Dis 1986; 133:264–268.

245. Harris LS, Greenstein SH, Bloom AF. Respiratory difficulties with betaxolol. Am J Ophthalmol 1986;102:274.

246. Orlando RG. Clinical depression associated with betaxolol. Am J Ophthalmol 1986;102:275.

247. Nelson WL, Kuristsky JN. Early post-marketing surveillance of betaxolol hydrochloride. Am J Ophthalmol 1987; 103:592.

248. Zabel R, MacDonald IA. Sinus arrest associated with betaxolol drops. Am J Ophthalmol 1987;104:431.

249. Krieglstein GK, Novack GD, Voepel E, et al. Levobunolol and metipranolol: Comparative ocular hypotensive efficacy, safety and comfort. Br J Ophthalmol 1987;71:250–253.

250. Ohrstrom A, Kattsstrom O. A combination of oral and topical beta-blockers with additive effects on intra-ocular pressure. Acta Ophthalmol 1983;61:1021–1028.

251. Williamson J, Young JDH, Atta H, et al. Comparative efficacy of orally and topically administered β-blockers for chronic simple glaucoma. Br J Ophthalmol 1985;65:41–45.

252. Doughty MJ, Lyle WM. The development of β-adrenergic blocking drugs for management of primary open angle glaucoma. Can J Optom 1987;49:195–202.

253. Bodor N, Elkoussi A. Novel "soft" β-blockers as potentially safe antiglaucoma agents. Curr Eye Res 1988;7:369–374.

254. Greef K, Schumann HJ. Zur pharmakologie des sympathicolyticums. 6-Actoxythymoxyaethyldimethylamin. Arzheim Forsch 1953;3:341–345.

255. Foster RW. The nature of the adrenergic receptors in the trachea of the guinea pig. J Pharmacol 1966;18:1–12.

256. Birmingham AT, Ernest K, Newcombe JF. Antagonism of the response of human isolated arteries to noradrenaline. Br J Pharmacol 1969;35:127–131.

257. Wand M, Grant WM. Thymoxamine hydrochloride: An alpha-adrenergic blocker. Surv Ophthalmol 1980;25:75–84.

258. Pau H. Sympathikolyse durch lokale konjuncktivale Opilon. Applikation am auge. Klin Monastbl Augenheil Kd 1955;126:171–176.

259. Turner P, Sneddon JM. Alpha receptor blockage by thymoxamine in the human eye. Clin Pharmacol Ther 1968;9:45–59.

260. Mayer GL, Stewart-Jones JH, Turner P. Influence of alpha adrenoceptor blockade with thymoxamine or changes in pupil diameter and accommodation produced by tropicamide and ephedrine. Curr Med Res Opinion 1977;4:660–664.

261. Susanna R, Drance S, Schulzer M, Douglas G. The effects of thymoxamine on anterior chamber depth in human eyes. Can J Ophthalmol 1978;13:250–251.

262. Saheb NE, Lorenzetti D, Salpeter-Carlton S. Effect of thymoxamine and pilocarpine on the depth of the anterior chamber. Can J Ophthalmol 1980;170–171.

263. Mapstone R. Mechanics of pupil block. Br J Ophthalmol 1968;52:19–25.

264. Mapstone R. Safe mydriasis. Br J Ophthalmol 1970;54:690–692.

265. Anastasi LM, Ogle KN, Kearns TP. Effect of pilocarpine in counteracting mydriasis. Arch Ophthalmol 1968;79:710–715.

266. Rutkowski PC, Fernandes JL, Galin MA, Halasa AM.

Alpha adrenergic receptor blockade in the treatment of angle-closure glaucoma. Trans Am Acad Ophthalmol Otolaryngol 1973;77:137–142.

267. Wand M, Grant WM. Thymoxamine hydrochloride: effects on the facility of outflow and intraocular pressure. Invest Ophthalmol 1976;15:400–403.

268. Lee DA, Brubaker RF, Nagataki S. Effect of thymoxamine on aqueous humor formation in the normal human eye as measured by fluorophotometry. Invest Ophthalmol Vis Sci 1981;21:805–811.

269. Campbell DG. Pigmentary dispersion and glaucoma: A new theory. Arch Ophthalmol 1972;97:1667–1672.

270. Marmion VJ. Actions and interactions of adrenergic-blocking drugs in the human eye. In: Pigott PV, ed. Evaluation of drug effects on the eye. London: JF Parsons, 1968;71–77.

271. Paterson GD, Paterson G. Drug therapy of glaucoma. Br J Ophthalmol 1972;56:288–294.

272. Lee DA, Brubaker RF, Nagataki S. Effect of thymoxamine on aqueous humor formation in the normal human eye as measured by fluorophotometry. Invest Ophthalmol Vis Sci 1981;21:805–811.

273. Dixon RS, Anderson RL, Hatt MU. The use of thymoxamine in eyelid retraction. Arch Ophthalmol 1979;97:2147–2150.

274. Grehn F. Intraocular thymoxamine for miosis during surgery. Am J Ophthalmol 1987;103:709–711.

275. Ellis PP. Ocular therapeutics and pharmacology. St. Louis: Mosby, 1985;Chap. 4.

276. Laws HW. Peripheral vasodilators in the treatment of macular degeneration changes in the eye. Can Med Assoc J 1964;97:325–330.

277. Iuglio N. Ocular effects of topical application of dapiprazole in man. Glaucoma 1984;6:110–116.

278. Reibaldi A. A new alpha blocking agent. Glaucoma 1984;6:255–257.

279. Brogliatti B, Rolle T, Messelod M, Carenini BB. A new alpha blocking agent in treatment of glaucoma: Dapiprazole. Glaucoma 1985;7:232–236.

280. Prosdocimo G, De Marco D. Intraocular dapiprazole to reverse mydriasis during extracapsular cataract extraction. Am J Ophthalmol 1988;105:321–322.

281. Bucci MG, D'Andrea D, Bettini A, DeGregorio M. Dapiprazole for reversal of mydriasis due to tropicamide. Glaucoma 1987;9:94–98.

282. Falter RT, Thompson HS. Mechanisms of guanethidine's sympatholytic action: a pupillographic demonstration. In: Blodi FC, ed. Current concepts in ophthalmology. St. Louis: C.V. Mosby Co, 1974;4:65–71.

283. Keates E, Krishna N, Leopold IH. Ocular effects of guanethidine and its use in glaucoma. Symposium on guanethidine. Memphis: University of Tennessee College of Medicine, 1960.

284. Jablonski J. Guanethidine (Ismelin) as an adjuvant in pharmacological mydriasis. Ophthalmologica 1974;168:27–38.

285. Jones DEP, Norton DA, Davies DJG. Low dosage combined adrenalin-guanethidine formulations in the management of chronic simple glaucoma. Trans Ophthalmol Soc UK 1977;97:192–195.

286. Romano J, Nogasubramanian S, Poinoosawny D. Double-

masked cross-over comparison of guanethidine 1% and adrenaline 0.2% with adrenaline 1% and with pilocarpine 1%. Br J Ophthalmol 1981;65:50–52.

287. Murray A, Glover D, Hitchings R. Low-dose combined guanethidine 1% and adrenaline 0.5% in the treatment of chronic simple glaucoma: A prospective study. Br J Ophthalmol 1981;65:533–535.

288. Hitchings RA, Clover D. Adrenaline 1% combined with guanethidine 1% versus adrenalin 1%. Br J Ophthalmol 1982;66:247–249.

289. Gay A, Welkenstein M. Topical guanethidine therapy for endocrine lid retraction. Arch Ophthalmol 1966;76:364.

290. Thoenen H, Tranzer JP. The pharmacology of 6-hydroxy-dopamine. Ann Rev Pharmacol 1973;13:169–180.

291. Holland MG, Mims JL. Anterior segment chemical sympathectomy by 6-hydroxydopamine. Invest Ophthalmol 1971;10:120–143.

292. Holland MG. Treatment of glaucoma by chemical sympathectomy with 6-hydroxydopamine. Trans Am Acad Ophthalmol Otolaryngol 1972;76:437–449.

293. Diamond JG. 6-Hydroxydopamine in treatment of open-angle glaucoma. Arch Ophthalmol 1976;94:41–47.

294. Talusan E, Schwartz B, Mandell AI, et al. 6-Hydroxydopamine in the treatment of open-angle glaucoma. Am J Ophthalmol 1981;92:792–798.

295. Watanabe H, Levene RZ, Bernstein M. 6-Hydroxydopamine therapy in glaucoma. Trans Am Acad Ophthalmol 1977;83:69–77.

296. Kitazawa Y, Nosi H, Horie T. Chemical sympathectomy with 6-hydroxydopamine in the treatment of primary open-angle glaucoma. Am J Ophthalmol 1975;79:98–103.

297. McEwen WK, Goodner EK. Secretion of tears and blinking. In: Davson H, ed. The eye. New York: Academic Press, 1969;3:341.

298. Zadunaisky JA, Spinowitz B. Drugs affecting the transport and permeability of the corneal epithelium. In: Dikstein S, ed. Drugs and ocular tissues. New York: Karger, 1977;69.

299. Michon J Jr, Kinoshita JH. Cholinesterase in the lens. Arch Ophthalmol 1967;77:807–808.

300. Scuderi G, Sborgia C, Sborgia G, et al. Acetylcholinesterase content in toto in the bovine crystalline lens. Boll Soc Ital Biol Spec 1972;48:811.

301. Michon J Jr, Kinoshita JH. Experimental miotic cataract II. Permeability, cation transport and intermediary metabolism. Arch Ophthalmol 1968;79:611–616.

302. DeRoetth A. Choline acetylase activity in ocular tissues. Arch Ophthalmol 1950;43:849–852.

303. Ross CD, McDougal BD Jr. The distribution of choline acetyltransferase activity in vertebrate retina. J Neurochem 1976;26:521–526.

304. Hutchins JB, Hollyfield JG. Cholinergic neurons in the human retina. Exp Eye Res 1987;44:363–375.

305. Dowling JE, Boycott BB. Organization of the primate retina: Electron microscopy. Proc R Soc Lond 1966;166:80.

306. Masland RH, Livinston CJ. Effect of stimulation with light on synthesis and release of acetylcholine by an isolated mammalian retina. J Neurophysiol 1976;39:1210.

307. Nicole CW, Hoelle GB. Acetylcholinesterases: Method for demonstration in amacrine cells of retina. Science 1967; 155:477–478.

308. Nichols CE, Koelle GB. Comparison of the localization of acetylcholine-esterase and non specific cholinesterase activities in mammalian and avian retinas. J Comp Neurol 1968;133:1.

309. Ross D, Cohen AJ, McDougal BD Jr. Choline acetyltransferase and acetylcholine esterase activities in normal and biologically fractionated mouse retinas. Invest Ophthalmol 1975;14:756.

310. Lund KR. Muscarinic receptor binding and the effect of atropine on the guinea pig iris. Exp Eye Res 1978;27:577–583.

311. Smith EL, Redburn DA, Harwerth RS, Maquire GW. Permanent alterations in muscarinic receptors and pupil size produced by chronic atropinization in kittens. Invest Ophthalmol Vis Sci 1985;25:239–243.

312. Akesson C, Swanson C, Patil PN. Muscarinic receptors of rabbit irides. Arch Pharmacol 1983;322:104–110.

313. Kaumann AJ, Hennekes R. The affinity of atropine for muscarine receptors in human sphincter pupillae. Arch Pharmacol 1979;306:209–211.

314. Hutchins JB, Hollyfield JG. Autoradiographic identification of muscarinic receptors in human iris smooth muscle. Exp Eye Res 1984;38:515–521.

315. Barany E, Berrie CP, Birdsall NJ, et al. The binding properties of the muscarinic receptors of the cynomolgus monkey ciliary body and the response to the induction of agonist subsensitivity. Br J Pharmacol 1982;77:731–739.

316. Konno F, Takayangi I. Muscarinic acetylcholine receptors in the rabbit ciliary body smooth muscle: Spare receptors and threshold phenomenon. Jpn J Pharmacol 1985;38:91–99.

317. Polansky JR, Zlock D, Brasier A, Bloom E. Adrenergic and cholinergic receptors in isolated non-pigmented ciliary epithelial cells. Curr Eye Res 1985;4:517–522.

318. Konno F, Takayanagi I. Comparison of the muscarinic cholinoceptors in the rabbit ciliary body and guinea pig ileum. Eur J Pharmacol 1986;132:171–178.

319. Lograno MD, Reibaldi A. Receptor responses in fresh human ciliary muscle. Br J Pharmacol 1986;87:379–385.

320. Huchins JB, Hollyfield JG. Acetylcholine receptors in the human retina. Invest Ophthalmol Vis Sci 1985;26:1550–1557.

321. Taylor P. Anticholinesterase agents. In: Gilman AG, Goodman LS, Rall TW, et al., eds. The pharmacological basis of therapeutics. New York: Macmillan Co, 1985;Chap. 6.

322. Wilson IB, Harison MA. Turnover number of acetylcholine esterase. J Biol Chem 1961;236:2292–2295.

323. Smith AA, Dancis J, Brienin G. Ocular responses to autonomic drugs in familial dysautonomia. Invest Ophthalmol 1965;4:358–361.

324. Andrade C. A peculiar form of peripheral neuropathy—familiar atypical generalized amyloidosis with special involvement of peripheral nerves. Brain 1952;75:408–411.

325. Sigsbee B, Torkelson R, Kadis G, et al. Parasympathetic denervation of the iris in diabetes mellitus—a clinical study. J Neurol Neurosurg Psychiatry 1974;37:1031–1039.

326. Gay AJ. Letter. Arch Ophthalmol 1969;81:601–602.

327. Taylor P. Cholinergic agonists. In: Gilman AG, Goodman LS, Rall TW, et al. eds. The pharmacological basis of therapeutics. New York: Macmillan Co, 1985;Chap. 5.

328. Krill AE, Newell FN. Effects of pilocarpine on ocular dynamics. Am J Ophthalmol 1964;57:34–41.

329. Harris LS, Galin MA. Dose response analysis of pilocarpine-induced ocular hypotension. Arch Ophthalmol 1970; 84:605–608.

330. Harris LS, Galin MA. Effect of ocular pigmentation on hypotensive response to pilocarpine. Am J Ophthalmol 1971;72:923–925.

331. Worthen DM. Effect of pilocarpine drops on diurnal intraocular pressure variation in patients with glaucoma. Invest Ophthalmol 1978;15:784–787.

332. Abramson DM, Chang S, Coleman J. Pilocarpine therapy in glaucoma. Arch Ophthalmol 1976;94:914–918.

333. Quigley HA, Pollack IP. Intraocular pressure control with twice-daily pilocarpine in two vehicle solutions. Ann Ophthalmol 1977;9:427–430.

334. Quigley HA, Pollack IP, Harbin TS. Pilocarpine Ocuserts. Long-term clinical trials and selected pharmacodynamics. Arch Ophthalmol 1975;93:771–775.

335. Brown HS, Meltzer G, Merrill RC, et al. Visual effects of pilocarpine in glaucoma. Arch Ophthalmol 1976;94:1716–1719.

336. Novak S, Stewart RH. The Ocusert system in the management of glaucoma. Tex Med 1975;71:63–65.

337. Stewart RH, Novak S. Introduction of the Ocusert ocular system to an ophthalmic practice. Am J Ophthalmol 1978; 3:325–30.

338. Krause K, Kuchle HJ, Baumgart M. Comparative studies of pilocarpine gel and pilocarpine eyedrops. Klin Monatsbl Augenheilkd 1984;187:178–183.

339. O'Connor Davies PH. The actions and uses of ophthalmic drugs. London: Butterworths, 1981;Chap. 7.

340. Gorin G. Angle-closure glaucoma induced by miotics. Am J Ophthalmol 1966;62:1063–1064.

341. Podos SM, Ritch R. Epinephrine as the initial therapy in selected cases of ocular hypertension. Surv Ophthalmol 1980;25:188–194.

342. Williams TD. Accommodative blur in pilocarpine-treated glaucoma. J Am Optom Assoc 1976;47:761–764.

343. Zimmerman TJ. Pilocarpine. Ophthalmology 1981;88:85–88.

344. Harris LS. Phenylephrine in miotic-treated eyes. Ann Ophthalmol 1972;10:861–870.

345. Sugar S. The ten commandments for management of primary open-angle glaucoma. Am J Ophthalmol 1979;5:783–791.

346. Schwartz B. Primary open-angle glaucoma. In: Duane TD, ed. Clinical ophthalmology. Hagerstown, MD: Harper & Row, 1981;3:1–45.

347. Kennedy RE, Roca PD, Platt DS. Further observations on atypical band keratopathy in glaucoma patients. Trans Am Ophthalmol Soc 1974;122:107–122.

348. Zimmerman TJ, Wheeler TM. Miotics. Side effects and ways to avoid them. Ophthalmology 1982;89:76–80.

349. Alpar JJ. Miotics and retinal detachment. Am J Ophthalmol 1979;3:395–401.

350. Greco JJ, Kelman CD. Systemic pilocarpine toxicity in the treatment of angle closure glaucoma. Ann Ophthalmol 1973;1:57–59.

351. Yamauchi DN, Patie PN. Relative potency of cholinomimetic drugs on bovine iris sphincter strips. Invest Ophthalmol 1973;12:80–83.

352. O'Brien CS, Swan KC. Carbamylcholine in the treatment of glaucoma simplex. Arch Ophthalmol 1942;27:253–263.

353. Lowenfeld IE. The iris as pharmacologic indicator. Arch Ophthalmol 1963;70:42–51.

354. Fincham EF. The proportion of ciliary muscular force required for accommodation. J Physiol 1953;128:99–112.

355. Duke-Elder S, ed. System of ophthalmology. St. Louis: C.V. Mosby Co, 1962;vol.7:Chap. 19.

356. Young SE, Ruiz RS, Falletta J. Reversal of systemic toxic effects of scopolamine with physostigmine salicylate. Am J Ophthalmol 1971;72:1136–1138.

357. El-Yousef MK, Janowsky DS, Davis JM, et al. Reversal of benztropine toxicity by physostigmine. JAMA 1972;220:125.

358. Arena JM. Poisoning. Springfield, IL: Charles C Thomas, 1974;3:414.

359. Riken WF Jr, Wescoe WC. The direct action of Prostigmin on skeletal muscle; its relationship to the choline esters. J Pharmacol Exp Ther 1946;88:58–63.

360. Walker MB. Case showing effect of Prostigmin on myasthenia gravis. Proc R Soc Med 1935;28:759.

361. Drance SM. Effect of demecarium bromide (BC-48) on intraocular pressure in man. Arch Ophthalmol 1959;62:673–678.

362. Osserman KE, Genkins G. Critical reappraisal of the use of edrophonium (Tensilon) chloride tests in myasthenia gravis and significance of clinical classification. Ann NY Acad Sci 1966;135:312–326.

363. Glaser JS. Tensilon tonography in the diagnosis of myasthenia gravis. Invest Ophthalmol 1967;6:135–140.

364. Van Dyk HJL, Laur F. The Tensilon test. A safe office procedure. Ophthalmology 1980;87:210–212.

365. Knapp P. Diagnostic drugs in strabismus. In: Srinivasan BD, ed. Ocular therapeutics. New York: Masson, 1980; 107–109.

366. Apt L. Toxicity of strong miotics in children. Newer observations. In: Leopold IH, ed. Symposium on ocular therapeutics. St Louis: C.V. Mosby Co, 1972;5:30–35.

367. Abraham SV. Intraepithelial cysts of the iris. Am J Ophthalmol 1954;37:327.

368. AMA Drug Evaluations. Littleton, Mass: PSG, 1980;4:Chap. 23.

369. Volle RL. Cholinomimetic drugs. In: DiPalma JR, ed. Drill's pharmacology in medicine. New York: McGraw-Hill, 1971;4:604.

370. Wade A, ed. Martindale, the extra pharmacopia. London: Pharmaceutical Press, 1978:995.

371. Klayman J, Taffets S. Low-concentration phospholine iodide therapy in open angle glaucoma. Am J Ophthalmol 1963;55:1233–1237.

372. DeRoetth A Jr. A reappraisal of phospholine iodide. In Srinivasan BD, ed. Ocular therapeutics. New York: Masson, 1980;157–158.

373. Van Buskirk EM. Hazards of medical glaucoma therapy in the cataract patient. Ophthalmology 1982;89:238–241.

374. Weiner N. Atropine, scopolamine and related antimuscarinic drugs. In: Gilman AG, Goodman LS, Rall TW, et al., eds. The pharmacological basis of therapeutics. New York: Macmillan Co, 1985;Chap. 7.

375. Kondritzer AA, Zvirblis P. Stability of atropine aqueous solution. J Am Pharmacol Assoc 1957;46:53–56.

376. Smith SE. Dose-response relationship in tropicamide-induced mydriasis and cycloplegia. Br J Clin Pharmacol 1974;1:37–40.

377. Janes RC, Stiles JF. The penetration of C^{14} labeled atropine into the eye. Arch Ophthalmol 1959;62:69–74.

378. Lussana F. Dell'azione e delle virtu terapeutiche dell' atropina e della belladonna. Ann Univ di Med 1852;140:514.

379. Feddersen IM. Beitrag zur Atropinvergiftung. Inaug Dissert Berlin; Francke O. 1884, as cited by: Manon J. Cycloplegia and mydriasis by use of atropine, scopolamine and homatropine-paredrine. Arch Ophthalmol 1940;23:340–350.

380. Wolf AV, Hodge HC. Effects of atropine sulfate, methylatropine nitrate (Metropine) and homatropine hydrobromide on adult human eyes. Arch Ophthalmol 1946;36:293–301.

381. Salazar M, Shimada K, Patie PN. Iris pigmentation and atropine mydriasis. J Pharmacol Exp Ther 1976;197:79–88.

382. Cauther SE, Ellis RD, Larrison SB, Kidd MR. Resolution, purification and characterization of rabbit serum atropinesterase and cocainesterase. Biochem Pharmacol 1976;25:181–185.

383. Mindel JS. Cholinergic pharmacology. In: Duane TD, Jaeger EA, eds. Biomedical foundations of ophthalmology. Philadelphia: Harper & Row 1982;3:Chap. 26.

384. Grimbel HV. The control of myopia with atropine. Can J Ophthalmol 1973;8:527–532.

385. Dyer JA. Role of cycloplegics in progressive myopia. Ophthalmology 1979;86:692–694.

386. Bedrossian RH. The effect of atropine on myopia. Ophthalmology 1979;86:713–717.

387. Sampson WG. Role of cycloplegia in the management of functional myopia. Ophthalmology 1979;86:695–697.

388. Gugersen E, Pontoppidan M, Rindziunski E. Optic drugs penalization and favouring in the treatment of squint amblyopia. Acta Ophthalmol 1974;52:60–72.

389. Von Noorden GK. Amblyopia caused by unilateral atropinization. Ophthalmology 1981;88:131–133.

390. Sugar HS. The provocative test in the diagnosis of the glaucomas. Am J Ophthalmol 1948;31:1193–1202.

391. Abraham S. Mydriatic glaucoma—a statistical study. Arch Ophthalmol 1933;10:757–762.

392. Cramp J. Reported cases of reactions and side effects of the drugs which optometrists use. Aust J Optom 1976;59:13–25.

393. Keller JT. The risk of angle closure from use of mydriatics. J Am Optom Assoc 1975;46:19–21.

394. Leopold IM, Comroe JH. Effects of intramuscular administration of morphine, atropine, scopolamine, and neostigmine on the human eye. Arch Ophthalmol 1948;40:285–290.

395. Mehra KS, Chandra P. The effects on the eye of premedication with atropine. Br J Anesth 1965;37:133–137.

396. Tammisto T, Castren JA, Marttila I. Intramuscularly administered atropine and the eye. Acta Ophthalmol 1964;42:408–417.

397. Eggers HM. Toxicity of drugs used in diagnosis and treatment of strabismus. In: Srinivasan DB, ed. Ocular therapeutics. New York: Masson, 1980;Chap. 15.

398. Scally CM. Poisoning after one instillation of atropine drops. Br Med J 1936;1:311.

399. Morton HG. Atropine intoxication: Its manifestations in infants and children. J Pediatr 1939;14:755–760.

400. Heath WE. Deaths from atropine poisoning. Br Med J 1950;2:608.

401. Shutt LE, Bowes JB. Atropine and hyoscine. Anesthesia 1979;34:476–490.

402. Smith SA. Factors determining the potency of mydriatic drugs in man. Br J Clin Pharmacol 1976;3:503–507.

403. Hoefnagel D. Toxic effects of atropine and homatropine eye drops in children. N Engl J Med 1961;264:168–171.

404. Marron J. Cycloplegia and mydriasis by use of atropine, scopolamine and homatropine-paredrine. Arch Ophthalmol 1940;23:340–350.

405. Freund M, Merin S. Toxic effect of scopolamine eye drops. Am J Ophthalmol 1970;70:637–639.

406. Priestly BS, Medine MM. A new mydriatic and cycloplegic drug. Am J Ophthalmol 1951;34:572–575.

407. Stolzar IH. A new group of cycloplegic drugs—further studies. Am J Ophthalmol 1953;36:110–111.

408. Gettes BD, Leopold IH. Evaluation of five new cycloplegic drugs. Arch Ophthalmol 1953;49:24–27.

409. Abraham SV. A new mydriatic and cycloplegic drug: Compound 75 GT. Am J Ophthalmol 1953;36:69–73.

410. Milder B, Riffenburgh R. An evaluation of Cyclogyl (compound 75 GT). Am J Ophthalmol 1953;36:1724–1726.

411. Merrill DL, Goldberg B, Zavell S. bis Tropicamide, A new parasympatholytic. Curr Ther Res 1960;2:43–50.

412. Gartner S, Billet E. Mydriatic glaucoma. Am J Ophthalmol 1957;43:975–976.

413. Harris LS. Cycloplegic-induced intraocular pressure elevations. A study of normal and open-angle glaucomatous eyes. Arch Ophthalmol 1968;79:242–246.

414. Simcoe CW. Cyclopentolate (Cyclogyl) toxicity. Arch Ophthalmol 1962;67:406–408.

415. Binkhorst RD, Weinstein GW, Baretz RM, Glahane MS. Psychotic reaction induced by cyclopentolate. Am J Ophthalmol 1963;56:1243–1245.

416. Praeger DL, Miller SN. Toxic effects of cyclopentolate (Cyclogyl). Am J Ophthalmol 1964;58:1060–1061.

417. Awan KJ. Adverse systemic reactions of topical cyclopentolate hydrochloride. Ann Ophthalmol 1978;8:695–698.

418. Shihab ZM. Psychotic reaction in an adult after topical cyclopentolate. Ophthalmologica 1980;181:228–230.

419. Kennerdell JS, Wucher FP. Cyclopentolate associated with two cases of grand mal seizure. Arch Ophthalmol 1972;87:634–635.

420. Gettes BD. Tropicamide, a new cycloplegic mydriatic. Arch Ophthalmol 1961;65:48–52.

421. Pollack SL, Hunt JS, Polse KA. Dose-response effects of tropicamide HCL. Am J Optom Physiol Opt 1981;58:361–366.

422. Huber MSE, Smith SA, Smith SE. Mydriatic drug for diabetic patients. Br J Ophthalmol 1985;69:425–427.

423. Gettes BC, Belmont O. Tropicamide: Comparative cycloplegic effects. Arch Ophthalmol 1961;66:336–340.

424. Milder B. Tropicamide as a cycloplegic agent. Arch Ophthalmol 1961;66:70–72.

425. Gettes BC. Tropicamide; comparative mydriatic effects. Am J Ophthalmol 1963;55:84–87.

426. Mordi JA, Lyle WM, Mousa GY. Does prior instillation of a topical anesthetic enhance the effect of tropicamide? Am J Optom Physiol Opt 1986;63:290–293.

427. Dillon JR, Tyhurst CW, Yolton RL. The mydriatic effect of tropicamide on light and dark irides. J Am Optom Assoc 1977;48:653–658.

428. Priestly BS, Medine MM, Phillips CC. Cyclomydril: a new mydriatic agent. Am J Ophthalmol 1960;49:1033–1034.

429. Jaanus SD, Saulles H, Col PR. A comparative study of diagnostic agents used for mydriasis (abstr.). Am Acad Optom 1979;15.

430. Brown C, Hanna C. Use of dilute drug solutions for routine cycloplegia and mydriasis. Am J Ophthalmol 1978;86:820–824.

431. Forman AR. A new low-concentration preparation for mydriasis and cycloplegia. Ophthalmology 1980;87:213–215.

432. Portney GL, Purcell TW. The influence of tropicamide on intraocular pressure. Ann Ophthalmol 1975;7:31–34.

433. Wahl JW. Systemic reaction to tropicamide. Arch Ophthalmol 1969;82:320–321.

434. Yolton DP, Kandel JS, Yolton RL. Diagnostic pharmaceutical agents: Side effects encountered in a study of 15,000 applications. J Am Optom Assoc 1980;51:113–117.

435. Applebaum J, Jaanus SD. Use of diagnostic pharmaceutical agents and incidence of adverse effects. Am J Optom Physiol Opt 1983;60:384–388.

436. Doughty MJ, Lyle W, Trevino R, et al. A study of mydriasis produced by topical phenylephrine 2.5% in young adults. Can J Optom 1988;50:40–60.

437. Geyer O, Lazar M. Allergic blepharoconjunctivitis due to phenylephrine. J Ocul Pharmacol 1988;4:123–126.

438. Alexander DW, Berson FG, Epstein DL. A clinical trial of timolol and epinephrine in the treatment of primary open-angle glaucoma. Ophthalmology 1988;95:247–251.

439. Schlecht LP, Brubaker RF. The effects of withdrawal of timolol in chronically treated glaucoma patients. Ophthalmology 1988;95:1212–1216.

440. Wandel T, Fishman D, Novack GD, et al. Ocular hypotensive efficacy of 0.25% levobunolol instilled once daily. Ophthalmology 1988;95:252–255.

441. Boozman FW, Carriker R, Foerster R, et al. Long-term evaluation of 0.25% levobunolol and timolol for therapy of elevated intraocular pressure. Arch Ophthalmol 1988;106:514–618.

442. Allen RC, Robin AL, Long D, et al. A combination of levobunolol and dipivefrin for the treatment of glaucoma. Arch Ophthalmol 1988;106:904–907.

443. Vogel R, Clineschmidt CM, Kulaga SK, et al. Comparison of the ocular tolerability of two beta-adrenergic antagonists: timolol and betaxolol. Glaucoma 1988;10:71–75.

444. Weinreb RN, Van Buskirk EM, Cherniack R, et al. Long-term betaxolol therapy in glaucoma patients with pulmonary disease. Am J Ophthalmol 1988;106:162–167.

445. Scoville B, Mueller B, White BG, et al. A double-masked comparison of carteolol and timolol in ocular hypertension. Am J Ophthalmol 1988;105:150–154.

446. Mandell AL, Bruce LA, Khalifa MA. Reduced cyclic myopia with pilocarpine gel. Ann Ophthalmol 1988;20:133–135.

447. Relf SJ, Gharagozloo NZ, Skuta GL, et al. Thymoxamine reverses phenylephrine-induced mydriasis. Am J Ophthalmol 1988;106:251–255.

448. Long DA, Johns GE, Mullen RS, et al. Levobunolol and betaxolol. A double-masked controlled comparison of efficacy and safety in patients with elevated intraocular pressure. Ophthalmology 1988;95:735–741.

CHAPTER 4

Local Anesthetics

Jimmy D. Bartlett

Siret D. Jaanus

Local anesthetics are drugs that block nerve conduction when applied locally to nerve tissue in appropriate concentrations.[1] Although a variety of factors can interfere with nerve conduction, including hypothermia, anoxia, and various chemical substances, the clinical advantage of local anesthetics is that their action is reversible. Nerve function recovers completely, with no evidence of structural damage to nerve fibers or cells. Another prominent clinical feature of local anesthesia is that loss of sensation occurs without loss of consciousness.[1,2] This chapter considers the pharmacologic properties of ophthalmic anesthetics in current clinical use, with emphasis on those that are topically applied.

Historical Perspective

The first documented use of local anesthesia was in approximately 800 AD, when cocaine-filled saliva, obtained by chewing the leaves of the shrub *Erythroxylon coca*, was placed on the skull for trephining operations.[3] The coca plant was considered sacred by the Inca Indians of South America, who chewed its leaves to overcome fatigue, thirst, hunger, and overwork at various extremes of temperature and high altitude.[3] Circumoral numbness was accepted as an unpleasant accompaniment to the central nervous system (CNS)-stimulating effects.[2,3] In 1860 Albert Niemann isolated the active alkaloid from the coca plant and named it

cocaine.[4] He also noted that cocaine numbed the tongue so that it became devoid of sensation to touch. In the late 1860s Charles Favel, a then-famous French laryngologist, used cocaine solution to anesthesize the pharynx. It remained, however, for Karl Koller to complete the discovery of local anesthesia. In the summer of 1884 he instilled a drop of cocaine solution into the eye of a frog. Within 1 minute the frog permitted its cornea to be touched. Koller subsequently tested the drug in other animals and finally in his own eye. He observed that his cornea was devoid of sensation when touched with a pin. He also noted that cocaine's local anesthetic effect was accompanied by a widening of the palpebral fissure, pupillary dilation, and a slight paresis of accommodation.[4] Within a year of Koller's discovery, cocaine was used not only in ophthalmic practice, but also in dentistry and had been administered by injection to produce nerve block and spinal anesthesia.[3]

The initial clinical success of cocaine anesthesia was soon dampened by reports of both acute and chronic adverse effects due to local and systemic toxicity and to cocaine's addicting properties.[2] As a result, an intense effort was made to develop local anesthetics with a more favorable therapeutic index. The chemical identification of cocaine as a benzoic acid ester led to the synthesis of procaine in 1905. An ester of para-aminobenzoic acid, procaine proved to possess an acceptable margin of safety for regional anesthesia, and soon numerous similar compounds were developed, including tetracaine in 1930.[2,5]

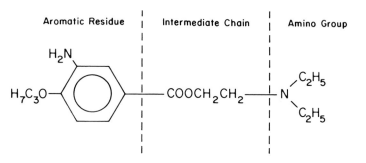

FIGURE 4.1 **Molecular structure of proparacaine, consisting of an aromatic residue, an intermediate alkyl chain, and an amino group.**

Pharmacologic Properties

Structural Features

Local anesthetics, except for cocaine, are synthetic, aromatic, or heterocyclic compounds. Nearly all local anesthetics in current clinical use are weakly basic tertiary amines. Their general configuration is shown in Figure 4.1. The structural components consist of an aromatic lipophilic portion, an intermediate alkyl chain, and a hydrophilic hydrocarbon chain containing nitrogen.[1,5] The intermediate chain, usually of 4 to 5 carbons, is linked to the aromatic group by either an ester or amide linkage, the nature of which determines certain pharmacologic properties of the molecule, including its metabolism.[1,5,6] All commonly used topical anesthetics are of the ester type (Table 4.1).

Physiochemical Characteristics

All local anesthetics exist in solution as the uncharged amine or as the positively charged substituted ammonium cation. In the amine form they tend to be only slightly soluble in water and are therefore usually formulated in solution in the form of their hydrochloride salt, which is water soluble.[1,5,7] Since the local anesthetics are weak bases, with a pK_a between 8.0 and 9.0, they tend to ionize in solution, thus enhancing their stability and shelf life.[1,5,7] On contact with more neutral or alkaline environments, such as tears, the uncharged form is liberated. In this form the drug can penetrate tissues, including the cornea.[1,5]

Mechanism of Action

Local anesthetics prevent both the generation and conduction of nerve impulses. Their main site of action appears to be the cell membrane, where they decrease or prevent the transient increase in membrane permeability to sodium ions.[1,5,7] They also reduce the permeability of resting nerve fibers to potassium as well as to sodium ions.[1] Debate about the pharmacologically active form of the anesthetic molecule seems to favor the cationic form, since in isolated mammalian nerve fibers, conduction is blocked at low pH.[1] There is also evidence, however, that both the cation and base form of the molecule possess anesthetic activity.[1]

The duration of action of local anesthetics is proportional to the drug contact time with nerve tissue. To prolong contact time of injectable local anesthetics, vasoconstrictors such as epinephrine may be added to their formulations.

Anesthetics in current clinical use have relatively low systemic and ocular toxicity. Compared with cocaine, they do not alter pupil size or affect accommodation. Their sufficiently long duration of action, low cost, stability in solution, and general lack of interference with actions of other drugs make them useful agents for such ocular procedures as tonometry, foreign body and suture removal, gonioscopy, and nasolacrimal duct irrigation and probing.

TABLE 4.1
Classification of Local Anesthetics

Ester linkage
  Esters of benzoic acid
    Cocaine
  Esters of meta-aminobenzoic acid
    Proparacaine
  Esters of para-aminobenzoic acid
    Procaine
    Chloroprocaine
    Tetracaine
    Benoxinate

Amide linkage (Amides of benzoic acid)
  Lidocaine
  Mepivacaine
  Bupivacaine
  Etidocaine

Injectable Anesthetics

A wide variety of ocular diagnostic and surgical procedures may be performed under local anesthesia. Many procedures, such as suture removal, removal of superficial foreign bodies in the cornea, nasolacrimal irrigation, and tonometry require only topical administration of a surface active anesthetic. However, when more extensive procedures are to be undertaken, it is necessary to administer the anesthetic by injection (Table 4.2). Facial nerve block, retrobulbar injection, or total tissue infiltration are widely used, and discomfort associated with these procedures may be reduced by preheating the anesthetic before injection.[8]

The required duration of a complete nerve block for a procedure is of great importance to the clinician in the selection of a suitable local anesthetic. The duration of the anesthetic effect is determined by the length of time the drug stays bound to the nerve protein. This is dictated by the chemical structure of the drug, the concentration and amount administered, and the rate of removal by diffusion and circulation. Various combinations of anesthetics are sometimes used in attempts to achieve both rapid onset and prolonged duration of anesthesia and akinesia produced by retrobulbar injections.[9] Use of bupivacaine, an extremely long-acting local anesthetic, reduces the need for postoperative analgesics and reduces eye movements that might compromise the healing process.[10]

The combination of epinephrine, a vasoconstrictor, with an injectable anesthetic prolongs the duration of anesthesia and decreases the rate of systemic absorption, thereby decreasing the risk of systemic toxicity. The duration of bupivacaine, however, an already long-acting anesthetic, cannot be significantly extended by adding epinephrine.[10] The epinephrine also decreases local bleeding. Effective vasoconstriction is obtained with a concentration of 1:100,000 or even 1:200,000. The usual concentrations of epinephrine used for ophthalmic procedures range from 1:50,000 to 1:200,000.

When epinephrine is subjected to heat, its potency is destroyed. As a result, solutions containing epinephrine should not be subjected to heat sterilization. Although epinephrine is widely used as an adjunctive agent in local anesthetics, undesirable effects on local tissue can occur. It has been found to delay wound healing and to cause occasional necrosis and intense vasoconstriction. It may also produce adverse systemic reactions such as apprehension, anxiety, restlessness, tremor, pallor, tachycardia, dyspnea, hypertension, palpitation, headaches, and precordial distress. A diagnosis of reaction to epinephrine rather than one due to the local anesthetic is indicated when subjective palpitation occurs with or without a throbbing headache, tachycardia, and hypertension. These reactions are temporary, but patients with cardiovascular disease may suffer cardiac irregularities, angina attacks, or cerebral ischemia.

Hyaluronidase (Wydase), an aqueous testicular extract, is often added to anesthetics for retrobulbar injection to enhance spread of the anesthetic through the retrobulbar tissues. This enzyme depolymerizes hyaluronic acid, which acts as tissue cement, thus causing the anesthetic to diffuse more rapidly through local tissues.[11] A more effective akinesia of the orbicularis and extraocular muscles is generally achieved with the concomitant use of hyaluronidase in retrobulbar injections of anesthetics.

Topical Anesthetics

The efficacy of topical anesthetics is usually determined by their ability to suppress corneal sensitivity. When a dose-response relationship is determined for various anesthetics, a concentration for each drug is obtained beyond which no further increase in activity occurs. The concentration at which this maximum efficacy occurs is termed the *maximum effective concentration*. Thus, increasing the concentration of the anesthetic

TABLE 4.2
Injectable Local Anesthetics

Generic Name	Trade Name	Dosage Form[a] (% solution)	Onset of Action (min)	Duration of Action (min)
Procaine hydrochloride	Novocain	1, 2, and 10	7–8	30–45 (60 with epinephrine)
Lidocaine hydrochloride	Xylocaine	0.5, 1, 1.5, 2, and 4	4–6	40–60 (120 with epinephrine)
Mepivacaine hydrochloride	Carbocaine	1, 1.5, and 2	3–5	120
Bupivacaine hydrochloride	Marcaine	0.25, 0.5, and 0.75	5–11	480–720 with epinephrine
Etidocaine hydrochloride	Duranest	1 and 1.5	4–6	300–600

[a]Some concentrations are commercially available with epinephrine. Hyaluronidase may be added to the retrobulbar injection to increase diffusion of the anesthetic.

beyond the maximum effective concentration serves no useful purpose yet increases the risk of local and systemic toxicity.

The maximum effective concentrations of proparacaine, tetracaine, and cocaine are 0.5%, 1%, and 20%, respectively. However, in clinical practice, the optimum effective concentration of the drug may be less than the maximum effective concentration. For instance, 0.5% tetracaine is less irritating to the eye than the maximum effective concentration of 1% and, thus, is better suited for clinical use. The topical application of a combination of two or more local anesthetics does not produce an additive effect, yet increases the risk of side effects. The use of combinations of anesthetics is therefore contraindicated. The commonly used topical anesthetics are listed in Table 4.3.

Cocaine

Cocaine is not commercially available in solution. For clinical use the salt form of cocaine, cocaine hydrochloride, must be specially formulated in aqueous solution. The usual concentration for topical ocular use is 1% to 4%,[12] but the 10% solution is often used as an adrenergic preparation for the diagnosis of Horner's syndrome. One drop of a 2% solution will produce excellent corneal anesthesia within 5 to 10 minutes.[13] Complete anesthesia lasts about 20 minutes, with incomplete surface anesthesia lasting for approximately 1 to 2 hours.[13] Anesthesia of the conjunctiva and insertions of the rectus muscles is sufficiently complete to permit painless grasping of the eye with forceps (in forced duction testing) for about 10 minutes.[14] Incomplete conjunctival anesthesia lasts for an additional 5 to 10 minutes.[14]

Cocaine is unique among the local anesthetic agents in its ability to cause vasoconstriction, thus retarding its own absorption. Hence, cocaine constricts the conjunctival and nasal vasculatures when applied topically to these mucous membranes. Because of this vasoconstrictor action, use of epinephrine with cocaine is not only unnecessary but may be harmful, since cocaine causes sensitization to exogenous epinephrine.[15] Although cocaine has not been compared with other topical anesthetics in well-controlled clinical studies, there is a strong clinical impression that use of cocaine as a topical anesthetic has several potential advantages[16]: (1) cocaine is considerably more effective and longer acting than the other available topical anesthetics for achieving anesthesia of the conjunctiva; (2) cocaine has a more prolonged action than the other topical anesthetics in anesthetizing the cornea, but the intensity of anesthesia is not greater; and (3) cocaine may loosen the corneal epithelium to a greater extent than other topically applied anesthetics, thus facilitating debridement of the corneal epithelium.

Cocaine is also used as a nasal spray or in a nasal pack during dacryocystorhinostomy (DCR). When applied to the nasal mucosa in a gauze pack, cocaine anesthetizes the contact area for an hour or longer.[15]

Because cocaine blocks reuptake of norepinephrine and has an adrenergic potentiating effect, its use is contraindicated in patients with systemic hypertension or patients taking adrenergic agonists.[15] The interaction between cocaine and catecholamines contraindicates cocaine's use in patients taking α-adrenergic modifying drugs such as guanethidine, reserpine, tricyclic anti-

TABLE 4.3
Topical Anesthetics

Generic Name	Trade Name (Manufacturer)	Dosage Form
Cocaine hydrochloride	Schedule II controlled substance	1%–10% solution, prepared from the bulk powder
Tetracaine hydrochloride	Pontocaine (Winthrop)	0.5% solution and ointment
Benoxinate hydrochloride with sodium fluorescein	Fluress (Barnes-Hind)	0.4% solution, combined with 0.25% sodium fluorescein
Proparacaine hydrochloride	AK-Taine (Akorn) Alcaine (Alcon) Ophthaine (Squibb) Ophthetic (Allergan)	0.5% solution
Proparacaine hydrochloride with sodium fluorescein	Fluorocaine (Akorn) Flurocaine (Medical Ophthalmics)	0.5% solution, combined with 0.25% sodium fluorescein

depressants, methyldopa, or monoamine oxidase in-hibitors (MAOs).[12,15] Conversely, pure adrenergic agonists such as phenylephrine are contraindicated with use of cocaine.[15] Systemic toxicity can be prevented by anticipating potential drug interactions or hypertensive crises. Furthermore, since cocaine has a mydriatic ef-fect, it is contraindicated in patients predisposed to angle-closure glaucoma.

The major side effect of cocaine is significant cor-neal epithelial toxicity. Grossly visible grayish pits and irregularities are readily produced by this drug.[12] These are followed by loosening of the corneal epithelium, which may result in large erosions.[12] Although this characteristic is generally considered to be an adverse side effect, it is clinically useful in cases requiring corneal epithelial debridement, as in treatment of her-petic ulcers. However, the corneal epithelial effects of cocaine contraindicate its use in any procedure requir-ing good visualization through the cornea, such as in retinal detachment surgery or in routine ophthalmos-copy or gonioscopy.

Since acute systemic cocaine toxicity may result from as little as 20 mg (10 drops of a 4% solution) of drug,[14] systemic side effects can potentially occur from the excessive topical application of the drug to the eye. Therefore, the total dose of cocaine should not exceed 3 mg/kg body weight. Typical manifestations of sys-temic toxicity include excitement, restlessness, head-ache, rapid and irregular pulse, dilated pupils, nausea, vomiting, abdominal pain, delirium, and convulsions.[17] The usual fatal dose is 1.2 g,[1] and death commonly results from respiratory failure.[18] Propranolol, a β-adrenergic blocking drug, has been reported to be an effective antagonist to the toxic cardiovascular effects of cocaine.[15]

Because of its potential ocular and systemic toxicity, cocaine has generally been replaced by the safer, syn-thetic local anesthetics. Nevertheless, it remains a drug of choice for topical anesthesia preceding corneal ep-ithelial debridement and forced duction testing. Its only nonanesthetic use in optometry and ophthalmol-ogy is in the pharmacologic diagnosis of suspected Horner's syndrome (see Chapter 18). Because of co-caine's strong abuse potential, its distribution and clin-ical use are subject to federal narcotic regulations under supervision of the Drug Enforcement Administration (DEA).[19]

Tetracaine

Tetracaine has been widely used for topical anesthesia of the eye. It is currently available in a 0.5% solution and a 0.5% ointment. Its onset, intensity, and duration of anesthesia are comparable to those of propar-acaine and benoxinate (Fig. 4.2). Onset of anesthesia sufficient to permit tonometry or other minor proce-dures involving the superficial cornea and conjunctiva is 10 to 20 seconds, and duration of anesthesia is 10 to 20 minutes. It has been reported, however, that the 1% solution produces anesthesia lasting nearly an hour.[20]

Tetracaine causes rapid surface anesthesia, but even repeated applications to the conjunctival surface may fail to achieve effective scleral anesthesia.[14] For ocular use as a local anesthetic, tetracaine should never be injected.[14] Moreover, since the 0.5% ointment pro-duces prolonged anesthesia, this formulation is pre-ferred for long-term topical anesthesia, which may be occasionally necessary for procedures such as electro-retinography (ERG), where reinstillation of the topical anesthetic solution during the procedure is impractical. The ointment formulation may be used following re-moval of corneal foreign bodies to allow prolonged comfort of the patched eye. Tetracaine ointment is also helpful following cauterization of corneal or con-junctival lesions requiring that the eye be pressure-patched. It is important to note, however, that the patient should *never* be allowed to self-administer this or any other topical anesthetic. Serious corneal com-plications may result (see Contraindications).

The practitioner is cautioned to consider tetracaine a potent and potentially toxic local anesthetic. Dan-gerous overdoses may occur if it is administered in doses higher than 1.5 mg/kg body weight.[12]

A variety of side effects often accompany the use of topical tetracaine. Tetracaine produces greater cor-neal compromise than proparacaine.[14,21] Perhaps the greatest objection, however, to the use of tetracaine is the moderate stinging or burning sensation that almost

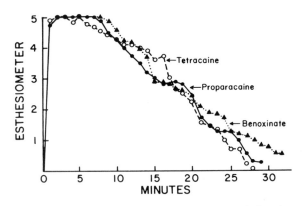

FIGURE 4.2 **Comparison of onset, intensity, and duration of anesthesia obtained with tetracaine 0.5%, proparacaine 0.5%, and benoxinate 0.4%. (Published with permission from The American Journal of Ophthalmology 40:697–704, 1955. Copyright by The Ophthalmic Publishing Company.)**

always occurs immediately following its topical instillation. This typically lasts 20 to 30 seconds following drug application. Another problem associated with use of tetracaine is allergic reactions. Although local allergy to tetracaine may develop because of repeated use (such as in tonometry of glaucoma patients), this is uncommon. The practitioner should suspect tetracaine allergy when the glaucoma patient complains of hyperemic, swollen, irritated, and itching eyelids that persist several days following the office visit during which tonometry was performed with tetracaine. Fortunately, tetracaine exhibits no cross-sensitivity with proparacaine.[17]

Benoxinate

Benoxinate is commercially available only in combination with sodium fluorescein 0.25% (Fluress). Benoxinate 0.4%, an ester of para-aminobenzoic acid (PABA), has an onset, intensity, and duration of anesthesia similar to those of tetracaine 0.5% and proparacaine 0.5% (see Fig. 4.2).[12,13,22]

Since benoxinate is available only in combination with sodium fluorescein, its primary clinical use is for applanation tonometry.[23]Although solutions of fluorescein serve as good culture media for *Pseudomonas aeruginosa*,[24] the benoxinate-sodium fluorescein combination has been shown to have substantial bactericidal properties.[13,25] Thus, the benoxinate-sodium fluorescein combination is ideal for use in applanation tonometry, since it does not have the same risk for *Pseudomonas* contamination characteristic of sodium fluorescein solutions.

When the anesthetic effect of low concentrations (0.1% and 0.2%) of benoxinate is compared with the commercially available 0.4% solution, the maximum increase in sensitivity threshold that can be measured following instillation of 50 µl of each concentration is 200 mg/mm².[26] All three anesthetic solutions produce this amount of decreased corneal sensitivity, although the lower concentrations have the shortest duration of anesthetic effect. Thus, lower concentrations of benoxinate than are commercially available may be sufficient for routine applanation tonometry and other procedures requiring only minimal superficial anesthesia.[26]

There are relatively few side effects associated with the clinical use of benoxinate as an ocular anesthetic. Topical instillation typically produces a sensation of stinging or burning that is greater than that produced by the instillation of proparacaine but less than that produced by tetracaine.[12,27] In addition, benoxinate appears to cause less corneal epithelial desquamation than proparacaine, but this has not been substantiated

by controlled clinical studies. Local allergic reactions to benoxinate are rare.[20] Since some patients who are allergic to tetracaine, another ester of PABA, may be safely administered benoxinate without allergic reactions, this suggests that the allergenic potential of benoxinate is extremely low.[28] There is no apparent cross-sensitivity between this agent and proparacaine.[17]

Proparacaine

Proparacaine is commercially available in an 0.5% solution, both with and without sodium fluorescein 0.25% (see Table 4.3). The onset, intensity, and duration of anesthesia from these preparations are similar to those of tetracaine 0.5% and benoxinate 0.4% (see Fig. 4.2).[12,22] Proparacaine, however, does not appear to penetrate into the cornea or conjunctiva as well as does tetracaine.[29]

When used without sodium fluorescein, proparacaine is widely employed as a general-purpose topical anesthetic. It produces little or no discomfort or irritation on instillation and is therefore readily accepted by most patients. Although unopened bottles may be stored at room temperature, once opened the bottles should be tightly capped and, ideally, refrigerated to retard discoloration.[13] Discolored solutions of proparacaine should be discarded (see Fig. 2.3).

Several investigators[26,27] have studied the anesthetic effects from low concentrations of proparacaine and found that 0.25% proparacaine is an effective anesthetic in all patients and that 0.125% proparacaine is effective in patients over age 40 years. Thus, as with benoxinate, lower concentrations of proparacaine than are commercially available may be sufficient for procedures requiring only minimal superficial anesthesia.

Proparacaine has few side effects. Although localized hypersensitivity reactions may develop, these are rare and occur less frequently with proparacaine than with tetracaine.[20] Allergic reactions to proparacaine may include corneal epithelial stippling with mild stromal edema appearing 5 to 10 minutes following drug instillation or may be characterized by conjunctival hyperemia and edema, edematous eyelids, and lacrimation.[21] Allergic systemic manifestations following topical ocular instillation in recommended doses are so rare as to be nonexistent. Topically instilled proparacaine has been reported to have had a possible role in the development of a hypersensitivity reaction resulting in exacerbation of Stevens-Johnson syndrome.[30]

Proparacaine does not exhibit cross-sensitivity with tetracaine.[14] However, since proparacaine and tetracaine both contain an ester linkage, it is theoretically possible for them to exhibit cross-sensitivity.[12]

Wilson and Fullard[321,32] have studied the effects of commercially prepared 0.5% proparacaine (Ophthaine) on the rate of corneal epithelial desquamation and observed that the drug initially reduces the rate of normal cell sloughing, but then there is apparently increased epithelial cell desquamation for at least 6 hours (Fig. 4.3). These investigators proposed that the proparacaine solution may cause desquamation by interfering with normal epithelial cell-membrane activity or by inhibiting a factor, released by functioning nerves, that mediates cell desquamation.

Side Effects

When used in recommended dosages, severe local reactions to topically applied anesthetics are exceedingly rare, and systemic reactions are even more uncommon. Although side effects can occur following use of topical anesthetics, adverse reactions are much more likely to

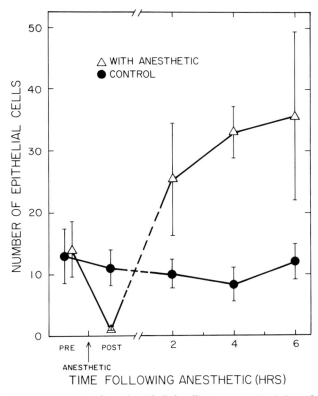

FIGURE 4.3 **Number of epithelial cells (mean ± SE) irrigated from precorneal tear film at different times. In the 2- to 6-hour period after instillation of 0.5% proparacaine, the number of cells was significantly greater with the anesthetic than with the control (*P* < 0.001, paired *t*-test). (From Wilson GS, Fullard RJ. Proparacaine sloughs cells. J Am Optom Assoc 1988;59:701–702.)**

occur with use of local anesthetics injected for infiltration or regional nerve block. Any use of local, including topically applied, anesthetics can cause systemic toxicity, but the vast majority of such systemic reactions occur as a result of overdosage of drug rather than true allergic hypersensitivity.[33] In general, patients who are particularly susceptible to the development of adverse reactions include those with known drug allergies, asthma, cardiovascular disease, and hyperthyroidism.[34] Elderly patients, debilitated patients, and infants are also more vulnerable.

Local reactions include relatively minor allergic or toxic involvement of the cornea, conjunctiva, or lids. Although the small amounts of anesthetic normally used in topical ocular applications are usually insufficient to cause toxic systemic effects,[35] systemic toxicity can potentially occur in any patient if the topical anesthetic is applied in dosages exceeding those normally recommended. There has been only one report of a severe systemic reaction to a topically applied ocular anesthetic. Cohn and Jocson[28] reported a case of grand mal seizures occurring in a 28-year-old patient following administration of a benoxinate-sodium fluorescein solution. These authors acknowledged that the anesthetic component, benoxinate, may not necessarily have been implicated, since the combination solution also contained sodium fluorescein as an indicator dye, polyvinylpyrrolidone as a vehicle, and chlorobutanol as a preservative. Furthermore, appropriate testing for a possible immune mechanism could not be performed. Because of the speed and severity of the reaction, the authors preferred to characterize the reaction as idiosyncrasy rather than as an immune response. There have been no other reports, however, of severe systemic toxic or allergic reactions to topically applied ocular anesthetics.[20,34] In general, all serious ocular or systemic side effects from local anesthetics have been associated with the use of cocaine or anesthetics for infiltration or regional nerve block or have developed as a result of prolonged use by self-administration.[34]

Toxicity

OCULAR

It is not uncommon for topically applied anesthetics, especially benoxinate and tetracaine, to cause mild local stinging or burning following initial instillation. As discussed previously, however, this will last only momentarily and requires no specific treatment other than patient reassurance.

In some patients, especially those over age 50 years, a localized or diffuse desquamation of corneal epithelium becomes evident (Fig. 4.4). This epithelial reac-

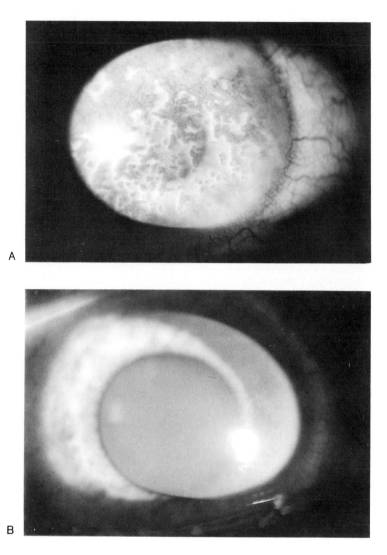

A

B

FIGURE 4.4   *(A)* **Severe toxic corneal epithelial des-quamation following instillation of proparacaine 0.5%.** *(B)* **Same cornea 24 hours later, demonstrating the rapidity with which healing occurs.**

tion usually develops within 2 to 5 minutes following instillation of the anesthetic, but sometimes it is not apparent for approximately 30 minutes. It is usually mild and of no clinical significance, but occasionally it can be extensive enough to reduce vision to 20/80 (6/24) to 20/200 (6/60). In its most severe form, it may be characterized by a diffuse, necrotizing, epithelial keratitis with filament formation and corneal edema, but this has been reported to occur in only 1 of every 1,000 patients receiving a topical ocular anesthetic.[34] The cornea can appear gray because of the epithelial and stromal edema, and folds may develop in Descemet's membrane.[34] The conjunctiva can be hyperemic, and the patient may complain of blurred vision or photophobia. There may be lacrimation and mild to intense ocular pain, but there tends to be little pain initially because of the corneal anesthesia. Treatment other than reassurance or mild ocular lubricating agents is usually not required because the corneal epithelium begins to spontaneously regenerate almost immediately (see Fig. 4.4)[20,34] In moderate to severe cases the episode should be treated as a superficial corneal abrasion, using a cycloplegic, antibacterial ointment, and pressure-patching (see Chapter 22). The patient should be administered systemic analgesics such as aspirin or ibuprofen and should be advised to use cold compresses for additional relief of local discomfort. Toxic reactions should be recorded in the patient's chart, and a different topical anesthetic should be used on subsequent patient visits.

The repeated administration of topical ocular anesthetics should be avoided because it may significantly retard healing of corneal epithelial wounds. Topical anesthetics are particularly dangerous when given to patients for self-administration. The diagnosis and treatment of severe corneal toxicity associated with the long-term administration of topical anesthetics is discussed later in this chapter.

SYSTEMIC

With the exception of one case of grand mal seizure possibly associated with the topical application of benoxinate,[28] there have been no cases of serious systemic reactions caused by topically instilled ocular anesthetics. However, since 98% or more of systemic reactions to local injectable anesthetics are due to drug overdose,[36,37] such systemic toxic reactions can potentially occur with the excessive administration of topical anesthetics to the eye. Topically applied anesthetics are rapidly absorbed into the systemic circulation, their blood level rising almost as rapidly as it does following an intravenous injection.[29,38] Systemic absorption of topical anesthetics can result in high blood levels of drug by any of the following mechanisms[36]: (1) too large a dosage of the local anesthetic; (2) unusually rapid absorption of the drug, as in patients with marked conjunctival hyperemia; (3) unusually slow drug detoxification, as in patients with liver disease; and (4) slow elimination of drug, as in patients with kidney disease.

Such high blood levels following the topical application of anesthetics may potentially cause systemic reactions similar to those reported for local injectable anesthetics.[17] Toxic effects may appear in the CNS, cardiovascular system, or respiratory system.[20] CNS toxicity appears initially as stimulation and may manifest itself clinically as nervousness, tremors, or convulsions. This is usually followed by CNS depression, observed clinically as loss of consciousness and depression of respiration. The earliest signs of cardiovascular involvement are hypertension, tachycardia, and, occasionally, cardiac irregularities.[17] Late cardiovascular signs are hypotension, absent pulse, and weak or absent heart beat.[17] The effects on the cardiovascular system can develop simultaneously with CNS depression, or they may develop alone.[17] If allowed to continue, such cardiac depression and resultant peripheral vasodilation is followed by secondary respiratory failure.[20] Fortunately, this syndrome is reversible if quickly recognized and appropriately treated. Administration of oxygen will usually rapidly restore normal CNS function.[36] The diagnosis and management of systemic toxicity associated with local anesthetics is discussed further in Chapter 31.

Hypersensitivity

OCULAR

Although local allergy to topical anesthetics can develop in some patients because of routine diagnostic use over many months or years, such as for tonometry, these reactions are extremely uncommon. Allergic episodes occur only with use of the ester groups of anesthetics, i.e., the commonly employed anesthetics for topical ocular use, and are virtually nonexistent with the use of the amide group of anesthetics for local injection, such as lidocaine, mepivacaine, and bupivacaine.[16] The usual clinical presentation following topical anesthesia is that of a mild, transient blepharoconjunctivitis characterized by conjunctival hyperemia and chemosis, swelling of the eyelids, lacrimation, and itching (Fig. 4.5).[14,21] These signs and symptoms usually appear 5 to 10 minutes following instillation of the anesthetic.[21] Such reactions may be treated with topical decongestants and cold compresses. The practitioner should record the event in the patient's chart and avoid using the same anesthetic on subsequent patient visits. Since there is apparently little cross-sensitivity between classes of local anesthetics, the practitioner can usually change from proparacaine to an ester of PABA, or vice versa, with little risk of local allergy.[17] Unfortunately, no topical anesthetics approved for ocular use have an amide linkage. Such anesthetics, because of their extremely low allergenic potential, would serve as ideal topical ocular anesthetics.

SYSTEMIC

Type I allergic reactions have been estimated to account for less than 1% of all adverse reactions to local anesthetics.[37] Moreover, there have been no reports of life-threatening allergic responses to anesthetics applied topically to the eye. The small amounts of anesthetic absorbed systemically following topical instillation are usually not sufficient to cause systemic reactions.[16] However, topical anesthetics can cause systemic reactions if enough drug is absorbed into systemic circulation. Most minor drug-induced systemic allergies are characterized by angioneurotic edema, urticaria (hives), bronchospasm, and hypotension. Joint pain and pruritus occur less commonly.[39,40] Treatment should be directed toward symptomatic relief by the use of systemically administered antihistamines, bronchodilators, or epinephrine.[17,40] Prophylaxis of this type of reaction may be difficult, since intradermal skin testing is not an entirely satisfactory method of detecting drug allergy. Prick testing followed by incremental subcutaneous provocative testing has been recommended in lieu of intradermal evaluation.[37] A

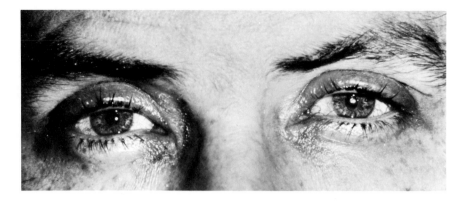

FIGURE 4.5 **Allergic blepharoconjunctivitis following instillation of proparacaine 0.5%. There is conjunctival hyperemia, swelling of the eyelids, lacrimation, and itching.**

history of extensive drug allergies should alert the practitioner to such a possible consequence of anesthetic administration, but Chandler and associates[37] found no evidence of immediate hypersensitivity reactions when patients with a history of anesthetic allergy were rechallenged, suggesting the relative safety of anesthetic use in such individuals.

Anaphylactoid reactions to local injectable anesthetics are extremely rare. Although these reactions are usually immediate, they may be delayed as long as 15 to 30 minutes.[33,34] Anaphylactoid reactions are characterized by a sudden circulatory collapse following drug administration. There is usually urticaria, respiratory distress, cyanosis, and hypotension.[33,40] Treatment directed at correcting the circulatory collapse and respiratory failure must be initiated promptly, since even a short delay can be fatal. The diagnosis and management of drug-induced systemic allergy, including anaphylaxis, is discussed in Chapter 31.

Psychomotor Reactions

Psychomotor reactions such as vasovagal syncope (fainting) may be readily mistaken for an adverse drug-related systemic reaction. However, such responses are not drug related and usually occur from anxiety related to the office visit.[20,34] Accordingly, they may occur before, during, or following drug administration. If fainting occurs, the patient should be reclined so that the head is low, tight clothing around the neck should be loosened, and the patient must be protected from falling or otherwise injuring himself or herself. Although recovery is usually spontaneous within a few seconds, aromatic spirits of ammonia, when inhaled by the patient, will usually hasten recovery. Respiration and cardiovascular status should be monitored to eliminate drug-induced anaphylaxis as a possible etiology of the collapse.

Prevention of Adverse Systemic Reactions

Although it is extremely unlikely that serious systemic reactions will occur from topical application of local anesthetics to the eye, the practitioner must limit the dosages of the drugs to those compatible with effective anesthesia without substantial risk of systemic toxicity. Although it is impossible to designate exact dosage limits of the local anesthetics, it has been suggested that the total dose applied topically to mucous membranes such as the conjunctiva should not exceed one-fourth of the maximum allowed for injection.[34] Table 4.4 shows suggested maximum dosages of topical anesthetics based on this formula. It has been reported[21,41] that the toxicity of local anesthetics increases in geometric rather than arithmetic progression with increases in concentration. Thus, while a given dose of a 1% solution would be 4 times as toxic as an equal amount of 0.5% solution, a 2% solution would be approximately 16 times as toxic as an equal dose of 0.5% solution. This necessitates that the practitioner always use the lowest concentration that permits effective anesthesia.

TABLE 4.4
Suggested Maximum Dosages of Topical Anesthetics

Anesthetic	Dosage (mg)
Cocaine	20 (about 5 drops to each eye of the 4% solution)
Tetracaine	5 (about 7 drops to each eye of the 0.5% solution)
Proparacaine	10 (about 14 drops to each eye of the 0.5% solution)

Modified from Lyle WM, Page C. Possible adverse effects from local anesthetics and the treatment of these reactions. Am J Optom Physiol Opt 1975;52:736–744.

Contraindications

The commonly employed topical anesthetics represent one of the safest groups of topically applied ocular drugs. They can generally be used with little risk of significant adverse local or systemic effects. The following specific contraindications should help to ensure the safe and effective ocular use of the topical anesthetics.

Hypersensitivity

Allergic reactions to local anesthetics, including those that are topically applied, are quite rare.[12,39,42] These reactions are virtually limited to the ester-linked anesthetics (see Table 4.1).[1,12] Allergy to the amide-linked anesthetics such as lidocaine is extremely rare. Unfortunately, intradermal skin tests as well as conjunctival and patch tests are not reliable for predicting the possibility of allergic reactions.[42] Thus, as a precaution before administering topical anesthetics, if a patient reports a history of hypersensitivity to a specific anesthetic, it is advisable to use a drug from a different chemical family. For example, an allergic reaction to a para-aminobenzoate drug such as procaine should alert the practitioner to avoid using a similar drug such as tetracaine or benoxinate.[43] In such cases proparacaine can usually be administered safely without causing an allergic reaction.[43] Although lidocaine, an amide-linked drug, may be used topically on the eye, it is not currently approved by the FDA for such use.

Hypersensitivity to benzalkonium chloride has been reported in association with the use of ophthalmic medications.[12] Since several of the commonly used topical ocular anesthetics contain benzalkonium as a preservative, it is reasonable to assume that some of the local allergic reactions to anesthetics may be due to this preservative.

Vital Staining of Ocular Tissues

When the use of sodium fluorescein or rose bengal is anticipated for the staining of ocular tissues, such as for evaluation of suspected dry eye syndromes or of patient complaints suggestive of anterior segment involvement, the practitioner must avoid instilling an anesthetic until after the vital staining and evaluation procedures have been performed. This is necessary because the topical anesthetic itself can induce corneal epithelial changes that may mask or otherwise confuse the corneal or conjunctival signs. In addition, the anesthetic-induced corneal epithelial changes can significantly alter the result obtained during evaluation of the tear breakup time (BUT).

Cultures

Whenever possible, culture specimens from the lid margins or conjunctiva should be obtained without the prior instillation of an anesthetic.[14,44] Topical anesthetics contain preservatives with antibacterial and antifungal properties. Moreover, the anesthetic agent itself is often toxic to microorganisms. Tetracaine 0.05% has been shown to inhibit the growth of *Staphylococcus aureus* and *Monilia*.[45] In a 0.5% concentration tetracaine is toxic to *Pseudomonas*.[46] Furthermore, proparacaine 0.5% and tetracaine 0.5% have been shown to have a greater inhibitory effect on bacterial growth than does benoxinate 0.4% or cocaine 5%.[47] Kleinfeld and Ellis,[44] however, have shown that proparacaine, when used without preservative, fails to inhibit the growth of *Staphylococcus albus, Pseudomonas aeruginosa,* and *Candida albicans.* Accordingly, these investigators have suggested that proparacaine, in single-dose containers without preservative, should be used when topical anesthesia is desired before obtaining material for culture. Although such a preparation is not commercially available, proparacaine would appear to be the best topical anesthetic for use before obtaining culture material.

Self-Administration of Topical Anesthetics

When evaluating an acute injury of the cornea, the practitioner is sometimes tempted to prescribe a topical anesthetic for administration at home by the patient for relief of ocular pain. This practice, however, is extremely dangerous and has led, in numerous instances, to severe infiltrative keratitis and even loss of the eye from anesthetic misuse or abuse by the patient.[48-51] *Topical anesthetics must be used only for the purpose of obtaining initial relief of ocular pain and never as part of a prolonged therapeutic regimen.* The potential corneal toxicity of topical anesthetics precludes their use as self-administered drugs.

A syndrome has been described resulting from the frequent use of topical anesthetics over prolonged periods ranging from 6 days to 6 weeks.[51] Severe corneal lesions and permanent reduction of visual acuity can occur in any eye that has been subjected to prolonged application of topical anesthetics as a means of relieving the pain of minor injuries. Although cocaine-induced corneal injury is well known, it is now recognized that virtually all topical ocular anesthetics can cause such corneal damage when used for prolonged periods.[49]

This syndrome has occurred in patients using topical anesthetics on their own initiative and in patients who have received prescriptions for anesthetics as part of their initial treatment. Most of these patients will continue to instill the drugs despite advice from the practitioner to discontinue their use. Furthermore, many of the patients in whom the syndrome has occurred have a medical or paramedical background. Of the 18 cases reported between 1968 and 1973, five were health professionals who had treated themselves for a few days up to 2 weeks,[48] and 3 of the 4 cases described in 1977 by Burns and associates[51] had such a medical background.

The numerous signs and symptoms characterizing the syndrome develop over days or weeks.[49–51] The continuous use of the anesthetic, even for only a few days, may cause loss of the corneal epithelium and inhibit the healing of existing epithelial defects. Loss of the epithelial microvilli results in instability and rapid breakup of the tear film, which compounds the drying effect from the decreased blinking secondary to the anesthetic-induced corneal hypoesthesia. Clinically, these changes result in a chronic, non-healing epithelial defect with a rolled edge. In the earliest stages, the cornea may take on an appearance similar to that observed in neuroparalytic keratitis.[49] As the condition progresses, deeper manifestations can include stromal edema with folds in Descemet's membrane, disciform cellular infiltrations into the corneal stroma, keratic precipitates, iridocyclitis, hypopyon, and hyphema. Additional findings may include eyelid edema, conjunctival hyperemia and papillary hypertrophy, mucopurulent discharge, and corneal vascularization. The primary sign allowing objective diagnosis of this disease appears to be a yellowish white, dense stromal ring surrounding the primary disease process (Fig. 4.6).[51] A history of topical anesthetic abuse, if obtainable, also serves to confirm the diagnosis, but

the patient often attempts to conceal the use of such drugs. In some cases patients may exhibit bizarre or combative behavior in efforts to maintain use of the anesthetic. Continued use of the anesthetic, however, serves only to accelerate the development of drug tolerance,[50] creating a cyclical problem of corneal damage, increased corneal pain, and then further corneal damage from the more frequent instillation of the drug but with progressively less effect on the relief of pain.[49] The drug-induced corneal changes create an environment that is susceptible to infection by opportunistic microorganisms. In addition to these manifestations of corneal toxicity, drug allergy may occur. Allergies of the immediate type are characterized by the relatively rapid onset of eyelid edema, conjunctival hyperemia and chemosis, and itching. Delayed hypersensitivity, on the other hand, becomes manifest as a slowly developing eczematoid contact dermatitis of the eyelids and surrounding skin.

The pathogenesis of these corneal changes remains speculative. It has been suggested, however, that the mechanism may involve depressed respiration and glycolysis, increased epithelial cell permeability, and damage to membranous cytoplasmic structures.[52] In addition, Gipson and Anderson[53] have suggested, using rat corneal epithelial cells, that topical anesthetics may disrupt the microfilament systems that are hypothesized to be responsible for generating the forces necessary to allow corneal epithelial cells to migrate to cover abrasions. This may also contribute to the inhibition of normal cell migration and mitosis following an epithelial abrasion. Because of the ring shape of the corneal stromal infiltration, a possible allergic mechanism has also been suspected.[51] This stromal lesion resembles a Wessely ring, which has been shown

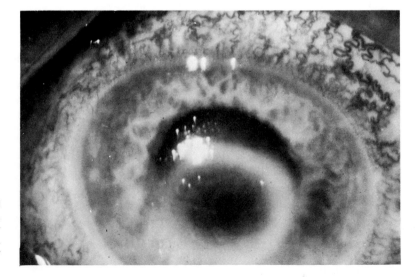

FIGURE 4.6   **Dense corneal stromal ring associated with abuse of topical anesthetics. (From Burns RP, Forster RK, Laibson P, Gipson IK. Chronic toxicity of local anesthetics on the cornea. In: Leopold IH, Burns RP, eds. Symposium on ocular therapy. New York: John Wiley & Sons, 1977;10:31–44.)**

in experimental animals to be of immune origin. However, eosinophils, which would suggest an immediate hypersensitivity reaction, have not been isolated from conjunctival or corneal scrapings taken from these patients.

Prevention of this disorder involves better education of the primary physician, who occasionally uses topical anesthetics, as well as of the optometrist and ophthalmologist, who routinely use these drugs.

Maurice and Singh,[54] using rabbit cornea, have shown that 0.05% proparacaine eyedrops can be used repeatedly to maintain anesthesia without causing corneal toxicity. This suggests that frequent instillation of dilute solutions of proparacaine may be of some value to obtain prolonged local anesthesia in selected patients.

Although the disease is easily treated once the etiology is known, its recognition may be delayed by deceit on the patient's part. The most important requirement in the management of such patients is discontinuation of the topical anesthetic. Treatment consists of cycloplegic agents such as 1% atropine, broad-spectrum antibiotics, and firm pressure-patching. Pain must be controlled with systemic analgesics. Occasionally therapeutic soft contact lenses may be required to promote corneal healing. In some cases of severe drug tolerance and serious corneal lesions, hospitalization may be required. Once the topical anesthetic has been discontinued, remarkable corneal clearing can occur for as long as 6 months.[50]

References

1. Ritchie JM, Green NM. Local anesthetics. In: Gilman AG, Goodman LS, Rall TW, et al., eds. The pharmacological basis of therapeutics, ed. 7. New York: Macmillan Co, 1985;302–321.
2. Covino BG, Vassalo HG. Chemical aspects of local anesthetic agents. In: Local anesthetics—mechanism of action and clinical uses. New York: Grune and Stratton, 1976,Chap. 1.
3. Altman AJ, Albert DM, Fournier GA. Cocaine's use in ophthalmology: Our 100-year heritage. Surv Ophthalmol 1985;29:300–306.
4. Liljestrand G. Carl Koller and the development of local anesthesia. Acta Physiol Scand 1967;30:252–303.
5. de Jong RH. Local anesthetics, ed. 2. Springfield, IL: Charles C Thomas, 1977.
6. Ritchie JM, Greengard P. On the mode of action of local anesthetics. Ann Rev Pharmacol 1966;6:405–430.
7. Bryant JA. Local and topical anesthetics in ophthalmology. Surv Ophthalmol 1969;13:263–283.
8. Bloom LH, Scheie HG, Yanoff M. The warming of local anesthetic agents to decrease discomfort. Ophthal Surg 1984;15:603.
9. Vettese T, Breslin CW. Retrobulbar anesthesia for cataract surgery: Comparison of bupivacaine and bupivacaine/lidocaine combinations. Can J Ophthalmol 1985;20:131–134.
10. Chin GN, Almquist HT. Bupivacaine and lidocaine retrobulbar anesthesia. A double-blind clinical study. Ophthalmology 1983;90:369–372.
11. Nicoll JMV, Treuren B, Acharya PA, et al. Retrobulbar anesthesia: The role of hyaluronidase. Anesth Analg 1986;65:1324–1328.
12. Smith RB, Everett WG. Physiology and pharmacology of local anesthetic agents. Int Ophthalmol Clin 1973;13:35–60.
13. Webster RB. Local anesthetics for ophthalmic use. Aust J Optom 1974;57:399–401.
14. Havener WH. Ocular pharmacology. St. Louis: C.V. Mosby Co, 1983;5:72–119.
15. Meyers EF. Cocaine toxicity during dacryocystorhinostomy. Arch Ophthalmol 1980;98:842–843.
16. Miscellaneous ophthalmic preparations. In: AMA drug evaluations. Chicago: American Medical Association, 1980;4:395–398.
17. Bryant JA. Local and topical anesthetics in ophthalmology. Surv Ophthalmol 1969;13:263–283.
18. Walsh FB. Clinical neuro-ophthalmology. Baltimore: Williams & Wilkins, 1957;2.
19. Bartlett JD, Wood JW. Optometry and the Drug Enforcement Administration. J Am Optom Assoc 1981;52:495–498.
20. Norden LC. Adverse reactions to topical ocular anesthetics. J Am Optom Assoc 1976;47:730–733.
21. Leopold IH, ed. Ocular therapy; complications and management. St. Louis: C.V. Mosby Co, 1966.
22. Linn JG, Vey EK. Topical anesthesia in ophthalmology. Am J Ophthalmol 1955;40:697–704.
23. Jose JG, Basta M, Cramer KJ, et al. Lack of effects of anesthetic on measurement of intraocular pressure by Goldmann tonometry. Am J Optom Physiol Opt 1983;60:308–310.
24. Vaughn DG. The contamination of fluorescein solutions, with special reference to *Pseudomonas aeruginosa (Bacillus pyocyaneus)*. Am J Ophthalmol 1955;39:55–61.
25. Yolton DP, German CJ. Fluress, fluorescein and benoxinate: Recovery from bacterial contamination. J Am Optom Assoc 1980;51:471–474.
26. Polse KA, Keener RJ, Jauregui MJ. Dose-response effects of corneal anesthetics. Am J Optom Physiol Opt 1978;55:8–14.
27. Jauregui MJ, Sanders TL, Polse KA. Anesthetic effects from low concentrations of proparacaine and benoxinate. J Am Optom Assoc 1980;51:37–41.
28. Cohn HC, Jocson VL. A unique case of grand mal seizures after Fluress. Ann Ophthalmol 1981;13:1379–1380.
29. Frayer WC, Jacoby J. Local anesthesia. In: Duane TD, ed. Clinical ophthalmology, vol. 5. Hagerstown, MD: Harper & Row, 1987;2:1–10.
30. Ward B, McCulley JP, Segal RJ. Dermatologic reaction in Stevens-Johnson syndrome after ophthalmic anesthesia with proparacaine hydrochloride. Am J Ophthalmol 1978;86:133–135.
31. Wilson GS, Fullard RJ. Proparacaine sloughs cells. J Am Optom Assoc 1988;59:701–702.
32. Fullard RJ, Wilson GS. Investigation of sloughed corneal

epithelial cells collected by non-invasive irrigation of the corneal surface. Curr Eye Res 1986;5:847–856.

33. Patterson RW, Yarberry H. Severe drug reactions and their emergency treatment as related to ophthalmology. Am J Ophthalmol 1964;58:1048–1054.

34. Lyle WM, Page C. Possible adverse effects from local anesthetics and the treatment of these reactions. Am J Optom Physiol Opt 1975;52:736–744.

35. Householder JR, Harris JE. Anesthetic drugs in ophthalmology. In: Leopold IH, ed. Ocular therapy, complications and management. St. Louis: C.V. Mosby Co, 1966;100.

36. Moore DC, Bridenbaugh LD. Oxygen: The antidote for systemic toxic reactions from local anesthetic drugs. JAMA 1960;174:102–107.

37. Chandler MJ, Grammer LC, Patterson R. Provocative challenge with local anesthetics in patients with a prior history of reaction. J Allergy Clin Immunol 1987;79:883–886.

38. Adriani J, Campbell D. Fatalities following topical application of local anesthetics to mucous membranes. JAMA 1956;162:1527–1530.

39. Cooley RL, Cottingham AJ. Ocular complications from local anesthetic injections. Gen Dent 1979;27:40–43.

40. Laskin DM. Diagnosis and treatment of complications associated with local anesthesia. Int Dent J 1984;34:232–237.

41. Sadove MS, Wyant GM, Gittelson LA, Kretchmer HE. Classification and management of reactions to local anesthetics. JAMA 1952;148:17–22.

42. Leopold IH. Advances in anesthesia in ophthalmic surgery. Ophthalmic Surg 1974;5:13–23.

43. Molinari JF. Adverse systemic drug reactions acquired from topical ocular drugs. South J Optom 1978;20:11–15.

44. Kleinfeld J, Ellis PP. Effects of topical anesthetics on growth of microorganisms. Arch Ophthalmol 1966;76:712–715.

45. Erlich H. Bacteriologic studies and effects of anesthetic solutions on bronchial secretions during bronchoscopy. Ann Rev Respir Dis 1961;84:414–421.

46. Murphy JT, Allen HF, Mangiaracine AB. Preparation, sterlization, and preservation of ophthalmic solutions: Experimental studies and a practical method. Arch Ophthalmol 1955;53:63–78.

47. Burns RP. Laboratory methods in diagnosis of eye infection. In: Infectious diseases of the conjunctiva and cornea (Symposium of the New Orleans Academy of Ophthalmology). St. Louis: C.V. Mosby Co, 1963;15.

48. Henkes HE, Waubke TN. Keratitis from abuse of corneal anesthetics. Br J Ophthalmol 1978;62:62–65.

49. Epstein DL, Paton D. Keratitis from misuse of corneal anesthetics. N Engl J Med 1968;279:369–396.

50. Michaels RH, Wilson FM, Grayson M. Infiltrative keratitis from abuse of anesthetic eyedrops. J Indiana State Med Assoc 1979;72:51–54.

51. Burns RP, Forster RK, Laibson P, Gipson IK. Chronic toxicity of local anesthetics on the cornea. In: Leopold IH, Burns RP, eds. Symposium on ocular therapy. New York: John Wiley & Sons, 1977;10:31–44.

52. Grant WM. Toxicology of the eye. Springfield, IL: Charles C Thomas, 1974;2:137–139.

53. Gipson IK, Anderson RA. Actin filaments in normal and migrating corneal epithelial cells. Invest Ophthalmol Vis Sci 1977;16:161–166.

54. Maurice DM, Singh T. The absence of corneal toxicity with low-level topical anesthesia. Am J Ophthalmol 1985;99:691–696.

CHAPTER 5

Anti-Inflammatory Drugs

Siret D. Jaanus

Since their introduction into clinical practice, corticosteroids have been useful in a variety of inflammatory and autoimmune disease states. Although their pharmacologic actions on ocular tissue remain an enigma, corticosteroids provide an important therapeutic tool for control of ocular inflammatory disorders. More recently another group of drugs, the nonsteroidal anti-inflammatory agents (NSAIAs) and cromolyn sodium have also proven effective in certain instances. This chapter considers the anti-inflammatory agents currently available, their mechanisms of action, clinical uses, and potential side effects.

Corticosteroids

The importance of the adrenal glands began to be appreciated following Addison's description in 1855 of the clinical syndromes associated with impaired function of these glands.[1] The following year, Brown-Sequard[2] published his classic experiments on the effects of removal of the adrenal glands and concluded that the adrenals are essential to life. Subsequent to that it was recognized that the adrenal glands consist anatomically of two distinct regions—an inner portion, the medulla, surrounded by an outer layer, the cortex.[3] By the 1930s, it was generally recognized that the adrenal cortex secretes at least two major types of physiologically important hormones, namely, glucocorticoids and mineralocorticoids.

Preparation of biologically active extracts from adrenal tissue resulted in the isolation of about 28 corticosteroids. By 1945 five of these had been demonstrated to be physiologically active.[3] Since then, further investigations into adrenal steroid biosynthesis and metabolism have led to the introduction of a host of synthetic compounds, some of which represent certain therapeutic advances compared with the naturally occurring hormones.[4]

At the same time other investigators turned their attention to the adenohypophysis, and it was established that impairment or removal of the pituitary gland results in adrenal cortical atrophy. Chemical fractionation of extracts from the gland led to the isolation of an active principle, later named adrenocorticotropin (ACTH), which exerts broad regulatory control over the adrenal cortex.[5]

Throughout the 1940s the intense interest in the physiologic effects of adrenocortical steroids and ACTH led to the appreciation that the body's response to noxious or stressful stimuli depends on the proper responses from the adrenal and pituitary glands.[6] Clinically it began to be appreciated that corticosteroids may be effective in diseases other than adrenocortical insufficiency. This resulted in the use by Hench and associates[7] in 1949 of one of the hormones, cortisone, in acute rheumatoid arthritis. The anti-inflammatory response obtained was dramatic. Soon the therapeutic application of corticosteroids, and later ACTH, was extended to other nonendocrine disease states. In 1950, Gordon and McLean[8] introduced corticosteroids and ACTH into ocular therapy.

To evaluate both the beneficial pharmacologic effects of corticosteroid hormones on the ocular tissues and the potential of these hormones to induce toxic effects, it is useful to consider some basic physiologic and pharmacologic principles involved in their actions.

The Adrenocortical System

Regulation of adrenal cortical function depends on a series of interactions between the adrenal cortex, adenohypophysis, and hypothalamus (Fig. 5.1).

ADRENAL CORTEX

As previously indicated, the adrenal gland is a complex organ, consisting of an inner portion, the medulla, surrounded by a three-layered structure, the cortex. In humans the medulla secretes epinephrine as well as smaller amounts of norepinephrine. The adrenal cortex secretes three general groups of steroid hormones. The outermost layer, the zona glomerulosa, produces mineralocorticoids, primarily aldosterone and deoxycorticosterone, which help to regulate salt and water metabolism. The inner two layers, the zona fasciculata and the zona reticularis, secrete glucocorticoids and small amounts of sex hormones. The physiologic role of the adrenal sex hormones is not well understood. It is thought that they supplement the actions of the androgens and estrogens secreted by the gonads. The glucocorticoids exhibit a variety of physiologic effects and, in addition, inhibit or suppress the processes accompanying inflammation. The principal glucocorticoid secreted by the human adrenal cortex is hydrocortisone, also known as cortisol. Small amounts of cortisone and corticosterone are also present in the systemic circulation.[3]

ADENOHYPOPHYSIS

The anterior pituitary secretes numerous tropic hormones that stimulate various glands to secrete their specific hormones.[3] Among these is ACTH, which stimulates the adrenal cortex to secrete glucocorticoids, mineralocorticoids, and androgenic steroids. Although ACTH can cause the release of the mineralocorticoid aldosterone, secretion of the latter is relatively independent of the anterior pituitary. Angiotensin, a plasma peptide formed by the action of renin released from the kidney in response to blood sodium levels, controls the secretion of aldosterone.[9]

In the absence of a functional pituitary, the adrenal cortex undergoes atrophy, and the secretion of glucocorticoids is markedly reduced. The tropic effect of ACTH determines both the size and the steroidogenic capacity of the adrenal gland. Lack of ACTH causes a rapid decline of adrenocortical function, particularly in plasma glucocorticoid levels. The zona glomerulosa, which is responsible for the synthesis of aldosterone, is least subject to atrophic changes associated with deficiencies of ACTH secretion.[3] The effects of ACTH on the adrenal cortex are mediated by adenosine 3'-5'-monophosphate (cyclic AMP).[10] As has been proposed for other hormones, ACTH is thought to interact with a specific site in the adrenal cell membrane. This results in the stimulation of activity of the enzyme, adenyl cyclase, and formation of cyclic AMP. The role of cyclic AMP as a mediator of hormone action has been viewed as a "second messenger." Its role in the production of adrenal corticosteroids is illustrated in Figure 5.2. There is also evidence that calcium is required for the action of ACTH on adrenal cortical hormone synthesis and release.[11,12]

HYPOTHALAMUS

A number of factors regulate the concentration of circulating ACTH and the consequent plasma concentrations of corticosteroids. The median eminence of the hypothalamus secretes a substance, corticotropin-releasing factor (CRF), which is transported through a series of vessels to the anterior pituitary gland. CRF serves as a positive modulator of ACTH synthesis and release. ACTH secretion is also subject to a negative feedback regulatory mechanism, since the levels of ACTH at any instant are determined by a balance of neural excitatory stimuli converging on the hypothalamus as well as plasma corticosteroid hormone inhibitory effects. The major site of glucocorticoid feedback appears to reside in the hypothalamus.[13]

General Physiologic and Pharmacologic Effects

The adrenal cortex has been termed the organ *par excellence* of homeostasis, allowing the body to adjust

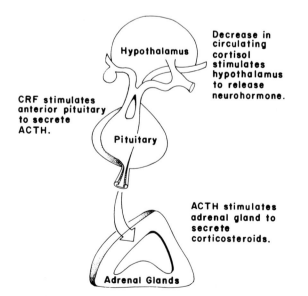

FIGURE 5.1 **Relationship of the adrenal cortex to the pituitary gland and hypothalamus. (Adapted from Leopold IH. Steroids and inflammation. Allergan Office Seminars in Ophthalmology, 1974.)**

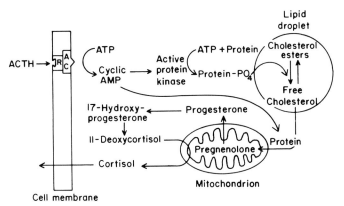

FIGURE 5.2 **The mechanism of action of ACTH on cortisol-secreting cells of the adrenal cortex. (AC, adenyl cyclase; R, receptor). (Adapted from Ganong WF. Review of medical physiology. Los Altos, CA: Lange, 1985; 12: Chap. 20.)**

to a constantly changing environment. In the absence of a functional adrenal cortex, survival can occur only under the most rigid of conditions. Temperature must be maintained within a narrow range. Food, water, and sodium chloride must be readily available. Moreover, the actions of the corticosteroids are related in a complex manner to many other hormones and physiochemical processes. This role of the corticosteroids has been termed their *permissive* action.[14]

Although clinically the glucocorticoids are used primarily for their anti-inflammatory and immunosuppressive effects, they also exhibit a wide variety of physiologic and pharmacologic actions. To understand the often complex signs and symptoms observed with systemic and topical corticosteroid therapy, a brief description of these effects is relevant.

CARBOHYDRATE AND PROTEIN METABOLISM

Administration of glucocorticoids causes elevation of blood sugar levels. This is most likely a result of increased glucose formation from protein. Liver glycogen storage is increased. Some inhibition of peripheral oxidation of glucose, along with an increased resistance to the effects of insulin, occurs. As a result of these effects on carbohydrate and protein metabolism, a diabeticlike state may ensue along with glycosuria and elevated blood sugar levels.[3,15] Thus, systemic steroid administration to patients with diabetes should be undertaken only with strict supervision of blood glucose levels.

LIPID METABOLISM

Pharmacologic doses of glucocorticoids cause a characteristic alteration in body fat distribution. There is an increased deposition of lipid in the back of the neck, supraclavicular area, and face. Fat is lost from the extremities. These same effects are seen with Cushing's syndrome, where the hypersecretion of cortisol is thought responsible for the "moon face" and "buffalo

hump." Although it has been shown that corticosteroids increase the production of lipid from protein, their mechanism of action in bringing about the abnormal distribution of fat is not well understood.[3,15]

CENTRAL NERVOUS SYSTEM

Administration of glucocorticoids can result in transient changes in mood. Reactions vary among patients, but euphoria, insomnia, restlessness, and enhanced motor activity can occur. A small number of patients become anxious, depressed, or psychotic. The reasons for these effects are not understood, but a direct action on the brain as well as tissue alteration in electrolyte concentrations and blood flow changes have been suggested as possible causes.[3,15]

BLOOD ELEMENTS

Glucocorticoids tend to increase the number of red blood cells and polymorphonuclear leukocytes in the blood and to reduce the number of circulating eosinophils, monocytes, and basophils.[3]

IMMUNE RESPONSE

Glucocorticoids modify the clinical course of a variety of diseases in which hypersensitivity is thought to play an important role.[3] Although there is no evidence that the titer of circulating antibodies that play a major role in the allergic state is altered, the symptoms of the disease often respond dramatically to use of corticosteroids.

ANTI-INFLAMMATORY EFFECTS

Corticosteroids can prevent or suppress the responses associated with inflammation, such as pain, redness, swelling, and local heat. At the cellular level they inhibit both the early and late manifestations of the inflammatory process including edema, fibrin deposition, capillary dilation, capillary and fibroblast proliferation, and deposition of collagen. Still later, cicatrization is also inhibited.[16–18]

The cellular mechanisms involved in the anti-inflammatory effects of steroids are not well established. However, the clinical actions of steroids on the disease process are almost always characteristic. The inflammatory response is inhibited whether its cause is mechanical, chemical, radiant, infectious, or immunologic. Since corticosteroids are effective following topical application to skin and mucous membranes, their anti-inflammatory effects are thought to depend on direct local actions, possibly on cells participating in the inflammatory process.[15–19] Corticosteroids induce a lymphocytopenia, with a greater reduction in T-cells than B-cells. The effect appears to be due to altered circulation or redistribution of blood lymphocytes rather than to cell lysis.[16] There is, however, no convincing evidence that the titer of circulating antibodies, either IgE or IgG, is affected by corticosteroid therapy. Serum complement levels also appear to be unaffected.[3,16] Migration of macrophages and neutrophils to inflamed areas is inhibited.[16] In addition, corticosteroids can inhibit prostaglandin synthesis by inhibition of phospholipase A_2.[3]

Although their effects on the inflammatory process make the corticosteroids a valuable therapeutic tool, *their use constitutes palliative therapy.* The inflammatory manifestations are suppressed while the underlying cause of the disease remains. The ability to suppress inflammation irrespective of cause has made the corticosteroids valuable, even lifesaving therapeutic agents, but with potential serious consequences.[16] The signs and symptoms of inflammation accompanying a disease are often useful expressions of the disease process and enable evaluation of treatment effectiveness. These inflammatory signs and symptoms are frequently suppressed or absent in patients treated with steroids. For example, an infectious process may continue to progress while, clinically, improvement is observed. Hench and associates[19] perhaps best described the dilemma with corticosteroid therapy: "It acts as a fire shield but never puts out the fire, nor acts as a carpenter to repair the fire's damage."

Glucocorticoid Receptors

General agreement exists that the effects of glucocorticosteroids are mediated by specialized intracellular receptors (Fig. 5.3). Circulating corticosteroid is thought to pass through the cell membrane and bind to a specific protein located in the cytoplasm. This is followed by an activation step that results in translocation of the corticosteroid-receptor complex into the cell nucleus. A series of steps, involving specific mRNA, leads to the

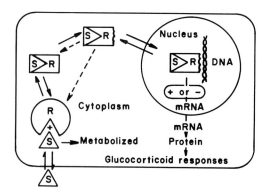

FIGURE 5.3 **Proposed sequence of corticosteroid hormone action. Following entry into cell, the hormone (S) combines with receptor (R) followed by a sequence of events resulting in synthesis of specific proteins that mediate steroid hormone responses. (Adapted from Polansky JR, Weinreb RN. Antiinflammatory agents. In: Sears ML, ed. Pharmacology of the eye. New York: Springer-Verlag, 1984;515.)**

production of specific proteins by which corticosteroids can influence a variety of target tissues. Most likely, the regulated production of specific proteins results in the diverse physiologic and pharmacologic effects observed following steroid administration.[20–22]

Synthetic and Metabolic Mechanisms

Cholesterol is the necessary intermediate in the biosynthesis of corticosteroids. Through a series of metabolic steps, the 27-carbon cholesterol is enzymatically converted to 21-carbon compounds in the adrenal cortex.[3] In addition to these corticosteroids produced endogenously by the adrenal cortex, several synthetic compounds have been developed since cortisone was synthesized in 1948 from an organic acid present in bile secretion.[3] The objective has been to obtain compounds with increased anti-inflammatory activity and reduced sodium retention effects. The chemical structures of cortisol and other corticosteroids in current clinical use are illustrated in Figure 5.4. A distinction is made between glucocorticoid and mineralocorticoid activity, but the separation is not absolute between the members of these two groups of steroids. Certain of the glucocorticoids exhibit varying degrees of mineralocorticoid effects (Table 5.1).

All biologically active corticosteroids have certain structural characteristics in common (see Fig. 5.4). A double bond between C 4,5 and the 3-ketone is necessary for adrenocortical activity. Alterations in molecular structure bring about changes in the ratio of anti-inflammatory to sodium-retaining potency (see

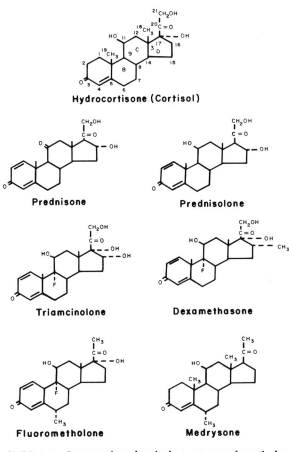

FIGURE 5.4 **Comparative chemical structures of cortisol and synthetic derivatives in current clinical use.**

Table 5.1). Introduction of a double bond at C 1,2, as in prednisone, enhances the ratio of carbohydrate-regulating potency to sodium-retaining activity. The presence of an oxygen function at C 11 appears essential for significant anti-inflammatory activity.[3]

Methylation at C 6, as in fluorometholone and medrysone, increases anti-inflammatory activity, whereas fluorination in the 9 alpha position enhances both glucocorticoid and anti-inflammatory effects.[3]

Since the fullest expression of anti-inflammatory activity requires the presence of the 17-hydroxy group,[3] nearly all anti-inflammatory steroids in current clinical use are 17 α-hydroxy compounds. An exception is medrysone.

Once synthesized, corticosteroids are not stored in the adrenal glands to any significant extent; rather, synthesis and release of hormones appear to be intimately related processes.[23] The average individual secretes about 25 mg cortisol and 5 mg corticosterone within a 24-hour period. The rate of secretion exhibits

diurnal fluctuations.[24] Plasma concentrations are usually highest between 6:00 and 8:00 AM. The lowest secretion level occurs about midnight[25] (Fig. 5.5).

In the plasma, corticosteroids are found as their native molecules and as derivatives of glucuronic acid. At a given time, both cortisol and corticosterone are about 95% bound to plasma protein. The unbound form is considered biologically active and appears to be involved in the regulatory control of steroid blood levels through the hypothalamus and the anterior pituitary.[3]

The liver, and to some extent the kidneys, are responsible for metabolic processes that convert the corticosteroid to water-soluble derivatives for excretion in the urine. Blood levels of free corticosteroid are therefore controlled by the degree of binding to plasma proteins, the metabolic activity of the liver, and the secretion of ACTH.[3]

Ocular Physiologic Effects

Several approaches have been used to study the effects of corticosteroids on ocular tissue, including correlation of ocular effects with diurnal variations of blood steroid levels as well as administration of steroids to normal and inflamed eyes.[26] The results are difficult to interpret due to differences in animal species, corticosteroids, dosages, and routes of administration. In addition, topical ocular application results in systemic absorption.[27,28]

CORNEA AND CONJUNCTIVA

An increase in corneal thickness has been reported with topical prednisolone and dexamethasone.[29,30] Uniocular administration to human volunteers with normal eyes has resulted in a small but statistically significant increase in corneal thickness in about 35% to 70% of the subjects tested. Although the increase was greatest in individuals who demonstrated the highest intraocular pressure elevation,[29] no significant correlation between corneal thickness and pressure change could be established.

Corticosteroids also affect conjunctival vessels. Topical administration to the eye causes arteriolar constriction. The vasoconstrictor effects of norepinephrine are potentiated.[31] The observed metabolic and vasoconstrictor effects may in part explain the decrease in corneal vascularization and the inhibition of neovascularization with corticosteroid therapy, which occur during various corneal and conjunctival diseases.[26]

Corticosteroids may also alter corneal metabolism. Corneal swelling under anoxic conditions is prevented by adding cortisone acetate to the bathing solution.[26] Corneal epithelial cell migration in partially denuded

TABLE 5.1
Relative Anti-Inflammatory Activity, Sodium-Retaining Activity, and Equivalent Doses of Currently Available Systemic Corticosteroids

Generic Name	Trade Name	Relative Anti-Inflammatory Activity	Relative Sodium-Retaining Activity	Equivalent Dose (mg)
Hydrocortisone (cortisol)	Cortef, Hydrocortone	1.0	1.0	20.00
Cortisone acetate	Cortisone, Cortone	0.8	0.8	25.00
Prednisone	Prednisone, Orasone, Deltasone, Meticorten	4.0	0.8	5.00
Prednisolone	Prednisolone, Delta-Cortef, Atolone	4.0	0.8	5.00
Triamcinolone	Aristocort, Kenacort	5.0	0.0	4.00
Methylprednisolone	Medrol	5.0	0.0	4.00
Paramethasone acetate	Haldrone	10.00	0.0	2.0
Fluprednisolone	Alphadrol	13.5	0.0	1.50
Dexamethasone	Decadron, Dexone	25.0	0.0	0.75
Betamethasone	Celestone	25.0	0.0	0.75

rabbit corneas does not appear to be inhibited by topical corticosteroid administration. However, corneal reepithelialization is significantly inhibited by prednisolone acetate, dexamethasone, and fluorometholone following complete corneal denudation.[32]

Recent studies with bovine corneal epithelial preparations indicate that corticosteroids inhibit adenylate cyclase activity.[33] Dose-response curves using clinically employed doses of dexamethasone, prednisolone, and hydrocortisone phosphate derivatives resulted in a non-competitive reversible inhibition of adenylate cyclase. Dexamethasone phosphate was the most potent inhibitor of the enzyme.

AQUEOUS AND VITREOUS HUMORS

Studies have indicated that corticosteroids are present in normal aqueous humor.[34] Moreover, their concentration increases following the administration of ACTH. Topical application to the eye or systemic administra-

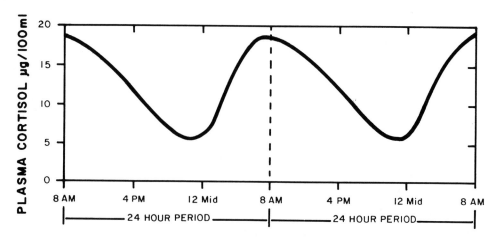

FIGURE 5.5 **The diurnal cycle of plasma cortisol levels. (Modified from Ney RL: Modern concepts of adrenocortical function. In: Thorn GW, ed. Steroid therapy: a clinical update for the 1970s. New York: Medcom, 1971.)**

tion can increase corticosteroid levels in the fluid compartments for extended periods following cessation of therapy. Protein and glucose levels may also rise, whereas urea and ascorbic acid may decrease.[26] Following systemic administration of ACTH, increases in mucopolysaccharide content of the vitreous have been observed. This is accompanied by an increase in relative viscosity of the vitreous.[35]

A clinically significant effect of corticosteroid use is an elevation of intraocular pressure in certain individuals.[36] This response is more pronounced with topical than with systemic administration of steroids. In addition, clinical evidence suggests that the tendency toward pressure elevation may be genetically determined, since patients with glaucoma, as well as those suspected of having glaucoma, may react to a greater extent than do healthy individuals.

Experimental evidence indicates that corticosteroid can reduce aqueous outflow facility.[37] More recent studies suggest that corticosteroids can bind with certain receptor sites on cultured human trabecular cells.[38] An effect on cells lining the aqueous outflow pathway could in part explain the observed pressure effects. It is also likely that corticosteroids exert effects on formation of aqueous and aqueous flow in the anterior chamber.[39]

LENS

Following the clinical observation by Black and associates[40] of increased incidence of lens opacities in patients on prolonged systemic corticosteroid therapy, numerous investigators have attempted to study this effect experimentally. Lenses of corticosteroid-treated subjects with and without associated lens opacities have been analyzed. Rats treated with systemic corticosteroids have shown a decrease in the number of mitotic counts in the lens epithelium, although no lens opacities were observed.[41,42] A shift in sodium and potassium content of lenses incubated with prednisolone has been reported. Incubated rabbit lenses demonstrated an increase in sodium and a decrease in potassium content. This was accompanied by an increase in lens hydration.[43] Glutathione and urea levels also appear to decrease.[26]

RETINA

Experimental evidence indicates that corticosteroids can influence retinal metabolism and vasomotor tone. A decrease in oxygen consumption and an increase in glycogen content has been reported following subconjunctival injection of cortisone.[25] Enzymatic activity is altered. Cortisone in vivo and in vitro inhibits pyruvic and succinic dehydrogenase activities of rabbit retina.[26] Relatively small concentrations of hydrocortisone in-

duce large increases of glutamine synthetase in the embryonic chick retina.[44]

Retinal capillaries, particularly near the fovea, can be affected. Vasoconstriction and a decrease in capillary pressure have been observed following subconjunctival cortisone.[26]

Ocular Pharmacologic Effects

More than 30 years following their introduction into ocular therapeutics, corticosteroids are still the most frequently used agents for control of ocular inflammatory disease. They have proven to be effective in protecting the delicate tissues of the eye from many of the deleterious effects accompanying the inflammatory response, in particular scarring and neovascularization.[18,45,46]

As demonstrated in other tissues,[3] corticosteroids do not appear to have specific effects on the inflamed eye but, rather, provide palliative therapy only. In general, ocular allergic reactions and uveal tract inflammations respond satisfactorily. Corticosteroids also appear to be more effective in acute than in chronic conditions. Degenerative diseases are usually completely refractory to corticosteroid therapy.[46] The primary ocular inflammatory disorders in which steroids have been reported to be beneficial are listed in Table 5.2.[47]

Corticosteroids are generally contraindicated in most ocular infections because they are not bactericidal, and they reduce resistance to many types of invading microorganisms, including bacteria, viruses, and fungi. In severe infections in which there is considerable ocular involvement and vision is threatened, their use must be accompanied by appropriate anti-infective therapy, since corticosteroids can mask evidence of progression of the infection.[45,46]

The beneficial effects of corticosteroids on ocular inflammation include a reduction in capillary permeability and cellular exudation, suppression of migration of polymorphonuclear leukocytes to the site of the injury,[19] and inhibition of fibroblast growth and release of hydrolytic enzymes from inflammatory cells.[46] Tissue infiltrates disappear, since the stimulus that attracts inflammatory cells to the injured area is inhibited. The anti-inflammatory effects of corticosteroids are nonspecific, occurring whether the etiology is allergic, traumatic, or infectious.[45,48]

Topical Ocular Corticosteroids

As previously indicated, corticosteroid preparations vary in their inherent anti-inflammatory potency.[48] Hydrocortisone (cortisol) has become the standard against

TABLE 5.2
Indications for Use of Corticosteroids in Ocular Disease

Eyelids
    Allergic blepharitis
    Contact dermatitis
    Herpes zoster dermatoblepharitis
    Chemical burns

Conjunctiva
    Allergic conjunctivitis
    Vernal conjunctivitis
    Herpes zoster conjunctivitis
    Chemical burns
    Mucocutaneous conjunctival lesions

Cornea
    Immune graft reaction
    Herpes zoster keratitis
    Disciform herpes simplex keratitis
    Marginal corneal ulcers
    Superficial punctate keratitis
    Chemical burns
    Acne rosacea keratitis
    Interstitial keratitis

Uvea
    Iritis, iridocyclitis
    Anterior uveitis
    Posterior uveitis
    Sympathetic ophthalmia

Sclera
    Scleritis
    Episcleritis

Retina
    Retinal vasculitis

Optic nerve
    Optic neuritis
    Temporal arteritis

Globe
    Endophthalmitis
    Hemorrhagic glaucoma

Orbit
    Pseudotumor
    Graves' ophthalmopathy

Extraocular muscles
    Ocular myasthenia gravis

which synthetic corticosteroids are measured. It is assigned a relative anti-inflammatory potency of 1. Except for cortisone, topical ocular steroids in current clinical use are more potent than cortisol. Their relative anti-inflammatory potencies are the same as those of the systemic corticosteroids (see Table 5.1). The data were compiled by Nelson[49] from reports in the literature on clinical observations as well as from animal studies and tissue culture models comparing the potencies of various steroids. These data can be criticized on the basis that each drug was not tested under the same experimental conditions. In addition, ocular effects were not studied in all instances. Moreover, data from other organ systems such as skin may not always apply to ocular tissue. Application of irritants to the eye and use of animal models with experimental uveitis may not simulate all aspects of the inflammatory process in humans.

An experimental system that could mimic the clinical course of inflammation and that could allow for the determination of dose-response curves would be desirable. However, such models are difficult to devise. A recent attempt to determine the ocular anti-inflammatory effectiveness of different corticosteroid preparations has been based on the measurement of the decrease in radioactivity of labeled polymorphonuclear leukocytes in rabbit corneas during keratitis.[48] This technique indicates that various topically administered corticosteroids differ in their ability to suppress the

inflammatory reaction (Table 5.3). These data indicate that prednisolone acetate 1% is the most effective of the preparations tested for suppressing corneal inflammation.

The derivative of the same corticosteroid base plays an important role in the drug's anti-inflammatory properties following topical administration to the eye.[48] In the rabbit cornea dexamethasone alcohol demonstrates greater anti-inflammatory activity than does dexamethasone phosphate (see Table 5.3). Similar experimental data also indicate that when comparable concentrations of prednisolone acetate and phosphate are tested, prednisolone acetate exhibits superior anti-inflammatory effects.[50,51] Similar data have been reported for fluorometholone. Leibowitz and associates[52] reported that the acetate derivative of fluorometholone was significantly more effective in suppressing external ocular inflammation than an equal concentration of the alcohol derivative. When fluorometholone acetate 0.1% was compared with prednisolone acetate 1%, no significant difference in clinical efficacy between the two steroids was observed.

Corticosteroid derivatives differ in their ability to penetrate the eye.[53,54] Their anti-inflammatory efficacy, however, does not appear to be directly proportional to the concentration of drug obtained at the site of inflammation. For example, data comparing corneal bioavailability and anti-inflammatory effectiveness for three different dexamethasones indicate that although

TABLE 5.3
Decrease in Corneal Inflammation following Topical Corticosteroid Therapy with Various Corticosteroid Derivatives

Corneal Epithelium Intact	% Decrease	Corneal Epithelium Absent	% Decrease
Prednisolone acetate 1.0%	51	Prednisolone acetate 1.0%	53
Dexamethasone alcohol 0.1%	40	Prednisolone sodium phosphate 1.0%	47
Fluorometholone alcohol 0.1%	31	Dexamethasone alcohol 0.1%	42
Prednisolone sodium phosphate 1.0%	28	Fluorometholone alcohol 0.1%	37
Dexamethasone sodium phosphate 0.1%	19	Dexamethasone sodium phosphate 0.1%	22
Dexamethasone sodium phosphate 0.05% (ointment)	13		

From Leibowitz HM, Kupferman A. Int Ophthalmol Clin 1980; 20:117–134.

the acetate achieves the lowest concentrations in the cornea, it produces the greatest anti-inflammatory effect[51] (Table 5.4).

The highly lipophilic character of the corneal epithelium compared with the stroma can also be expected to influence topical ocular drug absorption. Highly lipophilic agents tend to concentrate in the epithelial layer and may even reach a saturation concentration before passing through the hydrophilic layers of the cornea. Such a mechanism has been proposed for fluorometholone, which penetrates into and through the cornea in comparatively low concentration but produces moderate suppression of corneal inflammation.[55] Concentration of drug primarily in the corneal epithelium tends to reduce drug levels in the anterior chamber. It is not clear whether this is true for medrysone, a relatively weak anti-inflammatory agent clinically useful in minor conjunctival inflammatory conditions.[48]

The drug vehicle can affect the therapeutic efficacy of ophthalmic drugs. It is the general belief that ointments are superior to drops in terms of the effects achieved following topical application to the eye. Prolonged contact time of the drug due to the greater

viscosity of the ointment vehicle is presumed to result in higher ocular tissue drug concentration. Although ointment formulations exhibit greater potency for certain drugs (see Chapter 1), this does not seem to be the case for all steroid preparations. Dexamethasone phosphate in solution can reach comparatively higher concentration in the anterior segment than does the ointment form.[56] Rate of release of drug particles from the vehicle (suspension) and the drug's solubility in the precorneal tear film are additional factors that influence corneal penetration and therapeutic results.

High-viscosity gels have been formulated to enhance ocular bioavailability and pharmacologic effects of corticosteroids. Prednisolone acetate delivered to rabbit eyes in carboxy-poly-methylene gel produces higher drug concentrations in the cornea and aqueous humor than do comparable concentrations of commercially available ophthalmic suspensions.[57] In the rabbit cornea the gel preparation has demonstrated a prolongation of the anti-inflammatory effects of prednisolone acetate.[58] Gel preparations for human use have met with limited success due to toxicity.

Under clinical conditions, the principal means of

TABLE 5.4
Corneal Bioavailability and Anti-Inflammatory Effectiveness of Different Dexamethasones

Corticosteroid	Anti-Inflammatory Effect (%)	Corneal Bioavailability (μg-min/g)
Epithelium intact		
Dexamethasone acetate 0.1%	55	111
Dexamethasone alcohol 0.1%	40	543
Dexamethasone sodium phosphate 0.1%	19	1068
Epithelium absent		
Dexamethasone acetate 0.1%	60	118
Dexamethasone alcohol 0.1%	42	1316
Dexamethasone sodium phosphate 0.1%	22	4642

From Leibowitz HM, Kupferman A. Int Ophthalmol Clin 1980; 20:117–134.

TABLE 5.5
Anti-Inflammatory Effect of Different Dosage Schedules for Topical Administration of Prednisolone Acetate 1%

Treatment Regimen	Total No. of Doses Delivered	Decrease in Corneal Inflammation (%)
1 drop every 4 hours	6	11
1 drop every 2 hours	10	30
1 drop every hour	18	51
1 drop every 30 minutes	34	61
1 drop every 15 minutes	66	68
1 drop each minute for 5 minutes every hour	90	72

From Leibowitz HM, Kupferman A. Int Ophthalmol Clin 1980; 20:117–134.

regulating the dosage of topical ocular corticosteroid, in addition to varying the concentration, is by altering the frequency of application (Table 5.5). The type and the severity of inflammatory condition most likely play a major role in the therapeutic response obtained with a particular steroid preparation.[25] Table 5.6 lists the common topical ocular preparations currently available.

Principles of Corticosteroid Therapy

Following more than three decades of clinical experience with ocular corticosteroid therapy, the use of ocular steroids remains largely empirical. Over this time, certain observations have been made, and from these some general therapeutic principles have emerged[59]:

- The specific type and location of the inflammation determine if topical, systemic, periocular or multiple routes of administration are appropriate.
- Treatment should be instituted immediately when indicated, and the dose should be high enough to suppress the inflammatory response.
- The appropriate dose for a specific disease is largely determined by clinical experience and must be reev-

TABLE 5.6
Topical Ocular Corticosteroids

Corticosteroid Base	Derivative	Formulation	Concentration (%)	Trade Name
Prednisolone	Acetate	Suspension	0.125	Econopred (Alcon) Pred Mild (Allergan)
			1.0	Econopred Plus (Alcon) Pred Forte (Allergan) AK-Tate (Akorn)
Prednisolone	Sodium phosphate	Solution	0.125	Inflamase Mild (Iolab) AK-Pred (Akorn)
			0.5	Metreton (Schering)
			1.0	Inflamase Forte (Iolab) AK-Pred (Akorn)
Dexamethasone	Alcohol	Suspension	0.1	Maxidex (Alcon)
Dexamethasone	Sodium phosphate	Solution	0.1	Decadron Phosphate (MSD)
		Ointment	0.05	Decadron Phosphate (MSD) Maxidex (Alcon)
Fluorometholone	Alcohol	Ointment	0.1	FML (Allergan)
		Suspension	0.1	FML (Allergan)
			0.25	FML Forte (Allergan)
Medrysone	Alcohol	Suspension	1.0	HMS (Allergan)

aluated at frequent intervals during the course of treatment.

- Long-term, high-dosage therapy should not be discontinued abruptly; rather, the dose should be gradually reduced over time.
- Short-term, low-dosage topical ocular therapy generally does not produce significant systemic side effects.

Ideally the minimal effective dose should be used for the shortest time necessary to secure the desired clinical response. The dosage should be individualized as much as possible to the patient and the severity of the condition. The patient's general health must be considered and close supervision maintained to assess the effects of steroid therapy on the course of the disease and possible adverse effects.[15,16]

With ocular disease the route of steroid administration is an important determinant of the pharmacologic and therapeutic effects observed. Topical ocular therapy is usually satisfactory for inflammatory disorders of the lids, conjunctiva, cornea, iris, and ciliary body. In severe forms of anterior uveitis, topical therapy may require supplementation with systemic or periocular (local injection) steroids.[15,16,18] Chorioretinitis and optic neuritis are generally treated with systemic or periocular steroids or both.

Since topical prednisolone, fluorometholone, and medrysone have proved efficacious and less toxic than other steroids, these should be used whenever possible. However, the severity and location of the disorder as well as the steroid's inherent anti-inflammatory activity are more important considerations in situations where vision is seriously threatened. In such cases other corticosteroid agents may be indicated despite their increased risk of toxic side effects.

TOPICAL OCULAR ADMINISTRATION

Shortly after the introduction of corticosteroids to ocular therapeutics, it was realized that local treatment was equal to or superior to systemic administration, providing that the diseased tissue could be brought in contact with sufficient steroid.[18,46] Generally speaking, whenever possible, topical administration is indicated for anterior segment disease. Ease of application, comparatively low cost, and relative absence of systemic complications make it the preferred route of steroid therapy. Selection of the particular corticosteroid and dosage varies with the severity of the inflammation.

There is evidence that fluorometholone and possibly medrysone do not penetrate the cornea as well as do other commonly employed steroids and, thus, are less likely to produce intraocular pressure elevations.[45,60,61] However, since fluorometholone does penetrate to a

certain degree, another possibility is that it may be metabolized more rapidly than are other corticosteroids. This may also contribute to the fact that it does not raise intraocular pressure as much as do dexamethasone and betamethasone. Fluorometholone and medrysone produce relatively moderate suppression of corneal inflammation compared with prednisolone and dexamethasone formulations.[48] Medrysone is generally reserved for relatively minor conjunctival inflammations, since clinical experience indicates it to be the weakest anti-inflammatory steroid available but the one least likely to produce rises in intraocular pressure.[60] Fluorometholone can be effective for treatment of chronic inflammatory conditions requiring extended periods of therapy.[48]

On an empirical basis, the dosage of topical steroid solution or suspension recommended for severe inflammation is 1 drop every 1 to 2 hours for the first 24 to 48 hours. Thereafter, application of drops 2 to 4 times per day is usually sufficient to control the disease process.[62]

Topical therapy should usually be continued at a reduced dosage for several days to several weeks after symptoms have disappeared, since there is danger of relapse, particularly with high dosages, if treatment is prematurely discontinued. Corticosteroids reduce the leukocytic elements of the blood. As therapy is discontinued, white cells proliferate. The immature cells can produce large quantities of antibodies to residual antigen in the ocular tissue. The resultant antigen-antibody reaction is followed by massive polymorphonuclear leukocytic reaction. This sequence of events, unless interrupted immediately, can lead to a recurring, serious, necrotizing inflammatory reaction.[46] Thus, depending on the response obtained and the dosage used, topical therapy should generally be tapered over several days to weeks.[15,59]

SYSTEMIC TREATMENT

Inflammations of the posterior segment, optic nerve, or orbit usually require systemic administration of steroids.[15] The selection of the particular corticosteroid preparation and the dosage remain an individual choice, but the tendency is to use compounds with minimal mineralocorticoid activity (see Table 5.1). In recent years prednisone and triamcinolone have become the agents of choice for oral administration.

Since adverse effects are more likely to occur with systemic therapy, dosage should be individualized for each patient. The minimal effective dose for the shortest possible time is advocated. When long-term therapy is necessary, the lowest possible dose to control the disease must be given.

Gordon[59] and others[17,62] have suggested some general therapeutic guidelines for systemic corticosteroid therapy. For most mild to moderate ocular inflammatory disorders, initial daily doses of 20 to 40 mg of prednisone or its equivalent are recommended. If triamcinolone is chosen instead, doses in the 6 to 12 mg range are usually effective.

For patients with severe inflammation, initial daily doses of 40 to 60 mg of prednisone or its equivalent should be used. If there is no improvement within 48 to 72 hours, an increase to 80 mg or more may be necessary.[62]

As soon as the clinical response occurs, the dosage should be decreased over days or weeks depending on the length of treatment. Reduction should be in graduated decrements, guided strictly by the clinical course of the disease, usually reducing the daily dosage 10 mg for larger doses and 2 to 5 mg for smaller doses at intervals of 3 to 4 days. Once a dosage level of 15 to 20 mg is reached, the patient should be maintained at that level for 1 to 2 weeks to prevent recurrent flare-up of the condition. If a given reduction is followed by exacerbation of the inflammation, the dose of steroid must be immediately raised to the initial level. As long as there is evidence of active disease, therapy must continue at a level that permits control of symptoms.

The individual corticosteroids vary both qualitatively and quantitatively in their ability to suppress the inflammatory response. The approximate equivalent doses of systemic corticosteroids in current use are shown in Table 5.1.

LOCAL INJECTION

Periocular steroids can be administered by subconjunctival, sub-Tenon's, or retrobulbar injection. A topical anesthetic is often instilled before injection of the corticosteroid. This route of administration can be effective during surgical procedures, to supplement topical and systemic steroids in cases of severe inflammation, and in patients who will not comply with the prescribed regimen.[63] Experiments using radiolabeled methylprednisolone acetate (Depo-Medrol) indicate that retrobulbar injection can deliver high concentrations of medication to sclera, choroid, retina, and vitreous for a week or longer.[64] Long-term repository vehicles of triamcinolone acetonide injected beneath Tenon's capsule have been reported to be of value in several chronic inflammatory conditions, including certain forms of anterior uveitis.[65] Locally injected steroids may also be effective in the treatment of chalazia.[66,67,198]

The use of periocular steroids has several limitations and complications. The injections are usually somewhat uncomfortable and thus are not preferred by patients. Adverse ocular effects have included retinal detachment, optic nerve atrophy, and preretinal membrane formation.[68] Intraocular pressure can rise, particularly since the drug may remain in the eye for several days to weeks. Some of the observed effects may be due to the vehicle rather than to the steroid itself. Intravitreal injection of triamcinolone acetonide suspended in balanced saline solution has demonstrated lack of ocular toxicity in rabbits.[69]

Periocular injection of steroids should be reserved for those situations in which it is necessary to obtain an anti-inflammatory effect greater than can be obtained by topical or systemic administration.[48] Concurrent administration of corticosteroid by both topical and subconjunctival route does appear to produce an additive therapeutic effect in severe inflammations, but periocular injection alone does not necessarily result in greater anti-inflammatory effects. Experiments comparing equal doses of corticosteroid applied topically or by injection indicate that there is a greater reduction in polymorphonuclear leukocyte invasion of the cornea following topical use compared with periocular injection.[70] These data suggest that topical administration should be the primary route of therapy for anterior segment inflammations. Table 5.7 compares the advantages and disadvantages of the three routes of corticosteroid administration.[63]

ALTERNATE-DAY THERAPY

In 1963 Harter and associates[71] reported that single-dose alternate-day systemic administration of corticosteroid can be as effective as divided-dosage daily treatment. With this regimen a patient receives the entire total dose that would be given over a 2-day period as a single dose every other morning. The rationale for this regimen is to permit metabolic recovery and to prevent toxic effects from becoming cumulative. Since the normal physiologic release of ACTH and cortisol is characterized by episodic secretion with highest levels at about 8:00 AM,[25] the drug should be given in the early morning hours.

The concept of alternate-day systemic therapy is applicable only to the shorter-acting systemic steroids such as prednisone. Triamcinolone and dexamethasone continue their activity on the off-treatment day.[62]

The alternate-day approach can be useful when long-term systemic therapy is required, such as in the treatment of chronic uveitis.[72] This approach has been recommended for treatment of chronic conditions in children because it minimizes growth suppression.[73] Note, however, that the alternate-day regimen has not been widely accepted, and modifications have been suggested. It is also thought that this treatment method is not as effective as divided, daily doses, particularly

TABLE 5.7
Advantages and Disadvantages of the Three Routes of Corticosteroid Administration

Topical	*Periocular*	*Systemic*
	Advantages	
Placed near where it is needed	Placed near where it is needed	Tablets are easy to take
Simple to apply	Can treat one eye and use the other as	May be better at reaching all parts of
Can treat uniocular disease	a control	the eye
Avoids most systemic effects	Can treat the worse of two eyes	
	Can treat uniocular diseases	
	Avoids most systemic effects	
	Of value if patient cannot be trusted to	
	take medication	
	Valuable at time of surgery to help	
	prevent flare-up	
	Disadvantages	
Occasionally patient will develop	Patient will probably develop some	Adrenal suppression
adrenal suppression	adrenal suppression	Systemic side effects more likely to
Will aggravate a dendritic ulcer	Discomfort with injection	occur
May leave white residue	Occasionally, white material is	
Epithelial keratopathy from frequent	cosmetically objectionable	
applications	Subconjunctival adhesions	
Occasional conjunctival infections	Allergy to diluent	
	Occasional orbital infection	
	Occasional intraocular injection of	
	steroid	
	Ulceration of conjunctiva after repeated	
	injections if not given behind the eye	
	Exophthalmos and rugae in fundus	
	Papilledema	

Adapted from Schlaegel TF. Depot corticosteroid by the cul-de-sac route. In: Kaufman HE, ed. Ocular anti-inflammatory therapy. Springfield, IL: Charles C Thomas, 1970; 3:117.

in severe ocular inflammatory conditions. Adrenal gland suppression and other side effects associated with systemic therapy can still occur with the alternate-day regimen.[62]

Ocular Therapeutic Uses

Corticosteroids are useful in a variety of ocular diseases with an inflammatory or immunologic component (see Table 5.2).

ALLERGY AND HYPERSENSITIVITY REACTIONS

Type I allergic reactions often respond rapidly to topical steroids. For milder reactions such as allergic conjunctivitis due to airborne allergens, cold compresses and vasoconstrictor drugs with or without antihistamines may be sufficient. Severe forms of vernal or atopic keratoconjunctivitis may respond to topical steroids such as fluorometholone or prednisolone with dramatic

improvement of symptoms. The lowest dosage and frequency necessary should be prescribed to avoid complications. Use of cromolyn sodium (see below) may decrease the need for prolonged steroid therapy.

Treatment of contact dermatitis of the eyelids may employ topically applied steroids, and preservative-induced blepharoconjunctivitis, if not responsive to discontinuation of the allergen, may benefit from local administration of steroids.

For certain allergic diseases, such as phlyctenular keratoconjunctivitis, specific antimicrobial therapy may also reduce the need for steroids, possibly by eliminating or blocking the antigenic stimuli.[22]

UVEITIS

In both anterior and posterior uveitis, corticosteroids can reduce inflammation, relieve pain, and prevent synechiae. Adjunctive medication such as cycloplegics and antiglaucoma drugs may be necessary. For posterior uveitis, periocular or oral steroids are often required along with specific antimicrobial or cytotoxic therapy.[22]

HERPES SIMPLEX KERATITIS

The use of corticosteroids in herpes simplex keratitis is controversial, since steroids can disseminate the infectious agent and thus contribute to a more destructive lesion. It is generally agreed that steroids be reserved for stromal involvement and that they be used only in the presence of an intact corneal epithelium. Antiviral coverage should always be provided. The possibility of superinfection must be considered.[22]

MISCELLANEOUS CONDITIONS

Corticosteroids can also be useful in episcleritis, initially following alkali burns, and along with appropriate antimicrobial therapy in interstitial keratitis associated with syphilis. Part III of this book considers many examples of steroid use in specific disease states.

Side Effects

Although the effectiveness of corticosteroids in the treatment of ocular inflammation has stood the test of time, these agents sometimes cause side effects. Toxic effects can occur with all routes of administration and all preparations currently available. There is now sufficient evidence that systemic absorption of corticosteroid occurs with topical use on the eyes, skin, and mucosa of the upper respiratory tract.[3,27,28]

The incidence of side effects appears to rise significantly as dosages are increased. However, short-term, high-dosage therapy for emergencies appears to cause fewer side effects than do prolonged courses with lower dosages.[3]

SYSTEMIC TOXICITY

As indicated, systemic side effects can occur following all routes of administration and with all of the currently available preparations, particularly with prolonged high-dosage therapy. The observed effects result from their action on metabolic processes including glucose metabolism, electrolyte balance, tissue repair, and an inhibitory effect on the secretion of corticotropin by the adenohypophysis.

Potential adverse systemic effects observed with steroid therapy are listed in Table 5.8. In ocular therapeutics many of these effects can be avoided by use of topical or periocular injection of the drug.[74]

Suppression of the Pituitary-Adrenal Axis. Prolonged steroid therapy suppresses secretion of ACTH and induces morphologic changes in the adenohypophysis. The adrenal cortex undergoes atrophy, and the endog-

TABLE 5.8
Systemic Side Effects of Corticosteroid Therapy

- Adrenal insufficiency
- Cushing's syndrome
- Peptic ulceration
- Osteoporosis
- Hypertension
- Muscle weakness or atrophy
- Inhibition of growth
- Diabetes
- Activation of infection
- Mood changes
- Delay in wound healing

enous rate of corticosteroid secretion is reduced. Topical ocular application of dexamethasone to humans can reduce plasma cortisol levels by as much as 50%.[28]

Dosage, duration of treatment, and individual patient variability appear to be the important factors in pituitary-adrenal suppression. Administration of ACTH does not apparently restore adrenal responsiveness.[3]

Symptoms of adrenal insufficiency may occur during periods of stress while the patient is being treated with corticosteroids or following cessation of a prolonged course of therapy. A sudden change in dosage or route of administration can also bring on a crisis. Characteristic symptoms of adrenal insufficiency include fever, myalgia, arthralgia, systemic hypotension, and malaise.[3]

Depending on the dosage and duration of treatment, adrenal function can become adequate for daily needs following cessation of therapy, but months are usually required for sufficient return of function to meet severe stress. Reduction of drug therapy should be gradual, since deaths have occurred from too sudden withdrawals. With long-term use of prednisone it is recommended that the daily dosage not be reduced by more than 0.5 to 1 mg every 2 to 3 weeks.[3]

Cushing's Syndrome. The cushingoid state comprises a variety of manifestations, including a characteristic distribution of body fat in the form of "moon face," enlargement of supraclavicular fat pads ("buffalo hump"), and truncal obesity. The extremities become relatively thin, and weakness and atrophy of the proximal musculature can occur. Purple striae of the skin, hirsutism, acne, and systemic hypertension are not infrequent and are often difficult to avoid or manage. The patient may also exhibit behavioral disturbances and psychopathic as well as suicidal tendencies. If corticosteroid therapy is discontinued on appearance of these symptoms, the symptoms may be reduced or reversed.[3]

Gastrointestinal Lesions.   Corticosteroids tend to both enhance and activate peptic ulcer formation. It has been proposed that corticosteroids alter the gastric mucosal defense mechanism. A higher incidence of hemorrhage and perforation occurs in patients with gastrointestinal problems, and the insidious development of these problems can make ulcers a distressful and serious side effect.[3]

Osteoporosis.   Bones with a high degree of trabecular structure—ribs and vertebrae—are more readily affected. Glucocorticoids inhibit osteoblast activity and enhance secretion of parathyroid hormone. This results in decreased formation and increased resorption of bone. Osteoporosis is usually an indication for cessation of steroid therapy.[3]

Electrolyte Imbalance.   Sodium retention and potassium depletion with resultant edema and muscle weakness is less frequent with the synthetic compounds such as prednisone, dexamethasone, betamethasone, and triamcinolone. However, the possibility of hypertension and, in extreme situations, cardiac failure exists. Careful monitoring of the patient, including proper diet, can help prevent such complications.

Effects on Growth.   Long-term studies in children have indicated that corticosteroids can retard skeletal maturation. Impairment in growth can occur with relatively small doses (e.g., 8 mg of prednisone daily).[75] Alternate-day therapy appears to affect growth less and is recommended when possible for treatment in children.

Miscellaneous Adverse Effects.   Precipitation or aggravation of diabetes mellitus, increased susceptibility to infections, delay in wound healing, thinning of the skin, pancreatitis, and thyrotoxicosis are other possible complications of corticosteroid therapy.

Ocular Complications

Ocular complications can develop following either local or systemic corticosteroid administration and range from actual physical damage to the ocular tissue to interference with healing and immune mechanisms (Table 5.9).

Cataract

More than a decade following the introduction of corticosteroids for rheumatoid arthritis, Black and associates[76,77] reported a high incidence of lens opacities in

TABLE 5.9
Ocular Side Effects of Corticosteroid Therapy

- Posterior subcapsular cataracts
- Glaucoma
- Secondary ocular infection
- Retardation of corneal epithelial healing
- Uveitis
- Mydriasis
- Transient ocular discomfort
- Ptosis

patients receiving long-term systemic therapy. In 44 rheumatoid patients treated with steroids, 17 (39%) developed bilateral posterior subcapsular (PSC) cataracts. Of interest was the observation that dosage and duration of therapy correlated with incidence of development of PSC. Patients who received prednisone therapy for 1 to 4 years showed an 11% incidence if the dosage range was less than 10 mg/day, a 30% incidence if the dosage was 10 to 15 mg/day, and an 80% incidence if the dosage was above 15 mg/day.[76]

These observations aroused much interest, and conflicting reports began to appear in the literature.[78] More convincing evidence became available, however, when several investigators observed increased incidence of PSC cataracts in children receiving systemic steroid therapy for rheumatoid arthritis, systemic lupus erythematosus, and the nephrotic syndrome.[79,80] Although in adults steroid-related PSC cataracts do not usually occur within the first year of therapy regardless of dose, children manifested lens changes at lower doses and within shorter periods.[81]

Topical ocular steroid administration has also been implicated in the development of cataract.[82] It is possible that the ocular disease itself could be a causative factor in the observed lens changes. However, two cases of cataract following topical ocular steroid use indicate that long-term therapy may indeed result in lens opacities. Two females, aged 17 and 20 years, used topical steroids for several years to eliminate redness associated with contact lens wear. Both developed PSC cataract as well as glaucoma and visual field loss.[83]

In the majority of cases, lens changes accompanying steroid therapy do not significantly impair visual acuity. Less than 10% of patients receiving long-term therapy have vision reduced to less than 20/60 (6/18) (Fig. 5.6).[74] Patients seldom complain of visual problems unless the practitioner makes a direct inquiry.[78] Photophobia and glare may be complaints. Once vision is affected, reduction or cessation of steroid therapy seldom resolves the opacity.[78]

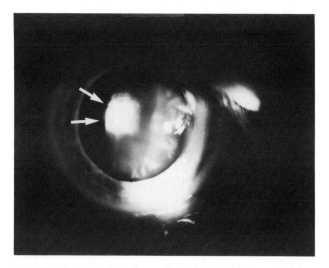

FIGURE 5.6   **Posterior subcapsular (PSC) cataract (arrows) in 48-year-old white man who had taken oral prednisone 7.5 mg daily for 13 years for treatment of rheumatoid arthritis. Visual acuity was 20/30 (6/9).**

Although it is now generally accepted that corticosteroids are cataractogenic, the mechanisms for development of the lens opacities have not been fully elucidated. It is possible that glucocorticoids cause cataract formation by gaining entry to the lens fiber cells. After reacting with specific amino groups of lens crystallins, a conformational change occurs within the cells, which exposes sulfhydryl groups. These are then free to form disulfide bonds, which subsequently lead to protein aggregation and finally to complexes that refract light.[78] The relationship of lens changes to total dose, duration of therapy, and individual susceptibility have been stressed as causative factors. A study compared PSC cataract formation in adult males with and without a history of systemic corticosteroid therapy.[84] Although the difference in prevalence of PSC cataract between the two groups was statistically significant, no significant correlation was found between lens opacities and total steroid dose, length of administration, or age of patient. The authors suggest that the most important factor in steroid-induced PSC cataract formation may be variability in individual susceptibility to side effects of corticosteroids. An ethnic susceptibility may also exist. Hispanics have been reported to be more predisposed to PSC cataract development than are whites or blacks.[81] Diabetic patients also appear to be more susceptible with topical steroid administration. In one study,[85] 9 of 11 patients developed cataract in the eye treated with 0.1% dexamethasone. The differences that appear to exist in patient response to dosage, duration of therapy, and age make inherent genetic factors a likely possibility.

Intraocular Pressure Elevation

Several years following the introduction of corticosteroids for ocular inflammatory disease, reports began to appear in the literature implicating topical steroid therapy as a cause for elevation in intraocular pressure.[86,87] However, it was not until Goldmann[88] reported his observation with topical steroid therapy in 1962 that it became generally accepted that these agents can produce the clinical picture of open-angle glaucoma.

Long-term systemic steroid therapy has also been implicated in intraocular pressure elevations. Bernstein and Schwartz[89] found that patients treated with systemic cortisone, 25 mg or its equivalent, for rheumatoid arthritis and collagen disease showed significantly higher mean applanation pressures compared with untreated individuals. They also observed lower facility of outflow and changes in ocular rigidity in steroid-treated patients. Other investigators[90] have also observed rises in pressure with systemic steroids. The intraocular pressure rose with administration of steroid and fell when intake was reduced or discontinued. If the dosage was raised or therapy reinstituted, the pressure elevations reoccurred.

More conclusive proof of the ability of steroids to raise intraocular pressure was provided in controlled studies in which patients showed reversible elevations of pressure with repeated use of topical steroids.[91,92] The hypertensive response can be elicited in both healthy and glaucomatous eyes and usually develops 2 to 8 weeks following initiation of therapy with dexamethasone, betamethasone, prednisolone, hydrocortisone, or triamcinolone. The effects on pressure and the reduction in outflow facility are generally reversible and return to their original levels within 1 to 3 weeks after steroid administration is discontinued. However, instances have been reported in which pressures have not reverted to pretreatment levels and glaucoma with accompanying vision loss has occurred. The pressure elevations are usually much greater in eyes with open-angle glaucoma and tend to be higher than normal in children of glaucoma patients.[92]

The work of Armaly[93] and Becker[94] has indicated that topically administered steroids tend to produce ocular hypertension in certain susceptible individuals. Statistical analysis of volunteers given topical dexamethasone 0.1% three times a day indicates 3 separate groups of responders in the general population. The largest group in the volunteer population responded with an average pressure elevation of 1.6 mm Hg after 4 weeks of topical dexamethasone. A second group responded with an average elevation of 10 mm Hg. Pressure elevations of 16 mm Hg or greater occurred in the third group. Of additional significance was the observation that there was also a difference in the time of pressure elevation. The second and third groups showed a continued and steady pressure elevation during the 4 weeks of observation compared with the first group with the small pressure increase that did not continue to rise during subsequent weeks of the study.

The degree of response to topical corticosteroid thus appears to be genetically determined. The response to topical steroids has been demonstrated to be inherited in Mendelian fashion. The offspring of matings of persons with various known degrees of response to topical steroids appear to fit the prediction of Mendelian inheritance.[94] Patients with primary open-angle glaucoma and their relatives show a remarkably high prevalence of pressure elevations with topical steroids. Information regarding patient or family history of glaucoma therefore becomes important when use of corticosteroids is considered.

An alternative to the Mendelian model of a single genetic locus representing steroid responsiveness has been offered by Schwartz.[95] Based on his studies in twins, Schwartz has proposed a multifactorial or polygenic model for the familial transmission of the ocular hypertensive response. In this model, high responders would not be confined to one locus or gene, but, rather, the hypertensive response to steroids would be due to a complex interaction of multiple genetic and perhaps environmental factors.

In addition to genetic tendencies, other factors can contribute to the pressure elevations resulting from topical steroid administration. These can include patient age, myopia of 5 diopters or more, Krukenberg's spindles, and diabetes.[99]

Corticosteroid-induced ocular hypertension relates not only to the individual patient, but the specific corticosteroid used may also play a role. In general, dexamethasone 0.1% and betamethasone 0.1% appear

more likely to induce significant pressure elevations than do prednisolone, fluorometholone, or medrysone.[93,94] In one study, 43 patients demonstrated pressure elevation with 0.1% dexamethasone sodium phosphate. Of these individuals, 15 had intraocular pressure increases of 5 mm Hg or more while receiving 0.1% fluorometholone, and 3 patients demonstrated pressure elevations greater than 15 mm Hg.[96] A masked study using male volunteers compared ocular pressure elevations with 0.1% dexamethasone phosphate, 0.1% fluorometholone, and 1% medrysone applied 4 times a day for 6 weeks. The relative ability of these steroids to raise intraocular pressure is shown in Figure 5.7. At the end of 6 weeks of treatment the mean pressure increases for dexamethasone, fluorometholone, and medrysone were 63.1%, 33.8%, and 8.3%, respectively.[97] Kass and associates[98] compared the effects of 0.25% fluorometholone suspension with 0.1% dexamethasone sodium phosphate solution in corticosteroid-responsive patients. Subjects received 1 drop of either drop in 1 eye 4 times daily for up to 6 weeks. Although both drugs elevated intraocular pressure, mean pressure increases from baseline in eyes treated with fluorometholone were significantly lower than those in eyes treated with dexamethasone at weeks 2, 4, and 6 (Fig. 5.8). In addition to the individual corticosteroid's tendency to raise intraocular pressure, it appears that concentration as well as length and frequency of administration are important factors in the observed pressure elevations.

It has been proposed that the steroid's ability to penetrate the anterior chamber may be a cause of the pressure elevation. Reduced ocular drug levels as well as plasma dilution may account for the lower incidence of pressure elevation with systemic therapy. The inherent anti-inflammatory potency of the corticosteroid formulations has also been implicated as a factor in

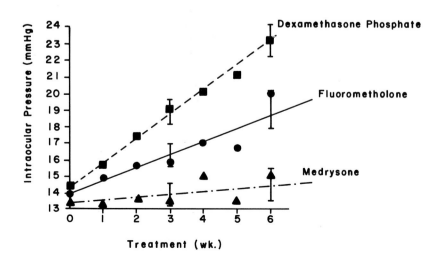

FIGURE 5.7 **Weekly intraocular pressure responses of eyes treated with 1% medrysone, 0.1% fluorometholone, and 0.1% dexamethasone phosphate. Each point represents a mean value (mm Hg) of 12 eyes. (From Mindel JS, Tovitian HO, Smith H, et al. Comparative ocular pressure elevations of topical corticosteroids. Arch Ophthalmol 1980;98:1578. Copyright 1980, American Medical Association.)**

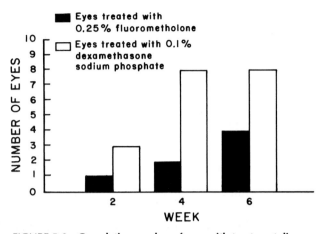

FIGURE 5.8 **Cumulative number of eyes with treatment discontinued because of increased intraocular pressure. (Published with permission from the American Journal of Ophthalmology 102:161, 1986. Copyright by the Ophthalmic Publishing Company.)**

intraocular pressure elevations.[95] At present none of the available corticosteroids seems to truly dissociate anti-inflammatory and ocular pressure effects. Data are also lacking on minimal concentrations of topical steroids that can produce effective control of inflammatory reactions without provoking significant elevations in intraocular pressure.

The molecular mechanism whereby corticosteroids induce pressure elevation is not fully understood. Receptors responsive to corticosteroids have been demonstrated in human trabecular cells.[100,101] It is therefore possible that alterations in outflow facility could be mediated by a direct action on meshwork cells. Electron microscopic studies of steroid-treated trabecular specimens have indicated the presence of extracellular materials including glycosaminoglycans (GAGS).[102] It has been suggested that their presence could obstruct the meshwork, thereby causing resistance to aqueous outflow.[103] Alternatively, the presence of excessive GAGS could result in fluid retention.[102]

Infection

Since corticosteroids reduce the immunologic defense mechanisms, resistance to many types of infection is lowered. In addition, by inhibiting the inflammatory response, symptoms of disease may be masked. There is evidence that steroid administration can increase susceptibility to viral, fungal, and bacterial infections.[46]

The course of an ocular or systemic bacterial infection can be adversely affected by corticosteroids. Latent tuberculosis may be activated by corticosteroid therapy.[3] Corticosteroids are generally contraindicated in systemic tuberculosis unless accompanied by appropriate antitubercular therapy. Bacterial corneal infections appear to react adversely to steroid therapy. Topical cortisone treatment of experimentally induced *Pseudomonas* corneal ulcers in rabbits has resulted in more extensive ulceration and scarring.[104] Treatment with antibiotic prevented the extension of corneal involvement both with and without cortisone. The use of corticosteroids in ocular infections requires caution so as not to interfere with the reparative processes. If the appropriate antibiotic is selected and if the course of therapy is relatively short, corticosteroids can help reduce inflammation and prevent possible scarring.[46] In general, however, steroids should be avoided in cases of routine bacterial infections of the lids and conjunctiva because no scarring is anticipated and because steroids provide relatively little benefit in the healing process.

The clinical course of dendritic keratitis caused by herpes simplex virus indicates that corticosteroids may prolong the disease.[105] Experiments with rabbits have added validity to these observations. Following inoculation with herpes simplex virus, the group treated with topical prednisolone developed a keratoconjunctivitis earlier that lasted longer and was more severe than that of the untreated animals.[106] Healing of experimental herpes simplex corneal infection is also retarded by corticosteroids. Dexamethasone, methylprednisolone, and triamcinolone instilled 3 times a day retarded healing of rabbit corneas inoculated with herpes simplex by as much as 2 weeks depending on the steroid used.[107]

Corticosteroids also increase the virulence of other viruses including vaccinia, mumps, and chicken pox.[46]

There is general agreement that topical use of steroids enhances ocular susceptibility to fungal infection. Minor ocular injuries treated with corticosteroids or corticosteroid-antibiotic combinations have resulted in fungal keratitis. Aggravation of fungal keratitis has also been demonstrated in animals. Inoculation of rabbit corneas with *Candida albicans* resulted in keratitis in 75% of eyes treated with cortisol 1%, while only 37% of eyes not treated with steroid developed the infection.[108]

There is also indirect evidence that corticosteroids decrease human resistance to fungal infections. Data from the Armed Forces Institute of Pathology indicate that fungal infection in cases of perforated corneal ulcers or penetrating wounds has increased 16-fold since the advent of corticosteroid therapy.[109]

The enhanced risk of superinfection by bacteria, fungi, and viruses emphasizes the need to maintain a balance between the steroid and the chemotherapeutic agent. While corticosteroids decrease the amount of tissue damage caused by the inflammatory response, the replicating organism must be simultaneously eradicated by specific anti-infective therapy to preserve the ocular structures.

Corneal Epithelial Healing

Both systemic and topical ocular steroid therapy can retard corneal healing. Persistent punctate staining of the cornea can indicate epithelial damage by the corticosteroid if the original disease has been eliminated.

In experimentally induced alkali corneal burns in rabbits, both topical and systemic steroid administration can increase by as much as 30% the time required for epithelial regeneration.[110] Effects on collagenase activity have been proposed as a possible mechanism whereby steroids affect corneal epithelial regeneration.[46]

Corticosteroid Uveitis

It seems paradoxical that the topical use of corticosteroids can lead to acute inflammation of the anterior segment. However, since the first report[111] of the development of anterior uveitis during provocative testing with steroids for glaucoma, additional cases have been reported during dexamethasone-induced pressure responses.[112] The incidence is higher in blacks (5.4%) than in whites (0.5%). Symptoms include pain, photophobia, blurred vision, and perilimbal (ciliary) hyperemia; anterior chamber flare and cells can be observed.

The cause appears to be the corticosteroid itself rather than the vehicle and does not appear to be related to a particular steroid preparation.

Mydriasis and Ptosis

Dilation of the pupil and ptosis have been observed with topical steroid administration.[91] Application of 0.1% dexamethasone in human volunteers has produced mydriasis as early as 1 week following its initial use. The average increase in pupillary diameter was about 1 mm. The effect disappears following cessation of drug therapy.[113]

The mydriatic effect of topically applied corticosteroids has been investigated in isolated intraocular muscle preparation[114] as well as in living monkey eyes.[115] The resting tension of the dilator muscle was increased and that of the sphincter decreased in the presence of steroids. Instillation of 0.1% dexamethasone (Decadron) produced pupillary dilation and ptosis as well as elevation of intraocular pressure in the monkey eyes.

When the steroids were tested without their vehicles, the effects on intraocular pressure, pupil size, and upper lid were not observed. Responses to the vehicle alone, however, were identical to steroid-containing drops, whereas corticosteroid in saline did not produce the observed changes. Thus, it has been suggested that a combination of agents in the vehicle mixture causes the effects.[114,115]

Other Side Effects

Transient ocular discomfort can ensue following topical application of steroids to the eye. Mechanical effects of the steroid particles in suspension, the vehicle itself, and the severity of the inflammatory condition can all be causative factors.

Occasional refractive changes, blurring of vision, and increases in corneal thickness have been described. A more recent observation following topical steroid use for the treatment of epidemic keratoconjunctivitis is the occurrence of dry eye syndrome in the postinfection period.[116] Systemic use of steroids has been implicated in cases of pseudotumor cerebri with papilledema and petechial conjunctival hemorrhages.

Precautions and Drug Interactions

Since the use of corticosteroids can be complicated by side effects, a careful history and certain tests may be advisable, particularly if systemic therapy is indicated.[46]

Corticosteroids should be used with great caution in patients with diabetes mellitus, infectious disease, chronic renal failure, congestive heart failure, and systemic hypertension. Systemic administration is generally contraindicated in patients with peptic ulcer, osteoporosis, and severe psychoses. Topical steroids must be used with caution and only when necessary in patients with glaucoma.

Patients receiving prolonged systemic therapy usually lack sufficient adrenal reserve to respond appropriately to such stresses as trauma or surgery. These individuals may need to be given supplementary corticosteroid to cover the period of stress.

Concurrent administration of other drugs may interfere with the metabolism and alter the effects of corticosteroids. It has been observed that rifampin, a drug used in the treatment of *Mycobacterium tuberculosis* infections, can interfere with the pharmacologic effects of corticosteroids. Loss of renal allograft function during rifampin therapy has been ascribed to decreased glucocorticoid activity. The effects appear to be due to increased metabolism of administered corticosteroid.[117] Other drugs, including barbiturates, phenylbutazone, and phenytoin, may also enhance metabolism and reduce the anti-inflammatory and immunosuppressive potential of systemic corticosteroids. Additionally, the response to anticoagulant therapy may be reduced by simultaneous administration of steroids.[3]

Patients receiving topical ocular steroids must be periodically examined for corneal, lens, and intraocular pressure changes. Slit-lamp examination for punctate, herpetic, or fungal keratitis is necessary. Patients receiving systemic therapy should be monitored for systemic hypertension, glaucoma, and cataracts. If prolonged systemic therapy is instituted, blood glucose levels should be evaluated at appropriate intervals.

Adrenocorticotropic Hormone

Adrenocorticotropic hormone (ACTH) from the anterior pituitary gland stimulates the synthesis of adrenal cortical hormones. Structurally it consists of 39 amino acid residues.

In the absence of ACTH, the adrenal cortex undergoes atrophy, and the rates of secretion of certain hormones, cortisol in particular, are reduced. In contrast, prolonged administration of large doses of ACTH induces hyperplasia and hypertrophy of the adrenal cortex, and the secretion of cortisol, corticosterone, and androgenic hormones is enhanced.[3]

ACTH is ineffective when given orally, since it is rapidly hydrolyzed by enzymes in the digestive tract. It is absorbed from parenteral sites, and the usual route of administration is by intramuscular injection. The dose is usually 40 to 80 units per day.

ACTH is also effective when administered by an intravenous drip. Twenty to 25 units of ACTH are placed in 1000 ml of solution. The therapeutic effect depends on the duration of the drip, which should usually last from 12 to 16 hours.

The hormone disappears rapidly from the circulation following intravenous infusion. In humans, the plasma half-life is approximately 15 minutes.[3]

Since ACTH exerts its effects indirectly through the release of adrenal corticosteroid hormones, it is ineffective when given topically. Its systemic administration, however, results in essentially the same effects as systemic administration of glucocorticoids and depends on a normally functioning adrenal cortex.[47]

At present, the most important clinical use of ACTH is as a diagnostic agent for disorders of the anterior pituitary gland and the adrenal cortex.[3] For these purposes ACTH is administered and the plasma cortisol concentration is determined.

The therapeutic uses of ACTH include adrenal cortical insufficiency and other disorders that are responsive to glucocorticoids. Its effectiveness in inflammatory conditions of the eye has been studied.[8] There is, however, no substantial evidence that ocular therapy with ACTH is superior to corticosteroids. In addition, the therapeutic effects of ACTH are less predictable. Furthermore, treatment with ACTH exposes the patient to a mixture of hormones secreted from the adrenal gland, in contrast to the conventional method of using only one particular corticosteroid. The use of ACTH is much less convenient, since ACTH cannot be given by the oral or topical route.

ACTH can cause toxic reactions. Since the secretion of mineralocorticoids may also be enhanced, salt and water retention can occur, primarily early in therapy. Hypersensitivity reactions ranging from mild fever to anaphylaxis have been reported.[3]

Nonsteroidal Anti-Inflammatory Agents

Since the usefulness of corticosteroids as anti-inflammatory agents can be limited by their side effects, efforts have been made to develop agents with fewer adverse reactions. The demonstration by Vane[118] that aspirin inhibits prostaglandin synthesis, along with the well-known observations that aspirin can have prominent anti-inflammatory actions, has resulted in development of other NSAIAs. Several chemical classes of compounds have demonstrated analgesic, antipyretic, and anti-inflammatory properties similar to those of aspirin (Table 5.10). All are thought to act in some manner on prostaglandin or leukotriene biosynthetic mechanisms.[119–122]

Ocular Actions of Prostaglandins

Prostaglandins are present in nearly every organ system, including the eye. Irides of various species contain the biosynthetic pathway for their manufacture. Release of prostaglandins from ocular tissue occurs in response to various stimuli, including stroking the iris, rubbing the fifth cranial nerve, and paracentesis.[118,123]

Historically, the link between prostaglandins and the eye originated from the demonstration that stimulation of the fifth cranial nerve in rabbits caused constriction of the pupil.[123] This observation suggested to Ambache[124] that a substance other than acetylcholine (ACh) may be responsible for the observed miosis. Subsequently, Ambache and his associates isolated an extract from rabbit irides, which they named *irin,* that

TABLE 5.10
Nonsteroidal Anti-Inflammatory Agents

Drug	Available Preparation
	Salicylates
Aspirin	Various manufacturers
	Indole Derivatives
Indomethacin	Indocin (MSD)
Ketorolac	Toradol (Syntex)
Sulindac	Clinoril (MSD)
Tolmetin	Tolectin (McNeil)
	Pyrazolon Derivatives
Phenylbutazone	Butazolidin (Geigy), Azolid (USV)
Oxyphenbutazone	Oxalid (USV), Tandearil (Geigy)
Apazone	Azapropazone
	Propionic Acid Derivatives
Carprofen	Rimadyl (Roche)
Fenoprofen	Nalfon (Dista)
Flurbiprofen	Ocufen (Allergen)
Ibuprofen	Motrin (Upjohn), Rufen (Boots), Advil (Whitehall), Nuprin (Bristol-Myers)
Ketoprofen	Orudis (Wyeth)
Naproxen	Naprosyn (Syntex), Anaprox (Syntex)
Suprofen	[a]
	Fenamates
Mefenamic acid	Ponstel (Parke-Davis)
Meclofenamate	Meclomen (Parke-Davis)
Flufenamic acid	[a]
Tolfenamic acid	[a]
Etofenamic acid	[a]
	Oxicam Derivatives
Piroxicam	Feldene (Pfizer)
	Miscellaneous
Cromolyn sodium	Opticrom (Fisons)
Dimethyl sulfoxide (DMSO)	Various manufacturers

[a]No preparations currently available.

caused pupillary constriction. Further studies showed that irin was a long-chain unsaturated hydroxy fatty acid that dilated blood vessels and caused miosis in several species. Moreover, the observed effects were not inhibited by atropine.[124–126] On the basis of more recent studies it must be assumed that irin contained other substances that were not known at the time and thus could not be identified. More recent investigations indicate that, in addition to prostaglandins, leukotrienes may have contributed to the effects initially observed with irin[127] (Fig. 5.9).

PROSTAGLANDINS

Chemically, prostaglandins are 20-carbon, unsaturated fatty acid derivatives, each containing a substituted cyclopentane ring structure. They are products of sev-

eral enzymatic reactions beginning with arachidonic acid, which is released from phospholipids through the action of phospholipase. The end products of the prostaglandin biosynthetic pathway include the prostaglandins as well as the prostacyclins and thromboxanes (see Fig. 5.9). In general, these substances are believed to play a role in platelet physiology, smooth muscle contraction, and in dilation of ocular blood vessels and elevation of intraocular pressure.[128,129]

Prostaglandins are subdivided into groups depending on the arrangement of ketone and hydroxyl groups. The members of each group are designated by the letters E, F, A, B, C, and D. The degree of unsaturation on the aliphatic chain of the molecule is indicated by a numerical suffix (Fig. 5.10). Their mechanism of action is not well defined. Wide tissue distribution, their lipid-acidic nature, and their diverse actions make

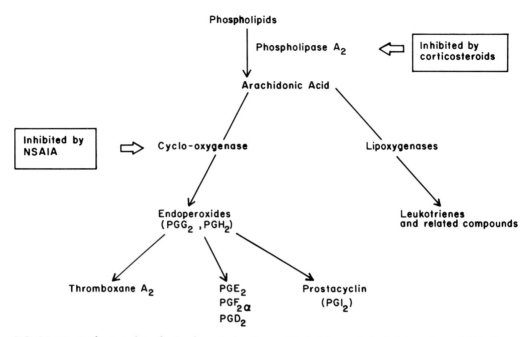

FIGURE 5.9   **Pathways of synthesis of prostaglandins and leukotrienes. (Adapted from Jampol LM. Pharmacologic therapy of aphakic cystoid macular edema. Ophthalmology 1982;89:894.)**

their pharmacologic actions difficult to interpret. Moreover, differences in actions between species of animals have been reported.[122,127,129]

Prostaglandins PGE₁, PGE₂, and PGF₂ₐ have been isolated from ocular tissue and aqueous humor. Analysis of aqueous for prostaglandin-like activity in untreated patients with uveitis has revealed substantial amounts of PGE₂ compared with aqueous samples taken from inflamed eyes treated with corticosteroids. Intradermal injection of PGE₁ and PGE₂ has produced inflammation in the eyes of several species.[120,128–130]

Prostaglandins have also been implicated in intraocular pressure elevations resulting from mechanical and chemical trauma to the eye.[121] Topical, systemic, or intracameral administration of PGE₁, PGE₂, and PGF₂ₐ is followed by a sustained rise in intraocular pressure.[131–133] Arachidonic acid, a precursor of PGE₂ synthesis, and prostacyclin, a major product of arachidonic acid metabolism, can also raise intraocular pressure when applied topically or injected intravenously in rabbits.[121]

Contrary to reports that prostaglandins are potent ocular hypertensive agents, several studies have demonstrated that PGF₂ has ocular hypotensive effects in several species, including healthy human eyes and in patients with exfoliation glaucoma.[135–138,199] In one study[138] the maximum reduction in intraocular pressure

occurred 7 hours following instillation of 200 μg into the eye. The hypotensive effect lasted for approximately 24 hours. No changes in pupil size or alteration of blood-aqueous barrier were observed, but conjunctival hyperemia was present in all subjects. The mechanism whereby PGF₂ lowers intraocular pressure has been investigated,[139,140] and there is evidence that an increase in uveoscleral outflow is the likely mechanism whereby this prostaglandin affects intraocular pressure.

Other effects of prostaglandins on the eye include miosis and vasodilation. The vascular response of the rabbit eye to prostaglandins has been studied using fluorescein iris angiography.[134] Following topical application of PGE₁, PGE₂, and PGF₂ₐ marked vasodilation of the iris vessels with leakage of the dye into the anterior chamber occurs. Fluorescein angiography carried out during an experimentally induced acute anterior uveitis also demonstrated vasodilation of iris vessels, with a dilated capillary network. Although these prostaglandins produce miosis and a cellular response in several species, this effect is minimal or absent in human eyes[127,137,138,141] following topical application of PGF₂ₐ.

At present, experimental evidence indicates an association among prostaglandins, ocular inflammation, and intraocular pressure. However, until our understanding of the complex events associated with inflam-

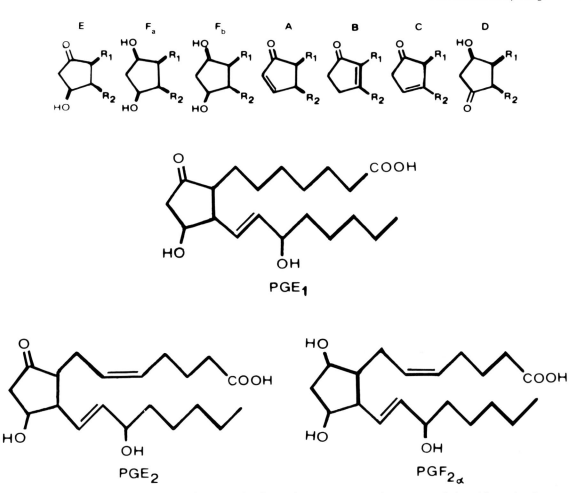

FIGURE 5.10   **Basic ring structures of the prostaglandins and some representative compounds found in ocular tissues.**

mation are better understood, the specific link for prostaglandins in the process will remain difficult to define.

LEUKOTRIENES

In addition to the cyclo-oxygenase pathway that leads to the formation of prostaglandins and thromboxane A_2, the lipoxygenase pathway is also active in ocular tissues.[122,127,140] The products of this pathway are called eicosanoids or leukotrienes (see Fig. 5.9). Kulkarni and Srinivasan[122] have reported the presence of leukotrienes LTB_4 and LTC_4 in rabbit aqueous humor following paracentesis. Intracameral injection of LTB_4 into the aqueous humor of the owl monkey has resulted in release of polymorphonuclear leukocytes into the anterior chamber.[122] LTB_4 has also been shown to be present in human tears during ocular allergy.[141] The exact role of the leukotrienes in ocular inflammation

needs further elucidation. If, indeed, the lipoxygenase pathway is involved in ocular inflammatory responses, it may imply that aspirin and other NSAIAs may be ineffective in some forms of ocular inflammation.[142]

Specific Nonsteroidal Anti-Inflammatory Agents

SALICYLATES

Salicylic acid was introduced in 1875 by Buss as an antipyretic and antirheumatic agent. A few years later, a less irritating derivative, aspirin, was synthesized. Aspirin has been shown to lower body temperature, relieve low to moderate pain, and have anti-inflammatory actions in many organ systems.[119] Until the advent of corticosteroid anti-inflammatory therapy, aspirin was also used to treat iritis and sympathetic ophthalmia.[143]

The increase in permeability of the blood-aqueous barrier that accompanies inflammation can be prevented by pretreatment with aspirin.[144] Experimentally it has been shown that the aqueous barrier can be disrupted by chemical, mechanical, and other irritative stimuli as well as by certain prostaglandins. Administration of aspirin before these stimuli prevents the disruption of the barrier. Paracentesis of the rabbit eye results in PGE_2-like activity in the aqueous. This is diminished by pretreatment with 200 mg/kg body weight of aspirin. The increased protein concentration in secondary aqueous that accompanies paracentesis or laser irradiation of the iris is also greatly reduced by pretreatment with aspirin.[145]

The mechanism of action of aspirin in the prevention or reduction of inflammation appears to be inhibition of prostaglandin biosynthesis by an irreversible acetylation of the cyclo-oxygenase enzyme.[121] Other mechanisms, however, may also be involved.

Salicylates have not been frequently used in the treatment of ocular inflammations. Their efficacy in ocular inflammation as compared to other NSAIAs (see below) has not been sufficiently studied, especially in human models. Two reports[146,147] have suggested that aspirin may be of value for intractable cases of vernal conjunctivitis. Patients who remained symptomatic following treatment with cromolyn sodium, corticosteroids, or both showed improvement in both symptoms and signs of the condition when aspirin was added to the therapeutic regimen.

Aspirin may be poorly tolerated, and its toxicity can take many forms. Many of the systemic side effects associated with salicylate use may be related to inhibition of prostaglandin synthesis. In addition to the well-known gastrointestinal intolerance to aspirin, hypersensitivity reactions, disturbance of renal function, abnormal results in liver function tests, and hearing loss are not uncommon.[119] These observations have stimulated the development of other aspirin-like anti-inflammatory, analgesic, and antipyretic drugs.

INDOLE DERIVATIVES

Of the available compounds in this group (see Table 5.10), indomethacin has been the most extensively studied and used in ocular inflammatory conditions. It has been administered both topically and systemically in experimental as well as in clinical cases of uveitis, to maintain mydriasis during cataract surgery, to prevent postoperative cystoid macular edema (CME), and to control inflammation following extracapsular cataract extraction and intraocular lens implantation.

Indomethacin, introduced in 1963 for treatment of rheumatoid arthritis and related disorders, is a product of laboratory research for aspirin-like drugs with anti-inflammatory properties. Two other indole derivatives,

sulindac and tolmetin, were developed later in an attempt to find less toxic congeners of indomethacin.[119] These agents are rapidly absorbed following oral administration. About 90% of the drug is bound to plasma proteins. Tissue binding is also extensive. Cerebrospinal fluid concentrations are low.

The effect of indomethacin on ocular inflammation was studied by Perkins and MacFaul in 1965.[148] In a double-blind clinical trial of unselected cases of uveitis, oral doses of 175 mg of indomethacin added daily to treatment with topical corticosteroids and mydriatics resulted in a 60% increase in the number of favorable patient responses. Other investigators have reported similar clinical results with systemic indomethacin. Beneficial effects have been reported in rheumatic uveitis and optic neuritis.[149] Ellis[62] has observed that indomethacin can be effective in mild anterior uveitis and episcleritis, but poor responses are obtained in more severe, well-established cases.

Attention has focused on the possible beneficial effects of indomethacin on postoperative inflammation and the prevention of cystoid macular edema (CME). Tenant[150] and Yannuzzi and Wallyn[152] have suggested that prostaglandin production by the iris during surgery may be a causative factor in CME. To test this possibility, several investigators[153,154] studied the effects of prophylactic topical and systemic indomethacin on patients undergoing intraocular surgical procedures. There is now general agreement that the incidence of angiographic CME is reduced or minimized by prophylactic administration of topical indomethacin. Systemic administration can also be useful, but it appears to be less effective and side effects are common.[155] Topical administration of one-fortieth of an oral dose resulted in higher aqueous levels and a better clinical response, with no detectable blood levels or toxic effects, in 1 group of patients scheduled for cataract surgery compared with another group receiving 25 mg of oral indomethacin 4 times daily.[156] Indomethacin by either route of administration has proved ineffective in chronic cases of CME.[154] Miyake and associates[157] have also reported that the incidence of angiographic CME in patients undergoing surgery to repair retinal detachment is reduced by topical prophylactic administration of indomethacin. No significant effects on short- or long-term visual acuity have been reported with prophylactic use.

The effects of indomethacin and other indole derivatives appear to be related to prostaglandin synthesis. They apparently inhibit cyclo-oxygenase, an important enzymatic step in prostaglandin synthesis (see Fig. 5.9). Indomethacin also affects the ocular actions of exogenously administered arachidonic acid. Topical application or intravenous administration of arachidonic acid to rabbits and monkeys elevates intraocular pressure and raises protein levels in the anterior chamber. Pretreatment with indomethacin 10 mg/kg or greater prevents the elevation of pressure and aqueous protein.[132]

In addition to their effect on prostaglandin synthesis, the indole derivatives may exert anti-inflammatory effects in other ways. In rats, indomethacin can interfere with migration of leukocytes into the inflammatory sites. There is evidence that prostaglandins can be largely concentrated in the inflamed site by migrating leukocytes. An effect on cyclic AMP-mediated cellular systems has also been postulated.[128]

The clinical usefulness of indomethacin is limited by the fact that a high percentage (35% to 50%) of patients experience adverse reactions. About 20% of patients must discontinue its use. The severity of the adverse effects appears to be dose related. Headache occurs in 50% of patients when the total daily dose exceeds 100 mg. Other central nervous system (CNS) manifestations such as dizziness, drowsiness, confusion, depression, depersonalization reactions, seizures, and syncope may occur in susceptible persons after ingestion of 25 mg. Gastrointestinal complaints and complications ranging from nausea and abdominal pain to ulceration are not infrequent. Hematopoietic and hypersensitivity reactions, including acute attacks of asthma, have been reported.[119]

Systemic use of indomethacin has been associated with possible ocular toxic effects. Both corneal opacities and pallor of the optic disc have been reported with indomethacin use.[151] However, more recent studies have failed to firmly support the ocular toxic effects of indomethacin.

The incidence of adverse effects appears to be somewhat less with sulindac and tolmetin. Sulindac is a prodrug. Both agents are less potent than indomethacin. This may explain, in part, the lower incidence of gastrointestinal, CNS, and hypersensitivity reactions.[119]

Although the indole derivatives have become an accepted part of the rheumatologist's armamentarium, the ocular anti-inflammatory usefulness of these agents appears to be minimal compared with present use of corticosteroids.

PYRAZOLON DERIVATIVES

Among this group, phenylbutazone, oxyphenbutazone, and apazone have been used to treat rheumatoid arthritis and allied inflammatory conditions. As a group, they share quite similar anti-inflammatory, antipyretic, and analgesic actions. In addition, these agents also exhibit uricosuric effects and thus are useful for the treatment of gout. In clinical use, one member of the group may be preferred over another because it may cause somewhat fewer side effects.[119]

Following oral administration, these agents are rapidly absorbed from the gastrointestinal tract and avidly bind to plasma proteins. Their half-life in the plasma varies from 24 hours for apazone to as long as 50 to 100 hours for phenylbutazone. They are excreted slowly in the urine as the parent compounds and their metabolites. The pharmacologic actions can, at least in part, be ascribed to their ability to inhibit prostaglandin synthetase.[119]

In 1935 Boeck and associates[158] demonstrated a reduced amount of protein in the secondary aqueous of rabbits following paracentesis when pretreated with pyrazolon derivatives. Since then, other investigators have reported their use in postoperative inflammation[159] as well as in various anterior segment inflammatory disorders such as iritis, keratitis, and chronic iridocyclitis.[160,161] Doses of 100 mg of oxyphenbutazone 4 times daily have been effective for control of anterior uveitis in humans.[161] Phenylbutazone has also been reported to have a beneficial effect on iritis in patients with rheumatoid arthritis.[161]

Use of topical ocular preparations of pyrazolon derivatives has met with mixed success. Clinical trials with oxyphenbutazone ointment for treatment of human uveitis, traumatic iritis, and postoperative uveitis have demonstrated little, if any, anti-inflammatory effects.[161] However, 2% oxyphenbutazone ointment has been shown to be effective in preventing the rise in aqueous protein and intraocular pressure elevation induced by arachidonic acid injection in rabbit eyes.[162] Further clinical trials in humans are necessary to determine the efficacy of pyrazolon derivatives for both topical and systemic therapy of ocular inflammatory conditions.

These agents are poorly tolerated by many patients. Side effects have been reported in 10% to 45% of patients, and the medication may need to be discontinued in 10% to 15%. Gastric irritation and skin rashes are the most frequently reported side effects. Death from aplastic anemia and agranulocytosis has been attributed to phenylbutazone.[119]

Ocular side effects are uncommon, but blurred vision has been reported.[119] Although oxyphenbutazone appears to penetrate the ocular tissues following topical application,[163] it does not induce cataracts or raise intraocular pressure in human eyes.[119]

Significant drug interactions can occur with pyrazolon derivatives, since these agents can displace other drugs from their binding sites on plasma proteins. Displacement of the anticoagulant agent, warfarin, and thyroid hormone from plasma proteins has been reported.[119]

PROPIONIC ACIDS

The propionic acids represent a newer group of aspirin-like anti-inflammatory agents. The members of this group vary in their clinical actions, but all exhibit anti-inflammatory, analgesic, and antipyretic activity. Their mechanism of action is similar to other NSAIAs. They inhibit both the cyclo-oxygenase enzyme in the pathway of prostaglandin synthesis and leukocyte migration in the eye.[122]

All members of this class of compounds are well absorbed following oral administration. Binding to plasma albumin occurs to varying degrees. The presence of food in the stomach may retard absorption and lower peak plasma concentrations. Certain other drugs such as aspirin and phenobarbital may also impair absorption of these agents, but the clinical significance of this has not been established.[119]

The propionic acid derivatives are useful for the symptomatic treatment of rheumatoid arthritis, osteoarthritis, and ankylosing spondylitis. They are also effective for symptomatic relief of pain associated with injury to soft tissues. There is evidence that these agents may be beneficial for relief of postoperative inflammation when administered following oral, ophthalmic, and other types of surgery. In addition to variable therapeutic responses obtained in the immediate postoperative period following various types of ocular procedures, they may be helpful in reducing anterior segment inflammation and in preventing aphakic CME.[164–166]

The experimental rabbit uveitis model has been used to compare the ocular anti-inflammatory activity of the propionic acids. Topical application of fenoprofen sodium and flurbiprofen has exhibited anti-inflammatory activity when applied either before or after the development of experimental uveitis.[165] Flurbiprofen inhibits hyperemia, flare, cells, and uveal congestion in rabbit eyes with experimental uveitis. Flurbiprofen has also been reported to be effective in human eyes. Oral flurbiprofen, 100 mg twice daily, has significantly diminished postoperative inflammatory responses in a group of patients undergoing cataract extraction.[167] Topical flurbiprofen 0.02% has reduced conjunctival injection but not the anterior chamber reactions in patients who received argon laser trabeculoplasty (ALT) to 180 degrees of the trabecular meshwork.[168]

The effects of the propionic acids on intraocular pressure have been studied in rabbits and, more recently, in humans.[165,168] Elevation of intraocular pressure and aqueous humor protein following topical administration of arachidonic acid to rabbit eyes is blocked by fenoprofen and flurbiprofen, but naproxen is apparently ineffective.[165] However, human glaucomatous eyes treated with 0.03% flurbiprofen have shown a significantly smaller reduction in intraocular pressure 1 day and 1 week after ALT compared with eyes receiving placebo treatment.[168]

Although indomethacin has been used topically on the eye in clinical trials, a commercial preparation is not presently available. Flurbiprofen is marketed as a topical ophthalmic formulation by Allergan Pharma-

ceuticals. Available as Ocufen, the formulation contains 0.03% flurbiprofen in the Liquifilm (polyvinyl alcohol 1.4%) vehicle. The solution is preserved with 0.005% thimerosol and edetate disodium. Ocufen is approved for use to inhibit miosis during surgical procedures such as cataract extraction and intraocular lens implantation. When used as indicated, Ocufen is reported not to raise intraocular pressure.[169] Ocufen is contraindicated in epithelial herpes simplex keratitis, since NSAIAs, like corticosteroids, tend to exacerbate ocular infections.

When used as a 1% solution, topically applied suprofen, a propionic acid derivative, has been shown to be superior to placebo therapy in contact-lens-associated giant papillary conjunctivitis.[200] In a randomized, double-masked comparison, suprofen provided a greater reduction of signs and symptoms such as papillae and mucous strands.

As a group the propionic acid derivatives are usually better tolerated following oral administration than are aspirin, indomethacin, and the pyrazolon derivatives. However, they can cause many of the detrimental effects of the other NSAIAs. Gastrointestinal side effects are common with all members of the group. CNS effects such as headache, dizziness, drowsiness, and fatigue may also occur. Other untoward reactions such as dermatologic problems and blood dyscrasia occur less frequently. Naproxen and fenoprofen have been reported to cause ototoxicity.[119]

Ocular side effects have been reported with ibuprofen. Blurred vision, diplopia, and several cases of reversible toxic amblyopia have reportedly occurred with the use of this agent.[170]

THE FENAMATES

The fenamates, anthranilic acid derivatives that exhibit aspirin-like activity, are well absorbed following oral administration. They affect prostaglandin synthesis due to their ability to inhibit cyclo-oxygenase and, in addition, reduce the activity of prostaglandins, possibly by blocking cellular receptor sites for certain of the prostaglandins.[171]

Mefenamic acid was the first member of the group to become available in the United States. All the fenamates exhibit varying degrees of anti-inflammatory, antipyretic, and analgesic properties. Mefenamic acid has been used to relieve pain arising from rheumatic conditions, soft-tissue injuries, musculoskeletal conditions, and dysmenorrhea. As an anti-inflammatory agent, it has been evaluated in the treatment of osteoarthritis and rheumatoid arthritis. Clinically, in most instances, mefenamic acid offers little advantage over other NSAIAs.[119,171]

The efficacy of the fenamates as ocular anti-inflammatory agents in humans must be evaluated. In rabbits meclofenamic acid suspensions inhibit the intraocular pressure rise in response to arachidonic acid.[130]

Side effects preclude their long-term use. Gastrointestinal problems, especially diarrhea, are relatively common and can be severe. Renal and hepatic toxicity have been noted. Other side effects include skin rashes, hemolytic anemia, and bronchospasm, particularly in asthmatics and patients sensitive to aspirin.[119,171]

The fenamates bind strongly to plasma proteins and can displace certain other drugs from their binding sites on plasma albumin. This has been confirmed with the concomitant use of warfarin anticoagulants.[119]

Among the various NSAIAs, only flurbiprofen has been approved in the United States for limited topical ocular use. Clinical trials are currently underway to test the anti-inflammatory effects of other NSAIAs. The efficacy of 0.5% tolmetin has been compared with prednisolone and betamethasone in acute nongranulomatous uveitis.[172,173] No statistically significant difference in effect was observed during a 21-day trial period. Another NSAIA, ketorolac tromethamine, has been compared to placebo treatment in patients with chronic, angiographically proven aphakic or pseudophakic CME.[174] A statistically significant improvement in distance visual acuity was observed in the ketorolac treatment group compared with the placebo group. Ketorolac 0.5% solution administered 3 times daily has also been reported to be more effective than a placebo solution in suppressing postoperative anterior segment inflammation after extracapsular cataract extraction and intraocular lens implantation.[201] More experimental studies and clinical trials are needed. A topical NSAIA that would be effective without adverse ocular and systemic effects would be desirable for long-term control of ocular inflammation.

Cromolyn Sodium (Disodium Cromoglycate)

Cromolyn sodium has become an important therapeutic agent for mast cell–related ocular and systemic diseases. Since the late 1960s, it has been a useful drug to control asthma. More recently it has also proven useful for such conditions as allergic rhinitis, certain food allergies, ulcerative colitis, and systemic mastocytosis.[175] Clinical experience with topical ocular cromolyn sodium has shown that this agent is also useful for control of certain inflammatory conditions of the eye in which degranulation of mast cells plays a major role.

Pharmacology

Cromolyn sodium was first synthesized in 1965 during a study of the biologic properties of khellin, an extract derived from the seed of an Eastern Mediterranean plant. Its chemical structure consists of two cromone rings joined by a flexible chain. Each ring contains two polar carboxylic acid groups[175] (Fig. 5.11).

Cromolyn acts primarily by stabilizing the mast cell[148] (Fig. 5.12). Several mechanisms may account for its effectiveness. Johnson[176] has proposed that antigen activation and inhibition must occur at the same time for cromolyn to inhibit release of mediators from mast cells. More recent studies suggest that cromolyn may selectively and rapidly phosphorylate a 78,000 Dalton protein in the mast cell membrane responsible for terminating secretion and restabilizing the mast cell after degranulation. Activating this naturally occurring stabilizer of the mast cell by administering cromolyn before antigen challenge may thus inhibit the degranulation process (see Fig. 5.12).

It has been suggested that cromolyn has another mode of action aside from stabilizing the mast cell membrane. In a study of 60 patients with noninfectious inflammatory reactions, Felius and van Bijsterveld[178] reported that cromolyn was effective despite the fact that several of the patients had neither laboratory evidence nor history to indicate atopic disease. They propose that, in the eye, cromolyn interacts with magnesium ions to produce thixotropic gels, which in turn protect the tear film against abnormal breakup. Administration of cromolyn in this study changed the mean tear film breakup time for all patients from a baseline of 5.95 seconds to a posttreatment 9.90 seconds, a 65% change (P <0.01). Mikuni[179] reported that cromolyn, in addition to improving subjective and objective allergic symptoms, also prevents the change in refractive index of tears seen in untreated eyes challenged with cedar pollen.

Ophthalmic drug disposition studies have been conducted with cromolyn sodium drops to determine the amount of ocular and systemic absorption.[180,181] When multiple doses of cromolyn sodium 4% were instilled into normal rabbit eyes, less than 0.07% of the administered dose was absorbed into the systemic circulation. The presumed route is by way of ocular tissue, nasal passages, buccal cavity, and gastrointestinal tract. Less than 0.01% was present in the aqueous humor. Plasma clearance was complete within 24 hours after stopping treatment. Likewise, in human studies, analysis of drug distribution indicates that approximately 0.03% of cromolyn sodium applied topically is absorbed into the

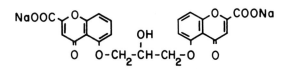

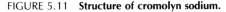

FIGURE 5.11   **Structure of cromolyn sodium.**

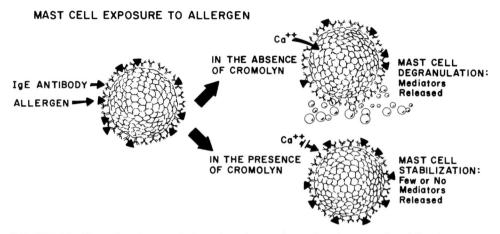

MAST CELL EXPOSURE TO ALLERGEN

FIGURE 5.12   **The major pharmacologic action of cromolyn sodium is mast cell stabilization. (From Ross RN. Opticrom 4% in clinical practice. Boston: Fisons Corporation, 1984;26.)**

eye.[180] Topical ocular application of cromolyn does not appear to accumulate in either daily wear or extended wear contact lenses.[202]

Cromolyn sodium is available as a 4% ophthalmic solution (Opticrom, Fisons Corporation). The formulation has a pH range of 4.0 to 7.0 and a tonicity of 123 mOsmol/liter. The diluent is purified water, and it is preserved with benzalkonium chloride 0.01% and ethylenediaminetetraacetic acid (EDTA) 0.10%. The shelf life is 36 months from date of manufacture. The preparation should be discarded within 4 weeks of opening. It should be protected from direct sunlight and stored below 30°C.[181]

Clinical Uses

Cromolyn sodium is effective in certain ocular allergic disorders such as vernal conjunctivitis and keratitis, allergic keratoconjunctivitis, and giant papillary conjunctivitis.[181,182] Other therapeutic modalities such as cold compresses, vasoconstrictor-antihistamine combinations, and corticosteroids may be used concomitantly with cromolyn sodium.

ALLERGIC CONJUNCTIVITIS

Of the four major types of hypersensitivity reactions, cromolyn sodium is most effective on the IgE-mediated type, also known as atopic allergy or immediate hypersensitivity reaction. Studies have indicated that the 4% solution is effective in relieving the ocular signs and symptoms of hay fever conjunctivitis and allergic conjunctivitis within 7 days of initiation of treatment 4 times daily in 92% to 96% of cases. The need for

supplementary oral antihistamines may be reduced or eliminated.[183]

In cases of chronic allergic conjunctivitis the therapeutic results with cromolyn sodium can be less satisfactory. A trial period of 10 to 14 days may be necessary before evaluating the effectiveness of therapy.[184]

VERNAL KERATOCONJUNCTIVITIS

Easty and associates[185] first demonstrated the usefulness of cromolyn sodium in vernal keratoconjunctivitis. Both subjective symptoms and objective signs may be alleviated (Fig. 5.13).[186,203] In many cases the drug may be effective when used alone. However, in patients with severe clinical symptoms, corticosteroids, vasoconstrictors, and other agents may also be required.[184] Cromolyn can decrease the need for corticosteroids in patients previously treated with steroids. Cromolyn and corticosteroids may be used together with good results in patients with severe disease or acute exacerbation of symptoms.[184]

GIANT PAPILLARY CONJUNCTIVITIS

Giant papillary conjunctivitis (GPC) is an iatrogenic disease that closely resembles vernal keratoconjunctivitis. It occurs in patients who wear contact lenses and ocular prostheses. Meisler and associates[187] reported relief of ocular discomfort in 5 patients with use of cromolyn sodium. Four of the 5 patients had less prominent giant papillae on the upper tarsal conjunctiva. Donshik and associates[188] studied 45 contact lens wearers with symptomatic GPC. For less severe cases, changing lenses was sufficient to control the condition.

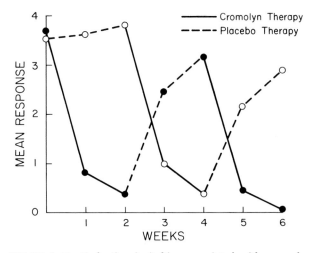

FIGURE 5.13 **Reduction in itching associated with cromolyn therapy in patients with vernal keratoconjunctivitis. (Adapted with permission from the American Journal of Ophthalmology 90:175–181, 1980. Copyright by the Ophthalmic Publishing Company.)**

For the more severe cases, however, addition of 2% cromolyn sodium provided significant improvement.

Further studies are needed to fully assess the effects of ocular cromolyn sodium in this condition.

Side Effects

Few side effects have been reported following topical ocular use of cromolyn sodium. Since systemic drug levels are extremely low, no adverse systemic reactions have been reported with ocular use.

The most frequently reported ocular reaction has been transient ocular stinging or burning.[181,185] Until recently, Opticrom 4% contained 2-phenylethanol as a preservative. Several investigators[189,190] have reported that the irritation following instillation of cromolyn sodium drops is significantly less marked when this preservative is omitted from the solution. In its present formulation, Opticrom does not contain 2-phenylethanol.

Other adverse reactions reported as infrequent events include conjunctival injection, watery or itchy eyes, dryness around the eyes, and styes.[181]

Dimethyl Sulfoxide

The clinical usefulness of dimethyl sulfoxide (DMSO) as an anti-inflammatory agent has been a subject of much debate. During the early 1960s it was first applied to the skin to alleviate symptoms associated with musculoskeletal inflammation. An additional use was as a solvent to aid absorption of various drugs through membranes, particularly the skin.[191,192]

DMSO is a colorless, highly polar, hydroscopic organic liquid. It exhibits solvent properties for a variety of substances. It is miscible with water, lipids, and numerous organic solvents. It has diverse industrial applications, including use as an antifreeze, as a solvent for dyes and pigments, and as a reactant for certain synthetic chemical reactions.[191]

Before 1970 hundreds of articles had been published on the clinical uses and pharmacologic and toxicologic effects of DMSO. In 1965 the Food and Drug Administration (FDA) ordered suspension of large-scale clinical trials with DMSO because of reported adverse ocular effects in certain experimental animals. Lenticular changes were first reported in dogs following oral or cutaneous application of DMSO. Initial ophthalmoscopic examination revealed a dark ring at the boundary between the lens nucleus and the cortex. As administration of DMSO continued, progressive lenticular myopia developed in the central zone with an increasing hyperopia in the periphery, resulting in a difference of as much as 20 diopters. These changes occurred within 9 weeks following administration of 5 mg/kg body weight daily orally or 8 g/kg body weight daily cutaneously.[193]

There is evidence, however, that dogs given smaller doses do not develop lens changes. Cutaneous application of 1 g/kg body weight for 5 days per week for 20 months has caused no evidence of ocular changes.[194]

The average human topical dose to the skin ranges from 0.1 to 0.2 g/kg daily. No drug-related lens changes in humans treated with DMSO have been reported. In rabbits, pigs, hamsters, and monkeys, lenticular changes have been reported with high doses, 5 to 10 g/kg daily, but few changes have been reported with doses closer to that used in humans. These observations suggest a possible dose-duration relationship to development of lens changes.[195]

It is always difficult to compare observations in animals to humans. Differences in species, age, dosage, and route of administration must be considered. Moreover, drug-induced lens changes in humans are characterized by posterior or anterior subcapsular lens opacities (see Chapter 31), whereas DMSO appears to affect the lens nucleus in animals.[195]

In humans, solutions of water and DMSO have been applied as eyedrops or administered as subconjunctival injections. Concentrations above 50% have generally been irritating, resulting in temporary stinging and burning. Lower concentrations (e.g., 10%) appear to cause no discomfort or ocular injury.[196]

Contrary to what has been reported for the skin,[191] DMSO does not appear to aid the penetration of drugs into the eye.[192] Jenkins[197] failed to demonstrate its effectiveness as a vehicle for ophthalmic agents. Moreover, its clinical usefulness as an anti-inflammatory agent in humans is questionable. DMSO appears to be ineffective in ocular allergic conditions, but it may be of some value in the treatment of episcleritis and postherpetic neuritis.[197] DMSO has been used in preservation of frozen corneas for transplantation.[191]

Following its application to the skin, DMSO is distributed to all tissues, including those of the eye. Apart from changes observed in the lenses of animals, no adverse effects have been reported for other ocular structures.[191]

Cutaneous use of DMSO does not appear to be systemically injurious. Since it can liberate histamine at the site of application, an initial dermatitis may occur, but the skin appears to become tolerant to the irritant effects on continuous exposure. DMSO is also mildly antifungal and antibacterial. Clinically, the principal adverse effect is an unpleasant odor of the breath.[192]

Unless further clinical observations prove otherwise, DMSO will continue to remain a pharmacologic enigma.

References

1. Addison T. On the constitution and local effects of disease of the suprarenal capsules. London: Samuel Highley, 1855.
2. Brown-Sequard CE. Recherches experimentales sur la physiologie et la pathologie des capsules surrenales. Arch Gen Med 1856;8:385–410.
3. Haynes RC, Murad F. Adrenocorticotropic hormone. Adrenocortical steroids and their synthetic analogs. In: Gilman AG, Goodman LS, Rall TW, et al., eds. The pharmacological basis of therapeutics, ed. 7. New York: Macmillan Co, 1985;1459–1485.
4. Reichstein T, Shopee CW. The hormones of the adrenal cortex. Vitam Horm 1943;1:346–413.
5. Foster GL, Smith PE. Hypophysectomy and replacement therapy in relation to basal metabolism and specific dynamic action in the rat. JAMA 1926;87:2151–2153.
6. Selye H. General adaptation syndrome and diseases of adaptation. J Clin Endocrinol Metab 1946;6:117–230.
7. Hench PS, Kendall EC, Slocumb CH, Polly HF. The effect of a hormone of the adrenal cortex and of pituitary adrenocorticotropic hormone on rheumatoid arthritis. Mayo Clin Proc 1949;24:181–197.
8. Gordon DM, McLean JM. Effects of pituitary adrenocorticotropic hormone (ACTH) therapy in ophthalmologic conditions. JAMA 1950;142:1271–1276.
9. Gross F, Möhring J. Renal pharmacology, with special emphasis on aldosterone and angiotensin. Ann Rev Pharmacol Toxicol 1973;13:57–90.
10. Haynes RC. The activation of adrenal phosphorylase by the adrenocorticotropic hormone. J Biol Chem 1958;233:1220–1222.
11. Bar HP, Hechter O. Adenylate cyclase and hormone action. III. Calcium requirement for ACTH stimulation of adenylate cyclase. Biochem Biophys Res Commun 1969;35:681–686.
12. Jaanus SD, Rubin RP. The effect of ACTH on calcium distribution in the perfused cat adrenal gland. J Physiol (Lond) 1971;213:581–589.
13. Ganong WF. The central nervous system and the synthesis and release of adrenocorticotropic hormone. In: Nalbandov AV, ed. Advances in Neuroendocrinology. Urbana, IL: University of Illinois Press 1963;92–149.
14. Ingle DS. Permissive action of hormones. J Clin Endocrinol Metab 1954;14:1272–1274.
15. Ellis PP. Pharmacological effects of corticosteroids. Int Ophthalmol Clin 1966;6:799–819.
16. Leopold IH. Pharmacology and toxicology. Arch Ophthalmol 1951;46:159–224.
17. Fauci AS. Immunosuppressive and antiinflammatory effects of glucocorticoids. In: Baxter JD, Roussea GG, eds. Glucocorticoid hormone action. Berlin: Springer, 1979.
18. Basu PK, Avaria M, Jankie R. Effect of hydrocortisone on the mobilisation of leucocytes in corneal wounds. Br J Ophthalmol 1981;65:694–698.
19. Hench PS, Kendall EC, Slocumb CH, Polley HF. Effects of cortisone acetate and pituitary ACTH on rheumatoid arthritis, rheumatic fever and certain other conditions. Arch Intern Med 1950;85:545–666.
20. Baxter JD, Rousseau GG. Glucocorticoid hormone action. An overview. In: Baxter JD, Rousseau GG, eds. Glucocorticoid hormone action. Berlin: Springer-Verlag, 1979; Chap. 1.
21. Lin MT, Eiferman RA, Wittliff JL. Demonstration of specific glucocorticoid binding sites in bovine cornea. Exp Eye Res 1984;38:333–339.
22. Polansky JR, Weinreb RN. Antiinflammatory agents. Steroids as antiinflammatory agents. In: Sears ML, ed. Pharmacology of the eye. Berlin: Springer-Verlag, 1984; Chap. 10a.
23. Rubin RP. The role of calcium in the release of neurotransmitter substances and hormones. Pharmacol Rev 1970; 22:389–415.
24. Peterson RE, Wyngaarden JB. The miscible pool and turnover rate of hydrocortisone in man. J Clin Invest 1956;35:552–561.
25. Ney RL. Modern concepts of adrenocortical function. In: Thorn GW, ed. Steroid therapy. A clinical update for the 1970s. New York: Medcom, 1971;14–21.
26. Schwartz B. Physiological effects of corticosteroids on the eye. Int Ophthalmol Clin 1966;6:753–797.
27. Janes RG, Stiles SF. The penetration of cortisol into normal and pathologic rabbit eyes. Am J Ophthalmol 1963;56:84–90.
28. Burch PG, Migeon CJ. Systemic absorption of topical steroids. Arch Ophthalmol 1968;79:174–176.
29. Miller D, Peczon JD, Whitworth CG. Corticosteroids and functions in the anterior segment of the eye. Am J Ophthalmol 1965;59:31–34.
30. Baum JL, Levene RZ. Corneal thickness after topical corticosteroid therapy. Arch Ophthalmol 1968;79:366–369.
31. Reis DS. Potentiation of the vasoconstrictor action of topical norepinephrine on human bulbar conjunctival vessels after topical application of certain adrenocortical hormones. J Clin Endocrinol 1960;20:445–456.

32. Srinivasan BD, Kulkarni PS. The effect of steroidal and nonsteroidal anti-inflammatory agents on corneal re-epithelialization. Invest Ophthalmol Vis Sci 1981;20:688–691.

33. Walkenbach RJ, LeGrand RD. Inhibition of adenylate cyclase activity in the corneal epithelium by anti-inflammatory steroids. Exp Eye Res 1982;34:161–168.

34. Green H, Leopold IH. Investigation of corticosteroids in aqueous humor of normal animal eyes. Am J Ophthalmol 1954;38:101–106.

35. Larsen G. The viscosity of the vitreous humor influenced by hormones. Arch Ophthalmol 1958;59:712–716.

36. Becker B. Intraocular pressure response to topical corticosteroids. Invest Ophthalmol 1965;4:198–205.

37. Armaly MF. Effects of corticosteroids on intraocular pressure and fluid dynamics. I. The effect of dexamethasone in the normal eye. Arch Ophthalmol 1963;70:482–491.

38. Weinreb RN, Bloom E, Baxter JD, et al. Detection of glucocorticoid receptors in cultured human trabecular cells. Invest Ophthalmol Vis Sci 1981;21:403–407.

39. Green K, Elijah D. Drug effects on aqueous humor formation and pseudofacility in normal rabbit eyes. Exp Eye Res 1981;33:239–245.

40. Black RL, Oglesby RB, Von Sallmann L, Bunim JS. Posterior subcapsular cataracts by corticosteroids in patients with rheumatoid arthritis. JAMA 1960;174:166–171.

41. Von Sallmann L, Caravaggio LL, Collin EM, Weaver K. Examination of lenses of steroid-treated rats. Am J Ophthalmol 1960;50:1147–1150.

42. Miki T. Fluctuations in mitosis count of lens epithelium: influence of age, season, and adrenal hormones. Acta Soc Ophthalmol Jap 1961;65:2207–2214.

43. Harris JE, Becker B. Cation transport of the lens. Invest Ophthalmol 1965;4:709–722.

44. Moscona AA, Piddington R. Stimulation by hydrocortisone of premature changes in the developmental pattern of glutamine synthetase in embryonic retina. Biochim Biophys Acta 1966;121:409–414.

45. Duke-Elder S, Ashton N. Action of cortisone on tissue reactions in inflammation and repair with special reference to the eye. Br J Ophthalmol 1951;35:695–707.

46. Leopold IH. The steroid shield in ophthalmology. Trans Am Acad Ophthalmol Otolaryngol 1967;71:273–289.

47. Ellis PP. Ocular therapeutics and pharmacology. St. Louis: C. V. Mosby Co, 1980.

48. Leibowitz HM, Kupferman A. Anti-inflammatory medications. Int Ophthalmol Clin 1980;20:117–134.

49. Nelson EL. Ophthalmic steroids. In: Kaufman H, ed. Symposium on ocular anti-inflammatory therapy. Springfield, IL: Charles C Thomas, 1970;17:217–233.

50. Leibowitz HM, Kupferman A. Bioavailability and therapeutic effectiveness of topically administered corticosteroids. Trans Am Acad Ophthalmol Otolaryngol 1975;79:78–88.

51. Leibowitz HM, Stewart RH, Kupferman A. Evaluation of dexamethasone acetate as a topical ophthalmic formulation. Am J Ophthalmol 1978;86:418–423.

52. Leibowitz HM, Hyndiuk RA, Lindsey C, Rosenthal AL. Fluorometholone acetate: Clinical evaluation in the treatment of external ocular inflammation. Ann Ophthalmol 1984;16:1110–1115.

53. Leopold IH, Sawyer JL, Green H. Intraocular penetration of locally applied steroids. Arch Ophthalmol 1955;54:916–921.

54. Leopold IH, Kroman HS. Methyl and fluoro-substituted prednisolones in the blood and aqueous humor of the rabbit. Arch Ophthalmol 1960;63:943–947.

55. Leibowitz HM, Kupferman A. Penetration of fluorometholone into the cornea and aqueous humor. Arch Ophthalmol 1975;93:425–427.

56. Cox WV, Kupferman A, Leibowitz HM. Topically applied steroids in corneal disease. II. The role of the drug vehicle in stromal absorption of dexamethasone. Arch Ophthalmol 1972;88:549–552.

57. Schoenwald RD, Boltralik JS. A bioavailability comparison in rabbits of two steroid formulations as high viscosity gels and reference aqueous preparations. Invest Ophthalmol Vis Sci 1979;18:61–66.

58. Kupferman A, Ryan WJ, Leibowitz HM. Prolongation of anti-inflammatory effect of prednisolone acetate. Influence of formulation in high viscosity gel. Arch Ophthalmol 1981;99:2028–2029.

59. Gordon DM. Diseases of the uveal tract. In: Gordon DM, ed. Medical management of ocular disease. New York: Harper & Row, 1964;245–271.

60. Becker B, Kolker AE. Intraocular pressure response to topical corticosteroids. In: Leopold IH, ed. Ocular therapy: complications and management. St. Louis: C. V. Mosby Co, 1967;79–83.

61. Fairbairn WD, Thorson JC. Fluorometholone: Anti-inflammatory and intraocular pressure effects. Arch Ophthalmol 1971;86:138–141.

62. Ellis PP. Corticosteroid therapy in ophthalmology. In: Adriani J, Bernstein HN, eds. Symposium on ocular pharmacology and therapy. St. Louis: C. V. Mosby Co, 1970;49–57.

63. Schlaegel TF. Depot corticosteroid by the cul-de-sac route. In: Kaufman HE, ed. Ocular anti-inflammatory therapy. Springfield, IL: Charles C Thomas, 1970;117–123.

64. Cloes RS, Krohn DL, Breslin H, Braunstein R. Depo-Medrol in treatment of inflammatory diseases. Am J Ophthalmol 1962;54:407–411.

65. Sturman RM, Laval J, Sturman MF. Subconjunctival triamcinolone acetonide. Am J Ophthalmol 1966;61:155–166.

66. Pizzarello LD, Jakobiec FA, Hofeldt AJ, et al. Intralesional corticosteroid therapy for chalazia. Am J Ophthalmol 1978;85:818–821.

67. Vidaurri LJ, Peer J. Intralesional corticosteroid treatment of chalazia. Ann Ophthalmol 1986;18:339–340.

68. Schlaegel TF. Nonspecific treatment of uveitis. In: Duane TD, ed. Clinical ophthalmology. Philadelphia: Harper & Row, 1980;4:43:1–12.

69. McCuen BW, Bressler M, Tano Y, et al. The lack of toxicity of intravitrally administered triamcinolone acetonide. Am J Ophthalmol 1981;91:785–788.

70. Leibowitz HM, Kupferman A. Periocular injection of corticosteroids. Arch Ophthalmol 1977;95:311–314.

71. Harter JG, Reddy WS, Thorn GW. Studies on intermittent corticosteroid dosage regimen. N Engl J Med 1963;269:591–596.

72. MacGregor RR, Sheagren HN, Lipsett MB, Wolff SM. Alternate day prednisone therapy. N Engl J Med 1969;280:1427–1431.

73. Gordon DM. Management of uveitis. Eye Ear Nose Throat Monthly 1966;45:72–81.

74. Becker B. The side effects of corticosteroids. Invest Ophthalmol 1964;3:492–497.

75. Sturge RA, Beardwell C, Hartog M, et al. Cortisol and growth hormone secretion in relation to linear growth. Br Med J 1970;3:547–551.

76. Black RL, Oglesby RB, Von Sallmann L, Bunim JJ. Posterior subcapsular cataracts induced by corticosteroids in patients with rheumatoid arthritis. JAMA 1960;174:166–171.

77. Oglesby RB, Black RL, Von Sallmann L, Bunim JJ. Cataracts in rheumatoid arthritis patients treated with corticosteroids. Arch Ophthalmol 1961;66:519–523.

78. Urban RC, Cotlier E. Corticosteroid-induced cataracts. Surv Ophthalmol 1986;31:102–110.

79. Havre DC. Cataracts in children on long-term corticosteroid therapy. Arch Ophthalmol 1965;73:818–821.

80. Braver DA, Richards RD, Good TA. Posterior subcapsular cataract in steroid treated children. Arch Ophthalmol 1967;77:161–169.

81. Loredo A, Rodriquez RS, Murillo L. Cataracts after short-term corticosteroid treatment. N Engl J Med 1972;286:160–163.

82. Becker B. Cataracts and topical corticosteroids. Am J Ophthalmol 1964;58:872–873.

83. Burde RM, Becker B. Corticosteroid-induced glaucoma and cataracts in contact lens wearers. JAMA 1970;213:2075–2078.

84. Skalka HW, Prchal JT. Effect of corticosteroids on cataract formation. Arch Ophthalmol 1980;98:1773–1777.

85. Yablonski ME, Burde RM, Kolker AE, Becker B. Cataracts induced by topical dexamethasone in diabetics. Arch Ophthalmol 1978;96:474–476.

86. Francois J. Cortisone et tension oculaire. Ann Oculistique 1954;187:805–816.

87. Linner E. Adrenocortical steroids and aqueous humor dynamics. Doc Ophthalmol 1959;13:210–222.

88. Goldman H. Cortisone glaucoma. Arch Ophthalmol 1962;68:621–626.

89. Bernstein HN, Schwartz B. Effects of long-term systemic steroids on ocular pressure and tonographic values. Arch Ophthalmol 1962;68:742–753.

90. Williamson J. A clinical evaluation of steroid cataract and steroid glaucoma with particular emphasis on systemic steroid therapy. In: Pigott A, ed. Evaluation of drug effects on the eye. Proc Royal Soc Med (Lond) May 1968.

91. Armaly MF. Effect of corticosteroids on intraocular pressure and fluid dynamics: I. The effect of dexamethasone in the normal eye. Arch Ophthalmol 1963;70:482–491.

92. Becker B, Mills DW. Corticosteroids and intraocular pressure. Arch Ophthalmol 1963;70:500–507.

93. Armaly MF. Genetic factors related to glaucoma. Ann NY Acad Sci 1968;151:861–875.

94. Becker B. The genetic problem of chronic simple glaucoma. Ann Ophthalmol 1971;3:351–354.

95. Schwartz B. The response of ocular pressure to corticosteroids. Int Ophthalmol Clin 1966;929–989.

96. Stewart RH, Kimbrough RL. Intraocular pressure response to topically administered fluorometholone. Arch Ophthalmol 1979;97:2139–2140.

97. Mindel JS, Tovitian HO, Smith H, Walker EC. Comparative ocular pressure elevations by medrysone, fluorometholone, and dexamethasone phosphate. Arch Ophthalmol 1980;98:1577–1578.

98. Kass M, Cheetham J, Duzman E, Burke PJ. The ocular hypertensive effect of 0.25% fluorometholone in corticosteroid responders. Am J Ophthalmol 1986;102:159–163.

99. Akingbekin T. Corticosteroid-induced ocular hypertension. J Cut Ocul Toxicol 1986;5:45–53.

100. Weinreb RN, Bloom E, Baxter JD, et al. Detection of glucocorticoid receptors in cultured human trabecular cells. Invest Ophthalmol Vis Sci 1981;21:403–407.

101. Hernandez MR, Wenk EJ, Weinstein BI, et al. Glucocorticoid target cells in human trabeculectomy specimens. Invest Ophthalmol Vis Sci (Suppl) 1981;20:23.

102. Francois J. Corticosteroid glaucoma. Ophthalmologica 1984;188:76–81.

103. Godel V, Rogenbogen L, Stein R. On the mechanism of corticosteroid-induced ocular hypertension. Ann Ophthalmol 1978;10:191–196.

104. Suie T, Taylor FW. The effect of cortisone on experimental pseudomonas corneal ulcers. Arch Ophthalmol 1956;56:53–56.

105. Leopold IH, Sery TW. Epidemiology of herpes simplex keratitis. Invest Ophthalmol 1963;2:498–503.

106. Kimura SJ, Okumoto M. The effect of corticosteroids on experimental herpes simplex keratoconjunctivitis in the rabbit. Am J Ophthalmol 1957;43:131–134.

107. McCoy G, Leopold IH. Simplex infections of the cornea. Am J Ophthalmol 1960;49:1355–1356.

108. Berson EL, Kobayaski GS, Becker B, Rosenbaum L. Topical corticosteroids and fungal keratitis. Invest Ophthalmol 1967;6:512–517.

109. Birge HL. Ocular aspects of mycotic infections. Arch Ophthalmol 1952;47:354–382.

110. Leopold IH, Maylath F. Intraocular penetration of cortisone and its effectiveness against experimental corneal burns. Am J Ophthalmol 1952;35:1125–1134.

111. Krupin T, LeBlanc RP, Becker B, et al. Uveitis in association with topically administered corticosteroid. Am J Ophthalmol 1970;70:883–885.

112. Martins JC, Wilensky JT, Asseth CF, et al. Corticosteroid-induced uveitis. Am J Ophthalmol 1974;77:433–437.

113. Spaeth GL. Effects of topical dexamethasone on intraocular pressure and the water drinking test. Arch Ophthalmol 1966;76:772–783.

114. Kern R, Marci FJ. Steroid eye drops and their components. Arch Ophthalmol 1967;78:794–802.

115. Newsome DA, Wong VG, Cameron TP, Anderson RR. "Steroid-induced" mydriasis and ptosis. Invest Ophthalmol 1971;10:424–429.

116. Trautzellel-Klosinski S, Sundmacker R, Wigand R. Die wirkung von steroiden bei keratoconjunctivities epidemica. Klin Monatsbl Augenheilk 1980;176:899–906.

117. Buffington GA, Dominguez JH, Piering WF, et al. Interaction of rifampin and glucocorticoids. JAMA 1976;236:1958–1960.

118. Vane JR. Inhibition of prostaglandin synthesis as a mechanism of action for aspirin-like drugs. Nature [New Biol] 1971;231:232–235.

119. Flower RJ, Moncada S, Vane JR. Analgesic-antipyretics

and anti-inflammatory agents. Drugs employed in the treatment of gout. In: Gilman AG, Goodman LS, Rall TW, et al., eds. The pharmacological basis of therapeutics, ed. 7. New York: Macmillan Co, 1985;674–715.

120. Waitzman MB. Possible new concepts relating prostaglandins to various ocular functions. Surv Ophthalmol 1970; 14:301–326.

121. Podos SM. Prostaglandins, nonsteroidal anti-inflammatory agents and eye disease. Trans Am Ophthalmol Soc 1976; 74:637–660.

122. Kulkarni PS, Srinivasan BD. Nonsteroidal antiinflammatory drugs in ocular inflammatory conditions. In: Lews AS, Furst DE, eds. Nonsteroidal antiinflammatory drugs. New York: Marcel Dekker, 1987; Chap. 7.

123. Neufeld AH, Sears ML. Prostaglandins and the eye. Prostaglandins 1973;4:157–168.

124. Ambache N. Irin, a smooth muscle contracting substance present in rabbit iris. J Physiol (Lond) 1955;129:65–66.

125. Ambache N. Further studies on the preparation, purification and nature of irin. J Physiol (Lond) 1959;146:255–294.

126. Ambache N, Reynolds M, Whiting J. Some differences in uveal reactions between cats and rabbits. J Physiol (Lond) 1966;182:110–130.

127. Bito LZ. Prostaglandins, other eicosanoids and their derivatives as potential antiglaucoma agents. In: Drance SM, Neufeld AH, eds. Applied pharmacology in medical treatments of glaucoma. New York: Grune & Stratton, 1984; Chap. 20.

128. Leopold IH. Advances in ocular therapy: Noncorticosteroid anti-inflammatory agents. Am J Ophthalmol 1974;78:759–773.

129. Moncada S, Flower RJ, Vane JR. Prostaglandins, prostacyclin and thromboxane A_2. In: Gilman AG, Goodman LS, Rall TW, et al., eds. The pharmacological basis of therapeutics. 7th ed. New York: Macmillan Co, 1985;660–673.

130. Mishima S, Masuda K. Clinical implications of prostaglandins and synthesis inhibitors. In: Leopold IH, Burns RP, eds. Symposium on ocular therapy. New York: John Wiley & Sons, 1977;10:1–19.

131. Waitzman MB, King CD. Prostaglandin influences on intraocular pressure and pupil size. Am J Physiol 1967;212:329–334.

132. Kelley RGM, Starr MS. Effects of prostaglandins and a prostaglandin antagonist on intraocular pressure and protein in the monkey eye. Can J Ophthalmol 1971;6:205–211.

133. Kass MA, Podos SM, Moses RA, Becker B. Prostaglandin E and aqueous humor dynamics. Invest Ophthalmol 1972;11:1022–1027.

134. Whitelocke RAF, Eakins KE. Vascular changes in the anterior uvea of the rabbit produced by prostaglandins. Arch Ophthalmol 1973;89:495–499.

135. Starr MS. Further studies on the effect of prostaglandin on intraocular pressure in rabbit. Exp Eye Res 1971;11:170–177.

136. Stern FA, Bito LZ. Comparison of the hypertensive and other ocular effects of prostaglandins E_2 and F_2 on cat and rhesus monkey eyes. Invest Ophthalmol Vis Sci 1982;22:588–598.

137. Villumsen J, Alm A. The effect of prostaglandin F_2 eye drops in open angle glaucoma. Invest Ophthalmol Vis Sci (Suppl) 1987;28:378.

138. Griffin G. The effects of prostaglandin F_2 in the human eye. Graefe's Arch Clin Exp Ophthalmol 1985;222:139–141.

139. Lee P, Podos SM, Severin C. Effect of prostaglandin F_2 on aqueous humor dynamics of rabbit, cat and monkey. Invest Ophthalmol Vis Sci 1984;25:1087–1093.

140. Crawford K, Kaufman PL. Pilocarpine antagonizes prostaglandin F_2-induced ocular hypotension in monkeys. Evidence for enhancement of uveoscleral outflow by prostaglandin F_2. Arch Ophthalmol 1987;105:1112–1116.

141. Bito LZ. Prostaglandins. Old concepts and new perspectives. Arch Ophthalmol 1987;105:1036–1039.

142. Bisggard H, Ford-Hutchinson AW, Charleson S. Presence of LTB_4 in human tears. Prostaglandins 1984;28:620–626.

143. Gifford H. On the treatment of sympathetic ophthalmia by large doses of salicylate of sodium aspirin or other salicylic compounds. Ophthalmoscope 1910;8:257–258.

144. Sears ML, Neufeld AH, Jampol LM. Prostaglandins. Invest Ophthalmol 1973;12:161–164.

145. Miller JD, Eakins K, Atwal M. The release of prostaglandin E_2-like activity into the aqueous humor after paracentesis and its prevention by aspirin. Invest Ophthalmol 1973;12:939–942.

146. Abelson MB, Butrus SI, Weston JH. Aspirin therapy for vernal conjunctivitis. Am J Ophthalmol 1983;95:502–505.

147. Meyer E, Kraus E, Zonis S. Efficacy of antiprostaglandin therapy in vernal conjunctivitis. Br J Ophthalmol 1987;71:497–499.

148. Perkins ES, MacFaul PA. Indomethacin in the treatment of uveitis; a double-blind trial. Trans Ophthalmol Soc UK 1965;85:53–58.

149. Tuovinen E, Esila R, Liesman M. Experience of the use of indomethacin in inflammatory eye diseases. Acta Ophthalmol 1966;44:585–589.

150. Tennant JL. Prostaglandins in ophthalmology. In: Emery JM, ed. Current concepts in cataract surgery. St. Louis: C. V. Mosby Co, 1978;360–362.

151. Burns CA. Indomethacin reduced retinal sensitivity and corneal deposits. Am J Ophthalmol 1968;66:825–835.

152. Yannuzzi LA, Wallyn RH. Cystoid macular edema. A controlled treatment using indomethacin. In: Emery JM, Paton D, eds. Current concepts in cataract surgery. St. Louis: C. V. Mosby Co, 1976;313–316.

153. Miyake K. Indomethacin in the treatment of postoperative cystoid macular edema. Surv Ophthalmol 1984;28:554–568.

154. Yannuzzi LA. A perspective on the treatment of aphakic cystoid macular edema. Surv Ophthalmol 1984;28:540–553.

155. Klein RM, Katzin HM, Yannuzzi LA. The effect of indomethacin pretreatment on aphakic cystoid macular edema. Am J Ophthalmol 1979;87:487–489.

156. Sanders DR, Goldstick B, Kraff C, et al. Aqueous penetration of oral and topical indomethacin in humans. Arch Ophthalmol 1983;101:164–1616.

157. Miyake K, Miyake Y, Maekubo K. Incidence of cystoid macular edema after retinal detachment surgery and the use of topical indomethacin. Am J Ophthalmol 1983;95:451–456.

158. Boeck J, Kaunitz H, Popper H. Effect of pyrazolon derivatives on the vessels. Arch Exp Pathol Pharmacol 1935; 179:170–176.

159. Junghannss K. Experiences with Tandearil in ocular surgery. Klin Monatsbl Augenheilkd 1966;149:512–518.

160. Werner LEJ. Hydroxyphenylbutazone (Tandearil) in the treatment of ocular disease. Br J Ophthalmol 1960;44:755–760.

161. Hunter PJL, Fowler PD, Wilkinson P. Treatment of anterior uveitis. Br J Ophthalmol 1973;57:892–896.

162. Podos SM, Becker B. Comparison of ocular prostaglandin synthesis inhibitors. Invest Ophthalmol 1976;15:841–844.

163. Wilhelmi E. Experimental and clinical investigation of a non-hormonal anti-inflammatory eye ointment. Ophthalmic Res 1973;5:253–289.

164. Harris LS, Kahanowicz Y, Hughes J. Ocular anti-inflammatory effects of fenoprofen. Arch Ophthalmol 1974;92:506–508.

165. Leopold IH, Murray D. Noncorticosteroidal anti-inflammatory agents in ophthalmology. Ophthalmology 1979;86:142–155.

166. Hillman JS, Frank S, Kheskani MB. Flurbiprofen and human intraocular inflammation. In: Samuellson B, Ramwell PW, Paolelti R, eds. Advances in prostaglandin and thromboxane research. New York: Raven Press, 1980;8:1723–1725.

167. Sabiston DW, Robinson IG. An evaluation of anti-inflammatory effect of flurbiprofen after cataract extraction. Br J Ophthalmol 1987;71:418–421.

168. Hotchkiss ML, Robin AL, Pollack I, Quigley HA. Nonsteroidal antiinflammatory agents after argon laser trabeculoplasty. Ophthalmology 1984;91:969–974.

169. Ocufen. Product information. Irvine, CA: Allergan Pharmaceuticals, 1986.

170. Colleen LMT, Bowen DI. Ocular side effects of ibuprofen. Br J Ophthalmol 1971;55:472–477.

171. Simon LS, Mills JA. Nonsteroidal anti-inflammatory drugs. N Engl J Med 1980;302:1237–1243.

172. Dunne JA, Jacobs N, Morrison A, Gilbert DJ. Efficacy of anterior uveitis of two known steroids and topical tolmetin. Br J Ophthalmol 1985;69:120–125.

173. Young BJ, Cunningham WF, Akingbehn T. Double-masked controlled clinical trial of 5% tolmetin versus 0.5% prednisolone, versus 0.9% saline in acute endogenous nongranulomatous anterior uveitis. Br J Ophthalmol 1982;66:389–391.

174. Flach AJ, Dolan BJ, Irvine AR. Effectiveness of ketorolac tromethamine 0.5% ophthalmic solution for chronic aphakic and pseudophakic cystoid macular edema. Am J Ophthalmol 1987;103:479–486.

175. Cox JSC. Cromolyn sodium. Pharmacol Biochem Properties of Drug Substances 1977;1:277–310.

176. Johnson HG. Cromoglycate and other inhibitors of mediator release. In: Middleton E, Reed CE, Ellis EF, eds. Allergic principles in practice. St. Louis: C.V. Mosby Co, 1983.

177. Theoharides TC, Sieghart W, Greengard P, Douglas WW. Antiallergic drug cromolyn may inhibit histamine secretion by regulating phosphorylation of mast cell protein. Science 1980;207:80–82.

178. Felius K, van Bijsterveld OP. Effect of sodium cromoglycate on tear film break-up time. Ann Ophthalmol 1987;17:80–82.

179. Mikuni I. Efficacy of 2% DSCG ophthalmic solution for allergic conjunctivitis from Japanese cedar pollinosin. Jpn J Clin Ophthalmol 1980;34:1655–1659.

180. Lee VHL, Swarbrick J, Stratford RE, Morimoto KW. Disposition of topically applied sodium cromoglycate in albino rabbit eye. Int J Pharmaceutics 1983;16:163–170.

181. Ross RW. Opticrom 4% in clinical practice. A monograph. Bedford, MA: Fisons Corporation, 1984.

182. Allansmith MR, Ross RN. Ocular allergy and mast cell stabilizers. Surv Ophthalmol 1986;30:229–244.

183. Greenbaum J, Cockroft D, Hargreave FE, et al. Sodium cromoglycate in allergic conjunctivitis. J Allergy Clin Immunol 1977;59:439–469.

184. Sorkin EM, Ward A. Ocular sodium cromoglycate. An overview of its therapeutic efficacy in allergic eye disease. Drugs 1986;31:131–148.

185. Easty DL, Rice NSA, Jones BR. Clinical trials of topical sodium cromoglycate in vernal keratoconjunctivitis. Clin Allergy 1972;2:99–107.

186. Ostler HB, Martin R, Dawson CR. The use of disodium cromoglycate in treatment of atopic ocular disease. In: Leopold IH, Burns RP, eds. Symposium on ocular therapy. New York: John Wiley & Sons, 1977;9:99–108.

187. Meisler DM, Berzins UJ, Krachmer JH, Stock EL. Cromolyn treatment in giant papillary conjunctivitis. Arch Ophthalmol 1982;100:1608–1610.

188. Donshik PC, Ballow M, Luistro A, Samartino L. Treatment of contact lens-induced giant papillary conjunctivitis. Contact Lens 1984;10:346–349.

189. Chin GN. Treatment of vernal keratoconjunctivitis with topical cromolyn sodium. J Pediatr Ophthalmol Strabismus 1978;15:326–329.

190. Inerfield CG, Million R, Singh MS. Cromoglycate eye drops in hay-fever conjunctivitis. A new formula appears to reduce stinging. Practitioner 1984;228:543–544.

191. Grant WM. Toxicology of the eye, ed. 2. Springfield, IL: Charles C Thomas, 1977;405–408.

192. Kligman AM. Topical pharmacology and toxicology of dimethyl sulfoxide. JAMA 1965;193:923–928.

193. Rubin L, Barnett KC. Ocular effects of oral and dermal application of dimethyl sulfoxide in animals. Ann NY Acad Sci 1967;141:333–345.

194. Jacob SW, Rosenbaum EE. The toxicology of dimethyl sulfoxide (DMSO). Headache 1966;6:127–136.

195. Gordon DM, Kleberger KE. The effects of dimethyl sulfoxide (DMSO) on animal and human eyes. Arch Ophthalmol 1968;79:423–427.

196. Gordon DM. Dimethyl sulfoxide in ophthalmology with special reference to possible toxic effects. Ann NY Acad Sci 1967;141:392–401.

197. Jenkins BH. Clinical tests with DMSO in ophthalmology (abstr.). Invest Ophthalmol 1966;5:329.

198. Garrett GW, Gillespie ME, Mannix B. Adrenocorticoid injection vs conservative therapy in the treatment of chalazia. Ann Ophthalmol 1988;20:196–198.

199. Kerstetter JR, Brubaker RF, Wilson SE, et al. Prostaglandin $F_{2\alpha}$-1-iso-propylester lowers 1OP without decreasing aqueous humor flow. Am J Ophthalmol 1988;105:30–34.

200. Wood TS, Steward RH, Bowman RW. Suprofen treatment of contact lens associated GPC. Ophthalmology 1988;96:822–826.

201. Flach AJ, Lavelle CJ, Orlander KW. The effect of ketorolac tromethamine solution 0.5% in reducing postoperative inflammation after cataract extraction and intraocular lens implantation. Ophthalmology 1988;95:1279–1284.

202. Iwasaki W, Kosaka Y, Momose T, et al. Absorption of topical disodium cromoglycate and its preservatives by soft contact lens. CLAO 1988;14:155–158.

203. Foster CS. Evaluation of topical cromolyn sodium in the treatment of vernal keratoconjunctivitis. Ophthalmology 1988;95:194–201.

CHAPTER 6

Anti-Infective Drugs

Diane P. Yolton

Humans are constantly exposed to a variety of microorganisms, including bacteria, viruses, and fungi. In most cases, these microorganisms do not produce infection because the skin and mucous membrane surfaces provide effective barriers against invasion. A few microorganisms, however, can invade directly through these barriers, and others can cause infection if introduced into the body through lesions such as those occurring during surgery or trauma. If microorganisms do penetrate the body's outer barriers, the immune system usually deals with them quite easily, but some types of microorganisms possess special properties that allow them to overcome this system. In addition, some patients' immune systems do not function optimally, and this allows microorganisms that would normally not pose a problem to cause an infectious disease. When the immune system is depressed, the term *immunocompromised* is used. Two of the many ways in which this can occur involve the use of drugs that depress the immune response (e.g., corticosteroids) and infection with human immunodeficiency virus (HIV), which causes acquired immunodeficiency syndrome (AIDS).

Over the years, many different compounds have been used to assist the body's immune system in killing microorganisms. An especially important property that an anti-infective drug must possess is selective toxicity. The drug must be more toxic for the microorganism than for the host. An ideal anti-infective drug would kill the microorganisms while causing minimal or no adverse reaction in the host.

Each of the major categories of microorganisms that cause disease (bacteria, viruses, and fungi) has a unique physical structure and metabolism. The differences among them are so wide that a drug that is toxic for organisms in one category will usually not be active

against members of the other two categories. Thus, anti-infective drugs are divided into antibacterial, antiviral, and antifungal groups.

Although an anti-infective drug is assigned to one group on the basis of its selective toxicity, it is usually toxic for only some species within that group. The species against which a drug shows intrinsic activity is referred to as the drug's "spectrum of activity." A narrow-spectrum anti-infective drug is active against only a few species, while a broad-spectrum drug is active against a wide variety of microorganisms. Knowledge of a drug's spectrum of activity is useful in determining clinical applications for the drug.

As the anti-infectives are used to treat diseases, microorganisms develop various strategies to resist them. Resistance occurs when a microorganism that was originally in an anti-infective drug's spectrum of activity is no longer sensitive to that drug. As more microorganisms become drug-resistant, new drugs that have the resistant microorganism in their spectrum must be isolated from other microorganisms or produced in the laboratory.

The purpose of this chapter is to describe the mechanisms of action, spectra of activity, resistances, and potential adverse reactions for each of the major antibacterial, antiviral, and antifungal drugs. This basic knowledge will provide a foundation for the appropriate clinical application of the anti-infective drugs in the treatment of ocular disease.

Guidelines for Effective Antimicrobial Therapy

The clinical process of selecting an anti-infective drug for treatment of disease can be complex, and many

TABLE 6.1
Guidelines for Effective Antimicrobial Therapy

- Establish accurate clinical and laboratory diagnosis
- Select anti-infective drug to which the microorganism is sensitive
- Select least toxic anti-infective drug
- Establish adequate drug levels at site of infection
  - Select optimum route(s) of administration
  - Use appropriate dosage regimen
  - Prescribe drug for appropriate length of time
- Augment drug therapy with physical procedures

factors must be considered (Table 6.1). First, the patient's history, symptoms, and signs must be evaluated to establish a tentative diagnosis, and then a best "guess" regarding the causative microorganism(s) must be made. Based on this "guess," an anti-infective agent (or combination of agents) can be selected and therapy planned. Appropriate patient care requires that samples of tissue or body fluids be obtained for laboratory culture and identification so that the clinician's "guess" can be confirmed and the susceptibility of the isolated microorganism(s) to the anti-infective drugs can be assessed. Unfortunately, laboratory identification and susceptibility testing can take days, and anti-infective therapy must often be initiated before the process is complete.

After a drug has been selected for use, the clinician must determine what route(s) of administration will best ensure a therapeutic concentration at the site of infection. For different types of ocular infections, topical application, subconjunctival injection, oral administration, and intravitreal injection may each be appropriate (Table 6.2). Topical instillation of anti-infective drugs is the most common route for local therapy. Use of drug solutions is usually preferred over ointments for adults because ointments tend to blur vision after application. Ointments, on the other hand, are often preferred in the therapy of infants and young children because of the prolonged contact time between the drug and the eye and the resistance to tear washout.

When planning drug therapy, the clinician should estimate the length of time that the drug should be administered, since an appropriate period will eradicate the microorganisms while minimizing adverse reactions; excessive use of topically applied anti-infective drugs can cause hypersensitivity or toxicity reactions. In addition, using an antibacterial drug longer than necessary to eradicate the microorganism or using it inappropriately facilitates the development of resistant strains of bacteria. The risk of superinfection, which is an overgrowth of microorganisms that are usually held in check by the normal flora, also exists with the use of any antibacterial drug and especially with excessive use of multiple antibacterial drugs.

A final factor to consider in developing a treatment plan is to determine what physical procedures might augment the drug therapy. Such procedures can be especially useful when appreciable quantities of purulent exudate or necrotic tissue are present and must be removed from the site of the infection. As examples, the application of hot compresses to improve circulation and to remove crusting deposits on the lashes is especially useful in the treatment of lid infections with staphylococci; local massage, such as meibomian gland expression, facilitates the drainage of inflammatory products and allows better penetration of antibacterial drugs; and mechanical debridement of infected corneal epithelial cells in cases of herpetic keratitis removes much of the virus and may allow better application of the antiviral drug.

When a patient with an ocular disease fails to respond to anti-infective therapy even though an appropriate treatment plan was developed and carried out, a variety of explanations are possible. These are outlined in Table 6.3.

Antibacterial Drugs

Bacteria are a diverse group of single-celled microorganisms that, in most cases, can produce their own energy and cellular components. The largest division of bacteria, the "true" bacteria, can be subdivided by shape and gram stain reaction. Although there are many species of "true" bacteria, only a few are pathogenic in humans. The most common pathogenic bacteria and the infections they cause are shown in Table 6.4.

In addition to these pathogenic "true" bacteria, several groups of bacteria that have a unique structural morphology or metabolism also include pathogens that can cause ocular disease. The *Rickettsia* and *Chlamydia* are bacteria that mimic viruses in that they are intracellular parasites that must grow and multiply inside other living cells. The *Rickettsia* occur as harmless parasites in insects such as lice, ticks, and mites but, when transmitted to humans through bites, cause dis-

TABLE 6.2
Antibacterial Drugs of Choice for Initial Treatment of Selected Ocular Infections

Ocular Disease	Antibacterial Drugs	Route of Administration
Blepharitis		
Acute and chronic staphylococcal	Bacitracin, erythromycin, or gentamicin	Topical
Angular	Bacitracin, erythromycin, gentamicin, or zinc sulfate	Topical
Seborrheic	Bacitracin, erythromycin, or sodium sulfacetamide	Topical (prophylactic)
Acne rosacea	Tetracycline[1]	Oral
Conjunctivitis		
Acute mucopurulent	Gentamicin and/or bacitracin-polymyxin B	Topical
Hyperacute purulent	Bacitracin or gentamicin and	Topical
	Penicillin G or	Parenteral
	Ampicillin	Oral
Chlamydial	Tetracycline or erythromycin	Oral
Hordeolum		
External	Bacitracin, gentamicin, erythromycin, or sodium sulfacetamide	Topical (prophylactic)
Internal	Erythromycin or tetracycline	Oral
Dacryocystitis		
Acute	Penicillin G or	Intramuscular
	Penicillin V, erythromycin, or ampicillin and	Oral
	Erythromycin, sodium sulfacetamide, or gentamicin[2]	Topical (prophylactic)
Neonatal	Gentamicin, or sodium sulfacetamide, or erythromycin[3]	Topical (prophylactic)
Preseptal Cellulitis	Methicillin, oxacillin or nafcillin, and penicillin G and gentamicin[4,5]	Intravenous
	Tetracycline, erythromycin, or ampicillin[5]	Oral
Keratitis	Cefazolin and gentamicin or tobramycin[6-8]	Topical or subconjunctival and intravenous[9-14]
Endophthalmitis	Cephaloridine or cefazolin and gentamicin and	Topical and subconjunctival
	Cephaloridine, gentamicin, and	Intravitreal
	Cefazolin or gentamicin[15]	Intravenous

[1]Brown SI, Shahinian L. Diagnosis and treatment of ocular rosacea. Ophthalmology 1978;85:779–786.
[2]Berkow R, ed. The Merck manual, ed. 14. Rahway, NJ: Merck & Co, 1982.
[3]Tabbara KF. Infections of the lacrimal apparatus. In: Tabbara KF, Hyndiuk RA, eds. Infections of the eye. Boston: Little, Brown, 1986;34:551–562.
[4]Baum J. Therapy for ocular infections. Trans Ophthalmol Soc UK 1986;105:69–77.
[5]Jones DB. Microbial preseptal and orbital cellulitis. In: Duane TD, Jaeger EA, eds. Clinical ophthalmology. Philadelphia: Harper & Row, 1986;4(25):1–19.
[6]Jones DB. Decision-making in the management of microbial keratitis. Ophthalmology 1981;88:814–820.
[7]Jones DB. A plan for antimicrobial therapy in bacterial keratitis. Ophthalmology 1975;79:95–103.
[8]Abbott RL, Abrams MA. Bacterial corneal ulcers. In: Duane TD, Jaeger EA, eds. Clinical ophthalmology. Philadelphia: Harper & Row, 1986;4(18):1–34.
[9]Woo FL, Johnson P, Insler MS, et al. Gentamicin, tobramycin, amikacin and netilmicin levels in tears following intravenous administration. Arch Ophthalmol 1985;103:216–218.
[10]Town AE, Hunt ME. Concentration of penicillin in the aqueous humor following systemic administration. Am J Ophthalmol 1946;29:171–175.
[11]Baum J, Barza M. Topical vs. subconjunctival treatment of bacterial corneal ulcers. Ophthalmology 1983;90:162–168.
[12]Leibowitz HM, Ryan WJ, Kupferman A. Route of antibiotic administration in bacterial keratitis. Arch Ophthalmol 1981;99:1420–1423.
[13]Kupferman A, Leibowitz HM. Topical antibiotic therapy of Pseudomonas aeruginosa keratitis. Arch Ophthalmol 1979;97:1699–1702.
[14]Davis SD, Sarff LD, Hyndiuk RA. Topical tobramycin therapy of experimental Pseudomonas keratitis. Arch Ophthalmol 1978;96:123–125.
[15]Forster RK, Abbott RL, Gelender H. Management of infectious endophthalmitis. Ophthalmology 1980;87:313–319.

eases such as typhus and Q fever. The *Chlamydia* are transmitted through direct contact with an infected person; *Chlamydia trachomatis* can cause venereal disease, inclusion conjunctivitis, and trachoma. The spirochetes, which have a special morphology consisting of flexible spirals, include *Treponema pallidum,* which can cause syphilis with possible ocular complications including interstitial keratitis, optic neuritis and atro-

TABLE 6.3
Reasons for Antimicrobial Failure

- Inaccurate diagnosis
- Resistant microorganism
- Inadequate drug dosage (size, frequency, or duration)
- Patient noncompliance
- Inadequate supplemental physical procedures
- Inadequate patient immune response

phy, chorioretinitis with pigmentary changes, iridocyclitis, and Argyll Robertson pupil. Another special group of bacteria, the mycobacteria, are characterized by large quantities of lipid contained in their cells. They exhibit acid-fast staining, have slow growth rates, and under certain growth conditions are able to form long filamentous forms. A member of this group, *Mycobacterium tuberculosis,* can cause tuberculosis with the ocular complications of granulomatous uveitis, phlyctenular keratoconjunctivitis, optic neuritis, and Eales' disease. The *Actinomyces* are bacteria but are characterized by filamentous branching that closely resembles the hyphae produced by fungi. This group includes *Actinomyces israelii,* which can cause chronic conjunctivitis and canaliculitis, and *Nocardia asteroides,* which can cause chronic corneal ulcers and endophthalmitis.

When antibacterial drugs are used to treat infections, bacteria may become resistant to them.[1] This resistance can be of chromosomal origin or can be transmitted by extrachromosomal plasmids. Spontaneous chromosomal mutations occur naturally in the bacterial population, and the presence of an antibacterial agent allows drug-resistant mutants to multiply. Extrachromosomal plasmids carry mutated genes that produce resistance, and these plasmids can easily be transferred from one bacterium to another. Drug resistance produced by chromosomal mutations or extrachromosomal plasmids may take many forms. Perhaps the most common form involves the bacterial production of enzymes that can inactivate the antibacterial drug itself—some bacteria actually produce substances that attack the drugs being used to fight them.

Because of bacterial drug resistance, information about a pathogen's pattern of resistance/susceptibility is essential to the choice of a successful antibacterial agent. For purposes of in vitro testing, an organism is generally considered susceptible if the concentration of antimicrobial agent necessary to inhibit its growth is lower than that attainable in body fluids, particularly blood. Two types of laboratory tests are available to determine resistance/susceptibility to antibacterial drugs.[2] In diffusion testing, filter-paper discs containing fixed amounts of the antibacterial drugs are applied to the surface of an agar plate that has been previously streaked with the test organism. The antibacterial drug diffuses into the medium and either inhibits the growth of or kills the organism. When done as a standardized test, the size of the inhibition zone can then be translated into 1 of 3 categories: susceptible, resistant, or intermediate in susceptibility. In the second type of susceptibility testing, the dilution test, serial dilutions of the antibacterial drug are inoculated with the test organism to determine the minimal inhibitory concentration (MIC), which is the lowest concentration without apparent growth. The MIC is directly compared with the concentration of the antibacterial drug attainable in body fluids to determine resistance or susceptibility. Since the results of these in vitro tests correlate closely with in vivo results, they are useful in determining the most appropriate antibacterial drug for a particular infection.

Several differences exist between bacterial and human cells, and these differences form the basis for selective toxicity of the antibacterial drugs (Fig. 6.1). First, bacteria have a unique outermost layer—a cell wall—that is not found in any other microorganism or in any human cell. The bacterial cell wall is necessary for the bacterium's structural integrity; without it the bacterium usually undergoes lysis and dies. Several antibacterial drugs act by inhibiting synthesis of the cell wall, thus causing death of the bacteria[a] (Table 6.5).

A second structure in which a potential difference may exist between bacterial and human cells is their cell membranes. Because the membranes of both cell types are so similar, only a few compounds have been found that can selectively disrupt bacterial cell membranes while leaving those of the host cell intact (see Table 6.5).

A third difference between bacterial and human cells involves their ribosomes. Bacterial ribosomes are not the same size, nor do they have exactly the same composition, as human ribosomes. Thus, drugs that bind more to bacterial than to mammalian ribosomes can inhibit bacterial protein synthesis and have a selective toxicity for these cells. Many antibacterial drugs fit into this category (see Table 6.5).

A fourth difference between bacterial and human cells involves specific biosynthetic pathways (intermediary metabolism). Bacterial cells usually synthesize their own folic acid, while humans receive folic acid preformed in their food. Thus, drugs that can inhibit folic acid synthesis are selectively toxic for bacteria;

---

[a]Drugs that kill bacteria are termed *bactericidal. Bacteriostatic* implies that growth of the bacteria is inhibited.

TABLE 6.4
The Most Common Pathogenic Bacteria and the Infections They Cause

Bacteria	Systemic Disease	Ocular Disease
Gram-positive cocci		
Staphyloccoccus aureus	Skin abscesses, impetigo, wound infections, pneumonia and other systemic infections; enterotoxin-producing strains cause food poisoning	Acute and chronic blepharitis (ulcerative blepharitis), angular blepharo-conjunctivitis, acute and chronic mucopurulent conjunctivitis, dacryoadenitis, dacryocystitis, external and internal hordeola, central and marginal corneal ulcers, preseptal and orbital cellulitis, endophthalmitis
Staphylococcus epidermidis	Wound and systemic infections	Acute and chronic blepharitis (ulcerative blepharitis), acute and chronic conjunctivitis, central corneal ulcers, endophthalmitis
Streptococcus pyogenes	Impetigo, erysipelas, sore throat, scarlet fever, puerperal fever, wound and burn infections	Dacryocystitis, pseudomembranous and membranous conjunctivitis, central corneal ulcers, preseptal and orbital cellulitis, endophthalmitis
Streptococcus pneumoniae	Pneumonia and other systemic infections	Acute mucopurulent conjunctivitis, central corneal ulcers, chronic dacryocystitis, preseptal and orbital cellulitis, endophthalmitis
Streptococcus faecalis (enterococcus)	Endocarditis, urinary tract infections	
Viridans group of streptococci	Chronic mucosal infections, endocarditis	Acute pseudomembranous and membranous conjunctivitis
Gram-positive rods		
Corynebacterium diphtheriae	Diphtheria	Pseudomembranous and membranous conjunctivitis
Gram-negative cocci		
Neisseria gonorrhoeae	Gonorrhea	Hyperacute, purulent conjunctivitis
Neisseria meningitidis	Meningitis	Hyperacute, purulent conjunctivitis
Gram-negative rods		
Moraxella lacunata		Chronic angular blepharoconjunctivitis, central and peripheral corneal ulcers
Haemophilus influenzae	Respiratory tract infections, infant meningitis	Acute mucopurulent conjunctivitis, dacryocystitis, preseptal and orbital cellulitis, endophthalmitis
Pseudomonas aeruginosa	Burn, wound, and systemic infections	Central corneal ulcers, endophthalmitis
Escherichia coli Enterobacter aerogenes Salmonella species Proteus mirabilis Klebsiella pneumoniae Serratia marcescens Shigella species Acinetobacter species	Gastrointestinal, urinary tract, wound, and respiratory tract infections	Chronic conjunctivitis, central corneal ulcers, endophthalmitis

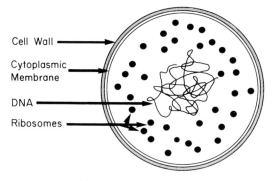

FIGURE 6.1 **Simplified diagram of a sphere-shaped bacterium showing cell wall, cytoplasmic membrane, ribosomes, and nuclear material. Bacteria do not have a nuclear membrane surrounding the DNA.**

several antibacterial drugs have been found to act in this way (see Table 6.5).

A fifth difference between bacterial and human cells involves the enzyme DNA gyrase. DNA gyrase mediates the supercoiling of DNA to enable this very long molecule to be enclosed by the cytoplasmic membrane. Drugs that selectively inhibit bacterial gyrase versus the corresponding human enzyme have a selective toxicity for bacteria. Several promising new drugs act in this manner (see Table 6.5).

Drugs Affecting Cell Wall Synthesis

Antibacterial drugs that affect bacterial cell wall synthesis include two large families, the penicillins and the cephalosporins, and two individual drugs, bacitracin and vancomycin (see Table 6.5).

Penicillins

PHARMACOLOGY

The penicillins act by inhibiting synthesis of the bacterial cell wall (Fig. 6.2). The rigid structure of the cell wall is due to peptidoglycan, which is a mucopeptide made up of linear, cross-linked polysaccharide chains. Bacterial cell wall synthesis is a complex process involving at least 30 enzymes.[3] Penicillins inhibit the terminal step in this process: the cross-linking of the polysaccharide chains through peptide bond formation (see Fig. 6.2). The cell walls thus develop abnormally, ultimately resulting in death of the organism. Penicillins exert their bactericidal effect most strongly on actively dividing cells that are synthesizing new cell walls.

TABLE 6.5
Classification of Antibacterial Drugs

Drugs affecting cell wall synthesis
  Penicillins
  Cephalosporins
  Bacitracin
  Vancomycin

Drugs affecting the cytoplasmic membrane
  Polymyxin B
  Colistin
  Gramicidin

Drugs affecting protein synthesis
  Aminoglycosides
    Streptomycin
    Neomycin
    Gentamicin
    Tobramycin
    Amikacin
    Kanamycin
  Tetracyclines
  Erythromycin
  Chloramphenicol
  Clindamycin

Drugs affecting intermediary metabolism
  Sulfonamides
  Pyrimethamine
  Trimethoprim

Drugs affecting bacterial DNA synthesis
  Nalidixic acid
  Quinolones
    Norfloxacin
    Ofloxacin
    Ciprofloxacin

The basic penicillin nucleus has been and continues to be chemically modified, so new penicillins with unique advantages frequently become available. Based on their spectra of antibacterial activity and their clinical applications, the penicillins can be divided into four categories (Table 6.6).

CLINICAL USES

Penicillins Highly Effective against Gram-Positive Bacteria. The two most important drugs in this category are penicillins G and V. The G form of the drug was originally derived from the fungus *Penicillium notatum,* while the V form is a semisynthetic derivative of penicillin G. Although penicillin G may be administered orally, its absorption is limited by its instability in gastric acid. Therefore, when therapy with an orally effective penicillin in this category is indicated, penicillin V is used. Both penicillins G and V are highly active against gram-positive cocci and are the antibiotics of choice for systemic infections caused by *Streptococcus pneumoniae, Streptococcus pyogenes,* and other

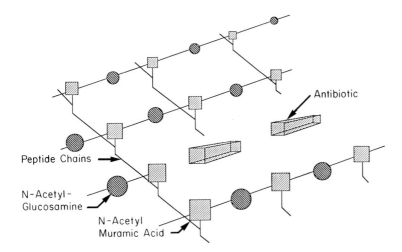

Peptide Chains

N-Acetyl-
Glucosamine

N-Acetyl
Muramic Acid

Antibiotic

FIGURE 6.2   **Structure of the peptidoglycan of the bacterial cell wall showing the mechanism of action of penicillin and cephalosporin antibacterial drugs.**

streptococci except enterococci. Since *Treponema pallidum* is sensitive to penicillin G, this antibiotic is the drug of choice for treatment of syphilis. Penicillin G is ineffective against gram-negative rod-shaped organisms such as *Pseudomonas* because it cannot penetrate their cell walls.[4]

The most important mechanism of acquired resistance to the penicillins is bacterial production of drug-inactivating enzymes such as β lactamases or penicillinases. Since most strains of *Staphylococcus aureus* produce penicillinase, penicillins G and V are not effective against this gram-positive bacterium. Penicillin G is usually active against gram-negative *Neisseria gonorrhoeae*, but penicillinase-producing strains of *N. gonorrhoeae* have now been isolated.[5] Although these resistant strains currently account for only a small per-

TABLE 6.6
Various Properties of Selected Penicillins

Drug	Route of Administration	Clinically Useful Spectrum of Activity
Penicillins highly effective against gram-positive bacteria		
Penicillin G	IV, IM	Most streptococci except enterococci, *Neisseria*, most
Penicillin V	PO	anerobes except *Bacteroides*, *Treponema*
Penicillins resistant to penicillinase		
Methicillin	IV, IM	*Staphylococcus aureus, Staphylococcus epidermidis*
Oxacillin	PO, IV, IM	
Cloxacillin	PO	
Dicloxacillin	PO	
Nafcillin	PO, IV, IM	
Penicillins with extended spectra of activity		
Ampicillin	PO, IV, IM	*Haemophilus influenzae*, streptococci including the viridans
Amoxicillin	PO	group, *Neisseria*
Penicillins with antipseudomonal activity		
Carbenicillin	IV	*Pseudomonas, Enterobacter, Proteus, Haemophilus influenzae,*
Ticarcillin		streptococci including the viridans group
Piperacillin	IV	*Pseudomonas, Enterobacter,* many *Klebsiella, Escherichia coli,*
Azlocillin		*Serratia, Proteus, Citrobacter*
Mezlocillin		

IV, intravenous; IM, intramuscular; PO, oral.

centage of gonococcal infections,[5] the number is increasing, and these strains pose a significant public health problem.

Topical use of the penicillins for the treatment of minor ocular infections such as blepharitis and conjunctivitis is limited by the high incidence of allergic reactions to the drug.[6] Because of this, other ocular antibacterial drugs, such as gentamicin, have replaced penicillin as agents of choice in the local treatment of minor, surface ocular infections. However, for the treatment of more serious ocular infections such as corneal ulcers caused by penicillin-sensitive staphylococci and micrococci, streptococci (including the pneumococcus), *Corynebacterium, Neisseria gonorrhoeae, Neisseria meningitidis,* and anaerobic gram-negative rods, penicillin G is still often administered in the form of fortified (concentrated) eyedrops, subconjunctival injection, and, if warranted, intravenous injection.[7] Although most strains of *Streptococcus pneumoniae* are sensitive to penicillin G, there is an increasing prevalence of resistant strains, and one such strain has been isolated from a bacterial keratitis.[8]

Penicillins Resistant to Penicillinase. Modification of the penicillin structure has produced a group of drugs including methicillin, oxacillin, cloxacillin, dicloxacillin, and nafcillin, which are not hydrolyzed by staphylococcal penicillinase. Their appropriate use is in the treatment of infections caused by strains of *Staphylococcus aureus* and *S. epidermidis* that produce penicillinase. These include the majority of the strains that have been isolated from hospital settings and the general community.[5] The initial therapy for infections in which *S. aureus* or *S. epidermidis* is a possible cause must therefore include a penicillinase-resistant penicillin or a cephalosporin. These drugs are usually administered concurrently with an antibiotic from the aminoglycoside family, which is active against gram-negative rods. The complementary spectra of the antibiotics in this combination cover most of the common pathogens.

Several ocular infections are treated with the penicillins in this category. Methicillin[9] or oxacillin[10] is injected subconjunctivally for the treatment of bacterial corneal ulcers caused by gram-positive cocci or penicillin-resistant staphylococci. Initial therapy for severe preseptal cellulitis is usually intravenous nafcillin or oxacillin and penicillin G plus an aminoglycoside to cover the gram-negative bacteria (see Table 6.2). If, however, only gram-positive bacteria are cultured from the infection site, treatment with methicillin, nafcillin, or oxacillin and penicillin G will usually be sufficient. For treatment of endophthalmitis, methicillin or dicloxacillin plus an aminoglycoside is often used as the initial therapy.[11]

Penicillins with Extended Spectra of Activity. Further modification of the basic penicillin structure has produced drugs including ampicillin and amoxicillin with broader spectra of activity than the original penicillins. Ampicillin and amoxicillin are less effective against bacteria that are sensitive to penicillin G, but their range of antimicrobial activity includes gram-negative bacteria such as *Haemophilus influenzae, Escherichia coli,* and *Proteus mirabilis.* Both drugs are destroyed by penicillinase and are thus ineffective against most staphylococci. Therapeutic indications for ampicillin and amoxicillin include gonococcal conjunctivitis, upper respiratory and urinary tract infections, bacterial meningitis, and *Salmonella* infections.

Penicillins with Antipseudomonal Activity. The chief advantage of the antipseudomonal penicillins—carbenicillin, azlocillin, mezlocillin, piperacillin, and ticarcillin—is that they are active against *Pseudomonas aeruginosa* and certain *Proteus, Enterobacter,* and *Acinetobacter* species not susceptible to most other penicillins. Patients with septicemia, burn infections, pneumonia, severe urinary tract disease, and meningitis caused by these organisms have often dramatically improved with use of carbenicillin, piperacillin, or ticarcillin. These three drugs are also used to treat patients with serious ocular infections caused by gram-negative bacteria, especially *Pseudomonas aeruginosa.* Carbenicillin or ticarcillin is used along with an aminoglycoside for the topical, subconjunctival, and, if necessary, intravenous treatment of bacterial corneal ulcers caused by gram-negative rods,[9,12] including *Pseudomonas aeruginosa.*[10]

SIDE EFFECTS

The major adverse reactions to the penicillins are hypersensitivity responses, with the incidence estimated at between 0.7% and 10%.[13] Manifestations of hypersensitivity include urticaria, angioedema and anaphylaxis (type I reaction), hemolytic anemia (type II reaction), interstitial nephritis, vasculitis and serum sickness (type III reaction), and contact dermatitis or Stevens-Johnson syndrome (type IV reaction). Once a patient has had a hypersensitivity reaction to any penicillin, it is probable, but not certain, that a reaction will occur with repeated exposure to the same penicillin or to any other penicillin.[5] Intradermal skin tests will predict whether a patient is at risk for developing a hypersensitivity reaction to the penicillin drugs.[5] If the results are positive, a penicillin drug should be used with considerable caution, if at all.

The penicillins, per se, are essentially nontoxic to humans. Most non-hypersensitivity reactions are caused by the irritant effects produced by excessive concentration in a small area of the body or by responses to another ingredient in the drug mixture. Most common among the irritative responses are pain and sterile inflammatory reactions at the site of intramuscular injection, with the severity of these reactions typically related to drug concentration. The most serious consequences of penicillin's irritant properties involve the nervous system. Accidental injection into a peripheral nerve can cause pain and dysfunction of the body part innervated by the affected nerve. High concentrations of penicillin in the central nervous system (CNS) can cause arachnoiditis, seizures, or fatal encephalopathy.[5]

Administration of large doses of any penicillin that is produced as a potassium salt may cause hyperkalemia, and large doses of other penicillins (most often carbenicillin and ticarcillin) can result in hypokalemia. Injection of penicillin G prepared with procaine may result in an immediate reaction characterized by dizziness, tinnitus, headache, hallucinations, and sometimes seizures due to the rapid liberation of toxic concentrations of procaine. Hematologic toxicity produced by penicillins is rare, but granulocytopenia has been encountered.[14] Large doses of carbenicillin and ticarcillin can prevent normal platelet aggregation, but significant bleeding disorders are relatively uncommon. Some individuals who receive penicillin intravenously develop phlebitis or thrombophlebitis.[5]

Penicillins alter the normal bacterial flora in areas of the body such as the respiratory and intestinal tracts. Many patients who take penicillin preparations by mouth experience nausea, vomiting, or diarrhea. This is usually of little clinical significance, since the normal microflora reestablish themselves quickly after cessation of therapy. However, a serious superinfection with resistant organisms such as *Pseudomonas, Proteus,* or *Candida* may follow long-term therapy with any penicillin. Superinfection with *Clostridium difficile* can lead to pseudomembranous colitis.[15]

CONTRAINDICATIONS

The reader should be aware of the drug-induced side effects, since they indicate contraindications to the use of penicillins.

Cephalosporins

PHARMACOLOGY

Penicillins and cephalosporins have similar mechanisms of action. They both interfere with the terminal step in bacterial cell wall formation by preventing proper cross-linking of the peptidoglycan (see Fig. 6.2). The cephalosporins also bind to enzymes associated with the cell membrane, and this triggers a complex series of reactions that may alter bacterial permeability, inhibit protein synthesis, and cause the bacteria to release autolysins. Some cephalosporins have a lytic effect, while others cause the bacteria to grow into long filamentous forms by preventing cellular division.

The important mechanisms of acquired resistance to cephalosporins include drug inactivation by β lactamases, to which the cephalosporins have variable susceptibility. For example, the β lactamases produced by *S. aureus* are considered to be true penicillinases and do not affect the cephalosporins.[16] Thus, the cephalosporins are usually active against penicillinase-producing *S. aureus*. In contrast, many of the cephalosporins are sensitive to inactivation by the β lactamases produced by gram-negative bacteria.

The parent cephalosporin compound has been extensively modified by adding different side chains to create a whole family of cephalosporin antibiotics. It is convenient to consider them as first-, second-, or third-generation compounds based on their spectra of bacterial activity and their clinical uses (Table 6.7).

CLINICAL USES

First-Generation Cephalosporins. First-generation cephalosporins include cephalothin, cefazolin, cephapirin, cephradine, cephalexin, cefadroxil, and cephaloridine. All have good activity against gram-positive bacteria and relatively modest activity against gram-negative bacteria. These drugs are, in addition, sensitive to many of the β lactamases produced by gram-negative bacteria, and this partially accounts for their somewhat limited range of clinical application.

Cephalosporins are frequently used clinically for surgical prophylaxis. Several first-generation cephalosporins have been successfully employed as prophylactic agents in certain cardiovascular, orthopaedic, head and neck, gastroduodenal, biliary tract, and gynecologic procedures.

Cefazolin has become a drug of first choice for treating bacterial corneal ulcers, either as part of a broad-spectrum approach[10] (see Table 6.2) or as a more specific treatment when gram-positive cocci are present.[7] Cefazolin is a drug of choice for several reasons.[10] First, its spectrum of activity encompasses penicillin-resistant staphylococci, *Proteus mirabilis,* streptococci including *S. pneumoniae,* and *E. coli.*[17] Second, it possesses greater activity against staphylococci and streptococci than other drugs such as bacitracin. Third, cefazolin is more soluble than cephaloridine, which is important in making the fortified solutions necessary for topical treatment of bacterial corneal ulcers, and, fourth, cefazolin may be used (with caution) in selected patients who are allergic to penicillin. Cefazolin may be administered both topically as fortified eyedrops or by subconjunctival injection.

TABLE 6.7
Various Properties of Selected Cephalosporins

Drug	Route of Administration	Clinically Useful Spectrum of Activity
First Generation		
Cephalothin	IV	Gram-positive cocci except enterococci, *Escherichia coli, Klebsiella, Proteus mirabilis*
Cefazolin	IV, IM	
Cephapirin	IV, IM	
Cephradine	PO, IV, IM	
Cephalexin	PO	
Cefadroxil	PO	
Cephaloridine	IV, IM	
Second Generation		
Cefamandole	IV, IM	Gram-positive cocci, *Haemophilus influenzae, Enterobacter, Proteus mirabilis, Escherichia coli, Klebsiella,* anaerobes especially *Bacteroides*
Cefoxitin	IV, IM	
Cefaclor	PO	
Ceforanide	IV, IM	
Cefuroxime	IV, IM	
Third Generation		
Ceftriaxone	IV, IM	*Escherichia coli, Klebsiella, Proteus, Haemophilus influenzae, Enterobacter, Serratia*
Ceftizoxime	IV, IM	
Cefotaxime	IV, IM	
Cefoperazone	IV, IM	All of the above plus *Pseudomonas*
Ceftazidime	IV, IM	

IV, intravenous; IM, intramuscular; PO, oral.

Cephaloridine, another first-generation cephalosporin, has sometimes been substituted for cefazolin in both the topical and subconjunctival treatment of bacterial corneal ulcers[7] (see Table 6.2). The recommended therapeutic regimen for the initial treatment of endophthalmitis also includes cephaloridine or cefazolin, along with an aminoglycoside[18] (see Table 6.2).

Second-Generation Cephalosporins. The second-generation cephalosporins include cefamandole, cefoxitin, cefaclor, ceforanide, and cefuroxime. These drugs are generally more active against gram-negative enteric bacteria than are first-generation analogs but are much less active against these organisms than are third-generation agents. For this reason, second-generation drugs have few current clinical applications.

Third-Generation Cephalosporins. Third-generation cephalosporins include ceftriaxone, ceftizoxime, cefotaxime, cefoperazone, and ceftazidime. These drugs are much more active against gram-negative organisms than are first- or second-generation drugs but are less active against gram-positive bacteria. Cefoperazone and ceftazidime are of particular value in treating ocular infections because they are also active against *Pseudomonas aeruginosa.*[17]

Second-generation cephalosporins, particularly cefoxitin, and most of the third-generation derivatives have been designed to be considerably more resistant to β lactamase activity than were the first generation drugs. Thus, they are especially useful for treating infections caused by gram-negative bacteria that produce β lactamase or that have become resistant to the aminoglycosides. These infections include gram-negative bacillary meningitis, pelvic and abdominal sepsis, lower respiratory tract infections, septicemia, and serious *Klebsiella* infections. Penicillinase-producing gonococcal infections can also be treated effectively with several of the penicillinase-resistant second- or third-generation cephalosporins.[19] Ophthalmia neonatorum caused by penicillinase-producing *Neisseria gonorrhoeae* has been treated successfully with a single intramuscular injection of ceftriaxone.[20,21]

SIDE EFFECTS

As with the penicillins, hypersensitivity reactions are the most common systemic adverse effects caused by cephalosporins. Maculopapular rash, urticaria, fever, bronchospasm, anaphylaxis and eosinophilia have all been associated with the use of cephalosporins. Because the structures of the penicillins and cephalosporins are very similar, patients who are allergic to penicillins may manifest a cross-reacting allergy when a cephalosporin is administered. Immunologic studies have found cross-reactivity in as many as 20% of penicillin-allergic patients,[22] but clinical reports suggest a lower range (5% to 10%) of cephalosporin reactions in penicillin-allergic patients.[23] This risk is greatly influenced by the severity of the prior reaction to penicillin. Therefore, a cephalosporin may be an effective substitute for penicillin in a patient who has an equivocal history of penicillin allergy (or a history of mild reactions), but one should not be used for a patient who has experienced a severe, immediate hypersensitivity reaction.

Like penicillins, cephalosporins alter the normal microflora of the body and can cause anorexia, nausea, vomiting, and diarrhea, with the diarrhea severe enough to warrant discontinuation of the drug in some cases. Antibiotic-associated pseudomembranous colitis due to *Clostridium difficile* can also occur with the cephalosporins[24,25]; it is important to consider this condition in the differential diagnosis of patients who develop diarrhea associated with cephalosporin use. Overgrowth of resistant organisms such as *Pseudomonas, Candida,* and enterococci can occur after long-term use of the cephalosporins. If the therapy is prolonged, patients should be closely monitored for signs of a superinfection, especially if the patient is severely ill or if invasive devices such as catheters have been used. In some patients, the third-generation cephalosporins destroy certain components of the intestinal microflora, and a vitamin K deficiency leading to bleeding episodes can result. This condition can be reversed by the administration of vitamin K.[26]

Reversible renal impairment has been reported following administration of cephalosporins,[27,28] and there may also be an additive nephrotoxicity when a cephalosporin and an aminoglycoside are administered concomitantly. This reaction is most likely to occur in the elderly and in patients with decreased renal function.

CONTRAINDICATIONS

The reader should be aware of the drug-induced side effects, since they indicate contraindications to the use of cephalosporins.

Bacitracin

PHARMACOLOGY

Bacitracin inhibits bacterial cell wall synthesis but acts at a different step in the process than do the penicillins and cephalosporins. It prevents the formation of polysaccharide chains that would normally be cross-linked to form the rigid peptidoglycan of the cell wall. The drug is bactericidal against gram-positive organisms such as staphylococci, streptococci and *Clostridium difficile* but is inactive against most gram-negative bacteria.

CLINICAL USES

Bacitracin is seldom used parenterally because renal necrosis has occurred after systemic use and because safer, more effective drugs with similar antibacterial spectra (such as the penicillins) are available. Bacitracin is primarily employed topically to treat skin and mucous membrane infections caused by gram-positive organisms because it is thought that only a few of these bacteria have become resistant to it.[29] A recent report,[30] however, has suggested that bacitracin may have poor activity against many strains of staphylococci and streptococci. If this finding is a widespread phenomenon, the general use of bacitracin for gram-positive infections should be reconsidered.

Bacitracin is available in topical preparations either as a single-entity product or as a component of fixed-combination products. Because bacitracin is unstable in solution, it is available only in ointment form in either type of product. The rationale for compounding drugs containing bacitracin along with other antibacterial agents, such as neomycin and polymyxin B, is that by judicious selection, combinations can be produced with complementary antibacterial spectra covering most of the common pathogens. The antibacterial spectrum of bacitracin is mostly gram-positive, while the spectrum of polymyxin B and neomycin is gram-negative. Thus, bacitracin complements either of the other two agents. Topical fixed-combination ointments containing bacitracin are very effective for a variety of dermatologic infections such as ulcers, external otitis, sycosis, and superficial folliculitis or impetigo. These topical combination products are also available as over-the-counter (OTC) preparations for use as skin prophylactics.

Topical ophthalmic preparations containing bacitracin (Tables 6.8 to 6.10) are effective for superficial infections of the eye, especially for staphylococcal blepharitis, since most staphylococci are still sensitive to bacitracin.[31] For treatment of staphylococcal blepharitis, warm compresses and lid scrubs are used to prepare the lid margin for the antibiotic. Bacitracin ophthalmic ointment is then placed on a sterile cotton applicator and rubbed along the base of the lashes. Initially this procedure may need to be performed several times daily, but the treatment can be reduced to once daily when the condition improves, usually after 1 to 2 weeks. Once the lids appear normal and symptoms have subsided, nightly treatments are often continued for an additional month or longer.

TABLE 6.8
Antibacterial Drugs for Topical Ocular Therapy

Generic Name	Formulation	Concentration	Trade Name (manufacturer)
Bacitracin	Ointment	500 U/g	Bacitracin (Various) AK-Tracin (Akorn)
Chloramphenicol	Solution	0.5%	Chloroptic (Allergan) Ophthochlor (Parke-Davis) Chlorofair (Pharmafair)
	Ointment	1%	Chloroptic S.O.P. (Allergan) Chloromycetin (Parke-Davis) Chlorofair (Pharmafair)
	Powder	25 mg/vial	Chloromycetin (Parke-Davis)
Chlortetracycline	Ointment	1%	Aureomycin (Lederle)
Erythromycin	Ointment	0.5%	AK-Mycin (Akorn) Ilotycin (Dista) Erythromycin (Various)
Gentamicin	Solution and ointment	0.3%	Gentak (Akorn) Genoptic (Allergan) Gentacidin (Iolab) Gentafair (Pharmafair) Garamycin (Schering)
Polymyxin B	Powder	500,000 U/vial	Polymyxin B Sulfate (Pfizer)
Tetracycline	Suspension and ointment	1%	Achromycin (Lederle)
Tobramycin	Solution and ointment	0.3%	Tobrex (Alcon)

TABLE 6.9
Combination Antibacterial Drugs for Topical Ocular Therapy

Generic Name	Concentration	Trade Name (manufacturer)
Solutions		
Polymyxin B Neomycin	16,250 U/ml 0.35%	Statrol (Alcon)
Polymyxin B Neomycin Gramicidin	10,000 U/ml 0.175% 0.0025%	Neosporin (Burroughs Wellcome) AK-Spore (Akorn) Neocidin (Major)
Ointments		
Polymyxin B Bacitracin	10,000 U/g 500 U/g	AK-Poly-Bac (Akorn) Polysporin (Burroughs Wellcome)
Polymyxin B Neomycin	10,000 U/g 0.35%	Statrol (Alcon)
Polymyxin B Oxytetracycline	10,000 U/g 0.5%	Terramycin w/Polymyxin (Pfipharmecs)
Polymyxin B Neomycin Bacitracin	10,000 U/g 0.35% 500 U/g	Mycitracin (Upjohn)
Polymyxin B Neomycin Bacitracin	10,000 U/g 0.35% 400 U/g	Neosporin (Burroughs Wellcome) AK-Spore (Akorn)

TABLE 6.10
Antibiotic-Steroid Combinations for Topical Ocular Therapy

Antibiotic	Steroid	Trade Name (manufacturer)
Solutions and Suspensions		
Neomycin 0.35%	Dexamethasone 0.1%	NeoDecadron (Merck)
Chloramphenicol 0.25%	Hydrocortisone 0.5%	Chloromycetin-Hydrocortisone (Parke-Davis)
Neomycin 0.35%	Hydrocortisone 0.5%	Neo-Cortef Suspension (Upjohn)
Neomycin 0.35% Polymyxin B 10,000 U/ml	Dexamethasone 0.1%	AK-Trol (Akorn) Maxitrol Suspension (Alcon) Dexacidin (Iolab) Dexasporin (Various)
Neomycin 0.35% Polymyxin B 10,000 U/ml	Hydrocortisone 1%	Bacticort (Rugby) Cortisporin (Burroughs Wellcome)
Neomycin 0.35% Polymyxin B 10,000 U/ml	Prenisolone 0.5%	Poly-Pred Suspension (Allergan)
Gentamicin 0.3%	Prednisolone 1%	Pred-G (Allergan)
Tobramycin 0.3%	Dexamethasone 0.1%	TobraDex (Alcon)
Ointments		
Neomycin 0.35%	Dexamethasone 0.05%	NeoDecadron (Merck)
Neomycin 0.35% Polymyxin B 10,000 U/g	Dexamethasone 0.1%	AK-Trol (Akorn) Maxitrol (Alcon) Dexacidin (Iolab) Dexasporin (Various)
Chloramphenicol 1% Polymyxin B 10,000 U/g	Hydrocortisone 0.5%	Ophthocort (Parke-Davis)
Neomycin 0.35% Bacitracin 400 U/g Polymyxin B 10,000 U/g	Hydrocortisone 1.0%	Cortisporin (Burroughs Wellcome)

For the initial treatment of bacterial corneal ulcers, bacitracin has been used in the form of fortified eyedrops.[9] Now, however, a penicillinase-resistant penicillin or cephalosporin is generally used in place of bacitracin to cover the gram-positive spectrum.[10]

SIDE EFFECTS

Hypersensitivity reactions, usually presenting as contact dermatitis, are rare but do occur when bacitracin is applied topically.[32] Superinfections have been observed after the use of mixtures containing bacitracin,[33] and this possibility should be considered if initial improvement is followed by a relapse of signs or symptoms.

CONTRAINDICATIONS

The reader should be aware of the drug-induced side effects of bacitracin, since they indicate the contraindications.

Vancomycin

PHARMACOLOGY

Like the other drugs discussed in this section, vancomycin acts by inhibiting biosynthesis of peptidoglycan during bacterial cell wall formation. It is highly active against gram-positive cocci (staphylococci and streptococci) as well as *Clostridium*, *Corynebacterium diphtheriae*, and *Neisseria gonorrhoeae*.

CLINICAL USES

Because of its toxicity, vancomycin is reserved for serious infections in which less toxic antibiotics are ineffective or not tolerated. Vancomycin, either alone or with an aminoglycoside, is used to treat bacterial endocarditis and for short-term prophylaxis against this condition in penicillin-allergic patients who are undergoing certain dental or surgical procedures. Vancomycin is an acceptable alternative to penicillins or cephalosporins for the treatment of serious infections caused by staphylococci, streptococci, or enterococci and is the drug of choice for treating infections caused by methicillin-resistant staphylococci. A case of blepharitis caused by a methicillin-resistant strain of *S. epidermidis* has resolved after treatment with topical vancomycin.[34] Oral vancomycin is also the drug of choice for treating patients with pseudomembranous colitis caused by *Clostridium difficile.*

SIDE EFFECTS

The use of vancomycin in large doses, with prolonged therapy, in concomitant or sequential use with other ototoxic or nephrotoxic drugs, or in patients with impaired renal function has caused permanent deafness and fatal uremia. Hearing and renal function should thus be monitored frequently when administering vancomycin.

CONTRAINDICATIONS

The reader should be aware of the drug-induced side effects, since they indicate the contraindications.

Drugs Affecting the Cytoplasmic Membrane

Antibacterial drugs that affect the bacterial cytoplasmic membrane include polymyxin B, colistin and gramicidin (see Table 6.5).

Polymyxin B and Colistin

PHARMACOLOGY

Of the large number of compounds that affect the bacterial cytoplasmic membrane, only a few have sufficient selective toxicity to be therapeutically useful. Polymyxin B and colistin (polymyxin E) are cationic detergents or surfactants that interact with the phospholipids of the cell's membranes, disrupting the osmotic integrity of the cell. This, in turn, increases the bacterial cells' permeability and causes leakage of intracellular molecules. The polymyxins are bactericidal and can kill non-dividing cells without necessarily lysing them.

CLINICAL USES

Both of these drugs are effective against gram-negative bacteria, but with the development of more effective, less toxic antibiotics, indications for the polymyxins have become limited. Currently, polymyxins are systemically administered primarily for serious infections caused by strains of *Pseudomonas aeruginosa* that are resistant to the antipseudomonal penicillins, the third generation cephalosporins, and the aminoglycosides. They are also used for gram-negative bacillary infections caused by organisms resistant to more preferred antibiotics or for patients who cannot tolerate the preferred drugs.

In combination with other antibacterial drugs or steroids, polymyxin B is useful for the prevention and treatment of skin infections and external otitis. It is also a popular antibiotic for treating common bacterial infections of the conjunctiva and lids. Polymyxin B is commercially available alone as an ophthalmic preparation (see Table 6.8) or in combination with other antibiotics (see Table 6.9) or with steroids (see Table 6.10). When prescribed for the treatment of bacterial conjunctivitis, an antibacterial combination containing polymyxin B should generally be used every 2 to 4 hours for 2 or 3 days or until the condition is controlled, and then 4 times a day for another week. Topical application or subconjunctival injection of polymyxin B has been used to treat corneal ulcers caused by *Pseudomonas aeruginosa,*[35] but the newer and less toxic penicillins or aminoglycosides are now the drugs of choice for this condition.

SIDE EFFECTS

The two most important side effects associated with systemic administration of polymyxins are neurotoxicity and nephrotoxicity. The incidence and severity of neurotoxicity produced by polymyxin B and colistin are essentially the same, but the risk of nephrotoxicity is greater with polymyxin B. Neurotoxic effects include dizziness, vertigo, ataxia, blurred vision, confusion, paresthesias, and numbness of the extremities. Muscular weakness, paresis, and complete paralysis also have been reported.[36] At appropriate systemic dosages, approximately 20% of patients experience nephrotoxicity as evidenced by a rising serum creatinine level, and 1% to 2% develop tubular necrosis. Anuria and tubular necrosis with serious renal failure are particularly common in patients who have received excessive doses or in whom drug use is continued despite impaired renal function.

Adverse reactions to topical application of poly-myxins, including irritation and allergic reactions of the eyelids and conjunctiva, are infrequent and typically mild. When administered by subconjunctival injection, polymyxin B may cause pain, chemosis, and tissue necrosis.

CONTRAINDICATIONS

The reader should be aware of the drug-induced side effects, since they indicate the contraindications for this drug.

Gramicidin

Gramicidin acts on bacteria in a fashion similar to polymyxin B and colistin in that it changes permeability characteristics of the cell membrane, killing the cell. However, in contrast to polymyxin B and colistin, gramicidin is effective against gram-positive bacteria and replaces bacitracin in some fixed-combination antibacterial solutions used topically for ocular infections (see Table 6.9).

Drugs Affecting Protein Synthesis

Antibacterial drugs that affect bacterial protein synthesis include the aminoglycoside family, the tetracycline family, and the single drugs erythromycin, chloramphenicol, and clindamycin (see Table 6.5).

Aminoglycosides

Since the isolation of streptomycin from *Streptomyces griseus* in the 1940s, one or another of the aminoglycosides has been a major antibiotic for the treatment of infections caused by gram-negative bacilli such as *P. aeruginosa, Proteus, Klebsiella, E. coli, Enterobacter,* and *Serratia.* Aminoglycosides are also effective against many strains of staphylococci but are not often used for systemic staphylococcal infections because a number of alternative antibiotics, such as penicillinase-resistant penicillins and cephalosporins, are effective and less toxic. In contrast to the other aminoglycosides, neomycin is a broad spectrum antibacterial drug active against many gram-positive as well as gram-negative bacteria. An important exception in its spectrum of activity is its ineffectiveness against *P. aeruginosa.*

PHARMACOLOGY

The aminoglycoside family of antibiotics includes streptomycin, neomycin, gentamicin, tobramycin, amikacin, and kanamycin. These drugs inhibit bacterial protein synthesis by binding to the 30S subunit of the bacterial ribosome (Fig. 6.3). The consequences of this interaction include inhibition of bacterial protein synthesis and an infidelity in correctly reading the genetic code.

Bacterial resistance to the aminoglycosides by gram-negative bacilli is widespread. This resistance is achieved by one or more of the following three mechanisms: alteration of the bacterial cell's ribosomes, decreased antibiotic uptake, and enzymatic inactivation of the drugs. Enzymatic inactivation is the most common and important type of resistance and results in production of a modified form of the drug that is not only inactive but that blocks further uptake of the active drug into the cell. There are many different aminoglycoside inactivating enzymes, with some enzymes inactivating certain drugs but not others. Cross-resistance among aminoglycosides that are susceptible to the same inactivating enzymes is often complete. For example, bacteria resistant to gentamicin are usually also resistant to tobramycin but, as an exception to this generalization, some gentamicin-resistant *Pseudomonas* strains remain sensitive to tobramycin.[37] Thus, known resistance patterns are helpful only in the initial selection of an aminoglycoside. The specific sensitivity to

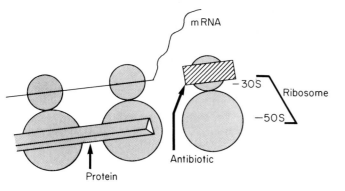

FIGURE 6.3 **Bacterial ribosomes showing the mechanism of action of the aminoglycosides, antibacterial drugs that inhibit protein synthesis.**

each drug must be determined for the individual pathogen.

The aminoglycosides are poorly absorbed from the gastrointestinal tract and must be given parenterally when used systemically. Note that penicillins may inactivate aminoglycosides if mixed together in the same solution for injection or for topical application, so each must be administered separately.

CLINICAL USES

Streptomycin.   Streptomycin is bactericidal against a variety of aerobic gram-negative bacilli and certain mycobacteria. More effective aminoglycoside antibiotics and other antituberculosis agents have replaced streptomycin except for the treatment of certain rare infections such as bacterial endocarditis, tularemia, plague, and the most serious forms of tuberculosis.

Neomycin.   Neomycin is the most toxic aminoglycoside antibiotic. It is available for oral, topical, and parenteral administration, but there are few or no indications for parenteral administration. Oral administration is employed chiefly to prepare the bowel for surgery and as an adjunct to hepatic coma therapy.

The most common form of neomycin administration is topical. The drug is available in combination with other antibiotics or steroids in numerous ophthalmic (see Tables 6.9 and 6.10), otic, and dermatologic preparations designed to treat a variety of skin and mucous membrane infections. Topical ocular application of neomycin frequently results in sensitization to the drug, which leads to contact dermatitis in about 4% of patients (Color Plate II).[33,38] Therefore, routine use of topical preparations containing neomycin is not recommended, and other individual drugs or combinations, such as bacitracin-polymyxin B, should be substituted.

Gentamicin.   Gentamicin remains a mainstay in the treatment of serious gram-negative bacillary infections. Systemic uses include complicated urinary tract infections, pneumonia, meningitis, and peritonitis in which the causal organism is a gram-negative bacillus sensitive to the drug.

Topical dermatologic preparations of gentamicin are most commonly used for the treatment of infected burns. Topical ophthalmic gentamicin (see Table 6.8) is used to treat a variety of bacterial infections of the external eye and adnexa such as conjunctivitis, blepharitis, keratoconjunctivitis, and dacryocystitis. Since most of the bacteria that cause these infections (staphylococci, *H. influenzae,* and gram-negative rods) are still sensitive to this antibiotic, gentamicin is efficacious for the treatment of these diseases. This has been substantiated in several clinical studies of external infections in which a favorable therapeutic response to a 0.3% solution or ointment was demonstrated.[39,40] In 1 study,[41] the clinical effectiveness (cured or improved) was 99% and the bacteriologic cure rate was 70%. Several investigators[42,43] have found gentamicin to be as effective as a combination of neomycin, bacitracin, and polymyxin B for treating external ocular infections. Currently it is generally recognized that gentamicin is an antibiotic of choice for the initial treatment of bacterial infections of the external eye (see Table 6.2). Treatment typically involves instilling 1 or 2 drops of gentamicin every 4 hours. In severe infections, dosage may be increased to as much as 2 drops every hour. If using the ointment, a small amount (one-quarter inch) is applied to the affected eye 2 to 3 times a day for 7 to 10 days.

For many years gentamicin has been an antibiotic of choice for the initial treatment of bacterial corneal ulcers (see Table 6.2).[10] In the treatment of these ulcers, it is usually used in combination with a penicillinase-resistant penicillin or cephalosporin. Gentamicin, sometimes in combination with a penicillin having antipseudomonal activity (such as carbenicillin or ticarcillin), is a specific treatment of choice for *Pseudomonas* corneal ulcers.[7,10]

Similar to the initial treatment of bacterial corneal ulcers, the initial treatment of bacterial endophthalmitis usually includes two antibiotics: a cephalosporin or a penicillin to which penicillinase-producing staphylococci are sensitive, and another drug, usually gentamicin, to which gram-negative bacilli are sensitive (see Table 6.2).[18] The practitioner may choose to use these antibiotics systemically, topically, subconjunctivally, or intravitreally.

The side effects encountered with topical gentamicin are rare but include occasional minor irritation, especially when the drug is first instilled, punctate epithelial keratopathy, delayed wound healing, and pseudomembranous conjunctivitis.[40] On rare occasions focal areas of bulbar conjunctival hyperemia that stain with sodium fluorescein may be seen.[44] One case has been reported of periocular skin and conjunctival paresthesia occurring after topical gentamicin application.[45] Allergic reactions to topical gentamicin are infrequent, but about 50% of patients who are allergic to neomycin are also allergic to gentamicin.[46]

Tobramycin.   Tobramycin is available as a topical ophthalmic solution and ointment (see Table 6.8) and as a powder for parenteral administration. Since the antibacterial activity and pharmacokinetic properties of tobramycin are very similar to those of gentamicin, its therapeutic uses are essentially identical to those for gentamicin (see Table 6.2).[47] However, tobramycin is more active against *P. aeruginosa,*[37,48] including some gentamicin-resistant strains,[37] and, in combination with an antipseudomonal penicillin (such as ticarcillin or carbenicillin), is usually preferred for infections caused by this organism. Tobramycin may also be less toxic than gentamicin when injected into the vitreous, and this may make it a more desirable drug for the treatment of bacterial endophthalmitis.[49] In contrast to *Pseudomonas,* cross-resistance between gentamicin and tobramycin for most strains of *Klebsiella, Enterobacter, E. coli,* and *Serratia* is common[37]; amikacin is usually effective for infections caused by organisms resistant to both gentamicin and tobramycin.

There is concern about the possibility that the widespread use of a clinically important antibacterial drug like tobramycin could facilitate the emergence of bacteria resistant to the drug, and it has therefore been suggested that tobramycin use should be limited. A number of reports[50,51] have correlated the development of progressive resistance to the aminoglycosides with greater aminoglycoside use, yet in other reports this association has not always been found.[52,53] In one study[53] the resistance to tobramycin closely paralleled gentamicin resistance despite limited and controlled use of tobramycin; the restricted use of tobramycin did not prevent or delay the development of resistance to it. Certainly, strategies that limit the emergence of bacterial strains resistant to the aminoglycosides must be considered, but it is not clear that restricting the use of tobramycin is a worthwhile strategy.

Topical administration of tobramycin can cause reversible tearing, burning, photophobia, eyelid edema, conjunctival hyperemia and chemosis, and punctate epithelial erosions.[47]

Amikacin. Amikacin was the first semisynthetic aminoglycoside marketed. Because a chemical modification present in amikacin protects the molecule from aminoglycoside-inactivating enzymes, it has become the preferred drug for the treatment of gram-negative bacillary infections in which resistance to gentamicin and tobramycin is encountered.[54] At the clinical level, however, there is little or no evidence for the superiority or inferiority of amikacin versus gentamicin or tobramycin as a treatment for infections caused by susceptible organisms.

Since amikacin is active against many gram-negative bacilli that are resistant to other aminoglycosides, it deserves consideration as a primary drug (along with a cephalosporin) for the treatment of bacterial endophthalmitis. Successful management of 4 cases of bacterial endophthalmitis with intravitreal amikacin in conjunction with cephalosporins has demonstrated the safety and effectiveness of this approach.[55] The aminoglycosides, especially amikacin, are the drugs of

choice for treating corneal ulcers due to infection with mycobacteria.[7]

Kanamycin. The use of kanamycin has declined in recent years due to limited spectrum of activity (it is inactive against *Pseudomonas* and most gram-positive bacteria) and the large number of strains resistant to it. Major remaining uses of kanamycin involve preparing the bowel for surgery and as an adjunct therapy in cases of hepatic coma.

SIDE EFFECTS

Both vestibular and auditory dysfunction resulting from progressive destruction of vestibular or cochlear sensory cells can follow systemic administration of any of the aminoglycosides. Initial symptoms of cochlear damage include tinnitus or a sensation of pressure or fullness in the ears. Vestibular dysfunction is manifest by nystagmus, vertigo, nausea, vomiting, or acute Meniere's syndrome. Patients receiving aminoglycosides must be carefully monitored for ototoxicity, since only the early symptoms may be reversible on discontinuation of the drug. If the drugs are used long enough or at high dosages, resultant toxicity can produce sensory cell death, and the dysfunction, in most cases, becomes irreversible. A dynamic illegible E test has been proposed as a sensitive screening procedure for detecting aminoglycoside ototoxicity.[56] During the test, the patient's best visual acuity is measured using the illegible E chart. The patient then oscillates his or her head from left to right and back at a frequency of 1 Hz and is asked to read the chart again. A deterioration in visual acuity suggests an infidelity of the vestibulo-ocular reflex that can be associated with aminoglycoside toxicity.

The very high concentrations of aminoglycosides that can accumulate in the kidney and urine are correlated with the potential for these drugs to cause nephrotoxicity in the form of acute tubular necrosis. Fortunately, early changes are usually reversible if the drug is discontinued.[57] Since the incidence and severity of nephrotoxicity and ototoxicity are directly related to the aminoglycoside concentration in the body and to the length of exposure to the drug, it is important to use these antibiotics only when less toxic antibiotics are not effective. Drug levels in the body should be monitored, and the dosage for patients with impaired renal function should be reduced. Although toxicity varies among the different aminoglycosides, it can be minimized by careful drug selection and control of plasma concentrations.

Systemic aminoglycoside administration has been associated with neuromuscular blockade.[47] This syndrome is characterized by respiratory depression with possible cardiac arrest. The pupils may become dilated, and a myasthenic effect may occur with generalized muscular weakness of the extremities, paralysis of the extraocular muscles, and ptosis.[59] Neuromuscular blockade can be reversed by calcium gluconate. Another rare, visually related side effect that has been produced by systemic gentamicin use is pseudotumor cerebri with secondary papilledema.[58]

CONTRAINDICATIONS

The reader should be aware of the drug-induced side effects of the aminoglycosides, since they indicate the contraindications.

Tetracyclines

PHARMACOLOGY

Tetracyclines are a family of antibiotics that have been isolated from species of *Streptomyces* or produced in the laboratory. Based on differences in their pharmacology, tetracycline analogs are usually divided into 3 groups: short-acting analogs (half-lives of 6 to 9 hours); intermediate-acting analogs; and long-acting analogs (half-lives of 17 to 20 hours) (Table 6.11). All the analogs are closely related chemically and generally have similar patterns of bacterial susceptibility and resistance. Tetracycline is the least expensive of the analogs and is usually preferred for oral administration. Doxycycline appears to be equally effective and is preferred to tetracycline when intravenous administration is required. One percent tetracycline suspension and ointment and 1% chlortetracycline ointment are available for topical ocular use (see Table 6.8) as is a fixed-combination ointment containing oxytetracycline and polymyxin B (see Table 6.9).

Tetracyclines enter bacteria by an energy-dependent process. Once inside, they bind to the 30S subunit of the ribosome, blocking the attachment of aminoacyl-tRNA to the receptor site on the messenger RNA-ribosome complex. The tetracyclines also inhibit protein synthesis in human cells but do not accumulate within these cells by an active process. This may explain the difference in degree of protein inhibition produced in host cells versus microorganisms. The difference in active transport, however, does not account for the high sensitivity of various intracellular bacteria such as *Chlamydia* and *Rickettsia* to the tetracyclines; other, as yet undiscovered factors appear to be involved.[60]

In addition to its antibiotic properties against pathogenic microorganisms, tetracycline appears to have other actions that can change the course of disease progression. When patients with acne vulgaris (a non-

infectious inflammatory disease) receive tetracycline, 2 changes occur: amelioration of their acne and a reduction in the composition of free fatty acids in their surface sebum.[61] Since the free fatty acids are probably produced by normal bacterial flora, this suggests that tetracycline is therapeutically effective in this disorder due to its antibiotic properties against normal bacteria, not against pathogens. In addition to its antimicrobial properties, anticollagenolytic activity has been demonstrated for tetracycline, and this action may be responsible for its effectiveness in treating certain noninfectious diseases.[62]

CLINICAL USES

The tetracyclines are broad-spectrum antibacterial drugs that are active against gram-positive, gram-negative, aerobic, and anaerobic bacteria as well as spirochetes, *Mycoplasma*, *Rickettsia*, *Chlamydia*, and some protozoa. Even though the tetracyclines are broad spectrum, their usefulness against some of the more common types of microbial pathogens, such as *S. aureus*, is decreasing due to resistance.[63,64] Because of this and the development of newer anti-infective drugs that are more effective for specific infections, the number of clinical indications for the tetracyclines has declined. Tetracyclines, however, remain the drugs of choice (or very effective alternative therapy) for a wide variety of infections caused by less common pathogens. These infections include brucellosis, rickettsial infections (such as Rocky Mountain spotted fever, typhus, and Q fever), *Mycoplasma* pneumonia, cholera, plague, *Ureaplasma* urethritis, and chlamydial infections (such as venereal disease, trachoma, and inclusion conjunctivitis).

Ophthalmic ointments containing a tetracycline or erythromycin are recommended by the Centers for Disease Control (CDC) as an effective alternative to silver nitrate for prophylaxis of gonococcal ophthalmia neonatorum.[65,66] A major advantage of using one of the tetracyclines is that they do not cause the chemical conjunctivitis typically produced by silver nitrate but do protect the eyes from infection with pathogenic microorganisms.[67]

Chlamydial ophthalmia neonatorum has been treated with topical tetracycline, but topical application may not be the most effective form of treatment because the *Chlamydia* are not always totally eradicated from the body.[68] Systemic tetracycline could be used but it causes side effects (discussed later) in children under age 8 years. For these reasons, oral erythromycin, an equally effective agent, is the drug of choice for this disease.[68,69]

In adults, tetracycline is the drug of choice for treating the chlamydial diseases, including chlamydial venereal disease, inclusion conjunctivitis, and trachoma.[60,70,71] The traditional treatment for adult inclu-

TABLE 6.11
Tetracyclines: Classes, Oral Doses, and Relative Costs

Generic Name	Trade Name	Oral Preparations	Usual Adult Dosage	Relative Cost Compared with Tetracycline (per capsule)
Short-acting				
Tetracycline	Tetracycline Achromycin V Cyclinex Cyclopar Nor-Tet Panmycin Retet Robitet Sumycin Tetra-C Tetracap Tetracyn Tetralan Tetram	100, 250, 500 mg capsules 250, 500 mg tablets	250–500 mg q.i.d.	250 mg—1
Oxytetracycline	Oxytetracycline E.P. Mycin Terramycin Uri-tet	250 mg capsules 250 mg tablets	250–500 mg q.i.d.	250 mg—2–3
Intermediate-acting				
Methacycline	Rondomycin	150, 300 mg capsules	150 mg q.i.d. or 300 mg b.i.d.	150 mg—90
Demeclocycline	Declomycin	150 mg capsules 150, 300 mg tablets	150 mg q.i.d. or 300 mg b.i.d.	150 mg—70
Long-acting				
Doxycycline	Doxycycline Doxy-Lemmon Doxychel Hyclate Vibramycin Vivox AK Ramycin Doxy-Caps Doryx AK Ratabs Vibra-Tabs	50, 100 mg capsules 50, 100 mg tablets	200 mg, then 100 mg q.d. or b.i.d.	100 mg—3–5
Minocycline	Minocin	50, 100 mg capsules 50, 100 mg tablets	200 mg, then 100 mg b.i.d.	100 mg—65

Modified from: Salamon SS. Tetracyclines in ophthalmology. Surv Ophthalmol 1985;29:265–275.
q.i.d., four times daily; b.i.d., twice daily; q.d., once a day.

sion conjunctivitis and trachoma is oral tetracycline, 1 g daily in 4 divided doses for 3 weeks. Two reports[72,73] suggest that doxycycline may be even more effective than tetracycline for treating these diseases, but this has not been substantiated in clinical trials. An effective dosage regimen for oral doxycycline is an initial dose of 300 mg on the first day followed by a daily dose of 100 mg for 2 weeks.[73] Topical treatment with oxytetracycline ointment, twice daily for 6 weeks, can also reduce trachomatous inflammation, but incomplete cure and subsequent disease transmission can result.[74] Therefore, oral tetracycline is still the most effective treatment for these conditions.

Some surface ocular infections, such as conjunctivitis and keratitis caused by susceptible microorganisms, respond well to topical tetracyclines. However, many of the organisms that cause infections of this type are either resistant or not responsive to tetracyclines. One-third or more of staphylococcal strains may be resistant, and *Pseudomonas aeruginosa* is rarely responsive.[63,75] Therefore, when the microorganism responsible for a surface ocular infection is unknown, a topical tetracycline is not usually the drug of choice.

Tetracycline can be an effective therapy for noninfectious conditions involving the eye. Oral tetracycline has been an effective treatment for recalcitrant (i.e., resistant to corticosteroid therapy) cases of nontuberculous phlyctenular keratoconjunctivitis.[76] The treatment resulted in rapid relief of symptoms and an apparent arrest of the disease. The dosage regimen consisted of 250 mg of tetracycline 2 to 3 times a day until 3 weeks after the patient was completely asymptomatic. The dosage was then decreased until the lowest possible maintenance dose was achieved. Phlyctenular keratoconjunctivitis is considered to be a delayed hypersensitivity reaction to foreign protein, especially the proteins associated with bacteria. The manner in which systemic tetracycline affects the ocular flora or alters the antigenically stimulated immune response remains unclear.

Oral tetracycline may also be effective for resolving noninfected corneal ulcers or "corneal melting" in which there is progressive necrosis of stromal tissue despite being culture negative.[77] This form of sterile ulceration is thought to be mediated by the action of tissue collagenases, and the anticollagenolytic activity of systemic tetracycline may explain its effectiveness.[62] Similarly, the anticollagenolytic activity of tetracycline may be clinically useful in treating persistent epithelial defects. Perry and associates[79] gave oral tetracycline (1 g daily divided into 4 doses) to 18 patients with persistent epithelial defects. The defects in 14 of the patients healed, while the other 4 showed either no improvement or worsened.

Tetracycline is effective in improving the ocular manifestations (irritation, blepharitis, keratitis, meibomianitis, and chalazia) of acne rosacea.[78] The suggested treatment regimen is 250 mg 4 times a day, reduced by 1 daily dose after every month of therapy, until a symptom-free maintenance dose level is determined. Some patients may be able to discontinue medication without recurrence of symptoms, but others must continue on low maintenance doses for extended periods. Brown and Shahinian[78] reported that many patients who had eyelid cultures positive for *S. aureus* at the initiation of tetracycline treatment continued to have positive cultures even though the signs and symptoms of ocular rosacea disappeared. This suggests that *S. aureus* does not have a prominent role in the etiology of this condition, even though the organism is often isolated from patients with the disease.

SIDE EFFECTS

Hypersensitivity reactions to tetracyclines, including anaphylaxis, urticaria, periorbital edema, and morbilliform rashes, can occur but are not common. Photosensitivity, manifest by an exaggerated sunburn reaction, is common in patients receiving demeclocycline but can occur with all analogs.[63,75]

All tetracyclines have relatively low toxicity at the usual dosage levels, but systemic use, especially oral administration, can produce varying degrees of gastrointestinal irritation in some patients. Anorexia, heartburn, nausea, vomiting, flatulence, and diarrhea are common. These reactions are not usually disabling but may become severe enough to require discontinuation or interruption of therapy. When diarrhea is severe or persistent, pseudomembranous colitis caused by *Clostridium difficile* must be considered. The administration of tetracyclines with food may ameliorate their irritative effects, but food can adversely affect their absorption. All tetracyclines can form complexes with cations, so their absorption is markedly decreased when administered with dairy products, iron-containing tonics, or antacids containing calcium, magnesium, or aluminum. Sodium bicarbonate also has an adverse effect on absorption.[80]

Tetracyclines can produce negative nitrogen balance and increased blood urea nitrogen (BUN) levels.[81] This is of little clinical importance when the usual doses are given to patients with normal renal function, but tetracyclines may cause azotemia in patients with impaired renal function. Thus, the only tetracycline that should be used with such patients is doxycycline because it is excreted mainly through the intestinal tract and not through the kidneys.

Tetracyclines are attracted to embryonic and growing bone tissue, in which they form a tetracycline-calcium orthophosphate complex, temporarily depressing bone growth. They can also cause changes in both deciduous and permanent teeth during the time of tooth development; these changes include dysgenesis, staining, and an increased tendency to caries. Discoloration may be progressive and can vary from yellowish brown to dark gray. Because of bone growth depression and tooth discoloration, tetracyclines should be avoided during the last half of pregnancy, in lactating women, or in children under 8 years of age.[82]

Intracranial hypertension (pseudotumor cerebri) secondary to use of many tetracycline analogs has been described in infants and adults.[83,84] When the antibiotic is discontinued, cerebral spinal fluid pressure, with accompanying visual and ophthalmoscopic changes, usually returns to normal over days or weeks.[83,84]

Atypically, tetracyclines can cause liver damage, which appears histologically as a fine droplet fatty metamorphosis and results in a high mortality. This type of hepatic damage has been associated with the intravenous administration of 2 g or more daily.[85] Administration of less than 2 g daily intravenously is not usually associated with liver dysfunction or injury except in pregnant women and in patients with excessive serum levels due to renal failure. Blood dyscrasias such as hemolytic anemia, thrombocytopenia, neutropenia, and eosinophilia have also been reported with tetracyclines, but these are rare.[63]

Vestibular toxicity is unique to minocycline.[63] Lightheadedness, loss of balance, dizziness, nausea, and tinnitus usually begin 2 to 3 days after starting therapy and occur in up to 70% of patients. Although these side effects are usually reversible after discontinuation of the drug, they have severely limited the use of minocycline.

Tetracyclines can interact in significant ways with other drugs, and these interactions should be considered when the patient is taking concomitant medications. Tetracyclines can potentiate the effects of the coumarin-type anticoagulants and seriously interfere with blood clotting. They may also interfere with the bactericidal action of the penicillins after concomitant parenteral administration, and such use should be avoided. Carbamazepine (Tegretol), diphenylhydantoin,[86] and barbiturates[87] decrease the normal half-life of doxycycline to almost half by increasing the hepatic metabolism of the antibiotic, so tetracycline dosages must be increased to compensate for this factor or a different antibiotic should be selected.

CONTRAINDICATIONS

The reader should be aware of the drug-induced side effects of the tetracylines, since they indicate the contraindications.

Erythromycin

PHARMACOLOGY

Erythromycin inhibits bacterial protein synthesis by binding to the 50S ribosomal subunit and preventing elongation of the peptide chain (Fig. 6.4). Its low toxicity is accounted for by the fact that it does not bind to mammalian ribosomes. At one time erythromycin was thought to be only bacteriostatic, but it is now considered to have bactericidal properties that depend on the organism and the drug concentration.

CLINICAL USES

Erythromycin has a limited antibacterial spectrum, being primarily effective against gram-positive bacteria. It is the drug of first choice for relatively few infections, but it does have a significant number of important applications as an alternative to penicillin. Among the few infections for which erythromycin is the drug of choice is legionnaires' disease, caused by *Legionella pneumophilia*. Primary atypical pneumonia caused by *Mycoplasma pneumoniae* may also be more responsive to erythromycin than to the tetracyclines, and erythromycin is therefore considered a drug of choice for this infection. Patients with diphtheria have been treated successfully with erythromycin and diphtheria antitoxin, with erythromycin being preferred for treating carriers of this disease. Erythromycin is also useful in acute, symptomatic *Campylobacter* enteritis, and erythromycin plus neomycin is the preferred prophylactic regimen for colorectal surgery.

Erythromycin is routinely employed as an alternative to penicillin for the treatment of streptococcal infections including pharyngitis, scarlet fever, cellulitis and erysipelas caused by *Streptococcus pyogenes,* and pneumonia and bronchitis caused by *Streptococcus pneumoniae*. It is also used as an alternative to penicillin for the prophylaxis of rheumatic fever recurrences and for preventing endocarditis resulting from dental procedures. Erythromycin is an alternative drug for

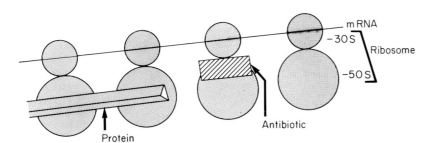

FIGURE 6.4 **Bacterial ribosomes showing the mechanism of action of erythromycin, an antibacterial drug that inhibits protein synthesis.**

acute otitis media due to *S. pneumoniae* or *S. pyogenes*, and erythromycin plus a sulfonamide can be used for children with otitis media caused by *H. influenzae*. The emergence of appreciable numbers of resistant strains of *S. aureus*, coupled with the availability of penicillinase-resistant penicillins and cephalosporins, has reduced the use of erythromycin for infections caused by this organism. Erythromycin is an alternative to penicillin for the treatment of anthrax, actinomycosis, *Listeria* infections, and certain anaerobic infections. It can also be used as an alternative for the treatment of syphilis and gonorrhea.

Staphylococcal infections of the eyelid are commonly treated with erythromycin ointment (see Tables 6.2 and 6.8) applied as a lid scrub. Supplemental therapy with warm, moist compresses followed by gentle shampooing of the lid margins with dilute baby shampoo should be done before application of the drug. Erythromycin ointment can be applied at bedtime or more often if the severity of the infection requires.

As discussed earlier, erythromycin and tetracycline ointments are recommended by the CDC as acceptable alternatives to the traditional use of silver nitrate for the prophylaxis of ophthalmia neonatorum.[65] Similar to silver nitrate, erythromycin is effective for prophylaxis of gonococcal ophthalmia neonatorum,[88,89] but, in contrast to silver nitrate, erythromycin is also effective for prevention of neonatal conjunctivitis due to *Chlamydia trachomatis*.[90] For prophylaxis, an approximately 0.5 to 1 cm ribbon of ointment is instilled into each conjunctival sac and is not flushed from the eyes following application.

Chlamydia trachomatis infections in infants and children are additional primary indications for the use of erythromycin. This antibiotic is as effective as the tetracyclines for chlamydial infections and is safer for pregnant women, nursing mothers, and children under 8 years of age. For infants with chlamydial ophthalmia neonatorum, effective therapy is provided by oral erythromycin, 25 mg/kg body weight every 12 hours for a minimum of 2 weeks.[69]

Erythromycin is also an effective alternative to tetracycline for the treatment of adult chlamydial venereal disease. Adults should receive 1 to 1.5 g of erythromycin daily in 4 divided doses for 2 to 3 weeks. Trachoma and inclusion conjunctivitis in the older child or adult can also be effectively treated with oral erythromycin with a 3-week course of 1 to 1.5 g daily in 4 divided doses.[91,92] Topical antimicrobial treatment with ophthalmic erythromycin ointment is not necessary for patients receiving full oral therapeutic doses of antibiotic. Topical treatment alone is extremely slow, is usually only partially effective in treating adult or neonatal chlamydial disease, and allows frequent relapses.[91,92]

SIDE EFFECTS

Erythromycin is one of the safest antibiotics in clinical use. Although irritative effects do occur, adverse reactions (except for pseudomembranous colitis associated with oral use) are rare and usually not life threatening. The most serious toxicity of erythromycin involves cholestatic hepatitis, which occurs chiefly in adults and only when the estolate preparation of erythromycin has been given.[93] Symptoms of nausea, vomiting, and abdominal pain followed by jaundice, fever, and abnormal liver function tests consistent with cholestatic hepatitis can begin after about 10 days of therapy. The abnormalities generally clear within days to a few weeks after discontinuation of the drug but may return rapidly on rechallenge. The syndrome appears to be a hypersensitivity reaction to the specific structure of the estolate compound, so, despite the rarity of this reaction, erythromycin estolate should be used with caution.

Mild allergic reactions such as urticaria and other rashes, fever, and eosinophilia have occurred occasionally. When given orally, erythromycin may produce mild gastrointestinal disturbances including nausea, vomiting, pyrosis and diarrhea, occurring most commonly with the enteric coated form of oral erythromycin.[94] This type of reaction is more common with higher doses but can be reduced by administering the drug with meals and by using the ethylsuccinate or stearate form of the drug. Sensorineural hearing loss, although extremely rare, has been reported following the use of large doses of erythromycin or the use of erythromycin in the presence of renal failure.[95] The hearing loss usually improves gradually on discontinuation of the drug.

CONTRAINDICATIONS

The reader should be aware of the drug-induced side effects, since they indicate contraindications to the use of erythromycin.

Chloramphenicol

PHARMACOLOGY

Chloramphenicol acts by binding to the 50S subunit of the bacterial ribosome and blocking peptidyl transferase, thereby inhibiting protein synthesis. This inhibition of protein synthesis produces a bacteriostatic effect on sensitive organisms.

CLINICAL USES

Chloramphenicol is active against most gram-positive and gram-negative bacteria, *Rickettsia*, *Chlamydia*, spirochetes, and *Mycoplasma*. However, despite its broad antibacterial spectrum, generally good tolerance by patients, and desirable pharmacokinetic characteristics, chloramphenicol's ability to cause fatal aplastic anemia limits its usefulness, even when administered topically to the eye. Indications for chloramphenicol include severe or life-threatening infections caused by susceptible organisms that are not responsive to less toxic drugs.[96] These infections include acute typhoid fever and other serious *Salmonella* infections such as bacteremia, for which chloramphenicol is the most effective antibiotic.

Chloramphenicol readily penetrates the blood-brain barrier, and it is often the preferred antibiotic for CNS infections; it is one of the drugs of choice for treating *Bacteroides* (especially *B. fragilis*) infections of the brain. Meningitis caused by *N. meningitidis* or *S. pneumoniae* generally responds to chloramphenicol, and this antibiotic is the preferred treatment for patients who are allergic to penicillin. Because isolates of ampicillin-resistant *H. influenzae* are becoming more common, chloramphenicol and ampicillin are often used together for the initial treatment of meningitis caused by *H. influenzae*. For infections outside the CNS that are caused by *H. influenzae*, chloramphenicol is reserved for ampicillin-resistant organisms.

The systemic use of chloramphenicol for ocular infections has been limited to the treatment of endophthalmitis following penetrating trauma or surgery. Chloramphenicol is able to cross the blood-aqueous barrier because of the drug's high lipid solubility, and since it has a reasonably broad spectrum, it would seem to be an ideal drug for treatment of endophthalmitis. However, concern about the toxic reactions that can occur with chloramphenicol use has shifted the drugs of choice for intraocular infections to a penicillinase-resistant penicillin or a cephalosporin combined with an aminoglycoside.[18]

Topical application of chloramphenicol ointment or solution (see Table 6.8) is effective against the majority of bacterial infections of the external eye.[97] However, because aplastic anemia has been reported following even topical ocular use of chloramphenicol,[98–100] its use should be limited to infections for which less toxic antibiotics are not effective.

SIDE EFFECTS

Chloramphenicol causes two types of hematopoietic abnormalities. The first is a dose-related toxic effect causing a reversible bone marrow depression associated with inhibition of mitochondrial protein synthesis. This toxicity is manifest by reticulocytopenia, anemia, elevated serum iron and iron-binding capacity, and decreased erythrocytic uptake of iron. It is more likely to occur in patients receiving 6 g or more daily or in patients with serum levels above 25 μg/ml, and it is usually reversible when the antibiotic is discontinued.[101]

A second, more serious type of bone marrow depression is aplastic anemia. Considered an idiosyncratic reaction rather than a drug toxicity, aplastic anemia occurs most commonly weeks to months following completion of therapy and is not dose-related. It can occur after either systemic or topical drug use[98,102] but is more common after systemic administration. In the most severe form of aplastic anemia, pancytopenia with an aplastic marrow is present. Prognosis is thus very poor, since the anemia is usually irreversible. The incidence of this condition is estimated to be approximately 1 in 25,000 patients who receive chloramphenicol.[103] Before administering chloramphenicol, even topically, baseline blood counts should be obtained. Thereafter, routine blood studies (every 48 hours) may reveal early changes, and the dosage of the drug can be reduced or the drug discontinued if bone marrow depression occurs.

A high plasma concentration of chloramphenicol in premature infants and neonates can occur because of the immature liver's inability to conjugate the drug or because the immature kidney cannot excrete the active form of the drug. This can cause a toxic reaction known as the "gray syndrome," which is characterized by abdominal distention, vomiting, flaccidity, cyanosis, circulatory collapse, and death. Because the gray syndrome can be fatal, administration of chloramphenicol to infants during the first 2 weeks of life is not recommended except under unusual circumstances.

Both mild and relatively severe neurologic complications have been observed following the use of systemic chloramphenicol. Confusion, depression, or delirium, sometimes associated with headache or mild fever, are not uncommon. Optic neuropathy resulting in decreased visual acuity has been described in patients receiving prolonged chloramphenicol therapy,[104,105] and the visual problems associated with the neuropathy did not always disappear on discontinuation of the drug.

Adverse gastrointestinal reactions following use of systemic chloramphenicol include nausea, vomiting, glossitis, stomatitis, diarrhea, and enterocolitis. Rash, angioedema, and urticaria have also been observed following administration of chloramphenicol. Sensitization to the drug can occur with topical ocular use, but hypersensitivity reactions to chloramphenicol are rare.

CONTRAINDICATIONS

The reader should be aware of the occasionally severe and life-threatening drug-induced side effects associated with chloramphenicol, since they indicate the contraindications to its use.

Clindamycin

PHARMACOLOGY

Like erythromycin and chloramphenicol, clindamycin binds to the 50S ribosomal subunit and inhibits protein synthesis. The drug is generally considered to be primarily bacteriostatic rather than bactericidal.

CLINICAL USES

Clindamycin can cause serious or even fatal pseudomembranous colitis. Coupled with the availability of safer alternative antibiotics, this limits the use of clindamycin to only a few conditions. It is effective for treatment of infections outside the CNS that involve *B. fragilis* or other penicillin-resistant anaerobic bacteria; usually these are intraabdominal or gynecologic/pelvic infections. Anaerobic bronchopulmonary infections are traditionally treated with penicillin G, but recent evidence suggests that clindamycin may be superior for treating some of these infections because an increasing number of anaerobic strains are becoming resistant to penicillin. Clindamycin is used as an alternative to penicillin for infections caused by *Clostridium perfringens* and *Actinomyces israeli* and has been effective in certain prophylactic regimens, especially in combination with an aminoglycoside for "dirty" colorectal and urologic surgical procedures. Topical clindamycin has also been effective for the treatment of acne.

Clindamycin may be useful for the treatment of ocular toxoplasmosis. The recurrent, necrotizing lesions of toxoplasmic retinochoroiditis are thought to be due to the multiplication of previously encysted *Toxoplasma gondii* in the ocular tissues,[106] and, although several antimicrobial drugs such as the sulfonamides and pyrimethamine can interfere with the growth of the proliferative form of the parasite, their efficacy against the encysted form is limited. Drugs that could destroy the parasite within the cysts would be of great value, since eradication of the encysted organisms would prevent recurrent episodes. Clindamycin may have this potential. An animal study[107] involving treatment of "healed" toxoplasmic retinochoroiditis has indicated that clindamycin is effective in reducing the number of cysts and viable organisms in the ocular structures. It did not, however, sterilize all the specimens obtained from chronically infected eyes.

Clindamycin alone or in combination with sulfadiazine also seems to be effective for the treatment of active recurrent toxoplasmic retinochoroiditis in humans. Ferguson[108] has reported that clindamycin ther-

apy produced rapid resolution of the inflamed toxoplasmic lesions and hastened healing. Final evaluation of clindamycin for the treatment of both active and healed ocular toxoplasmosis must, however, come from controlled, double-blind studies, since the active lesions usually heal even without treatment. Clindamycin is an expensive drug and has not yet been approved by the Food and Drug Administration (FDA) for treatment of toxoplasmosis.

SIDE EFFECTS

Clindamycin is usually well tolerated. A common gastrointestinal side effect is mild to moderate diarrhea.[109] A more serious concern with this antibiotic is that it can allow overgrowth of *Clostridium difficile* in the intestinal tract, causing potentially fatal pseudomembranous colitis.[110] If severe diarrhea occurs while a patient is taking clindamycin, the drug should be discontinued, and, if appropriate, the patient should be treated with vancomycin. Even though pseudomembranous colitis is treatable, is not unique to clindamycin, and is relatively uncommon, this drug should be prescribed only when specifically required and then with knowledge of the potential for this adverse reaction.

Hypersensitivity reactions have been reported during clindamycin treatment; pruritus, rash, and urticaria have been the most commonly observed manifestations. Transient changes in liver function have also occurred during clindamycin administration, but serious hepatotoxicity is rare.

CONTRAINDICATIONS

The reader should be aware of the drug-induced side effects of clindamycin, since they indicate the contraindications. Patients receiving clindamycin should be carefully monitored for indications of pseudomembranous colitis.

Drugs Affecting Intermediary Metabolism

Antibacterial drugs that affect the intermediary metabolism of bacteria include the family of sulfonamides and the individual drugs pyrimethamine and trimethoprim (see Table 6.5).

Sulfonamides

PHARMACOLOGY

Drugs in the sulfonamide family were the first effective chemotherapeutic agents to be used systemically for the prevention and treatment of bacterial infections in humans. They are broad-spectrum compounds effective against gram-positive and gram-negative bacteria as well as *Actinomyces, Chlamydia,* plasmodia, and *Toxoplasma.*

The sulfonamides act by inhibiting the synthesis of folic acid, a chemical required for bacterial growth. Because bacterial cells are impermeable to folic acid, the chemical must be synthesized internally from para-aminobenzoic acid (PABA). The sulfonamides are structural analogs of PABA; they competitively inhibit the first step in synthesis of folic acid—the conversion of PABA into dihydrofolic acid (Fig. 6.5). Since, in general, the sulfonamides exert only a bacteriostatic effect, cellular and humoral immune mechanisms must assume responsibility for eradicating the infecting bacteria. Because humans absorb preformed folic acid from food, sulfonamide inhibition has only a minimal effect on host cells.

Sulfonamide-induced inhibition of folic acid synthesis can be reversed by several antagonistic compounds, of which PABA is the most prominent. Certain local anesthetics, such as procaine, tetracaine, and benoxinate (which are esters of PABA), also antagonize these drugs in vitro and in vivo.[111] The antibacterial action of the sulfonamides can further be inhibited by blood, pus, and tissue breakdown products because the bacterial requirement for folic acid is reduced in media that contain purines and thymidine. Thus, sulfonamide therapy is contraindicated for infections with marked purulent exudation (Fig. 6.6).

Because acquired resistance to the sulfonamides is widespread, other antibacterial agents have replaced sulfonamides as drugs of first choice for the treatment of all but a few major infections. Mechanisms of resistance include an overproduction of PABA by the bacteria; decreased enzyme affinity for the sulfonamide; decreased bacterial permeability to the drug; and increased inactivation of the drug by the bacteria. Once resistance occurs for 1 sulfonamide, cross-resistance to other sulfonamides is common.

Clinically the sulfonamide family can be divided into 4 groups: short acting (administered every 4 to 6 hours), long acting (administered once or twice daily), poorly absorbed, and topically applied (Table 6.12).

CLINICAL USES

Short Acting Sulfonamides. The short acting sulfonamides include sulfisoxazole, sulfamethizole, sulfacytine, sulfamethoxazole, and sulfadiazine. Sulfamerazine and sulfamethazine can be combined with sulfadiazine in a short-acting mixture called trisulfapyrimidines. The advantage of a combination of sulfonamides involves their solubility. The older sulfonamides are less soluble than the newer ones and cause urinary tract injury due to precipitation of acetylated drug crystals. To circumvent this, sulfonamide mixtures were introduced. In the combination, each drug can coexist in solution without interfering with the solubility of the others. Thus, the total concentration of sulfonamides in the mixture is equal to a high dose of a single sulfonamide, but none of the individual drugs is in a high enough concentration to precipitate in the kidney. Because of the availability of the newer, more soluble sulfonam-

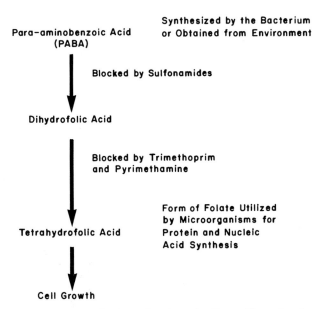

FIGURE 6.5 **Mechanism of action of sulfonamides, trimethoprim, and pyrimethamine.**

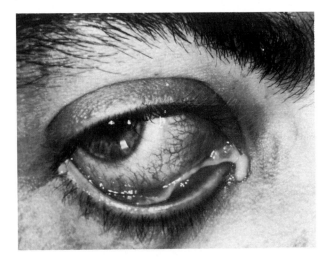

FIGURE 6.6 **Bacterial conjunctivitis with marked purulent exudation. The purulent exudation is a contraindication to topical sulfonamide treatment. (Courtesy Jimmy D. Bartlett, O.D.).**

TABLE 6.12
Clinical Uses of Selected Sulfonamides

Drug	Clinical Uses
Short Acting	
Sulfisoxazole	Urinary tract infections, *Nocardia*
Sulfamethizole	infections, prophylaxis of rheumatic
Sulfacytine	fever, trachoma, inclusion
Sulfamethoxazole	conjunctivitis, lymphogranuloma
Sulfadiazine	venereum, toxoplasmosis
Trisulfapyrimidines	
Sulfamerazine	
Sulfamethazine	
Sulfadiazine	
Long Acting	
Not currently marketed in the United States	
Poorly Absorbed	
Sulfasalazine	Ulcerative colitis, regional enteritis
Topically Applied	
Sulfacetamide	Blepharitis, conjunctivitis
Sulfisoxazole	
Silver Sulfadiazine	Prevention of infection of burns
Mafenide	

ides such as sulfisoxazole, combinations are now used infrequently.

Short acting sulfonamides are among the drugs of choice for acute, uncomplicated, first-episode urinary tract infections because the causative organism is usually *E. coli,* which is typically sensitive to sulfonamides. Sulfisoxazole is usually the sulfonamide chosen, but sulfamethizole, sulfacytine, and sulfamethoxazole are also used. For recurrent or chronic urinary tract infections, the infecting organism(s) may not be sensitive to sulfonamides, and therapy should be based on susceptibility tests.

Sulfonamides are sometimes used to treat chlamydial diseases. Topical sulfonamide therapy has occasionally been used to treat chlamydial neonatal conjunctivitis,[91] but this infection is best treated with systemic erythromycin.[69] The treatment of choice for adult inclusion conjunctivitis is oral tetracycline or erythromycin, with the sulfonamides being used as a distant third choice.[91] Local antimicrobial treatment of the eye with ophthalmic ointment is not necessary for patients receiving full oral therapeutic doses of any of these drugs.

Trachoma has been treated with oral sulfamethoxazole[112] and with oral or topical sulfacetamide,[112,113] but the preferred treatment is oral tetracycline, with oral erythromycin a close second choice.[92] Oral sulfonamides are also used to treat chlamydial venereal dis-

ease, but, again, oral tetracycline or erythromycin is the drug of choice.[70] Oral administration of a sulfonamide or tetracycline has been successful for the treatment of lymphogranuloma venereum and chancroid.[114]

The sulfonamides, particularly sulfadiazine and trisulfapyrimidines, can be used to treat toxoplasmic retinochoroiditis. The severe damage that affects the retina and adjacent tissues of patients with this infection can be attributed to several factors. Direct infection of retinal cells and multiplication of the parasite are probably the most important of these, but hypersensitivity reactions by the host to toxoplasmic antigens as well as to antigens released from the photoreceptors can also cause retinal damage.[115] Corticosteroids alone have been successfully used to treat this condition, but treatment with steroids may also weaken the host's natural cellular defenses and increase the risk of uncontrolled parasite proliferation. For this reason, steroids should not be used to treat toxoplasmic retinochoroiditis without the cover of at least 1 antitoxoplasmic agent.[116] Although pyrimethamine and sulfonamides constitute the classic agents for treatment of toxoplasmosis, newer drugs such as clindamycin may eventually substitute for them or be used concomitantly.[108,117] Some authors[118] consider that if only 1 drug is chosen, trisulfapyrimidines should be the first choice because of minimal expense, good tolerance, lack of spoilage, and simplicity of use.

Long Acting and Poorly Absorbed Sulfonamides. The long acting sulfonamides are not currently marketed in the United States because they have been frequently associated with hypersensitivity reactions such as Stevens-Johnson syndrome. The poorly absorbed sulfonamide, sulfasalazine, is used for prophylaxis before bowel surgery and for treating ulcerative colitis and regional enteritis but has few other common applications.

Topically Applied Sulfonamides. Topical ophthalmic preparations of sulfonamides include sodium sulfacetamide and sulfisoxazole (Table 6.13). Sodium sulfacetamide is available in 10%, 15%, and 30% solutions, in 10% ointment, and in combination with the steroids prednisolone acetate and prednisolone phosphate (Table 6.14). The 10% solution is the most common preparation for the treatment of routine bacterial conjunctivitis because the 30% concentration causes significant stinging on instillation.[119] The usual dose of sulfacetamide solution applied topically to the eye for treatment of conjunctivitis is 1 drop of the 10% solution every 2 hours for severe infections, or the same amount applied 3 or 4 times daily for chronic conditions. The ointment may be used instead of the solution, but it is typically

TABLE 6.13
Sulfonamide Preparations for Topical Ocular Therapy

Trade Name	Manufacturer
Sulfacetamide Solutions—10%	
Sodium Sulfacetamide	Various
AK-Sulf	Akorn
Bleph-10	Allergan
Sulten-10	Bausch & Lomb
Sulf-10	Iolab
Sodium Sulamyd	Schering
Sulfacetamide Solutions—15%	
AK-Sulf	Akorn
Isopto Cetamide	Alcon
Sulfair 15	Pharmafair
Sulfacetamide Solutions—30%	
Sodium Sulfacetamide	Various
AK-Sulf Forte	Akorn
Sodium Sulamyd	Schering
Sulfacetamide Ointments—10%	
Sodium Sulfacetamide	Various
AK-Sulf	Akorn
Cetamide	Alcon
Bleph-10 S.O.P.	Allergan
Sodium Sulamyd	Schering
Sulfisoxazole Solution and Ointment—4%	
Gantrisin	Roche

reserved for application at bedtime or for use in children. For the treatment of staphylococcal blepharitis, sulfacetamide ointment can be applied to the lids after they have been cleansed with warm compresses and lid scrubs. In mild cases, once daily at bedtime may be sufficient. In severe cases, 3 to 4 applications daily may be necessary to control the condition. Sulfisoxazole is available as a 4% ophthalmic solution and ointment, and it too can be used to treat conjunctivitis and blepharitis caused by a variety of bacteria.

Combinations of sulfacetamide and prednisolone acetate or phosphate are commercially available (see Table 6.14) and have been an effective treatment for chronic blepharitis. In a comparison study, Aragones[120] investigated patients with clinically diagnosed blepharitis (with an infectious component sensitive to sulfacetamide) who were treated using either sulfacetamide alone or the sulfacetamide-prednisolone combination. Results indicated that topical 10% sulfacetamide eliminated culturable evidence of the causative bacteria and cleared the patient's symptoms in approximately 6 to 8 days. Administration of anti-inflammatory therapy along with the anti-infective treatment reduced to one-half the time required for relief of symptoms without adversely affecting the anti-infective action of the combination. In addition, a few patients who had been treated with sulfacetamide alone had persistent symptoms of inflammation even after "bacteriologic cure."

TABLE 6.14
Sulfacetamide[a]-Steroid Combinations

Steroid	Trade Name (Manufacturer)
Solutions and Suspensions	
Prednisolone acetate 0.5%	AK-Cide (Akorn)
	Sulphrin (Bausch & Lomb)
	Predsulfair (Pharmafair)
	Metimyd Suspension (Schering)
Prednisolone phosphate 0.5%	Optimyd Solution (Schering)
Prednisolone acetate 0.25%	Isopto Cetapred Suspension (Alcon)
Prednisolone phosphate 0.25%	Vasocidin Solution (Iolab)
Prednisolone acetate 0.2%	Blephamide Suspension (Allergan)
Ointments	
Prednisolone acetate 0.5%	AK-Cide (Akorn)
	Vasocidin (Iolab)
	Predsulfair (Pharmafair)
	Metimyd (Schering)
Prednisolone acetate 0.25%	Cetapred (Alcon)
Prednisolone acetate 0.2%	Blephamide S.O.P. (Allergan)

[a]10% concentration.

These patients were treated with a steroid in addition to their antibiotic regimen and experienced dramatic improvement.[120]

Although the treatment of chronic blepharitis with sulfacetamide or with the combination of sulfacetamide and prednisolone seems ideal, an additional point must be considered. In a study of chronic blepharitis,[121] 50% of patients with clinical "staphylococcal blepharitis" were culture-positive for *S. aureus*. The remainder were positive for *S. epidermidis*. Possibly due to overuse of sulfonamides in the treatment of chronic blepharitis (most of the patients had been previously treated with the drug), only 29% of the *S. aureus* isolates and 33% of the *S. epidermidis* isolates were sensitive to sulfonamides. Initial treatment of chronic "staphylococcal blepharitis" should obviously include an anti-infective drug, but with so many strains of *S. aureus* and *S. epidermidis* resistant to sulfonamides, a sulfonamide alone or in combination with prednisolone no longer appears to be the most appropriate general therapy for this condition.

In contrast to the resistance found among isolates of *S. aureus* and *S. epidermidis,* two other bacteria that cause conjunctivitis, *Streptococcus pneumoniae* and *H. influenzae,* remain sensitive to the sulfonamides. Thus, topical sulfacetamide or sulfisoxazole is still useful for some forms of bacterial conjunctivitis presenting with minimal purulent discharge.

SIDE EFFECTS

The sulfonamides can produce a wide variety of side effects, and an adverse reaction to one sulfonamide frequently precludes the use of other sulfonamide derivatives. Anorexia, nausea, vomiting, and diarrhea are common side effects of systemic sulfonamide therapy. Blood dyscrasias such as acute hemolytic anemia, aplastic anemia, agranulocytosis, thrombocytopenia, and leukopenia occur only rarely, but the consequences of these conditions are potentially serious.[122] Because sulfonamides cross the placenta and compete with bilirubin for albumin binding, they can cause high levels of free bilirubin in infants born to mothers who have taken sulfonamides close to term. Sulfonamides are also excreted in breast milk, so use of sulfonamides for nursing mothers or for pregnant women close to term is not advisable.

Hypersensitivity reactions including urticaria and rashes (often accompanied by pruritus and fever) may result from sulfonamides administered by any route, including topical. Other hypersensitivity reactions include malaise and a serum sickness-like syndrome.[122] A case of an immune corneal ring formation after administration of sulfamethoxazole has been reported.[229] Contact dermatitis is common with topical application of these drugs, and they have also caused more serious dermatologic problems such as erythema nodosum, erythema multiforme (Stevens-Johnson syndrome), and exfoliative dermatitis. Rubin[123] reported a patient who experienced a skin reaction after taking an oral sulfonamide and who subsequently developed Stevens-Johnson syndrome after topical ophthalmic use of sodium sulfacetamide.

Perhaps the most common ocular side effect seen in patients taking systemic sulfonamides is transient myopia, with or without induced astigmatism.[124] The myopia is usually bilateral and may exceed several diopters, but the refractive state usually returns to normal when the serum drug level decreases.

In addition to hypersensitivity reactions, topical administration of sulfonamides can lead to other problems. When sulfonamide ointments are applied for treatment of staphylococcal blepharitis, local photosensitization may result in sunburning of the lid margins,[125] and this can mimic an allergic reaction. Topical use of sulfadiazine ointment for 1 year has caused formation of multiple small white concretions of sulfadiazine within cysts in the palpebral conjunctiva,[126] and topical use of sulfacetamide has caused white plaques to form on the cornea.[127] Topical sulfacetamide in the 30% concentration has been reported to produce a significant decrease in corneal sensitivity, while the 10% concentration produced no change compared with the control.[128]

Interactions between the sulfonamides and other drugs can include hypoglycemia occurring after sulfonamides are given to patients taking oral hypoglycemic drugs such as tolbutamide or chlorpropamide. Sulfonamides can also enhance the action of coumarin anticoagulants and should be used with caution in patients taking these drugs. PABA-containing compounds and PABA analogs, such as local anesthetics like procaine, may reduce the effectiveness of sulfonamides by allowing the bacteria to synthesize more folic acid.

CONTRAINDICATIONS

The reader should be aware of the drug-induced side effects, since they indicate the contraindications.

Pyrimethamine and Trimethoprim

PHARMACOLOGY

Both pyrimethamine and trimethoprim inhibit dihydrofolate reductase, which catalyzes the reduction of dihydrofolic acid to tetrahydrofolic acid (see Fig. 6.5). The dihydrofolate reductase of protozoa and some bacteria is affected by these drugs, but the human enzyme is not. This gives the drugs their selective action against microorganisms. A powerful synergism exists between either of these drugs and the sulfonamides; the sulfonamides inhibit the enzyme that converts PABA to dihydrofolic acid, while pyrimethamine and trimethoprim block a sequential step in the pathway—conversion of dihydrofolic acid to tetrahydrofolic acid (see Fig. 6.5). This sequential blockage of the same biosynthetic pathway results in a high degree of activity against a wide spectrum of microorganisms.

CLINICAL USES

Pyrimethamine and trimethoprim are 2 of many 2,4-diaminopyrimidines that were synthesized and tested for antimicrobial activity. Pyrimethamine was initially selected for its antimalarial properties; in combination with a sulfonamide such as sulfadiazine, it is useful for the treatment of acute attacks of chloroquine-resistant *P. falciparum* malaria, and it is also used as a prophylactic and suppressive drug for *P. vivax* malaria.

Administered concurrently with sulfadiazine or with triple sulfonamides (sulfadiazine, sulfamerazine, and sulfamethazine), pyrimethamine is beneficial for the treatment of toxoplasmosis.[118] The synergism of the combined drugs greatly enhances the therapeutic effect; combined therapy requires only one-eighth as much sulfonamide and one-twenty-fourth as much pyrimethamine as would be necessary if either drug were used alone.[129]

Trimethoprim, the other clinically useful diaminopyrimidine, is most often used in combination with sulfamethoxazole for the treatment of *Pneumocystis carinii* pneumonitis in the immunologically impaired patient and for treatment of adults with shigellosis, urinary tract infections, acute otitis media, and acute exacerbations of chronic bronchitis associated with *H. influenzae* or *S. pneumoniae*. It is also used alone in the treatment of initial episodes of uncomplicated urinary tract infections.

Although trimethoprim has been used systemically for many years, its use as a topical ophthalmic solution has only recently been evaluated. Nozik and associates[130] and Lamberts and associates[131] have compared the clinical and bacteriologic efficacy of an ophthalmic solution of trimethoprim-sulfacetamide-polymyxin B versus an ophthalmic solution of polymyxin B-neomycin-gramicidin in a group of patients having surface ocular bacterial infections such as acute blepharitis and acute conjunctivitis. Polymyxin B was included with the trimethoprim because *P. aeruginosa* is not sensitive to trimethoprim but is sensitive to polymyxin B.[132] The solution containing trimethoprim was as effective as the other drug combination in producing both clinical and bacteriologic cures of the infections.[130,131] The trimethoprim-sulfacetamide-polymyxin B solution was then compared with a trimethoprim-polymyxin B solution in another group of patients with surface ocular infections. There was no loss of effectiveness when the sulfacetamide was deleted from the solution, suggesting that the sulfonamide was not a necessary component. When the trimethoprim solution was used, there was a low incidence of adverse reactions, and those that did occur were mild.[131] The combination of trimethoprim and polymyxin B appears, therefore, to be an effective and safe topical antibacterial solution for the treatment of ocular surface infections.

SIDE EFFECTS

When the recommended dosage of 25 mg of pyrimethamine once weekly is used for prophylaxis of malaria, no significant toxic effects occur. Higher dosages, however, as needed for the treatment of toxoplasmosis, can result in white blood cell and platelet depression or megaloblastic anemia caused by drug-induced folic acid deficiency. When given in the recommended dosages, trimethoprim-sulfamethoxazole usually does not produce folate deficiency in normal individuals. If the patient is deficient in folic acid, however, this drug combination may precipitate hematologic reactions associated with a deficiency of this nutrient. The toxicity induced by pyrimethamine or trimethoprim may be counteracted by administration of folinic (*not* folic) acid. Use of folinic acid bypasses the need for dihydrofolate reductase by supplying the fully reduced folate.

Skin reactions typical of those produced by the sulfonamides have an increased incidence when trimethoprim-sulfamethoxazole is used compared with using just a sulfonamide.[133]

CONTRAINDICATIONS

The reader should be aware of the drug-induced side effects, since they indicate the contraindications.

Drugs Affecting Bacterial DNA Synthesis

Antibacterial drugs that inhibit bacterial DNA synthesis include a new generation of fluorinated quinolones structurally related to nalidixic acid: norfloxacin, ofloxacin, and ciprofloxacin (see Table 6.5).

PHARMACOLOGY

Nalidixic acid and the fluorinated quinolones inhibit DNA synthesis during bacterial replication. This effect is thought to be mediated through inhibition of DNA gyrase activity.[134] Supercoiling of bacterial DNA, mediated by DNA gyrase, is essential to enable bacteria to fit their very long chromosome within the cell. Bacterial gyrase, unlike the comparable human enzyme, is susceptible to inhibition by this group of antibacterial drugs, and this inhibition kills the bacteria.

CLINICAL USES

Oral nalidixic acid has been used for many years to treat urinary tract infections because it is bactericidal for most of the gram-negative bacteria that cause these infections. The drug is less active against gram-positive bacteria, and *Pseudomonas* is resistant. In contrast, the new fluoroquinolones are broad-spectrum antibacterial drugs with a greater potency than the parent compound, nalidixic acid. These drugs are active against most gram-negative bacteria including *Pseudomonas*, many gram-positive bacteria including *Staphylococcus*, and some anaerobes. In clinical trials, oral norfloxacin[135] and ofloxacin[136] have been effective in the treatment of urinary tract infections, including complicated and recurrent ones. Oral norfloxacin[135] has also been effective in the treatment of acute gastroenteritis due to common gastrointestinal pathogens such as enterotoxigenic *E. coli, Salmonella, Shigella,* and *Campylobacter.* Both norfloxacin[137,138] and ciprofloxacin[139] have been effective in the treatment of patients with gonorrhea, including those with extragenitourinary involvement and those infected with penicillinase-producing strains of *N. gonorrhoeae.*

The in vitro activity of norfloxacin against ocular pathogens has been compared with currently available antibacterial drugs such as bacitracin, erythromycin, and gentamicin.[30,140] In general, norfloxacin had the greatest potency and broadest spectrum of activity of the agents tested, being active against *S. aureus, P. aeruginosa, H. influenzae,* and most other gram-negative bacteria. In experimental trials, norfloxacin has been effective in the treatment of rabbit corneas infected with *P. aeruginosa.*[141] In clinical trials, 0.3% ofloxacin solution was clinically and bacteriologically effective for treating external ocular infections, including corneal ulcers.[230] Collectively, this evidence suggests that this group of antibacterial drugs has the potential for broad-spectrum, effective treatment of systemic and ocular bacterial infections.

SIDE EFFECTS

Oral nalidixic acid is usually well tolerated, but nausea, vomiting, and abdominal pain may occur. Allergic and toxic reactions affecting the blood cells and liver occur occasionally. In clinical trials, norfloxacin has been well tolerated with a low incidence (less than 3%) of drug-related adverse reactions.[135] The most common side effects include nausea, headache, dizziness, rash, bitter taste in the mouth, elevation of liver enzymes, and eosinophilia.[135,142]

CONTRAINDICATIONS

The reader should be aware of the drug-induced side effects of this class of drugs, since they indicate the contraindications.

Antiviral Drugs

Viruses are the smallest of the infectious organisms. They are obligate, intracellular organisms that can infect humans, animals, plants, and bacteria. Their simple structure consists of either DNA or RNA as genetic material and a protein coat called a capsid. For some viruses, the capsid is surrounded by an envelope composed of the nuclear or cell membrane of a previously infected cell (Fig. 6.7).

Viruses depend on host cells for multiplication. For a virus to replicate, it must invade (infect) a host cell and take over its metabolic machinery. After new viral nucleic acid and protein are produced, new viruses are released from the host cell to infect other host cells (Fig. 6.8). This type of infection produces an acute disease that is usually limited by the response of the patient's immune system. Alternatively, a few viruses are able to invade cells and then become latent. In these cases, the viral DNA becomes incorporated into the host cell's DNA and is thus protected from the host's immune system. At future times this viral DNA can be stimulated to produce new viruses that cause recurrent disease episodes.

Although the development of antibacterial drugs has progressed quickly over the last decades, the development of effective antiviral drugs has not been as rapid. This is due in large part to the nature of viruses themselves. Viruses grow and multiply inside host cells and are integrated into the metabolism of these cells. Because of this, it is difficult to find an antiviral drug that is selectively toxic for the virus while leaving the host cells unaffected. Many of the currently available antiviral drugs are antimetabolites that inhibit nucleic

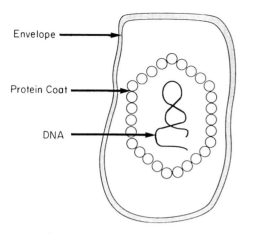

FIGURE 6.7 **A herpes virus particle showing the outer envelope and the nucleocapsid composed of the protein coat and DNA.**

acid synthesis; their usefulness is directly related to their ability to selectively block viral (as opposed to host) nucleic acid synthesis.

Because of ongoing development and testing of new antiviral drugs, consensus about the uses and therapeutic regimens for these drugs is not as complete as it is for the antibacterial drugs, and much of the work in this area is still in the investigational stage. The antiviral drugs now commercially available are used primarily for treatment of herpes infections. This virus group includes 4 distinct members: herpes simplex virus (HSV) , varicella-zoster virus (VZV), Epstein-Barr virus (EBV), and cytomegalovirus (CMV).

There are two types of HSV: type 1, which is associated with infections involving the eye, mouth, and skin above the waist; and type 2, which usually affects the skin including and surrounding the genitalia. A primary systemic infection with HSV-1 occurs in most children and is often subclinical with mild, flu-like respiratory symptoms. If the primary infection has ocular manifestations, they usually begin as a follicular conjunctivitis. Clusters of vesicles can occur on the periorbital and eyelid skin; corneal involvement in the form of diffuse epithelial keratitis or microdendrites may also be present. Generally, the primary infection is controlled by the immune system, but the virus usually becomes latent in the trigeminal ganglion, and this allows for later recurrences of the disease. During recurrent episodes, the viruses produced in the trigeminal ganglion move through the sensory nerves to the cornea and can infect the epithelial cells, producing a characteristic dendritic pattern. The virus can also cause stromal keratitis characterized by infiltration and necrosis or can cause disciform keratitis characterized by corneal edema. Besides affecting the eye, HSV-1 can cause recurrent herpes labialis with "cold sores" or "fever blisters" on the skin around the mouth. HSV-2 is a sexually transmitted disease that usually causes genital infection. As with HSV-1 infection, the primary HSV-2 infection allows the virus to become latent, and the disease usually becomes recurrent.

In the nonimmunized host, the primary infection with VZV produces chickenpox. Once this infection has occurred, the virus remains latent in sensory ganglia (e.g., the trigeminal ganglion) for the patient's life. When triggered by stress or other factors, the virus can reactivate, producing the syndrome of zoster (shingles). During a zoster episode, the virus replicates in the sensory ganglia and migrates along the sensory

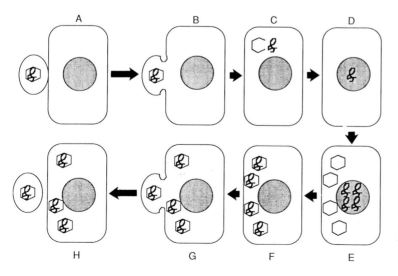

FIGURE 6.8 **Steps in herpes virus replication cycle. (A) Adsorption of the virus to the human cell. (B) Fusion of the viral envelope with the human cell membrane. (C) Release of the viral DNA. (D) Viral mRNA synthesis. (E) Viral protein and DNA synthesis. (F) Viral nucleocapsid assembly. (G) "Budding" of human cell membrane around viral nucleocapsid to produce infectious particle. (H) Replication process complete—new virus ready to infect another cell.**

nerves to the skin or eye. Signs and symptoms include vesicular eruption and neuralgic pain in the areas supplied by the sensory nerves from the affected ganglia.

Herpes zoster ophthalmicus usually first manifests as a severe, unilateral, disabling neuralgia in the region innervated by the trigeminal nerve. The virus then produces vesicles on the skin corresponding to the distribution of the nerve. Ocular complications include conjunctivitis, scleritis, keratitis, iridocyclitis, or glaucoma. Treatment should be aggressive, since the disease can have devastating consequences for the eye.[143]

The EBV probably causes some or all of the cases of infectious mononucleosis. Ocular involvement can include regional lymphadenopathy, uveitis, dacryocystitis, retinal periphlebitis, and, rarely, vitritis. Since the disease is usually limited by the immune system, treatment is primarily symptomatic.

CMV is the leading cause of congenital viral infections, but the majority of these infections do not manifest themselves clinically. Adults frequently show serologic evidence of previous CMV infections, but clinical illness is rarely recognized in healthy individuals. CMV can cause clinical disease, however, in immunocompromised adults and newborns. CMV retinitis is a necrotizing infection leading to full-thickness destruction of the retina that may result in total loss of vision. This infection is common in patients with AIDS; in one study,[144] 32% of AIDS patients had CMV retinopathy. CMV retinopathy is a poor prognostic sign; Holland and associates[144] found that no AIDS patient survived longer than 6 weeks after the development of retinopathy.

Idoxuridine

PHARMACOLOGY

Idoxuridine (IDU) is a halogenated pyrimidine that resembles thymidine (Fig. 6.9). This substituted nucleoside is phosphorylated by both viral and host cell (human) thymidine kinases to the active triphosphorylated derivative, which, in turn, is incorporated into both the viral and the host cell's DNA chains, thereby creating fraudulent DNA. The result is antiviral activity but with sufficient host cytotoxicity to severely limit systemic use. Such toxicity is not significant, however, when the drug is applied topically to the eye.

CLINICAL USES

HSV infection of the cornea is the primary clinical indication for treatment with IDU, which is commercially available as a 0.1% solution and an 0.5% ointment for topical ocular use (Table 6.15). The treatment of dendritic or geographic epithelial ulcers entails in-

stilling the 0.1% solution into the conjunctival sac every hour during the day and every 2 hours during the night until improvement is seen. After this, IDU is applied every 2 hours during the day and every 4 hours at night. An equivalent regimen involves instillation of the 0.5% ointment every 4 hours during the day and once before bedtime. Therapy is continued for 3 to 5 days after corneal healing is complete (as demonstrated by absence of fluorescein staining) to ensure that any virus released late in the recurrent episode does not initiate another active corneal infection. Therapy should not be continued for more than 21 days because prolonged treatment increases the risk of corneal toxicity.

Approximately 75% of patients with dendritic or geographic epithelial herpes are cured after 2 weeks of treatment with IDU,[145,146] but because idoxuridine does not eradicate the latent virus in the trigeminal ganglion, topical therapy with this drug does not decrease the recurrence rate of herpetic keratitis.[147] During recurrent episodes, the acute infection is often controllable, but corneal scarring can occur caused by the infectious process or by hypersensitivity reactions to the virus. When herpes epithelial keratitis fails to respond to antiviral therapy as evidenced by a lack of healing after 5 to 7 days or by an enlargement of the epithelial ulceration, several factors can be involved. In addition to the causes outlined in Table 6.3, a unique cause for the perceived failure of antiviral therapy in the treatment of herpes epithelial keratitis can occur.[148] In this situation, the disease process or drug toxicity can disrupt corneal epithelial healing. The result is a persisting epithelial defect or "ghost" dendrite that may mimic an active lesion. Thus, in many cases the corneal herpetic infection is cured, but the persisting lesion gives the appearance of treatment failure.

In addition to using idoxuridine for the treatment of recurrent dendritic keratitis, this drug can also be used to treat primary herpetic keratitis. The treatment regimen for the primary corneal infection is the same as outlined above for the recurrent disease.[149] In the absence of corneal ulceration, a prophylactic antiviral drug such as IDU should be administered until the follicular conjunctivitis or periocular skin lesions resolve. When skin lesions appear as part of the primary HSV infection, they are best treated by general cleanliness since IDU is not effective against HSV disease of the skin.[150]

IDU is relatively insoluble in water and does not penetrate into or through the cornea; it has no demonstrable effect on herpetic stromal disease or iritis.[151] However, treatment of herpetic stromal keratitis with high-dose steroids usually requires prophylactic use of an antiviral drug such as IDU to reduce the chance of recurrence of the epithelial disease. Unfor-

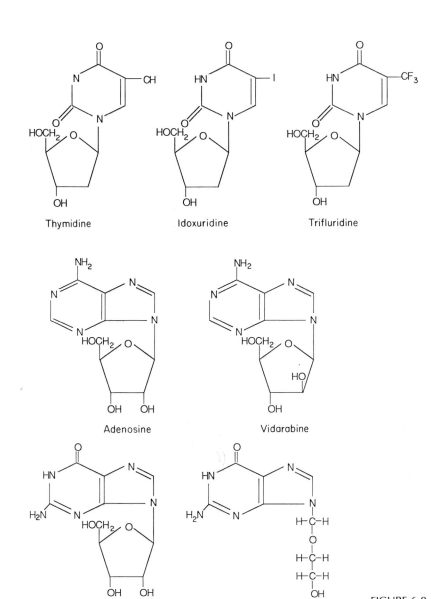

FIGURE 6.9 **Chemical structures of the antiviral drugs and the DNA nucleosides they resemble.**

TABLE 6.15
Antiviral Drugs for Topical Ocular Therapy

Generic Name	Concentration (%)	Formulation	Trade Name (manufacturer)
Idoxuridine	0.1	Solution	Herplex (Allergan)
			Stoxil (Smith Kline & French)
	0.5	Ointment	Stoxil (Smith Kline & French)
Vidarabine	3	Ointment	Vira-A (Parke-Davis)
Trifluridine	1	Solution	Viroptic (Burroughs Wellcome)

tunately, patients with herpetic stromal disease often require relatively long-term steroid treatment, and simultaneous use of an antiviral agent means substantial epithelial toxicity. Thus, when the antiviral drug is used prophylactically along with steroids, the dosage, tapering, and termination schedules of the antiviral drug remain controversial.[152,154]

SIDE EFFECTS

Although IDU is most active in virus-infected cells, the drug also affects the metabolism of normal cells. Toxic effects associated with the disruption of normal cellular DNA synthesis include changes in the cornea, conjunctiva, and lids. The cornea may show fine, superficial punctate keratopathy, corneal filaments, indolent ulceration, and the combination of slowed epithelial healing and superficial stromal opacification that can give a "ghost" dendrite. Inhibition of corneal stromal wound healing with IDU use is well established.[148] Conjunctival changes include chemosis, hyperemia, filaments, punctate staining, and follicles in the lower tarsus. Lid damage includes edema and plugging of the meibomian glands, as well as occlusion of the puncta.

CONTRAINDICATIONS

The reader should be aware of the drug-induced side effects of IDU, since they indicate the contraindications.

Vidarabine (Adenine Arabinoside)

PHARMACOLOGY

Vidarabine is an analog of the purine nucleoside adenosine (see Fig. 6.9). It is phosphorylated by both viral and host cell kinases to the corresponding active vidarabine phosphate. However, because the phosphorylated vidarabine is a more potent inhibitor of the herpes virus DNA polymerase than of host DNA polymerase, viral DNA synthesis is blocked at lower doses and a selective antiviral effect can be achieved. This drug is active against vaccinia virus, HSV, CMV, and VZV.

CLINICAL USES

The primary clinical indication for vidarabine is dendritic or geographic epithelial keratitis caused by HSV. For this infection, the 3% ointment (see Table 6.15) is usually applied 5 times daily for a maximum of 21 days, and treatment should be continued for 3 to 5 days after the cornea has healed. This regimen is ef-

fective for tne keratitis associated with both primary and recurrent infection.

Vidarabine is as effective as IDU for the treatment of HSV keratitis.[153,154] Treatment with vidarabine or IDU results in similar improvements in symptoms including lacrimation and photosensitivity and in similar rates and times for corneal reepithelialization. The time for reepithelialization of dendritic and geographic ulcers is often between 6 and 7 days with each of the drugs. Pavan-Langston and Buchanan[151] have shown that many patients whose ulcers do not respond to IDU have reepithelialization within 4 weeks of treatment with vidarabine, so vidarabine can be considered an effective alternative in cases of recurrent disease when the patient is intolerant of IDU or when the virus is resistant to that drug.

Vidarabine is an approved and effective drug for the treatment of HSV encephalitis.[155] It decreases overall mortality and debilitating neurologic sequelae, but comparison studies suggest that acyclovir is the drug of choice for treatment of this infection.[156] Like IDU, vidarabine has not proven useful for herpes simplex labialis or genitalis.

SIDE EFFECTS

Side effects associated with topical use of vidarabine are similar to those seen with IDU.[151] Symptoms include stinging, burning, irritation, lacrimation, and injection. Other reactions are follicular conjunctivitis, marked superficial punctate keratitis, corneal edema, corneal erosion, trophic epithelial defects, delay of corneal wound healing, and punctal occlusion. Compared with IDU, however, vidarabine is less toxic and less likely to provoke adverse reactions.[148] If a patient demonstrates a reaction to vidarabine, another antiviral should be used.

CONTRAINDICATIONS

The reader should be aware of the drug-induced side effects, since they indicate the contraindications.

Trifluridine

PHARMACOLOGY

Similar to idoxuridine, trifluridine (trifluorothymidine, F_3T) is also an analog of thymidine (see Fig. 6.9). It is an effective inhibitor of thymidine synthetase and therefore inhibits DNA synthesis in both virus-infected and normal host cells. Trifluridine is also incorporated into both viral and host DNA, producing a faulty DNA that does not allow replication of the virus.

CLINICAL USES

Like IDU and vidarabine, trifluridine is used to treat HSV keratitis. A 1% solution (see Table 6.15) is prescribed for use 9 times daily for 14 days or until re-epithelialization has occurred. The medication is then reduced to 1 drop every 4 hours while the patient is awake for an additional 7 days. Administration of trifluridine for more than 21 continuous days should be avoided because of the drug's potential for ocular toxicity. As with IDU and vidarabine, trifluridine is effective for both primary and recurrent epithelial keratitis.

When treatment of dendritic and geographic corneal ulcers with trifluridine was compared to treatment with idoxuridine, Wellings and associates[157] found trifluridine to be significantly superior. The mean time for healing of epithelial lesions with trifluridine was 6.3 days, which was significantly shorter than the 8.2 days with IDU. The number of treatment failures with trifluridine was also significantly less than with IDU, 7.5% with trifluridine compared to 39.5% with idoxuridine. Treatment of dendritic and geographic corneal ulcers with trifluridine has also been compared to treatment with vidarabine, and trifluridine has been shown to be significantly superior.[158,159] Pavan-Langston and Foster[146] demonstrated that when patients failed to respond to either IDU or vidarabine therapy (or manifested intolerance to either of these agents), substituting trifluridine resulted in healing in the majority of cases. Because of this superior clinical efficacy, trifluridine is now the drug of choice for the treatment of epithelial HSV keratitis.

Another possible use of trifluridine has been suggested by a report of 4 patients with Thygeson's superficial punctate keratitis who were successfully treated with this drug.[160]

SIDE EFFECTS

Adverse ocular reactions to trifluridine are often overlooked or assumed to be a worsening of the disease process. Corneal epithelial defects at a location other than the site of the active infection (dendritic or geographic ulceration) can be a sign of drug toxicity.[148] Additional side effects associated with trifluridine are mild transient burning or stinging on instillation, conjunctival hyperemia and edema, corneal erosion and edema, keratitis sicca, delayed corneal wound healing, and elevated intraocular pressure. The epithelial defects and other adverse reactions are generally reversible on discontinuation of the drug. However, some cases of ptosis and lacrimal punctal occlusion produced by trifluridine have been permanent.[161] Long-term use of this antiviral agent can also cause conjunctival scarring,[162] but compared with IDU and vidarabine, trifluridine causes the least amount of local irritation and toxicity.[148]

CONTRAINDICATIONS

The reader should be aware of the drug-induced side effects, since they indicate the contraindications.

Acyclovir (Acycloguanosine)

PHARMACOLOGY

Acyclovir, an analog of guanosine (see Fig. 6.9), is active against HSV and VZV. The selective action of acyclovir against these herpes viruses is a result of two major factors: the phosphorylation of acyclovir to the active phosphate moiety by the herpes-specified thymidine kinase, and the inhibitory action of acyclovir triphosphate against herpes-specified DNA polymerase, which results in viral DNA chain termination.[163] Acyclovir must be phosphorylated to be active in inhibiting DNA replication, and this takes place through the action of thymidine kinase, the enzyme that normally phosphorylates thymidine. Viral thymidine kinase, an enzyme specifically induced by the virus only in infected cells, readily phosphorylates acyclovir, but the uninfected host cell thymidine kinase appears to be more fastidious and does not phosphorylate acyclovir. Thus, acyclovir does not disrupt DNA synthesis nor interfere with the replication of normal cells, but it does disrupt viral DNA replication in virus-infected cells. This highly selective activity makes acyclovir a very potent and effective antiherpetic agent without the toxicity associated with other antiviral drugs.

CLINICAL USES

Acyclovir has been approved by the FDA for treatment of genital herpes. During initial episodes of this disease, oral acyclovir can decrease the duration of viral shedding from the genital lesions, reduce the development of new lesions, decrease the healing time of lesions, and decrease the severity of symptoms such as pain, adenopathy, dysuria, malaise, and headache.[164] Unfortunately, after discontinuation of treatment, the time to subsequent recurrence and the rate of recurrence are not altered by acyclovir,[164] and treatment of recurrent lesions with acyclovir is not as effective as is treatment of the initial infection.[164] However, this reduced effectiveness may reflect the milder expression of recurrent genital herpes. Acyclovir ointment is also approved for therapy of initial genital herpes[165]; intravenous acyclovir seems to be effective for severe initial episodes of this disease.[166]

Oral acyclovir has been studied to determine its effectiveness as a long-term suppressive agent to prevent recurrent episodes of genital herpes. This approach appears promising. In several studies,[167,168] fewer recurrences occurred and longer times from onset of treatment to recurrence were found for the acyclovir-treated groups compared with the placebo group. However, after acyclovir treatment was discontinued, the mean time to recurrence was similar for both groups,[167,168] indicating that the drug had no permanent effect on the latent virus. Acyclovir also seems to be effective in suppressing frequently recurring nongenital skin infections caused by HSV[169] and erythema multiforme occurring after recurrent HSV infections.[170]

Until recently, vidarabine was the drug used to treat biopsy-proven HSV encephalitis. Now, however, acyclovir is the treatment of choice for this infection because it causes less mortality and morbidity.[171]

Several studies[172,173] have demonstrated the value of acyclovir for the treatment of the ocular manifestations of HSV. In a double-blind clinical trial, Coster and associates[174] found that 1% IDU ointment and 3% acyclovir ointment allowed comparable healing rates and healing times when used to treat herpetic epithelial keratitis. The efficacy of 0.5% IDU was compared with 3% acyclovir in another double-blind clinical trial.[175] Collum and associates[175] showed that acyclovir was clearly superior for treating herpetic dendritic ulceration, with more rapid corneal healing (4.4 days versus 9.2 days) and an increased healing rate (100% versus 76%). These investigators[175] also demonstrated a higher incidence of toxicity in the form of superficial punctate epitheliopathy in the IDU-treated patients compared with the acyclovir-treated patients. In two studies,[176,177] topical acyclovir applied as a 3% ointment 5 times a day for 14 days was as effective for the treatment of HSV dendritic and geographic ulcers as was vidarabine ointment applied similarly. There was no significant difference in healing rates or times between the 2 patient groups in either study. Lau and associates[178] compared 3% acyclovir ointment to a 2% trifluridine ointment, both used 5 times per day. Although the rate of healing was similar, more of the dendritic ulcers treated with acyclovir healed within 14 days. These studies show that although acyclovir is effective for treating HSV epithelial keratitis, it has no clearly demonstrable superiority over the currently available antiviral drugs: IDU, vidarabine, or trifluridine.

The efficacy of acyclovir in treating stromal keratitis is not well established. Sanitato and associates[179] found that topical or oral acyclovir alone was not an effective treatment for either HSV disciform or stromal keratitis. When acyclovir was combined with a steroid for these diseases, however, treatment was significantly more effective. Topical acyclovir combined with betamethasone has been shown to be at least as effective as vidarabine combined with betamethasone for the treatment of herpetic disciform keratitis.[180]

In addition to being active against HSV, the drug is also active against VZV. A double-blind, placebo-controlled study[181] has found that oral acyclovir, 600 mg 5 times a day for 10 days, is successful for treatment of herpes zoster ophthalmicus. Treatment with acyclovir resulted in prompt resolution of signs and symptoms and shortened the duration of viral shedding, particularly for patients treated within 72 hours after onset of the skin lesions. The most dramatic effect of oral acyclovir was to decrease the incidence and severity of secondary ocular inflammatory disease. Episcleritis, anterior and posterior scleritis, stromal keratitis, and anterior uveitis were all found less frequently and in milder forms in patients treated with acyclovir. The postherpetic neuralgia was unaffected by acyclovir therapy.

Topical acyclovir also appears to be effective for the treatment of keratouveitis caused by VZV.[182] The corneal epithelial lesions resolved more quickly in acyclovir-treated patients than in patients treated with topical betamethasone, but there was no difference in the stromal, uveal, or scleral response between the two groups. Unlike the steroid-treated group, however, once the keratouveitis resolved and the acyclovir was tapered and discontinued, there were no recurrences. Recurrences did occur after steroid treatment, and some patients needed to continue receiving low-dose steroid maintenance therapy. These studies[181-183] suggest that treatment with oral or topical acyclovir, with avoidance of steroids, can eliminate many of the feared consequences of herpes zoster ophthalmicus.

Acute herpes zoster is a common cause of morbidity in immunocompromised patients, especially those with lymphoproliferative neoplasia or organ allografts. Intravenous acyclovir has halted the progression of both localized skin lesions and disseminated cutaneous zoster in a group of such patients,[184,185] but when the drug was discontinued, recurrences occurred.[186]

Acyclovir may have a role in the treatment of acute retinal necrosis syndrome, a disease characterized by the triad of acute confluent peripheral necrotizing retinitis, retinal arteritis, and vitritis in otherwise healthy adults. Treatment of 12 patients with acute retinal necrosis syndrome using intravenous acyclovir resulted in a regression of the retinal lesions and the lack of development of new lesions.[187] These results suggest that a randomized clinical trial to evaluate the efficacy of acyclovir in the treatment of this disease would be productive.

SIDE EFFECTS

Only minor side effects are associated with use of acyclovir. The most frequent adverse reactions during oral treatment are nausea, vomiting, diarrhea, head-ache, vertigo, and arthralgia. Less frequent reactions include skin rash, insomnia, fatigue, fever, menstrual abnormality, sore throat, acne, and lymphadenopa-thy.[188] The most frequent adverse reactions with intra-venous acyclovir are inflammation or phlebitis at the injection site, rash or hives, and transient elevations of BUN and creatinine. Elevated renal function test results typically occur when acyclovir is administered too rapidly or to dehydrated patients.[188] Slow infusion or increasing the patient's water intake can help pre-vent this reaction. Topical application of acyclovir can cause mild pain, burning, stinging, or pruritus.[188]

CONTRAINDICATIONS

The reader should be aware of the drug-induced side effects of acyclovir, since they indicate the contrain-dications.

Zidovudine (Azidothymidine, AZT, Retrovir)

Zidovudine has been approved by the FDA for treat-ment of patients with AIDS. It is a thymidine analog that inhibits HIV replication in vitro.[189] Zidovudine is phosphorylated by cellular enzymes, and, as the triphosphate, it inhibits reverse transcriptase and ter-minates viral DNA elongation.[190] Zidovudine admin-istration can decrease the frequency of opportunistic infections and mortality in selected AIDS patients.[191] The drug has been used successfully to treat CMV retinitis[231] and HIV-induced iridocyclitis and anterior uveitis[232] in patients with AIDS. Unfortunately, zido-vudine is a very toxic drug that can cause bone marrow hypoplasia and leave some patients more vulnerable to bacterial infections than they were before drug ther-apy.[192]

Experimental Drugs

Several compounds are undergoing investigation for use as antiviral drugs. Dihydroxy propoxymethyl guan-ine (Ganciclovir) is a relatively new cyclic nucleoside antiviral, similar in structure to acyclovir, with appar-ent activity against CMV. AIDS patients treated with Ganciclovir have shown regression or disappearance of the exudative, hemorrhagic, and periphlebitic lesions of CMV retinitis.[193–195]

Bromovinyldeoxyuridine (BVDU) has been shown to be an effective and safe compound for the treatment of HSV-1 and VZV ocular infections.[196] It acts in a manner similar to acyclovir in that both drugs are phosphorylated only by viral thymidine kinase.[197] Chlorethyldeoxyuridine, a compound chemically re-lated to BVDU, has also been found to be effective for the treatment of experimental HSV keratouveitis.[198]

Antifungal Drugs

The fungi (molds and yeasts) are an extremely large and diverse group of microorganisms ranging in size and complexity from simple unicellular yeasts (Fig. 6.10) to multicellular molds and mushrooms. The fungi are distinct from viruses and bacteria in size, structure, and chemical composition. The main structural com-ponent of a multicellular fungus is a filamentous tube containing cytoplasm with nuclei spaced at irregular intervals (see Fig. 6.10). In some fungi, these tubes are interrupted at numerous points by septations or cross-walls. An individual filament is called a hypha, and an entire mat of hyphae is referred to as mycelium. Some of the hyphae can differentiate into reproductive structures that produce reproductive cells called spores. The differentiation of the filamentous fungi into genera and species is based on the morphologic arrangement of the reproductive structures and spores.

Of the nearly 100,000 species of fungi, only a few cause infections in humans. Fungal infections are clas-sified as dermatophytic, mucocutaneous, or systemic. Dermatophytic infections are the most common types of fungal infection and involve the keratinized portions of the body: skin, hair, and nails. Species of *Epider-mophyton*, *Trichophyton* and *Microsporum* cause these infections, which are known collectively as tinea or ringworm.

Mucocutaneous infections are predominantly caused by the yeast *Candida*, which usually affects moist skin or mucous membranes such as in the oral cavity (thrush), gastrointestinal tract, or perianal or vulvo-vaginal areas. Patients with diabetes and those receiv-ing corticosteroids or broad-spectrum antibiotics are predisposed to candidiasis of the intertriginous skin folds and mucous membranes. These conditions, as well as pregnancy or use of oral contraceptives, pre-dispose patients to candidal vulvovaginitis.

Systemic mycoses may be either deep or subcuta-neous. Fungi causing deep mycoses usually enter the body by inhalation, and the infection may spread hem-atogenously to other tissues. Fungi causing subcuta-neous infections typically enter the body through the skin, usually by trauma, and the infection spreads di-

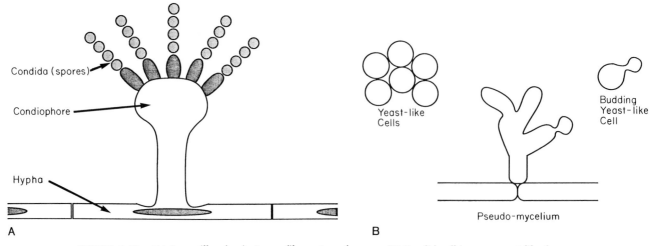

FIGURE 6.10   **(A) Aspergillus fumigatus, a filamentous fungus. (B) Candida albicans, a yeast-like fungus.**

rectly to contiguous tissues. Typical deep systemic mycoses are aspergillosis, blastomycosis, coccidioidomycosis, cryptococcosis, histoplasmosis, zygomycosis, candidiasis, and paracoccidioidomycosis. Major subcutaneous mycoses are chromomycosis, mycetoma, and sporotrichosis.

Two common fungal infections of the eye, fungal keratitis and endophthalmitis, occur most often after injury or surgery or when host resistance is decreased. The increased incidence of fungal corneal ulcers observed in recent years has been attributed to the widespread use of corticosteroids, which depress the immune system, and possibly to broad-spectrum antibiotic use. Although many types of fungi have been cultured from mycotic corneal ulcers, the most frequent are *Aspergillus, Fusarium solani, Candida albicans,* and *Acremonium* (formerly *Cephalosporium*).[199,200]

Because fungal infections of the cornea are comparatively rare, there is little incentive to develop new therapeutic agents specifically intended for topical use in the eye. Natamycin (pimaricin) is the only antifungal drug commercially available in the United States as a topical ophthalmic product, but dilute solutions or suspensions of some parenteral antifungal drugs such as amphotericin B, nystatin, and miconazole can be used for topical therapy. When administered either topically or systemically, most antifungal drugs penetrate the eye poorly.[201] Therefore, mycotic corneal ulcers are very difficult to treat successfully.

Amphotericin B

PHARMACOLOGY

Amphotericin B is a polyene antifungal drug (Table 6.16). The polyenes bind to a sterol moiety present in

the fungal cell membrane, and the polyene-sterol complex alters the selective permeability of the membrane, permitting leakage of essential intracellular constituents.[202] An organism's ability to bind amphotericin B depends on the presence of sterol in the cellular membrane, and, because bacterial membranes do not contain the sterol, they do not bind the drug. Bacteria are thus insensitive to amphotericin B.

CLINICAL USES

Amphotericin B is the drug of choice for the treatment of systemic infections resulting from *Coccidioides immitis, Histoplasma capsulatum, Cryptococcus neoformans, Blastomyces dermatitidis, Candida,* and many other less common fungi. The period of therapy is usually 6 to 10 weeks, but it can be as long as 3 to 4 months. When used for the treatment of these deep infections, amphotericin B is usually administered parenterally.

For many years, topically administered amphotericin B was the major antifungal therapy for keratomycoses. A 1% solution has been made from the commercial preparation intended for systemic use, but even though this therapy was effective, it was very toxic to the eye because of the drug concentration and also because of the desoxycholate present for solubilization purposes in the commercial preparation.[203] More recently, a 0.15% solution of amphotericin B has been found to be reasonably well tolerated and effective for the treatment of corneal ulcers caused by *Fusarium, Candida, Aspergillus,* and *Alternaria.*[204] The most common concentration of amphotericin B currently administered for the treatment of keratomycoses is between 0.10% and 0.25%.[205] The regimen for treatment of corneal ulcers involves topical administration of amphotericin B every hour throughout the day and every

TABLE 6.16
Antifungal Drugs Used for Ocular Therapy

Generic Name	Trade Name (Manufacturer)
Polyenes	
Amphotericin B	Fungizone (Squibb)
Nystatin	Nystatin (Various)
	Mycostatn (Squibb)
	Nilstat (Lederle)
	Nystex (Savage)
Natamycin (Pimaricin)	Natacyn (Alcon)
Pyrimidines	
Flucytosine	Ancobon (Roche)
Imidazoles	
Miconazole	Monistat (Janssen)
	Monistat (Ortho)
Ketoconazole	Nizoral (Janssen)

2 to 4 hours at night. Since the corneal epithelium is a significant barrier to the penetration of amphotericin B, drug efficacy is reduced if the epithelium is intact.[206]

Amphotericin B has also been injected subconjunctivally to treat fungal corneal ulcers. Subconjunctival injection can result in permanent yellowing of the cornea, and, at higher doses, can cause salmon-colored conjunctival nodules.[207]

Amphotericin B has been administered systemically, subconjunctivally, and, more recently, intravitreally to treat fungal endophthalmitis.[208] However, amphotericin B is a toxic drug and can cause retinal damage and ocular inflammation.[209] Another form of the drug, amphotericin B methyl ester, which is a water-soluble derivative of amphotericin B, appears to be less toxic and has been effective for treating experimental fungal infections in animals.[210]

SIDE EFFECTS

Unpleasant and potentially dangerous side effects are associated with the systemic use of amphotericin B. Headaches, chills, fever, and vomiting are common during infusion of the drug. Toxic reactions can result from the binding of amphotericin B to the sterol moiety of human renal tubular cells and erythrocytes; most patients receiving prolonged high doses of amphotericin B show renal damage, the extent of which depends on the total dose of the drug. Moderate anemia is also frequently encountered but usually disappears after therapy is discontinued. Other adverse effects include gastrointestinal cramps, hypomagnesemia, and hypokalemia. Because of these side effects, amphotericin B should be used only when the patient has a reasonably well-substantiated mycotic infection.

Nystatin

Nystatin is also a polyene (see Table 6.16) and works in a manner similar to that of amphotericin B. It is used for the treatment of *Candida* infections of the skin, mucous membranes, and intestinal tract. Oral, esophageal, gastric, and intestinal candidiasis usually respond to oral administration of nystatin. Vaginitis and stomatitis (thrush) caused by this organism are usually treated using topical therapy.

Topical application of nystatin ointment has also been used successfully to treat corneal infections caused by *Candida* and *Aspergillus*,[211-213] but there is no experimental or clinical evidence indicating that nystatin is more effective than amphotericin B against *Candida* or the filamentous corneal pathogens such as *Aspergillus* or *Fusarium*.

Since oral preparations of nystatin are poorly absorbed, adverse effects are uncommon, but mild and transient nausea, vomiting, and diarrhea may occur. Neither irritation of the skin or mucous membranes nor hypersensitivity reactions have been reported following topical application. No toxic effects on the blood or blood-forming organs have been noted.

Natamycin (Pimaricin)

Natamycin (pimaricin) is a small polyene (see Table 6.16) that acts in a manner similar to that of amphotericin B. Clinical trials of a 5% suspension have substantiated the effectiveness of natamycin for treatment of keratitis caused by *Acremonium* and other fungi.[214,215] Natamycin appears to have greater effectiveness than amphotericin B against *Fusarium*.[216] The 5% natamycin suspension is the only FDA-approved drug for topical treatment of ocular fungal infections; because of its broad spectrum of activity and its commercial availability, it is the drug of choice for initial therapy in fungal keratitis.[205]

Initial dosage for treatment of fungal corneal ulcers is 1 drop of the 5% suspension instilled into the conjunctival sac every 1 to 2 hours. The frequency of application can usually be reduced to 1 drop 6 to 8 times daily after the first 3 to 4 days. Therapy should generally be continued for 14 to 21 days, or until the active fungal infection resolves.

Because natamycin does not penetrate the cornea, conjunctiva, or other mucosal surfaces, topical application does not produce effective levels in the deep stroma or the anterior chamber. Toxic induration and lack of absorption preclude the subconjunctival use of natamycin.

Only a few adverse reactions have been reported. The suspension often adheres to areas of epithelial ulceration, and one case of conjunctival hyperemia and chemosis (thought to be allergic) has been reported.[188]

Flucytosine

Flucytosine is a fluorinated pyrimidine (see Table 6.16) related to fluorouracil. In fungal cells, it is converted to fluorouracil, which is metabolized to 5-fluorodeoxyuridylic acid, an inhibitor of thymidylate synthetase. Since there is no evidence that flucytosine is converted to fluorouracil in normal host cells, toxicity after oral administration is low.

Flucytosine is used orally to treat systemic infections caused by *Candida* or *Cryptococcus neoformans,* including *Candida* endophthalmitis.[217,218] Pretherapy resistance and the development of drug resistance during therapy is high; the drug is therefore usually used concomitantly with amphotericin B.

Flucytosine is readily absorbed after oral administration and can penetrate the blood-brain barrier. Side effects include bone marrow depression, hepatic damage, nausea, vomiting, diarrhea, and cerebral symptoms such as confusion and hallucinations.

Miconazole

Miconazole is an imidazole (see Table 6.16) having two distinct antifungal actions. A fungistatic effect is caused by inhibition of ergosterol synthesis in fungal cell membranes, which affects their permeability.[219] An additional fungicidal effect involves rapid membrane damage and appears unrelated to the imidazole-induced block in ergosterol synthesis.[219] Because in low doses miconazole is only fungistatic, prolonged treatment may be needed to ensure adequate eradication of the fungus.

Miconazole has a broad spectrum of activity against *Candida* and other yeasts, numerous genera of filamentous fungi, and the dermatophytes. Topical application of 2% miconazole ointment has been shown to be effective for treatment of dermatophytosis, *Candida* vulvovaginitis, and skin infections. Intravenous administration has been effective for treatment of deep infections caused by *Candida, Coccidioides, Cryptococcus, Paracoccidioides,* and *Pseudallescheria* organisms.

Miconazole has been used topically, subconjunctivally, and intravenously to treat fungal infections of the cornea.[220–222] For example, topical and subconjunctival miconazole have been used to treat keratomycoses caused by *Candida* and *Aspergillus.*[220] Progressive corneal ulceration stopped in each case, and clinical evidence of corneal infection disappeared. Topical and subconjunctival miconazole have also been combined with oral ketoconazole for successful therapy of keratomycosis.[221] For treatment of corneal infections, 1% drops are typically instilled in the eye every hour for several days; the dose is then decreased to 1 drop 6 times a day, depending on clinical response. Subconjunctival administration typically is 5 to 10 mg daily for 1 to 5 days. Intravitreal[223] injection of miconazole has been used to treat fungal endophthalmitis with beneficial results.

No major adverse reactions to miconazole have been reported, but minor side effects include pruritus, rash, chills, phlebitis, and gastrointestinal symptoms.

Ketoconazole

Ketoconazole is a recently developed antifungal imidazole (see Table 6.16). Similar to miconazole, ketoconazole affects the permeability of fungi by interfering with the biosynthesis of ergosterol and causing disorganization of the plasma membrane. Ketoconazole is an effective treatment for chronic superficial candidiasis and chronic dermatophytosis.[224] Limited data suggest that this antimycotic is also useful for the treatment of systemic (deep) mycoses caused by *Paracoccidioides, Candida,* and *Coccidioides.*[225,226]

Ketoconazole has been used to treat fungal infections of the cornea, with topical application effective for the treatment of keratitis due to *Aspergillus* and *Fusarium.*[227] A 1% solution does not irritate the conjunctiva or cornea even after prolonged use.[227] Oral ketoconazole alone,[228] and combined with topical and subconjunctival miconazole,[221] has been administered for the successful treatment of keratomycosis caused by *Fusarium, Aspergillus, Drechslera, Curvularia,* and *Candida.*

Side effects associated with ketoconazole include hepatic toxicity, which is usually reversible on discontinuation of the drug, but, in at least one case, the toxicity led to a fatality. Nausea and pruritus are the most common adverse effects, with headache, dizziness, abdominal pain, constipation, diarrhea, and nervousness occurring less frequently. Ketoconazole does not appear to produce ocular toxicity following systemic administration.

References

1. Murray BE, Moellering RC. Patterns and mechanisms of antibiotic resistance. Med Clin North Am 1978;62:899–919.
2. Rosenblatt JE. Laboratory tests used to guide antimicrobial therapy. Mayo Clin Proc 1987;62:799–805.
3. Mandell GL, Sande MA. Penicillins, cephalosporins, and other beta-lactam antibiotics. In: Gilman AG, Goodman LS, Rall TW, et al., eds. The pharmacological basis of therapeutics, ed. 7. New York: MacMillan Co, 1985;50:1115–1149.
4. Glasser DB, Hyndiuk RA. Antibacterial agents. In: Tabbara KF, Hyndiuk RA, eds. Infections of the eye. Boston: Little, Brown, 1986;13:211–238.
5. Wright AJ, Wilkowske CJ. The penicillins. Mayo Clin Proc 1987;62:806–820.
6. Noe CA. Penicillin treatment of eyelid infections. Am J Ophthalmol 1947;30:477–479.
7. Jones DB. Decision-making in the management of microbial keratitis. Ophthalmology 1981;88:814–820.
8. Sutphin JE, Pflugfelder, SP, Wilhelmus KR, et al. Penicillin-resistant *Streptococcus pneumoniae* keratitis. Am J Ophthalmol 1984;97:388–389.
9. Jones DB. A plan for antimicrobial therapy in bacterial keratitis. Ophthalmology 1975;79:95–103.
10. Baum JL. Initial therapy of suspected microbial corneal ulcers. I. Broad antibiotic therapy based on prevalence of organisms. Surv Ophthalmol 1979;24:97–116.
11. Abel R, Binder PS, Bellows R. Postoperative bacterial endophthalmitis: III. Ann Ophthalmol 1976;8:1253–1265.
12. Abbott RL, Abrams MA. Bacterial corneal ulcers. In: Duane TD, Jaeger EA, eds. Clinical ophthalmology. Philadelphia: Harper & Row, 1986;4(18):1–34.
13. Ullman RF, Cunha BA. Antibiotic selection in penicillin allergic patients. Int Med 1986;7:100–105.
14. Vanarsdel PP, Gilliland BC. Anemia secondary to penicillin treatment: Studies on two patients with "non-allergic" serum hemagglutinins. J Lab Clin Med 1965;65:277–285.
15. Bartlett JG, Chang TW, Gurwith M, et al. Antibiotic-associated pseudomembranous colitis due to toxin-producing clostridia. N Engl J Med 1978;298:531–534.
16. Farrar WE, O'Dell NM. Comparative β-lactamase resistance and antistaphylococcal activities of parenterally and orally administered cephalosporins. J Infect Dis 1978;137:490–493.
17. Thompson RL. Cephalosporin, carbapenem and monobactam antibiotics. Mayo Clin Proc 1987;62:821–834.
18. Forster RK, Abbott RL, Gelender H. Management of infections endophthalmitis. Ophthalmology 1980;87:313–319.
19. Berg SW, Kilpatrick ME, Harrison WO, et al. Cefoxitin as a single-dose treatment for urethritis caused by penicillinase-producing *Neisseria gonorrhoeae*. N Engl J Med 1979;301:509–511.
20. Haase DA, Nash RA, Nsanze H, et al. Single-dose ceftriaxone therapy of gonococcal ophthalmia neonatorum. Sex Transm Dis 1986;13:53–55.
21. Laga M, Naamara W, Brunhan RC, et al. Single-dose therapy of gonococcal ophthalmia neonatorum with ceftriaxone. N Engl J Med 1986;315:1382–1385.
22. Levine BB. Antigenicity and cross reactivity of penicillins and cephalosporins. J Infect Dis 1973;128(Suppl):364–366.
23. Sher TH. Penicillin hypersensitivity—a review. Pediatr Clin North Am 1983;30:161–176.
24. Bartlett JG, Willey SH, Chang TW, et al. Cephalosporin-associated pseudomembranous colitis due to *Clostridium difficile*. JAMA 1979;242:2683–2685.
25. Tan J, Bayne LH, McLeod PJ. Pseudomembranous colitis. A fatal case following prophylactic cephaloridine therapy. JAMA 1979;242:749–750.
26. Bang NU, Kammer RB. Hematologic complications associated with beta-lactam antibiotics. Rev Infect Dis 1983; 5(Suppl 2):S380.
27. Barza M. The nephrotoxicity of cephalosporins: An overview. J Infect Dis 1978;137(Suppl):S60.
28. Pasternak DP, Stephens BG. Reversible nephrotoxicity associated with cephalothin therapy. Arch Intern Med 1975; 135:599.
29. Kanof NB. Bacitracin and tyrothricin. Med Clin North Am 1970;54:1291–1293.
30. Goldstein EJ, Citron DM, Bendon L, et al. Potential of topical norfloxacin therapy. Arch Ophthalmol 1987;105:991–994.
31. Bellows J, Farmer C. The use of bacitracin in ocular infections. Am J Ophthalmol 1948;31:1211–1216.
32. Binnick AN, Clendenning WE. Bacitracin. Contact Dermatitis. 1978;4:180–181.
33. Fraunfelder FT, Meyer SM. Drug-induced ocular side effects and drug interactions, ed. 2. Philadelphia: Lea & Febiger, 1982.
34. Khan JA, Hoover D, Ide CH. Methicillin-resistant *Staphylococcus epidermidis* blepharitis. Am J Ophthalmol 1984; 98:562–565.
35. Havener WH. Ocular pharmacology, ed. 5. St. Louis: C.V. Mosby Co, 1983.
36. Fekety FR, Norman PS, Cluff LE. The treatment of gram-negative bacillary infections. The toxicity and efficacy in 48 patients. Am Intern Med 1962;57:214.
37. Melby K, Midtvedt T, Dahl O. A comparison of the *in vitro* activity of tobramycin and gentamicin against 6042 clinical isolates. Chemotherapy 1979;25:286–295.
38. Wilson FM. Adverse external ocular effects of topical ophthalmic medications. Surv Ophthalmol 1979;24:57–88.
39. Magnuson RH, Suie T. Gentamicin sulfate in external eye infections. JAMA 1967;199:177–178.
40. Halasa AH. Gentamicin in the treatment of bacterial conjunctivitis. Am J Ophthalmol 1967;63:1699–1702.
41. Magnuson R, Suie T. Clinical and bacteriologic evaluation

of gentamicin ophthalmic preparations. Am J Ophthalmol 1970;70:734–738.

42. Fox SL. Some aspects in the diagnosis and management of external infections of the eye: Experiences of a new antibiotic, gentamicin. South Med J 1970;63:1047–1052.

43. Gordon DM. Gentamicin sulfate in external eye infections. Am J Ophthalmol 1970;69:300–305.

44. Nauheim R, Nauheim J. Bulbar conjunctival defects associated with gentamicin (letter). Arch Ophthalmol 1987; 105:1321.

45. Awan KJ. Mydriasis and conjunctival paresthesia from local gentamicin. Am J Ophthalmol 1985;99:723–724.

46. Records RE. Gentamicin in ophthalmology. Surv Ophthalmol 1976;21:49–58.

47. Wilhelmus KR, Gilbert ML, Osato MS. Tobramycin in ophthalmology. Surv Ophthalmol 1987;32:111–122.

48. Smolin G, Okumoto M, Wilson FM. The effect of tobramycin on *Pseudomonas* keratitis. Am J Ophthalmol 1973;76:555–560.

49. D'Amico DJ, Caspers-Velu L, Libert J, et al. Comparative toxicity of intravitreal aminoglycoside antibiotics. Am J Ophthalmol 1985;100:264–275.

50. Moellering RC, Wennersten C, Kunz LF, et al. Resistance to gentamicin, tobramycin and amikacin among clinical isolates of bacteria. Am J Med 1977;62:873–881.

51. Siebert WT, Moreland NJ, Williams TW. Resistance to gentamicin: A growing concern. South Med J 1977;70:289–292.

52. Duncan IBR, Rennie RP, Duncan NH. A long-term study of gentamicin-resistant *Pseudomonas aeruginosa* in a general hospital. J Antimicrob Chemother 1981;7:147–15.

53. Cross AS, Opal S, Kopecko DJ. Progressive increase in antibiotic resistance of gram-negative bacterial isolates. Arch Intern Med 1983;143:2075–2080.

54. Yu VL, Rhame FS, Pesanti EL, et al. Amikacin therapy. Use against infections caused by gentamicin- and tobramycin-resistant organisms. JAMA 1977;238:943–947.

55. Talamo JH, D'Amico DJ, Kenyon KR. Intravitreal amikacin in the treatment of bacterial endophthalmitis. Arch Ophthalmol 1986;104:1483–1485.

56. Longridge NS, Mallinson AI. A discussion of the dynamic illegible "E" test: A new method of screening for aminoglycoside vestibulotoxicity. Otolaryngol Head Neck Surg 1984;92:671–677.

57. Lerner AM, Reyes MP, Cone LA, et al. Randomized controlled trial of comparative efficacy, auditory toxicity, and nephrotoxicity of tobramycin and netilmicin. Lancet 1983; 1:1123–1125.

58. Argov Z, Mastaglia FL. Disorders of neurotransmission caused by drugs. N Engl J Med 1979;301:409–413.

59. Boe R, Conner CS. Pseudotumor cerebri. JAMA 1973; 226:567.

60. Tabbara KF. Chlamydial conjunctivitis. In: Tabbara KF, Hyndiuk RA, eds. Infections of the eye. Boston: Little, Brown, 1986;24:421–436.

61. Freinkel RK, Strauss JS, Yip SY, et al. Effect of tetracycline on the composition of sebum in acne vulgaris. N Engl J Med 1965;273:850–854.

62. Golub LM, Ramamurthy NS, McNamara TF, et al. Tetracyclines inhibit tissue collagenase activity: a new mechanism

in the treatment of periodontal disease. J Periodontal Res 1984;19:651–655.

63. Neu HC. Symposium on the tetracyclines: A major appraisal. Bull NY Acad Med 1978;54:141–155.

64. Gopalakrishna KV, Lerner PI. Increasing incidence and cross resistance to newer tetracyclines. Am Rev Respir Dis 1973;108:1007–1011.

65. Gonorrhea: CDC recommended treatment schedules. Sex Transm Dis 1979;6:38–40.

66. Clark SG, Culler AM. Aureomycin as prophylaxis against ophthalmia neonatorum. Am J Ophthalmol 1951;34:840–847.

67. Chapman KJ. A comparative study of Neo-Silvol and Terramycin as prophylactic treatments in the eyes of the newborn. Ohio State Med J 1956;1:591–592.

68. Chandler JW, Rotkis WM. Ophthalmia neonatorum. In: Duane TD, Jaeger EA, eds. Clinical ophthalmology. Philadelphia: Harper & Row 1986;4(6):1–7.

69. Sandstrom I. Neonatal conjunctivitis caused by *Chlamydia trachomatis*. Acta Otolaryngol (Stockh) 1984;407(Suppl):67–69.

70. Dunlop EM. Treatment of patients suffering from chlamydial infections. J Antimicrob Chemother 1977;3:377–383.

71. Handsfield HH. Nongonococcal urethritis. Cutis 1981;27: 268–277.

72. Hoshiwara I, Ostler B, Hanna L, et al. Doxycycline treatment of chronic trachoma. JAMA 1973;224:220–223.

73. Viswalingam ND, Darougar S, Yearsley P. Oral doxycycline in the treatment of adult chlamydial ophthalmia. Br J Ophthalmol 1986;70:301–304.

74. Darougar S, Jones BR, Viswalingam N, et al. Topical therapy of hyperendemic trachoma with rifampicin, oxytetracycline, or spiramycin eye ointments. Br J Ophthalmol 1980;64:37–42.

75. Finland M. The place of the tetracyclines in antimicrobial therapy. Clin Pharmacol Ther 1973;15:3–8.

76. Zaidman GW, Brown SI. Orally administered tetracycline for phlyctenular keratoconjunctivitis. Am J Ophthalmol 1981;92:178–182.

77. Perry HD, Golub LM. Systemic tetracyclines in the treatment of noninfected corneal ulcers: A case report and proposed new mechanism of action. Ann Ophthalmol 1985; 17:742–744.

78. Brown SI, Shahinian L. Diagnosis and treatment of ocular rosacea. Ophthalmology 1978;85:779–786.

79. Perry HD, Kenyon KR, Lamberts DW, et al. Systemic tetracycline hydrochloride as adjunctive therapy in the treatment of persistent epithelial defects. Ophthalmology 1986;93:1320–1322.

80. Barr WH, Adir J, Garrettson L. Decrease of tetracycline absorption in man by sodium bicarbonate. Clin Pharmacol Ther 1971;12:779–784.

81. Boston Collaborative Drug Surveillance Program. Tetracycline and drug attributed changes in blood urea nitrogen. JAMA 1972;220:377–379.

82. Committee on Drugs, American Academy of Pediatrics. Requiem for tetracyclines. Pediatrics 1975;55:142–143.

83. Giles CL, Soble AR. Intracranial hypertension and tetracycline therapy. Am J Ophthalmol 1971;72:981–982.

84. Pierog SH, Al-Salihi FL, Cinotti D. Pseudotumor cerebri—

a complication of tetracycline treatment of acne. J Adolesc Health Care 1986;7:139–140.

85. Lepper MH, Wolfe CK, Zimmerman HJ, et al. Effect of large doses of aureomycin on human liver. AMA Arch Intern Med 1951;88:271–283.

86. Penttila O. Neuvonen PJ, Aho K. Interaction between doxycycline and some antiepileptic drugs. Br Med J 1974;2:470–472.

87. Neuvonen PJ, Penttila O. Interaction between doxycycline and barbiturates. Br Med J 1974;1:535–536.

88. Wachter HE. Prophylaxis in the eyes of the newborn infants. Missouri Med 1956;53:187–190.

89. Christian JR. Comparison of ocular reactions with the use of silver nitrate and erythromycin ointment in ophthalmia neonatorum prophylaxis. J Pediatr 1960;57:55–60.

90. Hammerschlag MR, Chandler JW, Alexander ER, et al. Erythromycin ointment for ocular prophylaxis of neonatal chlamydial infection. JAMA 1980;244:2291–2293.

91. Dawson CR. Inclusion conjunctivitis. In: Fraunfelder FT, Roy FH, eds. Current ocular therapy, ed. 2. Philadelphia: W.B. Saunders Co, 1985;34–35.

92. Dawson CR. Follicular conjunctivitis. In: Duane TD, Jaeger EA, eds. Clinical ophthalmology. Philadelphia: Harper & Row, 1986;4(7):1–19.

93. Sande MA, Mandell G. Miscellaneous antibacterial agents, antifungal and antiviral agents. In: Gilman AG, Goodman LS, Rall TW, et al., eds. The pharmacological basis of therapeutics, ed. 7. New York: MacMillan Co, 1985;54:1170–1198.

94. Cater BL, Woodhead JC, Cole KJ, et al. Gastrointestinal side effects with erythromycin preparations. Drug Intell Clin Pharm 1987;21:734–738.

95. Karmody CS, Weinstein L. Reversible sensori-neural hearing loss with intravenous erythromycin lactobionate. Ann Otol Rhinol Laryngol 1977;86:9–11.

96. Kucers A. Current position of chloramphenicol chemotherapy. J Antimicrob Chemother 1980;6:1–9.

97. Roberts W. Topical use of chloramphenicol in external ocular infections. Am J Ophthalmol 1951;34:1081–1088.

98. Abrams SM, Degnan TJ, Vinciguerra V. Marrow aplasia following topical application of chloramphenicol eye ointment. Arch Intern Med 1980;140:576–577.

99. Rosenthal RL, Blackman A. Bone marrow hypoplasia following use of chloramphenicol eyedrops. JAMA 1965;191:136–137.

100. Fraunfelder FT, Bagby GC, Kelly DJ. Fatal aplastic anemia following topical administration of ophthalmic chloramphenicol. Am J Ophthalmol 1982;93:356–360.

101. Scott JL, Finegold SM, Belkin GA, et al. A controlled double-blind study of the hematologic toxicity of chloramphenicol. N Engl J Med 1965;272:1137–1142.

102. Best WR. Chloramphenicol-associated blood dyscrasias. A review of cases submitted to the American Medical Association Registry. JAMA 1967;201:99–106.

103. Wellerstein RO, Condit PK, Kasper CK, et al. Statewide study of chloramphenicol therapy and fatal aplastic anemia. JAMA 1969;208:2045–2050.

104. Cocke JG, Brown RE, Geppert LJ. Optic neuritis with prolonged use of chloramphenicol. J Pediatr 1966;68:27–31.

105. Joy RJT, Scaletter R, Sodee DB. Optic and peripheral neuritis. Probable effect of prolonged chloramphenicol therapy. JAMA 1960;173:1731–1734.

106. Frenkel JK, Jacobs L. Ocular toxoplasmosis. Arch Ophthalmol 1958;59:260–279.

107. Tabbara KF, Dy-Liacco J, Nozik RA, et al. Clindamycin in chronic toxoplasmosis. Effect of periocular injections on recoverability of organisms from healed lesions in the rabbit eye. Arch Ophthalmol 1979;97:542–544.

108. Ferguson JG. Clindamycin therapy for toxoplasmosis. Ann Ophthalmol 1981;13:95–100.

109. Lakhanpal V, Schocket SS, Nirankari VS. Clindamycin in the treatment of toxoplasmic retinochoriditis. Am J Ophthalmol 1983;95:605–613.

110. Tedesco FJ. Clindamycin and colitis: A review. J Infect Dis 1977;135(Suppl):95–99.

111. Lyle WM, Page C. Possible adverse effects from local anesthetics and the treatment of these reactions. Am J Optom Physiol Opt 1975;52:736–744.

112. Darougar S, Viswalingham N. Trachoma. In: Fraunfelder FT, Roy FH, eds. Current ocular therapy, ed. 2. Philadelphia: W.B. Saunders Co, 1985;35–36.

113. Agarwal LP, Saxena RP, Gupta BML. Antibiotic and chemotherapeutic agents in treatment of trachoma. Am J Ophthalmol 1955;40:553–556.

114. Mandell GL, Sande MA. Sulfonamides, trimethoprim-sulfamethoxazole, and urinary tract antiseptics. In: Gilman AG, Goodman LS, Rall TW, et al., eds. The pharmacological basis of therapeutics, ed. 7. New York: MacMillan Co., 1985;49:1095–1114.

115. O'Connor GR. The roles of parasite invasion and of hypersensitivity in the pathogenesis of toxoplasmic retinochoroiditis. Ocular Inflam Ther 1983;1:37–46.

116. O'Connor RG. Manifestations and management of ocular toxoplasmosis. Bull NY Acad Med 1974;50:192–210.

117. Tabbara KF, O'Connor GR. Treatment of ocular toxoplasmosis with clindamycin and sulfadiazine. Ophthalmology 1980;87:129–134.

118. Schlaegel TF. Toxoplasmosis. In: Fraunfelder FT, Roy FH, eds. Current ocular therapy, ed. 2. Philadelphia: W.B. Saunders Co, 1985;80–82.

119. Siniscal AA. The sulfonamides and antibiotics in trachoma. JAMA 1952;148:637–639.

120. Aragones JV. The treatment of blepharitis: A controlled double blind study of combination therapy. Ann Ophthalmol 1973;5:49–52.

121. McCulley JP, Dougherty JM, Deneau DG. Classification of chronic blepharitis. Ophthalmology 1982;89:1173–1982.

122. Parker CW. Drug therapy—drug allergy. I. N Engl J Med 1975;292:511–514.

123. Rubin Z. Ophthalmic sulfonamide–induced Stevens-Johnson syndrome. Arch Dermatol 1977;113:235–236.

124. Abramowicz M. Adverse ocular effects of systemic drugs. Med Lett Drugs Ther 1976;18:63–64.

125. Flach A. Photosensitivity to sulfisoxazole ointment. Arch Ophthalmol 1981;99:609–610.

126. Boettner EA, Fralick FB, Wolter JR. Conjunctival concretions of sulfadiazine. Arch Ophthalmol 1974;92:446–448.

127. Tabbara KF, Veirs ER. Corneal white plaques caused by

sulfacetamide eyedrops. Am J Ophthalmol 1984;98:378–380.

128. Chang FW, Reinhart S, Fraser NM. Effect of 30% sodium sulfacetamide on corneal sensitivity. Am J Optom Physiol Opt 1984;61:318–320.

129. Eyles DE, Coleman N. Synergistic effect of sulfadiazine and daraprim against experimental toxoplasmosis in the mouse. Antibiot Chemother 1953;3:483–490.

130. Nozik RA, Smolin G, Knowlton G, et al. Trimethoprim-polymyxin B ophthalmic solution in treatment of surface ocular bacterial infections. Ann Ophthalmol 1985;17:746–748.

131. Lamberts DW, Buka T, Knowlton GM. Clinical evaluation of trimethoprim containing ophthalmic solutions in humans. Am J Ophthalmol 1984;98:11–16.

132. Reiseberg B, Herzog J, Weinstein L. In vitro antibacterial activity of trimethoprim alone and combined with sulfonamides. Antimicrob Agents Chemother 1967;1:424–429.

133. Arndt KA, Jick H. Rates of cutaneous reactions to drugs. JAMA 1976;235:918–922.

134. Smith JT. The mode of action of 4-quinolones and possible mechanisms of resistance. J Antimicrob Chemother 1986;18:(Suppl D)21–29.

135. Wang C, Sabbaj M, Corrado M, et al. World-wide clinical experience with norfloxacin: efficacy and safety. Scand J Infect Dis (Suppl) 1986;48:81–89.

136. Monk JP, Campoli-Richards DM. Ofloxacin. A review of its antibacterial activity, pharmacokinetic properties and therapeutic use. Drugs (New Zealand) 1987;33:346–391.

137. Holmes B, Brogden RN, Richards DM. Norfloxacin: A review of its antibacterial activity, pharmacokinetic properties and therapeutic use. Drugs (New Zealand) 1985;30:482–513.

138. Crider SR, Colby SD, Miller LK, et al. Treatment of penicillin-resistant Neisseria gonorrhoeae with oral norfloxacin. N Engl J Med 1984;311:137–140.

139. Oriel JD. Ciprofloxacin in the treatment of gonorrhoea and non-gonococcal urethritis. J Antimicrob Chemother 1986; Suppl:129–132.

140. Shungu DL, Tutlane VK, Weinberg E, et al. In vitro antibacterial activity of norfloxacin and other agents against ocular pathogens. Chemotherapy 1985;31:112–118.

141. Darrell RW, Modak SM, Fox CL Jr. Norfloxacin and silver norfloxacin in the treatment of Pseudomonas corneal ulcer in the rabbit. Trans Am Ophthalmol Soc 1984;82:75–91.

142. Marble DA, Bosso JA. Norfloxacin: A quinoline antibiotic. Drug Intell Clin Pharm 1986;20:261–266.

143. Reuler JB, Chang MK. Herpes zoster: Epidemiology, clinical features, and treatment. South Med J 1984;77:1149–1156.

144. Holland GN, Pepose JS, Pettit TH, et al. Acquired immune deficiency syndrome. Ophthalmology 1983;90:859–872.

145. Collum LMT, Benedict-Smith A, Hillary IB. Randomized double-blind trial of acyclovir and idoxuridine in dendritic corneal ulceration. Br J Ophthalmol 1980;64:766–769.

146. Pavan-Langston D, Foster CS. Trifluorothymidine and idoxuridine therapy of ocular herpes. Am J Ophthalmol 1977;84:818–825.

147. Carroll JM, Martola EL, Laibson PR, et al. The recurrence of herpetic keratitis following idoxuridine therapy. Am J Ophthalmol 1967;63:103–107.

148. Rich LF. Toxic drug effects on the cornea. J Toxicol—Cut Ocular Toxicol 1982;1:267–297.

149. Hyndiuk RA, Glasser DB. Herpes simplex keratitis. In: Tabbara KF, Hyndiuk RA, eds. Infections of the eye. Boston: Little, Brown, 1986;20:343–368.

150. Juel-Jensen BE, MacCallum FO. Treatment of herpes simplex lesions of the face with idoxuridine: Results of double-blind controlled trial. Br Med J 1964;2:987–988.

151. Pavan-Langston D, Buchanan RA. Vidarabine therapy of simple and IDU-complicated herpetic keratitis. Trans Am Acad Ophthalmol Otolaryngol 1976;81:813–825.

152. Pavan-Langston D, Dohlman CH. A double blind clinical study of adenine arabinoside therapy of viral keratoconjunctivitis. Am J Ophthalmol 1972;74:81–88.

153. Pavan-Langston D. Clinical evaluation of adenine arabinoside and idoxuridine in the treatment of ocular herpes simplex. Am J Ophthalmol 1975;80:495–502.

154. Hirst LW. Ocular and periocular infections. Sights and sounds in ophthalmology, vol. 6. St. Louis: C.V. Mosby Co, 1985.

155. Whitley RJ, Soong RJ, Dolin R, et al. Adenine arabinoside therapy of biopsy-proved herpes simplex encephalitis: NIAID collaborative antiviral study. N Engl J Med 1977;297:289–294.

156. Whitley RJ, Alford CA, Hirsch MS, et al. Vidarabine versus acyclovir therapy in herpes simplex encephalitis. N Engl J Med 1986;314:144–149.

157. Wellings PC, Awdry PN, Bors FH, et al. Clinical evaluation of trifluorothymidine in the treatment of herpes simplex corneal ulcers. Am J Ophthalmol 1972;73:932–942.

158. McKinnon JR, McGill JI, Jones BR. A coded clinical evaluation of adenine arabinoside and trifluorothymidine in the treatment of ulcerative herpetic keratitis. In: Langston D, Buchanan RA, Alford CS, eds. Adenine arabinoside: an antiviral agent. New York: Raven Press, 1975.

159. Coster DJ, Jones BR, McGill JI. Treatment of amoeboid herpetic ulcers with adenine arabinoside or trifluorothymidine. Br J Ophthalmol 1979;63:418–421.

160. Nesburn AB, Lowe GH, Lepoff NJ, et al. Effect of topical trifluridine on Thygeson's superficial punctate keratitis. Ophthalmology 1984;91:1189–1192.

161. Lass JH. Antivirals. In: Lamberts DW, Potter DE, eds. Clinical ophthalmic pharmacology. Boston: Little, Brown, 1987;4:107–156.

162. Udell IJ. Trifluridine-associated conjunctival cicatrization. Am J Ophthalmol 1985;99:363–364.

163. Elion GB. The biochemistry and mechanism of action of acyclovir. J Antimicrob Chemother 1983;12(Suppl B):9–17.

164. Nilsen AE, Aasen T, Halsos AM, et al. Efficacy of oral acyclovir in the treatment of initial and recurrent genital herpes. Lancet 1982;2:571–573.

165. Corey L, Benedetti JK, Critchlow CW, et al. Double-blind controlled trial of topical acyclovir in genital herpes simplex infections. Am J Med 1982;73:326–334.

166. Corey L, Fife KH, Benediti JK, et al. Intravenous acyclovir for the treatment of primary genital herpes. Ann Intern Med 1983;98:914–921.

167. Thin RN, Jeffries DJ, Taylor PK, et al. Recurrent genital herpes suppressed by oral acyclovir: A multicentre double blind trial. Br J Antimicrob Chemother 1985;16:219–226.

168. Mindel A, Weller IVD, Faherty A, et al. Acyclovir in first attacks of genital herpes and prevention of recurrences. Genitourin Med 1986;62:28–32.

169. Thomas RHM, Dodd HJ, Yeo JM, et al. Oral acyclovir in the suppression of recurrent non-genital herpes simplex virus infection. Br J Dermatol 1985;113:731–735.

170. Lemak MA, Duvic M, Bean SF. Oral acyclovir for the prevention of herpes-associated erythema multiforme. J Am Acad Dermatol 1986;15:50–54.

171. Skoldenberg B, Forsgren M, Alestig K, et al. Acyclovir versus vidarabine in herpes simplex encephalitis: Randomised multicentre study in consecutive Swedish patients. Lancet 1984;2:707–711.

172. Jones BR, Coster DJ, Fison PN. Efficacy of acycloguanosine (Wellcome 248U) against herpes-simplex corneal ulcers. Lancet 1979;2:243–244.

173. Hung SO, Patterson A, Clark DI, et al. Oral acyclovir in the management of dendritic herpetic corneal ulceration. Br J Ophthalmol 1984;68:398–400.

174. Coster DJ, Wilhelmus KR, Michaud R, et al. A comparison of acyclovir and idoxuridine as treatment for ulcerative herpetic keratitis. Br J Ophthalmol 1980;64:763–765.

175. Collum LMT, Benedict-Smith A, Hillary IB. Randomized double-blind trial of acyclovir and idoxuridine in dendritic corneal ulceration. Br J Ophthalmol 1980;64:766–769.

176. Collum LMT, Logan P, McAuliffe-Curtin D, et al. Randomised double-blind trial of acyclovir (Zovirax) and adenine arabinoside in herpes simplex amoeboid corneal ulceration. Br J Ophthalmol 1985;69:847–850.

177. Jackson WB, Breslin CW, Lorenzetti DWC, et al. Treatment of herpes simplex keratitis: Comparison of acyclovir and vidarabine. Can J Ophthalmol 1984;19:107–111.

178. Lau C, Oosterhuis JA, Versteeg J, et al. Multicenter trial of acyclovir and trifluorothymidine in herpetic keratitis. Am J Med 1982;(Suppl):305–306.

179. Sanitato JJ, Asbell PA, Varnell ED, et al. Acyclovir in the treatment of herpetic stromal disease. Am J Ophthalmol 1984;98:537–547.

180. Collum LMT, O'Connor M, Logan P. Comparison of the efficacy and toxicity of acyclovir and of adenine arabinoside when combined with dilute betamethasone in herpetic disciform keratitis: Preliminary results of a double-blind trial. Trans Ophthalmol Soc UK 1983;103:597–599.

181. Cobo LM, Foulks GN, Liesegang T, et al. Oral acyclovir in the treatment of acute herpes zoster ophthalmicus. Ophthalmology 1986;93:763–770.

182. McGill J, Chapman C. A comparison of topical acyclovir with steroids in the treatment of herpes zoster keratouveitis. Br J Ophthalmol 1983;67:746–750.

183. Buchi ER, Herbort CP, Ruffieux C. Oral acyclovir in the treatment of acute herpes zoster ophthalmicus. Am J Ophthalmol 1986;101:531–532.

184. Balfour HH, Bean B, Laskin OL, et al. Acyclovir halts progression of herpes zoster in immunocompromised patients. N Engl J Med 1983;308:1448–1453.

185. Shepp DH, Dandliker PS, Meyers JD. Treatment of varicella-zoster virus infection in severely immunocompromised patients. A randomized comparison of acyclovir and vidarabine. N Engl J Med 1986;314:208–212.

186. Oblon DJ, Elfenbein GJ, Rand K, et al. Recurrent varicella zoster infection after acyclovir therapy in immunocompromised patients. South Med J 1986;79:256–257.

187. Blumenkranz MS, Culbertson WW, Clarkson JG, et al. Treatment of the acute retinal necrosis syndrome with intravenous acyclovir. Ophthalmology 1986;93:296–300.

188. Physicians desk reference, ed. 41. Oradell, NJ: Medical Economics, 1987.

189. Mitsuya H, Weinhold KJ, Furman PA, et al. 3′-azido-3′deoxythymidine (3 BW A509U): An antiviral agent that inhibits the infectivity and cytopathic effect of human T-lymphotropic virus type III/lymphadenopathy-associated virus in vitro. Proc Natl Acad Sci USA 1985;82:7096–7100.

190. St. Clair MH, Weinhold K, Richards CA, et al. Characterization of HTLV-III reverse transcriptase and inhibition by the triphosphate of BW A509U. In: Program and abstracts of the 25th interscience conference on antimicrobial agents and chemotherapy, Minneapolis, October 1985. American Society of Microbiology 1985;172:abstract.

191. Fischl MA, Richman DD, Grieco MH, et al. The efficacy of azidothymidine (AZT) in the treatment of patients with AIDS and AIDS related complex: a double-blind placebo-controlled trial. N Engl J Med 1987;317:185–191.

192. Richman DR, Fischl MA, Grieco MH, et al. The toxicity of azidothymidine (AZT) in the treatment of patients with AIDS and AIDS related complex: A double-blind placebo-controlled trial. N Engl J Med 1987;317:192–197.

193. Rosecan LR, Stahl-Bayliss CM, Kalman CM, et al. Antiviral therapy for cytomegalovirus retinitis in AIDS with dihydroxy propoxymethyl guanine. Am J Ophthalmol 1986;101:405–418.

194. Robinson MR, Streeten BW, Hampton GR, et al. Treatment of cytomegalovirus optic neuritis with dihydroxy propoxymethyl guanine. Am J Ophthalmol 1986;102:533–534.

195. Henry K, Cantrill H, Fletcher C, et al. Use of intravitreal Ganciclovir (dihydroxy propoxymethyl guanine) for cytomegalovirus retinitis in a patient with AIDS. Am J Ophthalmol 1987;103:17–23.

196. Maudgal PC, DeClercq E, Missotten L. Efficacy of bromovinyldeoxy-uridine in the treatment of herpes simplex virus and varicella-zoster virus eye infections. Antiviral Res 1984;4:281–283.

197. Descamps J, DeClercq E. Specific phosphorylation of E-5-(2-iodovinyl)-2′-deoxyuridine by herpes simplex virus-infected cells. J Biol Chem 1981;256:5973–5976.

198. Maudgal PC, DeClercq E, Bernaerts R, et al. Ocular penetration and efficacy of chloroethyldeoxyuridine against herpetic keratouveitis. Invest Ophthalmol Vis Sci 1986;27:1453–1458.

199. Polack FM, Kaufman HE, Newmark E. Keratomycosis. Medical and surgical treatment. Arch Ophthalmol 1971;85:410–416.

200. Kolodner H. Fungal corneal ulcers. Int Ophthalmol Clin 1984;24:17–24.

201. Green WR, Bennett JE, Goos RD. Ocular penetration of amphotericin B. Arch Ophthalmol 1965;73:769–775.

202. Butler WT. Pharmacology, toxicity, and therapeutic usefulness of amphotericin B. JAMA 1966;195:127–131.

203. Anderson B, Roberts S, Gozalez C, et al. Mycotic ulcerative keratitis. Arch Ophthalmol 1959;62:169–179.

204. Wood TO, Williford W. Treatment of keratomycosis with amphotericin B 0.15%. Am J Ophthalmol 1976;81:847–849.

205. Jones DB. Fungal keratitis. In: Duane TD, Jaeger EA, eds. Clinical ophthalmology. Philadelphia: Harper & Row, 1986;4(21):1–13.

206. O'Day DM, Ray WA, Head S, et al. Influence of the corneal epithelium on the efficacy of topical antifungal drugs. Invest Ophthalmol Vis Sci 1984;25:855–859.

207. Bell RW, Ritchey JP. Subconjunctival nodules after amphotericin B injection: Medical therapy for *Aspergillus* corneal ulcer. Arch Ophthalmol 1973;90:402–404.

208. Perraut LE, Perraut LE, Bleiman B, et al. Successful treatment of *Candida albicans* endophthalmitis with intravitreal amphotericin B. Arch Ophthalmol 1981;99:1565–1567.

209. Jones DB. Therapy of postsurgical fungal endophthalmitis. Ophthalmology 1978;85:357–373.

210. McGetrick JJ, Peyman GA, Nyberg MA. Amphotericin B methyl ester: Evaluation for intravitreous use in experimental fungal endophthalmitis. Ophthalmic Surg 1979;10:25–29.

211. Mangiaracine AB, Liebman SD. Fungus keratitis *(Aspergillus fumigatus):* Treatment with nystatin (mycostatin). Arch Ophthalmol 1957;58:695–698.

212. McGrand JC. Symposium on direct fungal infection of the eye: Keratomycosis due to *Aspergillus fumigatus* cured by nystatin. Trans Ophthalmol Soc UK 1969;89:799–803.

213. Roberts SS. Nystatin in monilia keratoconjunctivitis. Am J Ophthalmol 1957;44:108–109.

214. Forster RK, Rebell G. The diagnosis and management of keratomycoses. Arch Ophthalmol 1975;93:1134–1136.

215. Newmark E, Ellison AC, Kaufman HE. Pimaricin therapy of *Cephalosporium* and *Fusarium* keratitis. Am J Ophthalmol 1970;69:458–466.

216. Jones DB, Forster RK, Rebell G. *Fusarium solani* keratitis treated with natamycin (pimaricin): Eighteen consecutive cases. Arch Ophthalmol 1972;88:147–154.

217. Richard AB, Jones BR, Whitwell J, et al. Corneal and intraocular infection by *Candida albicans* treated with 5-fluorocytosine. Trans Ophthalmol Soc UK 1969;89:867–885.

218. Robertson DN, Riley FC, Hermans PE. Endogenous *Candida* oculomycosis: Report of two patients treated with flucytosine. Arch Ophthalmol 1974;91:33–38.

219. Sud IJ, Feingold DS. Mechanisms of action of the antimycotic imidazoles. Invest Dermatol 1981;76:438–441.

220. Foster CS. Miconazole therapy for keratomycosis. Am J Ophthalmol 1981;91:622–629.

221. Fitzsimons R, Peters AL. Miconazole and ketoconazole as a satisfactory first-line treatment for keratomycosis. Am J Ophthalmol 1986;101:605–608.

222. Ishibashi Y, Matsumoto Y. Intravenous miconazole in the treatment of keratomycosis. Am J Ophthalmol 1984;97:646–647.

223. Fowler BJ. Treatment of fungal endophthalmitis with vitrectomy and intraocular injection of miconazole. J Ocular Ther Surg 1984;3:43–47.

224. Hay RJ. Ketoconazole in the treatment of fungal infection: Clinical and laboratory studies. Am J Med 1983;74:16–19.

225. Graybill JR, Lundberg D, Donovan W, et al. Treatment of coccidioidomycosis with ketoconazole: Clinical and laboratory studies of 18 patients. Rev Infect Dis 1980;2:661–673.

226. Cuce LC, Wroclawski EL, Sampaio SAP. Treatment of paracoccidioidomycosis, candidiasis, chromomycosis, lobomycosis and mycetoma with ketoconazole. Int J Dermatol 1980;19:405–408.

227. Torres MA, Mohamed J, Cavazos-Adame H, et al. Topical ketoconazole for fungal keratitis. Am J Ophthalmol 1985; 100:293–298.

228. Ishibashi Y. Oral ketoconazole therapy for keratomycosis. Am J Ophthalmol 1983;95:342–345.

229. Gutt L, Feder JM, Feder RS, et al. Corneal ring formation after exposure to sulfamethoxazole. Arch Ophthalmol 1988;106:726–727.

230. Borrmann LR, Leopold IH. The potential use of quinolones in future ocular antimicrobial therapy. Am J Ophthalmol 1988,106:227–229.

231. Slavin ML, Margolis AJ. Resolution of cytomegalovirus retinitis with zidovudine therapy. Arch Ophthalmol 1981;106:1168–1169.

232. Farrell PL, Heinemann MH, Roberts CW, et al. Response of human-immunodeficiency virus-associated uveitis to zidovudine. Am J Ophthalmol 1988;106:7–10.

CHAPTER 7

Inhibitors of Aqueous Formation

Jeffrey A. Hiett

Glaucoma is a disease in which intraocular pressure is increased beyond physiologic limits. This pressure rise generally results from impaired outflow of aqueous humor; however, excessive secretion of aqueous may account for the elevation of intraocular pressure in a small number of patients. Furthermore, since the intricate balance between formation and outflow of aqueous determines the level of intraocular pressure, the clinical management of all types of glaucoma involves the use of drugs that either improve aqueous outflow or decrease the formation of aqueous. This chapter considers those drugs thought to act by inhibiting aqueous formation. Chapters 3 and 8 discuss other agents used in the treatment of glaucoma.

Aqueous Humor Formation

The ciliary processes of the ciliary body are continually producing aqueous humor at a rate of approximately 2.5 μl/min in the human eye.[1] The anatomic structure of these processes (Fig. 7.1) indicates that to reach the posterior chamber, plasma constituents must travel from the extensive capillary network within each process into the stromal tissue and through the pigmented and nonpigmented ciliary epithelium. The main barrier to movement of plasma constituents, as determined by tracer studies, is the tight junctions of the nonpigmented ciliary epithelium (Fig. 7.2).[2,3] The existence of a functional barrier is further supported by differ-

ences in composition of the aqueous humor and the plasma. These differences provide sufficient evidence to conclude that aqueous humor is not solely an ultrafiltrate of plasma and that active transport processes must be involved in the formation of aqueous.

Aqueous formation is generally agreed to depend on 3 physiologic processes: diffusion, ultrafiltration, and secretion.[4] Diffusion occurs because of random movement of molecules and acts to eliminate local concentration gradients by allowing certain substances to cross membranes in accordance with the existing transmembrane concentration gradients. Ultrafiltration is the pressure-dependent component of aqueous formation, which is governed by the osmotic and hydrostatic pressure differences that exist between the plasma in the capillaries of the ciliary processes and the aqueous in the posterior chamber. Secretion occurs as a result of transepithelial fluid movement that is linked with the $Na^+ - K^+$ adenosinetriphosphatase (ATPase) and carbonic anhydrase-dependent systems in the nonpigmented ciliary epithelium. Of these 3 processes, ultrafiltration and secretion are probably the most likely to be altered by drug-induced changes in aqueous humor formation.

There are two major intraocular sites where drugs can act to inhibit the formation of aqueous humor: the vasculature of the ciliary processes, and the ciliary epithelium. Since the hydrostatic pressure of the blood within the ciliary vasculature probably provides a significant driving force for the movement of plasma constituents toward the posterior chamber, drug-induced

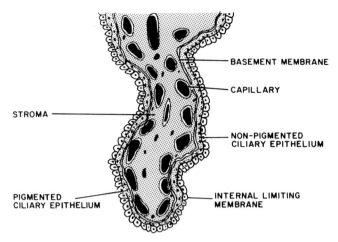

FIGURE 7.1   **Schematic diagram of the structure of a ciliary process (cross-section).**

changes in the rate of blood flow or in the pressure within the capillaries of the ciliary processes may alter the rate of aqueous formation. Blood flow through the anterior uveal vasculature of many species has been shown to be markedly reduced by either electrical stimulation of the sympathetic pathway to the eye[5–7] or topical application of adrenergic agonists.[8–10] Topical ocular application of α-receptor agonists, including phenylephrine, norepinephrine, and epinephrine, reduces uveal blood flow in the rabbit eye,[8] while topical epinephrine has a similar effect in the primate[9] and the human eye.[10] Decreased blood flow through the ciliary processes may reduce the rate of fluid movement toward the posterior chamber and can ultimately lead to a decreased rate of aqueous formation. Alterations in the uveal vascular resistance can also decrease the hydrostatic pressure within the ciliary vascular beds, thus reducing ultrafiltration. There is evidence to sup-

port the pressure dependence of aqueous humor formation. Using cats, Macri[11] showed that the rate of aqueous humor production is directly related to the ocular arterial perfusion pressure (blood pressure minus intraocular pressure). Furthermore, several investigators have found that systemic hypotension decreases intraocular pressure in animals[12,13] and in humans,[14] thereby illustrating the possible effect of decreasing the perfusion pressure to the eye. Therefore, drug-induced decreases in either the rate of blood flow to the ciliary processes or the perfusion pressure within the ciliary vascular beds may act to depress the rate of aqueous humor formation.

There is evidence to suggest that inhibition of active transport processes within the ciliary processes probably constitutes the most significant mechanism whereby drugs inhibit aqueous humor formation. Beta-adrenergic receptors have been localized to the ciliary proc-

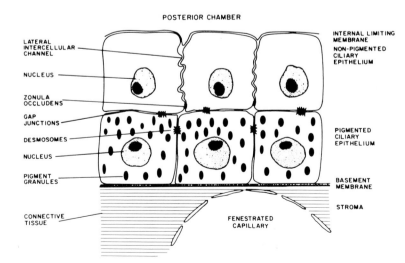

FIGURE 7.2   **The ciliary epithelia. Tight junctions between the epithelial cells act as the main barrier between the stromal fluid and the posterior chamber. Gap junctions and desmosomes provide a less restrictive barrier than the barrier created by the zonula occludens.**

esses in experimental animals[15,16] and humans,[17] and cytochemical studies[18] have shown that adenylate cyclase activity, a membrane-bound enzyme found in association with β receptors, is greatest on the lateral interdigitating membranes of the nonpigmented ciliary epithelium. When activated, the β receptor–adenylate cyclase complex produces increased levels of intracellular cyclic adenosine monophosphate (cAMP) in most tissues. Sears[19] has proposed that increased levels of intracellular cAMP may directly regulate the membrane permeability of the nonpigmented ciliary epithelium, or indirectly regulate aqueous formation by altering the rate at which sodium reaches the $Na^+ - K^+$ ATPase-dependent transport system. Since it is now generally accepted that both selective and nonselective β-receptor antagonists decrease intraocular pressure through a reduction in aqueous formation,[20–26] the site of action of these drugs is probably at the level of the ciliary epithelium.[27] Although cAMP certainly appears to be a common "second messenger" for many agents altering aqueous formation, the cascade of intracellular events produced by each agent, relative to their effects on intraocular pressure, are poorly understood. At present, the cellular actions of β-receptor antagonists as inhibitors of aqueous formation are unknown.

The unidirectional transepithelial movement of sodium and other ions probably plays a key role in aqueous formation. Since sodium transport is usually linked to $Na^+ - K^+$ ATPase,[28] it is not surprising that this membrane-bound enzyme has been demonstrated in the ciliary epithelium.[29] Carbonic anhydrase is an enzyme felt to be linked with transepithelial movement of sodium and bicarbonate ions, and it has been found in the ciliary epithelium of experimental animals[30–32] and humans.[32,33] Inhibition of either $Na^+ - K^+$ ATPase or carbonic anhydrase has been shown to decrease sodium movement into aqueous humor and results in a reduced rate of aqueous formation.[34]

Clinically useful drugs with ocular hypotensive actions attributable to inhibition of aqueous humor formation are listed in Table 7.1. Since their mechanisms are diverse, it is easiest to categorize these drugs by their pharmacologic properties rather than by their physiologic effects. Only a brief discussion of the topical adrenergic antagonists has been included in this chapter, since these agents are addressed in Chapter 3.

β-Adrenergic Blocking Agents

Intraocular pressure of both normal and glaucomatous human eyes is decreased following either systemic or topical ocular administration of β-adrenergic blocking

TABLE 7.1
Clinically Useful Inhibitors of Aqueous Humor Formation

Adrenergic antagonists
Atenolol
Betaxolol
Labetalol
Levobunolol
Metoprolol
Nadolol
Pindolol
Propranolol
Timolol
Carbonic anhydrase inhibitors
Acetazolamide
Methazolamide
Dichlorphenamide
Cannabinoids[a]
Cardiac glycosides[a]

[a]Of questionable clinical significance.

agents (β blockers). Although topical ocular application is the ideal route of administration for a drug designed to lower intraocular pressure, many patients may be receiving oral β blockers for treatment of a variety of unrelated conditions, including angina, systemic hypertension, arrhythmias, thyrotoxicosis, hypertrophic cardiomyopathies, and migraine headache. Eight β blockers have been approved for systemic administration (Table 7.2). Betaxolol, levobunolol, and timolol are available as ophthalmic drops for topical use in the treatment of glaucoma. The pharmacodynamic properties of the various β blockers are compared in Table 7.3.

Most studies[20–27] indicate that topical β blockers exert their primary ocular hypotensive action by inhibiting aqueous formation. Although some investigators[35,36] have reported that an increase in aqueous outflow also occurs following use of β blockers, others have shown that outflow is unchanged. Of the β blockers, timolol is the most widely investigated ocular hypotensive agent, but all β blockers may act by a similar mechanism(s). Neufeld[27] has postulated that timolol can act on secretion, ultrafiltration, or both. Since aqueous formation depends on blood flow and perfusion pressure within the ciliary vasculature, timolol may induce a net vasoconstriction by preventing β-receptor-mediated vasodilation of the afferent vessels in the ciliary processes. However, this vascular action of timolol has not been confirmed experimentally.[27] Consequently, Neufeld[27] has suggested that timolol reduces aqueous formation through a direct action on the ciliary epithelium. The intracellular effects of β-receptor blockade at the level of the nonpigmented ciliary epithelium are still unclear. At present, there is no evidence to suggest that sys-

TABLE 7.2
Systemic β Blockers Commercially Available in the United States

β Blocker	Trade Name (manufacturer)	Preparation
Acebutolol	Sectral (Wyeth)	200 and 400 mg capsules
Atenolol	Tenormin (ICI Pharma)	50 and 100 mg tablets
Labetalol	Normodyne; Trandate (Schering; Glaxo)	100, 200, and 300 mg tablets
Metoprolol	Lopressor (Geigy)	50 and 100 mg tablets
Nadolol	Corgard (Squibb)	20, 40, 80, 120, and 160 mg tablets
Pindolol	Visken (Sandoz)	5 and 10 mg tablets
Propranolol	Inderal (Ayerst)	10, 20, 40, 60, 80, and 90 mg tablets
Timolol	Blocadren (Merck)	5, 10, and 20 mg tablets

temic and topical β blockers decrease intraocular pressure by a different mechanism.

Topical β blockers have had a tremendous impact on the pharmacologic treatment of all types of glaucoma. Timolol was the first β blocker to be used extensively as an antiglaucoma agent, and the ocular hypotensive properties of all newly developed topical β blockers have been compared with those of timolol. Of the topical β blockers tested to date, none of these agents has been shown to be more effective in reducing intraocular pressure than timolol. Therefore, timolol has become the standard against which other topical β blockers are judged.

Although systemic β blockers are not approved for clinical use as ocular hypotensive agents, many drugs within this class are prescribed routinely for systemic conditions in doses that are known to reduce intraocular pressure. The ocular hypotensive action observed after systemic administration may be beneficial in patients with ocular hypertension or in the glaucoma patient controlled with antiglaucoma drugs other than epinephrine. Systemic β blockers are frequently overlooked as ocular hypotensive agents despite their ability to significantly reduce intraocular pressure. Table 7.4 illustrates the ocular hypotensive action of both systemic and topical β blockers. Therefore, the clini-

TABLE 7.3
Pharmacodynamic Properties of Systemic and Topical β Blockers

β Blocker	Potency (compared with propranolol)	Selectivity for β Receptors	Membrane-Stabilizing (local anesthetic) Activity	Partial β-Agonist Activity
Atenolol (T)	1	β₁ selective	−	−
Betaxolol (D)	1	β₁ selective	−	−
Labetalol (T)	0.06–0.7	Nonselective	+	±
Levobunolol (D)	6	Nonselective	−	−
Metoprolol (T)	0.5–2	β₁ selective	−	−
Nadolol (T)	1–6	Nonselective	−	−
Pindolol (T)	5–10	Nonselective	+	+
Propranolol (T)	1	Nonselective	+ +	−
Timolol (D, T)	6	Nonselective	−	−

T, available in tablet form for systemic use; D, available as ophthalmic drops for topical use; +, property present; −, property absent.

cian should not ignore systemic β blockers as useful ocular hypotensive agents. However, since systemic β blockers also reduce blood pressure, this route of administration may actually prove detrimental in certain glaucomatous patients. The decrease in the perfusion pressure to the optic nerve produced by decreased systemic blood pressure may offset the benefit derived from reducing the intraocular pressure. Despite this effect, patients with elevated intraocular pressure and systemic hypertension would appear to be ideal candidates for a therapeutic trial of oral β blockers to determine if both conditions can be adequately controlled with a single agent, thereby reducing the cost to the patient and hopefully improving compliance.

Atenolol

Atenolol (Tenormin) is a selective β_1-adrenergic receptor antagonist that lacks partial β-receptor agonist activity and membrane-stabilizing properties.[38] Atenolol is currently approved for the treatment of mild to moderate hypertension and is commercially available as 50 and 100 mg tablets. Because of its long plasma half–life, atenolol is administered once daily in the treatment of hypertension. The recommended initial adult dose of atenolol is 50 mg daily, either alone or with concurrent diuretic therapy. If after 1 or 2 weeks the desired blood pressure is not obtained, the dose is often increased to a single dose of 100 mg daily.[39] In elderly patients, the dosage changes are often made at 4- to 6-week intervals.[40] Further increases in dosage beyond 100 mg daily have not been found to be of any additional benefit.[41]

A single oral 50 mg dose of atenolol has been shown to decrease intraocular pressure in patients with ocular hypertension, open-angle glaucoma, and chronic angle-closure glaucoma.[42–45] A significant ocular hypotensive effect may occur for about 7 hours.[42] The average maximum reduction occurs 5 hours after ingestion, and the degree of reduction is about 35% of the initial intraocular pressure.[42] In patients with open-angle and chronic angle-closure glaucoma, a single oral 50 mg tablet of atenolol produces a significantly greater reduction in intraocular pressure than does a single dose of either propranolol (40 mg)[43] or acetazolamide (500 mg).[44] Oral doses of atenolol (50 mg twice daily) have also been reported to reduce intraocular pressure in nonglaucomatous eyes.[45] In this latter study, the initial pressure reduction was maintained throughout the 8 days of administration.

Topical ocular application of atenolol, as 1%, 2% and 4% drops, reduces intraocular pressure in patients with ocular hypertension.[46] The maximum pressure reduction occurs 2 to 3 hours after application, and the

intraocular pressure requires about 7 hours to return to pretreatment levels.[47] Four hours after topical administration, a single drop of atenolol 4% produces a 22% reduction of intraocular pressure (6.3 mm Hg) in eyes with primary open-angle glaucoma.[48] Atenolol 2% reduces intraocular pressure to levels comparable to pilocarpine 2%,[49] and atenolol 4% has been shown to have a greater ocular hypotensive effect than epinephrine 1%.[49] In a long-term study,[50] atenolol 4% reduced intraocular pressure in patients with either ocular hypertension or glaucoma; however, the effectiveness of atenolol's ocular hypotensive action decreases with long-term use in some patients. With long-term use, most patients seem to tolerate topical ocular administration of atenolol eyedrops without significant ocular side effects.[50]

Betaxolol

Betaxolol (Betoptic) is a selective β_1-adrenergic antagonist that lacks intrinsic sympathomimetic activity and membrane-stabilizing properties.[51] Betaxolol is approved for the treatment of elevated intraocular pressure, including ocular hypertension and open-angle glaucoma. It is commercially available as a 0.5% ophthalmic solution. For treatment of elevated intraocular pressure, betaxolol is administered in the affected eye(s) twice daily.

Since betaxolol is not commercially available for systemic administration, only its properties as an ocular agent are discussed in this chapter. Following topical ocular administration, betaxolol produces a dose-dependent reduction in intraocular pressure at concentrations up to 0.5%.[52–55] The onset of action is within 30 minutes, with the maximal effect noted at 2 hours after topical administration.[56] Betaxolol's ocular hypotensive action has a duration that is at least 12 hours.[57] The ocular hypotensive action of betaxolol has been attributed to reduced aqueous formation.[26] The reduction in intraocular pressure produced by betaxolol 0.5% is comparable to the ocular hypotensive response from timolol 0.5%.[58,59] Both drugs produce their maximum effect on intraocular pressure within the first week of therapy, and the degree of reduction remains relatively constant for at least 6 months.[59] At the end of a 6-month study, patients receiving betaxolol 0.5% showed a 28.9% reduction in intraocular pressure, while patients using timolol 0.5% exhibited a 33.2% reduction.[59] Although some studies have shown no statistically significant difference between the ocular hypotensive properties of betaxolol and timolol, other investigators have found betaxolol's ocular hypotensive efficacy to be slightly less than that of timolol.[59–61] An additional reduction in intraocular pressure can be pro-

TABLE 7.4
Ocular Hypotensive Action of Commercially Available β Blockers in Humans

β Blocker	Total Daily Dose	Reduction of IOP (%)
Systemic		
Acebutolol	—	—
Atenolol[43–45]	50 mg	35
Labetalol[a]	—	—
Metoprolol[81,82]	100–150 mg	32
Nadolol[89–92,292]	10–80 mg	21–41
Pindolol[a]	—	—
Propranolol[45,107]	80–160 mg	23–28
Timolol[110]	5–30 mg	20–25
Topical		
Betaxolol[59–62]	0.5% b.i.d.	26–29
Levobunolol[74,75]	0.5% b.i.d.	26–30
Timolol[58–60,74,75]	0.5% b.i.d.	28–33

[a]Limited information available. IOP, intraocular pressure; b.i.d., twice daily.

duced by adding betaxolol to a drug regimen including pilocarpine, epinephrine derivatives, or carbonic anhydrase inhibitors.[59,62,63]

Compared to nonselective β-adrenergic antagonists, the principal advantage to the clinical use of betaxolol is its ability to lower intraocular pressure with fewer systemic side effects attributed to β_2 blockade.[290] This feature is particularly important in glaucoma patients with bronchoconstrictive disorders. Betaxolol has been used in most glaucoma patients with asthma without exacerbation of pulmonary symptoms.[63] In addition, betaxolol has not been shown to reduce blood pressure or pulse rate significantly following prolonged ocular use for the treatment of glaucoma.[59] However, betaxolol has been documented to produce systemic side effects, including asthma and bradycardia, in a very small percentage of patients using it for antiglaucoma therapy.[64,290] A preliminary study[291] found that betaxolol may also produce fewer central nervous system side effects than timolol. The pharmacologic properties of betaxolol are discussed further in Chapter 3.

Labetalol

Labetalol (Normodyne, Trandate) is an adrenergic antagonist that has both selective α_1- and nonselective β-adrenergic blocking activity.[65] Labetalol is approved for the treatment of systemic hypertension. Available in 100, 200, and 300 mg tablets, labetalol is recommended in initial doses of 100 mg twice daily. The usual maintenance dosage of the drug is between 200 and 400 mg twice daily.

Studies using rabbits have shown that intravenous labetalol produces a dose-dependent decrease in intraocular pressure.[66] Although the action of systemic labetalol on intraocular pressure in humans has not been extensively studied, this agent would be expected to decrease intraocular pressure at clinically useful doses, since other oral β blockers share this property.

Topical labetalol has been found to be an extremely effective ocular hypotensive agent in normal rabbits and in two rabbit models of glaucoma.[67–69] Human studies, however, have shown that topically applied 0.5% and 1% labetalol, in aqueous solution, only moderately reduces intraocular pressure for about 5 hours.[67] In patients with open-angle glaucoma, topical labetalol was not found to be as effective an ocular hypotensive agent as timolol or nadolol.[69,70]

Levobunolol

Levobunolol (Betagan) is a nonselective β-adrenergic antagonist that lacks β-receptor agonist or membrane-stabilizing activity.[71] Available as a 0.5% ophthalmic solution, levobunolol is approved for the treatment of ocular hypertension and open-angle glaucoma. Because of its long duration of action, levobunolol may be administered once daily. If a satisfactory ocular hypotensive response is not achieved with once-daily administration, levobunolol should be administered twice daily.

Many of the pharmacologic properties of levobunolol are similar to those of timolol. Levobunolol and timolol are both very potent nonselective β blockers.[72]

Both drugs produce maximal ocular hypotensive response at 0.5% concentration.[73] No significant difference in the ocular hypotensive efficacy has been found in studies comparing 0.5% timolol and 0.5% levobunolol.[74,75] In addition, both drugs produce a contralateral effect on intraocular pressure.[76,77] Comparative studies, however, indicate that levobunolol has a longer duration of ocular hypotensive action than does timolol.[78] Levobunolol produces an ocular hypotensive response within 1 hour of instillation, and a significant reduction of intraocular pressure lasts up to 24 hours.[76] Following a 3-month trial of once-daily administration of 0.5% levobunolol, 1% levobunolol, and 0.5% timolol, satisfactory intraocular pressure was achieved in 72% of patients treated with 0.5% levobunolol, 79% of patients treated with 1% levobunolol, and 64% of patients treated with 0.5% timolol.[78] This study suggests that once-daily administration of levobunolol may provide adequate control of intraocular pressure in properly selected cases of ocular hypertension and open-angle glaucoma. With twice-daily administration, about 75% of patients with ocular hypertension or open-angle glaucoma achieve a satisfactory ocular hypotensive response with either 0.5% timolol or 0.5% levobunolol alone;[73] the remaining 25% must add other antiglaucoma agents to reach an acceptable level of intraocular pressure. Because of their pharmacologic similarities, the clinical applications, contraindications, and side effects of levobunolol are very similar to those of timolol. The pharmacologic properties of levobunolol are discussed further in Chapter 3.

Metoprolol

Metoprolol (Lopressor) is a selective β_1-adrenergic antagonist without partial β-receptor agonist activity and membrane-stabilizing properties.[38,79,80] Available in 50 and 100 mg tablets, metoprolol has its main clinical use in the treatment of mild to moderate hypertension. The initial recommended adult dosage is 50 mg given once daily. If blood pressure control is inadequate, the dose is usually increased by 50 mg increments separated by weekly intervals.[40] The adult dosage range is 100 to 400 mg daily in 2 divided doses.[39]

The dose-response relationship of metoprolol's ocular hypotensive action was studied by Alm and Wickstrom,[81] who found that single 25, 50, or 100 mg doses of metoprolol reduced intraocular pressure in healthy men and women. A maximum effect was noted 2 to 5 hours after oral administration of all doses. The duration and magnitude of the pressure reduction increased with increasing doses, but a significant ocular hypotensive effect that lasted the duration of the study (8 hours) was found only with the 100 mg dose. The

100 mg dose had a maximum effect 4 hours after administration and produced a 32% relative decrease in intraocular pressure from pretreatment levels. In a short-term study involving patients with previously untreated open-angle glaucoma, 50 mg of metoprolol, given every 8 hours for 24 hours, reduced intraocular pressure in the glaucomatous eyes from a mean pressure of 30.1 mm Hg to 20.6 mm Hg.[82]

Following topical ocular administration of metoprolol, the intraocular pressure reduction has been reported to be dose dependent at concentrations below 1%, while no significant increase in efficacy has been reported at higher concentrations.[83] Short-term topical administration of metoprolol tartrate 3% eyedrops applied twice daily has produced a 36% relative decrease (8.8 mm Hg) in the intraocular pressures of patients with ocular hypertension and glaucoma. While receiving this treatment regimen, these patients were monitored for 4 months, and their intraocular pressures were maintained at a level between 23% and 30% below pretreatment readings.[83] Pilocarpine 2% to 4% and metoprolol 3% have been found to reduce intraocular pressure to equivalent levels in patients with glaucoma and ocular hypertension.[84] Furthermore, in patients with glaucoma, metoprolol 3% has produced an ocular hypotensive effect comparable to that of timolol 0.5%.[85] However, other studies[86,87] have generally shown metoprolol 3% eyedrops to be less effective than timolol 0.5% as an ocular hypotensive agent.

Nadolol

Nadolol (Corgard) is a nonselective β-adrenergic antagonist that lacks β-receptor agonist or membrane-stabilizing activity.[38] Available in 20, 40, 80, 120, and 160 mg tablets, nadolol is approved for the treatment of angina and systemic hypertension. Because of its long half-life in plasma, nadolol is administered once daily. The usual adult daily dosage range is 80 to 240 mg once daily for the management of angina, while doses up to 320 mg may be used in the treatment of hypertension.[88]

Oral nadolol produces a dose-dependent ocular hypotensive response in humans with normal and elevated intraocular pressure.[89-92] In a study of patients with open-angle glaucoma, the ocular hypotensive effect of orally administered nadolol (20 and 40 mg once daily) was equivalent to 0.25% or 0.5% timolol eyedrops.[92] The ocular hypotensive effects of long-term nadolol were well maintained for the duration of the 2-year study. The investigators concluded that a 20 or 40 mg nadolol tablet, taken once daily, will control intraocular pressure in many patients with open-angle glaucoma.[92]

Topical nadolol has been studied specifically for its ocular hypotensive properties, and nadolol 2% eyedrops appears to be the concentration with the most potential for clinical use.[93,94] After short-term administration in patients with ocular hypertension and glaucoma, nadolol 2% has reduced intraocular pressure to levels comparable to those produced by 0.25% timolol.[94] However, with prolonged use nadolol has been shown to be less effective as an ocular hypotensive agent than is timolol.[94] Since the poor clinical efficacy was attributed to inadequate intraocular penetration, a prodrug analog, diacetyl nadolol, was produced and tested.[95] Diacetyl nadolol has a greater lipophilicity than its parent compound, and 30 minutes after topical application aqueous levels of drug have been demonstrated to be approximately 10 times greater than those of nadolol.[95] The majority of diacetyl nadolol undergoes hydrolysis to nadolol within ocular tissues during the first hour following administration.[95] In a study involving patients with open-angle glaucoma, diacetyl nadolol 2% produced a decrease in intraocular pressure similar in magnitude to that of timolol 0.5% during the first 8 hours following topical application.[95]

Pindolol

Pindolol (Visken) is a potent nonselective β-adrenergic antagonist. In binding to β-adrenergic receptors, pindolol produces slight receptor stimulation (partial β-agonist activity).[96] Pindolol also exerts very weak membrane-stabilizing activity; however, this action is not apparent at clinically useful plasma concentrations.[97] The drug is currently approved for use in the management of mild to moderate hypertension. Pindolol is available in 5 and 10 mg tablets, and the usual effective adult dosage range is approximately 15 to 30 mg daily. Pindolol therapy is often started at 5 mg twice daily, either alone or in combination with other antihypertensive agents. If an adequate blood pressure response is not obtained, the dose is adjusted, in 5 to 10 mg increments, up to 30 mg daily.[97]

Regarding the effects of systemic pindolol on intraocular pressure, only limited information is presently available. Smith and associates[98] administered intravenous pindolol to young healthy volunteers and found that intraocular pressure decreased to maximal levels within 1 hour. This study is of interest because these investigators compared the ocular hypotensive response and plasma concentrations of an intravenous dose of pindolol (1.13 mg) to an equivalent dose (2 drops of 1%) of pindolol applied topically to the eye. Both routes of administration produced equivalent pressure reductions (about 3 mm Hg). After topical ocular application to an eye, pindolol 1% produced a bilateral intraocular pressure reduction, although the untreated eyes exhibited a hypotensive response that was less than that of the treated eyes. Systemic absorption of topically applied pindolol was postulated to account for the reduction of intraocular pressure in the untreated eye. To support this contention, plasma pindolol concentrations were determined after topical ocular and intravenous administration of equivalent doses (2 drops of 1% and 1.13 mg, respectively). The plasma levels attained were much less after ocular instillation than the intravenous route (6.8 μmol/liter and 34.2 μmol/liter, respectively).

Topical pindolol 1% reduces intraocular pressure in normal and glaucomatous eyes, although, like other ocular hypotensive agents, the amount of reduction is greater in eyes with elevated intraocular pressure.[99] The pressure reduction has been shown to reach maximum 1 hour after topical instillation. In healthy eyes, the intraocular pressure slowly returns to pretreatment levels 24 hours after administration, while glaucomatous eyes maintain slightly reduced pressures beyond 24 hours. When added to a treatment regimen consisting of pilocarpine, guanethidine, and epinephrine, pindolol 0.5% reduces intraocular pressure 2.8 mm Hg (average) in patients with open-angle glaucoma.[100] Since facility of outflow is unaltered, the pressure reduction is attributable to decreased aqueous formation.[99]

When compared with timolol 0.5%, pindolol 0.25% has been demonstrated to reduce intraocular pressure to levels approximating those produced by timolol.[101] In patients with open-angle glaucoma, pindolol 0.25% twice daily was able to control intraocular pressure as effectively as timolol 0.5% twice daily.[101] At present, no long-term studies have evaluated topical pindolol in the treatment of glaucoma.

Propranolol

Propranolol (Inderal) is a nonselective β-adrenergic antagonist that is widely used for the treatment of systemic hypertension, angina, certain types of cardiac arrhythmias, hypertrophic cardiomyopathies, and migraine headache.[79] This drug does not exhibit partial β-receptor agonist activity, but it does possess membrane-stabilizing properties.[38] Propranolol is commercially available in 10, 20, 40, 60, 80, and 90 mg tablets. It is also available in 60, 80, 120, and 160 mg sustained-release capsules, and 1 mg/ml IV preparation. The recommended adult daily dosage range varies with the condition but is usually between 40 and 320 mg.

Systemic propranolol decreases intraocular pressure in healthy and glaucomatous eyes.[43,102–107] Since the ocular hypotensive effect of propranolol is dose-dependent, a greater pressure reduction has been noted when higher doses are given.[104] In 7 of 19 glaucomatous patients in one study, oral propranolol, in doses of 20 to 40 mg administered 3 to 4 times daily, reduced intraocular pressure to an acceptable level ($\leq$ 22 mm Hg) for up to 42 months.[105] Oral propranolol, 40 mg administered twice daily, reduces intraocular pressure to approximately the same level as acetazolamide 250 mg administered twice daily.[106]

Topical propranolol 1% also reduces intraocular pressure in glaucomatous eyes during long-term therapy, but a major disadvantage of this route of administration is the corneal anesthesia that accompanies topical ocular application.[108]

Timolol

Timolol maleate (Blocadren, Timoptic) is a potent, nonselective β-adrenergic antagonist. Timolol lacks both partial β-receptor agonist activity and membrane-stabilizing activity.[38] This latter property allows timolol to be applied topically to the eye with minimal alteration of corneal sensitivity. Oral timolol (Blocadren) is approved for the treatment of systemic hypertension and for prevention of myocardial ischemia in patients who have survived a myocardial infarction. Topical timolol (Timoptic) is currently approved for treatment of elevated intraocular pressure. Oral timolol is available in 5, 10 and 20 mg tablets, and the recommended adult daily dosage range is 20 to 60 mg.[39] For topical ocular administration, timolol is commercially available as ophthalmic drops in 0.25% and 0.5% solutions. In the treatment of elevated intraocular pressure, timolol is usually administered twice daily, although some patients may exhibit adequate control using timolol once daily.[109]

In nonglaucomatous eyes, the ocular hypotensive effect of oral timolol changes very little at doses above 5 mg daily, although higher doses would be expected to produce a more complete blockade of β receptors.[110] The dose-response relationship of oral timolol's ocular hypotensive effect has not been established for eyes with glaucoma. However, oral timolol (20 mg twice daily) produces a pronounced reduction of intraocular pressure in patients with open-angle glaucoma.[111] At these doses, an additional reduction in intraocular pressure does not occur following concomitant use of topical timolol.[111] At low doses (5 mg) of oral timolol, topical epinephrine produces an additional intraocular pressure reduction. Higher doses (20 mg) of oral timolol antagonize the ocular hypotensive action of epinephrine.[112] This antagonistic interaction has also been reported following use of topical timolol.[113–115] Since timolol produces a dose-dependent competitive blockade of β receptors, the higher doses of timolol appear

to antagonize the β-receptor-mediated increase in facility of outflow produced by epinephrine.[110]

When used alone as a topical ocular hypotensive agent, timolol is effective in reducing intraocular pressure by approximately 20% to 30% compared with pretreatment values.[23,116] Timolol is effective in reducing intraocular pressure in eyes with ocular hypertension, open-angle glaucoma, secondary glaucoma, angle-closure glaucoma, and congenital glaucoma.[37,117–120] The duration of the ocular hypotensive response following the instillation of a single drop is at least 24 hours, and dose-response studies have determined that the 0.5% concentration gives a maximum ocular hypotensive effect.[109]

In the treatment of open-angle glaucoma, the ocular hypotensive response following topical administration of timolol is greater than that of epinephrine and at least as great as that of pilocarpine.[23,116,121,122] In addition, timolol produces less variation in the diurnal intraocular pressure curve than does pilocarpine.[123] Topical timolol decreases intraocular pressure less effectively than does acetazolamide.[124,125] Although both timolol and acetazolamide decrease aqueous formation,[20,25,126,127] when used together they produce a greater intraocular pressure reduction than will either drug used alone.[124,125] Furthermore, timolol can produce an additional intraocular pressure reduction when added to a treatment regimen of miotics or maximum medical therapy.[128–131] Therefore, timolol may be used alone as the first drug in the treatment of open-angle glaucoma, or it may be added to a treatment regimen consisting of most other antiglaucoma agents. However, as previously mentioned, timolol and epinephrine should not be used concomitantly. Long-term concurrent use of topically applied timolol and epinephrine produces a reduction in intraocular pressure that is not significantly greater than that of either drug used alone.[134] In contrast to epinephrine, however, the addition of dipivefrin to timolol therapy does produce a small additional decrease (less than 2 mm Hg) in intraocular pressure after 1 month of combined therapy.[135] Since timolol and a miotic appear to be a particularly effective combination,[136] concurrent use of these two agents is often begun if either drug is ineffective when used alone. Unless systemic contraindications are present, timolol is generally incorporated into the treatment regimen before the addition of a carbonic anhydrase inhibitor.[120]

In patients with acute angle-closure glaucoma, instillation of timolol followed 3 hours later by 1 drop of pilocarpine 2% has been shown to be an effective means of reducing intraocular pressure to normal levels before surgery.[117] However, further studies must be done to determine if this approach has any advantages when compared with the conventional treatment consisting of pilocarpine, hyperosmotic agents, and carbonic anhydrase inhibitors.

Topical timolol further reduces intraocular pressure when given to patients already receiving oral β blockers for systemic hypertension.[137] Although some glaucomatous patients receiving systemic β-blocker therapy might benefit from the addition of topical timolol, topical timolol alone will produce maximum reduction in intraocular pressure.[137] Therefore, topical timolol is not contraindicated in patients already taking systemic β blockers, since intraocular pressure may decrease further.

In blacks, timolol is more effective as an ocular hypotensive agent than are other antiglaucoma drugs. Thus, timolol or another β blocker should be considered as the primary therapy for black patients with open-angle glaucoma.[138]

Carbonic Anhydrase Inhibitors

Mechanism of Action

In 1949, Friedenwald[139] proposed that bicarbonate formation was an essential component of aqueous production. His theory was supported by the discovery of a relatively high concentration of bicarbonate in aqueous humor obtained from the rabbit posterior chamber.[140] Wistrand[30] subsequently demonstrated the presence of carbonic anhydrase in the ciliary processes of the rabbit, and Becker,[141] in 1954, reported the ocular hypotensive properties of acetazolamide, a carbonic anhydrase inhibitor. Tonographic data obtained by Becker[141] suggested that the decrease in intraocular pressure induced by acetazolamide results from inhibition of aqueous humor production. Other studies[126,142] have confirmed this action of carbonic anhydrase inhibitors. Since the discovery of their ocular hypotensive properties, carbonic anhydrase inhibitors (Table 7.5)

have been widely used in the treatment of all types of glaucoma.

All commercially available carbonic anhydrase inhibitors are unsubstituted aromatic sulfonamides $(ARYL-SO_2NH_2)$.[143] The resonating heterocyclic side group confers a high inhibitory activity to these agents. Substitutions on the amino nitrogen produce compounds that are inactive as carbonic anhydrase inhibitors.[142] These compounds produce their primary pharmacologic effects through reversible, noncompetitive binding with the enzyme carbonic anhydrase.[144] Carbonic anhydrase catalyzes the first step (I) in the following reaction:

$$CO_2 + H_2O \overset{I}{\rightleftharpoons} H_2CO_3 \overset{II}{\rightleftharpoons} H^+ + HCO_3^- \quad (7.1)$$

Reaction II is an ionic dissociation reaction that occurs very rapidly and that is not under enzymatic control.[144] Therefore, carbonic anhydrase catalyzes the cellular production of H_2CO_3 and thus the formation of H^+ and HCO_3^-. Although several isoenzymes of carbonic anhydrase are present in body tissues, the C-type, sulfonamide-sensitive carbonic anhydrase, is the predominant isoenzyme found in the human ciliary processes.[32,33]

Inhibition of carbonic anhydrase activity in the ciliary processes is probably the mechanism responsible for decreased aqueous formation produced by carbonic anhydrase inhibitors. The production of bicarbonate in the ciliary epithelium appears to play a key role in the formation of aqueous humor. Although both bicarbonate and chloride are anions present in appreciable concentration in the aqueous humor, Zimmerman and associates[145] found that acetazolamide decreased bicarbonate entry into the posterior chamber of the dog by about 50%, while chloride entry was not significantly altered. From this finding, these investigators concluded that bicarbonate is the key anion associated

TABLE 7.5
Carbonic Anhydrase Inhibitors

Drug	Trade Name (manufacturer)	Preparation
Acetazolamide	Diamox (Lederle)	125 and 250 mg tablets 500 mg sustained-release capsules (Sequels) 500 mg vials for injection
Methazolamide	Neptazane (Lederle)	25 and 50 mg tablets
Dichlorphenamide	Daranide (Merck)	50 mg tablets

with the decrease in aqueous formation produced by inhibition of carbonic anhydrase. This conclusion has been further supported by similar findings in other species.[146,147]

Inhibition of carbonic anhydrase also produces decreased sodium entry into the posterior chamber.[34,148,149] Sodium, transported by $Na^+ - K^+$ ATPase, probably acts as the counter-ion for newly formed bicarbonate.[150] These two ions are linked such that inhibition of either carbonic anhydrase or $Na^+ - K^+$ ATPase reduces sodium movement into the posterior chamber.[34,149] However, inhibition of both carbonic anhydrase and $Na^+ - K^+$ ATPase produces a net effect on aqueous production that is not any greater than is inhibition of either enzyme individually.[34]

The transepithelial movement of several ions is essential for fluid movement from the stroma of the ciliary processes into the posterior chamber. Assuming that Na^+, HCO_3, and Cl^- are the major ions involved in secretion, Figure 7.3 illustrates how these ions may be involved in fluid movement across the nonpigmented ciliary epithelium and into the posterior chamber. Sodium is thought to enter the epithelium from the stromal side either by diffusion or by a Na^+/H^+ exchange system.[151] The intracellular sodium concentration is maintained, since Na^+ is also being transported extracellularly into the lateral intercellular channels of the nonpigmented epithelium by a $Na^+ - K^+$ ATPase-dependent system. HCO_3 is formed from the hydration of CO_2, a process catalyzed by carbonic an-

hydrase. Cl^- enters the lateral intercellular channel and thereby balances a portion of the transported Na^+. Cl^- enters the lateral intercellular channel by a mechanism that is not understood. Because of the entry of ions into the lateral intercellular channel, a hypertonic fluid is produced that results in an osmotic water flux.[151] Because of restrictions by the stromal end of the channel, fluid moves by bulk flow toward the posterior chamber. In addition to their ability to decrease bicarbonate formation, carbonic anhydrase inhibitors may also alter the intracellular pH so that ATPase activity is modified and Na^+ movement is inhibited.[151] Therefore, it is reasonable to postulate that inhibition of carbonic anhydrase in the ciliary processes probably acts to decrease bicarbonate, sodium, and fluid movement into the posterior chamber, with the net result being decreased aqueous humor formation.

The reduction of intraocular pressure produced by the carbonic anhydrase inhibitors has been attributed, at least in part, to the accompanying metabolic acidosis that occurs secondary to the renal effects of these agents.[152,153] This theory receives support from the clinical observation that diabetics in ketoacidosis often have "soft" eyes. In addition, acidosis produced following administration of ammonium chloride has also been shown to decrease intraocular pressure.[154,155] Using nephrectomized rabbits, which prevents metabolic acidosis and diuresis, Becker[155] has shown that acetazolamide reduces intraocular pressure, thereby illustrating that its renal effects do not contribute significantly to

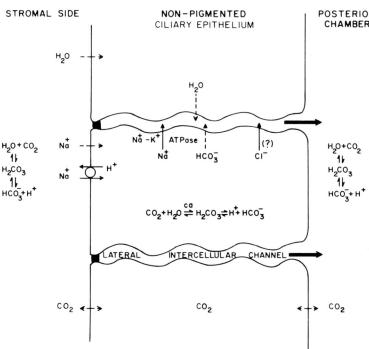

FIGURE 7.3 **Ion and fluid movement in the nonpigmented ciliary epithelium. Na^+ enters the nonpigmented ciliary epithelium from the stromal side either by diffusion or by Na^+/H^+ exchange. Na^+, the main cation involved in aqueous formation, is transported extracellularly into the lateral intercellular channel by a Na^+-K^+ ATPase-dependent transport system. HCO_3^- is formed from the hydration of CO_2, a reaction catalyzed by carbonic anhydrase. HCO_3^-, the major anion involved in aqueous formation, balances a portion of the Na^+ being transported into the lateral intercellular channel. Cl^- enters the intercellular space by a mechanism that is not understood. This movement of ions into the lateral intercellular space creates a hypertonic fluid, and water enters by osmosis. Because of the restriction on the stromal side of the channel, the newly formed fluid moves toward the posterior chamber. A rapid diffusional exchange of CO_2 allows for its movement into the posterior chamber. (Adapted from Cole DF. Secretion of aqueous humor. Exp Eye Res (Suppl) 1977;25:161–176.)**

acetazolamide's ocular hypotensive action. A more recent study[153] using nephrectomized rabbits has confirmed this finding. These investigators demonstrated that acetazolamide (5 mg/kg body weight) can reduce intraocular pressure without altering arterial pH, bicarbonate, or pCO_2. However, doses producing metabolic acidosis (> 15 mg/kg) further reduced intraocular pressure. Of the carbonic anhydrase inhibitors, acetazolamide has the greatest effect on acid-base balance. Therefore, these experiments have shown that metabolic acidosis produced by carbonic anhydrase inhibitors contributes only slightly to their maximal ocular hypotensive effect.

Carbonic anhydrase is present in most tissues in quantities that exceed physiologic requirements. Because of this excess, it has been estimated that at least 99% of carbonic anhydrase activity must be inhibited before aqueous production is significantly depressed.[148,156] Drug levels sufficient to reduce aqueous humor formation are readily achieved following systemic administration of carbonic anhydrase inhibitors.[141] However, systemic use has the disadvantage that the activity of carbonic anhydrase throughout the body is also significantly inhibited.

Topically active carbonic anhydrase inhibitors would have the advantage of producing decreased intraocular pressure without the severe side effects that are associated with inhibition of carbonic anhydrase in nonocular tissues. Unfortunately, many studies[157–159] have shown that topical and subconjunctival administration of carbonic anhydrase inhibitors does not produce a significant or prolonged reduction in intraocular pressure. The inability of topically applied carbonic anhydrase inhibitors to decrease intraocular pressure may stem from the poor corneal penetration.[293] Maren and associates[160] have demonstrated that acetazolamide, ethoxzolamide, and methazolamide do not readily penetrate the rabbit cornea. Several researchers, however, have recently demonstrated the ocular hypotensive action of certain topically applied carbonic anhydrase inhibitors. Friedman and associates[161] found that high-water-content soft contact lenses soaked in acetazolamide and methazolamide 2.5% solution delivered a sufficient concentration of the drugs to lower intraocular pressure in rabbits. Flach[162,163] showed that topical acetazolamide 10% solution alone, and combined with systemic acetazolamide, significantly reduced the intraocular pressure rise in water-loaded pigmented rabbits. In another study,[164] a single application of dichlorphenamide sodium 10% produced a significant reduction in intraocular pressure in rabbits with alpha-chymotrypsin-induced ocular hypertension.

In an attempt to develop agents with improved corneal penetration, trifluormethazolamide, a halogenated derivative of methazolamide, has been studied.

Topically applied trifluormethazolamide has been shown to enter the anterior chamber and ciliary body in concentrations sufficient to inhibit carbonic anhydrase.[160] In several studies[165,166] using topically applied trifluormethazolamide, this agent has been found to decrease aqueous formation and to lower intraocular pressure in cats and rabbits.[160]

Among the most promising new carbonic anhydrase inhibitors include the analogs of ethoxzolamide. Several investigators have evaluated analogs of ethoxzolamide for their ocular hypotensive properties following topical administration.[167–169] In a study[170] using ocular hypertensive humans, 3% aminozolamide gel produced a 26.3% reduction in intraocular pressure. The onset of action occurred between 1 and 2 hours after application, and the ocular hypotensive action following a single application lasted more than 8 hours.[170] Additional studies on the dose-response relationship of aminozolamide gel, its duration of action, the long-term response, and its toxicity are currently underway.[170] These studies indicate that topically applied carbonic anhydrase inhibitors may be used clinically as ocular hypotensive agents in the near future.

The future clinical usefulness of topical carbonic anhydrase inhibitors is promising. If marketed as gel preparations, these agents would most likely be administered at bedtime to reduce the diurnal variation in intraocular pressure. Another possible use for the topical agents would be to supplement systemic carbonic anhydrase inhibitor therapy, thereby allowing reduction of the systemic dose. This latter approach would have great appeal, since it would produce fewer systemic side effects from chronic carbonic anhydrase inhibitor therapy. However, before widespread clinical use, further research is needed to evaluate the effects of long-term topical carbonic anhydrase inhibitor therapy on corneal metabolism. Since several new water-soluble carbonic anhydrase inhibitors have been recently developed,[294] this group of agents will probably become available for clinical use in the near future.

Of the currently available carbonic anhydrase inhibitors (see Table 7.5), acetazolamide is the prototype drug and has been studied extensively. Other agents within this class include methazolamide and dichlorphenamide. Becker[142] has shown that systemic administration of any of these agents produces a 45% to 55% inhibition of aqueous formation in humans.

Acetazolamide

PHARMACOLOGY

In the treatment of all types of glaucoma, acetazolamide (Fig. 7.4) is the most widely used carbonic anhydrase inhibitor. Acetazolamide (Diamox) is com-

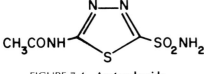

FIGURE 7.4 **Acetazolamide.**

mercially available as 125 and 250 mg tablets, 500 mg sustained-release capsules (Diamox Sequels), and a 500 mg vial formulated for parenteral administration. In long-term antiglaucoma therapy in adults, acetazolamide is usually administered in doses of 250 mg every 6 hours or a single 500 mg sustained-release capsule twice daily. The recommended acetazolamide dose for children is 5 to 10 mg/kg body weight, administered every 4 to 6 hours.[171]

Acetazolamide has also been formulated in a gastrointestinal therapeutic system that delivers the drug at an essentially constant rate of 15 mg/hr.[172] Although not commercially available, this drug delivery system offers the advantage of decreased fluctuations in plasma concentration compared with acetazolamide tablets and, as a result, a lower incidence of side effects.[172]

Bioavailability studies have shown generic acetazolamide tablets to be equivalent to brand-name acetazolamide (Diamox) tablets.[173] Therefore, generic acetazolamide may be used, when available, at a reduced cost to the patient.

Acetazolamide is readily absorbed from the gastrointestinal tract after oral administration.[174,175] Following ingestion of acetazolamide tablets, peak drug levels are reached within 2 to 4 hours and are maintained for 4 to 6 hours.[176] Drug levels are higher after ingesting acetazolamide tablets than after an equivalent dose of the time-release preparation. The time-release capsules produce maximum drug levels in 3 to 4 hours, and levels of 10 μg/ml are maintained for about 10 hours.[177]

The time course of acetazolamide's ocular hypotensive effect parallels its plasma concentration.[178] Oral acetazolamide tablets, in dosages greater than 63 mg, produce a significant ocular hypotensive response within 2 hours, and the effects last beyond 6 hours[178] (Table 7.6). The ocular hypotensive effect of the sustained-release capsules begins within 2 hours, and the maximum reduction in intraocular pressure occurs 6 to 18 hours after oral administration.[179] Although a 500 mg capsule administered once daily produces a substantial decrease in intraocular pressure lasting at least 24 hours, the magnitude of the pressure drop is greater when the drug is administered twice daily.[180] The sustained-release capsules, administered in dosages of 500 mg twice daily, are as effective in reducing intraocular pressure as are 250 mg acetazolamide tablets administered every 6 hours.[180]

Plasma levels sufficient to decrease intraocular pressure occur only minutes after intravenous administration of acetazolamide,[181,182] but this route of administration is generally reserved for situations, such as in acute angle-closure glaucoma, when vomiting precludes the oral route. The duration of acetazolamide's action after intravenous administration is about 4 hours.[183]

In humans, 90% to 95% of acetazolamide in the blood is bound to plasma proteins.[156] Therefore, relatively large dosages of acetazolamide are required to produce a significant plasma level of the unbound drug. At plasma pH (7.4), half the unbound acetazolamide ($pK_a = 7.4$) exists in the un-ionized form (Table 7.7). It is the un-ionized drug that penetrates tissues and inhibits carbonic anhydrase.

TABLE 7.6
Pharmacokinetic Properties of Carbonic Anhydrase Inhibitors

Drug	Dose	Onset of Ocular Hypotensive Action	Maximum IOP Reduction	Duration of Ocular Hypotensive Action
Acetazolamide tablet	65–250 mg q.i.d.	½–1 hr	2–4 hr	4–6 hr
Acetazolamide capsule	500 mg b.i.d.	1–2 hr	8–12 hr	10–18 hr
Acetazolamide IV	500 mg IV	1 min	20–30 min	4 hr
Methazolamide	25–100 mg b.i.d., t.i.d.	1 hr	7–8 hr	10–14 hr
Dichlorphenamide	25–50 mg b.i.d., t.i.d., q.i.d.	½ hr	2–4 hr	6–12 hr

IOP, intraocular pressure; b.i.d., twice daily; t.i.d., three times daily; q.i.d., four times daily.
Adapted from Flach AJ. Topical acetazolamide and other carbonic anhydrase inhibitors in the current medical therapy of the glaucomas. Glaucoma 1986;8:20–27.

TABLE 7.7
Pharmacologic Properties of Carbonic Anhydrase Inhibitors

Drug	% Bound to Plasma Proteins	pK_a	% Un-ionized in Plasma (pH 7.4)
Acetazolamide	95	7.4	50
Methazolamide	55	7.2	39
Dichlorphenamide	—	8.3	89

Adapted from Wistrand PJ, Rawls JA, Maren TH. Sulfonamide carbonic anhydrase inhibitors and intraocular pressure in rabbits. Acta Pharmacol Toxicol 1960; 17:337–355.

Acetazolamide is not metabolized; it is excreted, primarily by tubular secretion, into the urine.[175] Due to its action on the kidney, acetazolamide increases urinary excretion of HCO_3 and produces an alkaline urine. This alteration of urinary pH favors excretion of acetazolamide, since more drug exists in the water-soluble, ionized form.

Acetazolamide therapy is often difficult to optimize due to pharmacokinetic variables and differences in responsiveness.[184] The plasma levels necessary for effective glaucoma therapy have been reported to range from 5 to 20 μg/ml.[172,178,180,184] Furthermore, after a given dose, large interindividual variations in plasma levels are often obtained. Alm and associates[184] studied plasma concentrations after oral acetazolamide doses of 187.5, 375, 750, and 1000 mg. At all doses, large variations in the plasma levels attained were observed. When the plasma levels achieved following a 1000 mg dose of acetazolamide were analyzed with respect to age, patients older than 80 years exhibited drug levels that were approximately 2 to 3 times higher than patients younger than 60 years (21.6 and 8.3 μg/ml, respectively). Therefore, older patients seem to attain higher serum levels and may require modifications in their doses, especially if renal function is decreased, which may impair excretion.

CLINICAL USES

In the treatment of primary open-angle glaucoma, acetazolamide is almost always added to the treatment regimen after topical agents alone do not control intraocular pressure satisfactorily (see Fig. 29.28). Acetazolamide produces an additional decrease in intraocular pressure when added to drug regimens including miotics,[184,185] epinephrine,[186] or β blockers.[124,125] Although timolol and acetazolamide both inhibit aqueous formation, they produce nearly additive effects on intraocular pressure reduction when administered concurrently.[124,125]

In acute angle-closure glaucoma, oral or parenteral acetazolamide is often administered soon after the diagnosis is made. The combination of acetazolamide, hyperosmotic agents, a β blocker, and pilocarpine usually reduces the intraocular pressure sufficiently to permit a laser iridotomy or surgical peripheral iridectomy. Use of acetazolamide in the management of acute angle-closure glaucoma is frequently limited to the preoperative period, since many patients require no further medication or can be managed with topical agents following surgery.

For many years certain secondary glaucomas were treated using a combination of oral acetazolamide and topical epinephrine. The availability of topical β blockers, however, has lessened the use of acetazolamide for the treatment of secondary glaucoma.

An additional clinical use of acetazolamide is unrelated to its ocular hypotensive properties. In a recent study,[295] acetazolamide, 500 mg daily administered for 2 weeks, was found to produce either a partial or complete resolution of macular edema in many patients with Irvine-Gass syndrome, retinitis pigmentosa, and chronic intermediate uveitis (pars planitis). Macular edema produced by primary retinal vascular diseases (branch and central retinal vein occlusion and macular telangiectasia) did not respond to acetazolamide therapy. The role of acetazolamide in the resolution of certain types of macular edema is unclear.

SYSTEMIC SIDE EFFECTS

Although acetazolamide is frequently effective as an ocular hypotensive agent, its clinical usefulness is often limited by a significant number of side effects (Table 7.8). Maximal doses of carbonic anhydrase inhibitors produce intolerable side effects in 30% to 80% of patients.[179,188–190] The incidence of side effects varies with the dose and the preparation; however, when all side effects are considered, the incidence probably approaches 100% in patients taking acetazolamide tablets or the 500 mg sustained-release capsules. Lichter and associates[190] have shown that only 26% of patients were able to tolerate acetazolamide tablets beyond 6 weeks, while 58% of patients were able to tolerate prolonged

TABLE 7.8
Side Effects of Acetazolamide

Systemic
    Numbness and tingling of extremities and perioral region[a]
    Metallic taste[a]
    Symptom complex[a]
        Decreased libido
        Depression
        Fatigue
        Malaise
        Weight loss
    Gastrointestinal irritation[a]
    Metabolic acidosis[a]
    Hypokalemia
    Renal calculi
    Blood dyscrasias
    Dermatitis
Ocular
    Transient myopia

[a]Common.

use of the time-release preparation. Becker and Middleton[191] have observed a lower incidence of side effects in blacks receiving long-term acetazolamide therapy than in whites.

Numbness and tingling of the fingers, toes, and perioral region are among the most common side effects resulting from use of carbonic anhydrase inhibitors.[183] This loss of sensitivity may be quite disconcerting to some patients, but rarely is it intolerable, and it is usually transient. Another common, but tolerable, side effect is an alteration in gustation, resulting in a metallic taste.[183]

Epstein and Grant[189] have described a symptom complex consisting of malaise, fatigue, weight loss, depression, anorexia, and often decreased libido as the side effects most likely to require discontinuation of carbonic anhydrase inhibitors. In addition, impotence has been reported in some patients taking acetazolamide.[296] These symptoms may take several months to become manifest and appear to be at least partially related to serum drug levels.[189,192] The symptom complex also appears to occur more commonly in patients exhibiting marked acidosis.[189] Therefore, sodium bicarbonate (up to 80 mEq/day) has been used in an attempt to decrease the level of acidosis.[189,192] In some patients, supplemental sodium bicarbonate may improve drug tolerance, but this finding has not been associated with significant changes in the level of acidosis.[189,193] Leopold and associates[193] found that sodium chloride supplements also decrease the side effects associated with acetazolamide therapy.

Symptoms indicating gastrointestinal irritation, including abdominal cramps, nausea, and diarrhea, have been reported following use of acetazolamide.[189] In

some patients, these symptoms may be improved by administering the tablets with food or by changing from acetazolamide tablets to the sustained-release capsules.[189] Other patients have obtained relief from gastrointestinal symptoms by using sodium bicarbonate tablets.[189,192] These symptoms, if persistent, can be intolerable and may require an alternative means of intraocular pressure control.

Carbonic anhydrase inhibitors alter renal function primarily by inhibiting carbonic anhydrase in the proximal tubule, which results in decreased bicarbonate reabsorption. Inhibition of intracellular carbonic anhydrase also affects both the distal tubule and the collecting duct. These effects produce decreased secretion of hydrogen ions and increased excretion of sodium, potassium, and bicarbonate ions. The net effect of the renal actions of acetazolamide therapy is alkalinization of the urine and metabolic acidosis. Metabolic acidosis results from the initial bicarbonate loss. Because carbonic anhydrase is inhibited at the level of the distal tubule, normal acidification does not recur. Thus, a mild metabolic acidosis persists with continued acetazolamide use. Severe acidosis is prevented by the reabsorption of bicarbonate independent of carbonic anhydrase.[194] Initially, acetazolamide produces diuresis, but urinary output decreases with the development of metabolic acidosis.[195] In addition, decreased urinary citrate excretion is produced following acetazolamide therapy and has been attributed to the metabolic acidosis it produces.[196] High urinary pH and low urinary citrate concentration are conducive to precipitation of calcium phosphate in both the renal papillae and the urinary tract.[197,297]

Although acetazolamide therapy increases urinary excretion of potassium, problems associated with hypokalemia are rare.[189,198] However, this potassium-depleting action may become significant if the patient is also taking a thiazide diuretic[189] or digitalis derivative. Concomitant use of acetazolamide and a thiazide diuretic can lead to drug-induced hypokalemia, and potassium supplementation may be required in these patients.[189] Since decreased potassium levels also increase the possibility of digitalis toxicity, potassium levels should be monitored closely in patients taking acetazolamide in addition to digitalis derivatives and thiazide diuretics.

The most serious side effects associated with acetazolamide are blood dyscrasias. Thrombocytopenia, agranulocytosis, and aplastic anemia have all been found in patients taking acetazolamide; however, drug-induced blood dyscrasias are extremely rare.[199] Therefore, Fraunfelder and associates[200] have made the following recommendations: (1) complete blood counts should be performed before starting treatment with carbonic anhydrase inhibitors and at intervals of every

6 months thereafter; (2) patients receiving carbonic anhydrase inhibitor therapy should be advised to report a persistent sore throat, fever, fatigue, pallor, easy bruising, epistaxis, purpura, or jaundice; and (3) a decrease in the level of any single, formed blood element should result in immediate termination of carbonic anhydrase inhibitor therapy. Although strongly recommended by the drug manufacturers and by Fraunfelder and associates,[200] the usefulness of routine hematologic evaluations in patients receiving chronic carbonic anhydrase inhibitor therapy has been questioned because of its high cost relative to its low detection rate of drug-induced hematologic adverse reactions.[201,298]

OCULAR SIDE EFFECTS

Drug-induced transient myopia has been reported with several sulfonamides.[202–204] Acetazolamide, an unsubstituted heterocyclic sulfonamide, has also been associated with myopic shifts in refractive error.[205–208] Shallowing of the anterior chamber has been shown to be the only parameter that could be documented to change in eyes exhibiting this increase in myopia following sulfonamide therapy.[209] Myopia probably results from ciliary body edema that produces a forward displacement of the lens-iris diaphragm.[202,209] The myopia subsides upon reducing or discontinuing acetazolamide therapy.

CONTRAINDICATIONS

Since long-term use of acetazolamide is usually associated with a significant number of side effects, acetazolamide should be avoided in patients who are particularly susceptible to its side effects (Table 7.9). Because of the significant structural differences between the antibacterial and the carbonic anhydrase inhibiting sulfonamides, Friedland and Maren[210] believe there is little evidence to suggest overlapping sensitivities between the two classes of drugs. However, hypersensitivity reactions including exfoliative dermatitis, nonthrombocytopenic purpura, hepatitis, nephropathy, and transient myopia have all been cited by Fraunfelder and associates[200] as being linked with

TABLE 7.9
Contraindications for Use of Acetazolamide

- Clinically significant liver disease
- Severe chronic obstructive pulmonary disease
- Certain secondary glaucomas[a]
- Renal disease, including kidney stones[a]
- Pregnancy
- Known hypersensitivity to sulfonamides

[a]See text for discussion.

sulfonamide compounds and their derivatives. Therefore, patients with known hypersensitivity reactions to sulfonamides should not take carbonic anhydrase inhibitors.

Since acetazolamide is excreted unchanged in the urine,[175] patients with impaired renal function may require substantially lower doses and should be monitored closely for side effects. Acetazolamide must be used with caution in patients taking potassium-depleting diuretics because of the possibility of drug-induced hypokalemia. Since patients taking digitalis preparations are at greater risk of developing digitalis toxicity secondary to hypokalemia, acetazolamide must be used with caution or avoided in these individuals.

Patients with cirrhosis of the liver are particularly sensitive to toxicity associated with acetazolamide use. Alkalinization of the urine decreases urinary trapping of NH_4^+ and may result in increased levels of ammonia in the systemic circulation.[211] An increased level of ammonia in the circulation may contribute to the development of hepatic encephalopathy.[211] Therefore, acetazolamide is contraindicated in patients with clinically significant liver disease.

Acetazolamide should be avoided in patients with severe chronic obstructive pulmonary disease. These patients may be unable to increase their alveolar ventilation enough to compensate for the acid-base alterations induced by acetazolamide. In some patients, especially those with severe pulmonary disease, increased CO_2 gradients or acidosis may lead to acute respiratory failure. However, if acetazolamide is essential to the successful management of glaucoma in such patients, the lowest effective dose should be used to reduce intraocular pressure without completely inhibiting renal or red blood cell carbonic anhydrase activity.[212]

Since medical therapy is often completely ineffective in the management of the closed-angle stage of neovascular glaucoma[213,214] and other secondary glaucomas characterized by severe impairment of aqueous outflow,[215] acetazolamide should not be used routinely because of the systemic side effects it produces.[214] In addition, it is important to remember that carbonic anhydrase inhibitors reduce aqueous formation only by 45% to 55%.[142] In glaucomas arising from severe impairment of outflow, as in chronic angle-closure glaucoma, aqueous production will not be inhibited enough to allow long-term control of intraocular pressure. Therefore, the clinician may derive a false sense of security from the decrease in intraocular pressure produced by carbonic anhydrase inhibitors, while the underlying ocular condition progresses.

Black patients with sickle cell hemoglobinopathies and hyphema-induced secondary glaucomas should be administered acetazolamide with caution.[216] Acetazolamide increases the ascorbate concentration in aqueous humor and reduces plasma pH.[216] Both actions can promote sickling of red blood cells in the anterior chamber and within small blood vessels perfusing intraocular structures. Hyphemas containing sickled red blood cells resolve more slowly and elevate intraocular pressure more than do hyphemas containing nonsickled red blood cells.[217] Therefore, all black patients with hyphemas should be screened for sickle cell hemoglobinopathies before acetazolamide treatment, as should any black patient requiring long-term acetazolamide therapy.

Since it has been estimated that 5% to 10% of patients receiving long-term acetazolamide therapy either pass urinary calculi or have symptoms indicative of calculi,[218] acetazolamide may precipitate calculi formation in predisposed individuals. Therefore, acetazolamide should not be used in patients with bacteriuria, previous bladder surgery, or a history suggestive of previous calculus formation.[218] Furthermore, since high urinary pH and low urinary citrate concentration are conducive to calculus formation, concurrent use of acetazolamide and sodium bicarbonate may increase the risk of calculus formation.[197] In addition, other forms of renal disease should be excluded before long-term acetazolamide therapy. If standard doses of acetazolamide are given to patients with diabetic nephropathy, severe acidosis may result[219,220]; therefore, these patients should have serum electrolytes monitored closely to prevent this complication.

Acetazolamide has been found to be teratogenic in experimental animals.[221] Although it has not been linked with birth defects in humans, acetazolamide use should be avoided during pregnancy.

DRUG INTERACTIONS

Drug interactions attributable to acetazolamide therapy are uncommon. However, the metabolic acidosis and alkalinization of the urine may alter the activity of several drugs. Amphetamines, quinidine, and tricyclic antidepressants have a prolonged effect and enhanced activity in alkaline urine due to increased renal tubular reabsorption.[222] Another important interaction stems from the increased serum levels of un-ionized salicylic acid that result when aspirin and acetazolamide are used concurrently. The acidosis produced by acetazolamide allows more salicylic acid to become unionized and thereby enhances penetration into the central nervous system (CNS).[223] Therefore, a potential hazard exists in patients with glaucoma who are taking high doses of aspirin for arthritis; arthritic patients requiring carbonic anhydrase inhibitor therapy should be given low doses of methazolamide, which has a minimal effect on the acid-base balance, and these patients should be monitored closely for salicylate intoxication.[224]

Methazolamide

PHARMACOLOGY

During the last several decades, acetazolamide has been considered the carbonic anhydrase inhibitor of choice in the treatment of glaucoma. More recently, however, the properties of methazolamide have been reevaluated, and several studies[196,225,226] indicate possible advantages to its use as an ocular hypotensive agent.

Methazolamide (Neptazane) is commercially available in 25 and 50 mg tablets. The adult dosage range is 25 to 100 mg 3 times daily.

Methazolamide (Fig. 7.5) is structurally similar to acetazolamide. The structure of methazolamide was designed to decrease ionization and thereby improve its intraocular penetration.[196] After oral administration, methazolamide is well absorbed from the gastrointestinal tract. Average serum levels peak in 2 to 3 hours after an oral 100 mg dose and are maintained nearly constant for at least 8 hours.[226] Methazolamide has higher lipid and water solubilities than does acetazolamide.[227] These properties favor renal tubular reabsorption and increase both its half-life and plasma concentration.[227] Methazolamide has a plasma half-life of about 14 hours, compared with 5 hours for acetazolamide.[196] Since only 25% of methazolamide is excreted unchanged in the urine, the remaining 75% is probably metabolized to an inactive form, although its fate is unknown.[196]

Only 55% of methazolamide is bound to plasma proteins, compared with 90% to 95% of acetazolamide.[196] Since only the unbound portion of the drug dose is pharmacologically active, methazolamide can be given at lower doses than acetazolamide to achieve comparable effects. Methazolamide ($pK_a = 7.2$) is 39% unionized at plasma pH.

The dose-response studies of methazolamide's ocular hypotensive effect have shown that intraocular pressure is decreased in a dose-dependent manner for doses of 25, 50, and 100 mg given every 8 hours; the mean decreases in intraocular pressure at these doses were 3.3, 4.3, and 5.6 mm Hg, respectively.[226]

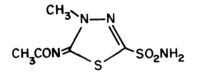

FIGURE 7.5 **Methazolamide.**

CLINICAL USES

Methazolamide, like the other carbonic anhydrase inhibitors, may be added to the treatment regimen of patients with primary open-angle glaucoma and secondary glaucomas when topical antiglaucoma agents alone provide inadequate pressure control. Because of its ability to decrease intraocular pressure with less alteration of acid-base balance, methazolamide is probably a better drug to use in patients with severe obstructive pulmonary disease.[212] Methazolamide also alters urinary citrate excretion less than does acetazolamide, and it therefore is recommended for use in patients predisposed to renal calculus formation who require carbonic anhydrase inhibitors.[218]

The advantages of methazolamide are numerous enough that many authorities believe it should be the first carbonic anhydrase inhibitor used for systemic glaucoma therapy.[225,228,229] Zimmerman[228,229] has recommended that the initial dose should be 25 mg orally administered twice daily. This dose usually produces a 4 to 5 mm Hg decrease in intraocular pressure with minimal side effects. If after one week the intraocular pressure remains at an unacceptable level, the dose should be increased to 50 mg orally administered twice daily. The level of intraocular pressure reduction should again be evaluated after 1 week; if the pressure is still not at the desired level, the medication should be changed to acetazolamide 500 mg sequels orally administered twice daily. Lichter and associates[190] reported that about 75% of patients can be expected to tolerate either methazolamide (50 mg every 6 hours) or acetazolamide sequels (500 mg twice daily) beyond 6 weeks.

SIDE EFFECTS

Methazolamide is one of the best tolerated carbonic anhydrase inhibitors, especially at low doses.[190,225] However, administration of this drug poses the same general risk as does administration of acetazolamide, and the side effects associated with methazolamide use are essentially those associated with acetazolamide. Compared with acetazolamide, methazolamide generally produces less acidosis and has less effect on urinary citrate levels.[196] Thus, patients who are intolerant of acetazolamide may tolerate methazolamide therapy without difficulty.

Methazolamide is particularly useful in patients predisposed to develop renal calculi.[218] Methazolamide interferes less with excretion of urinary citrate, which may explain why kidney stones have only rarely been associated with its use.[230,231]

Compared with acetazolamide, methazolamide generally causes less paresthesia but often causes more drowsiness.[190] Although extremely rare, aplastic anemia and agranulocytosis have been reported as complications of methazolamide therapy.[200,232]

CONTRAINDICATIONS

Contraindications to the use of methazolamide are essentially those associated with the use of acetazolamide. Methazolamide, however, can be used more safely in patients with a history of kidney stones or renal impairment. Patients with chronic obstructive pulmonary diseases may tolerate methazolamide better than acetazolamide, since the metabolic acidosis is less pronounced.

Dichlorphenamide

PHARMACOLOGY

Dichlorphenamide (Daranide) is a potent carbonic anhydrase inhibitor. The structure of carbonic acid (H_2CO_3), the substrate for carbonic anhydrase, spatially resembles the sulfonamide portion of those compounds known to inhibit carbonic anhydrase.[142] Since dichlorphenamide (Fig. 7.6) has two sulfamyl ($-SO_2NH_2$) groups, this configuration probably accounts for its unwanted chloruretic effect.[210] Dichlorphenamide is available in 50 mg tablets for oral use. The usual adult dosage range is 25 to 100 mg administered 3 times daily.

Dichlorphenamide is readily absorbed from the gastrointestinal tract after oral administration. Dichlorphenamide ($pK_a = 8.3$) is largely un-ionized at plasma pH. The fate of absorbed dichlorphenamide is not known. After oral administration, the decrease in intraocular pressure begins within 30 minutes, reaches maximum within 2 hours, and has a duration of about 6 hours.[233] The maximum intraocular pressure response during dichlorphenamide therapy is equivalent to that of acetazolamide, although dichlorphenamide produces this effect at lower dosages.[233,234]

CLINICAL USES

The main ocular use for dichlorphenamide is in the treatment of primary open-angle glaucoma and some

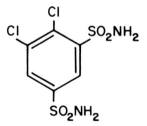

FIGURE 7.6 **Dichlorphenamide.**

secondary glaucomas. Dichlorphenamide is generally added to the treatment regimen when the intraocular pressure cannot be adequately controlled with topical antiglaucoma agents alone. Patients intolerant of acetazolamide and methazolamide may be able to tolerate dichlorphenamide.[233] However, Lichter and associates[190] have reported that only about 20% of patients are able to tolerate dichlorphenamide beyond 6 weeks. The relatively limited number of patients who can tolerate dichlorphenamide therapy limits the usefulness of this agent.

SIDE EFFECTS

The side effects of dichlorphenamide are similar to those produced by acetazolamide. In addition, dichlorphenamide produces more confusion and anorexia than do other carbonic anhydrase inhibitors.[190] The frequency and severity of systemic side effects following dichlorphenamide therapy is greater than with acetazolamide therapy.[190,233]

Unlike acetazolamide, the diuresis produced by dichlorphenamide is not self-limiting. Because dichlorphenamide causes less acidosis, its diuretic action persists with chronic use. Some authors believe that, compared with other carbonic anhydrase inhibitors, dichlorphenamide has the greatest potential to deplete potassium.[171,235] The potassium loss associated with dichlorphenamide is linked with its chloruretic effect, a characteristic shared with thiazide diuretics.[210,236] Hence, electrolytes should be monitored in patients taking dichlorphenamide to detect drug-induced hypokalemia. Potassium supplementation does not alter the drug's effectiveness on intraocular pressure.[215]

Cannabinoids

The popularity of marijuana as a recreational drug has increased dramatically during the last several decades. Therefore, it is not surprising that a significant amount of research has been directed toward understanding the pharmacology of derivatives obtained from the marijuana plant, *Cannabis sativa*. Among the chemical constituents of marijuana are a number of related compounds collectively known as cannabinoids. In 1964, Gaoni and Mechoulam[237] isolated and identified Δ^9-tetrahydrocannabinol (Δ^9-THC) (Fig. 7.7) as the primary pharmacologically active ingredient of marijuana. Subsequent studies have revealed that at least 20 other constituents of marijuana exist, and many of these compounds have now been synthesized.[238]

The observation that marijuana smoking produces conjunctival hyperemia probably aroused much curiosity relative to its actions on ocular physiology. How-

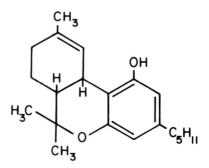

FIGURE 7.7 **Δ^9-tetrahydrocannabinol (Δ^9-THC).**

ever, it was not until 1971 that the action of marijuana on intraocular pressure was reported. In this preliminary study, Hepler and Frank[239] found that intraocular pressure was reduced in 9 of 11 young human subjects after they inhaled the smoke from 2 g of high-grade marijuana. A similar effect was observed following intravenous administration of Δ^9-THC.[240,241] The reduction of intraocular pressure was found to be dose-related and resulted in a 37% decrease from baseline values following an intravenous dose of Δ^9-THC (0.044 mg/kg body weight).[241] Several other studies[242,243] have confirmed the acute ocular hypotensive response produced by Δ^9 = THC in healthy human subjects. Long-term studies with marijuana and Δ^9-THC in healthy subjects have revealed a consistent decrease in intraocular pressure that persists 4 to 5 hours after inhalation; no tolerance to the ocular hypotensive response has been reported.[244–246] These preliminary studies stimulated much interest in the possible use of cannabinoids in the treatment of glaucoma.

Routes of Administration

Various cannabinoids and synthetic congeners have been administered orally, topically, and by inhalation with the hopes of finding an effective means of reducing intraocular pressure in the glaucomatous patient. The earliest investigations studied marijuana smoking for its potential ocular hypotensive effects. In 1976, Hepler and Petrus[245] reported an ocular hypotensive effect in glaucomatous patients who smoked or ingested marijuana. Merritt and associates[247] described the ocular hypotensive response of 18 patients with either primary open-angle glaucoma or secondary glaucoma following inhalation of a single 900 mg marijuana cigarette (2% THC by weight). The maximal hypotensive response appeared 60 to 90 minutes after inhalation (Fig. 7.8). The duration of the pressure reduction was approximately 4 hours, although a longer hypotensive effect was observed in several subjects. These

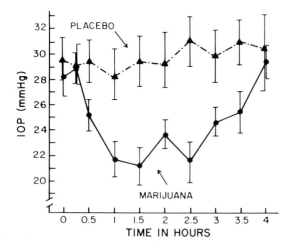

FIGURE 7.8   **Intraocular pressure (mean ± SE) in 31 glaucomatous eyes after marijuana and placebo inhalations. (From Merritt JC, Crawford WJ, Alexander PC, et al. Effect of marijuana on intraocular and blood pressure in glaucoma. Ophthalmology 1980; 87:222–228. Used with permission of the authors and publisher.)**

TABLE 7.10
Common Systemic Side Effects following Marijuana Inhalation

Cardiovascular
   Postural hypotension
   Tachycardia
Central Nervous System (Altered Mental Status)
   Anxiety
   Drowsiness
   Euphoria
   Hunger
   Thirst

Adapted from Merritt JC, Crawford WJ, Alexander PC, et al. Effect of marihuana on intraocular and blood pressure in glaucoma. Ophthalmology 1980; 87:222–228.

investigators also found a disconcerting number of side effects, the most significant being systemic hypotension. Although other studies[248] have confirmed the ocular hypotensive actions of Δ^9-THC inhalation in glaucomatous patients, the frequency and severity of systemic side effects (Table 7.10) make marijuana inhalation an unrealistic route of administration for the patient with glaucoma.

Oral cannabinoids have also been shown to have ocular hypotensive properties.[249–251] Merritt and associates[250] found a 7.8 mm Hg decrease in intraocular pressure of glaucomatous eyes following oral administration of synthetic Δ^9-THC. Doses of 20 mg and 25 mg THC reduced pressures to equivalent levels, and both had a duration of action that exceeded 10 hours. However, at these doses adverse reactions were frequent and included acute panic reactions, paranoiac tendencies, and depersonalization.

Synthetic cannabinoids have been tested to determine if the ocular hypotensive response could be produced without the concomitant psychotropic and cardiovascular effects.[252,253] Newell and associates[253] reported that in 18 patients with open-angle glaucoma, oral nabilone (0.5 to 2.0 mg) produced a 28% reduction (average) of intraocular pressure. The maximum decrease in intraocular pressure occurred 2 to 6 hours following nabilone administration, and the reduction seemed to be independent of changes in outflow facility. Long-term administration of 0.5 mg nabilone in a patient resulted in a maintained ocular hypotensive response after 21 days.[253] Patients generally tolerated the drug at these dosage levels.

The least toxic route of administration for an ocular hypotensive agent would be topical ocular application. However, since cannabinoids are lipid soluble, aqueous-based solutions cannot be used for topical administration. Consequently, Green and associates[254] studied a variety of potentially useful vehicles for topical use. The finding of these investigators using radioactive Δ^9-THC indicates that a low-viscosity mineral oil vehicle produces the greatest intraocular penetration in the rabbit. This vehicle, when applied topically to human eyes, appears to be well tolerated.[255]

Topical administration of Δ^9-THC and many other cannabinoids has been shown to reduce intraocular pressure in experimental animals by as much as 40%.[254,256-262] However, many of these experiments were performed with different drug vehicles, and it is therefore difficult to make a direct comparison of the effectiveness of the particular compounds.

To identify a concentration of topical Δ^9-THC that would reduce intraocular pressure without altering blood pressure, Merritt and associates[263] studied the effects of multiple dose administration of topical Δ^9-THC in a mineral-oil vehicle in 8 patients with glaucoma and systemic hypertension. Although 0.01% Δ^9-THC failed to produce a change in intraocular pressure, both 0.05% and 0.1% Δ^9-THC decreased intraocular pressure in the treated eye and the untreated fellow eye. Intraocular pressures were reduced 4.8 mm Hg and 5.4 mm Hg following topical ocular application of 0.05% and 0.1% Δ^9-THC, respectively. The 0.1% concentration also produced a 12 mm Hg decrease in systolic blood pressure, while a systemic hypotensive effect was not found following application of either 0.05% or 0.01% Δ^9-THC. In this study, no significant adverse cardiovascular or psychological alterations were associated with the topical administration of Δ^9-THC.

In contrast, Jay and Green[264] found that 1% THC in light mineral oil, administered 4 times a day for 1 week, did not significantly reduce intraocular pressure in healthy, nonglaucomatous eyes. In addition, 4 of 28 subjects developed lid swelling, and 1 developed severe burning during the study. These side effects were attributed to the light mineral oil or to the preservatives used in the preparation. Another study[262] has also shown topical Δ^9-THC to be ineffective in reducing intraocular pressure in humans with glaucoma. These studies have led Green[265] to conclude that topical ocular Δ^9-THC does not reduce intraocular pressure.

Water-soluble derivatives of marijuana have been reported to reduce intraocular pressure in experimental animals.[266] Therefore, it is possible that this newer group of compounds may solve some of the problems encountered with Δ^9-THC.

Clinical Uses

Although orally administered cannabinoids are now available for the treatment of nausea and vomiting associated with cancer chemotherapy, the use of cannabinoids for the treatment of glaucoma is still investigational. Systemic side effects following either inhalation or oral administration prevent the cannabinoids from being clinically useful as ocular hypotensive agents. Topical ocular application of these agents seems to be the most promising route of administration. However, topical administration of the currently available cannabinoids has not been shown to be effective in reducing intraocular pressure in humans. Thus, the ocular hypotensive properties of cannabinoids must be further evaluated before any definite conclusions can be reached regarding their potential as antiglaucoma agents.

Mechanism of Action

Possible mechanisms for the ocular hypotensive action of Δ^9-THC include: (1) decreased capillary pressure in the ciliary body resulting in a reduction of the rate of aqueous formation,[257,267] (2) increased outflow of aqueous humor,[259] and (3) a centrally mediated effect.[256,258] The molecular basis for these actions has not been elucidated.

Other Ocular Effects

In addition to its ocular hypotensive properties, inhalation of marijuana smoke produces several other ocular changes in humans. Reduced tear production, conjunctival hyperemia, and photophobia have all been associated with both acute and chronic use of marijuana.[268,269]

Cardiac Glycosides

The action of the cardiac glycosides, primarily digitalis derivatives and ouabain, on intraocular pressure has been of interest for many years. The physiologic effects of these agents are produced by their ability to inhibit Na^+-K^+ ATPase, and a ouabain-sensitive Na^+-K^+ ATPase has been demonstrated to exist in the ciliary epithelium.[29] In the ciliary nonpigmented epithelium, like other types of secretory epithelium, Na^+-K^+ ATPase is thought to be responsible for the active transport of sodium, a process necessary for secretion to occur. Therefore, numerous studies have investigated cardiac glycosides as potential ocular hypotensive agents.

Animal experiments have shown that ouabain reduces intraocular pressure following intravitreal injection and systemic administration.[34,270-274] Tonographic data imply that the reduction of intraocular pressure associated with ouabain administration occurs through inhibition of aqueous formation, since outflow is not significantly altered.[271] Using anesthetized cats, Garg and Oppelt[34] found that intravenous ouabain (67 μg/kg) significantly reduced the rate of aqueous formation and the transport of Na^+ and Cl^- from plasma to aqueous humor. These investigators found that outflow facility was not significantly changed. Furthermore, digitalis derivatives have been reported to inhibit Na^+-K^+ ATPase in the cat ciliary body in vivo and in vitro.[270] Thus, these findings indicate that the decrease in aqueous humor formation found following use of cardiac glycosides probably results from inhibition of Na^+-K^+ ATPase in the ciliary epithelium.

Cardiac glycosides, when administered systemically, reduce intraocular pressure in humans. Systemic digoxin therapy has been shown to reduce intraocular pressure by 14% in glaucomatous human eyes.[270] Another study[275] reported that aqueous formation was decreased by 45% after several days of digoxin therapy. However, patients with uncontrolled intraocular pressures, despite maximum medical therapy, have been shown to remain uncontrolled after digitalization.[276] Therefore, systemic cardiac glycosides may reduce intraocular pressure to some degree in glaucomatous and nonglaucomatous eyes, but they are unlikely to produce adequate control of intraocular pressure when maximum medical therapy has failed to achieve this goal. In addition, cardiac glycosides have a low margin of safety and are frequently associated with toxicity. Gastrointestinal disturbances, fatigue, and visual complaints are among the more common side effects encountered with cardiac glycosides.[277] Although all types of arrhythmias have been associated with cardiac glycoside toxicity, ventricular arrhythmias are of particular concern, since they may be life-threatening due to decreased cardiac output. For this reason, it is unlikely that systemic cardiac glycosides will ever have a place in the therapy of glaucoma.

Theoretically, a sufficient concentration of an inhibitor of Na⁺-K⁺ ATPase delivered intraocularly after topical administration should reduce aqueous production. In humans, topical ocular application of 5% digitoxin ointment significantly reduces intraocular pressure that lasts for several days.[278] Unfortunately, such ocular application of digitoxin drops and ointment produces a painful keratopathy characterized by diffuse epithelial edema and large vertical folds in Descemet's membrane.[278] Since Na⁺-K⁺ ATPase is present in both the corneal epithelium and endothelium,[279] inhibition of corneal Na⁺-K⁺ ATPase is probably responsible for digitalis keratopathy. These corneal changes preclude the topical administration of inhibitors of Na⁺-K⁺ ATPase to human eyes.

Other Inhibitors of Na⁺-K⁺ ATPase

Vanadate, an ubiquitous element, is a potent reversible inhibitor of Na⁺-K⁺ ATPase.[280] When applied topically to unanesthetized rabbit eyes, vanadate (0.5% or 1.0%) reduces intraocular pressure without altering episcleral venous pressure or facility of outflow.[281] Tonographic findings suggest that aqueous production is reduced by 32%.[281] Topical vanadate also significantly reduces intraocular pressure in monkey eyes.[281] The mechanism for this ocular hypotensive effect appears to be inhibition of Na⁺-K⁺ ATPase in the ciliary epithelium.[280,281]

Recent Developments

New classes of drugs with ocular hypotensive properties are constantly being tested. Recently, topical ocular application of forskolin, a diterpene, was reported to lower intraocular pressure in rabbits, monkeys, and humans.[282,283] The reduction in intraocular pressure was attributed to decreased aqueous production. In the rabbit, intraocular pressure has been shown to be significantly reduced following topical ocular application of 0.05% and 0.1% forskolin.[283] In contrast, ocular hypertension has been noted following topical application of 0.2% and 0.5% forskolin.[283] Human studies using a topical suspension of 1% forskolin have been equally inconclusive. One study[284] demonstrated a marked reduction in intraocular pressure, while another study[285] found that topical 1% forskolin did not significantly affect aqueous flow.

Forskolin appears to increase intracellular cAMP levels, without receptor stimulation, by acting directly upon adenylate cyclase.[286] Since β-adrenergic agonists increase intracellular cAMP levels through stimulation of membrane-bound β receptors coupled to adenylate cyclase, the net cellular effects of forskolin would be expected to be similar to those of β-adrenergic agonists. Although topical ocular application of β-adrenergic agonists, such as isoproterenol, has been documented to reduce intraocular pressure in humans, these agents have not been clinically useful because of the cardiac side effects that result on systemic absorption.[287] Furthermore, animal studies[286,288] have suggested that increased cAMP levels in the anterior chamber produce increased aqueous outflow. Therefore, more studies are needed to establish the effects of forskolin on both aqueous formation and outflow.

Apraclonidine 1% ophthalmic solution (Iopidine, Alcon) has been recently marketed in 0.25 ml unit-dose dispensers for use in controlling or preventing the rapid rise in intraocular pressure frequently associated with argon laser trabeculoplasty and argon laser iridotomy. When 1 drop of apraclonidine 1% is instilled into the operative eye 1 hour prior to the laser procedure and a second drop is instilled immediately following the procedure, the frequency of post-laser intraocular pressure spikes is greatly reduced.[299] Apraclonidine, an α-adrenergic agonist, lowers intraocular pressure almost 40% in nonglaucomatous humans.[300] A slight reduction in intraocular pressure has also been noted in the untreated fellow eye.[301] Following instillation of 1 drop of apraclonidine 1%, intraocular pressure drops at least 20% during the first hour, with a maximum reduction being noted within 3 to 5 hours. The duration of apraclonidine's ocular hypotensive effect appears to be at least 7 hours.[301] Since apraclonidine does not alter the coefficient of outflow, the drug's ocular hypotensive action probably results from decreased aqueous formation.[301] Eyelid retraction, conjunctival blanching, and mydriasis frequently occur with short-term use of apraclonidine.[301]

References

1. Brubaker RF, Nagataki S, Townsend DJ, et al. The effect of age on aqueous humor formation in man. Ophthalmology 1981;88:283–288.
2. Smith RS, Rudt LA. Ultrastructural studies of the blood-aqueous barrier. II. The barrier to horseradish peroxidase in primates. Am J Ophthalmol 1973;76:937–947.
3. Uusitalo R, Palkama A, Stjernschantz J. An electron microscopical study of the blood-aqueous barrier in the ciliary body and iris of the rabbit. Exp Eye Res 1973;17:49–63.
4. Richardson KT. Cellular response to drugs affecting aqueous dynamics. Arch Ophthalmol 1973;89:65–84.
5. Alm A. The effect of sympathetic stimulation on blood flow

through the uvea, retina and optic nerve in monkeys (Macaca irus). Exp Eye Res 1977;25:19–24.

6. Bill A. Autonomic nervous control of uveal blood flow. Acta Physiol Scand 1962;56:70–81.

7. Cole DF, Rumble R. Response of iris blood flow to stimulation of the cervical sympathetic in the rabbit. Exp Eye Res 1970;10:183–191.

8. Morgan TR, Green K, Bowman K. Effects of adrenergic agonists upon regional ocular blood flow in normal and ganglionectimized rabbits. Exp Eye Res 1981;32:691–697.

9. Alm A. The effect of topical l-epinephrine on regional ocular blood flow in monkeys. Invest Ophthalmol Vis Sci 1980;19:487–490.

10. Yermakova VN. Investigation of some mechanisms of sympathicomimetic drugs' hypotensive action. Arch Klin Exp Ophthalmol 1974;192:331–338.

11. Macri FJ. The pressure dependence of aqueous humor formation in the anesthetized cat. Ophthalmic Res 1982;14:279–283.

12. Kaskel A, Baumgart W, Metzler U, Fink H. Blood pressure, blood flow and intraocular pressure. Ophthalmic Res 1974;6:338–345.

13. Barany E. The influence of local arterial blood pressure on aqueous humor and intraocular pressure. Acta Ophthalmol (Copenh) 1947;25:189–193.

14. Levy N, Rawitscher R. The effect of systemic hypotension during cardiopulmonary bypass on intraocular pressure and visual function in humans. Ann Ophthalmol 1977;9:1547–1552.

15. Dafna Z, Lahav M, Melamed E. Localization of beta-adrenoceptors in the anterior segment of the albino rabbit eye using a fluorescent analog of propranolol. Exp Eye Res 1979;29:327–330.

16. Lahav M, Melamed E, Dafna Z, Atlas D. Localization of beta receptors in the anterior segment of the rat eye by a fluorescent analogue of propranolol. Invest Ophthalmol Vis Sci 1978;17:645–651.

17. Nathanson JA. Human ciliary process adrenergic receptor: Pharmacological characterization. Invest Ophthalmol Vis Sci 1981;21:798–804.

18. Tsukahara S, Maezawa N. Cytochemical localization of adenylate cyclase in the rabbit ciliary body. Exp Eye Res 1978;26:99–106.

19. Sears ML. Autonomic nervous system: Adrenergic agonists. In: Sears ML, ed. Pharmacology of the eye. New York: Springer-Verlag, 1984;193–248.

20. Yablonski ME, Zimmerman TJ, Waltman SR, Becker B. A fluorophotometric study of the effect of topical timolol on aqueous humor dynamics. Exp Eye Res 1978;27:135–142.

21. Coakes RL, Brubaker RF. The mechanism of timolol in lowering intraocular pressure in the normal eye. Arch Ophthalmol 1978;96:2045–2048.

22. Zimmerman TJ, Harbin R, Pett M, Kaufman HE. Timolol and facility of outflow. Invest Ophthalmol Vis Sci 1977;16:623–624.

23. Sonntag JR, Brindley GO, Shields MB, et al. Timolol and epinephrine. Comparison of efficacy and side effects. Arch Ophthalmol 1979;97:273–277.

24. Schenker HI, Yablonski ME, Podos SM, Linder L. Fluo-

rophotometric study of epinephrine and timolol in human subjects. Arch Ophthalmol 1981;99:1212–1216.

25. Vareilles P, Lotti VJ. Effect of timolol on aqueous humor dynamics in the rabbit. Ophthalmic Res 1981;13:72–79.

26. Reiss GR, Brubaker RF. The mechanism of betaxolol, a new ocular hypotensive agent. Ophthalmology 1983;90:1369–1372.

27. Neufeld AH. Experimental studies on the mechanism of action of timolol. Surv Ophthalmol 1979;23:363–370.

28. Sweadner KJ, Goldin SM. Active transport of sodium and potassium ions: mechanism, function, and regulation. N Engl J Med 1980;302:777–783.

29. Riley MV. The sodium-potassium-stimulated adenosine triphosphate of rabbit ciliary epithelium. Exp Eye Res 1964;3:76–84.

30. Wistrand PJ. Carbonic anhydrase in the anterior uvea of the rabbit. Acta Physiol Scand 1951;24:144–148.

31. Bhattacherjee P. Distribution of carbonic anhydrase in the rabbit eye as demonstrated histochemically. Exp Eye Res 1971;12:356–359.

32. Dobbs PC, Epstein DL, Anderson PJ. Identification of isoenzyme C as the principal carbonic anhydrase in human ciliary processes. Invest Ophthalmol Vis Sci 1979;18:867–870.

33. Wistrand PJ, Garg LC. Evidence of a high-activity C type of carbonic anhydrase in human ciliary processes. Invest Ophthalmol Vis Sci 1979;18:802–806.

34. Garg LC, Oppelt WW. The effect of ouabain and acetazolamide on transport of sodium and chloride from plasma to aqueous humor. J Pharmacol Exp Ther 1970;175:237–247.

35. Obstbaum SA, Galin MA, Katz IM. Timolol: Effect on intraocular pressure in chronic open-angle glaucoma. Ann Ophthalmol 1978;10:1347–1351.

36. Lin LL, Galin MA, Obstbaum SA, Katz I. Long-term timolol therapy. Surv Ophthalmol 1979;23:377–380.

37. Sonntag JR, Brindley GO, Shields MB. Effects of timolol therapy on outflow facility. Invest Ophthalmol Vis Sci 1978;17:293–296.

38. Wood, AJJ. How the β-blockers differ: A pharmacologic comparison. Drug Ther 1983;13:59–71.

39. Frishman WH. Atenolol and timolol, two new systemic β-adrenoceptor antagonists. N Engl J Med 1982;306:1456–1462.

40. Gifford RW. Management of systolic hypertension in the elderly. In: Vidt DG, ed. Cardiovascular therapy. Philadelphia: F.A. Davis Co, 1982;69–77.

41. Heel RC, Brogden RN, Speight TM, Avery GS. Atenolol: A review of its pharmacological properties and therapeutic efficacy in angina pectoris and hypertension. Drugs 1979;17:425–460.

42. Elliot MJ, Cullen PM, Phillips CI. Ocular hypotensive effect of atenolol. Br J Ophthalmol 1975;59:296–300.

43. Macdonald MJ, Cullen PM, Phillips CI. Atenolol versus propranolol. Br J Ophthalmol 1976;60:789–791.

44. Macdonald MJ, Gore SM, Cullen PM, Phillips CI. Comparison of ocular hypotensive effects of acetazolamide and atenolol. Br J Ophthalmol 1977;61:345–348.

45. Wettrell K, Pandolfi M. Effect of oral administration of various beta-blocking agents on the intraocular pressure in healthy volunteers. Exp Eye Res 1975;21:451–456.

46. Wettrell K, Pandolfi M. Effect of topical atenolol on intra-ocular pressure. Br J Ophthalmol 1977;61:334–338.

47. Ros FE, Dake CL, Offerhaus L, Greve EL. Atenolol 4% eye drops and glaucoma. Arch Klin Exp Ophthalmol 1977;205:61–70.

48. Wettrell K, Wilke K, Pandolfi M. Topical atenolol versus pilocarpine: A double-blind study of the effect on ocular tension. Br J Ophthalmol 1978;62:292–295.

49. Phillips CI, Gore SM, Gunn PM. Atenolol versus adrenaline eye drops and an evaluation of these two combined. Br J Ophthalmol 1978;62:296–301.

50. Phillips CI, Gore SM, Macdonald MJ, Cullen PM. Atenolol eye drops in glaucoma: A double-masked, controlled study. Br J Ophthalmol 1977;61:349–353.

51. Cavero I, Lefevro-Borg F, Manoury P, Roach AG. In vitro and in vivo pharmacological evaluation of betaxolol, a new, potent, and selective β_1-adrenoceptor antagonist. In: Morelli PL, ed. Betaxolol and other β_1-adrenoceptor antagonists. New York: Raven Press, 1983;1:31–42.

52. Berrospi AR, Leibowitz HM. Betaxolol: A new β-adrenergic blocking agent for treatment of glaucoma. Arch Ophthalmol 1982;100:943–946.

53. Radius RL. Use of betaxolol in the reduction of elevated intraocular pressure. Arch Ophthalmol 1983;101:898–900.

54. Caldwell DR, Salisbury CR, Guzek JP. Effects of topical betaxolol in ocular hypertensive patients. Arch Ophthalmol 1984;102:539–540.

55. Feghali JG, Kaufman PL. Decreased intraocular pressure in the hypertensive human eye with betaxolol, a β_1-adrenergic antagonist. Am J Ophthalmol 1985;100:777–782.

56. Ward RL, Smith JP, Lumsden JB, Thoms PH. Safety study of betaxolol ophthalmic solution in normal volunteers. Alcon Clinical Monitor's Report 1980;021:3430:0880.

57. Drake MM, Beasley CH. Betaxolol duration of action study. Alcon Clinical Monitor's Report 1984;012:3432:0484.

58. Levy NS, Boone L, Ellis E. A controlled comparison of betaxolol and timolol with long-term evaluation of safety and efficacy. Glaucoma 1985;7:54–62.

59. Berry DP, Van Buskirk ME, Shields MB. Betaxolol and timolol: A comparison of efficacy and side effects. Arch Ophthalmol 1984;102:42–45.

60. Stewart RH, Kimbrough RL, Ward RL. Betaxolol vs timolol: A six-month double-blind comparison. Arch Ophthalmol 1986;104:46–48.

61. Allen RC, Hertzmark E, Walker AM, Epstein DL. A double-masked comparison of betaxolol vs timolol in the treatment of open-angle glaucoma. Am J Ophthalmol 1986;101:535–541.

62. Smith JP, Weeks RH, Newland EF, Ward RL. Betaxolol and acetazolamide: Combined ocular hypotensive effect. Arch Ophthalmol 1984;102:1794–1795.

63. Van Buskirk EM, Weinreb RN, Berry DP, et al. Betaxolol in patients with glaucoma and asthma. Am J Ophthalmol 1986;101:531–534.

64. Nelson WL, Kuritsky JN. Early postmarketing surveillance of betaxolol hydrochloride, September 1985–September 1986. Am J Ophthalmol 1987;103:592.

65. Brogden RN, Heel RC, Speight TM, Avery GS. Labetalol: A review of its pharmacology and therapeutic use in hypertension. Drugs 1978;15:251–270.

66. Kogure H, Hosaka A, Abiko Y. Hypotensive effect of labetalol on intraocular pressure in rabbits: In relation to its alpha- and beta-adrenergic blocking action on the cardiovascular system. Arch Intern Pharmacodyn 1981;250:109–122.

67. Leopold IH, Murray DL. Ocular hypotensive action of labetalol. Am J Ophthalmol 1979;88:427–431.

68. Murray DL, Podos SM, Wei CP, Leopold IH. Ocular effects in normal rabbits of topically applied labetalol. Arch Ophthalmol 1979;97:723–726.

69. Bonomi L, Perfetti S, Bellucci R, et al. Ocular hypotensive action of labetalol in rabbits and human eyes. Arch Klin Exp Ophthalmol 1981;217:175–181.

70. Krieglstein GK, Kontic D. Nadolol and labetalol: Comparative efficacy of two beta-blocking agents in glaucoma. Arch Klin Ophthalmolol 1981;216:313–317.

71. Robson RD, Kaplan HR. The cardiovascular pharmacology of bunolol, a new beta-adrenergic blocking agent. J Pharmacol Exp Ther 1970;175:157–167.

72. Weiner N. Drugs that inhibit adrenergic nerves and block adrenergic receptors. In: Gilman AG, Goodman LS, Rall TW, et al. eds. The pharmacologic basis of therapeutics. New York: Macmillan Co, 1985; 194.

73. Zimmerman T, Spaeth G, Novack G, et al. Minimum concentration of levobunolol required to control intraocular pressure in patients with primary open-angle glaucoma or ocular hypertension. Am J Ophthalmol 1985;99:18–22.

74. Cinotti A, Cinotti D, Grant W, et al. Levobunolol vs timolol for open-angle glaucoma and ocular hypertension. Am J Ophthalmol 1985;99:11–17.

75. Berson FG, Cohen HB, Foerster RJ, et al. Levobunolol compared with timolol for long-term control of elevated intraocular pressure. Arch Ophthalmol 1985;103:379–382.

76. Partamian LG, Kass MA, Gordon M. A dose-response study of the effect of levobunolol on ocular hypertension. Am J Ophthalmol 1983;95:229–232.

77. Kwitko GM, Shin DH, Ahn BH, Hong YJ. Bilateral effects of long-term monocular timolol therapy. Am J Ophthalmol 1987;104:591–594.

78. Wandel T, Charap AD, Lewis RA, et al. Glaucoma treatment with once-daily levobunolol. Am J Ophthalmol 1986;101:298–304.

79. Frishman WH. β-adrenoceptor antagonists: New drugs and new indications. N Engl J Med 1981;305:500–506.

80. Kock-Weser J. Metoprolol. N Engl J Med 1979;301:698–703.

81. Alm A, Wickstrom CP. Effects of systemic and topical administration of metoprolol on intraocular pressure in healthy subjects. Acta Ophthalmol 1980;58:740–747.

82. Alm A, Wickstrom CP, Ekstrom C, Ohman L. The effect of metoprolol on intraocular pressure in glaucoma. Acta Ophthalmol 1979;57:236–242.

83. Krieglstein GK. The long-term ocular and systemic effects of topically applied metoprolol tartrate in glaucoma and ocular hypertension.. Acta Ophthalmol 1981;59:15–20.

84. Nielsen PG, Ahrendt N, Buhl H, Byrn E. Metoprolol eye-drops 3%, a short-term comparison with pilocarpine and a five-month follow-up study. Acta Ophthalmol 1982;60:347–352.

85. Nielsen NV, Eriksen JS. Timolol and metoprolol. A diurnal

study of the ocular and systemic effects in glaucoma patients. Acta Ophthalmol 1981;59:517–525.

86. Nielsen NV, Eriksen JS. Timolol and metoprolol in glaucoma. A comparison of the ocular hypotensive effect, local and systemic tolerance. Acta Ophthalmol 1981;59:336–346.

87. Alm A, Wickstrom CP, Tornquist P. Initial and long-term effects of metoprolol and timolol on the intraocular pressure. A comparison in healthy subjects. Acta Ophthalmol 1981;59:510–516.

88. Heel RC, Brogden RN, Pakes GE, et al. Nadolol: A review of its pharmacological properties and therapeutic efficacy in hypertension and angina pectoris. Drugs 1980;20:1–23.

89. Duff GR. The effect of twice daily nadolol on intraocular pressure. Am J Ophthalmol 1987;104:343–345.

90. Rennie IG, Smerdon DL. The effect of a once-daily oral dose of nadolol on intraocular pressure in normal volunteers. Am J Ophthalmol 1985;100:445–447.

91. Williamson J, Atta HR, Kennedy PA, Muir JG. Effect of orally administered nadolol on the intraocular pressure in normal volunteers. Br J Ophthalmol 1985;69:38–40.

92. Williamson J, Young JD, Atta H, et al. Comparative efficacy of orally and topically administered β blockers for chronic simple glaucoma. Br J Ophthalmol 1985;69:41–45.

93. Krieglstein GK. Nadolol eye drops in glaucoma and ocular hypertension: A controlled clinical study of dose response and duration of action. Arch Klin Exp Ophthalmol 1981;217:309–314.

94. Krieglstein GK, Mohamed J. The comparative multiple-dose intraocular pressure response of nadolol and timolol in glaucoma and ocular hypertension. Acta Ophthalmol 1982;60:284–292.

95. Duzman E, Chen C, Anderson J, et al. Diacetyl derivative of nadolol. I. Ocular pharmacology and short-term ocular hypotensive effect in glaucomatous eyes. Arch Ophthalmol 1982;100:1916–1919.

96. Levy JV. Cardiovascular effects of pindolol (LB-46), a potent beta-adrenergic receptor antagonist. J Clin Pharmacol 1971;11:249–260.

97. Golightly LK. Pindolol: A review of its pharmacology, pharmacokinetics, clinical uses, and adverse effects. Pharmacotherapy 1982;2:134–147.

98. Smith SE, Smith SA, Reynolds R, Whitmarsh VB. Ocular and cardiovascular effects of local and systemic pindolol. Br J Ophthalmol 1979;63:63–66.

99. Bonomi L, Steindler P. Effect of pindolol on intraocular pressure. Br J Ophthalmol 1975;59:301–303.

100. Smith RJH, Blamires T, Nagasubramanian S, et al. Addition of pindolol to routine medical therapy: A clinical trial. Br J Ophthalmol 1982;66:102–108.

101. Andreasson S, Jensen KM. Effect of pindolol on intraocular pressure in glaucoma: Pilot study and randomized comparison with timolol. Br J Ophthalmol 1983;67:228–230.

102. Phillips CI, Howitt G, Rowlands DJ. Propranolol as ocular hypotensive agents. Br J Ophthalmol 1967;51:222–226.

103. Pandolfi M, Ohrstrom A. Treatment of ocular hypertension with oral beta-adrenergic blocking agents. Acta Ophthalmol 1974;54:464–467.

104. Wettrell K, Pandolfi M. Early dose response analysis of ocular hypotensive effects of propranolol in patients with ocular hypertension. Br J Ophthalmol 1976;60:680–683.

105. Ohrstrom A, Pandolfi M. Long-term treatment of glaucoma with systemic propranolol. Am J Ophthalmol 1978;86:340–344.

106. Wettrell K, Pandolfi M. Propranolol vs acetazolamide. Arch Ophthalmol 1979;97:280–283.

107. Borthne A. The treatment of glaucoma with propranolol (Inderal): A clinical trial. Acta Ophthalmol 1976;54:291–300.

108. Vale J, Gibbs ACC, Phillips CI. Topical propranolol and ocular tension in the human. Br J Ophthalmol 1972;56:770–775.

109. Zimmerman TJ, Kaufman HE. Timolol: Dose response and duration of action. Arch Ophthalmol 1977;95:605–607.

110. Ohrstrom A. Dose response of oral timolol combined with adrenaline. Br J Ophthalmol 1982;66:242–246.

111. Batchelor ED, O'Day DM, Shand DG, Wood AJ. Interaction of topical and oral timolol in glaucoma. Ophthalmology 1979;86:60–65.

112. Ohrstrom A. Dose-related interaction between timolol and adrenaline. Arch Klin Exp Ophthalmol 1981;216:55–59.

113. Thomas JV, Epstein DL. Study of additive effect of timolol and epinephrine in lowering intraocular pressure. Br J Ophthalmol 1981;65:596–602.

114. Ohrstrom A, Pandolfi M. Regulation of IOP and pupil size by beta-blockers and epinephrine. Arch Ophthalmol 1980;98:2182–2184.

115. Goldberg I, Ashburn FS Jr, Palmberg PF, et al. Timolol and epinephrine: A clinical study of ocular interactions. Arch Ophthalmol 1980;98:484–486.

116. Radius RL, Diamond GR, Pollack IP, Langham ME. Timolol: A new drug for management of chronic simple glaucoma. Arch Ophthalmol 1978;96:1003–1008.

117. Airaksinen PJ, Saari KM, Tiainen TJ, Jaanio EAT. Management of acute closed-angle glaucoma with miotics and timolol. Br J Ophthalmol 1979;63:822–825.

118. Kaufman HE. Timolol maleate. Ophthalmology 1980;87:164–168.

119. Wilson RP, Kanal N, Spaeth GL. Timolol: Its effectiveness in different types of glaucoma. Ophthalmology 1979;86:43–50.

120. Wilson RP, Spaeth GL, Poryzees E. The place of timolol in the practice of ophthalmology. Ophthalmology 1980;87:451–454.

121. Boger WP, Steinert RF, Puliafito CA, Pavan-Langston D. Clinical trial comparing timolol ophthalmic solution to pilocarpine in open-angle glaucoma. Am J Ophthalmol 1978;86:8–18.

122. Moss AP, Ritch R, Hargett NA, et al. A comparison of the effects of timolol and epinephrine on intraocular pressure. Am J Ophthalmol 1978;86:489–495.

123. Hass I, Drance SM. Comparison between pilocarpine and timolol on diurnal pressures in open-angle glaucoma. Arch Ophthalmol 1980;98:480–481.

124. Berson FG, Epstein DL. Separate and combined effects of timolol maleate and acetazolamide in open-angle glaucoma. Am J Ophthalmol 1981;92:788–791.

125. Kass MA, Korey M, Gordon M, Becker B. Timolol and acetazolamide: A study of concurrent administration. Arch Ophthalmol 1982;100:941–942.

126. Dailey RA, Brubaker RF, Bourne WM. The effects of

timolol maleate and acetazolamide on the rate of aqueous formation in normal human subjects. Am J Ophthalmol 1982;93:232–237.

127. Brubaker RF, Nagataki S, Bourne WM. Effect of chronically administered timolol on aqueous humor flow in patients with glaucoma. Ophthalmology 1982;89:280–283.

128. Zimmerman TJ, Gillespie JE, Kass MA. Timolol plus maximum-tolerated antiglaucoma therapy. Arch Ophthalmol 1979;97:278–279.

129. Sonty S, Schwartz B. The additive effect of timolol on open angle glaucoma patients on maximal medical therapy. Surv Ophthalmol 1979;23:381–388.

130. Smith RJ, Nagasubramananian S, Watkins R, Poinoosawmy D. Addition of timolol maleate to routine medical therapy: A clinical trial. Br J Ophthalmol 1980;64:779–781.

131. Ashburn FS, Gillespie JE, Kass MA, Becker B. Timolol plus maximum tolerated antiglaucoma therapy: A one year followup study. Surv Ophthalmol 1979;23:389–394.

132. Keates EU. Evaluation of timolol maleate combination therapy in chronic open-angle glaucoma. Am J Ophthalmol 1979;88:565–571.

133. Zimmerman TJ, Canale P. Timolol—further observations. Ophthalmology 1979;86:166–169.

134. Korney MS, Hodapp E, Kass MA, et al. Timolol and epinephrine. Long-term evaluation of concurrent administration. Arch Ophthalmol 1982;100:742–745.

135. Tsoy EA, Meekins BB, Shields MB. Comparison of two treatment schedules for combined timolol and dipivefrin therapy. Am J Ophthalmol 1986;102:320–324.

136. Zimmerman TJ. Ophthalmol Audio Digest 1979;17.

137. Maren N, Alvan G, Calissendorff BM, et al. Additive intraocular pressure reducing effect of topical timolol during systemic β-blockade. Acta Ophthalmol 1982;60:16–23.

138. Katz IM, Berger ET. Effects of iris pigmentation on response of ocular pressure to timolol. Surv Ophthalmol 1979;23:395–398.

139. Friedenwald JS. The formation of the intraocular fluid. Am J Ophthalmol 1949;32:9–27.

140. Kinsey VE. A unified concept of aqueous humor dynamics and the maintenance of intraocular pressure: An elaboration of the secretion-diffusion theory. Arch Ophthalmol 1950;44:215–235.

141. Becker B. Decrease in intraocular pressure in man by a carbonic anhydrase inhibitor, Diamox: A preliminary report. Am J Ophthalmol 1954;37:13–15.

142. Becker B. Carbonic anhydrase and the formation of aqueous humor. Am J Ophthalmol 1959;47:342–361.

143. Maren TH. Relations between structure and biological activity of sulfonamides. Ann Rev Pharmacol Toxicol 1976;16:309–327.

144. Mudge GH. Diuretics and other agents employed in the mobilization of edema fluid. In: Gilman AG, Goodman LS, Gilman A, et al. eds. The pharmacological basis of therapeutics. New York: Macmillan Co, 1980;6:896–899.

145. Zimmerman TJ, Garg LC, Vogh BP, Maren TH. The effect of acetazolamide on the movements of anions into the posterior chamber of the dog eye. J Pharmacol Exp Ther 1976;196:510–516.

146. Kinsey VE, Reddy DVN. Turnover of carbon dioxide in the aqueous humor and the effect thereon of acetazolamide. Arch Ophthalmol 1959;62:78–83.

147. Maren TH, Wistrand P, Swensen ER, Talalay ABC. The rates of ion movement from plasma to aqueous humor in the dogfish, Squalus ascanthias. Invest Ophthalmol 1975;14:662–673.

148. Maren TH. The rates of movement of Na+, Cl−, and HCO3 from plasma to posterior chamber: Effect of acetazolamide and relation to treatment of glaucoma. Invest Ophthalmol 1976,15:356–364.

149. Maren TH. Ion secretion into the posterior aqueous humor of dogs and monkeys. Exp Eye Res (Suppl) 1977;25:245–247.

150. Maren TH. HCO3 formation in aqueous humor: Mechanism and relation to treatment of glaucoma. Invest Ophthalmol 1974;13:479–484.

151. Cole DF. Secretion of aqueous humor. Exp Eye Res (Suppl) 1977;25:161–176.

152. Bietti G, Virno M, Pecori-Giraldi J, Pellegrino N. Acetazolamide, metabolic acidosis, and intraocular pressure. Am J Ophthalmol 1975;80:360–369.

153. Friedman Z, Krupin T, Becker B. Ocular and systemic effects of acetazolamide in nephrectomized rabbits. Invest Ophthalmol Vis Sci 1982;23:209–213.

154. Langham ME, Lee PM. Action of Diamox and ammonium chloride on formation of aqueous humor. Br J Ophthalmol 1957;41:65–92.

155. Becker B. The mechanism of the fall in intraocular pressure induced by the carbonic anhydrase inhibitor, Diamox. Am J Ophthalmol 1955;39:177–182.

156. Maren TH. Carbonic anhydrase: chemistry, physiology, and inhibition. Physiol Rev 1967;47:595–781.

157. Foss RH. Local application of Diamox: an experimental study of its effect on the intraocular pressure. Am J Ophthalmol 1955;39:336–339.

158. Green H, Leopold IH. Effects of locally administered Diamox. Am J Ophthalmol 1955;40:137–139.

159. Kimura R. Effect of long-term subconjunctival administration of Diamox (acetazolamide) on the ocular tension in rabbit. Arch Klin Exp Ophthalmol 1978,205:221–227.

160. Maren TH, Jankowska L, Sanyal G, Edelhauser HF. The transcorneal permeability of sulfonamide carbonic anhydrase inhibitors and their effect on aqueous humor secretion. Exp Eye Res 1983;36:457–480.

161. Friedman Z, Allen RC, Raph SM. Topical acetazolamide and methazolamide delivered by contact lenses. Arch Ophthalmol 1985;103:963–966.

162. Flach AJ, Peterson JS, Seligmann KA. Local ocular hypotensive effect of topically applied acetazolamide. Am J Ophthalmol 1984;98:66–72.

163. Flach AJ. Topical acetazolamide and other carbonic anhydrase inhibitors in the current medical therapy of the glaucomas. Glaucoma 1986;8:20–27.

164. Lotti VJ, Schmitt CJ, Gautheron PD. Topical ocular hypotensive activity and ocular penetration of dichlorphenamide sodium in rabbits. Arch Klin Exp Ophthalmol 1984;222:13–19.

165. Maren TH, Jankowska L, Sanyal G, Edelhauser H. Reduction of aqueous humor secretion by topical carbonic anhydrase inhibitors (abstr.). Invest Ophthalmol Vis Sci (Suppl) 1982;22:39.

166. Stein A, Pinke R, Krupin T, et al. The effect of topically administered carbonic anhydrase inhibitors on aqueous hu-

mor dynamics in rabbits. Am J Ophthalmol 1983;95:222–228.

167. Schoenwald RD, Eller MG, Dixson JA, Barfknecht CF. Topical carbonic anhydrase inhibitors. J Med Chem 1984;27:810–812.

168. Lewis RA, Schoenwald RD, Eller MG, et al. Ethoxzolamide analogue gel: A topical carbonic anhydrase inhibitor. Arch Ophthalmol 1984;102:1821–1824.

169. Sugrue MF, Gautheron P, Schmitt C, et al. On the pharmacology of L-645,151: A topically effective ocular hypotensive carbonic anhydrase inhibitor. J Pharmacol Exp Ther 1985;232:534–540.

170. Lewis RA, Schoenwald RD, Barfknecht CF, Phelps CD. Aminozolamide gel: A trial of a topical carbonic anhydrase inhibitor in ocular hypertension. Arch Ophthalmol 1986;104:842–844.

171. Kolker AE, Hetherington J Jr. Becker-Shaffer's diagnosis and therapy of the glaucomas. St Louis: C. V. Mosby Co, 1976;339.

172. Theeuwes F, Bayne W, McGuire J. Gastrointestinal therapeutic system for acetazolamide. Arch Ophthalmol 1978;96:2219–2221.

173. Ellis PP, Price PK, Kelmenson R, Rendi M. Effectiveness of generic acetazolamide. Arch Ophthalmol 1982;100:1920–1922.

174. Maren TH, Mayer E, Wadsworth BD. Carbonic anhydrase inhibitors. I. The pharmacology of Diamox,2-acetylamino-1,3,4,-thiadiazole-5-sulfonamice. Bull Johns Hopkins Hosp 1954;95:199–243.

175. Maren TH, Robinson B. The pharmacology of acetazolamide as related to cerebrospinal fluid and the treatment of hydrocephalus. Bull Johns Hopkins Hosp 1960;106:1–24.

176. Yakatan GJ, Frome EL, Leonard RG, et al. Bioavailability of acetazolamide tablets. J Pharm Sci 1978;67:252–256.

177. Bayne WF, Rogers G, Crisologo N. Assay for acetazolamide in plasma. J Pharm Sci 1975;64:402–404.

178. Friedland BR, Mallonee J, Anderson DR. Short-term dose response characteristics of acetazolamide in man. Arch Ophthalmol 1977;95:1809–1812.

179. Garner LL, Carl EF, Ferwerda JR. Advantages of sustained-release therapy with acetazolamide in glaucoma. Am J Ophthalmol 1963;55:323–327.

180. Berson FG, Epstein DL, Grant WM, et al. Azetazolamide dosage forms in the treatment of glaucoma. Arch Ophthalmol 1980;98:1051–1054.

181. Linner E, Wistrand P. The initial drop of intraocular pressure following intravenous administration of acetazolamide in man. Acta Ophthalmol 1959;37:209–214.

182. Nissen OI. The immediate response in applanation pressure to intravenous acetazolamide in primary glaucomas and glaucoma suspects. Acta Ophthalmol 1975;53:537–552.

183. Shields BM. A study guide for glaucoma. Baltimore: Williams & Wilkins, 1982;429–430.

184. Alm A, Berggren L, Hartvig P, Roosdorp M. Monitoring acetazolamide treatment. Acta Ophthalmol 1982;60:24–34.

185. Kupfer C, Lawrence C, Linner E. Long-term administration of acetazolamide (Diamox) in the treatment of glaucoma. Am J Ophthalmol 1955;40:673–680.

186. Becker B, Ley AP. Epinephrine and acetazolamide in the therapy of the chronic glaucomas. Am J Ophthalmol 1958;45:639–643.

187. Leopold IH, Carmichael PL. Prolonged administration of Diamox in glaucoma. Trans Am Acad Ophthalmol Otolaryngol 1956;60:210–214.

188. Becker B. Use of methazolamide (Neptazane) in the therapy of glaucoma: Comparison with acetazolamide (Diamox). Am J Ophthalmol 1960;49:1307–1311.

189. Epstein DL, Grant WM. Carbonic anhydrase inhibitor side effects. Serum chemical analysis. Arch Ophthalmol 1977;95:1378–1382.

190. Lichter PR, Newman LP, Wheeler NC, Beall OV. Patient tolerance to carbonic anhydrase inhibitors. Am J Ophthalmol 1978;85:495–502.

191. Becker B, Middleton WH. Long-term acetazolamide (Diamox) administration in the therapy of glaucomas. Arch Ophthalmol 1955;54:187–192.

192. Epstein DL, Grant WM. Management of carbonic anhydrase inhibitor side effects. In: Leopold IH, Burns RP, eds. Symposium on ocular therapy. New York: John Wiley & Sons, 1979;11:51–64.

193. Leopold IH, Eisenberg IJ, Yasuna J: Experience with Diamox in glaucoma. Am J Ophthalmol 1955;39:885–888.

194. Maren TH. Chemistry of the renal reabsorption of bicarbonate. Can J Physiol Pharmacol 1974;52:1041–1050.

195. Stitzel RE, Irish JM III. Water, electrolyte metabolism, and diuretic agents. In: Craig CR, Stitzel RE, eds. Modern pharmacology. Boston: Little, Brown, 1982;328–329.

196. Maren TH, Haywood JR, Chapman SK, Zimmerman TJ. The pharmacology of methazolamide in relation to the treatment of glaucoma. Invest Ophthalmol Vis Sci 1977;16:730–742.

197. Parfitt AM. Acetazolamide and sodium bicarbonate induced nephrocalcinosis and nephrolithiasis. Arch Intern Med 1969;124:736–740.

198. Spaeth GL. Potassium, acetazolamide, and intraocular pressure. Arch Ophthalmol 1967;78:578–582.

199. Grant WM. Antiglaucoma drugs: problems with carbonic anhydrase inhibitors. In: Leopold IH, ed. Symposium on ocular therapy. St Louis: C. V. Mosby Co, 1973;6:19–38.

200. Fraunfelder FT, Meyer SM, Bagby GC, Dreis MW. Hematologic reactions to carbonic anhydrase inhibitors. Am J Ophthalmol 1985;100:79–81.

201. Zimran A, Beutler E. Can the risk of acetazolamide-induced aplastic anemia be decreased by periodic monitoring of blood cell counts? Am J Ophthalmol 1987;104:654–658.

202. Granstrom K. Transient myopia following the administration of sulphonamides. Acta Ophthalmol 1949;27:59–68.

203. Mattson R. Transient myopia following the use of sulfonamides. Acta Ophthalmol 1952;30:385–398.

204. Hook SR, Holladay JT, Prager TC, Goosey JD. Transient myopia induced by sulfonamides. Am J Ophthalmol 1986;101:495–496.

205. Back M. Transient myopia after use of acetazolamide (Diamox). Arch Ophthalmol 1956;55:546–547.

206. Halpern AE, Kulvin MM. Transient myopia during treatment with carbonic anhydrase inhibitors. Am J Ophthalmol 1959;48:534–535.

207. Galin MA, Baras I, Zweifach P. Diamox-induced myopia. Am J Ophthalmol 1962;54:237–240.

208. Garland M, Sholk A, Guenter K. Acetazolamide-induced myopia. Am J Obstet Gynecol 1962;84:69–71.

209. Bovino JA, Marcus DF. The mechanism of transient myopia

induced by sulfonamide therapy. Am J Ophthalmol 1982; 94:99–102.

210. Friedland BR, Maren TH. Carbonic anhydrase: Pharmacology of inhibitors and treatment of glaucoma. In: Sears ML, ed. Pharmacology of the eye. New York: Springer-Verlag, 1984;279–309.

211. Warnock DG. Diuretics. In: Katzung BG, ed. Basic and clinical pharmacology. Los Altos: LANGE Medical Publications, 1982;157–158.

212. Block ER, Rostand RA. Carbonic anhydrase inhibition in glaucoma: Hazard or benefit for the chronic lunger? Surv Ophthalmol 1978;23:169–172.

213. Nissen SH. Acetazolamide in the treatment of haemorrhagic glaucoma. Ophthalmologica 1979;179:286–290.

214. Weber PA. Neovascular glaucoma. Current management. Surv Ophthalmol 1981;26:149–153.

215. Havener WH. Ocular pharmacology. St Louis: C. V. Mosby Co, 1978;475–496.

216. Goldberg MF. Sickled erythrocytes, hyphema, and secondary glaucoma: The effect of vitamin C on erythrocyte sickling in aqueous humor. Ophthalmic Surg 1979;10:70–77.

217. Goldberg MF. The diagnosis and treatment of secondary glaucoma after hyphema in sickle cell patients. Am J Ophthalmol 1979;87:43–49.

218. Rubenstein MA, Bucy JG. Acetazolamide-induced renal calculi. J Urol 1975;114:610–612.

219. Siklos P, Henderson RG. Severe acidosis from acetazolamide in a diabetic patient. Curr Med Res Opin 1979;6:284–286.

220. Gabay EL. Metabolic acidosis from acetazolamide therapy. Arch Ophthalmol 1983;101:303–304.

221. Maren TH. Teratology and carbonic anhydrase inhibition. Arch Ophthalmol 1971;85:1–2.

222. Leopold IH, Gordon B. Drug interactions. In: Leopold IH, ed. Symposium on ocular therapy. St Louis: C. V. Mosby, 1973;6:103.

223. Hill JB. Experimental salicylate poisoning: Observations on the effects of altering blood pH on tissue and plasma salicylate concentrations. Pediatrics 1971;47:658–665.

224. Anderson CJ, Kaufman PL, Sturm RJ. Toxicity of combined therapy with carbonic anhydrase inhibitors and aspirin. Am J Ophthalmol 1978;86:516–519.

225. Stone RA, Zimmerman TJ, Shin DH, et al. Low-dose methazolamide and intraocular pressure. Am J Ophthalmol 1977;83:674–679.

226. Dahlen K, Epstein DL, Grant WM, et al. A repeated dose-response study of methazolamide in glaucoma. Arch Ophthalmol 1978;96:2214–2218.

227. Vogh BP, Doyle AS. The effect of carbonic anhydrase inhibitors and other drugs on sodium entry to cerebrospinal fluid. J Pharmacol Exp Ther 1981;217:51–56.

228. Zimmerman TJ. Acetazolamide and methazolamide. Ann Ophthalmol 1978;10:509–510.

229. Zimmerman TJ. Basic pharmacology of some glaucoma drugs. Ophthalmic Optician 1981;21:286–289.

230. Ellis PP. Urinary calculi with methazolamide therapy. Doc Ophthalmol 1973;34:137–142.

231. Sheilds MB, Simmons RJ. Urinary calculus during methazolamide therapy. Am J Ophthalmol 1976;81:622–624.

232. Werblin TP, Pollack IP, Liss RA. Blood dyscrasias in pa-

tients using methazolamide (Neptazane) for glaucoma. Ophthalmology 1980;87:350–353.

233. Gonzales-Jimeney E, Leopold IH. Effect of dichlorphenamide on the intraocular pressure of humans. Arch Ophthalmol 1958;60:427–436.

234. Garrison L, Roth A, Rundle H, Christensen RE. A clinical comparison of three carbonic anhydrase inhibitors. Trans Pac Coast Oto-ophthalmol Soc 1967;48:137–143.

235. Heilmann K. Special pharmacology. In: Heilmann K, Richardson KT, eds. Glaucoma. Conceptions of a disease. Pathogenesis, diagnosis, therapy. Philadelphia: W. B. Saunders Co, 1978;284.

236. Beyer KH, Baer JE. Physiological basis of action of newer diuretic agents. Pharmacol Rev 1961;13:517–562.

237. Gaoni Y, Mechoulam R. Isolation, structure and partial synthesis of active constituent of hashish. J Am Chem Soc 1964;86:1646–1647.

238. Lemberger L. Potential therapeutic usefulness of marijuana. Ann Rev Pharmacol Toxicol 1980;20:151–172.

239. Helper RS, Frank IM. Marihuana smoking and intraocular pressure. JAMA 1971;217:1392.

240. Purnell WD, Gregg JM. Δ⁹-Tetrahydrocannabinol, euphoria and intraocular pressure in man. Ann Ophthalmol 1975; 7:921–923.

241. Cooler P, Gregg JM. Effect of delta-9-tetrahydrocannabinol on intraocular pressure in humans. South Med J 1977;70:951–954.

242. Hepler RS, Frank IM, Ungerleider JT. Pupillary constriction after marijuana smoking. Am J Ophthalmol 1972;74:1185–1190.

243. Flom MC, Adams AJ, Jones RT. Marijuana smoking and reduced pressure in human eyes: Drug action or epiphenomenon? Invest Ophthalmol 1975;14:52–55.

244. Hepler RS, Frank IM, Petrus R. Ocular effects of marihuana smoking. In: Braude MC, Szara S, eds. The pharmacology of marihuana. New York: Raven Press, 1976;815–824.

245. Hepler RS, Petrus R. Experiences with administration of marihuana to glaucoma patients. In: Cohen S, Stillman RC, eds. The therapeutic potential of marihuana. New York: Plenum Press, 1976;63–76.

246. Green K. Current status of basic and clinical marijuana research in ophthalmology. In: Leopold IH, Burns RP, eds. Symposium on ocular therapy. New York: John Wiley & Sons, 1979;11:37–49.

247. Merritt JC, Crawford WJ, Alexander PC, et al. Effect of marihuana on intraocular and blood pressure in glaucoma. Ophthalmology 1980;87:222–228.

248. Crawford WJ, Merritt JC. Effects of tetrahydrocannabinol on arterial and intraocular hypertension. Int J Clin Pharm Biopharm 1979;17:191–196.

249. Green K, Kim K. Acute dose response of intraocular pressure to topical and oral cannabinoids. Proc Soc Exp Biol Med 1977;154:228–231.

250. Merritt JC, McKinnon S, Armgstron JR, Hatem G, Reid LA. Oral Δ⁹-tetrahydrocannabinol in heterogeneous glaucomas. Ann Ophthalmol 1980;12:947–950.

251. Green K, Symonds CM, Oliver NW, Elijah DR. Intraocular pressure following systemic administration of cannabinoids. Curr Eye Res 1982;2:247–253.

252. Newell FW, Jay WM, Sternberg P. Use of cannabinoid derivatives in glaucoma. Trans Ophthalmol Soc UK 1979; 99:269–271.

253. Newell FW, Stark P, Jay WM, Schanzlin DJ. Nabilone: A pressure-reducing synthetic benzopyran in open-angle glaucoma. Ophthalmology 1979;86:156–160.

254. Green K, Bigger JF, Kim K, Bowman K. Cannabinoid penetration and chronic effects on the eye. Exp Eye Res 1976;24:197–205.

255. Green K, Roth M. Ocular effects of topical administration of Δ^9-tetrahydrocannabinol in man. Arch Ophthalmol 1982;100:265–267.

256. Green K, Kim K. Mediation of ocular tetrahydrocannabinol effects by adrenergic nervous system. Exp Eye Res 1976;23:443–448.

257. Green K, Kim K. Interaction of adrenergic blocking agents with prostaglandin E_2 and tetrahydrocannabinol in the eye. Invest Ophthalmol 1976;15:102–112.

258. Green K, Bigger JF, Kim K, Bowman K. Cannabinoid action on the eye as mediated through the central nervous system and local activity. Exp Eye Res 1977;24:189–196.

259. Green K, Wynn H, Padgett D. Effect of Δ^9-tetrahydrocannabinol on ocular blood flow and aqueous formation. Exp Eye Res 1978;26:65–69.

260. Green K, Wynn H, Bowman KA. A comparison of topical cannabinoids on intraocular pressure. Exp Eye Res 1978;27:239–246.

261. Green K, Sobel RE, Fineberg E, et al. Subchronic ocular and systemic toxicity of topically applied Δ^9-tetrahydrocannabinol. Ann Ophthalmol 1981;13:1219–1222.

262. Merritt JC, Perry DD, Russell DN, Jones BF. Topical Δ^9-tetrahydrocannabinol and aqueous dynamics in glaucoma. J Clin Pharmacol 1981;21:457S–471S.

263. Merritt JC, Olsen JL, Armstrong JR, McKinnon SM. Topical Δ^9-tetrahydrocannabinol in hypertensive glaucomas. J Pharm Pharmacol 1981;33:40–41.

264. Jay WM, Green K. Multiple-drop study of topically applied 1% Δ^9-tetrahydrocannabinol in human eyes. Arch Ophthalmol 1983;101:591–593.

265. Green K. Physiology and pharmacology of aqueous humor inflow. Surv Ophthalmol 1984;29:208–214.

266. Deutsch HM, Green K, Salkow LH. Isolation of ocular hypotensive agents from Cannabis sativa. J Clin Pharmacol 1981;21:479S–485S.

267. Liu JH, Dacus AC. Central nervous system and peripheral mechanisms in ocular hypotensive effect of cannabinoids. Arch Ophthalmol 1987;105:245–248.

268. Shapiro D. The ocular manifestations of cannabinols. Ophthalmologica 1974;168:366–369.

269. Korozyn AD. The ocular effects of cannabinoids. Gen Pharmacol 1980;11:419–423.

270. Simon KA, Bonting SL, Hawkins NM. Studies on sodium-potassium-activated adenosine triphosphatase. II. Formation of aqueous humour. Exp Eye Res 1962;1:253–261.

271. Becker B. Ouabain and aqueous humor dynamics in the rabbit eye. Invest Ophthalmol 1963;2:325–331.

272. Bonting SL, Becker B. Studies on sodium-potassium activated adenosinetriphosphatase XIV. Inhibition of enzyme activity and aqueous humor flow in the rabbit eye after intravitreal injection of ouabain. Invest Ophthalmol 1964; 3:523–533.

273. Langham ME, Eakins KE. The influence of the cardiac glycoside ouabain on the intraocular pressure and dynamics of the rabbit and cat. J Pharmacol Exp Ther 1964;144:421–428.

274. Ferraiolo BL, Pace DG. Digoxin-induced decrease in intraocular pressure in the cat. Eur J Pharmacol 1979;55:19–22.

275. Simon K, Bonting SL. Possible usefulness of cardiac glycosides in the treatment of glaucoma. Arch Ophthalmol 1962;68:227–234.

276. Peczon JD. Clinical evaluation of digitalization in glaucoma. Arch Ophthalmol 1964;71:500–504.

277. Lely AH, van Enter CHJ. Large scale digitoxin intoxication. Br Med J 1970;3:737–740.

278. Smith JL, Mickatavage RC. The ocular effects of topical digitalis. Am J Ophthalmol 1963;56:889–894.

279. Waltman SR. The cornea. In: Moses RA, ed. Adler's physiology of the eye. Clinical application. St Louis: C. V. Mosby Co, 1981;50.

280. Becker B. Vanadate and aqueous humor dynamics. Invest Ophthalmol Vis Sci 1980;19:1156–1165.

281. Krupin T, Becker B, Podos SM. Topical vanadate lowers intraocular pressure in rabbits. Invest Ophthalmol Vis Sci 1980;19:1360–1363.

282. Capriolli J, Sears M. Forskolin lowers intraocular pressure in rabbits, monkeys, and man. Lancet 1983;1:958–960.

283. Smith BR, Gaster RN, Leopold IH, Zeleznick LD. Forskolin, a potent adenylate cyclase activator, lowers rabbit intraocular pressure. Arch Ophthalmol 1984;102:146–148.

284. Sears ML. Regulation of aqueous flow by the adenylate cyclase receptor complex in the ciliary epithelium. Am J Ophthalmol 1985;100:194–198.

285. Brubaker RF, Carlson KH, Kullerstrand LJ, McLaren JW. Topical forskolin (colforsin) and aqueous flow in humans. Arch Ophthalmol 1987;105:637–641.

286. Seamon KB, Daly JW. Forskolin: A unique diterpene activator of cyclic AMP-generating systems. J Cyclic Nucl Res 1981;7:201–224.

287. Ross RA, Drance SM. Effects of topically applied isoproterenol on aqueous dynamics in man. Arch Ophthalmol 1970;83:39–46.

288. Neufeld AH, Dueker DK, Vegge T, Sears ML. Adenosine 3′, 5′-monophosphate increases the outflow of aqueous humor from the rabbit eye. Invest Ophthalmol 1975;14:40–42.

289. Neufeld AH, Sears ML. Adenosine 3′, 5′-monophosphate analogue increases the outflow facility of the primate eye. Invest Ophthalmol 1975;14:688–689.

290. Weinreb RN, van Buskirk ME, Cherniack MD, et al. Long-term betaxolol therapy in glaucoma patients with pulmonary disease. Am J Ophthalmol 1988;106:162–167.

291. Lynch MG, Whitson JT, Brown RH, et al. Topical beta-blocker therapy and central nervous system side effects. A preliminary study comparing betaxolol and timolol. Arch Ophthalmol 1988;106:908–911.

292. Duff GR, Watt AH, Graham PA. A comparison of the effects of oral nadolol and topical timolol on intraocular pressure, blood pressure, and heart rate. Br J Ophthalmol 1987;71:698–700.

293. Edelhauser HF, Maren TH. Permeability of human and sclera to sulfonamide carbonic anhydrase inhibitors. Arch Ophthalmol 1988;106:1110–1115.

294. Ponticello GS, Freedman MB, Habecker CN, et al. Thienothiopyran-2-sulfonamides: a novel class of water-soluble carbonic anhydrase inhibitors. J Med Chem 1987;30:591–597.

295. Cox SN, Hay E, Bird AC. Treatment of chronic macular edema with acetazolamide. Arch Ophthalmol 1988;106:1190–1195.

296. Epstein RJ, Allen RC, Lunde MW. Organic impotence associated with carbonic anhydrase inhibitor therapy for glaucoma. Ann Ophthalmol 1987;19:48–50.

297. Ahlstrand C, Tiselius HG. Urine composition and stone formation during treatment with acetazolamide. Scand J Urol Nephrol 1987;21:225–228.

298. Mogk LG, Cyrlin MN. Blood dyscrasias and carbonic anhydrase inhibitors. Ophthalmology 1988;95:768–771.

299. Brown RH, Stewart RH, Lynch MG, et al. ALO 2145 reduces the intraocular pressure elevation following anterior segment laser surgery. Ophthalmology 1988;95:378–384.

300. Abrams DA, Robin AL, Pollack IP, et al. The safety and efficacy of topical 1% ALO 2145 (p-aminoclonidine hydrochloride) in normal volunteers. Arch Ophthalmol 1987;105:1205–1207.

301. Robin AL. Short-term effects of unilateral 1% apraclonidine therapy. Arch Ophthalmol 1988;106:912–915.

CHAPTER 8

Hyperosmotic Drugs

Siret D. Jaanus

Osmotherapy was introduced into ocular therapeutics by Cantonnet in 1904 with use of oral hypertonic saline to reduce intraocular pressure.[1] Since then, systemically administered hyperosmotic agents have proved effective in several forms of glaucoma, surgery to repair detached retina, cataract extraction, keratoplasty, and corneoscleral lacerations. Topical ocular application of such drugs can be of considerable value in the treatment of corneal edema.

This chapter considers agents currently available for topical and systemic ocular osmotherapy.

Corneal Hydration

The cornea, a 5-layered avascular structure, is bathed on its anterior surface by the tear film and on its posterior surface by the aqueous humor. Under normal physiologic conditions, the cornea is about 78% hydrated. When placed in contact with water, an excised piece of cornea will imbibe water and reach a hydration level of 98%.[2] The water is taken up primarily by the mucopolysaccharide matrix of the thickest part of the cornea, the stroma.[3]

Among the factors controlling corneal hydration are the epithelium, the endothelium, and the intraocular pressure. The multilayered epithelium covering the anterior surface of the cornea prevents water from moving from the tears to the corneal stroma.[4]

The endothelium plays a key role in maintaining normal corneal deturgescence, since it bars fluid movement into the cornea from the anterior chamber. It also provides an active transport system for the flow of water from the stroma to the aqueous.[4] When the cornea is exposed to certain drugs, such as ouabain, which affect this transport mechanism, the cornea takes up water and swells.[5]

Intraocular pressures within the normal limits exert minimal influence on corneal thickness. However, with a sudden elevation of intraocular pressure, the stroma becomes compressed and water moves toward the epithelium. The relatively high resistance of the epithelium to water flow, compared with that of stroma and of endothelium, causes retention of water, resulting in epithelial edema.[4]

In addition to intraocular pressure effects, the eyelids and tear film influence epithelial hydration. Changes in corneal thickness occur with the eyelids open and closed.[4] The tear film contributes to the optical surface of the cornea by interaction with the epithelial microvilli. It also influences the state of corneal hydration, since when the lids are open, the tear film becomes hypertonic, and the resultant osmotic gradient allows the outward flow of water from the cornea across the epithelium[6]

Causes of Corneal Edema

A variety of clinical situations can give rise to corneal edema[7,8] (Table 8.1). Since the endothelium is the main structure involved in maintaining normal corneal deturgescence, it must play a role in stromal hydration and compensate for the driving force of intraocular pressure. Also, the active transport system involved in the movement of water and electrolytes from the cornea to aqueous must be maintained to prevent fluid retention. Endothelial failure will result in corneal edema, and this can occur due to defects in the trans-

TABLE 8.1
Causes of Corneal Edema

Endothelial decompensation
  Birth trauma
  Congenital hereditary corneal dystrophy
  Fuch's dystrophy
  Keratoconus and hydrops
  Mechanical trauma
  Surgical trauma
  Inflammation
Increased intraocular pressure
  Acute angle-closure glaucoma
  Chronic glaucoma

Adapted from Boruchoff SA. Clinical causes of corneal edema. Int Ophthalmol Clin 1968;8:581–600.

port system or stromal compression due to elevation of intraocular pressure, resulting in water movement toward the epithelium.[4,7]

Whenever swelling takes place, transparency is lost in the region where the edema is present.[7] Since the corneal epithelium constitutes the most anterior optical surface of the eye, epithelial edema may exert a major detrimental influence on vision. It is clinically useful to consider corneal edema as epithelial, stromal, or a combination of both.[9] In general, epithelial edema is more responsive to topical hyperosmotic therapy.[10]

The following discussion considers the pharmacologic properties of hyperosmotic agents available for topical use. The clinical uses of topical osmotherapy in the diagnosis and management of conditions characterized by corneal edema are discussed in detail in Chapter 22.

Topical Hyperosmotic Agents

The clinical objective of topical osmotherapy is to increase the tonicity of the tear film and thereby enhance the rate of movement of fluid from the cornea. All the currently available hyperosmotic preparations are hyperosmolar to the ocular tissue fluid. When they are applied to the eye, water is drawn from the cornea to the more highly osmotic tear film and is eliminated through the usual tear flow mechanisms. Patients with minimal to moderate epithelial edema often achieve subjective comfort and improved vision with use of these agents.[7,9,10]

Various agents have been used to reduce corneal edema, including corn syrup, glucose, gum cellulose, sodium chloride, and glycerin.[9] Only a few have proved clinically useful and acceptable to most patients. Among those presently available, sodium chloride and glycerin

TABLE 8.2
Topical Hyperosmotic Preparations

Trade Name (manufacturer)	*Composition*
Sodium Chloride	
Adsorbonac Solution, 2% and 5% (Alcon)	NaCl, povidone and other water soluble polymers, thimerosal 0.004%, EDTA 0.1%
Muro-128 Solution, 2% and 5% (Bausch & Lomb)	NaCl, hydroxypropyl methylcellulose, methylparaben, propylparaben, boric acid
Muro-128 Ointment, 5% (Bausch & Lomb)	NaCl, anhydrous lanolin, mineral oil, white petrolatum
AK-NaCl 5% Ointment (Akorn)	NaCl, anhydrous lanolin, mineral oil, white petrolatum
Glycerin (Glycerol)	
Ophthalgan[a] (Ayerst)	Anhydrous glycerin, chlorobutanol 0.55%
Glucose	
Glucose-40 Ophthalmic Ointment[a] (CooperVision)	Glucose 40%, white petrolatum, anhydrous lanolin, methylparaben, propylparaben

[a]Available only by prescription. EDTA, ethylenediamine tetraacetic acid.

(Table 8.2) are the most widely used in clinical practice.

Sodium Chloride

Sodium chloride is a component of all body fluids, including tears. A solution of 0.9% is approximately isotonic with tears.[4]

Cogan and Kinsey[6] were the first investigators to demonstrate the clinical usefulness of sodium chloride for corneal dehydration. Of the various concentrations tested, the 5% formulation proved the most effective and with an irritation level acceptable to most patients.

Subsequent studies comparing various hyperosmotics in human subjects have confirmed the usefulness of hypertonic sodium chloride solutions in the treatment of corneal edema. Luxenberg and Green[11] studied a series of hyperosmotic preparations including sodium chloride in various formulations. These investigators concluded that 5% sodium chloride in ointment form with petrolatum and lanolin was most effective in reducing corneal thickness and improving vision. A maximum reduction in corneal thickness of about 20% was observed 3 to 4 hours following instillation of the ointment (Fig 8.1). Marisi and Aquavella[12] studied the effect of 5% sodium chloride in a water-soluble polymer base (Adsorbonac) in a series of patients with corneal edema. All patients continued their use of ancillary medications or hydrophilic bandage contact lenses. Visual acuity was used as the sole parameter of therapeutic efficacy. Although this study showed a high degree of individual variability, improvement in visual acuity was reported in 61% of the patients. There were, however, no controls in the study, nor was the study masked. Since all patients continued their original therapy at the time the sodium chloride was added to the therapeutic regimen, the results of the study are difficult to interpret.

The usefulness of sodium chloride solutions in edematous corneas with a traumatized epithelium appears to be limited. The intact corneal epithelium exhibits limited permeability to inorganic ions.[9] In the absence of an intact epithelium, however, the cornea imbibes salt solutions, thereby reducing the osmotic effect. Thus, in the management of corneal edema associated with traumatized epithelium, hypertonic saline solutions may be of only limited value due to their increased ability to penetrate the epithelial barrier.

CLINICAL USES

Sodium chloride is commercially available in 2% and 5% solutions and as 5% ointment (see Table 8.2). In clinical practice the 5% concentration appears to be somewhat more effective.[11]

Sodium chloride is useful for reducing corneal edema of various etiologies, including bullous keratopathy. Generally, 1 to 2 drops are instilled in the eye every 3 to 4 hours.[13] Sodium chloride ointment requires less frequent instillation and is generally reserved for nighttime use in patients with good vision.[7]

The way in which hyperosmotic preparations are administered may affect the clinical results.[7,9] Since vision is usually worse on arising, several instillations during the first waking hours can be helpful. On hot, dry days less medication may be needed, since tear film evaporation is enhanced.

Sodium chloride, especially in the 5% concentration, can cause discomfort upon instillation. Stinging, burning, and irritation are common complaints, but patients generally tolerate the therapy, especially if vision is improved. A case of epistaxis has been associated with use of 2% NaCl solution. The patient complained that the drops irritated the nasolacrimal system, but changing to the ointment form overcame the problem.[39]

Hypertonic saline is nontoxic to the cornea and conjunctiva, and allergic reactions are uncommon.[7]

Glycerin (Glycerol)

Glycerin is a clear, colorless, syrupy liquid with a sweet taste. It is miscible with both water and alcohol. When in contact with water, glycerin will absorb water and thereby exert an osmotic effect.[14] When placed on the eye its hydroscopic action will clear the haze of corneal epithelial edema.[14] Topical application of full strength (100%) glycerin to human and rabbit eyes produces no significant tissue damage.[14,15] The osmotic effects of

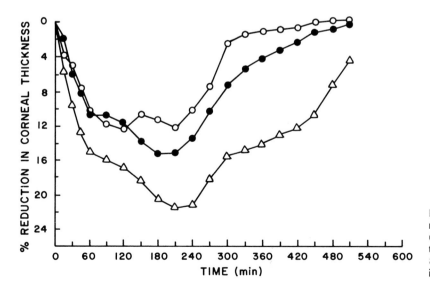

FIGURE 8.1 **Percent reduction in corneal thickness following application of 5% NaCl ointment (Δ, central; ○, nasal; ●, temporal). (Modified from the American Journal of Ophthalmology 71:847–853, 1971. Copyright by The Ophthalmic Publishing Company.)**

topically applied glycerin are transient. Since the molecules mix readily with water, the osmolality of the applied solution decreases rapidly as water is imbibed from the cornea.[15]

CLINICAL USES

Glycerin is useful to permit ophthalmoscopic and gonioscopic examination of the eye in such clinical conditions as acute angle-closure glaucoma, bullous keratopathy, and Fuch's endothelial dystrophy.[13] Significant reduction of edema occurs within 1 to 2 minutes. Since application to the eye is painful, a topical anesthetic must be instilled before use.

Because its action is transient and its application to the eye painful, glycerin is used primarily for diagnostic purposes. It is valuable for permitting gonioscopy and ophthalmoscopy through edematous corneas when used in concentrations of 50% to 100%. In acute angle-closure glaucoma, additional glycerin may be used as the gonioscopic bonding solution to prolong the hyperosmotic effect during gonioscopy.[13]

Glucose

Glucose solutions ranging from 30% to 50% have been used topically on the eye to treat corneal edema. The clinical effectiveness of 40% glucose is comparable to that of 5% sodium chloride.[10]

CLINICAL USES

The dehydrating action of a 30-minute glucose bath eliminates corneal epithelial edema and reduces corneal thickness. The effect lasts 3 to 4 hours. The bath can be repeated 2 to 3 times per day.[16]

Glucose frequently causes transient irritation of the conjunctiva. It is also difficult to maintain sterility of the solution unless a preservative is added. A commercial preparation containing 40% glucose, preserved with methylparaben and propylparaben, is available as an ophthalmic ointment (see Table 8.2).

Systemic Osmotherapy

Hyperosmotic agents administered by the oral and intravenous routes are particularly useful in the initial management of acute angle-closure glaucoma and before intraocular surgery to reduce intraocular pressure.[17]

Following systemic administration, a relatively rapid increase in serum osmolality occurs. The osmotic gradient induced between the ocular fluids (aqueous and vitreous) and the plasma causes fluid to move from the eye into the hyperosmotic plasma, manifested by a decrease in intraocular pressure. The decrease of pressure depends on the degree to which it is elevated and the osmotic gradient induced. When the intraocular pressure is elevated, volume changes induced in the eye by loss of water to the hyperosmotic plasma result in a greater effect than when the pressure is at normal levels. Since their mechanism of action is thought to be primarily an osmotic phenomenon, the difference in osmotic pressure between the ocular fluids and the blood will determine the degree of reduction of intraocular pressure.[17,18] Most hyperosmotic agents effectively lower intraocular pressure when the serum osmolality is increased by 20 to 30 mOsmol/liter.[17] Factors determining the osmotic gradient are listed in Table 8.3. Rates of ocular penetration and method of administration play a major role. Agents that enter the eye rapidly produce less of an osmotic gradient than those that penetrate slowly or not at all. In addition, the state of the ocular tissue influences penetration. Inflammation may enhance intraocular penetration of the hyperosmotic agents and decrease the osmotic gradient, thereby reducing the pressure-lowering effect[19] (Fig. 8.2).

Systemic Hyperosmotic Agents

Among the agents of current interest are urea, mannitol, glycerin, isosorbide, sodium ascorbate, and ethyl alcohol (Table 8.4). The two most commonly used agents are glycerin, which is widely used in office practice, and mannitol, which is usually reserved for pre-surgical use.

These agents can have serious and potentially fatal side effects. The type of agent used, dose, and route of administration should be individualized as much as possible to the patient's needs. For these reasons intelligent clinical use requires an understanding of the

TABLE 8.3
Factors Determining the Osmotic Gradient Induced between Plasma and Ocular Fluids

Molecular weight and concentration
Dose administered
Rate of absorption
Distribution in body water
Ocular penetration
Rate of excretion
Nature of diuresis

Adapted from Becker B, Kolker AE, Krupin T. Hyperosmotic agents. In: Leopold IH, ed. Symposium on ocular therapy. St. Louis: C.V. Mosby Co, 1968.

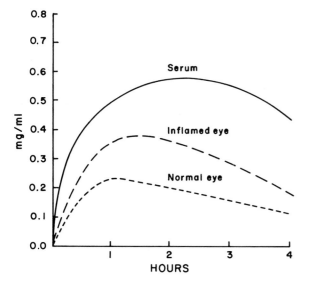

FIGURE 8.2 **Glycerol concentration in serum and aqueous of normal and inflamed rabbit eyes after administration of oral glycerol. (Published with permission from the American Journal of Ophthalmology 62:629–634, 1966. Copyright by The Ophthalmic Publishing Company.)**

factors involved in their action on ocular as well as on other body fluids.[18]

UREA

Urea was introduced for ocular osmotherapy in the late 1950s by Javid.[20] It is easily soluble in water and exerts a relatively strong osmotic effect.[21] Following its administration, urea is distributed in all body fluids including the eye. Osmotic alterations occur in both aqueous humor and the vitreous body, which can cause the anterior chamber to deepen by as much as 0.2 mm.[22] The ability of urea to penetrate cells can result in a rebound effect on intraocular pressure if the serum

level falls below that of the vitreous.[23] Urea is not metabolized, and it is excreted unchanged in the urine.[17,21]

Clinical Uses. At present, urea is rarely used in clinical practice. Solutions for intravenous infusion must be freshly prepared, since urea decomposes to ammonia on standing. Urea is administered as a 30% solution in 10% invert sugar to prevent hemolysis of red blood cells.[24] Intravenous infusion of 2 to 7 ml/kg body weight reduces intraocular pressure within 30 to 45 minutes, with a return to pretreatment levels in 5 to 6 hours.[23] During infusion the site of administration should be frequently observed, since urea can cause tissue sloughing and phlebitis if the needle becomes dislodged.[21,23]

The administration of urea causes frequent systemic complications.[23] All patients experience a rapid diuresis. Severe headache and arm pain are common. About one-third of patients experience nausea, and some patients will experience confusion and disorientation.

MANNITOL

A larger molecule than urea, mannitol is one of the most effective agents for reducing intraocular pressure. Its distribution is confined to the extracellular fluid compartment.[17] Unlike urea, mannitol is stable in solution and can be stored without deterioration. However, the solution should be warmed before use to dissolve crystals that may form during storage. Mannitol is also less irritating than urea and does not cause tissue necrosis if the infusion extravasates.[17,21]

Since mannitol penetrates little into all cells, including those of the eye, it generally reduces intraocular pressure significantly. In addition, since it is confined to the extracellular water, it may produce a greater cellular dehydration and diuresis than does urea.[17,21] It

TABLE 8.4
Systemic Hyperosmotic Agents

Drug	Dosage (g/kg body weight)	Route of Administration	Onset of Effect (min)
Urea (30% IV, 50% oral)	0.5–2	IV, Oral	30–45 (IV) 120 (Oral)
Mannitol 20%	1.5–2.5	IV	30–60
Glycerol 50%	1–1.5	Oral	15–30
Isosorbide 45%	1.5–2	Oral	30–60
Ascorbate 20%	0.5–1	IV, Oral	40–90
Alcohol 40–50%	0.8–1.5	Oral	60–120

Adapted from Becker B, Kolker A, Krupin T. Hyperosmotic agents. In: Leopold IH, ed. Symposium on ocular therapy. St Louis: C.V. Mosby Co, 1968.

is not metabolized and is excreted in the urine.[17] Thus, it may be safely used in diabetic patients.

Clinical Uses.   Mannitol is the hyperosmotic agent of choice for intravenous administration. It is available as a 20% solution in water. Intravenous administration in doses of 2.5 to 10 ml/kg body weight reduces intraocular pressure within 20 to 30 minutes. The effect can last for 4 to 10 hours.[17,21] Since mannitol is not absorbed from the gastrointestinal tract, oral administration does not reduce intraocular pressure.

Mannitol is generally less toxic than urea. It is less irritating to tissues should the intravenous infusion extravasate.[17,21] However, diuresis, headache, chills, and chest pain may occur during infusion.[17] Mannitol should be administered with caution in patients with renal disease.[17] A case of acute oliguric renal failure has been attributed to mannitol administration for acute angle-closure glaucoma.[40]

GLYCERIN (GLYCEROL)

Since 1963 when Virno and associates[25] reported the intraocular pressure effects of oral glycerin in patients with various types of glaucoma, glycerin has become the most commonly used hyperosmotic agent for the initial management of acute angle-closure glaucoma.

Chemically glycerin is a trivalent alcohol. It is metabolized by the body in a manner analogous to other carbohydrates and produces 4.32 Kcal/g.[25] When glycerin is administered in recommended dosages, the resulting calories do not usually cause any significant problems. However, since hyperglycemia and glycosuria can result following glycerin administration, its caloric value must be considered when repeated administration is necessary. Caution should therefore be exercised when glycerin is administered to patients with diabetes—the drug-induced hyperglycemia may require treatment.[17,21]

Following oral administration, glycerin is confined to the extracellular fluid and penetrates the eye poorly.[17] However, aqueous levels of glycerin are higher in the inflamed eye due to the breakdown of the blood-aqueous barrier, which allows for greater intraocular penetration of the osmotic agent[26] (see Fig. 8.2).

Clinical Uses.   The use of glycerin provides a clinical advantage in that oral administration results in rapid systemic absorption. Although the reduction in intraocular pressure is somewhat slower than with intravenous agents, doses of 1.5 to 3.0 ml/kg body weight of a 50% solution reduce pressure within 30 to 60 minutes. The effect can last for several hours.[26] Figure 8.3 compares the effects of oral glycerin with intravenous urea and mannitol.

Although oral administration simplifies its use, glycerin has several characteristics that may limit its clinical use in acute angle-closure glaucoma and before and after surgery. Glycerin cannot be administered to patients who are nauseated or vomiting.[17] Extreme caution must be exercised with diabetic patients, since in addition to hyperglycemia, ketoacidosis may be induced. Since glycerin has a sweet taste, it may induce nausea and vomiting on administration. The resultant increase in serum osmolality following administration can cause dehydration, confusion, and disorientation.[13]

Glycerin is commercially available as a 50% solution (Osmoglyn). The formulation is lime flavored and preserved with potassium sorbate 0.05%.[13] For clinical administration, the glycerin solution should be administered chilled or over ice to reduce potential nausea or vomiting.

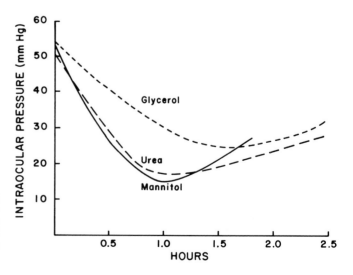

FIGURE 8.3   **A comparison of the intraocular pressure–lowering effects of intravenous urea (1 g/kg body weight), intravenous mannitol (3 g/kg), and orally administered glycerol (1.5 ml/kg) in humans. (Published with permission from the American Journal of Ophthalmology 62:629–634, 1966. Copyright by The Ophthalmic Publishing Company.)**

ISOSORBIDE

Although it resembles mannitol chemically, isosorbide is readily absorbed from the gastrointestinal tract and therefore can be given orally.

In contrast to glycerin, isosorbide is not metabolized. About 95% of an administered dose is excreted unchanged in the urine.[17] It therefore provides no calories and can be administered to diabetic patients without altering the insulin requirement.[27] However, isosorbide does penetrate cells, and it enters the aqueous humor.

Clinical Uses.   Administration of isosorbide reduces intraocular pressure within 30 to 60 minutes. The effects last for as long as 5 to 6 hours[13,27] (Fig. 8.4).

Compared with glycerin, the incidence of nausea and vomiting on administration may be lower.[28] Headache, confusion, and disorientation may occur.[27,28] Rare occurrences of gastric discomfort, dizziness, thirst, and lethargy have been reported.[13]

Isosorbide is available as a 45% solution in a vanilla-mint flavored vehicle (Ismotic). Clinical indications for use are the same as for glycerin.[13]

SODIUM ASCORBATE

An infrequently used hyperosmotic agent, ascorbate is physiologically present in relatively high concentrations in ocular tissue. The original reports indicated that it was effective in lowering intraocular pressure following oral or intravenous administration.[29–31] A 20% intravenous solution at pH 7.2 to 7.4 in dosages of 0.5 to 1.0 g/kg body weight lowered intraocular pressure within 40 to 90 minutes. The effect lasted 2 to 4 hours.[29]

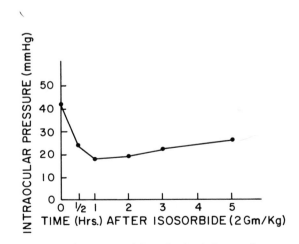

FIGURE 8.4   Time course of the reduction in intraocular pressure in a patient with secondary glaucoma following oral administration of isosorbide 2 g/kg. (From Becker B, Kolker AE, Krupin T. Isosorbide: an oral hyperosmotic agent. Arch Ophthalmol 1967; 78:150. Copyright 1967, American Medical Association.)

Oral administration of a 20% solution flavored with orange juice was effective in reducing pressure in various types of glaucoma. In the mid 1960s, Virno and associates[30] reported that dosages of 0.5 g/kg, divided into 3 to 4 daily administrations, lowered intraocular pressure in patients with open-angle glaucoma. More recent evidence, however, has failed to demonstrate a clinically significant effect on intraocular pressure.[41,42] Oral administration of 3 g 3 times daily for 4 weeks produced no significant difference between intraocular pressure response to the ascorbic acid and placebo.[42]

When given exogenously, ascorbate is distributed in total body water and is transported into the eye. It is both metabolized by the body and excreted in the urine. There appears to be somewhat less diuresis with ascorbate than with other hyperosmotic agents.[17] Solutions of ascorbate are unstable and must be prepared just before administration.

Side effects are not uncommon. Gastric disorders together with diarrhea, especially early in treatment, are frequent.[30] Adverse effects occur less frequently with the intravenous route and can be kept to a minimum with oral use if doses are divided into 3 to 4 daily administrations. Ascorbic acid can also interfere with many laboratory tests, including fecal and urinary occult blood tests.[43]

ETHYL ALCOHOL (ETHANOL)

The oral administration of ethyl alcohol can reduce intraocular pressure in both normal and glaucomatous eyes.[32,33] The usual dosage is 2 to 3 ml/kg body weight of a 40% to 50% solution of ethyl alcohol in fruit juice or a straight 80 to 100 proof whiskey.[17] The hypotensive effect is slower in onset than with other hyperosmotic agents. The maximum effect occurs in 1 to 2 hours.[33]

Ethyl alcohol is distributed in total body water and penetrates the eye very rapidly. However, penetration of the vitreous is somewhat slower than penetration of the aqueous. This lag results in a sufficient osmotic gradient between plasma and vitreous to draw fluid out of the eye.[33] However, this may not entirely explain the mechanism of drug action in lowering intraocular pressure. Ethyl alcohol also inhibits the secretion of antidiuretic hormone (ADH).[34] A hypotonic diuresis is produced following its administration, and it has been suggested that this contributes to the increase of serum osmolality induced by ethyl alcohol.[32,33] Ethyl alcohol is metabolized, and the excess caloric production is similar to that found with glycerol.[17]

Although ethyl alcohol is easy to administer and is stable in solution, it has several disadvantages compared with other oral hyperosmotic agents. In addition to the slower onset of action, it produces a more profound diuresis and causes both early and delayed central nervous system (CNS) effects. Intoxication, headache, nausea, and vomiting are not uncommon. Because of its frequent side effects, ethyl alcohol is seldom used for osmotherapy.[17]

Side Effects

With few exceptions, use of systemic hyperosmotic agents results in side effects and complications, as summarized in Table 8.5. All these agents can produce headache, nausea, and vomiting. Excessive thirst is common following intravenous infusion of hyperosmotic agents. Patients will experience varying degrees of diuresis depending on the agent used. Since potassium deficiency can accompany the diuresis, patients with cardiac, hepatic, or renal disorders should be carefully monitored and given supplements as necessary.[17]

In addition to these generalized effects common to all the systemic hyperosmotic agents, each of the agents can exhibit a variety of other side effects that can vary in severity and type of symptoms observed. Intravenous infusion of urea can cause severe arm pain, phlebitis, confusion, and disorientation. Fever, although a rare complication, may last for several hours. Death from subdural hematoma has been reported as a complication of urea-induced dehydration.[23]

Mannitol, in general, has fewer side effects than urea. It causes less local tissue irritation, thrombophlebitis, and necrosis than does urea.[17] Since it is not metabolized to any significant degree, metabolic problems in diabetic patients are not often encountered.[17] However, chills during mannitol infusion, angina-like chest pains, and precipitation of pulmonary edema and congestive heart failure in elderly patients have been reported.[35] An acute allergic reaction to mannitol infusion in a patient allergic to penicillin, procaine, and various agents in ophthalmic drops was reported by

Spaeth and associates.[36] A skin test for mannitol hypersensitivity was positive.

Use of oral glycerin generally causes few problems. Headache and nausea are the major side effects.[37] Gastrointestinal upset may occur, but diuresis is less common.[38] Glycerin should be used cautiously in diabetic patients, since hyperglycemia and glycosuria can occur as well as more serious effects such as diabetic acidosis.[38] Confusion and disorientation may result from drug-induced dehydration in elderly patients. Glycerin should be used cautiously in patients with congestive heart disease.

Isosorbide produces the same general side effects as do all other hyperosmotic agents. Such side effects include headache, dehydration, diuresis, and disorientation in the elderly. According to some authors, isosorbide seems to cause less nausea than does glycerin. Cardiac and renal disease may contraindicate its use.[27,28]

Hyperosmotic agents are clinically useful in ocular therapeutics for both topical and, in particular, systemic osmotherapy. Although the topical agents are safe and usually effective when used in recommended dosages, the systemic hyperosmotic agents, because of their tendency to cause adverse effects, should be used in the smallest possible doses consistent with their clinical efficacy and under close supervision.

References

1. Cantonnet A. Essai de traitement du glaucome par les substances osmotiques. Arch D'Ophtalmol 1904;24:1–25.
2. Waltman SR. The cornea. In: Moses RA, ed. Adler's physiology of the eye. 7th ed. St Louis: C. V. Mosby Co, 1981;Chap 3:38–62.
3. Maurice DM. The structure and transparency of the cornea. J Physiol 1957;136:263–286.
4. Mishima S, Hedbys BO. Physiology of the cornea. Int Ophthalmol Clin 1968;8:527–560.
5. Brown SI, Hedbys BO. The effect of ouabain on the hydration of the cornea. Invest Ophthalmol 1965;4:216–221.
6. Cogan DG, Kinsey VE. The cornea. V. Physiologic aspects. Arch Ophthalmol 1942;28:661–669
7. Levenson JE. Corneal edema: Cause and treatment. Surv Ophthalmol 1975;20:190–204.
8. Boruchoff SA. Clinical causes of corneal edema. Int Ophthalmol Clin 1968;8:581–600.
9. Lamberts DW. Topical hyperosmotic agents and secretory stimulants. Int Ophthalmol Clin 1980;20:163–169.
10. Payrau P, Dohlman CH. Medical treatment of corneal edema. Int Ophthalmol Clin 1968;8:601–610.
11. Luxenberg MN, Green K. Reduction of corneal edema with topical hypertonic agents. Am J Ophthalmol 1971;71:847–853.
12. Marisi A, Aquavella JV. Hypertonic saline solution in corneal edema. Ann Ophthalmol 1975;7:229–233.

TABLE 8.5
Side Effects of Systemic Osmotherapy

Headache
Pain in upper extremities
Nausea and vomiting
Diuresis
Dehydration
K^+ deficiency
Vertigo
Fever
Confusion and disorientation
Congestive heart failure
Subdural hematoma

13. Physicians Desk Reference for Ophthalmology. Oradell, NJ: Medical Economics Co, 1989.

14. Cogan DG. Clearing of edematous corneas by glycerine. Am J Ophthalmol 1943;26:551.

15. Hine CH, Anderson HH, Moon HD, et al. Comparative toxicity of synthetic and natural glycerin. Arch Ind Hyg 1953;7:282–291.

16. Bietti GB, Pecori J. Topical osmotherapy of corneal edema. Ann Ophthalmol 1969;1:40–49.

17. Becker B, Kolker AE, Krupin T. Hyperosmotic agents. In: Leopold IH, ed. Symposium on ocular therapy. St Louis: C. V. Mosby Co, 1968;3:42–53.

18. Kolker AE. Hyperosmotic agents in glaucoma. Invest Ophthalmol 1970;9:418–423.

19. Galin MA, Davidson R. Hypotensive effect of urea in inflamed and noninflamed eye. Arch Ophthalmol 1962;68:633–635.

20. Javid M. Urea—new use of an old agent; reduction of intracranial and intraocular pressure. Surg Clin North Am 1958; 38:907–928.

21. Becker B. Use of hyperosmotic agents in the treatment of the glaucomas. Trans New Orleans Acad Ophthalmol 1967; 170–174.

22. Duncan LS, Hostetter T, Ellis PP. Vitreous osmolality changes following administration of hyperosmotic agents (abstr.). Invest Ophthalmol 1969;8:353.

23. Tarter RC, Linn JG. A clinical study of the use of intravenous urea in glaucoma. Am J Ophthalmol 1961;52:323–331.

24. Galin MA, Aizawa F, McLean JM. A comparison of intraocular pressure reduction following urea and sucrose administration. Arch Ophthalmol 1960;63:281–286.

25. Virno M, Cantore P, Bietti C, Bucci MG. Oral glycerol in ophthalmology: A valuable new method for the reduction of intraocular pressure. Am J Ophthalmol 1963;55:1133–1142.

26. Galin MA, Davidson R, Shachter N. Ophthalmological use of osmotic therapy. Am J Ophthalmol 1966;62:629–634.

27. Becker B, Kolker AE, Krupin T. Isosorbide: An oral hyperosmotic agent. Arch Ophthalmol 1967;78:147–150.

28. Wisznia KI, Lazar M, Leopold IH. Oral isosorbide and intraocular pressure. Am J Ophthalmol 1970;70:630–634.

29. Virno M, Bucci MG, Pecori-Giraldi J, Canatore G. Intravenous glycerol—vitamin C (sodium salt) as osmotic agents to reduce intraocular pressure. Am J Ophthalmol 1966;62:824–833.

30. Virno M, Bucci MG, Pecori-Giraldi J, et al. Oral treatment of glaucoma with vitamin C. Eye Ear Nose Throat Monthly 1967;46:1502–1508.

31. Bietti GB. Further contributions of the value of osmotic substances as means to reduce intra-ocular pressure. Trans Ophthalmol Soc Aust 1967;26:61–71.

32. Peczon JD, Grant WM. Glaucoma, alcohol, and intraocular pressure. Arch Ophthalmol 1965;73:495–501.

33. Krupin T, Kolker AE, Becker B. Alcohol and intraocular pressure. Invest Ophthalmol 1967;6:559–560.

34. Houle RE, Grant WM. Alcohol, vasopressin and intraocular pressure. Invest Ophthalmol 1967;6:145–154.

35. Smith EW, Drance SM. Reduction of human intraocular pressure with intravenous mannitol. Arch Ophthalmol 1962;68:734–737.

36. Spaeth Gl, Spaeth EB, Spaeth PG, Lucier AC. Anaphylactic reaction to mannitol. Arch Ophthalmol 1967;78:583–584.

37. McCurdy DK, Schneider B, Scheie H. Oral glycerol: The mechanism of intraocular hypotension. Am J Ophthalmol 1966;61:1244–1249.

38. D'Alena P, Ferguson W. Adverse effects after glycerol orally and mannitol parenterally. Arch Ophthalmol 1966;75:201–203.

39. Kushner FH. Sodium chloride eye drops as a cause of epistaxis. Arch Ophthalmol 1987;105:1634.

40. Weaver A, Sica A. Mannitol-induced acute renal failure. Nephron 1987;45:233–235.

41. Fishbein SL, Goodstein S. The pressure lowering effect of ascorbic acid. Ann Ophthalmol 1972;4:487–491.

42. Feldman RM, Steinmann WC, Spaeth GL, et al. Oral ascorbic acid therapy in glaucoma. Glaucoma 1987;9:181–183.

43. Jaffe RM, Lawrence L, Young DS, et al. False negative stool occult blood tests caused by ingestion of ascorbic acid. Ann Intern Med 1975;83:824–826.

CHAPTER 9

Irrigating Solutions

David R. Whikehart

Originally, the term *irrigating solution* in clinical practice referred to any aqueous solution that could be used to cleanse a tissue while maintaining its moisture. Although extraocular irrigating solutions achieve this purpose, intraocular irrigating solutions must also be able to supply nutrients to the anterior segment, particularly the sensitive corneal endothelium. Accordingly, extraocular solutions may be referred to as true irrigators, while intraocular solutions take on the role of perfusion media. An understanding of these two kinds of irrigating solutions and their respective functions depends on knowledge of the physiologic chemistry of the cornea, lens, uvea, and retina.

Desirable Properties of Irrigating Solutions

Nearly any aqueous medium can, in theory, be used to wash debris from the eye. However, the physiologic limitations of ocular tissues must be considered in the design of an appropriate solution. Consequently, the osmolality, pH, and sterility of such solutions are important. Moreover, irrigating solutions must have a sufficiently low concentration of any chemicals that might be toxic to the eye.[1] Nutrient components must be supplied to dependent tissues when irrigation takes place over an extended period, as occurs with intraocular surgery.[2,3]

Metabolic Demands of Anterior Segment Ocular Tissues

CORNEA

The cornea consists of 3 cellular and 2 noncellular layers. The most anterior cellular layer, the epithelium, is composed of epithelial cells that are normally 5 to 6 deep across the entire cornea. These cells act as a barrier to the external environment for the cornea and are nourished by glucose primarily from the aqueous humor and secondarily from the limbal vessels.[4] In contrast, the oxygen supply for cells of the epithelium originates from atmospheric air dissolved in the precorneal tear film. Although epithelial cells are superficially located in the cornea, it appears peculiar that they do not also receive glucose from the precorneal tear film. Evidence against this, however, stems from the paucity of glucose in the tear film compared with that in the aqueous. Glucose is generally present in a ratio of about 1:12 to 1:15 of tear film to aqueous in humans.[4,5] Glucose flux across the cornea from the endothelium toward the epithelium, as studied in rabbits, is reduced to less than 10% when the posterior corneal surface is blocked with silicone.[6] Glucose metabolism in epithelial cells normally does not depend on high amounts of oxygen due to the predominantly anaerobic use of glucose in these cells,[4,7,8] as shown in Table 9.1. These cells are also known to store glucose in the form of glycogen. The corneal epithelium, therefore, can survive quite well with extraocular irrigating solutions that do not contain glucose. During ocular surgery the epithelium can also rely on its store of glycogen and on communication with those limbal vessels with which contact remains intact.

The metabolism of stromal keratocytes, the second cellular layer of the cornea, has been difficult to study. This is due, in part, to the great bulk of collagen and proteoglycans present in the stroma, which interfere with a direct comparison of other corneal tissues on the basis of wet weight and protein. Keratocytes occupy only about 10% of the volume of the stroma.[9] Waltman[10] has stated that if correction factors are ap-

TABLE 9.1
Glucose Metabolism in Corneal Epithelial Cells[4,7,8]

Pathway	%
Aerobic glycolysis	8
Anaerobic glycolysis	57
Pentose shunt	35

plied to allow for the small percentage of keratocytes in stroma, then the metabolic rate of the stroma would be comparable to that of the epithelium. Present evidence indicates that these cells participate in both aerobic and anaerobic glycolysis; however, a key enzyme involved in pentose shunt metabolism is missing.[7] Since glucose destined for the epithelium passes through the stroma, the amount is sufficient for the needs of the stromal cells. Oxygen partial pressure varies from 40 to about 120 mm Hg depending on relative anterior-posterior location.[11] This is adequate for the small percentage of cells present in this layer. Keratocytes would likewise not depend on a glucose-containing extraocular fluid (irrigating fluid). Despite the above, their dependence on a glucose-containing intraocular irrigating fluid during surgery has yet to be established.

The most posterior cellular layer of the cornea, the endothelium, has a comparatively higher percentage of aerobic glycolysis than does the epithelium. Although not specifically measured, this is suggested from the pentose shunt studies of Geroski and associates.[12] These investigators concluded that 63% of all glucose metabolism occurs by glycolysis in the endothelium compared with 34% in the epithelium. In both cases the remaining CO_2 is formed through the pentose shunt. Riley,[13] by comparison, suggests that 93% of all glucose is processed through the Embden-Meyerhof pathway, of which 23% is aerobic. Endothelial cells can also be inferred to have a high rate of aerobic glycolysis by their numerous mitochondria, more than those of any other cell type except retinal photoreceptors.[14] The endothelium receives both glucose and oxygen directly from the aqueous, which bathes the apical cellular membranes. Gaasterland and associates[15] have reported an average value of 53 mg/dL (2.94 mM) of glucose in the aqueous of fasting Rhesus monkeys. The partial pressure of oxygen in the aqueous is approximately 50 mm Hg.[11] The endothelial layer causes a drop of about 10 mm Hg as oxygen diffuses past into the stroma.

Endothelial cells are especially vulnerable to interruptions in their source of nourishment. This is unfortunate, since this cellular layer is dominant in controlling the relative hydration and clarity of the cornea.[16,17] Accordingly, these cells may be affected by the nature of the intraocular irrigating solution used in the course of anterior segment surgery.[18]

CONJUNCTIVA

The conjunctiva generally contains several layers of epithelial cells whose number of mitochondria exceeds that of the corneal epithelial cells.[4] Goblet cells, which secrete tear film mucus, are also present. Conjunctival cells as well as goblet cells receive their supply of glucose and oxygen directly from numerous supporting conjunctival vessels.[19] Consequently, their metabolic needs do not depend on any irrigating solution.

LENS

The lens as a whole has a low metabolic rate.[20] Fiber cells, which make up the bulk of the lens, are largely devoid of both nuclei and mitochondria. Glucose is processed in these cells anaerobically. Epithelial cells and the very superficial fiber cells of the lens are, by contrast, quite active metabolically. However, these are found only on the surface of the lens. Although the lens can survive quite well anaerobically,[21] the deprivation of glucose may ultimately lead to the formation of cataracts. The time course of this process in humans as well as the detailed mechanism remain unknown. However, Chylack and Schaefer[22] have shown that in rat lens an irreversible shift of lens hexokinase from the soluble to the insoluble form takes place after 8 hours. This drastically reduces the ability of the metabolically active surface cells to phosphorylate glucose and essentially shuts down glucose metabolism. The lens, like the corneal endothelium, receives both glucose and oxygen solely from the aqueous. However, an intraocular deprivation of glucose is not a matter of concern in surgery, and, apparently, the presence of glucose in an irrigating solution is of no import for the lens. In the diabetic state, however, the osmotic stress due to changes in glucose metabolism is important. This will be considered later.

UVEA

All tissues of the uvea—iris, ciliary body, and choroid—are nourished directly from ocular blood vessels. Consequently, their metabolism does not depend on an intraocular irrigating solution.

RETINA

All tissues of the retina are also nourished from ocular blood vessels. However, some evidence[23,24] suggests that perfused glucose is important for maintaining amplitude of the electroretinogram (ERG) when the vitreous is surgically removed.

Physiologic Constraints of the Anterior Segment

Both extraocular and intraocular irrigating solutions must be formulated to fall within the physiologic limitations of the cells with which they come in contact. A hypertonic solution will cause cell shrinkage due to water loss, while a hypotonic solution causes swelling and even destruction of cells. Normally at 37°C extracellular and intracellular fluids exert equivalent forces of 5.79×10^3 mm Hg at a chemical activity of 300 mOsm.[25] Despite this, Edelhauser and associates[26] have been able to show that the vulnerable corneal endothelium can withstand a perfusion medium with a range from 200 to 400 mOsm of chemical activity. Figures 9.1 to 9.4 demonstrate effects on the endothelium over a range of 200 to 500 mOsm. A 100 mOsm range above or below 300 mOsm implies a negative or positive pressure on these cells as high as 193 mm Hg. However, tolerance to these pressures exists only in the presence of ions known to strengthen cellular adhesion, particularly calcium. Solutions and drugs have been formulated, especially for use within the eye, with an osmolality between 78 and 440 mOsm. Consequently, the practitioner or surgeon should be cautioned about using agents that introduce cellular stress to ocular regions. Corneal edema has been reported, for exam-

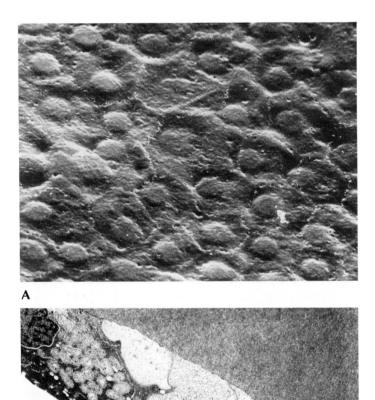

FIGURE 9.1   *(A)* **Scanning electron microscopy of human corneal endothelium following 2-hour perfusion with 200 mOsm salt solution. Nuclear bulges are prominent, and endothelial cells are swollen at junctions (×1,000).** *(B)* **Transmission electron microscopy of same cornea. There is dilation of intracellular spaces and vacuolization and swelling of cytoplasm (×9,500). (From Edelhauser HF, Hanneken AM, Pederson HJ, VanHorn DL. Osmotic tolerance of rabbit and human corneal endothelium. Arch Ophthalmol 1981;99:1281–1287. Copyright 1981, American Medical Association.)**

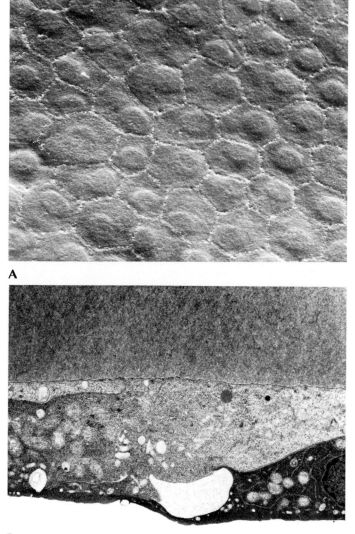

FIGURE 9.2 *(A)* Scanning electron microscopy of human corneal endothelium perfused with balanced salt solution (BSS Plus) (300 mOsm) for 3 hours. Normal mosaic-like pattern of endothelial cells is present (×1,000). *(B)* Transmission electron microscopy of same cornea showing intact junctions, normal cell organelles, and some intracellular and extracellular vacuoles (×10,300). (From Edelhauser HF, Hanneken AM, Pederson HJ, VanHorn DL. Osmotic tolerance of rabbit and human corneal endothelium. Arch Ophthalmol 1981;99:1281–1287. Copyright 1981, American Medical Association.)

ple, when acetylcholine (ACh) was used for miosis after delivery of the lens in cataract surgery. The osmolality of ACh when reconstituted with sterile saline is in the high range of 388 to 440 mOsm.[27] Virtually all commercial ophthalmic irrigating solutions, both intraocular and extraocular, are isotonic; that is, they are formulated with an osmolality of 300 mOsm. A recent report by Briggs and McCartney,[62] however, found an exception. Although the composition of salts used is not critical at a chemical activity of 300 mOsm for extraocular irrigating solutions, it is important with solutions used for intraocular surgery that specific salts be added not only to maintain cells but also to maximize cell adhesion, cell-to-cell junctions, and cellular transport during surgery. The salts included should

contain ions of sodium, potassium, calcium, magnesium, chloride, and bicarbonate.[3,18,28] Topical hypertonic or hyperosmolar preparations are available to reduce corneal edema, but such preparations should not be considered as physiologic irrigants,[29] and their use should be regarded with the above-mentioned precautions.

Another important physiologic limitation is the hydrogen ion concentration, commonly expressed as pH. Normal serum or plasma extracellular pH is 7.4, with a tolerable range of 7.35 to 7.45.[30] The precorneal tear film has a pH of 7.4 with a range of 7.3 to 7.7,[31] while the aqueous (in Rhesus monkeys) has been reported at 7.49.[15] Gonnering and associates[32] have shown that both structural and functional alterations occur to the

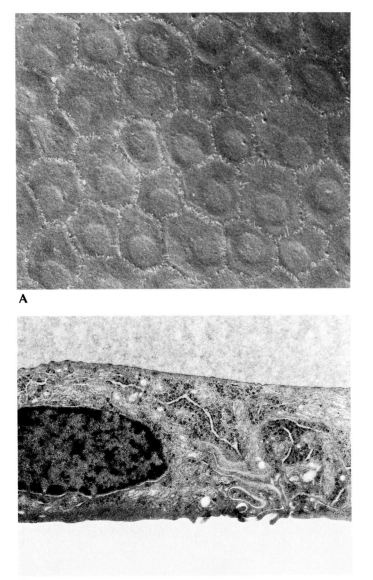

A

B

FIGURE 9.3   *(A)* Scanning electron microscopy of human corneal endothelium after 2-hour perfusion of 400 mOsm salt solution. Cells are intact, and tight junctions are present ($\times$1,000). *(B)* Transmission electron microscopy of same cornea. Intercellular junctions are intact, cytoplasm is condensed, and cell organelles are normal ($\times$14,350). (From Edelhauser HF, Hanneken AM, Pederson HJ, VanHorn DL. Osmotic tolerance of rabbit and human corneal endothelium. Arch Ophthalmol 1981;99:1281–1287. Copyright 1981, American Medical Association.)

human corneal endothelium outside of the pH range 6.5 to 8.5. These alterations consist of swelling, pits at cellular junctions, as well as loss of plasma membrane and recognizable subcellular components (i.e., cell death), as shown in Figures 9.5 to 9.8. A normal corneal endothelium is shown in Figure 9.7 after perfusion at pH 7.2. As mentioned previously regarding osmotic pressure anomalies, drugs and vehicles that are made up without regard to pH buffering capacity, or that are buffered outside the physiologic range, can also destroy ocular tissue. This statement is qualified, however, by the consideration that some drugs must be formulated outside the normal pH range (e.g., pilo-

carpine HCl) to remain stable before topical administration. The amount of vehicle contact time in topical administration is so small that it involves only momentary discomfort (e.g., stinging) to the patient. When an irrigating solution for intraocular surgery is used, especially for prolonged periods, the potential for cellular destruction exists if the solution is either unbuffered or buffered in preference to a particular medication. Although the pH values of commercially available extraocular irrigating solutions are not stated,[27,33] these solutions are generally either neutral or buffered toward neutrality and constitute virtually no pH risk for the outer ocular surface. Intraocular

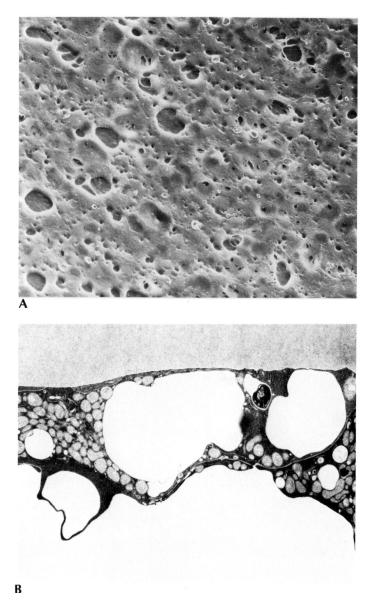

FIGURE 9.4 *(A)* Scanning electron microscopy of human corneal endothelium after 2-hour perfusion of 500 mOsm salt solution. Mosaic-like pattern has disappeared, and cells are pulling apart (×1,000). *(B)* Transmission electron microscopy of same cornea. Posterior surface is wavy, and large intercellular vacuoles are present. Junctions between cells are connected by thin bridges of cytoplasm, and cytoplasm is condensed (×8,100). (From Edelhauser HF, Hanneken AM, Pederson HJ, VanHorn DL. Osmotic tolerance of rabbit and human corneal endothelium. Arch Ophthalmol 1981;99:1281–1287. Copyright 1981, American Medical Association.)

irrigating solutions are designated as being either pH adjusted or at approximately pH 7.4. Briggs and McCartney,[62] however, have noted one exception.

The Use of Preservatives

Antimicrobial agents are used in irrigating solutions to prevent microbial growth and to preserve the composition of the solutions from microbial attack. As such they are often designated as preservatives[34] or disinfectants.[35] Their use is limited to extraocular irrigants due to their toxic effects on intraocular tissues. Coles[36] has shown that 12 different commonly used therapeutic antimicrobial agents (antibiotics) have some deleterious effects on rabbit corneal endothelia. This was manifested as increasing corneal thickness and interference with cell membrane or junctional integrity (Fig. 9.9). Lower limits for toxicity have apparently not been adequately demonstrated. Although Leopold[37] has suggested dosage schedules for therapeutic agents that are injected into the anterior chamber, the risks are great. Havener[38] states that irrigation of the anterior chamber with antibiotics can produce endothelial cell death with concomitant corneal opacity, destructive iritis with neovascularization, and cataract induction.

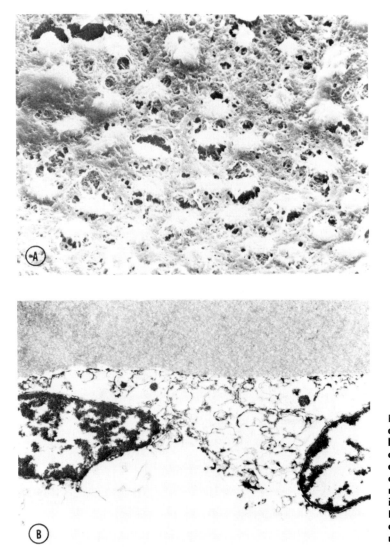

FIGURE 9.5   *(A)* **Scanning electron micrograph of the endothelium of a human cornea perfused at pH 5.50 for 1 hour. The nuclei of most cells are exposed due to the collapse of the outer plasma membrane (×1000).** *(B)* **Transmission electron micrograph of endothelial cells from the same cornea displaying completely necrotic cells. There are no recognizable organelles, and the outer plasma membrane is completely disrupted (×11,200). (From Gonnering R, Edelhauser HF, VanHorn DL, Durant W. The pH tolerance of rabbit and human corneal endothelium. Invest Ophthalmol Vis Sci 1979;18:373–390.)**

The preservatives used in extraocular irrigating solutions should ideally be effective against both gram-negative and gram-positive bacteria without ocular toxicity. Furthermore, they should not compromise the components of the solution. Practically, irrigating solutions are formulated to make the best compromise between antimicrobial action and corneal epithelial deterioration. Table 9.2 gives an overview of the preservatives and their use in extraocular irrigating solutions. In general, the preservatives are used at concentrations that are bacteriostatic rather than bactericidal. Assuredly the prevention of bacterial growth is aided by refrigerating these solutions.

Summary

Irrigating solutions used on the outer surface of the eye do not require metabolic nutrients, while intraocular irrigating (perfusion) solutions should contain nutrients, especially for use during prolonged ocular surgery. Ideally, irrigating solutions should be isotonic, although the eye will tolerate moderate departures from normal tonicity. The desirable pH of all solutions is 7.4. Cellular stress and death occur with prolonged exposure below pH 7 and above pH 8. Antimicrobial agents are used in extraocular solutions as preservatives. Their usual concentrations make them bacterio-

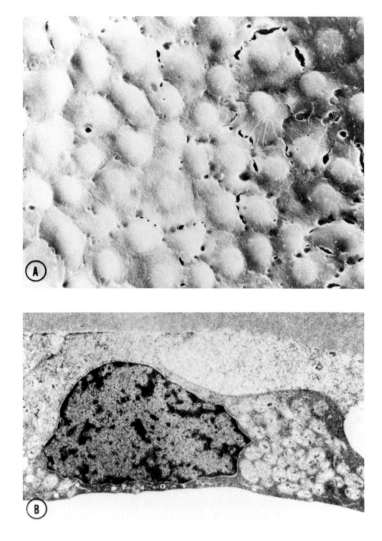

FIGURE 9.6   *(A)* Scanning electron micrograph of the endothelium of a human cornea perfused at pH 6.50 for 3 hours. The cells appear to be swollen, and pits are present at many of the junctions (×1000). *(B)* Transmission electron micrograph of endothelial cells from the same cornea displaying both cytoplasmic and mitochondrial swelling and some clumping of the nuclear chromatin. The junctional complexes have partially broken down, leaving large spaces between many cells (×8600). (From Gonnering R, Edelhauser HF, VanHorn DL, Durant W. The pH tolerance of rabbit and human corneal endothelium. Invest Ophthalmol Vis Sci 1979;18:373–390.)

static. No antimicrobial agents should be used in intraocular solutions due to their toxic effects, particularly to the corneal endothelium.

Extraocular Irrigating Solutions

The previous section has demonstrated that extraocular irrigating solutions must be physiologically balanced with respect to pH and osmolality but do not require nutrients or specific ions. Their short-term use and the fact that cells with which they come in contact obtain nutrients elsewhere render them quite safe as formulated. Their role is primarily that of clearing away unwanted materials from the outer ocular surface.

Components

A general and detailed discussion of the components of both kinds of irrigating solutions appears in the previous section. Table 9.3 lists the components of three typical extraocular irrigating solutions.

Clinical Uses

These solutions are used primarily for washing away debris and liquids that are foreign to the extraocular surface. The solutions are available over the counter, without prescription, and so may be used by patients and practitioners alike. In the practitioner's office they are useful following tonometry (removal of fluores-

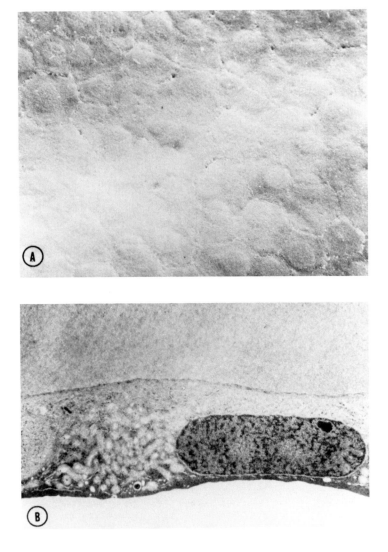

FIGURE 9.7 *(A)* **Scanning electron micrograph of the endothelium of a human cornea perfused at pH 7.2 for 3 hours. The normal mosaiclike cellular pattern is preserved (× 1000). *(B)* Transmission electron micrograph of endothelial cells from the same cornea displaying normal ultrastructure except for some clarification of the cytoplasm between the nucleus and Descemet's membrane (× 8600). (From Gonnering R, Edelhauser HF, VanHorn DL, Durant W. The pH tolerance of rabbit and human corneal endothelium. Invest Ophthalmol Vis Sci 1979;18:373–390.)**

cein), gonioscopy (removal of methylcellulose), foreign body removal, and for the removal of routine, diagnostic fluorescein. They serve an important function in diagnostic nasolacrimal duct irrigation in patients with chronic epiphora. These solutions have further use in washing out mucus or purulent discharge. They are also used at the hospital bedside to clean out eyes between dressing changes.[33]

Irrigating solutions should not be used with contact lenses in place. The solutions tend to cause contact lens irritation by reducing natural, lubricating mucin and, in the case of rigid lenses, by reducing the hydrophilicity of the lens surface.[34] The absorption of benzalkonium chloride and phenylmercuric acetate by hydrogel lenses can potentially lead to corneal epithelial damage if sufficient amounts of preservative are

released to the eye. Although irrigating solutions may be used to wash out the eyes after contact lens wear, these solutions have no value as contact lens solutions per se for wetting, cleansing, or cushioning.

First-Aid Irrigating Solutions

There is no doubt that one of the worst ocular disasters is a chemical insult to the outer ocular surface. Penetrating chemicals require that the eyes be given an immediate copious lavage and that the patient be transported to an emergency room or appropriate treatment facility as soon as possible. Although the ideal irrigating solution for the immediate accident is physiologic saline, water is very nearly the only available sub-

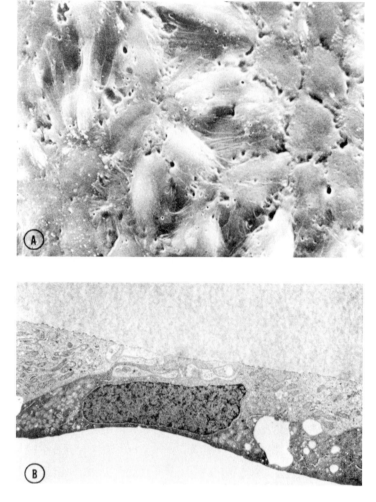

FIGURE 9.8   *(A)* Scanning electron micrograph of the endothelium of a human cornea perfused at pH 8.50 for 3 hours. Some of the cells appear to be swollen, whereas others appear quite normal. Pits are present at many of the cellular junctions (×1000). *(B)* Transmission electron micrograph of the endothelial cells from the same cornea showing normal ultrastructure except for varying degrees of cytoplasmic swelling. The junctional complexes have partially broken down, leaving large spaces between many cells (×6800). (From Gonnering R, Edelhauser HF, VanHorn DL, Durant W. The pH tolerance of rabbit and human corneal endothelium. Invest Ophthalmol Vis Sci 1979; 18:373–390.)

stance. Alkali burns are particularly harmful to the cornea, since they cause the saponification and dissociation of cell membrane fatty acids, hydrolysis of proteoglycans, and swelling of collagen fibers[41,42] accompanied by rapid penetration to the aqueous with possible similar damage to other ocular tissues. Paterson and associates[43] studied the effects of alkali on the pH of rabbit aqueous humor. They found that with the application of 100 μl of 2N sodium hydroxide, the aqueous pH rose to 12 within 5 minutes and fell to only 11 after 90 minutes. A similar rapid penetration was shown with enucleated human eye-bank eyes. When rabbit eyes were topically irrigated 2 minutes after the alkali burn with physiologic saline at a rate of 30 drops per minute, the aqueous pH dropped to only 10 after 90 minutes, indicating the inadequacy of this procedure alone for treating alkali burns. The use of paracentesis of the anterior chamber combined with the intracameral injection of buffer for enhanced treatment will be discussed in the next section.

Intraocular Irrigating Solutions

History

Ophthalmologists once used normal saline routinely as an intraocular irrigating solution in surgery. Merrill and associates,[44] however, showed in 1960 that such solutions are inadequate for the physiologic well-being of isolated iris and conjunctival tissues after a 35-minute perfusion. A balanced salt solution was reported to be significantly less traumatic. One serious problem that occurs with the use of saline is corneal swelling, which results from rapidly developing abnormalities of the endothelium.[45] In fact, Edelhauser and associates[3] were able to demonstrate that lactated Ringer's solution, used in some vitrectomy surgery, and Plasma-Lyte 148, used in some phacoemulsification surgery, are also unacceptable as irrigating solutions for intraocular tissues. The principal effect of both solutions is early breakdown of corneal endothelial cells. These irrigating solutions lack ions of

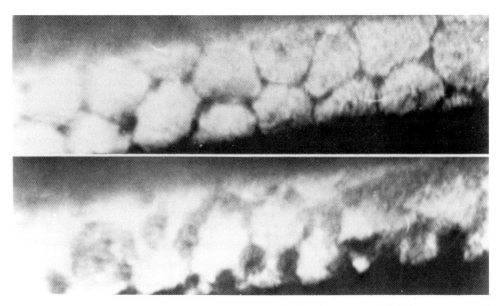

FIGURE 9.9   **Rabbit corneal endothelium showing examples of enlarging intercellular spaces seen with erythromycin and bacitracin. The upper segment represents early changes and the lower segment late changes. Intercellular swelling seems to have pushed the cell substance to the side. Eventually there was complete loss of recognizable cell morphology. (From Coles WH. Effects of antibiotics on the in vitro rabbit corneal endothelium. Invest Ophthalmol 1975;14:246–250.)**

either calcium, magnesium, or both, which have been previously indicated in this chapter as being important for cell adhesion and cell-to-cell junctions. A balanced salt solution (BSS, Alcon) containing calcium and magnesium was made available as early as 1960 for intraocular surgery.[46]

Although a balanced salt solution is apparently acceptable for short-term intraocular surgery,[47] it is only marginally acceptable for protracted intraocular surgery. Some corneal swelling continues to occur.[3] Recently, Glasser and associates[48] have shown the development of polymegathism and pleomorphism in

TABLE 9.2
Preservatives Used in Some Extraocular Irrigating Solutions

Preservative	Epithelial Toxicity Level[a]	Antimicrobial Level[b]		Irrigating Solution Level[c]	
Benzalkonium chloride (BAK)	0.01%[1] 0.02%[39] 0.01%[34]	0.0029%	*Staphylococcus aureus*[34] *Salmonella typhosa* *Candida albicans*	0.013% ? 0.013%	AK-Rinse Dacriose[d,e] Eye Stream
		0.0025%	*Escherichia coli*	0.005%	Lavoptik
		0.0014%	*Cryptococcus neoformans*	0.01%	Murine
		0.0011%	*Streptococcus pyogenes*	0.01%	Ocu-Drop
		0.02%	*Pseudomonas aeruginosa* (may be partially resistant)		
Thimerosal	>0.01%[1] >2.0 %[39]	0.01%	*Pseudomonas aeruginosa*[40] *Staphylococcus aureus* *Candida albicans*	<0.002% 0.004%	Collyrium M/Rinse
Phenylmercuric acetate	Unknown	0.004%	*Pseudomonas aeruginosa*[34] (may be partially resistant)	0.004%	Blinx

[a]Concentration at which epithelial cell damage has been reported.
[b]Concentration necessary to be bacteriostatic against the named microorganisms.
[c]Concentration used in the following commercial preparations.
[d]Concentration not given in pharmacology literature.
[e]In combination with ethylenediaminetetraacetic acid (EDTA).

TABLE 9.3
Components of Some Commercial Extraocular Irrigating Solutions

Solution	Components	
Eye-Stream	0.49%	sodium chloride
	0.075%	potassium chloride
	0.03%	magnesium chloride
	0.048%	calcium chloride
	0.39%	sodium acetate
	0.17%	sodium citrate
	0.013%	benzalkonium chloride
Murine Regular Formula	a	sodium chloride
	a	potassium chloride
	a	sodium phosphate
	a	glycerin
	0.01%	benzalkonium chloride
	0.05%	EDTA
Ocu-Bath Eye Lotion	0.38%	potassium chloride
	0.014%	sodium carbonate
	1.2%	boric acid
	0.01%	benzalkonium chloride
	0.05%	EDTA

aPercentage not specified. EDTA, ethylenediaminetetraacetic acid.
Data from Kastrup EK, Olin BR, Covington TR, et al., eds. Facts and comparisons. St. Louis: J.B. Lippincott Co, 1988.

cat corneal endothelial cells after 1 hour in a balanced salt solution. Araie[49] has indicated that endothelial barrier function is compromised with a solution containing only salts. Several investigations during the 1970s had already indicated the need for other components in intraocular irrigating solutions. Hodson[50] demonstrated a need for bicarbonate ions. Dikstein and Maurice[51] showed that glucose, adenosine, and glutathione were each able to thin a swollen cornea, albeit to different degrees. It has never been adequately explained how bicarbonate ions work. Hodson[52] proposed that bicarbonate ions were pumped into the aqueous to aid deturgescence. However, neither Riley and Peters[53] nor Whikehart and Soppet[54] were able to locate a bicarbonate transporting ATPase in the plasma membranes of the corneal endothelial cells. Whikehart and Soppet[55] were able to show stimulation of membrane bound Na^+-K^+ ATPase in these cells by glutathione, but not by adenosine. Zagrod and Whikehart[56] recently demonstrated that adenosine may act as a substitute for glucose by supplying metabolic intermediates via the pentose shunt. In the retina, work by Winkler and associates[28] has shown the importance of bicarbonate in maintaining both the retinal ERG and lactate production. This finding has been supported by other researchers.[23,24,57] However, the mechanism is still elusive.

Edelhauser and associates[45] prepared and perfused rabbit corneas with a modified basic salt solution ("GBR") containing bicarbonate, glucose, adenosine, and glutathione and found essentially no swelling of rabbit corneas over a 3- to 6-hour period. This compared effectively with earlier preparations and with partial components of GBR[2,3] in which corneas were always observed to swell in various amounts. When Christiansen and associates[58] prepared fresh solutions of D5W and sodium bicarbonate with either lactated Ringer's or Ringer's injection solution and used them in studies of the monkey lens, they found it difficult to control pH with lactated Ringer's solution.

Attempts to prepare this and similar formulations fresh for use in the operating room were met with the same instability. Moreover, the preparations were somewhat less stabilizing to the lens as well in preventing cataractogenesis during vitrectomies. A commercial formulation (BSS Plus, Alcon) appeared in 1981 that contained bicarbonate, glucose and glutathione in addition to balanced salts.[46] Adenosine was not included due to problems of maintenance in storage. This commercial formulation has been successful in stabilizing both the cornea and the lens in nondiabetic patients during long-term ocular surgery (1 to 3 hours).

Components

Table 9.4 lists the formulations of some commercial intraocular irrigating solutions, past and present, for comparative purposes. However, even present formulations have limitations, as discussed in the next section. BSS Plus has its components divided into 2 containers and must be premixed before use. Once mixed, it has the composition given in Table 9.4 and is stable for 24 hours.

Surgical Uses

Two intraocular irrigating solutions that are currently available have been formulated for short-term (BSS) and long-term (BSS Plus) surgery, respectively. The latter solution is intended to be used for pars plana vitrectomy, phacoemulsification, extracapsular cataract extraction, anterior segment reconstruction, and other sophisticated ocular surgery requiring 1 to 3 hours of perfusion with large volumes of solution. There is virtually no corneal swelling and no endothelial changes during that time with the more complete medium. However, other factors must be considered in the use of intraocular irrigating solutions. An abnormal endothelium predisposes toward bullous keratopathy with the use of the less complete solution (BSS). Berger and associates[59] have even recommended that no intraocular irrigation be performed during cataract extraction when an abnormal endothelium is present. Such

TABLE 9.4
Components of Some Commercial Intraocular Irrigating Solutions

Component (mM/liter)	Physiologic Saline[3] mOsm = 308 pH = 7.0	Lactated Ringer's[3] mOsm = 277 pH = 6.6	Plasmalyte 148[3] mOsm = 299 pH = 7.4	BSS[3] mOsm = 270 pH = 7.4	BSS Plus[46] mOsm = 305 pH = 7.4	Surgisol[29] mOsm = 300 pH = 7.4
Sodium chloride	154	102	85.9	83.8	122.2	109.5
Potassium chloride		4	5	10.1	5.1	10.1
Calcium chloride[a]		3		4.3	1.1	3.3
Magnesium chloride[b]			1.5	1.5	1	1.5
Sodium phosphate[c]					3.5	
Sodium bicarbonate					25	
Glucose					5.1	
Glutathione disulfide					.3	
Sodium acetate			2.7	28.6		28.7
Sodium citrate				5.8		5.8
Sodium lactate		28				
Sodium gluconate			16.9			

[a]Dihydrate.
[b]Hexahydrate.
[c]Calculated as the monobasic salt but not mentioned in Alcon's literature.[46]

a caveat would not apply to the use of a long-term irrigating solution that was adequately formulated[a] with the components previously mentioned (see Table 9.4, BSS Plus).

A different problem that occurs with pars plana vitrectomy is the development during surgery of a posterior subcapsular lens opacification in diabetic patients. The opacification blocks the appearance of both vitreous cavity and retina. A lensectomy to clear the view may, in turn, double the risk of postoperative neovascular glaucoma. An investigation by Haimann and associates[60] demonstrated that a long-term intraocular irrigating solution was not able to protect against cataract formation in diabetic rabbits. It was found, however, that glucose fortification of the solution to 335 mOsm prevented cataract formation during perfusion while performing vitrectomies on rabbits. Perfusions were carried out for 2 hours. The increased osmolarity acts as a guard against osmotic stress, which is worsened with the use of solutions of normal osmolarity. The reason for this is that diabetic lenses have trapped within their cells polyols that cause osmotic stress.[61] This is ameliorated by the high glucose content of a diabetic aqueous.

First-Aid Irrigating Solutions

A continuation of the study by Paterson and associates,[43] mentioned earlier in this chapter, showed that para-

centesis of the rabbit anterior chamber following the application of 100 μl of 2N sodium hydroxide to the corneal surface reduced aqueous pH from 12 to 10 in 5 minutes. This is compared with the same drop in pH over 90 minutes with external irrigation using physiologic saline. The same workers, furthermore, demonstrated that the simultaneous introduction of pH 7.2 phosphate buffer, intracamerally injected, can lower aqueous pH to 8.5 in 30 minutes. The pH at 30 minutes with paracentesis alone was still at 10. It may be recalled that Gonnering and associates[32] reported structural and functional alterations to the human corneal endothelium outside of the pH range 6.5 to 8.5. This indicates that immediately following extraocular lavage of an alkali burn the two-fold techniques of paracentesis and intracameral buffer may be able to restore the aqueous to a pH nearly acceptable to the cornea and other ocular tissues. These procedures have been recommended[42,43] in cases of moderately severe and severe alkali burns, using sterile phosphate buffer or other compatible irrigating solutions. In view of the preceding discussions, the solution of choice should be a complete physiologic solution.

References

1. Pfister RR, Burstein N. The effects of ophthalmic drugs, vehicles, and preservatives on corneal epithelium: A scanning electron microscope study. Invest Ophthalmol 1976;15:246–259.

[a]Personal communication, Henry F. Edelhauser, Ph.D.

2. Whikehart DR, Edelhauser HF. Glutathione in rabbit corneal endothelia: The effects of selected perfusion fluids. Invest Ophthalmol Vis Sci 1978;17:455–464.

3. Edelhauser HF, VanHorn DL, Schultz RO, Hyndick RA. Effects of intraocular irrigating solutions on the cornea. In: Leopold IH, Burns RP, eds. Symposium on ocular therapy. New York: John Wiley & Sons, 1977;10:45–60.

4. Friend J. Biochemistry of ocular surface epithelium. Int Ophthalmol Clin 1979;19:73–91.

5. Daum KM, Hill RM. Human tear glucose. Invest Ophthalmol Vis Sci 1982;22:509–514.

6. Thoft RA, Friend J. Corneal epithelial glucose utilization. Arch Ophthalmol 1971;88:58.

7. Edelhauser HF, VanHorn DL, Records RE. Cornea and sclera. In: Records RE, ed. Physiology of the human eye and visual system. Hagerstown, MD: Harper & Row, 1979;68–97.

8. Kinoshita JH. Some aspects of the carbohydrate metabolism of the cornea. Invest Ophthalmol 1962;1:178.

9. Kaye GI. Stereologic measurement of cell volume fraction of rabbit corneal stroma. Arch Ophthalmol 1969;82:792–794.

10. Waltman SR. The cornea. In: Moses RA, ed. Adler's physiology of the eye. St. Louis: C. V. Mosby Co, 1981;47.

11. Fatt I. Physiology of the eye. Boston: Butterworths, 1978;160–161.

12. Geroski DH, Edelhauser HF, O'Brien WJ. Hexose-monophosphate shunt activity in the component layers of the cornea: Its response to thiol oxidation. Exp Eye Res 1978;26:611–619.

13. Riley MV. Transport of ions and metabolites across the corneal endothelium. In: McDevitt DS, ed. Cell biology of the eye. New York: Academic Press, 1982;53–95.

14. Hogan MJ, Alvarado JA, Weddel JE. Histology of the human eye. Philadelphia: W. B. Saunders Co, 1971;102–109.

15. Gaasterland DE, Pederson JE, MacLellan HM, Reddy VN. Rhesus monkey aqueous humor composition and a primate ocular perfusate. Invest Ophthalmol Vis Sci 1979;18:1139–1150.

16. Maurice D. The location of the fluid pump in the cornea. J Physiol 1972;221:43–54.

17. Green K. Ion transport in isolated cornea of the rabbit. Am J Physiol 1965;209:1311–1316.

18. Edelhauser HF, VanHorn DL, Schultz RO, Hyndick RA. Comparative toxicity of intraocular irrigating solutions on the corneal endothelium. Am J Ophthalmol 1976;81:473–481.

19. Records RE. Conjunctiva and lacrimal system. In: Records RE, ed. Physiology of the human eye and visual system. Hagerstown, MD: Harper & Row, 1979;25–46.

20. Zagrod ME, Whikehart DR. Cyclic nucleotides in anatomical subdivisions of the bovine lens. Curr Eye Res 1981;1:49–52.

21. Kinoshita JH, Kern HL, Merola LO. Factors affecting the cation transport of calf lens. Biochem Biophys Acta 1961;47:458.

22. Chylack LT, Schaefer FL. Mechanism of "hypoglycemic" cataract formation in the rat lens. II. Further studies on the role of hexokinase instability. Invest Ophthalmol 1976;15:519–528.

23. Negi A, Honda Y, Kawano S-I. Effects of intraocular irri-

gating solutions on the electroretinographic B-wave. Am J Ophthalmol 1981;92:28–37.

24. Textorious O, Nilsson SEG, Anderson B-E. Effects of intraocular perfusion with two alternating irrigation solutions on the simultaneously recorded electroretinogram of albino rabbits. Doc Ophthalmol 1986;63:349–358.

25. Jensen D. The principles of physiology. New York: Appleton-Century-Crofts, 1980.

26. Edelhauser HF, Hanneken AM, Pederson HJ, VanHorn DL. Osmotic tolerance of rabbit and human corneal endothelium. Arch Ophthalmol 1981;99:1281–1287.

27. Fraunfelder FT. National drug registry of drug-induced ocular side effects. Case reports 1545, 1878, 2016, 2226. Portland: University of Oregon, 1980.

28. Winkler BS, Simson V, Benner J. Importance of bicarbonate in retinal function. Invest Ophthalmol Vis Sci 1977;16:766–768.

29. Kastrup EK, Olin BR, Covington TR, et al, eds. Facts and comparisons. St. Louis: J.B. Lippincott Co, 1988.

30. Siggaard-Anderson O. Blood gases. In: Tietz NW, ed. Fundamentals of clinical chemistry. Philadelphia: W. B. Saunders Co, 1976:854–944.

31. Milder B. The lacrimal apparatus. In: Moses RA, ed. Adler's physiology of the eye. St Louis: C. V. Mosby Co, 1981;16–37.

32. Gonnering R, Edelhauser HF, VanHorn DL, Durant W. The pH tolerance of rabbit and human corneal endothelium. Invest Ophthalmol Vis Sci 1979;18:373–390.

33. Henkind P, Walsh JB, Berger AW, eds. Physicians desk reference for ophthalmology. Oradell, NJ: Medical Economics, 1982.

34. Hales RH. Contact lenses. A clinical approach to fitting. Baltimore: Williams & Wilkins, 1978:32–50.

35. Harvey SC. Antiseptics and disinfectants; fungicides; ectoparasiticides. In: Gilman AG, Goodman LS, Rall TW, et al., eds. The pharmacological basis of therapeutics. 7th ed. New York: Macmillan Co, 1985;959–979.

36. Coles WH. Effects of antibiotics on the in vitro rabbit corneal endothelium. Invest Ophthalmol 1975;14:246–250.

37. Leopold IH. Antibiotics and antifungal agents. Invest Ophthalmol 1964;3:510–511.

38. Havener WH. Ocular pharmacology. St Louis: C. V. Mosby Co, 1983.

39. Zand LM. Review: The effect of non-therapeutic ophthalmic preparations on the cornea and tear film. Aust J Optom 1981;64:44.

40. Wade A, ed. Martindale, the extra pharmacopoeia. London: Pharmaceutical Press, 1977.

41. Grayson M. Diseases of the cornea. St Louis: C. V. Mosby Co, 1979.

42. Pfister RR, Koski J. Alkali burns of the eye: Pathophysiology and treatment. South Med J 1982;75:417–422.

43. Paterson CA, Pfister RR, Levinson RA. Aqueous humor pH changes after experimental alkali burns. Am J Ophthalmol 1975;79:414–419.

44. Merrill DL, Fleming TC, Girard LJ. The effects of physiologic balanced salt solutions and normal saline on intraocular and extraocular tissues. Am J Ophthalmol 1960;49:895–989.

45. Edelhauser HF, VanHorn DL, Hyndiuk RA, Schultz RO.

Intraocular irrigating solutions. Arch Ophthalmol 1975;93:648–657.

46. Alcon Laboratories. A brief history of intraocular irrigating solutions. (Form No. 098116A). Fort Worth, TX: Alcon Laboratories, 1981.

47. Rosenfeld SI, Waltman SR, Olk RJ, Gordon M. Comparison of intraocular irrigating solutions in pars plana vitrectomy. Ophthalmology 1986;93:109–115.

48. Glasser DB, Matsuda M, Ellis JG, Edelhauser HF. Effects of intraocular irrigating solutions on the corneal endothelium after in vivo anterior chamber irrigation. Am J Ophthalmol 1985;99:321–328.

49. Araie M. Barrier function of corneal endothelium and the intraocular irrigating solutions. Arch Ophthalmol 1986;104:435–438.

50. Hodson S. Evidence for a bicarbonate-dependent sodium pump in corneal endothelium. Exp Eye Res 1971;11:20–29.

51. Dikstein S, Maurice DM. The metabolic basis to the fluid pump in the cornea. J Physiol 1972;221:29–41.

52. Hodson S. The bicarbonate ion pump in the endothelium which regulates the hydration of rabbit cornea. J Physiol 1976;263:563–577.

53. Riley MV, Peters MI. The localization of the anion-sensitive ATPase activity in corneal endothelium. Biochim Biophys Acta 1981;644:251–256.

54. Whikehart DR, Soppet DR. Activities of transport enzymes located in the plasma membranes of corneal endothelial cells. Invest Ophthalmol Vis Sci 1981;21:819–825.

55. Whikehart DR, Soppet DR. The effects of glutathione and adenosine on plasma membrane ATPases of the corneal endothelium. An hypothesis on the stimulatory mechanism of perfused glutathione upon deturgescence. Curr Eye Res 1981;1:451–455.

56. Zagrod ME, Whikehart DR. Adenosine-stimulated production of sugar-phosphates in bovine corneal endothelium. Invest Ophthalmol Vis Sci 1985;26:1475–1483.

57. Moorhead LC, Redburn DA, Merritt J, Garcia CA. The effects of intravitreal irrigation during vitrectomy on the electroretinogram. Am J Ophthalmol 1979;88:239–245.

58. Christiansen JM, Kollarits CR, Fukui H, et al. Intraocular irrigating solutions and lens clarity. Am J Ophthalmol 1976;82:594–597.

59. Berger BB, Emery JM, Brown NV, et al. The lens, cataract, and its management. In: Peyman GA, Sanders DR, Goldberg MF, eds. Principles and practice of ophthalmology. Philadelphia: W. B. Sanders Co, 1980;585.

60. Haimann MH, Abrams GW, Edelhauser HF, Hatchell DL. The effect of intraocular irrigating solutions on lens clarity in normal and diabetic rabbits. Am J Ophthalmol 1982;94:594–605.

61. Kinoshita JH, Kador P, Catiles M. Aldose reductase in diabetic cataracts. JAMA 1981;246:257–261.

62. Briggs RB, McCartney DL. Balanced salt solution infusion alert. Arch Ophthalmol 1988;106:718.

CHAPTER 10

Lubricants and Other Preparations for the Dry Eye

Siret D. Jaanus

Dryness of the eyes has been recognized since the time of Hippocrates as a condition often difficult to alleviate. During the eighth century AD, Paul of Aegina suggested bathing the eye with warm water, applying egg white or goose fat, and observing healthy living conditions as a cure for dryness of the eye. Galen and his contemporaries, and later Boerhave in 1750, used elixirs of herbs boiled in wine or vinegar to ameliorate dry eye conditions.[1]

During the 19th century aqueous salt solutions, glycerin, and various oils came into use. Early in this century a more balanced salt solution, Locke's solution, to which gelatin was added to impart viscosity, became a popular remedy.[2] Gelatin and other natural products used to provide more viscous solutions proved to be chemically unstable and served as good media for growth of microorganisms. The introduction of a synthetic cellulose ether, methylcellulose, by Swan[3] proved to be a major advance in the search for a suitable substitute for ocular secretions lubricating the eye. Over the years, other synthetic colloids have been used to enhance viscosity of artificial tear solutions. Although ocular retention time of tear substitutes is enhanced by the addition of viscous agents, high viscosity itself does not provide relief for all dry eye conditions.[4] Thus, other less viscous hydrophilic substances such as polyvinyl alcohol (PVA) and polyvinylpyrrolidone (PVP) have been included as the polymeric ingredients of many artificial tear formulations.[5]

Although advances have been made in understanding the mechanisms involved in tear film formation and rupture, the role of tears in maintaining a normal conjunctival and corneal surface is not completely understood.[6] The availability of synthetic polymers suitable for ocular use has resulted in the development of various artificial tear solutions and other formulations to help alleviate dryness of the ocular surface.

Products in current use appear to be more compatible with the precorneal tear film and ocular tissues, but similarities between the ancient and the more recent artificial tear formulations remain. Use of water-soluble polymer solutions and bland ointments remains the mainstay of therapy for the dry eye, but other products such as solid water-soluble inserts (Lacrisert) and punctal plugs have also proven to be of value in some patients.

Tear Film Physiology

Through the Middle Ages, tears were thought to be excrements of the brain. About 45 years ago Eugene Wolff[7] described in clinical terms the basic concepts governing tear film composition and structure. The tear film is usually described as a 3-layer structure consisting of a superficial lipid layer, a middle aqueous layer, and a deep mucoid layer (Fig. 10.1). This relatively thin fluid film covering the cornea and conjunctiva is about 7 μm thick and is commonly referred to as the precorneal tear film.[8]

The lipids of the outermost layer are fluid at body temperature and consist primarily of low-polarity lipids such as waxy and cholesteryl esters. This layer is de-

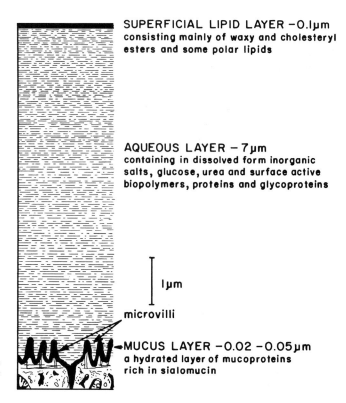

SUPERFICIAL LIPID LAYER −0.1μm
consisting mainly of waxy and cholesteryl
esters and some polar lipids

AQUEOUS LAYER − 7μm
containing in dissolved form inorganic
salts, glucose, urea and surface active
biopolymers, proteins and glycoproteins

1μm

microvilli

MUCUS LAYER −0.02 −0.05μm
a hydrated layer of mucoproteins
rich in sialomucin

FIGURE 10.1   **Structure and composition of the tear film. (Modified from Holly FJ, Lemp MA. Tear physiology and dry eyes. Surv Ophthalmol 1977;22:70.)**

rived from the meibomian glands and covers the entire free surface of the tear fluid. An intact lipid layer prevents evaporation of the underlying aqueous component of the precorneal tear film, and interacts with the aqueous layer to promote tear film stability.[8,9]

The aqueous layer, supplied by the main and accessory lacrimal glands, constitutes the thickest portion of the precorneal tear film. Dissolved in this layer are inorganic salts, glucose, urea, some trace elements, and various surface active biopolymers in the form of proteins and glycoproteins.[8–12] Lactoferrin and lysozyme are the main protein constituents in human tears. Both are considered to play important roles in defense against bacteria.[12] The presence of proteins and bicarbonate ions adds buffering capacity to the tears.[8,9] The aqueous layer also contains immunoglobulins, primarily IgA, lactate dehydrogenase, and several inhibitors of proteolytic activity.[10–12]

The most posterior layer of the precorneal tear film consists of mucus, which coats the superficial epithelium of the cornea and conjunctiva. Although the origin of the mucus is not clear, conjunctival goblet cells are most likely one source of the mucoid material. The motion of blinking distributes the material over the preocular surface. The mucus layer is the thinnest layer

of the tear film, being only a few hundredths of a micrometer thick in the healthy eye. Being a highly hydrated, semisolid layer of glycoproteins of varying molecular weight, it is thought to play a vital role in tear film stability through its interactions with both the epithelial surface of the cornea and conjunctiva and the overlying tears.[13] Mucin has at least a two-fold function in controlling tear film stability. First, it lowers the surface tension of the tear fluid and the interfacial tension of the tear-epithelium boundary by providing a layer capable of hydrogen bond formation with water. Mucin, therefore, acts as a wetting as well as a stabilizing agent for the thin precorneal tear film between blinks. Second, it plays a role in the removal of excessive lipid contaminants in the form of mucus threads and fibrils.[2,9]

Currently the only clinical measurement reflecting relative stability of the tear film is tear breakup time (TBUT or BUT).[2] This test requires instillation of sodium fluorescein and measures the time elapsed between the last complete blink and the appearance of the first randomly formed dry spot on the corneal surface.[14] It is thought to reflect the functional integrity of the tear film. The clinical procedure and uses of the test are discussed further in Chapter 20.

Tear Film Abnormalities

Based on our present knowledge of tear film physiology and clinical observations of dry eye states, clarification of tear film abnormalities has become possible. The various dry eye conditions may be divided into 5 groups according to the type of abnormality responsible for the clinical symptoms.[2,8,15] An understanding of these abnormalities is essential to appreciate the therapeutic role of the clinically useful artificial tear formulations and bland, nonmedicated, ophthalmic ointments (Table 10.1).

Aqueous Deficiency

Continuous production and drainage of the aqueous tear layer maintains the corneal and conjunctival epithelium in a moist state, supplies nutrients and bacteriostatic agents, and clears the ocular surface by the flushing action of tear movement.[16] Deficiencies in the aqueous tear layer can be partial or absolute. Symptoms can progress from mild foreign body sensation to constant burning or irritative sensation of such degree that the patient can be debilitated by the condition.[8] Clinically this condition is most commonly referred to as keratoconjunctivitis sicca (KCS) and is diagnosed primarily by rose bengal staining and determination of the TBUT (see Chapter 20). Instillation of tear sub-

TABLE 10.1
Classification of Tear Film Abnormalities and the Possible Role of Lubricants and Other Dry Eye Preparations

Tear Film Abnormality	Treatment Options
Aqueous tear deficiency	Acetylcysteine Artificial tears Sodium hyaluronate Lacrisert Punctal plug
Mucin deficiency	Artificial tears Lacrisert
Lipid abnormality	Artificial tears Ointments
Impaired lid function	Artificial tears Ointments
Epitheliopathy	Artificial tears Ointments Vitamin A

Adapted from Farris RL. The dry eye: Its mechanism and therapy, with evidence that contact lens is the cause. CLAO 1986;12:234–246.

stitutes to enhance fluid volume of the eye is presently the mainstay in the treatment of aqueous deficiencies.[2,69]

Mucin Deficiency

Diminished secretion of soluble surfactant mucin despite sufficient aqueous volume results in an unstable tear film.[14] Mucin deficiency usually arises from a reduction of goblet cells in the conjunctiva. Conditions that alter goblet cell function affect the integrity of the mucin layer overlying the cornea, resulting in the appearance of nonwetting areas on the corneal and conjunctival surfaces.[8] The most important clinical sign of mucin deficient dry eye is an abnormally rapid breakup of the tear film (TBUT). In normal patients without ocular disease the TBUT usually ranges between 15 and 45 seconds. Breakup times of less than 10 seconds are considered to be clinically significant. Conditions that diminish goblet cell density such as hypovitaminosis A, ocular pemphigoid, Stevens-Johnson syndrome, and chemical burns all result in an unstable tear film as indicated by decreased TBUT.[8]

Lipid Abnormality

Alterations in lipid composition of tears have been associated with chronic blepharitis.[8] Evidence has accumulated indicating that certain microbes can secrete the enzyme lipase that hydrolyzes meibomian lipids to more polar-free fatty acids. These polar lipids are highly surface active, spreading so rapidly as to cause instantaneous dry spot formation in the preocular tear film.[17] A characteristic of avid lipid-mucin interaction is a decrease in the rate of spreading of the tear film, resulting in a rapid TBUT. A rapid TBUT has been demonstrated in chronic blepharitis as well as in acne rosacea.[2]

Impaired Lid Function

Shear forces produced by the moving lids play a vital role in the maintenance of a normal tear film.[13,14] Compromise of normal lid-globe contact or an abnormality in the blinking process can adversely affect mucus distribution and turnover.[13] Seventh cranial nerve paresis and symblepharon formation are among the conditions that can restrict lid movement, resulting in exposure keratitis due to localized nonwetting of the corneal epithelium.[8]

Epitheliopathy

Alterations in normal epithelial morphology have been shown to affect tear film stability. Electron microscopic studies appear to indicate an intimate relationship between the microvilli of the corneal epithelium and the mucus layer[18] (see Fig. 10.1). Clinically it has been observed that the tear film becomes thin and retracts near areas of epithelial irregularity.[8] Dry, nonwetting areas are commonly found associated with both old and active corneal lesions, producing an irregular epithelial surface. It has been suggested that nervous innervation plays a role in corneal epithelial integrity. The presence of acetylcholine (ACh) and cholinesterase has been demonstrated in the corneal epithelium.[19] Such neurohumoral influences have been shown to play an important role in regulating epithelial turnover.[8] This may explain, in part, the role of certain drugs and chemicals in causing dry eye syndromes.

Composition of Tear Substitutes

Ideally the ingredients of artificial tear formulations should fulfill the physiochemical role of a normal tear film. This implies compatibility with the natural components of tears and no alteration in the clarity of the aqueous layer. An effective tear substitute should lower the surface tension of the tear film, aid in the formation of a hydrophilic layer that is compatible with adsorbed mucin, and enhance tear volume when necessary. In the absence of functional mucin, it should be able to form a hydrophilic layer and exhibit the functional properties of a normal mucin layer.[2] Preferably, the topical application of a well-formulated tear substitute and lubricating agent should provide relief for both aqueous and mucin deficient dry eyes. Moreover, functions associated with the lipid layer of the precorneal tear film should not be altered by artificial tears. In addition, minor epitheliopathies may be aided if the tear substitute also thickens the tear film.[2,20] Lubricants currently available include preparations formulated as solutions, ointments, or artificial tear inserts.

Artificial Tear Solutions

Lubricants formulated as solutions consist of inorganic electrolytes to achieve tonicity and maintain pH, preservatives to prevent bacterial growth, and water-soluble polymeric systems. The polymers can alter viscosity of the solution and decrease the wetting angle of saline solution on a mucin-free but polymer-coated cornea in vitro. The reduction in wetting angle can be resistant to saline rinsing, suggesting possible adsorption of polymer to the corneal surface.[21] Table 10.2 lists representative formulations currently available. They are usually administered in dosage frequencies of 3 to 4 times daily but, depending on the patient's clinical needs and response to therapy, may be administered as often as hourly or only occasionally. Since the role of electrolytes and preservatives in ophthalmic preparations is discussed in Chapter 1, emphasis here will be placed on the polymeric ingredients found in the various artificial tear solutions.

SUBSTITUTED CELLULOSE ETHERS

Since their introduction for ophthalmic use, methylcellulose (MC) and other substituted cellulose ethers such as hydroxyethylcellulose (HEC), hydroxypropylcellulose (HPC), hydroxypropylmethylcellulose (HPMC), and carboxymethylcellulose (CMC) have been used as artificial tear formulations.[2] These colloids dissolve in water to produce colorless solutions of varying viscosity. They have the proper optical clarity and a refractive index similar to the cornea, and they are nearly inert chemically.[3,4] In the past, the most frequently used representative of this group was methylcellulose.

Methylcellulose is a synthetic, granular white substance that forms a viscous solution when added to water. It is stable in the pH range tolerated by the eye and seems unaffected by light or aging of the solution. High temperatures (100°C or above) produce coagulation, but on cooling the methylcellulose redissolves. Heat sterilization is therefore possible. Solutions containing only pure methylcellulose do not support growth of microorganisms. Methylcellulose is available in varying degrees of viscosity. For ocular use a concentration range of 0.25% to 1.0% is preferred. At concentrations above 2%, methylcellulose becomes sufficiently viscous to be classified as an ointment.[3]

Over the years, the other substituted cellulose ethers, particularly hydroxyethylcellulose and hydroxypropylmethylcellulose, have become frequently used. They are somewhat less viscous than methylcellulose but possess cohesive and emollient properties equal or superior to those of methylcellulose. Like methylcellulose, these ethers also mix well with other polymers and substances present in artificial tear formulations and are compatible with many drugs and chemicals used on the eye.

In addition to their use as tear substitutes, cellulose ethers are also used to moisten contact lenses (see Chapter 13); also, as discussed in Chapter 1, they are added to ophthalmic drug formulations to prolong contact time of the drug with the eye.[4] More viscous solutions are also used for application of gonioscopic

TABLE 10.2
Composition of Various Artificial Tear Preparations

Trade Name (manufacturer)	Active Ingredient	Preservative
Adsorbotear (Alcon)	HEC, povidone	Thimerosal 0.004%, EDTA 0.1%
Akwa Tears (Akorn)	PVA, NaCL	Benzalkonium chloride 0.01%, EDTA
Artificial Tears Solution (Rugby)	PVA 1.4%	Chlorobutanol, EDTA
Hypotears (Iolab)	PVA 1%, PEG-8000 dextrose	Benzalkonium chloride, EDTA
Isopto Tears (Alcon)	HPMC	Benzalkonium chloride 0.01%
Lacril (Allergan)	HPMC, gelatin A	Chlorobutanol 0.5%
Lacrisert[a] (Merck)	HPC (solid)	None
Liquifilm Forte (Allergan)	PVA 3%	Thimerosal 0.002%, EDTA
Liquifilm Tears (Allergan)	PVA 1.4%	Chlorobutanol 0.5%
Lyteers (Bausch & Lomb)	HEC	Benzalkonium chloride 0.01%, EDTA 0.05%
Moisture Drops (Bausch & Lomb)	HPMC, dextran 0.1%	Benzalkonium chloride 0.01%, disodium EDTA
Muro Tears (Bausch & Lomb)	HPMC, dextran 40	Benzalkonium chloride 0.01%, EDTA
Murocel (Bausch & Lomb)	MC, propylene glycol	Parabens
Neo-Tears (Barnes-Hind)	PVA, HEC, PEG-300	Thimerosal 0.004%, EDTA 0.02%
Refresh (Allergan)	PVA 1.4%, povidone 0.6%	None
Tear Gard (Medtech)	HEC, lecithin	Sorbic acid, edetate disodium
Tearisol (Iolab)	HPMC	Benzalkonium chloride, EDTA
Tears Naturale (Alcon)	HPMC, dextran 70	Benzalkonium chloride 0.01%, EDTA 0.05%
Tears Naturale II (Alcon)	HPMC, dextran 70	Polyquaternium 0.001%, EDTA
Tears Plus (Allergan)	PVA 1.4%, povidone	Chlorobutanol 0.5%
Tears Renewal (Akorn)	HPMC, dextran 70	Benzalkonium chloride 0.05%, EDTA
Ultra Tears (Alcon)	HPMC	Benzalkonium chloride 0.01%
Vit-A-Drops (Vision Pharmaceuticals)	5000 IU Vitamin A, polysorbate 80	None

CMC, carboxymethylcellulose; HEC, hydroxyethylcellulose; HPMC, hydroxypropylmethylcellulose; HPC, hydroxypropyl cellulose; MC, methylcellulose; PVA, polyvinyl alcohol; EDTA, ethylenediaminetetraacetic acid.
[a]Available only by prescription.

and fundus contact lenses to the eye (Table 10.3). The viscous properties of the colloid aid in contact of the lens with the cornea and also prevent damage to the corneal epithelium.[18] When used for this purpose the solution is often referred to as *goniogel*. Goniogels should be allowed to slowly flow into the bowl of the gonioscope or fundus contact lens to minimize annoying bubbles that may subsequently interfere with the diagnostic procedure. Storing goniogels inverted also reduces bubble formation (see Fig. 2.2).

Although the cellulose ethers enhance viscosity and prolong the ocular retention time of solutions, they

TABLE 10.3
Lubricants Used with Gonioscopic Prisms

Trade Name (manufacturer)	Composition
Goniosol (Iolab) Gonak (Akorn)	Hydroxypropylmethylcellulose 2.5%, boric acid, EDTA, benzalkonium chloride 0.01%
Gonioscopic Prism Solution (Alcon)	Hydroxyethylcellulose, thimerosal 0.004%, EDTA 0.1%

EDTA, ethylenediaminetetraacetic acid.

may also exert other effects, less well understood. It has been proposed that cellulose ethers and other water soluble polymers may adsorb at the cornea-aqueous tear layer interface, thereby stabilizing a thicker layer of fluid adjacent to the adsorbing surface.[6,20,21] The observation that TBUT can be prolonged by these compounds supports such assumptions.[23,24] Norn[23] reported that in the presence of methylcellulose the precorneal film seemed thicker, and wetting time was prolonged by 5 to 42 seconds. Lemp and associates[25] tested the effects of commercial artificial tear solutions on TBUT. A significant increase in TBUT was observed with several of the preparations tested. However, this study was performed with normal subjects with no clinical symptoms of tear deficiencies. Thus, it is possible that the observed effects may not apply in all cases of dry eye syndromes.

The cellulose ethers are generally nonirritating and nontoxic to the ocular tissues.[70] Pfister and Burstein[26] observed no effects on plasma membranes following application of 0.5% methylcellulose in normal saline to rabbit eyes. Healing of corneal epithelial wounds appears not to be inhibited by concentrations of methylcellulose as high as 2%.[27]

Their relative lack of toxicity, their viscous properties, and their beneficial effects on tear film stability have made cellulose ethers useful components of artificial tear preparations.

POLYVINYL POLYMERS

Polyvinyl alcohol (PVA) is a suspending agent and emulsifier. It has been used in topical ocular solutions to enhance ocular contact time of ophthalmic medications and as a wetting and coating agent for contact lenses (see Chapter 13). Most frequently used in a 1.4% concentration, it is much less viscous than methylcellulose. A 0.5% solution of methylcellulose has a viscosity of 50 centipoise as compared to 1.4% PVA with a viscosity of 4 centipoise. It lowers the surface tension of water 46 degrees/cm as compared to 47 to 53 degrees/cm for methylcellulose. The refractive index approximates that of distilled water. Like methylcellulose, PVA is transparent and colorless in solution.[5,18]

Solutions of PVA can be easily sterilized, since they can withstand high temperatures. They can also be autoclaved or filter sterilized through a millipore filtering system. Moreover, heating and subsequent cooling to room temperature does not affect the clarity of the solution, since it does not coagulate or precipitate with temperature changes.[22]

At the concentration used in ophthalmic preparations, PVA is nonirritating to the eye.[28] Moreover, it does not appear to interfere with normal plasma membrane integrity[26] or corneal epithelial regeneration.[5]

Like methylcellulose and hydroxypropylmethylcellulose, PVA may also enhance the stability of the precorneal tear film.[5,9,28] Norn and Opauszki[29] reported that 1.4% PVA increased TBUT by a factor of 1.89. Higher concentrations of PVA further prolonged TBUT. With 3% PVA a 2.96 increase in TBUT occurred. A maximum increase in TBUT was observed with 10.0% PVA. At this concentration the TBUT was prolonged by a factor of 7.16.

Although PVA is compatible with many commonly used drugs and preservatives, certain agents can thicken or gel solutions containing PVA. Compounds that can cause these reactions include sodium bicarbonate, sodium borate, and the sulfates of sodium, potassium, and zinc.[5] The reasons for these reactions are not well understood. It is important, therefore, to be somewhat cautious in the clinical use of solutions containing PVA with solutions containing any of these agents to avoid incompatibility. For example, some extraocular irrigating solutions containing sodium borate have been known to cause such a reaction when used to irrigate from the eye contact lens wetting solutions containing PVA.

OTHER POLYMERIC SYSTEMS

Polyvinylpyrrolidone (povidone, PVP) exhibits surface active properties similar to the cellulose ethers. However, its ability to lower the interfacial tension at a water-oil interface appears to be less than that of the cellulose ethers.[30] Nevertheless, in contrast to the cellulose ethers, PVP appears capable of forming hydrophilic coatings in the form of adsorbed layers.[21,30] Since conjunctival mucin is thought to interact with the ocular surface in a manner that results in the formation of an adsorbing surface for aqueous tears, the formation of a hydrophilic layer by artificial means, which would mimic conjunctival mucin (mucomimetic), would seem clinically desirable. Since the wetting ability of the corneal surface would be enhanced, both mucin- and aqueous-deficient dry eyes would benefit.[21,31]

As previously mentioned, evaluations of commercial artificial tear formulations in humans have indicated that TBUT can be prolonged.[25,31] Lemp and Hamill[31] evaluated the effect of 12 artificial tear preparations on TBUT in normal subjects. Significant prolongation of TBUT was observed with Adapt, Adapette, Adsorbotear, and Tears Naturale. Certain preparations in current use, such as Neo-Tears and Hypotears, were not tested. Geeting and Bakar[24] evaluated 4 artificial tear solutions (Hypotears, Liquifilm Tears, Neo-Tears, Tears Naturale) in 8 patients having an initial TBUT of not more than 8 seconds. All 4 preparations prolonged TBUT for approximately 60 to 90 minutes. The greatest mean increase in TBUT was observed with Neo-Tears, which also had the longest duration of action, prolonging TBUT for nearly 2 hours.

Other parameters of surface chemistry that have been evaluated—surface tension, interfacial tension at the water-oil interface, contact angle of solutions on clean cornea or polymethylmethacrylate (PMMA)—show similarities among cellulose ethers, PVA, and the polymeric systems.[29,30] Surface tension measurements indicate that all are less surface active than mucin.[13,30] Moreover, with artificial tear preparations exhibiting surface activity, their action was found to be due to the presence of other ingredients, particularly the preservative benzalkonium chloride.[21,27] These observations indicate that subtle interactions may occur between the various ingredients present in artificial tear formulations. The effects could further extend to interactions among synthetic polymers, preservatives, tear film constituents, and the epithelial surface. Questions remaining are numerous and can be answered only as better and less ambiguous testing procedures, both in vitro and in vivo, are developed. Clinical results as well as patient acceptance remain the final criteria of in vivo efficacy of specific artificial tear solutions. No single formulation has yet been identified that universally provides improvement in clinical signs and symptoms while allowing patient comfort and acceptance.

Vitamin A Derivatives

Vitamin A deficiency can affect a variety of epithelial-lined organs, including the eye. Epidermal keratinization and squamous metaplasia of the mucus membranes, including the cornea and conjunctiva, respond to both oral and topical vitamin A therapy.[32,33] Recent evidence suggests that retinol is secreted by the lacrimal gland and is metabolized in the cornea to retinoic acid.[71] Topical use of both tretinoin (all-trans retinoic acid) and retinol, the alcohol form of vitamin A, has been advocated for treatment of various dry eye disorders.[34–38].

Tseng and associates[34,35] evaluated in a noncontrolled fashion the clinical efficacy of tretinoin ointment in various dry eye disorders including keratoconjunctivitis sicca, Stevens-Johnson syndrome, pemphigoid, and surgery- or radiation-induced dry eye. Depending on severity of the condition, doses of 0.01% or 0.1% were applied to affected eyes 1 to 3 times daily for 2 months. Patients continued to use their previous medications as prescribed. All patients in this study showed clinical improvement in symptoms, including visual acuity, rose bengal staining, and Schirmer testing. Impression cytology performed before and after treatment indicated that vitamin A reversed the squa-

mous metaplastic changes of the surface epithelium observed before treatment. Use of artificial tears and lubricants could be reduced or discontinued. The therapeutic efficacy observed in these patients has been attributed to the restoration of cellular differentiation, with goblet cell regeneration and enhanced mucin production, whereby the interaction between epithelial cell surface and tear film are normalized.[37]

Soong and associates[75] recently evaluated in a controlled study the efficacy and safety of topical tretinoin ointment 0.01% and found it to be ineffective in improving symptoms and clinical signs in patients with noncicatricial dry eyes. The drug, however, was able to reverse conjunctival keratinization in patients with conjunctival cicatricial diseases although clinical symptoms and signs showed no significant improvement with tretinoin therapy compared with placebo. The presence of squamous metaplasia thus appears to be a requirement for potentially treatable cases.[37]

Side effects associated with use of topical tretinoin ointment include transient hyperemia, irritation, or burning. Ocular pharmacokinetic studies in rabbits show low levels of drug in the aqueous humor, approximately $1/1000$ that of tears, following topical application of [^{3}H]-tretinoin. Major tissue uptake occurs in the surface epithelium and the iris.[38]

Retinol, the alcohol form of vitamin A, is available over the counter in solution form as Vit-A-Drops. The preparation contains 5000 IU of vitamin A and polysorbate 80.

Controlled clinical trials are presently lacking regarding the usefulness of retinol solution in dry eye disorders. Preliminary studies[a] claim possible benefit in conjunctival hyperemia, superior limbic keratitis,[72] corneal staining, and giant papillary conjunctivitis. Until more definitive data become available, however, the benefits of vitamin A solution in dry eye disorders remain unknown.

Viscoelastic Agents

SODIUM HYALURONATE

A polysaccharide polymer (glycosaminoglycan), hyaluronate is a structural component of vertebrate connective tissue matrices. It is also present in the vitreous and aqueous humor of the eye. At physiologic pH, it is a viscoelastic solution, with a viscosity of over 500,000 times that of physiologic saline. Sodium hyaluronate has been used with success in intraocular surgical procedures such as cataract extraction, intraocular lens

---

[a]Rengstorff RH. Personal Communication, 1988.

implantation, corneal transplantation, glaucoma filtration, and procedures to repair retinal detachment.[39,40]

Polack and McNiece[41] first studied the effects of a 0.5% solution in patients with severe dry eye syndromes. They observed a decrease in pain shortly following instillation, improved vision, and reduced redness within the first week of treatment in patients for whom conventional artificial tear preparations had failed. Since then other investigators have reported similar results in clinical trials with a 0.1% concentration.[42–45,73] A variety of dry eye syndromes, including keratoconjunctivitis sicca, show subjective as well as objective improvement including decreased itching and burning, reduced foreign body sensation, and reduction of mucus strands.

Rose bengal staining of cornea and conjunctiva is reduced, and corneal luster appears to be increased. Tear film stability may be improved[42] or significantly increased.[44] The beneficial effects of sodium hyaluronate have been attributed to its viscoelastic properties, which lubricate as well as protect the ocular surface.[43] Most patients achieve control of symptoms with topical instillation up to 4 times daily. Subjective relief of symptoms such as burning and "grittiness" is usually immediate following drug instillation, and these effects can last up to 60 minutes or more.

Sodium hyaluronate is synthesized from rooster coombs and is commercially available as Amvisc or Healon. It is supplied in a disposable glass syringe as a 1% (10 mg/ml) sterile preparation of sodium hyaluronate dissolved in physiologic sodium chloride-phosphate buffered solution with a pH range of 7.0 to 7.5. When prepared as a 0.1% saline solution (Healon tears) it must be vigorously shaken before use. Current limitations to its use as an artificial tear are the absence of a commercial preparation for the dry eye, and its cost, which makes it considerably more expensive than other dry eye preparations for long-term use.

Sodium hyaluronate appears to be free of adverse ocular or systemic effects when used topically on the eye at the 0.1% concentration. It is nonantigenic and does not cause inflammatory or foreign body reactions.[45]

CHONDROITIN SULFATE

A polysaccharide of D-glucuronic acid and N-acetyl-galactosamine, chondroitin sulfate is 350,000 times as viscous as saline. Limberg and associates[46] compared solutions of hyaluronic acid 0.1%, chrondoitin sulfate 1%, and a mixture of chondroitin sulfate 0.38% and hyaluronic acid 0.3% with an artificial tear solution containing PVA and polyethylene glycol. All solutions were instilled at 2-hour intervals for 2 weeks. All 4 solutions appeared to be equal in alleviating symptoms of itching, burning, and foreign body sensation in pa-

tients with keratoconjunctivitis sicca. However, patients with low Schirmer test scores uniformly preferred a solution containing chondroitin sulfate. Since only 20 patients took part in this study, it may be premature to conclude that patients with severe dry eyes derive greater benefit from frequent instillation of chrondroitin sulfate compared with other viscous agents present in artificial tear products.

Chondroitin sulfate is commercially available as Viscoat, a mixture of sodium chondroitin sulfate 40 mg/ml and sodium hyaluronate 30 mg/ml.

Mucolytic Agents

ACETYLCYSTEINE

An N-acetyl-derivative of the naturally occurring amino acid L-cysteine, acetylcysteine has been clinically useful as a mucolytic agent in acute and chronic bronchopulmonary conditions. It is believed to exert its action by opening up disulfide linkages in mucus, thereby lowering the viscosity of mucus.[47]

Available as Mucomyst in a 10% or 20% solution as the sodium salt of acetylcysteine, it is usually administered by nebulization for its local effect on the bronchopulmonary tree. Since the product also contains disodium edetate and sodium hydroxide, a slight odor can accompany its administration. Adverse effects may include stomatitis, nausea, and rhinorrhea. Asthmatics may experience bronchospasm with use of nebulized acetylcysteine.[48]

Absolon and Brown[49] compared the effects of an artificial tear solution with a 20% solution of acetylcysteine in a double-blind study in patients with keratoconjunctivitis sicca. They observed a greater objective improvement in signs such as conjunctival and corneal staining, mucus threads and filaments by slit-lamp examination in patients using the acetylcysteine solution. However, no subjective differences between the two groups were observed. The acetylcysteine solution produced a stinging sensation on instillation, which may in part explain the subjective results.

When used on the eye, Mucomyst can dissolve mucus threads as well as decrease tear viscosity.[49] A commercial artificial tear preparation containing acetylcysteine is presently not available, but it is commonly prepared for topical ocular use by diluting the commercial preparation to 2% to 5% in artificial tears or physiologic saline.

Lipid-Containing Formulations

In recent years the importance of a normal lipid layer in tear film stability has been emphasized.[50] This has led to the incorporation of lipid compounds into several artificial tear preparations. One such product, Tear Gard, is formulated by incorporating a phospholipid into an aqueous solution of hydroxyethylcellulose and inorganic buffers. Although the manufacturer claims that this product replaces all 3 layers of the tear film, controlled clinical trials in human subjects with dry eye syndromes are lacking, and the claims remain unsubstantiated.

Non-Preserved Tear Preparations

A major advance in artificial tear preparations is the introduction of preservative-free formulations. For patients who are sensitive to preservatives such as benzalkonium chloride and thimerosal, unit-dose packages of artificial tear solutions (see Table 10.2) or preservative-free ointments (Table 10.4) can be useful. The clinical disadvantages of such formulations is that the cost of unit-dose preparations is usually higher, and they can be easily contaminated by the patient during use. Strict hygienic procedures for instillation must be followed, and any excess solution must be discarded. Tips of ointment tubes should not come in contact with the eyes during instillation.

Bland Ointment Formulations

Another approach for lubrication and stabilization of the precorneal tear film is the use of nonmedicated, semisolid preparations of petrolatum and mineral oil to which lanolin may be added (see Table 10.4). Although these preparations melt at the temperature of the ocular tissue and disperse with the tear fluid, they appear to be retained longer than other ophthalmic vehicles.[51,52]

Several explanations have been offered as to why ointments are retained longer in the tear fluid. Because of their molecular size, petrolatum and mineral oil are not as easily removed by the lacrimal drainage system by blinking. Another significant factor appears to be the physiochemical relationship between the components of the ointment and the cornea. The fact that the precorneal tear film and the ointment bases both have nonpolar components may allow the adsorption of the oil bases to the cornea.[53] It has further been suggested that ointment droplets are trapped by mucus and often form a mucus thread along the inferior fornix.[51] If this is indeed true, the integrity of the mucin layer would be enhanced. Both mucin and aqueous deficient eyes may therefore benefit from the application of lubricating ointments.

TABLE 10.4
Composition of Bland Ointments

Trade Name (manufacturer)	Composition
Akwa Tears (Akorn)	White petrolatum, mineral oil, lanolin (preservative free)
Duolube (Bausch & Lomb)	White petrolatum, mineral oil (perservative free)
DuraTears (Alcon)	White petrolatum, anhydrous liquid lanolin, mineral oil, methylparaben, propylparaben
DuraTears Naturale (Alcon)	White petrolatum, anhydrous liquid lanolin, mineral oil (preservative free)
HypoTears (Iolab)	White petrolatum, light mineral oil (preservative free)
Lacri-Lube S.O.P. (Allergan)	White petrolatum, mineral oil, nonionic lanolin derivatives, chlorobutanol
Lacri-Lube NP (Allergan)	White petrolatum, mineral oil, petrolatum/lanolin alcohol (preservative free)
Ocu-Lube (Bausch & Lomb)	White petrolatum, mineral oil (preservative free)
Refresh PM (Allergan)	White petrolatum, sodium chloride, mineral oil, petrolatum/lanolin alcohol (preservative free)

Ointment formulations are usually administered in dosage frequencies of twice daily, but depending on the patient's clinical needs and the response to therapy, they may be administered as often as every few hours or only occasionally as needed. Bedtime instillation of ointments is often helpful in the treatment of exposure keratopathy secondary to nocturnal lagophthalmos.[51,53]

Patient acceptance of ointment preparations is highly variable. Blurred vision is a frequent complaint following the daytime instillation of ointment. This problem can usually be resolved by decreasing the amount instilled.[54] Ointment preparations are generally nonirritating to ocular tissue. In addition, ointment vehicles presently used do not appear to interfere with corneal or conjunctival wound healing. Ointment use, however, should be avoided in eyes with impending corneal perforations, deep or flap-like corneal abrasions, or severe corneal lacerations because of the possibility of ointment entrapment[54] (see Chapter 2).

Artificial Tear Inserts

A more recent approach to the treatment of moderate to severe dry eye syndromes has been the use of water-soluble inserts that provide a constant release of polymer.[55–57] When placed in the inferior cul de sac, these solid inserts dissolve over a period of hours while releasing their polymeric contents.

The artificial tear insert (Lacrisert, Merck) is a cylindrical rod approximately 1 mm wide and 4 mm long containing 5 mg of hydroxypropylcellulose without preservative. When placed in the inferior cul de sac it imbibes fluid and swells to several times its original volume (Fig. 10.2). Following the initial swelling, the insert dissolves over 6 to 8 hours.[58] It is designed to be replaced every 24 hours, although some patients require more frequent replacement.[58]

Measurement of the TBUT in rabbit and human subjects indicates that the insert prolongs breakup time. The effect lasts longer than with tear substitutes applied as drops.[59] It produces a tear film that is clinically thicker than normal and which appears to retain fluid within it.[60,61]

Clinical studies indicate that the insert can be beneficial in the treatment of certain dry eye syndromes such as keratitis sicca.[61,62] Some patients may experience relief of symptoms of burning, photophobia, and foreign body sensation. Corneal abnormalities may also be decreased, and rose bengal staining of cornea and conjunctiva may be reduced.[61,62]

The device is generally comfortable and well accepted by many patients, but some disadvantages are associated with its use. A moderate amount of dexterity is required to properly place the insert into the lower cul de sac. The most common patient complaint is blurred vision associated with the intense release of polymer after the first 4 to 6 hours following instillation, resulting in a thickened tear film.[61,62] Adding fluid such as drops of 0.9% NaCl or artificial tear solution can reduce the tear film viscosity and minimize the visual complaints.[61,62] As the insert dissolves, debris is released that can also blur vision and cause irritation. Most patients with only mild signs and symptoms of dry eye do not appreciate improvement with use of the insert compared with use of conventional artificial tear solutions. In fact, complaints of blurred vision and foreign body sensation often limit usefulness of the insert. In addition, absence of measurable tear secretion, as detected by a very low Schirmer test, seems to predict treatment failure with artificial tear inserts.[74]

Punctal Plugs

Occlusion of the lacrimal puncta has been used to preserve existing tears since Beetham[63] first advocated electrocautery of the canaliculi in 1936. Since cautery may be an irreversible procedure, punctal plugs have been developed to block tear drainage and thus prolong the action of natural tears as well as artificial tear preparations.

Two types of punctal plugs have become clinically acceptable. A silicone-based plug was evaluated by Freeman[64] in 1975, and more recently a temporary absorbable collagen implant has been introduced by Herrick.[65]

The Freeman Punctum Plug (Eagle Vision, Memphis, TN) is usually inserted directly into both inferior puncta. The method requires only topical anesthesia

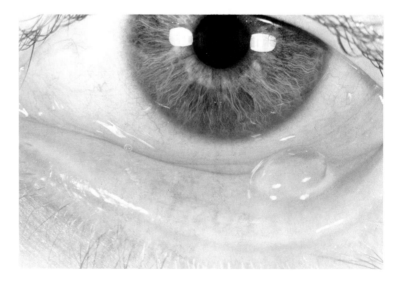

FIGURE 10.2   **Artificial tear insert (Lacrisert). Following placement of insert into inferior conjunctival sac with specially designed applicator (see Fig. 2.18), the insert swells to several times its original volume and begins to release the nonmedicated polymer to the eye.**

and expansion of the punctal opening with a punctal dilator. The plug is inserted to the base of the domed head, with the head of the plug resting outside the opening of the punctum. Insertion can be difficult, and the plugs are prone to expulsion, especially if the eyelid is rubbed by the patient or if ointments are used after placement.

The Temporary Intracanalicular Collagen Implant (Lacrimedics, Rosemead, CA) consists of 0.2, 0.3, or 0.4 mm diameter collagen implants packed on the edge of a foam strip (see Fig. 20.12). The implant is grasped from the package with a jeweler's forcep and, with the aid of magnification, is placed halfway into the punctal opening. It is then nudged until it is flush with the punctum and then further advanced into the horizontal canaliculus. Topical anesthetics may be used to minimize eyelid reaction, but the procedure can be performed without anesthesia. The aqueous environment of the canaliculus causes the collagen implant to swell, impeding tear flow by as much as 60% to 80%. Tear drainage can be blocked for up to 14 days before the implants are totally absorbed.

Punctal occlusion can benefit patients whose symptoms of dryness or other ocular abnormalities are not relieved by topical therapy alone.[66–68] Although rare, punctal occlusion can lead to epiphora. Tearing secondary to chronic dacryocystitis with mucopurulent discharge is a contraindication to the use of punctal plugs. Chapter 20 considers in further detail the use of punctal occlusion in dry eye syndromes.

References

1. Boerhave H. De morbis oculum. Gottingen, 1750.
2. Holly FJ. Artificial tear formulations. Int Ophthalmol Clin 1980;20:171–184.
3. Swan KC. Use of methylcellulose in ophthalmology. Arch Ophthalmol 1945;33:378–380.
4. Blaug SM, Canada AT. Relationship of viscosity, contact time, and prolongation of action of methyl-cellulose-containing ophthalmic solutions. Am J Hosp Pharm 1965;22:662–666.
5. Krishna N, Brow F. Polyvinyl alcohol as an ophthalmic vehicle: Effect on regeneration of corneal epithelium. Am J Ophthalmol 1964;57:99–106.
6. Lemp MA. Recent developments in dry eye management. Surv Ophthalmol 1987;94:1299–1304.
7. Wolff E. The muco-cutaneous junction of the lid-margin and the distribution of the tear fluid. Trans Ophthalmol Soc UK 1946;66:291–308.
8. Holly FJ, Lemp MA. Tear physiology and dry eyes. Surv Ophthalmol 1977;22:69–87.
9. Mishima S. Some physiological aspects of the precorneal tear film. Arch Ophthalmol 1965;73:233–241.
10. MacKay C, Abramson DH, Ellsworth RM, et al. Lactate dehydrogenase in tears. Am J Ophthalmol 1980;90:385–387.
11. Anderson JA, Leopold IH. Antiproteolytic activities found in human tears. Ophthalmology 1981;88:82–84.
12. Smolin G. The role of tears in the prevention of infections. Int Ophthalmol Clin 1987;27:25–26.
13. Holly FJ, Patten JT, Dohlman CH. Surface activity of aqueous tear components in dry eye patients and normals. Exp Eye Res 1977;24:479–491.
14. Holly FJ. Formation and rupture of the tear film. Exp Eye Res 1973;15:515–525.
15. Holly FJ. Tear film physiology. Int Ophthalmol Clin 1987;27:2–6.
16. Duke-Elder S. System of ophthalmology. IV. Physiology of the eye and vision. London: Kimptom, 1968;419–423.
17. McDonald JE. Surface phenomena of tear films. Trans Am Ophthalmol Soc 1968;66:905–939.
18. Pfister RR. The normal surface of the corneal epithelium. A scanning electron microscopic study. Invest Ophthalmol Vis Sci 1973;12:654–668.
19. Van Alphen GWHM. Acetylcholine synthesis in corneal epithelium. Arch Ophthalmol 1957;58:449–451.
20. Benedetto DA, Shah DO, Kaufman HE. The instilled fluid dynamics and surface chemistry of polymers in the preocular tear film. Invest Ophthalmol Vis Sci 1975;14:887–902.
21. Lemp MA, Szymanski ES. Polymer adsorption at the ocular surface. Arch Ophthalmol 1975;93:134–136.
22. Havener WH. Ocular pharmacology, ed. 5. St. Louis: C. V. Mosby Co, 1983;628–630.
23. Norn MS. Desiccation of the precorneal film. I. Corneal wetting time. Acta Ophthalmol 1969;47:865–880.
24. Geeting DG, Bakar SR. In vivo comparison of ocular lubricants in patients having reduced tear film break-up times. J Am Optom Assoc 1980;8:757–780.
25. Lemp MA, Goldberg M, Roddy MR. Effect of tear substitutes on tear film breakup time. Invest Ophthalmol 1975;14:225–258.
26. Pfister RR, Burstein N. The effects of ophthalmic drugs, vehicles, and preservatives on corneal epithelium. A scanning electron microscope study. Invest Ophthalmol 1976;15:246–259.
27. Alexander CM, Newell FW. The effect of various agents on corneal epithelialization. Am J Ophthalmol 1959;48:210–211.
28. Krishna N, Mitchell B. Polyvinyl alcohol as an ophthalmic vehicle: Effect on ocular structures. Am J Ophthalmol 1965;59:860–864.
29. Norn MS, Opauszki A. Effects of ophthalmic vehicles on the stability of the precorneal film. Acta Ophthalmol 1977;55:23–34.
30. Lemp MA, Holly FJ. Ophthalmic polymers as ocular wetting agents. Ann Ophthalmol 1972;4:15–20.
31. Lemp MA, Hamill JR. Factors affecting tear film breakup in normal eyes. Arch Ophthalmol 1973;89:103–105.
32. Sommer A, Green WR. Goblet cell response to vitamin A treatment for corneal xerophthalmia. Am J Ophthalmol 1982;94:213–215.
33. Sommer A. Treatment of corneal xerophthalmia with topical retinoic acid. Am J Ophthalmol 1983;95:349–352.
34. Tseng SCG, Maumenee AE, Stark WS, Maumenee IH, et al. Topical retinoid treatment of various dry-eye disorders. Ophthalmology 1985;92:717–727.

35. Tseng SCG. Topical retinoid treatment for dry eye disorders. Trans Ophthalmol Soc UK 1985;104:489–495.

36. Wright P. Topical retinoic acid therapy for disorders of the outer eye. Trans Ophthalmol Soc UK 1985;104:869–874.

37. Tseng SCG. Topical tretinoin treatment for dry-eye disorders. Int Ophthalmol Clin 1987;27:47–53.

38. Vidaurri LJ, Huang ASW, Tseng SCG. Pharmacokinetics of topical tretinoin in normal rabbit eyes. Invest Ophthalmol Vis Sci 1986;27:24.

39. Pape LG, Balazs EA. The use of sodium hyaluronate (Healon) in human anterior segment surgery. Ophthalmology 1980;87:699–705.

40. Miller D, Stegman R. Healon: A comprehensive guide to its use. In: Ophthalmic surgery, New York: John Wiley & Sons, 1983.

41. Polack RM, McNiece MT. The treatment of dry eyes with Na hyaluronate (Healon). Cornea 1982;1:133–136.

42. DeLuise VP, Peterson WS. The use of topical Healon tears in the management of refractory dry-eye syndrome. Ann Ophthalmol 1984;16:823–824.

43. Stuart JC, Linn JG. Dilute sodium hyaluronate (Healon) in the treatment of ocular surface disorders. Ann Ophthalmol 1985;17:190–192.

44. Mengher LS, Pandher KS, Bron AJ, et al. Effect of sodium hyaluronate (0.1%) on break-up time (NIBUT) in patients with dry eyes. Br J Ophthalmol 1986;70:442–447.

45. Richter W, Ryde M, Zetterstrom O. Nonimmunogenicity of a purified sodium hyaluronate preparation in man. Int Arch Appl Immunol 1979;59:45–48.

46. Limberg MB, McCaa C, Kissling GE, et al. Topical application of hyaluronic acid and chondroitin sulfate in treatment of dry eyes. Am J Ophthalmol 1987;103:194–197.

47. Webb WR. Clinical evaluation of a new mucolytic agent acetylcysteine. J Thorac Cardiovasc Surg 1962;44:330–335.

48. Mucomyst. Physicians Desk Reference. Oradell, NJ: Medical Economics Co, 1988;752.

49. Absolon MJ, Brown CA. Acetylcysteine in keratoconjunctivitis sicca. Br J Ophthalmol 1968;52:310–316.

50. Holly FJ. Surface chemical evaluation of a novel lipid containing tear substitute. Contacto 1982;26:5–7.

51. Norn MS. Role of vehicles in local treatment of the eye. Acta Ophthalmol 1964;42:727–734.

52. Hardberger R, Hanna C, Boyd CM. Effect of drug vehicles on ocular contact time. Arch Ophthalmol 1975;93:42–45.

53. Stenbeck A, Ostholm I. Ointments for ophthalmic use. Acta Ophthalmol 1954;43:405–423.

54. Hanna C, Fraunfelder FT, Cable M, Hardberger RE. Effect of ophthalmic ointments on corneal wound healing. Am J Ophthalmol 1973;76:193–200.

55. Bloomfield SE, Dunn MW, Miyata T, et al. Soluble artificial tear inserts. Arch Ophthalmol 1977;95:247–250.

56. Beslin CW, Katz J, Kaufman HE, Katz I. Slow release artificial tears. In: Leopold IH, Burns RP, eds. Symposium on ocular therapy. New York: John Wiley & Sons, 1977;10:77–83.

57. Katz MK, Blackman WM. A soluble sustained-release ophthalmic delivery unit. Am J Ophthalmol 1977;83:728–734.

58. Lamberts DW, Langston DP, Chu W. A clinical study of slow-releasing artificial tears. Ophthalmology 1978;85:794–800.

59. Gautheron PD, Lotti YJ, Le Douraree JC. Tear film breakup time prolonged with unmedicated cellulose polymer inserts. Arch Ophthalmol 1979;97:1944–1947.

60. Katz JI, Kaufman HE, Breslin C, Katz IM. Slow-release artificial tears and the treatment of keratitis sicca. Ophthalmology 1978;85:778–793.

61. Werblin TP, Rheinstrom SD, Kaufman HE. The use of slow-release artificial tears in the long-term management of keratitis sicca. Ophthalmology 1981;88:78–81.

62. Hording G, Aasred H. Slow-release artificial tears (SRAT) in dry eye disease. Acta Ophthalmol 1981;59:842–846.

63. Beetham WP. Filamentary keratitis. Trans Am Ophthalmol Soc 1936;33:413–435.

64. Freeman JM. Punctal plug: Evaluation of a new treatment for dry eyes. Trans Am Acad Ophthalmol Otolaryngol 1975;79:874–879.

65. Herrick RS. Collagen implants said to help Dx of keratoconjunctivitis sicca. Ophthalmol Times 1985;10:3.

66. Dohlman CH. Punctal occlusion in keratoconjunctivitis sicca. Ophthalmology 1978;85:1277–1281.

67. Tuberville AW, Frederick WR, Wood TO. Punctal occlusion in tear deficiency syndromes. Ophthalmology 1982;89:1170–1172.

68. Willis RM, Folberg R, Krachmer JH, Holland EJ. The treatment of aqueous-deficient dry eye with removable punctal plugs. Ophthalmology 1987;94:514–518.

69. Holly FJ. Dry eye and artificial tear formulations. Contact Lens Forum 1988;13:30–38.

70. Bigar F, Gloor B, Schimmelpfennig B, et al. Die verträglichkeit von hydroxypropylmethylcellulose bei der implantation von hinterkammer-linsen. Klin Monatsbl Augenheilk 1988;193:21–24.

71. Ubels JL, Foley KM, Rismondo V. Retinol secretion by the lacrimal gland. Invest Ophthalmol Vis Sci 1986;27:1261–1262.

72. Ohasi Y, Watanabe H, Kinoshita S, et al. Vitamin A eyedrops for superior limbic keratoconjunctivitis. Am J Ophthalmol 1988;105:523–527.

73. Nelson JD, Farris RL. Sodium hyaluronate and polyvinyl alcohol artificial tear preparations. A comparison in patients with keratoconjunctivitis sicca. Arch Ophthalmol 1988;106:484–488.

74. Lindahl G, Calissendorff B, Carle B. Clinical trial of sustained-release artificial tears in keratoconjunctivitis sicca and Sjogren's syndrome. Acta Ophthalmol 1988;66:9–14.

75. Soong HK, Martin NF, Wagoner MD, et al. Topical retinoid therapy for squamous metaplasia of various ocular surface disorders. A multicenter, placebo-controlled, double-masked study. Ophthalmology 1988;95:1442–1446.

CHAPTER 11

Antihistamines

Sally L. Hegeman

Antihistamines are used to block the actions of endogenously produced histamine. Histamine has a number of effects on cells and tissues, especially when released from mast cells in large quantities as part of a type I allergic reaction. Some of the associated clinical manifestations, such as anaphylactic shock, are life-threatening, while other effects, such as rhinitis, tearing and redness of the eye, and itching, are benign although disturbing to the patient.

The two classes of antihistaminic drugs, H_1 and H_2, are so designated because of the nature of the histamine receptor to which they bind. H_1 antihistamines, developed in the 1940s, prevent histamine-H_1 receptor interaction and thus provide symptomatic relief from histamine activity. H_1 antihistamines have a variety of pharmacologic actions that impart to this class of drugs a wide range of therapeutic uses in addition to the symptomatic relief of allergic reactions. H_2 antihistamines, developed in the 1960s, prevent histamine interaction with the H_2 receptor.

This chapter considers the pharmacologic actions of histamine and the antihistaminic agents of clinical importance in the therapy of allergic ocular disease.

Hypersensitivity Reactions

A hypersensitivity reaction is a pathologic condition caused by an exaggerated response of the immune system to an antigen, or foreign substance, to which the immune system has been previously exposed. Hypersensitivity reactions are divided into types I, II, III, and IV,[1,2] based essentially on the pathology involved, nature of the immune response, and sites of interaction of antibody and antigen.

Type I Reactions

Type I hypersensitivity reactions, also known as anaphylactic, immediate, or IgE-mediated reactions, occur when an antigen such as a drug or pollen is reintroduced into an individual who has previously been exposed to the antigen. The first exposure produces IgE antibodies that attach to mast cells and make the cells susceptible to rupture when the antigen is reintroduced. Disruption of mast cells causes release of large quantities of pharmacologically active chemicals that may, within minutes after exposure to the antigen, cause anaphylactic shock, asthma, urticaria, angioedema, or gastrointestinal disturbance. Type I reactions occur in hay fever, allergic conjunctivitis, some aspects of vernal conjunctivitis, asthma, and reactions to penicillin, bee stings, and many other chemicals and toxins.

Type II Reactions

Type II reactions, also known as cytotoxic or cell-stimulating reactions, or cytolytic complement-dependent cytotoxicity reactions, are characterized by an exogenous antigen combining with cell surfaces, making the cells susceptible to attack by the body's immunologic system. Antibodies bind to the attached antigens, and the complex initiates activation of the complement system, which ultimately causes either phagocytosis or lysis of the affected cell. Examples of type II reactions are found in mismatched blood transfusions, early stages of graft rejection in kidney and other transplants, and penicillin-induced hemolytic anemia.

Type III Reactions

Type III reactions, also known as toxic complex reactions, soluble-complex or immune-complex reactions, occur when circulating antibody-antigen complexes precipitate out in tissues, causing an acute inflammatory reaction. Tissues that are especially involved are joints, the kidney glomerulus, and lung. Serum sickness, due to agents such as serum, venom, and drugs, is partly caused by a type III reaction, as are some of the symptoms of rheumatoid arthritis, systemic lupus erythematosus (SLE), acute glomerulonephritis, and hypersensitivity pneumonitis.

Type IV Reactions

Type IV reactions, also known as tuberculin type, cellular, cell-mediated, or delayed reactions, differ from the other three types of hypersensitivity reactions in that sensitized T-lymphocytes, rather than antibodies, interact with antigen. The interaction of the T-lymphocyte and antigen injures tissue by either a direct toxic effect or by causing release of lymphokines from the T-lymphocyte. Lymphokines[3] are a group of biologically active chemicals, some of which are involved in the acute inflammatory response. Contact dermatitis, the Mantoux tuberculin test, and allograft rejection are believed to be due to type IV reactions. In ocular tissues, vernal conjunctivitis, atopic keratoconjunctivitis, and preservative-induced blepharoconjunctivitis in contact lens wearers are mediated, at least in part, by type IV reactions.[4]

Histamine

Histamine is synthesized and stored in nearly all tissues, with especially high concentrations in the lungs, skin, stomach, duodenum, and nasal mucosa.[5] In normal, nonhuman ocular tissues, histamine is found in highest concentrations in the surface portions of the eye, namely, the lids, conjunctiva, subconjunctiva, episclera, and limbus. The uveal tissues have low but measurable concentrations of histamine, while the lens, aqueous humor, retina, and other internal ocular structures have essentially none.[6] Human ocular tissues, enucleated because of trauma, uncontrolled glaucoma,

or endophthalmitis, were studied by Nowak and Nawrocki,[7] who found histamine in the iris, ciliary body, choroid, retina, sclera, and optic nerve, with the highest levels in the uvea and the lowest levels in the retina and sclera. Tissues from traumatized eyes contained less histamine than eyes with endophthalmitis, although the pattern of high histamine content in the uvea and low histamine content in the sclera and retina was consistent in all groups. Histamine content was intermediate in tissues from eyes with glaucoma.

Histamine is produced by the conversion of the amino acid, histidine, to histamine by the enzymes histidine decarboxylase and L aromatic amino acid decarboxylase (Fig. 11.1A). Some of the histamine is stored, along with a number of other biologically active chemicals, in tissue mast cells and blood basophils, while a quantity of histamine, referred to as nascent histamine, is synthesized de novo and is used according to the cells' needs. Metabolism of histamine is shown in Figure 11.1B and involves two pathways, with diamine oxidase (histaminase) and monoamine oxidase (MAO) as the principal metabolic enzymes.[5]

Mast Cell Histamine

It has been difficult to ascribe a physiologic function to mast cell histamine, which, when released, produces adverse nonphysiologic symptoms such as severe headache, urticaria (hives), angioneurotic edema, bronchospasm, and anaphylactic shock. However, studies[4,8] suggest that mast cell histamine may be an important modulator of many aspects of the immune response and that the adverse symptoms associated with histamine release occur only when the histamine receptor is somehow deficient or abnormal.

Although many chemical and physical agents are known to degranulate mast cells, from a therapeutic point of view the most important histamine-releasing agents are certain drugs and allergens.[9] Drugs, or physical agents such as heat, often cause release of histamine by a direct action on the mast cell. Drugs are most likely to induce histamine release when administered intravenously, and signs and symptoms of histamine release usually occur within minutes after drug injection. Drugs that cause release of histamine by a direct action on the mast cell include morphine, codeine, atropine, curare, hydralazine, and meperidine.[10]

Drugs may also be allergens and cause histamine release by allergen-induced sensitization of mast cells.[3] When an allergen (drug, pollen, dander) enters the body, the immune system is stimulated to produce specific antibodies to the allergen. When the antibody is of the IgE variety, the potential for mast cell sensitization is established. The IgE antibodies attach to

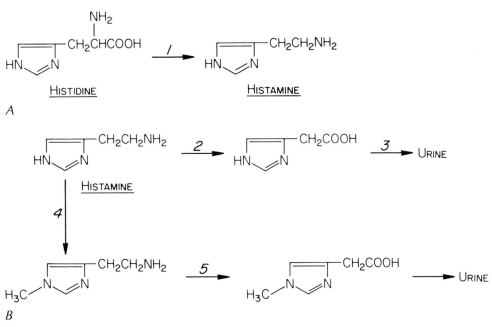

FIGURE 11.1 *(A)* **Synthesis of histamine from the amino acid, histidine. 1 (histidine decarboxylase).** *(B)* **Metabolism of histamine. 2 (diamine oxidase), 3 (elimination as either imidazole acetic acid or as the riboside conjugate), 4 (N-methyltransferase), 5 (monoamine oxidase).**

the mast cell, and when the allergen is reintroduced, the allergen will interact with the IgE mast cell (Fig. 11.2). This causes degranulation of the mast cell, with the release of histamine, leukotrienes (formerly known as slow-reacting substance of anaphylaxis, SRS-A), and other inflammatory mediators into the blood (type I hypersensitivity reaction). Penicillin most frequently induces histamine release by this mechanism, but procaine, salicylates, folic acid, and thiamine, and a variety of protein drugs such as insulin, ACTH, and heparin, commonly do so as well.[9]

Nonmast Cell (Nascent) Histamine

A number of physiologic roles have been proposed for nonmast cell histamine—histamine that is synthesized according to cellular demands. Since an increase in the rate of synthesis of histamine occurs during growth and repair of tissue, it has been proposed that histamine is involved in tissue growth and repair processes.[11] Because nonmast cell histamine is associated with certain capillary beds, a role in regulation of capillary permeability has also been suggested.[12] There is some evi-

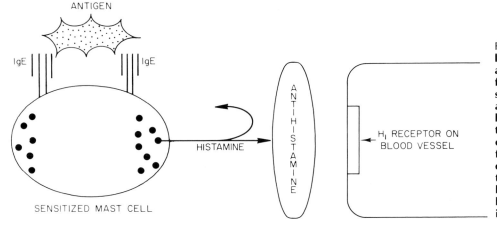

FIGURE 11.2 **Sensitized mast cell liberates histamine, leukotriene, and many other mediators of inflammation and the immune response on interaction of specific antigen and IgE antibodies (type I hypersensitivity reaction). IgE antibodies are antibodies to the specific antigen and are produced and fixed on mast cells during a prior exposure to the antigen. Antihistamines reversibly bind to the histamine receptor and prevent histamine and histamine receptor interaction.**

dence that histamine may serve as a central nervous system (CNS) neurotransmitter,[13] and it is well established that histamine is a regulator of gastric acid secretion.[14] Nonmast cell histamine is probably not involved in the clinical manifestations (anaphylaxis, urticaria) associated with mast cell histamine release.

Histamine Receptors

Two types of histamine receptors have been described: H_1, or classic, and H_2. The distinction between the two is based on the chemical structure of the antihistamine that binds to the receptor and on the type of histamine agonist (Fig. 11.3). For example, a methyl group on the C_2 position of the imidazole ring confers H_1 agonist selectivity, while a methyl group on the C_4 position of the imidazole ring confers H_2 agonist selectivity. H_1 receptors are found in many tissues, including the smooth muscle of bronchi, blood vessels, and intestine. Antihistamines commonly used to treat allergies, such as diphenhydramine, are effective blockers of the H_1 receptor. H_2 receptors are present in gastric parietal cells, the heart, pulmonary blood vessels, cells of the immune system, and other tissues. Many tissues contain both H_1 and H_2 receptors, and the effects of simultaneously stimulating both may be antagonistic or complementary, depending on the specific tissue. H_2 receptor action is blocked by the antihistamines cimetidine, ranitidine, nizatidine, and famotidine, drugs used extensively for the treatment of peptic ulcers. The distribution of H_1 and H_2 receptors and their common antagonists are summarized in Table 11.1.

Pharmacologic Actions of Histamine

Histamine is essentially ineffective when administered orally. When parenterally administered, however, or when there is massive mast cell disruption, histamine causes significant vascular effects including transient flushing of the face and neck, reduced blood pressure, and edema. Blood vessels contain H_1 and H_2 histamine receptors that, when stimulated, dilate the small precapillary blood vessels and constrict the larger venules, which causes passive capillary dilatation, pooling of blood, and hypotension. In addition, histamine causes edema by constricting the cells of the small venules, thus exposing the basement membrane, which allows plasma to pass into extracellular space. The triple response of Lewis,[15] produced when a small amount of histamine (10 μg) is injected intradermally, illustrates such dilatation and edema. Initially there is local redness caused by a direct vasodilator action of histamine, then a neuronally mediated diffuse redness, followed

by a wheal at the site of the initial localized erythema caused by increased capillary permeability. A reaction similar to this triple response is observed with both allergic and physical injury to the skin.

Heart rate and force of contraction increases with histamine administration. H_2 receptor activation causes increased rate and force of contraction, while H_1 receptors produce increased force of contraction and decreased AV conduction. Although histamine also stimulates the heart by releasing norepinephrine from adrenergic nerve terminals, the precise role of histamine in cardiac physiology is not understood.

Bronchial smooth muscle constriction is another consequence of histamine injection or mast cell degranulation. Stimulation of the H_1 receptors, in particular, produces constriction, while stimulation of H_2 receptors produces relaxation. In non-asthmatic individuals histamine produces only slight constriction due to the balancing effects of both receptors. In asthmatics, however, histamine injection can provoke severe bronchospasm, probably because the H_2 receptors are either deficient or abnormal in such individuals.[8] Although there is no question that injected histamine will produce some bronchospasm, histamine is not believed to be the only bronchoconstrictor involved during an asthmatic attack, since antihistamines will not terminate the attack. Other mast cell substituents, including leukotrienes, are considered to be more important mediators of asthma. Some leukotrienes derived from prostaglandins have been purified and shown to be 100 to 1000 times more potent than histamine in constricting the bronchial tree.[16]

Subcutaneous doses of histamine stimulate gastric acid secretion by parietal cells but produce no other obvious pharmacologic effects. Gastrin and an intact vagus nerve are required for maximal gastric acid secretion. Cimetidine and other H_2 blockers will inhibit gastric acid secretion whether it is caused by increased vagal activity, histamine, food, or gastrin. Histamine appears, therefore, to have a key role in gastric secretion either by allowing hormones or transmitters to function or by being the final stimulator of the parietal cell.

In the eye histamine release produces the characteristic symptoms of ocular allergy: itching, redness, tearing, and chemosis. Signs of ocular allergy include conjunctival and lid edema, dilation of conjunctival blood vessels, and evidence of a papillary reaction.[4]

In animal studies topically administered or injected histamine produces hyperemia and edema in the uvea and conjunctiva, increased intraocular pressure, mild pupillary constriction, and, in some cases, leaking of the blood-aqueous barrier.[6] Blood vessels dilate and leak in structures such as the iris, conjunctiva, and ciliary processes. Histamine, however, has no effect on retinal blood vessels.

RECEPTOR   COMPOUND

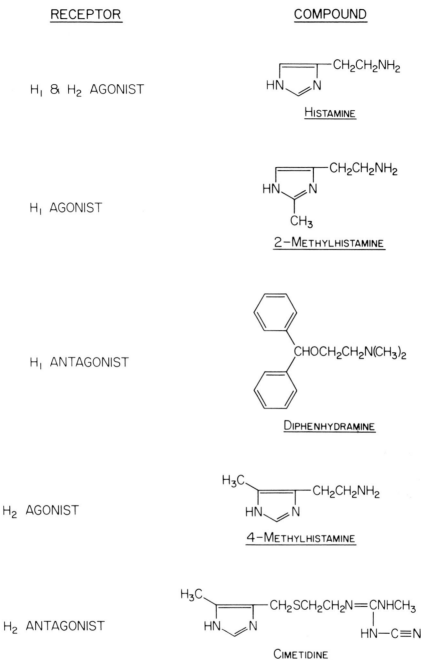

H_1 & H_2 AGONIST

HISTAMINE

H_1 AGONIST

2-METHYLHISTAMINE

H_1 ANTAGONIST

DIPHENHYDRAMINE

H_2 AGONIST

4-METHYLHISTAMINE

H_2 ANTAGONIST

CIMETIDINE

FIGURE 11.3   **Structures of representative H_1 and H_2 agonists and antagonists.**

H_1 Antihistamines

Pharmacology

The pharmacologic diversity of the H_1 antihistamines can be explained by the variety of chemical structures in this class of agents. Figure 11.4 shows the general structure of an H_1 antihistamine. By altering the aryl X group of the general structure, H_1 antihistamines with quite different pharmacologic properties can be synthesized. Thus, the practitioner may choose from the many H_1 antihistamines the agent most suited to the patient's needs.

The H_1 antihistamines are rapidly and completely

TABLE 11.1
Distribution of H₁ and H₂ Receptors[a]

Histamine Receptor	Tissue	Representative Antagonists
H₁	Bronchial smooth muscle Heart CNS Mucous membranes Eye (blood vessels) Blood vessels	Phenoxybenzamine Diphenhydramine Chlorpheniramine Pyrilamine maleate Promethazine Dimenhydrinate Antazoline Cyclizine Terfenadine
H₂	Gastric parietal cells Heart Blood vessels Mast cells Eye (blood vessels) Bronchial smooth muscle CNS White blood cells	Cimetidine Ranitidine Famotidine

[a]Refs. 5, 8, 13, 14, 29.

absorbed after oral administration. Drug effects are observed within 30 minutes, and peak effects are present from 1 to 2 hours. Drug action lasts approximately 4 to 6 hours. Since the H₁ antihistamines are lipid soluble, they readily penetrate the blood-brain, blood-placental, and blood-ocular barriers. The H₁ antihistamines that have been studied are completely metabolized by the liver, and the metabolites are excreted in the urine.

The site of action of the H₁ antihistamines is shown in Figure 11.2. The antihistamines reversibly bind to the histamine receptor, thus preventing histamine-receptor interaction.

In addition to histamine-blocking actions, the H₁ antihistamines have important antimuscarinic, local anesthetic, and CNS effects. The histamine-blocking properties of the H₁ antihistamines are predictable based on an appreciation of the biologic actions of histamine. Histamine-induced capillary dilatation, increase in capillary permeability, and the associated itching and pain are blocked by the H₁ antihistamines. If the dilatation and edema have already occurred, administration of such drugs will prevent further histamine action but will usually not reverse those clinical manifestations already present.

Considerable therapeutic use is made of H₁ antihistamines in the symptomatic relief of allergen-induced urticaria, mucosal congestion, and itching. However, H₁ antihistamines are not useful in preventing or terminating an asthmatic attack because histamine is only marginally involved in the pathogenesis of bronchospasm. Although anaphylactic shock and angioedema, which are histamine mediated and often life threatening, may be relieved by antihistamines, the slow onset of antihistaminic action is such that these emergencies necessitate subcutaneous administration of the physiologic antagonist, epinephrine. H₁ antihistamines are useful, however, as adjuncts to prevent additional symptoms from developing.

Anticholinergic actions are often observed in varying degrees with use of H₁ antihistamines; pyrilamine has few anticholinergic effects while diphenhydramine and promethazine have considerable anticholinergic action.[17] Although the anticholinergic actions of H₁ antihistamines are usually considered annoying side effects, therapeutic advantage is taken of their atropine-like effects in the treatment of Parkinson's disease and motion sickness. H₁ antihistamines such as dimenhydrinate, cyclizine, and meclizine are used alone, or in combination with scopolamine, in the treatment of motion sickness, a motion-induced disturbance of the vestibular apparatus of the ear, which has a cholinergic component in its central control mechanism. Even though antihistamines with the greatest anticholinergic action are effective in the treatment of motion sickness, other noncholinergic mechanisms may be important in the antiemetic properties of this class of drugs.

Although the CNS can be depressed or stimulated by the H₁ antihistamines, depression is the more common action. Sedation, a common side effect of many H₁ receptor antagonists, may have an anticholinergic basis, but other central mechanisms are presumed to be involved as well. Therapeutic use is made of the sedative properties of diphenhydramine in over-the-counter (OTC) sleeping medications and of promethazine in prescription sedatives. Terfenadine, on the other hand, is useful because it lacks sedative properties and can be used to relieve mild symptoms of seasonal allergic rhinitis and conjunctivitis in those patients for whom sedation would be dangerous or interfere with activity.[18,19] Not all patients, however, obtain relief with terfenadine, and it appears to be useful only when symptoms are mild to moderate.[20]

Local anesthetic properties probably explain some of the antipruritic effects of topically applied H₁ antihistamines. Topical administration provides therapeutically effective control of allergic symptoms in the

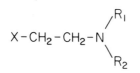

FIGURE 11.4   **General structure of an H₁ antihistamine.**

skin, but since the risk of sensitization is high, this route of administration should be used conservatively.

Clinical Uses

H$_1$ antihistamines, administered systemically or topically, are indicated for the relief of symptoms of mild to moderate allergic conjunctivitis or irritation (see Chapter 21), where the symptoms are caused by disruption of mast cells and the release of histamine. However, when the symptoms are severe or the degree of inflammation is high, corticosteroid therapy is usually required. Additional indications for antihistamines include lid myokymia (see Chapter 19) and prevention of histamine-induced miosis during cataract surgery.[19]

Three H$_1$ antihistamines are currently available for the topical treatment of ocular allergic reactions; pyrilamine maleate, pheniramine maleate, and antazoline phosphate.[20] Although these agents may be applied alone, they are commercially available only in combination with a vasoconstrictor, either phenylephrine or naphazoline (Table 11.2). The combination of an antihistamine and a vasoconstrictor is superior for relief of conjunctival signs and symptoms than is either drug used alone.[21,22]

One or 2 drops every 3 to 4 hours is the recommended dosage regimen for each of the available antihistaminic preparations. The warnings, precautions, and adverse effects are similar for all preparations. Since systemic effects can occur with topically administered drugs, the addition of phenylephrine or naphazoline to such topical antihistamines can, by its adrenergic agonist actions, exacerbate cardiovascular disease, hypertension, and diabetes, especially in elderly patients. Mydriasis and elevated intraocular pressure are potential ocular side effects caused by both the vasoconstrictor and the antihistamine. Accordingly, administration of these preparations may precipitate acute angle-closure glaucoma in susceptible individuals. With long-term use local hypersensitivity reactions may also occur, attributable primarily to the antihistaminic component.

Ocular allergic symptoms of itching, redness, and tearing are often successfully controlled by oral administration of antihistamines. Many oral preparations are available OTC. Representative oral preparations, dosage regimens, and side effects are listed in Table 11.3.

Side Effects

Sedation and depression of reflexes and sensory input are the most worrisome side effects of all antihistam-

TABLE 11.2
Antihistaminic-Vasoconstrictor Preparations for Topical Ocular Use

Trade Name (manufacturer)	Composition	Concentration (%)
Albalon-A (Allergan)	Antazoline phosphate Naphazoline HCl	0.5 0.05
Vasocon-A (Iolab)	Antazoline phosphate Naphazoline HCl	0.5 0.05
Naphcon-A (Alcon)	Pheniramine maleate Naphazoline HCl	0.3 0.025
Prefrin-A (Allergan)	Pyrilamine maleate Phenylephrine HCl	0.1 0.12
AK-Vernacon (Akorn)	Pheniramine maleate Phenylephrine HCl	0.5 0.125
AK-Con-A (Akorn)	Pheniramine maleate Naphazoline HCl	0.3 0.025
Muro's Opcon-A (Bausch & Lomb)	Pheniramine maleate Naphazoline HCl	0.3 0.025

ines, especially in those patients who drive or operate hazardous machinery. Sedation can be minimized by careful drug dosage, or by changing to another antihistaminic preparation. *ALCOHOL (OR OTHER CNS DEPRESSANTS) AND ANTIHISTAMINES DO NOT MIX.* Serious accidents occur because of the synergistic sedative actions of alcohol and H$_1$ antihistamines. Because of the many sites of action of the H$_1$ antihistamines, a large number of other drug interactions occur. In addition to increasing the actions of CNS depressants, H$_1$ antihistamines are additive with the anticholinergics, adrenergic agonists, phenothiazines, and MAO inhibitors. The actions of adrenergic blockers, corticosteroids, and phenylbutazone, on the other hand, are decreased.[21]

Bothersome systemic side effects include palpitations; drying of secretions in the throat and bronchi; and gastrointestinal and urinary tract disturbances such as anorexia, nausea, vomiting, diarrhea or constipation, urinary frequency, and dysuria. Several of these effects can be minimized by taking the agents with meals. Adjustment of dose or change of drug may also decrease or eliminate these effects.

Ocular side effects relate primarily to the anticholinergic properties of the H$_1$ antihistamine. Accordingly, one can anticipate mydriasis with the potential of acute angle-closure glaucoma, decreased secretion of tears and mucus, and, with continued use, anisocoria, decreased accommodation, and decreased vision. These atropine-like effects are not common, and usually the antihistaminic therapy can be continued, since these effects typically diminish with time.[21]

Cyclizine and structurally related compounds, which are used in the treatment of motion sickness, are associated with teratogenic effects in animals.[26] Therefore, these agents should not be administered during pregnancy.

Allergic reactions to H_1 antihistamines may occur with oral administration but are much more likely following topical use.[27] The ocular allergic signs and symptoms are similar to the conditions for which the antihistamine was prescribed. The allergic condition has two etiologic factors—the original allergy and the allergic response to the H_1 antihistamine. Because of the structural diversity of H_1 antihistamines, an allergic reaction to one agent does not imply hypersensitivity to another H_1 drug. Accordingly, the practitioner can change to another, structurally different H_1 antihistamine.

When used in recommended dosages, antihistamines are reasonably safe drugs. Acute toxicity following massive doses is characterized by marked CNS stimulation (convulsions) in children and depression (coma) followed by stimulation (convulsions) in adults. Coma, cardiorespiratory failure, and death follow convulsions in cases of severe toxicity. Treatment is supportive.

Phenobarbital or diazepam therapy may be attempted during the convulsive phase.[28]

Contraindications

H_1 antihistamines are contraindicated if there is a known hypersensitivity reaction to the agent. Oral preparations are also contraindicated in nursing mothers and in the third trimester of pregnancy because the H_1 antihistamines are secreted in milk and because infants and neonates appear to be more susceptible to these drugs' adverse effects.[17] As with all medication, extreme caution should be used in prescribing antihistamines to women in the first 3 months of pregnancy, when the risk of fetal malformation is very high.[9] Antihistamines with a strong anticholinergic component should be avoided in patients with peptic ulcer disease, prostatic hypertrophy, and bladder or pyloroduodenal obstruction and in patients who have the potential for acute angle-closure glaucoma.[17] The antihistamines and CNS drugs such as sedatives, MAO inhibitors, antianxiety agents, and narcotic analgesics are additive, and their concomitant use should be discouraged.[17,21,30] Because of the number of H_1 antihistamines and their diverse pharmacologic properties, and because of po-

TABLE 11.3
Representative Orally Administered H₁ Antihistamines

Drug	Strength (mg)	Dosage Form[a]	Adult Daily Dose (mg)[b]	Rx/ OTC	Trade Name	Antihistaminic Activity[c]	Sedation[c]	Anticholinergic Activity[c]
Diphenhy-dramine	25,50 12.5/5 ml	Capsule Elixir, syrup	25-50 q 4-6 h	OTC	Benadryl	+ +	+ + +	+ + +
Tripelenna-mine	25,50 100	Tablet Tablet (TR)	25-50 q 4-6 h 1 tab q 8-12 h	Rx Rx	PBZ PBZ SR	+ to + +	+ +	±
Chlorpheni-ramine	4,2/5 ml	Tablet, syrup	4 q 4-6 h	OTC	Chlor-Trimeton	+ + to + + +	+	+ to + +
	8, 12	Tablet (TR), Capsule (TR)	1 tab q 8-12 h	OTC Rx/ OTC	Chlor-Trimeton			
Dexchlor-phenira-mine	2,2/5 ml	Tablet, syrup	2 q 4-6 h	Rx	Polaramine	+ + +	+	+ +
	4, 6	Tablet (TR)	1 tab q 8-10 h	Rx	Polaramine			
Brompheni-ramine	4,2/5 ml 8,12	Tablet, elixir Tablet (TR)	4 q 4-6 h 1 tab q 8-12 h	OTC OTC	Dimetane Dimetane Extentab	+ + +	+	+ +
Triprolidine	2.5	Tablet	2.5 q 4-6 h	OTC	Actidil	+ + to + + +	+	+ +
	1.25/5 ml	Syrup	2.5 q 4-6 h	OTC	Actidil			
Terfenadine	60	Tablet	60 q 12 h	Rx	Seldane	+ + to + + +	±	±

[a]TR, Timed release.
[b]For dosage recommendations in children 2–6 and 6–12, consult the package literature.
[c]+ + + + = very high; + + + = high; + + = moderate; + = low; ± = low to none.
Modified from Covington TR. Rational antihistamine therapy. Facts and Comparisons Drug Newsletter 1988;7:65–67.

tentially dangerous interactions with many medications, the clinician prescribing antihistamines should fully understand the actions and side effects of these agents.

H$_2$ Antihistamines

H$_2$ antihistamines, such as cimetidine (Tagamet), block the actions of H$_2$ histamine receptors located in the heart, eye, vascular and respiratory smooth muscle, and parietal cells of the stomach, but they are useful therapeutically only for their action on stomach parietal cells. Cimetidine and the newer H$_2$ blockers, ranitidine, nizatidine, and famotidine, are remarkably effective for the treatment of peptic ulcers, Zollinger-Ellison syndrome, and other diseases associated with increased gastric acid secretion.

H$_2$ antagonists produce relatively few adverse side effects. Agranulocytosis was observed with some of the older H$_2$ antagonists, but almost never with cimetidine, ranitidine, nizatidine, or famotidine. Skin rashes, headache, muscle pain, gynecomastia, constipation, or diarrhea may occur. Although some CNS dysfunction may occur in the elderly, it is unusual in other age groups because of poor blood-brain barrier penetration.

Cimetidine was the first H$_2$ blocker commercially available in the United States. In the treatment of peptic ulcers, 300 mg of the drug is administered orally 4 times a day with meals. Because it is a polar drug, only 70% is absorbed. Peak blood levels occur in 1 hour, and drug effects last 6 to 8 hours.

References

1. Gell PGH, Coombs RRA, eds. Clinical aspects of immunology, ed. 2. Oxford: Blackwell Scientific, 1968.
2. Barber HRK. Immunobiology for the clinician. New York: John Wiley & Sons, 1977:75–83.
3. David JR, David RR. Cellular hypersensitivity and immunity. Inhibition of macrophage migration and the lymphocyte mediators. Prog Allergy 1972;16:300–449.
4. Allansmith MR, Ross RN. Ocular allergy and mast cell stabilizers. Surv Ophthalmol 1986;30:229–244.
5. Van Arsdel PP Jr, Beall GN. The metabolism and functions of histamine. Arch Intern Med 1960;106:714–733.
6. Stjernschantz J. Autocoids and neuropeptides. In: Sears ML, ed. Pharmacology of the eye. Handbook of experimental pharmacology, Vol. 69 Berlin: Springer-Verlag, 1984;311–332.
7. Nowak JJ, Nawrocki J. Histamine in the human eye. Ophthal Res 1987;19:72–75.
8. Chand N. Distribution and classification of airway histamine receptors: The physiological significance of histamine H$_2$ receptors. Adv Pharmacol Chemother 1980;17:103–131.
9. Cluff LE, Caranasos GJ, Stewart RB. Clinical problems with drugs. Philadelphia: W. B. Saunders Co, 1975.
10. Lagunoff D, Martin TW. Agents that release histamine from mast cells. Ann Rev Pharmacol Toxicol 1983;23:331–345.
11. Kahlson G, Rosengren E. Biogenesis and physiology of histamine. London: Arnold, 1971.
12. Schayer RW. Induced synthesis of histamine, microcirculatory regulation and the mechanism of action of the adrenal glucocorticoid hormones. Prog Allergy 1963;7:187–212.
13. Schwartz JC. Histaminergic mechanisms in brain. Ann Rev Pharmacol Toxicol 1977;17:325–339.
14. Soll A, Walch JH. Regulation of gastric acid secretion. Ann Rev Physiol 1979;41:35–53.
15. Lewis T. The blood vessels of the human skin and their responses. London: Shaw and Sons, 1927.
16. Lewis RA, Austen KF, Drazen JM, et al. Slow-reacting substances of anaphylaxis: Identification of leukotrienes C$_1$ and D from human rat sources. Proc Natl Acad Sci USA 1980;77:3710–3714.
17. Facts and Comparisons. St Louis: J. B. Lippincott Co, 1988; 188a–194.
18. Kemp JP, Buckley CE, Gershwin ME, et al. Multicenter, double-blind, placebo-controlled trial of terfenadine in seasonal allergic rhinitis and conjunctivitis. Ann Allergy 1985;54:502–509.
19. Johansen LV, Bjerrum P, Illum P. Treatment of seasonal allergic rhinitis—a double-blind, group comparative study of terfenadine and dexchlorpheniramine. Rhinology 1987;25:35–40.
20. Choice of antihistamines for allergic rhinitis. Med Lett 1987;29:105–108.
21. Fraunfelder FT, Meyer SM. Drug-induced ocular side effects and drug interactions. Philadelphia: Lea & Febiger, 1982;297–305.
22. Havener WH. Ocular pharmacology. St Louis: C. V. Mosby Co, 1978.
23. Physicians' desk reference for ophthalmology. Oradell, NJ: Medical Economics, 1988.
24. Miller J, Wolf EH. Antazoline phosphate and naphazoline hydrochloride, singly and in combination for the treatment of allergic conjunctivitis—a controlled, double-blind clinical trial. Ann Allergy 1975;35:81–86.
25. Abelson MB, Allansmith MR, Friedlaender MH. Effects of topically applied ocular decongestant and antihistamine. Am J Ophthalmol 1980;90:254–257.
26. Sadusk JF Jr, Palmisano PA. Teratogenic effect of meclizine, cyclizine, and chlorcyclizine. JAMA 1965;194:987–989.
27. Mosko MM, Peterson WL. Sensitization to antistine. J Invest Dermatol 1950;14:1–2.
28. Friedman PA. Common poisons. In: Isselbacher KJ, Adams RD, Braunwald E, et al., eds. Harrison's principles of internal medicine, ed. 9. New York: McGraw-Hill, 1981;953–954.
29. Abelson MB, Udell IJ. H$_2$ receptors in the human ocular surface. Arch Ophthalmol 1981;99:302–304.

CHAPTER 12

Dyes

Siret D. Jaanus

The application of dyes as ophthalmic diagnostic agents has been greatly expanded since Baeyer first synthesized fluorescein in 1871.[1] Other staining agents such as rose bengal, methylene blue, indocyanine green, trypan blue, alcian blue, and, more recently, a large-molecular derivative of fluorescein, fluorexon, have also proved clinically useful for topical ocular or intravenous use.

Fluorescein and Derivatives

Fluorescein Sodium

Fluorescein has been used as a diagnostic agent since Ehrlich's discovery in 1882 that it can enter the anterior chamber of the eye following subcutaneous injection.[2] Ehrlich further observed that following intravenous administration, the dye appears in the anterior chamber as a vertical yellow-green line behind the cornea, and he later used this observation to study aqueous secretion. It was, however, Straub[3] who in 1888 popularized the clinical application of fluorescein for the detection of corneal ulcers. In 1910 Burk[4] first reported the use of fluorescein to detect retinal disease.

PHARMACOLOGY

Fluorescein is a yellow acid dye of the xanthene series. Its molecular weight is 376, and its solubility in water at 15°C is 50%. It is generally formulated as its sodium salt[5] (Fig. 12.1).

When exposed to light, fluorescein absorbs certain wavelengths and emits fluorescent light of a certain longer wavelength. The absorbed and emitted wavelengths of light can be measured spectrophotofluorimetrically. The resultant excitation and emission spectra are illustrated in Figure 12.2. There is an overlap between the wavelengths of light that can be absorbed and those that are emitted. For dilute concentrations of fluorescein, light of wavelength 530 nm produces the maximum intensity of fluorescence.[5]

Since fluorescein is a weak acid, it can exist, depending on the pH of the solution, in various ionic states. Below pH 2, the cationic form predominates and a weak blue-green fluorescence is seen. Between pH 2 and 4, the cations dissociate to neutral molecules. At pH 7, negative ions prevail and are associated with a brilliant yellow-green fluorescence.[5]

Several factors can alter the activity of fluorescein in solution. Its concentration, the pH of the solution, the presence of other substances, and the intensity and wavelength of the absorbed light can affect its fluorescence. Increasing the concentration to a maximum of about 0.001% results in increased intensity. Likewise,

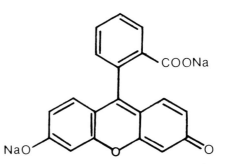

FIGURE 12.1 **Molecular structure of fluorescein sodium.**

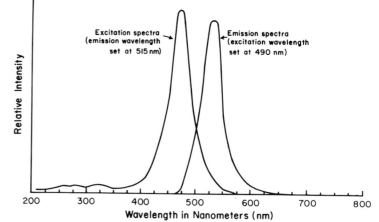

FIGURE 12.2 **Excitation and emission spectra of a 0.00005% solution of sodium fluorescein in KH₂PO₄-K₂HPO₄ buffer at pH 8. (From Romanchuk KG. Fluorescein. Physiochemical factors affecting its fluorescence. Surv Ophthalmol 1982;26:269–283.)**

the intensity of fluorescence increases with increasing pH, reaching a plateau at approximately pH 8. Thus, at physiologic pH the fluorescence is nearly maximum. Further increases in pH above 8 reduce the intensity of fluorescence.[5,6]

CLINICAL USES

Fluorescein may be applied topically to the eye in the form of a solution or by fluorescein-impregnated filter paper strips (Table 12.1). It is also available in injection form for intravenous use (Table 12.2).

Fluorescein in solution is highly susceptible to bac-terial contamination, especially by *Pseudomonas aeruginosa*.[7] This organism grows easily in the presence of fluorescein. Several methods have been devised to reduce the possibility of bacterial growth. Kimura[8] developed fluorescein-impregnated filter paper strips. On wetting the strip, the dye is released and can be applied to the eye. Commercially available fluorescein strips have proved clinically useful for applanation tonometry, contact lens fitting, and other ocular diagnostic procedures requiring topical fluorescein.

The need for sterile fluorescein has also resulted in the development of sterile, combination fluorescein-anesthetic solutions.[9,10] An example of such a preparation is Fluress, which was developed in 1967 (see Table 12.1). Fluress is a combination of sodium fluorescein and a local anesthetic, benoxinate hydrochloride. Chlorobutanol 1% is added as a preservative. The solution is buffered with boric acid to pH 5.[11]

Fluress has been shown to be remarkably resistant to bacterial contamination.[8–10,12] Bacteriologic studies to determine the bacteriostatic and bactericidal activity, as well as self-sterilization rate of the solution, have been carried out. Using select organisms to de-

TABLE 12.1
Fluorescein Preparations for Topical Ocular Use

Fluorescein Sodium Solutions

Fluorescein sodium (Various manufacturers)	2%; 1, 2, 15 ml
Fluress (Barnes-Hind)	0.25% with 0.4% benoxinate HCl, boric acid, povidone, 1% chlorobutanol; 5 ml
Fluoracaine (Akorn)	0.25% with 0.5% proparacaine HCl, povidone, glycerin, 0.01% thimerosal

Fluorescein Strips

Ful-Glo (Barnes-Hind)	0.6 mg; sterile
Fluor-I-Strip (Ayerst)	9 mg; with buffers, 0.5% chlorobutanol, polysorbate 80
Fluor-I-Strip-A.T. (Ayerst)	1 mg, with buffers, 0.5% chlorobutanol, polysorbate 80

Fluorexon

Fluoresoft (Holles)	0.35% in 0.5 ml pipettes

TABLE 12.2
Fluorescein Preparations for Intravenous Use

Fluorescite (Alcon)	10% in buffered sterile solution; 5 ml ampules
Funduscein-10 (Iolab)	10% in sterile water; 5 ml ampules
AK-Fluor (Akorn)	10% in sterile water; 5 ml ampules 25% in sterile water; 2 ml ampules
Fluorescite (Alcon)	25% in buffered sterile solution; 2 ml ampules
Funduscein-25 (Iolab)	25% in sterile water; 3 ml ampules

termine maximum dilution for bacteriostatic and bactericidal activity, Fluress has been found to be bactericidal against hazardous organisms known to infect ocular tissues[10] (Table 12.3). The self-sterilization rate of Fluress has been studied by inoculation of the solution with various microorganisms.[12,14] Quickert[9] observed resterilization times of 5 to 120 minutes, depending on the concentration and type of organisms used. There was also a tremendous reduction in the bacterial count from the moment the inoculum was added to the Fluress. Yolton and German[12] reported that no organisms could be recovered in even the zero-time sample of Fluress incubated with *P. aeruginosa* or *Staphylococcus aureus*. Figure 12.3 shows the results with *P. aeruginosa*. No detectable bacteria were present in the zero-time sample. Similar data were reported with *S. aureus*. In addition, no microorganisms have been recovered from open bottles of Fluress in routine clinical use for 1 month or more.[13]

The preservatives used to prevent growth of microorganisms in fluorescein solutions include chlorobutanol and thimerosal. Others, such as benzalkonium chloride, are inactivated by fluorescein and a precipitate is formed. Since fluorescein solutions can support the growth of bacteria,[7] care must be exercised with nonpreserved preparations. Sterile single-dose vials of fluorescein solutions or filter paper strips are recommended for topical use if a preservative is clinically contraindicated. Solutions of fluorescein may be sterilized by autoclaving.

TOPICAL OCULAR APPLICATIONS

Detection of Corneal Lesions. Fluorescein is frequently used in clinical practice to detect lesions of the corneal epithelium. Because of its high degree of ionization at physiologic pH, fluorescein does not penetrate the intact corneal epithelium, nor does it form a firm bond with any vital tissue.[6,89] Breakdown of the epithelium allows for stromal penetration, and, depending on the extent of the lesion, fluorescein may appear in the anterior chamber as a greenish "flare."[15]

Instillation of the dye in the cul de sac allows detection of corneal lesions such as abrasions, ulcers, and edema and aids in the detection of foreign bodies. When observed with the cobalt blue filter of the slit lamp, the epithelial defect is usually outlined in vivid green fluorescence, since the yellow-orange dye diffuses freely through the intercellular spaces and accumulates in the defect.[6] It is important to recognize that fluorescein does not actually stain tissues but rather, demonstrates its green coloration because of its fluorescent properties.[5] The reason for the observed color change from orange-yellow to green is not fully understood. Havener[15] suggests that a break in the epithelial barrier permits penetration of fluorescein into Bowman's layer and stroma whereby the dye makes contact with an alkaline interstitial fluid derived from the aqueous, and the fluorescein turns bright green due to its pH indicator properties. Romanchuk,[5] however, believes that the change in color of fluorescein when

---

TABLE 12.3
Resterilizing Time Studies for Fluress

Organisms	Range of Organisms Inoculated Per Tube	Time (min) Required to Kill All Organisms (range)
Klebsiella	$6.8 \times 10^4 - 1.7 \times 10^6$	15–120
Pseudomonas aeruginosa μ-21-A	$1.9 \times 10^5 - 1.9 \times 10^6$	15–60
P. aeruginosa 7700	$4.2 \times 10^4 - 7.7 \times 10^5$	5–120
Escherichia coli K-12	$2.6 \times 10^4 - 7.5 \times 10^5$	30–120
E. coli 931	$5.7 \times 10^4 - 1.3 \times 10^6$	30–120
Staphylococcus aureus FDA-209	$1.8 \times 10^4 - 2.9 \times 10^5$	120–180[a]
S. aureus 6538P	$8.4 \times 10^3 - 6.8 \times 10^4$	90–>180[a]
Proteus vulgaris	$6.1 \times 10^4 - 7.7 \times 10^5$	30–120
Candida albicans	$1.5 \times 10^4 - 1.1 \times 10^5$	75–120[a]

[a]In some experiments the exposure time required exceeded 180 minutes. In these instances specific kill times were not determined. However, the organisms were all killed when examined at 24 hours.

From Quickert MH. A fluorescein-anesthetic solution for applanation tonometry. Arch Ophthalmol 1967; 77:736. Copyright 1967, American Medical Association.

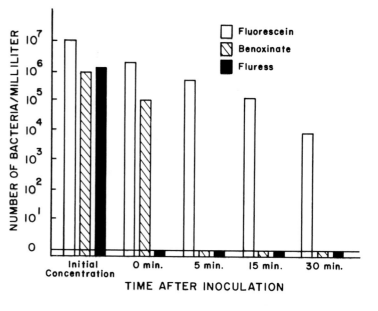

FIGURE 12.3   **Number of** *Pseudomonas aeruginosa* **present at various times following contamination of fluorescein, benoxinate, and Fluress. (Adapted from Yolton DP, German CJ. J Am Optom Assoc 1980;51:471–474.)**

applied following cataract extraction is due to its dilution by the leaking of aqueous from the anterior chamber. He further suggests that the staining seen with corneal lesions could be due to fluorescence of the intracellular contents of groups of cells after fluorescein has gained entry into a damaged cell and is then transferred to the interior of adjacent cells. The exact mechanism of staining of corneal lesions by fluorescein requires further study before a definitive conclusion can be reached.

Fluorescein is useful during corneal surgical procedures such as corneal transplantation.[15] Topical administration of the dye during trephining can detect aqueous leakage from the anterior chamber. When the cornea has been penetrated and the aqueous begins to leak, the dye appears bright green. The dye may also be used to perform Seidel's test,[16] in which a drop of fluorescein is placed on the superior bulbar conjunctiva in an attempt to detect a surgical wound leakage following cataract extraction. If a leak is present, a bright green rivulet of aqueous flows through the fluorescein on the cornea. This line of fluorescence can be traced to its origin and is best seen with cobalt blue light or the cobalt blue filter of the slit lamp.[5]

Contact Lens Fitting and Management.   Vital staining of the tear film is a major aid in the fitting of rigid gas-permeable contact lenses.[90] Following topical application of fluorescein to the eye, the tear layer becomes visible, with a characteristic pattern of green fluorescence. By observing the fluorescein-stained tear film with an ultraviolet light or the cobalt blue filter of the slit lamp, the fit of the lens may be determined.

Areas where the lens makes corneal contact show a thin (blue) fluorescence or absence of the fluorescein dye[15] (Fig. 12.4).

In addition to its usefulness during the contact lens fitting procedures, fluorescein is essential for assessing the integrity of the cornea in contact lens wearers. Since fluorescein penetrates the corneal epithelium only at sites of interrupted epithelial integrity, the dye will disclose areas where the contact lens may be disrupting the corneal epithelium.[17]

Lacrimal System Evaluation.   Topical ocular fluorescein can be used to evaluate the integrity of the precorneal tear film[18–20] and the patency of the lacrimal drainage system.[21,22]

Assessment of tear breakup time (TBUT), defined as the interval between the last complete blink and the development of the first randomly distributed dry spot in the tear film, is commonly used for determining tear film stability.[19] A wet fluorescein strip is applied to the superior or superotemporal aspect of the bulbar conjunctiva. Using the cobalt blue filter of the slit lamp, the cornea is scanned during the interval from the last complete blink to the appearance of the first dry spot (see Fig. 20.5). TBUTs of less than 10 seconds suggest an unstable tear film.[23] The determination of TBUT is used clinically as a diagnostic aid in dry eye syndromes and for testing the efficacy of tear replacement products. However, the clinical validity of the test has been questioned, since wide variations in TBUT have been reported.[18] The volume and concentration of fluorescein administered, the properties of the precorneal tear film itself, and problems inherent in the technique of

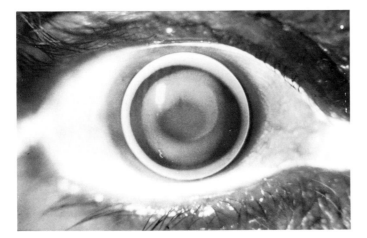

FIGURE 12.4   Contact lens fluorescein pattern in eye with keratoconus. Central, dark area reflects absence of fluorescein, indicating central contact lens bearing (touch). There is also bearing in the intermediate area surrounded by peripheral clearance indicated by the pooling of fluorescein. (Courtesy A. Christopher Snyder, O.D.)

measuring TBUT may contribute to the lack of reproducibility in the TBUT.[24,25]

Fluorescein is also useful clinically in evaluating epiphora. Fluorescein testing for lacrimal obstruction usually involves instilling the dye into the conjunctival cul de sac followed by observing for the presence of fluorescein in the nose. Appearance of the dye in the nose or posterior oropharynx indicates that the lacrimal drainage system of that eye is functional.[21,22] Generally a 2% fluorescein solution is used, and this test can be employed in conjunction with other procedures for diagnosis of lacrimal obstruction (see Chapter 20).

Applanation Tonometry.   The use of topical fluorescein is an important component in the measurement of intraocular pressure with the Goldmann applanation tonometer. The dye permits accurate visualization of the 3.06 mm² applanated area.[26]

Measurement of intraocular pressure with the Goldmann applanation tonometer requires that the meniscus of tear fluid surrounding the flattened corneal surface be sufficiently stained with fluorescein so that the apex of the wedge-shaped meniscus is visible. If the fluid apex is not visible, intraocular pressure will be underestimated.[27]

The measurable thickness of a wedge of fluorescein-containing fluid is inversely proportional to the concentration of fluorescein and directly proportional to the concentration of a substance that can suppress fluorescence.[4] Moses[27] measured the thickness of a minimally visible fluorescent solution at varying concentrations of fluorescein. The vehicle for dilution of the dye was either (1) normal saline alone, (2) equal parts of saline with the anesthetics benoxinate (Novesine) or proparacaine (Ophthaine), or (3) anesthetic solution combined with fluorescein solution. The data indicate that at low fluorescein concentrations the fluid

apex becomes less visible. Although both topical anesthetics impaired fluorescence in a concentration-dependent manner, the quenching effect was least with 0.1% benoxinate (Fig. 12.5).

The effect of anesthetics on the fluorescence of fluorescein can be explained in part by the acidity of the anesthetic solutions (pH 4 to 4.5), since fluorescein loses its ability to fluoresce in acid solutions.[28] However, since fluorescence is only slightly greater in the presence of a buffer, the anesthetic base must also be able to reduce the fluorescence to some degree.

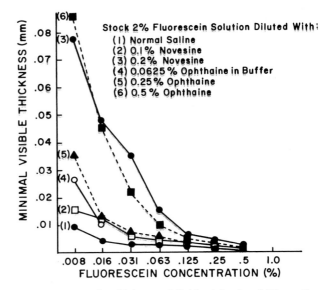

FIGURE 12.5   The thickness of fluid minimally visible as fluorescent for different fluorescein concentrations and solvents. (Published with permission from the American Journal of Ophthalmology 49: 1149–1155, 1960. Copyright by The Ophthalmic Publishing Company.)

The concentration of fluorescein that is most satisfactory for applanation tonometry appears to be 0.25% solution.[29] Previous instillation of an anesthetic does not interfere with the fluorescence, provided the anesthetic has been absorbed and is not present in the cul de sac.[9]

It has been suggested that Goldmann applanation tonometry can be performed without fluorescein.[30,31] With the white light of a biomicroscope, intraocular pressure can be measured following the application of an anesthetic alone, when the two mires are aligned to the point of touch. However, several investigators have compared ocular tension measurements with Goldmann applanation tonometry in the presence and absence of fluorescein.[32–34] The results indicate that readings using white light without fluorescein are significantly lower than those obtained using cobalt blue light with fluorescein. Roper[32] found an underestimation of 5.62 mm Hg when fluorescein was not used. Bright and associates[34] found that readings without fluorescein were lower by an average of 7.01 mm Hg (Table 12.4). The mean reading with Fluress was 18.03 mm Hg as compared to 11.02 mm Hg with the anesthetic Ophthetic in the absence of fluorescein. By performing a regression analysis these investigators further suggested that the difference in intraocular pressure readings with and without fluorescein becomes even greater as the intraocular pressure rises.

The lower readings observed in the absence of fluorescein can be due to difficulties in viewing the applanated area. The apex of the tear film meniscus, which defines the applanated area, is not clearly visible without fluorescein. The applanated area may be less than 3.06 mm^2, thus resulting in underestimation of intraocular pressure (Fig. 12.6).[34]

Although there could be certain advantages to performing Goldmann applanation tonometry without fluorescein, including avoidance of possible contamination of the eye or soft contact lens, the differences in the readings at higher intraocular pressure can present significant clinical problems.

INTRAVENOUS APPLICATIONS

The introduction of fluorescein angiography by Novotny and Alvis[35] in 1961 provided a useful method for studying various parameters of ocular function. Intravenous fluorescein is used extensively to delineate vascular abnormalities of the fundus and occasionally to determine ocular blood and aqueous flow.

Fluorescein Angiography. In the bloodstream fluorescein is excited by a wavelength of 465 nm and emits a wavelength of 525 nm. Circulating fluorescein is bound to albumin and red blood cells. It is also metabolized to a weakly fluorescent conjugate, fluorescein monoglucoronide, which exhibits less plasma protein binding than fluorescein. The amount of binding can affect the penetration of fluorescein through blood-ocular barriers.[36] Following injection of 10 ml of a 5% solution in the antecubital vein, the dye usually appears in the central retinal artery within 13 seconds.[37] Both circulation time and integrity of the retina and choroid may be examined.

Fluorescein angiography shows retinal blood vessels in high contrast. Nonvascularized, pigmented retinal and subretinal lesions may be recognized as dark areas against the green fluorescing background.[38] The abnormal fluorescence of various retinal and choroidal lesions has been explained by several mechanisms, including (1) some abnormalities in the retina allow for greater visibility of choroidal fluorescence; (2) neovascularization produces enhanced fluorescence due to new vascular channels, and (3) pathologic processes resulting in enhanced capillary permeability allow for leakage of fluorescein into the lesions.[39] These types of abnormalities may often be differentiated by time of onset of fluorescence. Choroidal fluorescence appears early and usually precedes the arterial phase. Depending on the origin of the new vessels, neovascular fluorescence coincides with the arteriolar or venous phase of fluorescence. Enhanced capillary permeability (leakage) delays fluorescence, followed

TABLE 12.4
Results of Intraocular Pressure Readings (mm Hg) from $N = 100$ Eyes for Ophthetic and Fluress

	Mean Tonometric Readings (mm Hg)	*Standard Deviation*	*Standard Error*	*R*	*Regression*
Fluress	18.03	4.27	0.427	0.552	y = 0.45 + 0.59x
Ophthetic	11.02	4.53	0.453		

From Bright DC, Potter JW, Allen DC, et al. Goldmann applanation tonometry without fluorescein. Am J Optom Physiol Optics 1981; 58:1120–1126, with permission of the authors and publisher.

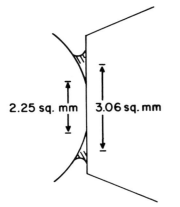

2.25 sq. mm | 3.06 sq. mm

FIGURE 12.6 **Cornea partially flattened by applanation tono-meter. The apices of the fluorescein-stained wedges above and below the flattened area are too dilute to be visible. The 3.06 mm² end point of applanation appears to have been reached but in reality consists of a smaller flattened area. (Modified from Moses RA. Fluorescein in applanation tonometry. Am J Ophthalmol 1960; 49:1149–1155.)**

by a slow increase in fluorescence as the dye recirculates and stains the affected tissues.

Fluorescein angiography has proved helpful in the diagnosis of a variety of pathologic conditions of the fundus. Various macular lesions, central serous choroidopathy,[40] diabetic retinopathy,[41] and disciform macular degeneration show typical fluorescein patterns.

Fluorescein angiography can also differentiate early papilledema from pseudopapilledema. In papilledema, fluorescein angiography shows capillary dilation, microaneurysms, and leakage of the dye into extravascular tissue. The abnormal fluorescence may persist for hours. In contrast, no leakage is seen in pseudopapilledema, and the residual fluorescence is insignificant after 10 minutes.[42]

Malignant melanomas, metastatic tumors, and hemangiomas of the choroid also fluoresce. However, since the pattern is similar for choroidal melanomas and hemangiomas, these conditions cannot be differentiated by fluorescein angiography alone.[43]

The clinical procedure and interpretation of fluorescein angiography is discussed in Chapter 25.

Circulation Time. Fluorescein can be used to evaluate arm-to-retina circulation time. A fluorescein solution is rapidly injected into the antecubital vein. The appearance of the dye in the central retinal artery of each eye is observed by indirect ophthalmoscopy and is recorded with stopwatches.[44,45]

The normal arm-to-retina circulation time is 11 to 13 seconds, depending on speed of injection, cardio-vascular factors, and intraocular pressure.[45] The time should not differ by more than 1 second between the 2 eyes. A prolonged circulation time indicates occlusive carotid disease.

The determination of circulation time requires 3 experienced observers and can therefore be subject to technical error. However, the determination of circulation time can yield information in support of other clinical and ophthalmodynamometric findings.

Iris Angiography. Intravenous injection of fluorescein can be useful for visualization of iris tumors and vessel infarcts.

Following injection into the antecubital vein, the dye first appears in the radial vessels of the iris between 9 and 20 seconds.[46] The amount of iris pigmentation as well as the pattern of its distribution affects the amount of detail observed in a normal iris angiogram. Blue irides generally show the vessels in greater detail than do brown ones.[46] More recently, an adapter mounted in front of a fundus camera lens has made it possible to visualize the vascular structure more completely in heavily pigmented irides.[47]

Aqueous Flow. Changes in the concentration of fluorescein in the anterior chamber following intravenous injection were first measured by Goldmann in 1950.[48] Using a slit-lamp fluorophotometer, the time course of the fluorescence in the circulating blood and the anterior chamber was determined in humans. The rate of aqueous flow was calculated by Goldmann to be about 1.5% to 2% of the volume of the anterior chamber per minute. Since then several other methods have been devised to measure aqueous turnover. All have given comparable results.[49]

Vitreous Fluorophotometry. Vitreous fluorophotometry (VFP) is a noninvasive quantitative method for measuring small amounts of fluorescein in various ocular compartments. This technique was first introduced by Cunha-Vaz and associates[50] to study the blood-retinal barrier. It is based on the slit-lamp fluorophotometer method designed by Maurice[51] in 1963.

Since the normal blood-retinal barrier resists various substances, including fluorescein, a functional breakdown of this barrier should be detectable by the presence of fluorescein in the vitreous. Although physiologic factors and instrument artifacts can influence vitreous fluorescence, this technique has been used to detect retinal vascular disease, especially in diabetes.[50,52,53] The procedure has also been used to study integrity of the blood-retinal barrier in various other diseases, including retinitis pigmentosa,[54] optic neuritis,[55] and essential hypertension.[56]

ORAL FLUORESCEIN ANGIOSCOPY

Since the integrity of the normal ocular physiologic barriers to fluorescein depends less on dye administration velocity than on certain other parameters, such as retinal circulation time, fluorescein has also been administered by mouth to study certain lesions of the fundus.[57–62] The oral procedure in adults usually involves administration of 1 to 2 g of fluorescein powder or 3 vials of 10% injectable fluorescein mixed in a citrus drink over ice.[57,61] In children, fruit juice containing 1 ml of a 10% fluorescein solution/20 ml juice/ 5 kg body weight has been used to determine macular leakage following removal of congenital cataracts.[59] The dye begins to appear in the fundus in approximately 15 minutes, but maximal fluorescence is not obtained until 45 to 60 minutes following ingestion.[57] Fasting can enhance the serum concentration of the dye.[61]

Oral fluorescein has been used to study disorders characterized by late leakage of dye, such as cystoid macular edema in both children and adults,[57,59–61] and has been used to study retinal vascular abnormalities in young diabetic patients.[62] It is also useful to document other disorders characterized by late leakage, such as retinal pigment epithelial detachment, central serous choroidopathy, and optic disc edema.[61] In the diagnosis of these conditions the arterial and early venous phases of the angiogram are not critical. It is important to note that the late leakage of dye can be shown by the oral use of fluorescein even in mild cases.[57] Oral fluorescein, however, does not clearly outline critical vascular details such as may be needed for photocoagulation.[57]

The use of oral fluorescein thus appears to be a feasible method for evaluating certain clinical conditions in both children and adults. The oral route of administration has the advantage that side effects are rare.[61,62,91]

SIDE EFFECTS

Studies in humans indicate that about 10% of patients receiving intravenous fluorescein experience adverse effects.[63,64] The most common reaction is nausea, accompanied less frequently by vomiting. The nausea usually occurs 15 to 30 seconds following injection and subsides within several minutes. The incidence of nausea appears to be higher in women. Schatz and Farkos[65] reported that in 400 consecutive patients undergoing intravenous fluorescein angiography, 9.4% of the females experienced nausea compared with 6.1% of male patients. The incidence of postinjection nausea may be related to the concentration of fluorescein used.[66] Intravenous injection of 25% fluorescein resulted in nausea in 23% of patients. Only 11% were nauseated with 10% fluorescein. With 5% fluorescein the incidence of nausea was only 2%. The speed of injection may also play a role. A slower injection permits more protein binding of the fluorescein in the plasma and thereby reduces the bolus of free fluorescein.[67] The incidence of nausea has been reported to be reduced in susceptible patients by administration of 50 mg promethazine orally 1 hour before injection of the dye.[65]

Allergic reactions have also occurred, including urticaria and pruritus. Less frequently, more serious respiratory effects such as laryngeal or pulmonary edema have been reported.[68,69]

Cardiovascular toxicity in the form of severe hypotension and shock as well as myocardial infarction and basilar artery ischemia have rarely occurred.[69] Other adverse effects reported with intravenous use of fluorescein include pain at the site of injection, dizziness with rare episodes of fainting, and paresthesia of the tongue and lips.[68]

Patients should be advised that both skin and urine will be temporarily discolored by intravenous fluorescein.

Several investigators have studied the possible mechanisms associated with the pathophysiologic changes observed during administration of intravenous fluorescein. An allergic reaction of the immediate hypersensitivity type (type I) resulting from an immunologic response of the host to a hapten (drug)-protein combination or the release of histamine have been proposed as causative factors.[68,70] Studies for cell-mediated immunity reactions have given negative results with fluorescein.[68]

Following infusion of fluorescein, plasma histamine concentrations increase within the first few minutes and persist up to 10 minutes.[70] Increased histamine has been found in 66% of patients with adverse reactions to fluorescein and in 15% of patients with no reactions. Possibly the occurrence of reactions to fluorescein depends not on the concentration of histamine but, rather, on the individual's susceptibility to respond to histamine in the circulation.[70] Fluorescein is also detectable in breast milk for up to 76 hours following intravenous administration.[92]

Because of the possibility of adverse reactions, a family and personal history of allergies should be obtained from every patient who is to undergo fluorescein angiography. Appropriate medications such as epinephrine (1:1000 ampules) should be available in case of allergic responses.[15,70] Other recommended safety precautions include a pressure ventilation device, an airway, corticosteroids, and sedatives[15,67] (see Chapter 31).

Adverse effects associated with topical fluorescein and anesthetic-fluorescein combinations are usually limited to transient irritation of the cornea or conjunc-

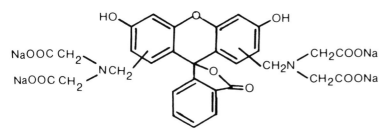

FIGURE 12.7 **Molecular structure of fluorexon.**

tiva.[10,71] Fluress has been associated with vasovagal responses in 3 young adults during applanation tonometry. Loss of consciousness was not associated with any other symptoms.[72]

A unique case of grand mal seizure following instillation of Fluress has been reported in 1 patient.[73] Less than 1 minute following instillation of Fluress into each conjunctival cul de sac the patient lost consciousness and had a generalized clonic seizure, lasting less than 1 minute. He was placed on the floor and regained consciousness. While lying supine, he had another seizure lasting about 1 minute and again regained consciousness. No erythema or edema of the lids or conjunctiva was noted. The patient showed normal findings on follow-up neurologic examination. Note, however, that the fluorescein could not be definitely implicated as the causative factor, since Fluress also contains benoxinate as the anesthetic and a preservative, chlorobutanol. Hypersensitivity testing with each of these ingredients was not performed.

Since the topically administered dye will discolor soft contact lenses, they should not be reinserted until the dye has left the eye, usually after 1 to 2 hours. Alternatively, the lenses may be reinserted immediately following irrigation of the dye from the eye.

Fluorexon

Since fluorescein sodium can penetrate into soft contact lenses, the lenses become discolored, which is cosmetically objectionable. In addition, the boundary between lens and tears becomes obscured, which precludes the use of fluorescein in soft contact lens fitting. Fluorexon, a molecule similar to that of fluorescein, is less readily absorbed by the soft lens material, which makes it more useful in fitting and evaluating soft lenses.[74]

PHARMACOLOGY

Fluorexon, N,N-bis(carboxymethyl)-aminoethylfluorescein tetrasodium salt, has a molecular weight of 710 (Fig. 12.7).[74] Compared with fluorescein sodium it yields a paler, yellow-brown color. Its staining properties are similar to those of fluorescein sodium. The dye stains epithelial defects but, unlike fluorescein sodium, it does stain devitalized tissue.[75]

Fluorexon, like fluorescein sodium, is vulnerable to bacterial contamination.[74] It, however, appears to support bacterial growth longer than a comparable solution of fluorescein sodium (Table 12.5). For clinical use it is therefore dispensed in single-dose sterile pipettes (see Table 12.1).

CLINICAL USES

Fluorexon can aid in the fitting of soft contact lenses. It can be applied to the eye with the lens in place, but it is more effective when placed in the posterior bowl of the lens before insertion. Fluorexon will stain the soft lens if it remains in contact with the lens for more than a few minutes. However, repeated rinsing with saline will usually remove the dye from the lens. Note that fluorexon is not recommended for use with highly hydrated soft lenses with water content of 60% or higher. In such cases absorption of dye by the lens is much more difficult to rectify.

Topical application to the eye may produce a mild stinging sensation. Occasional conjunctival injection

TABLE 12.5

Time Course of Contamination of Fluorexon and Fluorescein following Inoculation with *Pseudomonas aeruginosa*

Contaminant: P. aeruginosa	1 hr	2 hr	24 hr	Meat Broth 24 hr
Control	+[a]	+	+	+
Fluorescein 0.25%	+	+	−[a]	−
Fluorescein 0.25% with benoxinate 0.4%	−	−	−	−
Fluorescein 2.2%	+	+	−	−
Fluorexon 0.25% in normal saline	+	+	+	+

[a] + means positive culture for organism; −, no growth.
From Refojo MF, Miller D, Fiore AS. A new fluorescent stain for soft hydrophilic lens fitting. Arch Ophthalmol 1972; 87:277. Copyright 1972, American Medical Association.

has been reported.[74] In clinical use fluorexon has proved to be nontoxic to ocular tissue, but it is not widely employed because the observation of dye-stained tears in the evaluation of soft contact lens fitting is not significantly more effective than simple evaluation of the lens without dye.[75] In addition, a special yellow filter is required to enhance observation of the fluorescence, which makes the procedure cumbersome.

Rose Bengal

Rose bengal, unlike fluorescein sodium, stains devitalized corneal and conjunctival epithelium a readily visible red color. In addition, it will also stain mucus strands within the precorneal tear film.[75,76]

PHARMACOLOGY

Rose bengal is a fluorescein derivative (4,5,6,7-tetrachloro-2′,4′,5′,7′-tetraiodo fluorescein sodium) (Fig. 12.8). The dye is readily soluble in water.[76] It can be applied as a 1% solution or as a moistened filter paper strip.

CLINICAL USES

In 1914 Romer and associates reported the use of rose bengal to treat an ocular pneumococcal infection. A few years later, Kleefeld used the dye as a vital stain for a corneal ulcer.[78] Extensive clinical use since then has shown that rose bengal is of value in the diagnosis of exposure keratitis, keratoconjunctivitis sicca, corneal abrasions, and in the detection of corneal foreign bodies.[12,76,77,79,80] However, its most frequent clinical use is in the evaluation of epithelial lesions associated with keratoconjunctivitis sicca. Punctate staining of the exposed part of the cornea and conjunctiva, which includes the lower two-thirds of the cornea and the adjacent triangular sections of the bulbar conjunctiva nasally and temporally, indicates dessication of the epithelium.[76]

Rose bengal has also been shown to inhibit various microorganisms in vitro.[79] Roat and associates[80] eval-

uated the antiviral activities of rose bengal and fluorescein sodium against herpes simplex virus type I (HSV-1) in both an in vitro direct neutralization assay and in a mouse keratitis model. The results of the in vitro assay demonstrated that rose bengal significantly inhibits HSV-1 when compared with fluorescein sodium. The LD_{50} for rose bengal was 16 μg/ml compared with an LD_{50} of 460 μg/ml for fluorescein. In the mouse herpetic model, rose bengal reduced ocular surface virus, as measured by swabs, 1 million-fold, whereas fluorescein had no clinically significant antiviral effect. Thus, since rose bengal appears to be a potent antiviral agent, its diagnostic use before viral cultures in an inflamed eye may preclude a positive result.

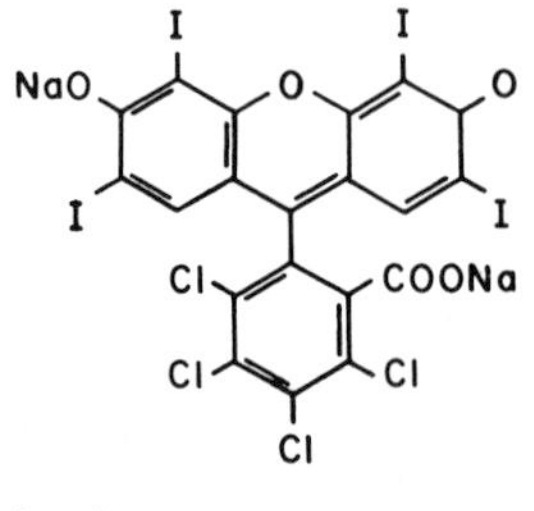

Irritation and discomfort are more marked with rose bengal than with fluorescein sodium and are usually proportional to the degree of epithelial involvement and conjunctival injection.[77] A topical anesthetic may be applied before instillation of the stain, but the anesthetic can cause sufficient epithelial lesions to give false positive staining. If the amount of rose bengal applied is not excessive, there is little or no patient discomfort, and an anesthetic is therefore not required.

Thorough irrigation is recommended to remove excessive dye, since discoloration of the skin around the eyes is more pronounced than with fluorescein sodium.

Methylene Blue

This vital stain has properties similar to those of rose bengal. It can stain devitalized cells as well as mucus and corneal nerves. It is not a specific stain when applied to the eye because the blue areas may be either cells or mucus. Norn,[76] therefore, does not recommend its use on the cornea due to its lack of specificity. Methylene blue is also useful for staining the lacrimal sac before dacryocystorhinostomy (DCR).[15]

Pharmacology

Methylene blue is an aniline dye. It has some bacteriostatic properties against microorganisms.[77] The dye is usually employed as a 5% solution, and benzalkonium chloride may be added to the dye solution to enhance sterility. Methylene blue precipitates in alkaline solutions.

Clinical Uses

Vital staining of corneal nerves requires up to 3 instillations at 5-minute intervals.[15] The bluish ocular discoloration may remain for 24 hours.

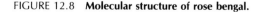

FIGURE 12.8   **Molecular structure of rose bengal.**

For staining of the lacrimal sac before surgery, the sac is irrigated with methylene blue. The dye should remain in the sac for several minutes. Before beginning surgery the dye should be washed out of the sac, since it could spill out on incision and stain the surrounding tissues.[15]

When topically applied, methylene blue can be quite irritating to ocular tissue. A topical anesthetic may be used, since it enhances penetration of the drug at the same time as it relieves the discomfort.[77]

Indocyanine Green

Indocyanine green selectively stains devitalized corneal endothelial cells.[81] Its ocular uses have included the study of choroidal circulation and the assessment of viability of corneal endothelial cells to ensure the success of keratoplasty.[82–84]

Pharmacology

Indocyanine green has an absorption spectrum in the near infrared region because it peaks near 800 nm. This allows for better visualization of the choroidal vasculature, since fluorescein has absorption and emission spectra in the range of the pigment epithelium (490 nm and 520 nm). Indocyanine green is highly soluble in water and binds avidly to protein.[83] The dye selectively stains dead corneal endothelial cells, and exposure to 1% indocyanine green solution also appears to damage living endothelial cells.[83]

Clinical Uses

Following intravenous injection of the dye, visualization of choroidal vessels becomes possible with infrared absorption angiography. Thus, choroidal circulatory activity can be studied under various intraocular conditions such as high intraocular pressure.[82,84] No toxic effects have been associated with intravenous use of the dye.[83]

To date only rabbit corneas have been stained with the topically applied dye.[83] Further work is necessary to demonstrate the efficacy of this stain on human corneal endothelium.

Trypan Blue

This stain has also proved useful as an indicator of corneal endothelial integrity.

Pharmacology

Trypan blue is an anionic acid dye. It appears to stain only damaged or dead endothelial cells.[85]

Clinical Uses

Vital staining with trypan blue has been advocated for determining the suitability of human donor corneal material for grafting.[85,86] The dye has also been injected as a 1% solution into the human anterior chamber during cataract extraction to identify corneal endothelial damage.[87] It appears to be free of any adverse effects on human corneal cells.

Alcian Blue

This dye is a specific vital stain for mucus. It can be used to differentiate mucus deposits from normal epithelial cells.[88]

Pharmacology

Alcian blue is a cationic dye of complex composition containing copper. It does not stain normal epithelial cells but will stain mucus-producing goblet cells, mucus fibrils of mucus threads in the inferior conjunctival fornix, and mucus flakes.[88]

Clinical Uses

The dye has proved clinically useful and nontoxic as a 1% solution applied topically to the eye. At this concentration it will stain degenerated epithelial cells and mucus on the surface of the eye, but it will not stain normal epithelial cells. Alcian blue is not recommended for staining corneas with serious injuries of the epithelium, since it will cause prolonged discoloration of the tissue.[88]

References

1. Baeyer A. Uber eine neue klasse von farbstoffen. Ber Deutsch Chem Ges 1871;4:555–558.
2. Ehrlich P. Uber provozierte fluorescenz serscheinungen am auge. Deutsch Med Wochnschr 1882;8:35–36.
3. Straub A. 1888. As quoted by Campbell FW, Boyd TAS. Use of sodium fluorescein in assessing the rate of healing in corneal ulcers. Br J Ophthalmol 1950;34:545–549.

4. Burk A. Die klinische physiologische und pathologische Bedeutung der Fluoreszenz in Auge nach Darreichung von Uranin. Klin Montagsbl Augen-heilkund 1910;48:445–454.

5. Romanchuk KG. Fluorescein: Physicochemical factors affecting its fluorescence. Surv Ophthalmol 1982;26:269–283.

6. Maurice DM. The use of fluorescein in ophthalmological research. Invest Ophthalmol 1967;6:464–477.

7. Vaughan DG. The contamination of fluorescein solutions—with special reference to Pseudomonas aeruginosa. Am J Ophthalmol 1955;39:55–61.

8. Kimura SJ. Fluorescein paper; a simple means of insuring the use of sterile fluorescein. Am J Ophthalmol 1951;34:446–447.

9. Hales RH. Combined solution of fluorescein and anesthetic. Am J Ophthalmol 1967;64:158–160.

10. Quickert MH. A fluorescein-anesthetic solution for applanation tonometry. Arch Ophthalmol 1967;77:734–739.

11. Physicians desk reference for ophthalmology. Oradell, NJ: Medical Economics, 1987.

12. Yolton DP, German CJ. Fluress, fluorescein and benoxinate: Recovery from bacterial contamination. J Am Optom Assoc 1980;51:471–474.

13. Lee H. Prolonged antibacterial activity of a fluorescein-anesthetic solution. Arch Ophthalmol 1972;88:385–387.

14. Clague C. Experimental contamination of minims of fluorescein by Pseudomonas aeruginosa. Br J Ophthalmol 1986;70:507–509.

15. Havener WH. Ocular pharmacology. St Louis: C. V. Mosby Co, 1978; Chap. 17.

16. Seidel E. Weitere experimentelle utersuchungen uber die quelle und den verlauf der intraokularen saftromung XII. Uber den manometrischen nachweis des physiologischen druckfalles zwischen voderkammer und schlemmschen kanal. Arch Ophthalmol 1921;107:101–104.

17. Norn MS. Micropunctate fluorescein staining of the cornea. Acta Ophthalmol 1970;48:108–118.

18. Norn MS. Dessication of the precorneal tear film. I. Corneal wetting time. Acta Ophthalmol 1969;47:865–880.

19. Lemp MA, Hamill JR. Factors affecting tear breakup in normal eyes. Ophthalmology 1973;89:103–105.

20. Benedetto DA, Clinch TE, Laibson PR. In vivo observation of tear dynamics using fluorophotometry. Arch Ophthalmol 1984;102:410–412.

21. Jones LT. The lacrimal secretory system and its treatment. Am J Ophthalmol 1966;62:47–60.

22. Flach A. The fluorescein appearance test for lacrimal obstruction. Ann Ophthalmol 1979;11:237–242.

23. Lemp MA, Dohlman CH, Kuwabarat T, et al. Dry eye secondary to mucus deficiency. Trans Am Acad Ophthalmol Otol 1971;75:1223–1227.

24. Vanley GT, Leopold IH, Gregg TH. Interpretation of tear film breakup. Arch Ophthalmol 1977;95:445–448.

25. Mengher LS, Bron AJ, Tonge SR, Gilbert DJ. Effect of fluorescein instillation on the pre-corneal tear film stability. Curr Eye Res 1985;4:9–12.

26. Goldmann H. Applanation tonometry. In: Newell FW, ed. Glaucoma. New York: Josiah Macy, Jr. Foundation 1956;167–220.

27. Moses RA. Fluorescein in applanation tonometry. Am J Ophthalmol 1960;49:1149–1155.

28. The Merck Index, ed. 9. Rahway, NJ: Merck & Co. Inc., 1967;4042–4043.

29. Grant WM. Fluorescein for applanation tonometry: More convenient and uniform application. Am J Ophthalmol 1963;55:1252–1253.

30. Smith R. Applanation tonometry without fluorescein. Am J Ophthalmol 1979;87:583.

31. Weinstock FJ. Applanation tonometry without fluorescein. Ophthalmology 1979;84:797.

32. Roper DL. Applanation tonometry with and without fluorescein. Am J Ophthalmol 1980;90:668–671.

33. Rosenstock T, Breslin CW. The importance of fluorescein in applanation tonometry. Am J Ophthalmol 1981;92:741.

34. Bright DC, Potter JW, Allen DC, Spruance RD. Goldmann applanation tonometry without fluorescein. Am J Optom Physiol Optics 1981;58:1120–1126.

35. Novotny HR, Alvis DL. A method of photographing fluorescence in circulating blood in human retina. Circulation 1961;24:82–86.

36. Nagataki S, Matsunaga I. Binding of fluorescein monoglucuronide to human serum albumin. Invest Ophthalmol Vis Sci 1985;26:1175–1178.

37. Smith J, Lawton D, Noble J, et al. Hemangioma of the choroid. Arch Ophthalmol 1963;69:51–54.

38. Lebensohn JE. Fluorescein in ophthalmology. Am J Ophthalmol 1969;67:272–274.

39. Kearns TP, Hollenhorst RW. Chloroquine retinopathy. Arch Ophthalmol 1966;76:378–384.

40. Norton EWD, Gutman F. Fluorescein in the study of macular disease. Trans Am Acad Ophthalmol Otol 1965;69:631–642.

41. Norton EWD, Gutman F. Diabetic retinopathy studied by fluorescein angiography. Ophthalmologica 1965;150:5–17.

42. Kearns TP. Neuro-ophthalmology. Arch Ophthalmol 1966;76:729–755.

43. Norton EWD, Gutman F. Fluorescein angiography and hemangiomas of the choroid. Arch Ophthalmol 1967;78:121–125.

44. David NJ, Saito Y, Heyman A. Arm to retina fluorescein appearance time. A new method of diagnosis of carotid artery occlusion. Arch Neurol 1961;5:165–170.

45. Pernberton JW, Britton WA. The arm-retina circulation time. Arch Ophthalmol 1964;71:364–370.

46. Kottow MH. Fundamentals of angiographic interpretation: the normal anterior segment fluorescein angiogram. In: Anterior segment fluorescein angiography. Baltimore: Williams & Wilkins; Chap. 3.

47. D'Anna SA, Hochheimer BF, Joondeph HC, Graebner KE. Fluorescein angiography in the heavily pigmented iris and new dyes for iris angiography. Arch Ophthalmol 1983;101:289–293.

48. Golmann H. Uber fluorescein in der menschlichen vorderkammer. Das kammer-wasser-minutenvolumen des menschen. Ophthalmologica 1950;120:65–79.

49. Coakes RL, Brubaker RF. Method of measuring aqueous humor flow and corneal endothelial permeability using a fluorophotometry nomogram. Invest Ophthalmol Vis Sci 1979;18:288–302.

50. Cunha-Vaz J, De Abreu JRF, Campos AJ. Early breakdown of the blood-retinal barrier in diabetes. Br J Ophthalmol 1975;59:649–656.

51. Maurice DM. A new objective fluorophotometer. Exp Eye Res 1963;2:33–48.
52. Cunha-Vaz J. The blood ocular barriers. Surv Ophthalmol 1979;23:279–296.
53. Waltman SR. Sequencial vitreous fluorophotometry in diabetes mellitus. A five year prospective study. Trans Am Ophthalmol Soc 1984;82:827–849.
54. Fishman GA, Cunha-Vaz J, Salazano T. Vitreous fluorophotometry in patients with retinitis pigmentosa. Arch Ophthalmol 1981;99:1202–1206.
55. Braude LS, Cunha-Vaz JG, Goldberg MF, et al. Diagnosing acute retrobulbar neuritis by vitreous fluorophotometry. Am J Ophthalmol 1981;91:764–773.
56. Kayazawa F, Miyake K. Ocular fluorophotometry in patients with essential hypertension. Arch Ophthalmol 1984;102:1169–1170.
57. Kelley JS, Kincaid M. Retinal fluorography using oral fluorescein. Arch Ophthalmol 1979;97:2331–2332.
58. Hunter JE. Oral fluorography in a retinal pigment epithelial detachment. Am J Optom Physiol Opt 1982;59:908–910.
59. Morgan KS, Franklin RM. Oral fluorescein angioscopy in aphakic children. J Pediatr Ophthalmol Strabismus 1984;21:33–36..
60. Noble MJ, Cheng H, Jacobs PM. Oral fluorescein and cystoid macular edema: Detection in aphakic and pseudophakic eyes. Br J Ophthalmol 1984;68:221–224.
61. Potter JW, Bartlett JD, Alexander LJ, et al. Oral fluorography. J Am Optom Assoc 1985;56:784–792.
62. Nuzzi G, Vanelli M, Venturini I, et al. Vitreous fluorophotometry in juvenile diabetes after oral fluorescein. Arch Ophthalmol 1986;104:1630–1631.
63. Marcus DF, Etienne C. Adverse effects of sodium fluorescein as used in fluorescein angiography. Presented at the Ocular Toxicology Symposium, Little Rock, Arkansas, 1977.
64. Yannuzzi LA, Rohrer KT, Tindel LJ, et al. Fluorescein angiography complications survey. Ophthalmology 1986;93:611–617.
65. Schatz H, Farkos WS. Nausea from fluorescein angiography. Am J Ophthalmol 1982;93:370–371.
66. Willerson D, Tate GW, Baldwin HA, Hernsberger PL. Clinical evaluation of fluorescein 25%. Ann Ophthalmol 1976;8:833–842.
67. Charzan BI, Balodimos ML, Konez L. Untoward effects of fluorescein retinal angiography in diabetic patients. Ann Ophthalmol 1971;3:42–49.
68. Stein MF, Parker CW. Reactions following intravenous fluorescein. Am J Ophthalmol 1971;72:861–868.
69. Hess JB, Pacuraria RI. Acute pulmonary edema following intravenous fluorescein angiography. Am J Ophthalmol 1976;82:567–570.
70. Arroyave CM, Wolbers R, Ellis PP. Plasma complement and histamine changes after intravenous administration of sodium fluorescein. Am J Ophthalmol 1979;84:474–479.
71. Applebaum M, Jaanus SD. A study of utilization of diagnostic pharmaceutical agents and incidence of adverse effects. Am J Optom Physiol Optics 1983;60:384–388.
72. National registry of drug-induced ocular side effects. Case reports 404a, 4046, 421. Portland: University of Oregon Health Sciences Center, 1979.
73. Cohn CH, Jocson VL. A unique case of grand mal seizures after Fluress. Ann Ophthalmol 1981;13:1379–1380.
74. Refojo MF, Miller D, Fiore AS. A new fluorescent stain for soft hydrophilic lens fitting. Arch Ophthalmol 1972;87:275–277.
75. Norn MS. Fluorexon vital staining of cornea and conjunctiva. Acta Ophthalmol 1973;51:670–678.
76. Norn MS. External eye. Methods of examination. Copenhagen: Scriptor, 1974; Chap. IV.
77. Passmore JW, King JH. Vital staining of conjunctiva and cornea. Arch Ophthalmol 1955;53:568–574.
78. Norn MS. Rose bengal vital staining. Acta Ophthalmol 1970;48:546–559.
79. Marsh RJ, Fraunfelder FT, McGill JI. Herpetic corneal disease. Arch Ophthalmol 1976;94:1899–1902.
80. Roat MI, Romanowski E, Acaullo-Cruz T, Gordon YL. The antiviral effects of rose bengal and fluorescein. Arch Ophthalmol 1987;105:1415–1417.
81. Cherrick GR, Stein SW, Leery CM. Indocyanine green: Observation on its physical properties, plasma decay, and hepatic function. J Clin Invest 1960;39:592–601.
82. Flower RW, Hochheimer BF. A clinical technique and apparatus for simultaneous angiography of the separate retinal and choroidal circulation. Invest Ophthalmol 1973;12:248–261.
83. McEnerney JK, Peyman GA. Indocyanine green. A new vital stain for use before penetrating keratoplasty. Arch Ophthalmol 1978;96:1445–1447.
84. Hayashi K, Hasegawa Y, Tokoro T. Indocyanine green angiography of central serous chorioretinopathy. Int Ophthalmol Clin 1986;9:37–41.
85. Stocker FW, King EH, Lucas DO, Georiade N. Clinical test for evaluating donor corneas. Arch Ophthalmol 1970;84:2–7.
86. Taylor MS, Hunt CJ. Dual staining of corneal endothelium with trypan blue and alizarin red S: Importance of pH for the dye-lake reaction. Br J Ophthalmol 1981;65:815–819.
87. Norn MS. Preoperative trypan blue vital staining of corneal endothelium. Eight year's follow-up. Acta Ophthalmol 1980;58:550–555.
88. Norn MS. Specific double vital staining of the cornea and conjunctiva with rose bengal and alcian blue. Acta Ophthalmol 1964;42:84–96.
89. Bourne WM. The permeability of the corneal endothelium to fluorescein in normal human eye. Curr Eye Res 1984;3:509–513.
90. Young G. Fluorescein in rigid lens fit evaluation. Int Cont Lens Clin 1988;15:95–100.
91. Nayak BK, Ghose S. A method for fundus evaluation in children with oral fluorescein. Br J Ophthalmol 1987;71:907–909.
92. Maguire AM, Bennett J. Fluorescein elimination in human breast milk. Arch Ophthalmol 1988;106:718–719.

CHAPTER 13

Preparations Used with Contact Lenses

Gerald E. Lowther

Numerous formulations have been developed for use with contact lenses. New products are continually being developed to overcome specific problems and to be compatible with new lens polymers. To prescribe the correct solutions and to diagnose problems that they may cause, the practitioner must understand the products in current use, their formulation strategies, interactions, sensitivities, and toxicities.

The safety of solutions and lens care systems is of constant concern. In the United States the Food and Drug Administration (FDA) regulates contact lens solutions for new lens polymers. Most new contact lens solutions, except those used with polymethylmethacrylate (PMMA) lenses, must undergo laboratory tests, including toxicology studies and clinical trials, before being placed on the market. This does not mean, however, that they are safe and effective for all patients and under all conditions. Therefore, the practitioner must understand the solutions, their potential shortcomings, and their possible abuses by patients.

Physiochemical Properties of Contact Lens Solutions

To understand the uses, problems, and interactions of solutions, it is important to consider the chemical properties of these solutions.

Osmolarity (Tonicity)

The osmotic pressure of a solution affects the water flow across a semipermeable membrane. For example, if a hypotonic solution is placed on the cornea, water will flow from the solution, which has a low concentration of ions, into the cornea, which has a higher ion concentration. This will cause corneal swelling (edema). Likewise, if the solution has a higher concentration of ions (is more hypertonic) than the corneal tissue, water will be drawn from the cornea into the solution, causing the cornea to deturgesce. To maintain normal corneal thickness, contact lens solutions should be isotonic with the normal tear film. With the eye open, the tear film has a tonicity of 0.95% to 1.0% equivalent NaCl.[1-3] With the eye closed, as during sleep, the tonicity drops to 0.9% equivalent NaCl or less.[1] Variations from 0.5% to 2.0% equivalent NaCl solutions usually do not cause discomfort if placed directly onto the eye.

With hydrogel lenses, the tonicity of the solution in which the lens is soaked will affect the lens dimensions. If a hydrogel lens is placed in distilled water, a very hypotonic solution, the lens will swell.[4] Conversely, if it is placed in a hypertonic solution, it will shrink. In addition, if a hydrogel lens is soaked in either a hypertonic or a hypotonic solution and placed on the eye, the lens will adhere to the cornea. The greater the difference in tonicity between the lens and cornea, the tighter will be the adhesion.[5] If the patient then attempts to remove the lens, corneal epithelium may be removed. However, if the patient waits a few minutes after placing the lens on the eye before attempted removal, the tears will have time to equilibrate with the solution in the lens, ensuring easy removal.

Because of the tonicity effect on the integrity of ocular tissue, contact lens solutions should be adjusted to a tonicity of 0.9% to 1.0% equivalent NaCl by adding an appropriate amount of a salt, such as sodium or potassium chloride. Contact lens solutions, however, may have tonicity values from 0.14% to 1.4% equivalent NaCl.[6]

Hydrogen Ion Concentration

The concentration of hydrogen (H^+) or hydroxyl (OH^-) ions in a contact lens solution is important. This property is specified by the notation pH, where the pH is the logarithm of the inverse of the hydrogen ion concentration. If the pH is 7.0, the solution is considered neutral; if less than 7.0, it is acidic; and if greater than 7.0, it is alkaline. A change in pH of 1.0 unit is a 10 times change in H^+ concentration. The average pH of the normal tear film is about 7.35, with most being between 7.0 and 7.4. With the eye closed the pH often decreases by 0.1 to 0.3 pH units.

A solution that is too acidic (pH $\leq$ 6.6) or too alkaline (pH $\geq$ 7.8) may cause ocular discomfort.[7] Some of the problems might be tearing, burning for the first few minutes after lens placement, conjunctival injection, stringy mucus formation, and lens filming.[8]

The optimum effectiveness of preservatives is related to a solution's pH. Certain preservatives, such as chlorobutanol, are most effective and stable at an acidic pH. Others, like benzalkonium chloride (BAK), exert their maximum antibacterial effect in an alkaline environment. Thus, fluctuations in pH can inactivate a preservative and increase the chance of microbial contamination. Such changes can occur if CO_2 from the air diffuses into the solution, forming carbonic acid. CO_2 can diffuse through polyethylene storage bottles or the rubber stoppers used on some hydrogel lens vials. Such decreases in pH may cause ocular discomfort and indicate the importance of using buffers to maintain solution pH.

The pH values of contact lens solutions vary from 4.2 to 8.6,[6] which may explain why some patients complain of discomfort on initial lens placement and why patients often prefer one brand of solution to another.

Buffering

Buffers are used to maintain a solution at a desired pH. The more strongly a solution is buffered, the more acid or base can be added before the pH changes.

Buffers are either acid or alkaline salts and include phosphates, borates, citrates, acetates, and bicarbonates. Bicarbonates, acetates, and citrates are relatively volatile and unstable and may be incompatible with other compounds.[9] The type of buffer used often depends on the preservative. For example, borate buffer is incompatible with the common preservative benzalkonium chloride.[10] Likewise, if borates are used with alkaline contact lens solutions or solutions containing polyvinyl alcohol (PVA), a gel or gummy deposit can form.[9] This points out the importance of not mixing solutions that may be incompatible. For example, using a wetting solution from 1 manufacturer with a soaking solution from a different manufacturer may result in such an untoward reaction.

If a contact lens solution requires an acidic pH to maintain an active preservative or to prevent the breakdown of other compounds while stored in the bottle, it may be buffered at the optimum pH. However, since the tear film is basic, the application of a highly buffered acidic solution to the eye might cause discomfort or corneal damage. Thus, any solution that is destined for the eye and requires an acidic environment should either not be buffered or be only minimally buffered so that the tear film's buffering capacity can bring the solution to the tear film pH. If the solution has an alkaline pH near 7.3 to 7.4, it can be strongly buffered, since the pH will not have to change when the solution is introduced into the eye.

Preservatives and Disinfectants

The major concern with contact lens fitting is maintaining ocular health. A potential problem is ocular infection from contaminated lenses. Likewise, accessory solutions for use with lenses can become contaminated in the bottle if these solutions are not properly packaged or preserved. Due to contamination from the environment and favorable growth factors offered by the nutrients from the tear film, if a lens is removed from the eye and placed in water or unpreserved saline, organisms usually thrive (Fig. 13.1).

In an attempt to overcome the problem of microorganism contamination, a number of procedures and chemicals have been used. This section will discuss some of the chemicals, often called preservatives. Other methods of preventing growth or killing organisms are considered later in this chapter.

Benzalkonium Chloride

Benzalkonium chloride (BAK), known by a number of proprietary names including Zephiran Chloride and

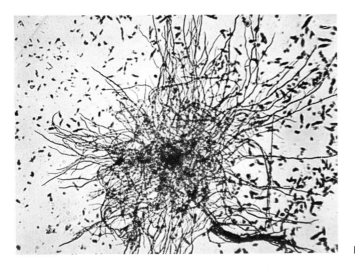

FIGURE 13.1   **Fungal and bacterial organisms on a hydrogel lens.**

Roccal, is a quaternary ammonium compound. It is used extensively in solutions for use with PMMA contact lenses. This surface-active agent is a cationic detergent compound with a hydrophilic end group and a hydrophobic (lipophilic) end group (Fig. 13.2). Thus, it acts as a soap and attaches to surfaces, such as lens and cell surfaces, and acts at lipid-water interfaces. A detrimental effect of this compound is that the hydrophilic end groups align on the lens surface, allowing the lipophilic end groups to be exposed. This causes the lens to become hydrophobic. Thus, an effective wetting agent must be used with this preservative to maintain lens wettability.[11]

BAK acts against microorganisms by adsorbing on the cell membrane and increasing its permeability, with eventual rupture of the cell membrane. In addition, the compound may penetrate the cell wall and precipitate respiratory and glycolytic enzymes.[12] It is used in concentrations of 0.001% (1:100,000) to 0.1% (1:10,000). As with any preservative, there must be a high enough concentration to prevent microbial growth but not cause significant toxicity to the eye. A number of studies[11,13] have shown that BAK can cause corneal damage in concentrations as low as 0.005%, although it may require a longer exposure time than would normally occur with a solution used on a rigid contact lens.[14,15] At concentrations of 0.0075% to 0.01%, major corneal epithelial damage can occur within several minutes of continuous exposure.

Since hydrogel lenses absorb and concentrate significant amounts of BAK,[9,16–18] it cannot be used in soaking solutions for these lenses.

BAK is most effective at an alkaline pH of approximately 8.0.[19] Phospholipids will inactivate this preservative, and it is strongly absorbed by organic matter, rubber, fibers, and sponge material.[20] Therefore, it is important to clean all tear film debris from the lens before placing the lens in a storage solution containing BAK and not to use cases that contain absorbent material. Likewise, since soap inactivates BAK,[21] soap must be well rinsed off the hands before handling lenses.

Ions such as those of magnesium, calcium, and potassium have a detrimental effect on the action of BAK by competing for active sites on the cell membranes. To overcome this problem, the chelating agent, ethylenediaminetetraacetic acid (EDTA), is usually used with BAK to increase its effectiveness.[11,19]

Even though BAK is still widely used in contact lens solutions and other ophthalmic preparations, its use is decreasing because of its incompatibility with new lens materials, especially with hydrogels, and its detrimental effect on the cornea.

Chlorobutanol

Chlorobutanol is a preservative that has been incorporated into some solutions for use with PMMA lenses. A volatile compound with a characteristic odor, it is easily lost from solution.[22] Chlorobutanol is effective at acidic but not at alkaline pH.[23] It is also easily deactivated by heat. Because of its instability and slow kill rate, it is seldom used.[24] When used, concentrations of 0.3% to 0.5% are common. It is used in combination with other preservatives such as BAK. Chlorobutanol cannot be used with hydrogel lenses.

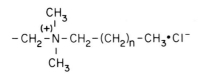

FIGURE 13.2   **Chemical structure of benzalkonium chloride.**

Phenylmercuric Nitrate

This compound has slow antimicrobial activity but has been used to a limited extent in some rigid contact lens solutions in combination with other preservatives. It can be maintained in an acid solution without precipitation.

Thimerosal

Thimerosal is an organic mercury compound (Fig. 13.3) used in both rigid and hydrogel lens solutions. It apparently does not bind significantly to hydrogel lenses,[25] but the negatively charged ion may bind with proteins.[26]

Thimerosal must be maintained in a neutral or alkaline pH, since it may precipitate in an acid environment. In addition, it should be stored in an opaque container, since light breaks it down.[20] It acts by forming covalent bonds with SH-groups of microbial cell enzymes. This inhibits enzyme function and kills microorganisms. Thimerosal also inhibits cell membrane processes by this mechanism.[12]

Thimerosal is usually used in concentrations of 0.001% to 0.2% in combination with other preservatives such as EDTA or chlorhexidine. It is not chemically compatible with BAK.

One problem with thimerosal is the development of sensitivity to the compound, which occurs in as many as 25% to 50% of patients wearing hydrogel lenses.[27] This is discussed in greater detail in Chapter 14.

Thimerosal does not seem to have as great an effect on corneal metabolism as does BAK,[28] but it may be absorbed into the corneal tissue, at least under some conditions, causing corneal damage.[29]

Chlorhexidine

Chlorhexidine (Fig. 13.4) is used as a preservative in hydrogel lens solutions. Chlorhexidine digluconate and chlorhexidine diacetate have both been employed, with the former causing less ocular irritation. Chlorhexidine does bind to hydrogel lenses and is only slowly released.[18,30–32] It also binds to proteins and other tear film substances. This adherence to surface deposits on lenses may cause some of the observed sensitivities.

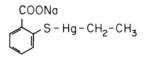

FIGURE 13.3   **Chemical structure of thimerosal.**

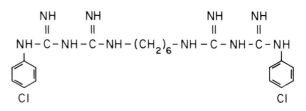

FIGURE 13.4   **Chemical structure of chlorhexidine.**

This preservative can cause ocular damage but not to the extent demonstrated by BAK.[15]

Chlorhexidine acts by attacking and rupturing cell membranes. It inhibits both cation transport and membrane-bound adenosine triphosphate (ATP) in the cell membrane.[12] It is less stable in alkaline than acidic solutions and should be maintained in a neutrally buffered solution. Since chlorhexidine is very effective against bacteria but not fungi, it is usually used in combination with another preservative, such as thimerosal.[33]

Ethylenediaminetetraacetic Acid

EDTA (Fig. 13.5) is a chelating agent that binds bivalent or trivalent metal ions. Since bacteria need trace amounts of metal ions, this compound slows or prevents cell growth. EDTA is not an effective antimicrobial agent when used alone and is therefore used only in combination with other preservatives. When used with other preservatives, there is a synergistic effect that increases the combination's effectiveness. EDTA or disodium edetate is used in nearly all contact lens preparations.

Disodium Edetate

Disodium edetate (Na_2 EDTA) is a chelating agent very similar in structure and function to EDTA. Many manufacturers use it in place of EDTA.

Sorbic Acid

Sorbic acid (Fig. 13.6) or its salt, sorbate, is a preservative commonly used in hydrogel contact lens solu-

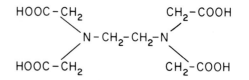

FIGURE 13.5   **Chemical structure of EDTA.**

$$CH_3-CH=CH-CH=CH-COOH$$

FIGURE 13.6 **Chemical structure of sorbic acid.**

tions. Its greatest advantage is that it can be used with hydrogel lenses, since it is associated with a very low incidence of allergic or toxic reactions. Sorbic acid is most effective at a pH of 4.5 and is not effective above a pH of 6.5.[34] It is usually used in concentrations of 0.1% to 0.2% and is employed in combination with EDTA. Sorbic acid is a weak preservative. As a bacteriostatic agent it can be used as a preservative in saline for heat disinfection or as a lens rinse but not as a chemical disinfecting solution.

Tris (2-hydroxyethyl) Tallow Ammonium Chloride

This preservative has been used in conjunction with thimerosal as a hydrogel lens disinfecting solution, since it is not sufficiently strong to be used alone as a disinfectant. The solution (Allergan Hydrocare Cleaning and Disinfection Solution) contains other polymeric compounds to aid in the formation of micelles, large groups of molecules that minimize absorption of the preservatives into the lens and thus decrease allergic or toxic reactions.

Polyquad

Polyquad is a high molecular weight quaternary compound. Because of its large molecular size (Fig. 13.7), it is not absorbed into most hydrogel lenses, and thus toxic or allergic reactions are rare. However, the first formulation using this preservative did cause toxic re-

actions when used with high water ionic lenses. It is a strong enough disinfectant to have been approved for cold disinfection of hydrogel lenses.

Polyhexamethylene Biguanide (Dymed)

This compound was developed for use with hydrogel lenses to overcome the toxic and allergic reactions common with solutions containing thimerosal and chlorhexidine. The molecule consists of chains of 6-carbon groups with biguanide groups between them (Fig. 13.8), resulting in a long chain molecule. The positive charge surrounding the molecule reacts with the negatively charged phospholipid groups in the cell walls of microorganisms, causing damage to the membrane and cell death. It is used in very low concentrations (0.00005%). Polyhexamethylene biguanide is from the same family of compounds as chlorhexidine, but polyhexamethylene biguanide does not have the parachloroaniline end group that may degrade, causing the toxic problem occasionally found with chlorhexidine.

Hydrogen Peroxide

Use of hydrogen peroxide was one of the earliest methods for disinfecting hydrogel lenses.[35] It has been used extensively for years as a disinfectant for hydrogel lenses outside the United States. Because of the multiple steps required to neutralize the low pH (3 to 5) of the hydrogen peroxide with sodium bicarbonate, and questions about its stability, it was not approved in the United States until 1983. Today, due to better methods for neutralization, hydrogen peroxide has become the system of choice for many practitioners.

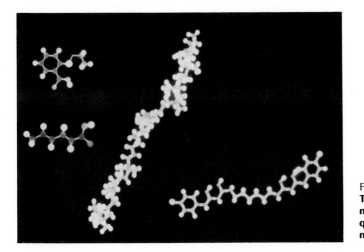

FIGURE 13.7 **Relative molecular sizes of different preservatives.** Thimerosal *(upper left)*; sorbic acid *(left)*; alkyl triethanol ammonium chloride *(lower right)*; and Polyquad *(center)*. The Polyquad molecule is shown at one-quarter the size of the other molecules. (Courtesy Alcon Laboratories, Inc.)

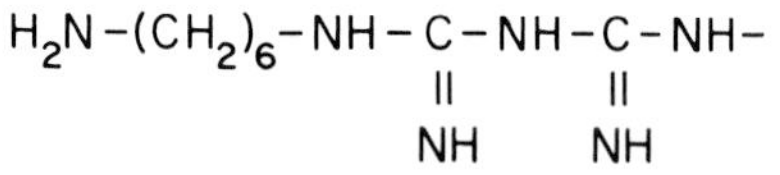

$$H_2N-(CH_2)_6-NH-C-NH-C-NH-$$

FIGURE 13.8   **Chemical structure of polyhexamethylene biguanide (Dymed).**

$$2 H_2O_2 \longrightarrow 2 H_2O + O_2$$

FIGURE 13.9   **Chemical reaction for the breakdown of hydrogen peroxide.**

Hydrogen peroxide is a highly reactive oxidizing agent with the advantage that it can be broken down into water and oxygen (Fig. 13.9). It apparently kills organisms by the oxidizing action of the free radicals that form. Its effectiveness is related to its concentration and time of exposure to the organism. It is a very reactive substance that can decompose in the bottle if not properly stabilized. Most hydrogen peroxides used with contact lenses are stabilized with small quantities of inorganic sodium stannate and sodium nitrate. Some hydrogen peroxides not specifically formulated for contact lenses may be stabilized with other compounds that can cause brownish, pink, yellow, or other lens discolorations.

Numerous methods of neutralizing hydrogen peroxide are available.[61] One of the first commercially viable methods was the use of a platinum catalyst to accelerate the breakdown of hydrogen peroxide to water and oxygen. A small amount of platinum is coated on a plastic disk. When the hydrogen peroxide contacts the disk, it is neutralized but the platinum is not consumed in the reaction. However, with time the disk may become coated, requiring replacement. Some time is required for all the hydrogen peroxide to come in contact with the catalytic disk, since the hydrogen peroxide must diffuse from the lens and through the so-lution to the disk. The first catalytic disk system to become commercially available in the United States (Septicon) used a 10-minute soak in hydrogen peroxide. The lens was then removed from hydrogen peroxide and placed in saline along with the catalytic disk. The hydrogen peroxide was diluted with the saline, and the remainder broken down by the disk. Figure 13.10 shows the time for neutralization to occur assuming 3000 parts per million (ppm) carry-over of the hydrogen peroxide from the 3% (30,000 ppm) disinfecting solution.[36] It takes several hours for the hydrogen peroxide level to reach a low value. Patients' sensitivity to hydrogen peroxide varies, but if the level is less than 30 to 60 ppm, most patients will have no discomfort.[36-38]

The more recently developed catalytic system (AOSept) eliminates the step of removing the lens from the hydrogen peroxide and placing it in a second solution of saline for neutralization. The lens and 3% hydrogen peroxide are placed in the case with the catalytic disk. Since it takes some time for the hydrogen peroxide to break down (Fig. 13.11), it is present long enough to kill most organisms. Up to 3 hours after the beginning of neutralization, the level of hydrogen peroxide is still higher than with the Septicon system, since with AOSept the starting level is 30,000 ppm and with Septicon it was about 3000 ppm.

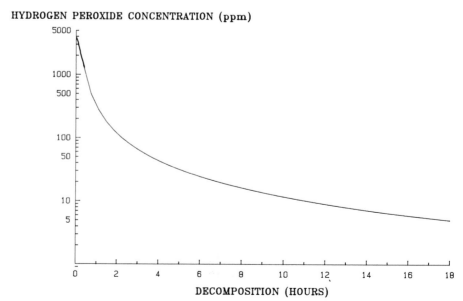

HYDROGEN PEROXIDE CONCENTRATION (ppm)

DECOMPOSITION (HOURS)

FIGURE 13.10   **Rate of decomposition of hydrogen peroxide after lens is removed from 3% hydrogen peroxide and placed in saline with the catalytic disk. (Modified from Janoff LE. The Septicon system: A review of pertinent scientific data. Int Cont Lens Clin 1984; 11:274–279.)**

PPM HYDROGEN PEROXIDE

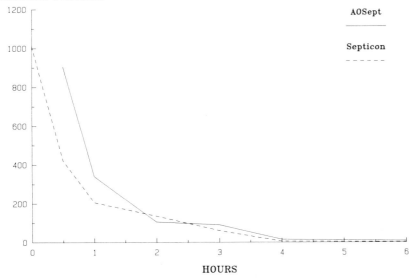

FIGURE 13.11 **Rate of decomposition of hydrogen peroxide when 3% hydrogen peroxide is placed with the catalytic disk (AOSept system) and when lens is removed and placed in saline with the catalytic disk (Septicon system). (Modified from Gyulai P, Dziabo A, Kelley W, et al. Relative neutralization ability of six hydrogen peroxide disinfection systems. Contact Lens Spectrum 1987; 2:61–66.)**

Another system of neutralization is the use of an enzyme, catalase, which breaks down the hydrogen peroxide.[39] Catalase, derived from bovine liver, is used in the OxySept and the Lensept system. The hydrogen peroxide is neutralized in about 1 minute (Fig. 13.12).

Sodium pyruvate, another agent, neutralizes hydrogen peroxide in 5 to 6 minutes (see Fig. 13.12).

Sodium sulfite is another compound used to rapidly break down hydrogen peroxide. The chemical reaction is shown in Figure 13.13. Sodium thiosulfate, used in the Consept system, will also neutralize hydrogen peroxide (Fig. 13.14) but apparently takes longer to do so than catalase and sodium pyruvate (see Fig.13.12).

The concentration of hydrogen peroxide can also be decreased by dilution (see Fig. 13.12). Multiple rinses with saline will decrease the levels of hydrogen peroxide enough for some patients not to notice stinging on lens placement, but this technique is not sufficient for many patients.

Sodium Dichloroisocyanurate

Sodium dichloroisocyanurate has been used for disinfection of hydrogel lenses. It is supplied in the form of effervescent tablets (Softab, Alcon). A tablet is

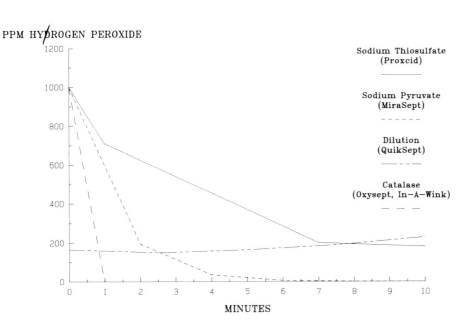

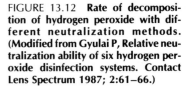

FIGURE 13.12 **Rate of decomposition of hydrogen peroxide with different neutralization methods. (Modified from Gyulai P, Relative neutralization ability of six hydrogen peroxide disinfection systems. Contact Lens Spectrum 1987; 2:61–66.)**

$$Na_2SO_3 + H_2O_2 \rightarrow Na_2SO_4 + H_2O$$

FIGURE 13.13   **Sodium sulfite neutralization of hydrogen peroxide.**

$$2[S_2O_3]^{-2} + H_2O_2 \rightarrow [S_4O_6]^{-2} + 2[OH]^{-1}$$

FIGURE 13.14   **Thiosulfate neutralization of hydrogen peroxide.**

placed in saline with the lens and breaks down, giving off chlorine, which is an oxidative disinfectant. It takes 2 to 4 hours for disinfection to occur. Following disinfection the lenses must be thoroughly rinsed with saline.

Alcohol

Alcohol is a good disinfectant as well as a cleaner. Some solutions use alcohol as a cleaner (MiraFlow) and have enough alcohol to reduce microbial growth. If the solution is not sufficiently rinsed off the lens, it will cause considerable discomfort. Benzyl alcohol in low concentrations (0.1%) in conjunction with other preservatives is also used.

Trimethoprim

This compound is an antibiotic used in urinary tract and other systemic disorders.[40] It has been evaluated for use as a contact lens "preservative," but due to concerns about microbial resistance occurring with its use, it has not been approved for use in the United States.

Effectiveness of Preservatives

Many factors can influence the effectiveness of a preservative against microorganisms. These must be taken into account in clinical practice. For example, with time many compounds decompose. Therefore, solutions beyond their expiration date should not be used. Increased heat—for example, if a patient keeps solutions on a heater or leaves them in a hot car for a period of time—will accelerate the decomposition. Leaving the container open, allowing evaporation, can affect the concentration of the solution. Some preservatives are adsorbed to the bottle surfaces and to any organic contaminates that get into the bottle or lens case, decreasing the amount of preservative available to work against microorganisms.

The amount of preservative in a solution does not necessarily determine the solution's antimicrobial activity. Other components in the system, such as viscosity-increasing agents, wetting agents, buffers, salts, and other ingredients, can affect the activity. Figure 13.15 shows the effect of 2 formulations of 0.001% chlorhexidine against *Staphylococcus aureus*.[41]

Preservatives are absorbed and adsorbed by hydrogel lenses. Figure 13.16 shows the effect of having lenses present in a solution of 0.001% chlorhexidine

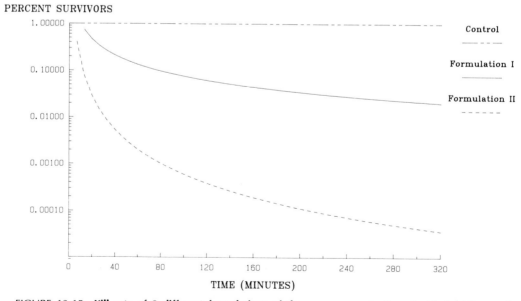

FIGURE 13.15   **Kill rate of 2 different formulations of the same concentration of chlorhexidine against *Staphylococcus aureus*. (Modified from Meakin BJ. Contact lens solutions in the United Kingdom. J Br CL Assoc 1984;7:192–203.)**

PERCENT SURVIVORS

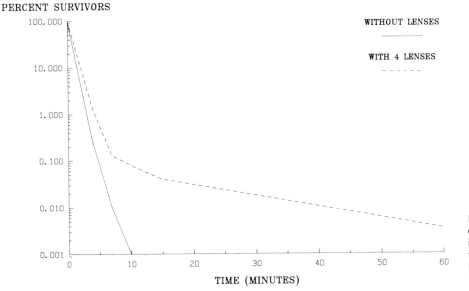

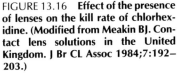

FIGURE 13.16 **Effect of the presence of lenses on the kill rate of chlorhexidine. (Modified from Meakin BJ. Contact lens solutions in the United Kingdom. J Br CL Assoc 1984;7:192–203.)**

on the time required to kill *S. aureus*.[41] The kill time is considerably increased due to the presence of the lenses.

The temperature in which the disinfection occurs can also be a factor. Some patients may soak lenses in solutions in very warm climates or bathrooms, while others may soak them in much cooler locations and climates. Figure 13.17 shows the difference in kill times on *S. aureus* between two very feasible environmental temperatures.[41]

In addition to solution composition and environ-

mental factors influencing solutions' effectiveness is the question of the relative effectiveness of different preservatives and systems. Likewise, the time required to effectively kill organisms is important clinically. In the United States, the FDA requires a number of tests for new solutions and preservatives. These include the effectiveness against a challenge of a series of bacteria at a level of 10^6 colony forming units (CFU)/ml of challenge solution, and a rechallenge after 2 weeks to see if the disinfectant remains effective. The ability of the preservative to kill organisms is often reported as

SURVIVING FRACTION

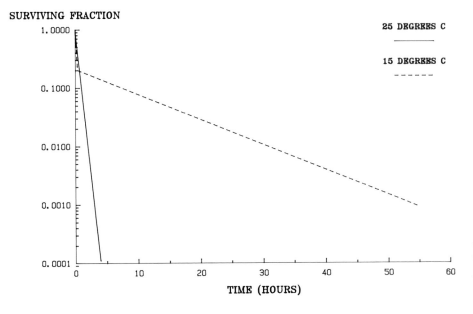

FIGURE 13.17 **Effect of temperature of 0.001% chlorhexidine against *Staphylococcus aureus*. (Modified from Meakin BJ. Contact lens solutions in the United Kingdom. J Br CL Assoc 1984;7:192–203.)**

LOG REDUCTION IN ORGANISMS

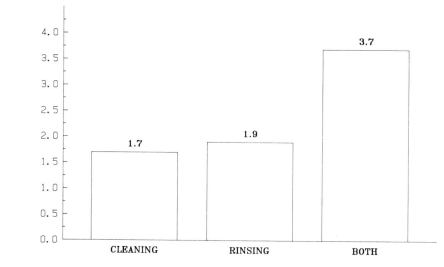

FIGURE 13.18 **Effect of cleaning and rinsing a lens prior to disinfection as related to removal of microorganisms. (Modified from Houlsby RD, Ghajar M, Chavez G. Microbiological evaluation of soft contact lens disinfecting solutions. J Am Optom Assoc 1984;55:205–211.)**

a D-value. The D-value is the time required to decrease the number of organisms 1 log unit, i.e., to kill 90% of the organisms present. Therefore, the shorter the D-value, the more effective is the solution at killing the organism.

Not only must the preservative itself be tested, but the effect of the entire disinfecting system must be taken into account. This can result in different effectivenesses being reported for the same preservative. For example, the cleaning and rinsing of a lens before placing the lens in the disinfecting solution is important. If a lens is taken from a solution of organisms and cleaned with a contact lens cleaner and rinsed with saline, many organisms are removed before beginning disinfection. Figure 13.18 shows the effect of cleaning

and rinsing.[42] Thus, it is important to educate the patient about proper cleaning and rinsing not only for preventing deposits, but also to help prevent infections. Since many patients may not clean lenses before disinfecting, a system reported as being safe may not be in actual use.

Different compounds and systems have different kill rates. Figure 13.19 shows the effect of three different preservative systems on three different organisms.[42] Another study[43] performed under different conditions showed somewhat different kill times but the same general relationship (Fig. 13.20).

Bacteria are killed more quickly than are fungi. In 1 study[42] the D-value for *Candida albicans* was 3.7 minutes for a solution of chlorhexidine-thimerosal, 27.9

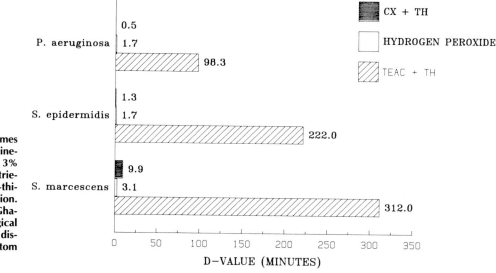

FIGURE 13.19 **Relative kill times of 3 organisms for a chlorhexidine-thimerosal (CX+TH) solution, 3% hydrogen peroxide, and alkyl triethanol ammonium chloride–thimerosal (TEAC+Th) solution. (Modified from Houlsby RD, Ghajar M, Chavez G. Microbiological evaluation of soft contact lens disinfecting solutions. J Am Optom Assoc 1984;55:205–211.)**

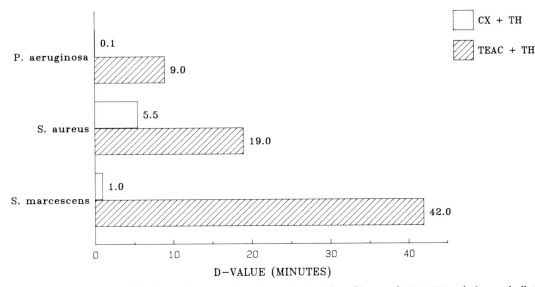

FIGURE 13.20   **Relative kill times of 3 organisms for a chlorhexidine-thimerosal (CX + TH) solution and alkyl triethanol ammonium chloride–thimerosal (TEAC + TH) solution. (Modified from Penley CA, Schlitzer RL, Adhearn DG, et al. Laboratory evaluation of chemical disinfection of soft contact lenses. Contact Intraocular Lens Med J 1981;7:101–110.)**

for hydrogen peroxide, and 98.3 for the tallow ammonium chloride and thimerosal solution. For *A. fumigatus* it was 25.1 minutes for hydrogen peroxide, 215 minutes for alkyl triethanol ammonium chloride and thimerosal solution, and undetermined for the chlorhexidine-thimerosal solution due to a nonlinear disinfection rate. Penley and associates[43] found that the chlorhexidine-thimerosal and the alkyl triethanol ammonium chloride–thimerosal solutions gave adequate disinfection against three different fungi, but that a 3 ppm chlorine tablet solution—the dichloroisocyanurate dihydrate tablets giving about 27 ppm chlorine—and a povidone-iodine system did not give adequate disinfection.

Another area of concern and controversy has been the effective disinfection time for hydrogen peroxide. With the AOSept system the hydrogen peroxide starts to be neutralized immediately on placement in the case and then decreases, reaching less than 400 ppm after 1 hour compared with the 30,000 ppm initially. With the chemical neutralization methods the disinfection is ended within seconds or minutes after the neutralizer is introduced. The question remaining is whether the 10- or 20-minute recommended time is sufficient to kill organisms that may be present. Studies[36,44] have indicated that bacteria such as *Pseudomonas aeruginosa*, *S. aureus*, and *Staphylococcus epidermidis* have D-values less than 5 minutes, so a 10- or 20-minute soak will usually suffice. On the other hand, most fungi require much longer D-values in 3% hydrogen peroxide. Fig-

ure 13.21 shows the D-values for several fungi. Note that the tests were done with high levels of fungi, but, on the other hand, the D-value is the time to kill 90% of all organisms, not 100% of the organisms. Seldom would one expect to have such high levels of organism on patients' lenses if they are cared for properly. However, to be safe, longer disinfecting times could be recommended. In general, no adverse effects on lenses occur with 1-hour or overnight disinfection, but some high water, ionic lenses will have a temporary change in parameters.

There has been particular concern about the possibility of transmitting the human immunodeficiency virus (HIV), which causes acquired immunodeficiency syndrome (AIDS), through contaminated contact lenses, especially diagnostic lenses used in the office on more than 1 patient. A 5- to 10-minute soak in 3% hydrogen peroxide will kill the virus on both hydrogel and rigid lenses.[45] Likewise, standard heat disinfection as used by patients with hydrogel lenses will kill the virus. Vogt and associates[46] have shown that using solutions preserved with chlorhexidine (Boston solutions for rigid, and Softmate Disinfection Solution for hydrogels) following normal cleaning also kills the virus. Simply rinsing with saline alone does not affect the virus.

During the last decade there has been a dramatic increase in reported cases of *Acanthamoeba* keratitis, the majority of which have occurred in wearers of hydrogel contact lenses.[47,48] However, the number of

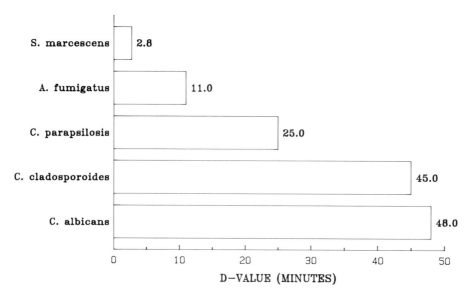

FIGURE 13.21 **Kill rates (minutes) for different organisms in 3% hydrogen peroxide. (Modified from Penley CA, Llabres C, Wilson LA, et al. Efficacy of hydrogen peroxide disinfection systems for soft contact lenses contaminated with fungi. CLAO 1985;11:65–68.)**

cases of *Acanthamoeba* infection is very small. A significant problem has been the lack of effective drug therapy, with most cases progressing to partial or complete corneal destruction. *Acanthamoeba,* a free-living protozoan, can exist in 2 forms, the motile trophozoite form and a dormant cyst. Standard heat disinfection kills both forms.[49] Alkyl triethanol ammonium chloride–thimerosal and 3% hydrogen peroxide chemical disinfection systems have been ineffective against the organism. The chlorhexidine-thimerosal system has been effective against some strains of *Acanthamoeba* but not against others. Since most cases of the disease have involved patients improperly using salt tablet saline, a primary method of prevention would be to discontinue the use of salt tablet prepared saline and to discontinue the use of distilled water for enzymatic cleaning. Likewise, lenses should not be rinsed in anything except prepared, sterile, or preserved contact lens solutions.

Wetting Agents

Solutions used with contact lenses can be placed into general categories based on their function. With rigid contact lenses some type of wetting solution is normally used. Such a solution forms a uniform film over the lens surface so that when the lens is placed on the cornea, the lens will be compatible with the ocular tissue. If the lens surface is dry when the eyelid moves over the lens, it will be quite irritating and cause tearing. Likewise, tear film breakup on the front of the lens will cause blurred vision. If the relative wettability of the surface is adequate, a thin mucoid layer

will form on the lens surface after the lens has been on the eye a few minutes, and the tear film will wet the lens. This natural wetting by the tears is necessary, since any solution placed on the lens dissipates within a few minutes. If the polymer surface is quite hydrophobic, the tear film will not form and the lens becomes unwearable. On the other hand, a hydrophilic surface will be wetted with a uniform film.

With nonhydrogel lenses a wetting or viscosity-increasing agent is helpful to initially obtain a liquid film over the hydrophobic lens surface to improve comfort and vision following lens placement. Pharmaceutical companies have taken 2 approaches to overcoming the hydrophobic surface: (1) to use a wetting agent that interacts with the surface, and (2) to use a viscosity agent that coats the surface simply by thickening the tear film.

The most commonly used wetting agent is PVA. It adheres to the surface of the lens and reportedly remains on the lens considerably longer than do viscosity-increasing agents.[50] PVA is a synthetic, long-chain polymer with a very low viscosity. Partially acetylated PVA is often used because it has better surface-wetting properties. However, partially acetylated PVA will hydrolyze to yield PVA and acetic acid if the pH of the solution is in the alkaline range. Excessive acetic acid will act as a buffer and will prevent the pH of the solution from adjusting to the pH of the tears, thus causing stinging.[51] Therefore, solutions with PVA must be kept at an acidic pH (5 to 6).

PVA is compatible with most preservatives. It also does not retard corneal epithelial healing.[13,50] The use of solutions of PVA may lessen the symptoms of some patients who produce an excessive amount of mucus.[10]

Polysorbate 80 is another wetting agent used in some contact lens wetting solutions. It is an oleic acid ester of sorbitol. Because of the ester linkage, insoluble oleic acid and several alcohol species may result from hydrolytic breakdown of wetting solutions containing polysorbate 80.[51]

Lubricants

Other solutions may also be used in conjunction with contact lens wear. One category is the lubricating, comfort, or rewetting solutions that are placed onto the eye while the lenses are being worn. Sometimes lens surfaces dry, particularly in low humidity or windy conditions. These solutions are designed to rewet the surface and, in some cases, to help prevent and remove surface deposits. They may make the lenses temporarily more comfortable and extend wearing time. Solutions with high viscosity tend to coat a lens surface heavily and stay on the lens until mechanically wiped or washed off the lens by lid action and tearing. Since these substances are inert, there is no chemical interaction between the solutions and the lens.

The most common lubricants used in contact lens solutions are the substituted cellulose ethers, including methylcellulose and its derivatives, hydroxyethylcellulose and hydroxypropylcellulose. Solutions of these compounds form a thicker film on the lens than does PVA, but there is no correlation between the contact angle (measure of the wettability of the lens material) and the film thickness.[52] Increased film thickness may be detrimental, since a thick film can cause blurred vision and a sticky sensation and may coat the lid margins and dry, forming a white coating on the lids.

Polyvinylpyrrolidone (povidone, PVP) is another lubricant finding increasing use in contact lens solutions. A polymer, it can be produced in varying molecular weights.

Soaking (Storage) Agents

In the early years of rigid contact lens fitting there was controversy over whether contact lenses should be stored dry or in solution when not being worn. At that time only water or poorly preserved solutions were available for lens storage. Thus, if the lenses were maintained in these media, there was an increased chance of microbial contamination and ocular infection. Organisms will not normally thrive on a clean, dry surface. However, if lenses are stored dry, the dimensions, particularly the base curve radius, will change as the lens rehydrates, even though only about 1.5% water is absorbed.[53,54] Moreover, the dry surface will not wet well, even if a wetting solution is used, until the surface layers of the polymer become hydrated. Since solutions are currently formulated to prevent growth of organisms, soaking solutions are now universally used. Not only do they keep the lens hydrated, but they also prevent tear film debris from drying on the lens surface.

Soaking solutions are used with hydrogel lenses to maintain needed lens hydration and softness. Since growth of microorganisms is also a concern with these lenses, any solution used must contain a chemical agent to prevent microbial growth, or another method of killing contaminating organisms, such as heat, must be used. It is not necessary to use a separate wetting agent with hydrogel lenses due to the hydrophilic nature of the lens material. The same solution used for soaking is usually used on the lens before placement on the eye. In some cases, a rinsing solution, with less or no preservative, is used before lens placement to decrease the amount of preservative introduced onto the eye.

Cleaning Agents

Since proteins, mucus, and lipids from the tear film, and foreign material such as oils, hand creams, and make-up can contaminate the lens surface (Fig. 13.22), cleaning solutions must be used. These help to maintain a clean, wettable surface and good optics. Coatings develop on both rigid and soft lenses, and they are usually more difficult to remove from soft lenses. To prevent coating, daily cleaning is necessary. More effective cleaning methods or surface polishing may be required periodically.

One method of cleaning, used either alone or in combination with a special cleaning formulation, is mechanical rubbing of the lens surface. Simply rubbing the lens with the fingers, using water or saline, will remove some coatings, but this method is usually not sufficient. The practitioner may rub or polish the lens surface with a polishing compound such as Silvo (for PMMA lenses) or with a special polish such as XPAL in water (for rigid or hydrogel lenses).[55,56] Such procedures are not routinely recommended for patient use because of possible lens damage.

The daily use of surfactant cleaners is routinely recommended for all daily lens wearers of either rigid or soft lenses. Surfactant cleaners reduce surface tension, emulsify lipids, and solubilize other contaminants. Mechanical rubbing of the lens with the surfactant is required. Nonionic surfactants are often used so that there is no interaction between the solution and the

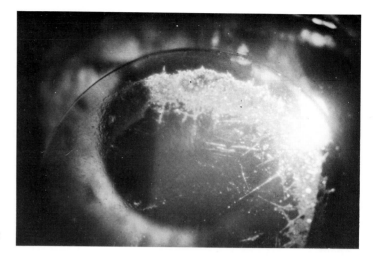

FIGURE 13.22   **Rigid lens (PMMA) with coating of foreign material.**

lens. Octoxynol, a macrogel ether, is an example of a surfactant. Such cleaners often have a high pH because proteins are more soluble in alkaline solutions. Chelating agents may also be used to remove ionic materials. Mild abrasive compounds have been added to some surfactant cleaners to enhance cleaning. Isopropyl and other alcohols have been incorporated into some cleaners to remove lipids. Other surfactant cleaners are formulated to be hypertonic to help remove deposits from hydrogel lenses. The osmotic pressure is thought to force water out of the lens, lifting debris from the lens surface.

Anionic surfactants (detergents) have been used with rigid lenses. The rationale is that since lens surfaces are negatively charged, positively charged debris attaches to the surface. Negatively charged (anionic) cleaners, therefore, should remove the debris. However, the cleaner may adhere to the lens surface, forming an insoluble film.

Patients and some practitioners have used household cleaners such as dishwashing compounds, laundry soaps, shampoos, toothpaste, scouring compounds, and skin cleaners. These should not be used because many contain anionic detergents, perfuming agents, solvents, reoiling agents, or abrasives. Such compounds may form insoluble films, craze or scratch the lens surface, and thereby adversely affect the cornea. Anionic detergents are not compatible with cationic preservatives such as BAK.[51]

Strong oxidizing agents have been used to clean hydrogel lenses. These are often effective but with repeated use may damage the lens. Some oxidizing agents are extremely acidic or alkaline and can cause severe ocular damage if the lens is accidentally placed on the eye without the proper neutralization.

A variety of enzymatic cleaners in the form of tablets are used to remove deposits from hydrogel lens surfaces. Papain, derived from the papaya, was the first enzyme used with hydrogel lenses and acts by breaking peptide bonds in the proteins.[57–60,62] The tablets contain an activator that gives the resulting solution a characteristic odor. Cysteine hydrochloride is added to the tablet (Allergan Enzymatic and Extenzyme) to act as a substrate modifier. Cysteine breaks disulfide bonds in the denatured lysozyme, which should then expose more of the peptide bonds to the proteolytic action. The enzyme is deactivated by heat and hydrogen peroxide. Another enzyme in common use is the pancreatic enzyme (from the hog pancreas). It contains lipase and amylase as well as protease.

Subtilisin A and B (produced by microorganisms) is now being used extensively. It is formulated to use with heat disinfection by placing the tablet in the case and enzyme treating the lenses at the same time as the lenses are heat disinfected (ReNu Thermal Enzymatic Cleaner, Bausch and Lomb). Likewise, it is used separately in an effervescent formulation, as are papain or pancreatic enzyme. Since it is not deactivated quickly in hydrogen peroxide (Fig. 13.23), it can be used during hydrogen peroxide disinfection, decreasing the number of steps required in lens care (Ultrazyme, Allergan). The enzyme's cleaning ability is apparently enhanced in the hydrogen peroxide compared with use of the enzyme in saline (Fig. 13.24). It has also been shown that the microbiologic effectiveness of hydrogen peroxide is enhanced by the enzyme (Fig. 13.25). Most of the enzyme formulations contain an effervescent compound for more rapid dissolving of the tablets. Since these enzymes degrade in the presence of moisture, they are supplied in foil wrappers. The significant ad-

% PROTEIN REMOVAL CAPACITY

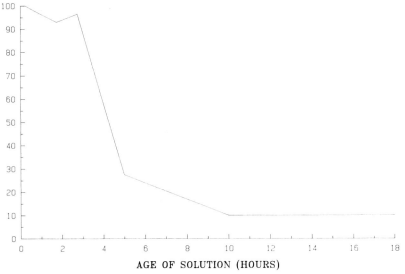

FIGURE 13.23 **Cleaning capacity of subtilisin in 3% hydrogen peroxide. (Courtesy Allergan Pharmaceuticals.)**

vantage of enzymatic cleaners is that they will remove denatured proteins, whereas most surfactant cleaners will not.

Polishing Compounds

A number of different polishing compounds have been used to clean and polish contact lenses. One of the most common polishes used in office practice is Silvo (RT French Co, Rochester, NY), which is formulated as a polish for silver. It performs well as a polish for PMMA lenses, but it should not be used with many of the new polymers because the ammonia in it can damage these materials. Other polishes such as tin oxide and precipitated calcium carbonate are commonly used by contact lens laboratories. One commercial product is XPAL (WR Grace Co, Davison Chemical Division, Pompton Pines, NJ), which is available from most contact lens laboratories that finish rigid lenses. The commercially available powder is mixed with water for

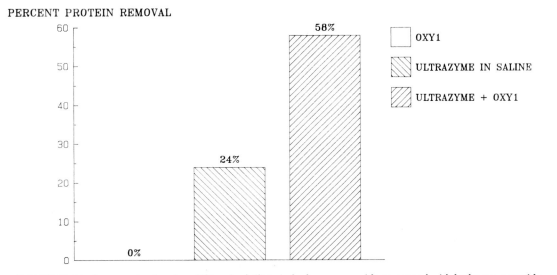

FIGURE 13.24   **Increase in cleaning ability of subtilisin in hydrogen peroxide compared with hydrogen peroxide alone or subtilisin alone. (Courtesy Allergan Pharmaceuticals.)**

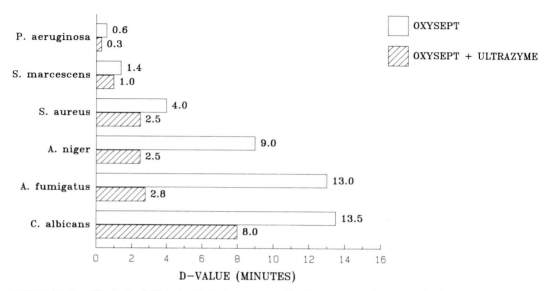

FIGURE 13.25   **Effect of subtilisin in 3% hydrogen peroxide (Oxysept) on shortening the kill times for various organisms. (Courtesy Allergan Pharmaceuticals.)**

use as a lens polish. Sil-O₂-Care (Optacryl Inc, 2890 S. Tejon, Englewood, CO 80110) and Boston Polish (Polymer Technology, 33 Industrial Way, Wilmington, MA 01887) are polishes formulated for use with rigid gas-permeable lenses. These polishes can be used on the newer gas-permeable lenses except for the Silcon lens, which cannot be polished because of its surface treatment.

Decongestant Agents

Ocular decongestants such as phenylephrine or naphazoline are occasionally used with contact lens wear. In some cases they may be justified, but they should not be used routinely because they may mask irritation and signs of a poorly performing lens. The underlying cause of persistent redness and irritation should be diagnosed and corrected.

References

1. Terry J, Hill RM. Human tear osmotic pressure. Arch Ophthalmol 1978;96:120–122.
2. Mishima S. Corneal thickness. Surv Ophthalmol 1978;13:57–96.
3. Hill RM. Osmotic vulnerability. Int Contact Lens Clin 1977;4:31–33.
4. Gumpelmayer T. Absorption and diffusion of small molecules in hydrophilic materials. Optician 1976;Spec Suppl 44–48.
5. Mandell RB. Sticking of gel contact lenses. Int Contact Lens Clin 1975;2:28–29.
6. Hill RM, Young WH. Ophthalmic solutions. J Am Optom Assoc 1973;44:263–270.
7. Moses RA, ed. Adler's physiology of the eye: Clinical application, ed. 6. St Louis: C. V. Mosby Co, 1975.
8. Alder I, Wlodyga RJ, Rope SJ. The effects of pH on contact lens wearing. J Am Optom Assoc 1968;39:1000–1001.
9. MacKeen DG, Bulle K. Buffers and preservatives in contact lens solutions. Contacto 1977;21:33–36.
10. Philips AJ. Contact lens plastics, solutions and storage: Some implications. Ophthal Optician 1968;8:1058,1075–1076.
11. Dabezies DH. Contact lenses and their solutions: A review of basic principles. Eye Ear Nose Throat Month 1966;45:39–44,68–72,82–84.
12. Kreiner CF. Biochemical aspects of ophthalmic preservatives. Contacto 1979;23:10–14.
13. Zand ML. The effect of non-therapeutic ophthalmic preparation on the cornea and tear film. Aust J Optom 1981;64:44–67.
14. Burstein NL, Klyce SD. Electrophysiologic and morphologic effects of ophthalmic preparations on rabbit corneal epithelium. Invest Ophthalmol Vis Sci 1977;18:899.
15. Burstein NL. Preservative cytotoxic threshold for benzalkonium chloride and chlorhexidine digluconate in cat and rabbit corneas. Invest Ophthalmol Vis Sci 1980;19:308–313.
16. Ganju S, Cordrey P. Proceedings: Reversible uptake of preservatives by soft contact lenses. J Pharm Pharmacol 1975; 27 Suppl 2:25.
17. McTaggart C. Care of soft contact lenses. Optician 1980; 180:15–20.
18. Kaspar H. Binding characteristics and microbiological effectiveness of preservatives. Aust J Optom 1976;59:4–9.
19. Weir NW. Do the varying pHs of contact lens solutions affect their bacterial action against *Pseudomonas aeruginosa?* Ophthal Optician 1977;17:311–313.

20. Riegelman S. Bacterial testing of contact lens solutions. Am J Ophthalmol 1967;64:485–486.

21. Stone J. Notes on the after-care of contact lens patients. Ophthal Optician 1967;10:966–976.

22. Hopkkins CJ. Contact lens solutions and preservatives. Ophthal Optician 1980;20:626.

23. Troy G. Contact lens solutions: Your first aid to a successful fit. Optom Management 1975;11:49–75.

24. Bailey W. Preservatives for contact lens solutions. Contact Lens Soc Am J 1972;6:33–39.

25. Sibley MJ, Yung G. A technique for the determination of chemical bindings to soft contact lenses. Am J Optom Physiol Opt 1973;50:710–714.

26. Krezanoski JZ. The significance of cleaning hydrophilic contact lens. J Am Optom Assoc 1972;43:350–357.

27. Kline LN, Deluca TJ. Thermal vs chemical disinfection. Int Contact Lens Clin 1978;5:23–31.

28. Burton GD, Hill RM. Aerobic responses of the cornea to ophthalmic preservatives, measured in vivo. Invest Ophthalmol Vis Sci 1981;21:842–845.

29. Winder AF, Astbury NJ, Sheraidah GAK, et al. Penetration of mercury from ophthalmic preservatives into the human eye. Lancet 1980;2:237–239.

30. Refojo M. Reversible binding of chlorhexidine gluconate to hydrogel contact lenses. Contact Intraocular Lens Med J 1976;2:47–56.

31. Mackeen D, Green K. Chlorhexidine kinetics of hydrophilic contact lens. J Pharm Pharmacol 1978;30:678–682.

32. Riedhammer TM. A simple chemical test for chlorhexidine in hydrophilic contact lenses. Int Contact Lens Clin 1979;6:26–30.

33. Wechsler S, George NC. Disinfection of hydrophilic lenses. J Am Optom Assoc 1981;52:179–186.

34. Lum VJ, Lyle WM. Chemical components of contact lens solutions. Can J Optom 1981;43:136–151.

35. Isen A. The Griffin lens. J Am Optom Assoc 1972;43:275–286.

36. Janoff LE. The Septicon system: A review of pertinent scientific data. Int Cont Lens Clin 1984;11:274–279.

37. Gyulai P, Dziabo A, Kelley W, et al. Relative neutralization ability of six hydrogen peroxide disinfection systems. Contact Lens Spect 1987;2:61–66.

38. Janoff LE. The effective disinfection of soft contact lenses using hydrogen peroxide. The Optician Aug. 28–30, 1979;24–30.

39. Gyulai P, Dziabo A, Kelley W, et al. Efficacy of catalase as a neutralizer of a hydrogen peroxide disinfecting solution for soft contact lenses. Intern Eyecare 1986;2:418–422.

40. Feldman GL. The trimethoprim solution. Contact Lens Forum 1985;10:40–41.

41. Meakin BJ. Contact lens solutions in the United Kingdom. J Br Contact Lens Assoc 1984;7:192–203.

42. Houlsby RD, Ghajar M, Chavez G. Microbiological evaluation of soft contact lens disinfecting solutions. J Am Optom Assoc 1984;55:205–211.

43. Penley CA, Schlitzer RL, Adhearn DG, et al. Laboratory evaluation of chemical disinfection of soft contact lenses. Contact Intraoc Lens Med J 1981;7:101–110.

44. Penley CA, Llabres C, Wilson LA, et al. Efficacy of hydrogen peroxide disinfection systems for soft contact lenses contaminated with fungi. CLAO 1985;11:65–68.

45. Centers for Disease Control. Recommendations for preventing possible HTLV-III/LAV virus from tears. MMWR 1985;34:1429.

46. Vogt MW, Ho DD, Sherwyne AR, et al. Safe disinfection of contact lenses after contamination with HTLV-III. Ophthalmology 1986;93:771–774.

47. Moore MB, McCulley JP, Luckenbach M, et al. *Acanthamoeba* keratitis associated with soft contact lenses. Am J Ophthalmol 1985;100:396–403.

48. Dornic DI, Wolf T, Dillon WH, et al. *Acanthamoeba* keratitis in soft contact lens wearers. J Am Optom Assoc 1987;58:482–486.

49. Ludwig IH, Meisler DM, Rutherford I, et al. Susceptibility of *Acanthamoeba* to soft contact lens disinfection systems. Invest Ophthalmol Vis Sci 1986;27:626–628.

50. Krishna N, Brown F. Polyvinyl alcohol as an ophthalmic vehicle: Effect on regeneration of corneal epithelium. Am J Ophthalmol 1964;57:99–106.

51. Krezanoski J. Contact lens products. J Am Pharm Assoc 1970;10:13–18.

52. Benedetto D, Shah D, Kaufman H. The dynamic film thickness of cushioning agents on contact lens materials. Ann Ophthalmol 1978;10:437–442.

53. Gordon S. Dimensional stability of contact lenses. J Am Optom Assoc 1971;42:239.

54. Pearson RM. Dimensional stability of several hard contact lens mateials. Am J Optom Physiol Opt 1977;54:826–833.

55. Bailey N. Cleaning of coated soft lenses. J Am Optom Assoc 1974;45:1049–1052.

56. Bier N, Lowther GE. Contact lens correction. Boston: Butterworths, 1976:410–424.

57. Lloyd DJ. Enzyme cleaners: The structure, properties and mode of action of enzymes. Ophthal Optician 1979;19:833–839.

58. Phillips AJ. The cleaning of hydrogel contact lenses. Ophthal Optician 1980;20:375–388.

59. Josephson JE, Caffery BE. Selecting an appropriate hydrogel lens care system. J Am Optom Assoc 1981;52:227–234.

60. Kleist FD. Soft lens cleaners compared. Contact Lens Forum 1980;5:47–51.

61. Sibley MJ. Hydrogen peroxide residues: A comparison between chemical and osmotic extraction. Contact Lens Spectrum 1988;3:39–43.

62. Dea D, Huth SW. The effect of reducing agents on enzymatic cleaning efficacy. Int Contact Lens Clin 1988;15:256–259.

PART III

Ocular Drugs in Clinical Practice

Experience is the best teacher.

—Anonymous

CHAPTER 14

Contact Lens Solutions in Clinical Practice

Gerald E. Lowther

The proper use of contact lens solutions is important to the success of lens wear. If a patient does not use the proper procedures, he or she may discontinue lens wear because of discomfort or deposit-laden or damaged lenses. Even worse, a serious infection might result. Practitioners should be familiar with the clinical uses of the many care systems employed with both rigid and soft contact lenses. This chapter considers the most commonly used care systems as they are employed in clinical practice.

Solutions Used with Nonhydrogel Lenses

Nonhydrogel Lens Materials

Until the late 1970s polymethylmethacrylate (PMMA) was the only rigid contact lens material routinely used. It has a number of desirable qualities for use as a contact lens, since it is transparent, stable, easily manufactured, easy to modify, and generally nontoxic to ocular tissue. Its surface wettability as measured by the Sessile drop technique is 60 to 70 degrees, about the same as the cornea. Therefore, the tears can form a film over the lens unless there is a contaminated surface. PMMA absorbs about 1.5% water, which can cause some parameter changes, particularly of the base curve radius, but this is usually not a major problem. It does not absorb significant amounts of chemicals from solutions. Thus, allergic or toxic reactions from

preservatives are rare, since any solution on the lens when placed on the eye is rapidly washed away. The primary disadvantage of PMMA material is impermeability to oxygen.

Due to PMMA's lack of oxygen permeability, other polymers have come into wide clinical use. Oxygen-permeable materials minimize or eliminate corneal edema and spectacle blur. These rigid materials include cellulose acetate butyrate (CAB), PMMA-silicone copolymers, fluoropolymers, and pure rigid and soft silicone, among others. Although all these have the advantage of increased oxygen permeability, other problems complicate their use in practice.

CAB is not as stable as PMMA, so many lenses warp. This is partially because CAB material absorbs 2% to 3% water on hydration. To counteract the base curve changes, CAB lenses are made thicker, which increases fitting problems and edge discomfort. Debris from the tear film tends to collect on the front of the lens (Fig. 14.1), blurring vision. This is accelerated if foreign material such as hand oil or cream is on the lenses. It is therefore crucial that an effective cleaner be used before placing the lens on the eye. There has been some controversy over which solutions can be used with CAB lenses. Benzalkonium chloride (BAK), at least in high concentrations, adversely affects CAB[1] and alters the lens surface, allowing fluorescein to penetrate the lens and discolor it yellow.[2] With the low concentration of BAK encountered in rigid lens solutions, it is doubtful that any adverse effects would occur, yet it is probably best to avoid this preservative with CAB.

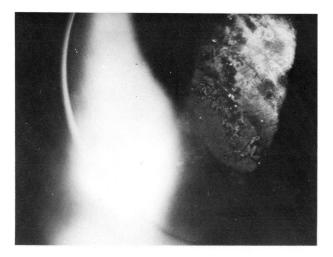

FIGURE 14.1   **Rigid gas-permeable lens (CAB) with surface debris from the tear film.**

Many PMMA-silicone copolymer lenses are being used. The percentage of silicone varies, as do the physical properties, but in general the copolymer lenses perform similarly. Since this material is more stable than CAB, it can be made thinner, which improves fitting, comfort, and oxygen permeability. Due to the silicone the surface wettability may be less than with PMMA lenses. The silicone attracts and holds lipid materials, and the monomers such as methacrylic acid and HEMA added to increase wettability attract proteins. Thus, there is surface debris buildup that appears very similar to that seen with CAB lenses. The lenses must be very clean before placement. This can be ensured by the daily use of effective surfactant cleaners. PMMA-silicone copolymers are easily modified and polished, but Silvo should not be used for this purpose because of the ammonia and cleaners present. Ammonia, alcohol, and other nonaqueous cleaners can break down the polymer and adhere to the surface. Heat will warp these lenses and should be avoided. As with CAB, controversy exists over which preservatives to use with these lenses, but numerous ones are routinely used.[3]

A number of recently developed materials have fluorine compounds added to increase wettability and oxygen permeability. Most of these fluoropolymers are silicone-acrylate-based materials. The oxygen permeabilities of these materials are considerably higher than previous rigid materials and are the major lens materials for extended wear. A disadvantage can be lens stability. With time some of these materials may change base curve radius or become distorted.

Rigid silicone lenses (Silcon Resin, Conforma Laboratories, Inc.) are slightly more flexible than silicone-

acrylate lenses. To obtain surface wettability they must be modified by the addition of ⁻OH groups. This means that the lens cannot be polished or modified, since the surface will become hydrophobic and the lens unwearable. The lens is very stable with respect to heat and can be heat disinfected, as with hydrogel lenses. The thimerosal-preserved solutions have been approved for use with this lens, but other solutions appear to be compatible.

Soft silicone lenses are unique in that they do not absorb water but are very flexible. They have the highest oxygen permeability of all lens materials. Since silicone is very hydrophobic, the surface is treated as with rigid silicone. It is an elastomer and thus has inherent elasticity, which can affect the way it is fitted. This lens is quite tough, does not absorb solutions, and can be disinfected with heat or chemicals. The thimerosal solutions have been approved for its chemical disinfection. Quaternary ammonium compounds should not be used with silicone, since corneal epithelial compromise and lens discoloration may occur. The surfaces of soft silicone lenses are susceptible to deposits, as with hydrogel lenses. Thus, surfactant and enzyme cleaners should be routinely used. Since silicone does not absorb water, distilled water alone can be used with heat disinfection.

Wetting Solutions

A wetting solution (Table 14.1) should be used on a hydrophobic lens surface (any rigid lens) before lens placement. This provides a film on the surface that increases lens comfort and provides good visual acuity following lens placement. Such solutions must be formulated to be comfortable and compatible with ocular tissues. This requires that they be nearly isotonic and pH compatible. This can usually be achieved with sodium chloride or potassium chloride salts. The pH of the solution should be near physiologic pH or only lightly buffered so that the pH will rapidly adjust to that of the tear film. A borate or phosphate buffer is commonly used. If polyvinyl alcohol (PVA) is used as the wetting agent, the pH will be in the acidic range but the solution will not be highly buffered. As discussed in Chapter 13, either a wetting agent is used with or without a viscosity agent, or a viscosity agent only is used to obtain the surface coating on the lens. If a wetting agent only (e.g., PVA) is used, the solution will not be viscous but will be very thin, like water. To increase the thickness of the solution a viscosity agent is often incorporated even though it is not needed to wet the surface. In cases in which only a viscosity agent is used, the solution will be thick. In addition to these ingredients, preservative(s) must be used to prevent contamination.

TABLE 14.1
Wetting Solutions for Rigid Lenses

Trade Name	Manufacturer	Wetting Agent (viscosity agent)	Preservative and Other Ingredients
Akwa-Tear	Akorn	Polyvinyl alcohol	Benzalkonium chloride, disodium edetate
Charter Labs Wetting	Charter Labs	(not given)	Benzalkonium chloride, disodium edetate
Contique Wetting	Alcon	Polyvinyl alcohol (hydroxypropylmethylcellulose)	Benzalkonium chloride (0.004%), disodium edetate (0.025%)
Liquifilm	Allergan	Polyvinyl alcohol (hydroxypropylmethylcellulose)	Benzalkonium chloride (0.004%), disodium edetate (0.2%)
Barnes-Hind Wetting Solution	Barnes-Hind	Polyvinyl alcohol (hydroxyethylcellulose)	Benzalkonium chloride (0.004%), disodium edetate (0.2%)
hy-Flow	CooperVision	Polyvinyl alcohol (hydroxyethylcellulose)	Benzalkonium chloride (0.01%), disodium edetate (0.025%), NaCl, KCl, sodium hydroxide
OWS Blue	Danker	Hydroxypropylmethylcellulose	Chlorobutanol
O-3	Danker	Hydroxypropylmethylcellulose	Benzalkonium chloride
Visalens	Leeming	Polyvinyl alcohol (hydroxypropylmethylcellulose)	Benzalkonium chloride (0.01%), disodium edetate (0.1%)
Stay-Wet	Sherman	Polyvinyl alcohol (cellulose derivatives)	Benzalkonium chloride (0.01%), disodium edetate (0.025%), NaCl, KCl, sodium carbonate
Sereine	Optikem	Polyvinyl alcohol (hydroxypropylmethylcellulose)	Benzalkonium chloride (0.01%), disodium edetate (0.1%)
Wet-Cote	Danker	Polyvinyl alcohol (hydroxyethylcellulose)	Benzalkonium chloride (0.01%), disodium edetate (0.025%), NaCl, KCl
Lobob	Lobob	Polyvinyl alcohol (methylcellulose)	Benzalkonium chloride (0.01%), sodium edetate (0.025%)

In using the wetting solution, the patient should remove the lenses from the soaking solution, place a few drops of the wetting solution on the lens, and gently rub the lens surfaces between the thumb and forefinger. Some patients will put a drop or two of the solution on the lens before placement. A problem with this method is that excessive solution often spills onto the lids and lashes and then dries, leaving a white residue, especially with solutions containing methylcellulose or one of its derivatives. When indicated, lightly rinsing the lens with a saline solution before placement will prevent this problem.

Some patients will report that a certain wetting solution stings or burns immediately following lens placement. Patients have different sensitivities to the pH, tonicity, and preservatives used in solutions. Therefore, patients having mild discomfort following lens placement should be instructed to change to another wetting solution. If a solution with a low pH is being used, substituting another with a higher pH or lower buffering capacity may eliminate the problem. A solution with a different preservative may be re-

quired if the patient has a sensitivity to the preservative. In some cases corneal infiltrates will occur with rigid lens wetting solutions if the patient has a hypersensitivity to the solution.[4] Aging of solutions can result in breakdown of compounds, pH changes,[5] and changes in tonicity.[6]

Prosthetic eyes are manufactured from PMMA, and solutions formulated for rigid lenses can be used on them. Enuclene (Alcon) is specifically formulated for use with prosthetic eyes. It contains BAK (0.02%), hydroxpropylethyl cellulose, tyloxapol (0.25%), boric acid, and sodium phosphate.

Soaking Solutions

A soaking solution (Table 14.2) is necessary to maintain lens hydration, to prevent contamination of the lens with microorganisms, and to help maintain a clean lens by solubilizing debris from the surface. This solution is not intended for instillation into the eye, but it nevertheless must not cause ocular damage, since it

TABLE 14.2
Soaking Solutions for Rigid Lenses

Trade Name	Manufacturer	Preservatives and Other Ingredients
Soakare	Allergan	Benzalkonium chloride (0.01%), edetate disodium (0.25%), sodium hydroxide
Soquette	Barnes-Hind	Benzalkonium chloride (0.01%), edetate disodium (0.2%), polyvinyl alcohol
Lobob	Lobob	Benzalkonium chloride (0.013%), sodium edetate (0.25%)

might accidentally be used as a wetting solution. The soaking solution should not be viscous, since this hampers solubilization of surface debris. Likewise, it should have a high enough concentration of preservatives to prevent the growth of microorganisms if a relatively large number are introduced into the solution with the lens or if considerable organic matter, such as tear film debris, is introduced.

Patients should be instructed to clean the lenses well following removal, using a cleaning solution, and then to place the lenses in the storage case with fresh soaking solution. The importance of using fresh soaking solution each day must be emphasized, since the preservative's effectiveness is rapidly lost when it becomes bound to proteins and other debris.

Controversy exists over the use of BAK-preserved solutions with gas-permeable lenses, especially silicone-acrylate materials. Some reports[7,8] have indicated that BAK is adsorbed to the lenses and can create clinical problems. Others,[9-11] however, indicate that the adsorption of BAK with these materials is no greater than with PMMA lenses. Solutions containing BAK have been used by many patients wearing silicone-acrylate lenses with no problems. However, some patients may develop sensitivity problems, and the clinician should not hesitate to change to solutions not containing BAK if the patient reports discomfort or itching. Likewise, if hyperemia, superficial punctate keratitis, or infiltrates are encountered, a solution with a different preservative may alleviate the problem.

Cleaning Solutions

These solutions contain cleaners that are usually nonionic surfactants (Table 14.3). Ethylenediaminetetraacetic acid (EDTA) may be used not only to enhance the antimicrobial activity of other preservatives, but also to soften the water by removing ions, thereby enhancing the solution's cleaning action. Mild abrasive compounds may also be added. Because of their nature and the fact that they are not intended for instillation into the eye, these compounds will usually cause considerable discomfort if inadvertently used as a wetting solution. Punctate epithelial keratitis may occur.

Patients should be instructed to clean the lenses well on removal, using the surfactant cleaners by placing each lens in the palm of the clean hand along with a few drops of the cleaner. The lens should then be rubbed, both front and back surfaces, for several seconds. The cleaner should be thoroughly rinsed from the lens, using soaking solution or water, before the lens is placed in fresh soaking solution for storage. Often deposits will build up on the back surface of the lens and not be sufficiently cleaned with normal rubbing. Such coating can cause superficial punctate keratitis and discomfort. Patients developing this problem should be taught to clean the back surface of the lens by rubbing it with a cotton-tipped applicator coated with the surfactant cleaner.

If it can be avoided, the lens should not be cleaned with the surfactant cleaner in the morning before placement or during a break in wearing during the day. By overnight soaking, any residual cleaner will be diluted by the soaking solution and will not cause discomfort.

Some cleaners contain abrasive particles (e.g., Opti-Clean I and II, Boston Cleaner, and SLC Cleaner) that enhance cleaning. These products are suspensions and should therefore be shaken to ensure adequate suspension of particles. Patients must be particularly careful to rub and rinse the cleaner from the lens because it can cause discomfort if left on the lens. Alcohol is a good solvent for lipid and other nonaqueous deposits and is present in Miraflow cleaner. One must be cautious in using this with silicone-acrylate and fluoropolymer lenses and instruct patients not to soak lenses in it. If accidentally soaked in this solution for several hours, the lens will swell and the base curve will change.[12] Minus lenses will steepen initially and then flatten (Fig. 14.2). They may also become toric (Fig. 14.3) or distorted and not return to the original dimensions when returned to the proper solution (Fig. 14.4).

Enzymatic cleaners can also be effective in removing protein deposits from rigid lenses and, thus, increase wearing time and comfort.[13] The same enzymes used with hydrogel lenses can be used with rigid lenses. One enzyme cleaner, PROFREE/GP (Allergan), is a papain enzyme specifically packaged for rigid lens patients. Enzyme cleaning once a week is usually

TABLE 14.3
Cleaning Solutions for Rigid Lenses

Trade Name	Manufacturer	Preservative	Other Ingredients
Contique Cleaning	Alcon	Benzalkonium chloride (0.002%), disodium edetate (0.025%)	
Clens	Alcon	Benzalkonium chloride (0.02%), disodium edetate (0.1%)	Polyoxane derivatives, sodium phosphate
Opti-Clean	Alcon	Thimerosal (0.004%), edetate disodium (0.1%)	Tween 21, polymeric cleaning agents, hydroxyethylcellulose
Opti-Clean II	Alcon	Polyquad (0.01%), disodium edetate (0.01%)	Tween 21, polymeric cleaning agents, hydroxyethylcellulose
Easy Clean/GP	Allergan	None	
LC-65	Allergan	Thimerosal (0.001%), disodium edetate	Cleaning agent
Concentrated Cleaner	Bausch & Lomb	None	Anionic and other surfactants, friction-enhancing agents, sodium chloride
Gel-Clean	Barnes-Hind	Thimerosal (0.004%)	Thixotropic gel, nonionic surfactants
Titan	Barnes-Hind	Benzalkonium chloride (0.01%), disodium edetate (2.0%)	Nonionic surfactants
Titan II Weekly Cleaner	Barnes-Hind	Thimerosal (0.001%), edetate disodium (0.1%)	Cleaning agents
Gas Permeable Daily Cleaner	Barnes-Hind	Thimerosal (0.004%), edetate disodium (2.0%)	Nonionic cleaning agents, buffers
Duracare	Blairex	Thimerosal (0.0004%), EDTA (0.1%)	Detergents, salt buffers
Hard Contact Lens Cleaner	Blairex	None	Nonionic cleaners
Charter Lab Cleaner	Charter Lab	Sorbic acid, edetate disodium	Poloxamine, hydroxypropylmethylcellulose
d-Film	CooperVision	Benzalkonium chloride (0.025%), trisodium edetate (0.25%)	Nonionic detergent, poloxamer 407
HGP Cleaner	CooperVision	None	Anionic sulfate surfactant, friction-enhancing agents, sodium chloride
Mira-Flow	CooperVision	Isopropyl alcohol (20%)	Poloxamer 407 (15%), amphotoric 10
Obrite	Danker	(not given)	Miranol H2M, antistatic and defogging agents
Lobob	Lobob	None	Nonionic surfactant
Murine Daily Contact Lens Cleaner	Ross Labs	Sorbic acid (0.25%), edetate disodium (0.5%)	Poloxamine, borate buffer, sodium chloride, hydroxypropylethylcellulose
SLC Hard Lens Cleaner	Ocular Pharm	Sorbic acid (0.1%), EDTA (0.1%)	Surfactants, abrasives
Sereine	Optikem	Benzalkonium chloride (0.1%), EDTA (0.1%)	Surfactants, viscosity agents
Boston Lens Cleaner	Polymer Tech	None	Sodium chloride, anionic sulfate surfactant, friction-enhancing agents
Sila Clean	Professional Supplies	Benzalkonium chloride, edetate disodium	
Stay-Brite	Sherman	Benzalkonium chloride (0.01%), disodium edetate (0.25%)	Nonionic detergents
Hard Contact	Rynco Scientific	Benzalkonium chloride	

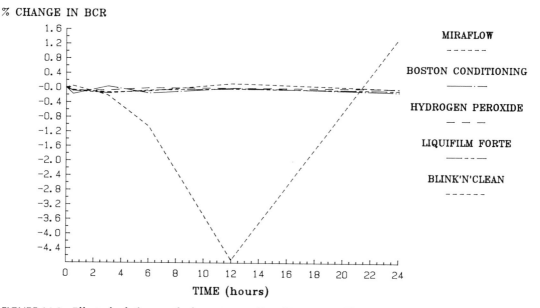

FIGURE 14.2   **Effect of solutions on the base curve radius of Boston IV (silicone-acrylate) lenses following a 24-hour soak. Miraflow was the only solution to change the base curve radius. A similar change occurred with Equalens (fluorosiloxane-acrylate) lenses. (From Lowther G. Effect of some solutions on HGP contact lens parameters. J Am Optom Assoc 1987;58:188–192.)**

sufficient. More frequent use does not adversely affect the lens.

Combination Solutions

For patient convenience manufacturers have developed combinations of solutions. These can be wetting-soaking (Table 14.4), cleaning-soaking (Table 14.5), or wetting-soaking-cleaning (Table 14.6) combinations. The problem with combination solutions is that compromises in function must usually be made.

With a wetting-soaking solution the combination may be more viscous than desired for a soaking solution, and thus it will not solubilize and clean the lens surface or be as effective against microorganisms as will a separate soaking solution. The concentration of preservative and buffering capacity may not be as ad-

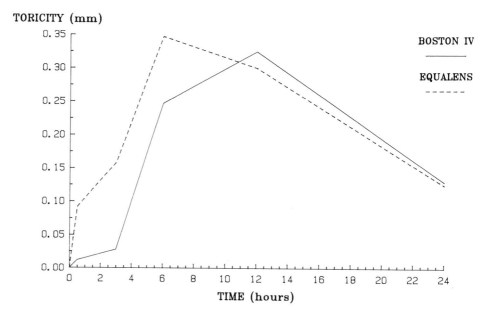

FIGURE 14.3   **Effect of solutions on the base curve radius of Boston IV and Equalens lenses showing the toricity created as the lenses were swollen. Miraflow was the only solution to cause this change. (From Lowther G. Effect of some solutions on HGP contact lens parameters. J Am Optom Assoc 1987; 58:188–192.)**

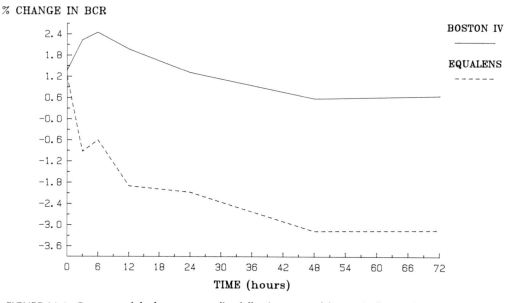

FIGURE 14.4 Recovery of the base curve radius following removal from Miraflow and soaking in saline. (From Lowther G. Effect of some solutions on HGP contact lens parameters. J Am Optom Assoc 1987; 58:188–192.)

equate as a separate soaking solution because the combination solution must be capable of being placed on the eye without discomfort. Furthermore, the combination solution may be formulated with less viscosity than is a separate wetting solution.

The soaking-cleaning solution may represent less of a compromise, since neither of the separate solutions is intended for placement on the eye. However, the strength of the cleaner must be compromised, since

some of the soaking solution is likely to get into the eye if it is not fully rinsed from the lens with wetting solution. With the combination there is no soaking solution to dilute the stronger cleaner.

The all-in-one solutions require the greatest compromise. These solutions cannot be as effective a cleaner as a separate cleaner because the combination must be formulated to be compatible with ocular tissue. It must contain a wetting or viscosity agent if it is to act as a

TABLE 14.4
Wetting and Soaking Combinations for Rigid Lenses

Trade Name	Manufacturer	Preservative	Other Ingredients
Soaclens	Alcon	Thimerosal (0.004%), disodium edetate (0.1%)	Buffers
Wet-N-Soak	Allergan	Benzalkonium chloride (0.004%), disodium edetate	Polyvinyl alcohol, buffers
GP Wetting & Soaking	Barnes-Hind	Thimerosal (0.002%), chlorhexidine (0.003%), edetate disodium (0.02%)	Polyvinyl alcohol
Wetting & Soaking	Bausch & Lomb	Chlorhexidine (0.006%), EDTA (0.05%)	Hydrophilic polyelectrolyte, polyvinyl alcohol, hydroxyethylcellulose, other hydrophilic polymers
HGP Conditioning Solution	CooperVision	Chlorhexidine (0.005%), edetate disodium (0.05%)	Polyvinyl alcohol, hydroxyethylcellulose
Sereine Wetting & Soaking	Optikem	Benzalkonium chloride (0.1%), EDTA (0.1%)	Viscosity agents
Boston Lens Conditioning Solution	Polymer Tech	Chlorhexidine (0.006%), EDTA (0.05%)	Hydrophilic polyelectrolyte, polyvinyl alcohol, hydroxyethylcellulose, other hydrophilic polymers

TABLE 14.5
Cleaning and Soaking Combinations for Rigid Lenses

Trade Name	Manufacturer	Preservative	Other Ingredients
Contique Cleaning & Soaking	Alcon	Benzalkonium chloride (0.02%), disodium edetate (0.1%)	Triethanolamine (0.5%), detergents
Clean-N-Soak	Allergan	Phenylmercuric nitrate (0.004%)	Cleaning agent, buffers
Cleaning-Soaking	Barnes-Hind	Benzalkonium chloride (0.01%), disodium edetate (0.2%)	
Clear/Clean	Contex	None	Surfactant
Ova-Nite	Danker	Benzalkonium chloride (0.02%), disodium edetate (0.25%)	Nonionic surface-active agents
Sereine Soaking & Cleaning	Optikem	Benzalkonium chloride, edetate disodium	Surfactants
duo-Flow	CooperVision	Edetate trisodium (0.25%)	Poloxamer 188 (0.5%)
Visalens	Leeming	Benzalkonium chloride (0.02%), disodium edetate (0.1%)	
de-Stat Cleaning/ Soaking	Sherman	Benzalkonium chloride (0.01%), EDTA (0.25%)	Lauryl sulfate salt of imidazoline, octylphenoxypolyethoxyethanol
Stay-Brite	Sherman	Benzalkonium chloride (0.01%), disodium edetate (0.25%)	Buffers, 3 surfactants

wetting solution, and these agents interfere with the soaking and cleaning functions.

The practitioner or patient using combination solutions must realize that such solutions represent a compromise situation and must be willing to change to separate solutions if problems develop. If patient compliance can be expected, separate solutions are preferred.

Lubricating (Rewetting or Comfort) Solutions

Occasionally while wearing contact lenses the patient will experience dehydration of the lens surface, causing blurred vision or drying of the peripheral cornea and conjunctiva. This may lead to burning, stinging, conjunctival hyperemia, and ocular discomfort. When this occurs, the practitioner must first attempt to find and alleviate the underlying cause. Potential causes include a poorly fitted lens, inadequate lens oxygen permeability, or a poorly shaped or thick edge causing infrequent blinking. If none of these problems exists, and the signs and symptoms appear to be due to low humidity or a dry eye, then lubricating drops may be used.

Lubricating solutions (Table 14.7) are usually isotonic or slightly hypertonic to enable water to be removed from the cornea in cases of edema. It has been

TABLE 14.6
Wetting-Soaking-Cleaning Combinations for Rigid Lenses

Trade Name	Manufacturer	Wetting Agent (viscosity agent)	Preservative
Lens-Mate	Alcon	Polyvinyl alcohol (hydroxypropylmethylcellulose)	Benzalkonium chloride (0.01%), disodium edetate (0.1%)
Total	Allergan	Polyvinyl alcohol	Benzalkonium chloride, edetate disodium
One-Solution	Barnes-Hind	Polyvinyl alcohol	Benzalkonium chloride (0.01%), disodium edetate (0.03%)
Lensine-5	CooperVision	Polyvinyl alcohol (polyethylene glycol, hydroxyethylcellulose, poloxamer 407)	Benzalkonium chloride (0.01%), disodium edetate (0.05%)

TABLE 14.7
Lubricating-Rewetting Solutions

Trade Name	Manufacturer	Preservative	Other Ingredients
Adapettes for Sensitive Eyes[a]	Alcon	Sorbic acid, edetate disodium	Absorbase
Adapt	Alcon	Thimerosal (0.004%), EDTA (0.05%)	Hydroxyethylcellulose (0.55%), Adsorbobase
Opti-Tears[a]	Alcon	Polyquad (0.1%), edetate disodium (0.1%)	Hydroxypropylmethylcellulose, dextran, NaCl, KCl
Blink-N-Clean	Allergan	Chlorobutanol (0.5%)	Polyoxyl 40 stearate, polyethylene glycol 300
Lens Fresh Lubricating & Rewetting[a]	Allergan	Sorbic acid (0.1%), edetate disodium (0.2%)	Hydroxyethylcellulose, NaCl, sodium borate, boric acid
Lens Plus Rewetting Drops[a]	Allergan	None	Boric acid, NaCl
Lens-Wet[a]	Allergan	Thimerosal (0.002%), disodium edetate (0.01%)	Polyvinyl alcohol, sodium phosphates, NaCl
Pre-Sert	Allergan	Benzalkonium chloride (0.004%)	Polyvinyl alcohol (3%)
Comfort Drops	Barnes-Hind	Benzalkonium chloride (0.005%), disodium edetate (0.02%)	Nonionic surfactant
Soft Mate Comfort Drops[a]	Barnes-Hind	Thimerosal (0.004%), disodium edetate (0.1%)	NaCl, borate buffer
Soft Mate ps Comfort Drops[a]	Barnes-Hind	Potassium sorbate (0.13%), EDTA (0.1%)	NaCl, borate buffer
Sterile Lens Lubricant[a]	Bausch & Lomb	Thimerosal (0.004%), disodium edetate (0.1%)	Polyoxyethylene, Adsorbobase
Sensitive Eyes Drops[a]	Bausch & Lomb	Sorbic acid (0.1%), edetate disodium	NaCl, borate buffer
Lens Lubricant[a]	Blairex Lab	Sorbic acid (0.25%), edetate disodium (0.1%)	Hydroxypropylmethylcellulose, glycerin, borate buffer, NaCl
Charter Lens Lubricant for Sensitive Eyes[a]	Charter Labs	Sorbic acid, thimerosal (0.001%), edetate disodium	Poloxamer 407, hydroxyethylcellulose, sodium borate, NaCl, KCl
Ciba Vision Drops[a]	Ciba	Sorbic acid (0.1%), edetate disodium (0.2%)	Hydroxyethylcellulose, sodium borate, boric acid, NaCl
Clerz[a]	CooperVision	Sorbic acid (0.1%), disodium edetate (0.1%), thimerosal (0.001%)	Poloxamer 407, sodium borate (0.22%), hydroxyethylcellulose, NaCl, KCl
Clerz 2[a]	CooperVision	Sorbic acid, edetate disodium	Hydroxyethylcellulose, polxomer 407, NaCl, KCl, sodium borate, boric acid
Boston Reconditioning Drops	Polymer Tech.	Chlorhexidine (0.006%), EDTA	Hydrophilic polyelectrolyte, polyvinyl alcohol, hydroxyethylcellulose, other hydrophilic polymers
Murine Lubricating & Rewetting Drops[a]	Ross Labs	Sorbic acid (0.1%), edetate disodium (0.2%)	Hydroxyethylcellulose, boric acid, sodium borate, NaCl
Stay-Wet "In-Eye" Lubricant	Sherman Labs	Benzalkonium chloride (0.01%), EDTA (0.25%)	Polyvinyl alcohol, hydroxyethylcellulose, PVP

[a]For use with hydrogel lenses.

suggested that a 1% NaCl solution alone will provide a longer effect than will the usual lubricating solutions.[14] Lubricating solutions usually contain a viscosity or wetting agent to keep the eye moist as long as possible between instillations. The solutions also contain preservatives to prevent contamination.

These preparations should not be used excessively due to the detrimental effects of preservatives and other compounds on the cornea.[15] In addition, the patient may have or develop a sensitivity to an ingredient in the solution. The practitioner should determine if the patient is using such drops when other solutions are changed in response to a suspected solution reaction. If the patient continues to use the lubricating drops after discontinuing other solutions, the signs and symptoms may continue.

Solutions and Systems Used with Hydrogel Lenses

Hydrogel lenses present unique problems in care, cleaning, and disinfection. Since hydrogel lenses are hydrophilic and absorb water and water-soluble substances, compounds in solutions used with these lenses are also absorbed. If the absorbed substances are toxic, such as preservatives in sufficient concentration, then corneal and ocular damage might occur during lens wear because the preservative is released onto the cornea. The situation is made worse if the preservative is concentrated in the lens. In some cases the concentration of preservative in the lens may be much higher than is its concentration in the solution in which the lens is soaked. For this reason many preservatives, especially BAK and chlorobutanol, cannot be used with hydrogel lenses.

The water content of the hydrogel lens may also be a factor in the method of care or solution used. High-water-content lenses, 60% or higher, often must be treated differently than lower-water-content lenses. Most high-water-content lenses are more susceptible to deterioration from heating. Likewise, they may absorb or adsorb more foreign material such as preservatives. Some cleaning systems, such as enzymes, might cause a toxic reaction when used with high-water-content lenses due to absorption of the enzyme, which may remain active if the lens is not disinfected with heat or hydrogen peroxide. The FDA has classified hydrogel lenses into 4 categories (Table 14.8) for purposes of testing new solutions and care systems. This classification can be useful clinically. If a patient is incurring deposits, discoloration, or solution problems with a lens, the practitioner should change to a lens in a different class instead of to another one in the same group to minimize chances of recurrence.[16]

The use of improper solutions can also result in discolored, coated, or otherwise damaged lenses. If a hydrogel lens is heat disinfected in some solutions formulated for rigid lenses[17,18] or solutions formulated for cold disinfection, the lens may become white due to crystallization of material in the lens. The use of water contaminated with certain salts or minerals will cause crystal formation on and in the lenses.[19–21]

Since the solution in which hydrogel lenses are soaked is absorbed into the lens, the solution must be compatible with the eye. The tonicity must be near that of the tear film to maintain proper lens parameters and to prevent an osmotic pressure difference between the lens and the cornea. If there is a significant difference, the lens may adhere to the eye and be uncomfortable. To maintain proper tonicity, a sterile saline solution, either unpreserved or preserved, is used.

Saline solution is an effective medium for growth of microorganisms and can be the source of ocular infection.[22,23] If lenses are stored in saline without disinfection or preservatives, growth of bacteria or fungi is common. To prevent this the lenses must be disinfected by heat or chemicals. With disinfection all vegetative organisms are killed, but spores may be spared. Thus, if lenses remain in the solution for several days, it is possible that spores present may become vegetative. In the case of sterilization (usually by heating to 120°C under a pressure of 15 lb/sq in. for 15 minutes) all organisms are killed. As long as the container remains sealed, the lenses should remain sterile indefinitely.

Heat Disinfection

One of the advantages of disinfecting lenses with heat is that preservatives that cause toxic or allergic reactions can be avoided. Saline is used with no preservatives or only sufficient preservative to prevent contamination of the solution in the bottle. The heat system is effective even in the presence of considerable contaminating organic matter such as tear film components or exceptionally large numbers of organisms. In such cases chemical systems may be ineffective because the chemicals will bind to organic material and will not be available to act against organisms. Heat kills the organisms very rapidly, usually within 15 to 20 minutes, whereas many chemical systems may require several hours for disinfection to occur. Heat disinfection systems are usually relatively inexpensive compared with chemical systems.

The primary disadvantage of heat disinfection compared with chemical systems is that it may shorten the useful lens life. Heat denatures proteins and other contaminants and crystallizes materials on the lens surface that may not be removed with cleaners. Heat

TABLE 14.8
Classification of Hydrogel Lenses

Group 1	Group 2	Group 3	Group 4
Low Water (<50% H₂O) Nonionic Polymers	High Water (>50% H₂O) Nonionic Polymers	Low Water (<50% H₂O) Ionic Polymers	High Water (>50% H₂O) Ionic Polymers

Low Water ($<50\%$ H_2O)
Nonionic
Polymers

High Water ($>50\%$ H_2O)
Nonionic
Polymers

Low Water ($<50\%$ H_2O)
Ionic
Polymers

High Water ($>50\%$ H_2O)
Ionic
Polymers

Group 1	Group 2	Group 3	Group 4
Tefilcon (38%) 　AO Multivue 　Cibasoft 　Cibathin 　Torisoft 　Weicon 　Weico tinted 　Softint 　Bisoft	Lidofilcon B (79%) 　CW 79 　Sauflon PW	Etafilcon (43%) 　Hydromarc	Bufilcon A (55%) 　Hydrocurve II₅₅ 　Hydrocurve II Bifocal
Tetrafilcon A (43%) 　AO Soft 　AO Soft Super Thin 　Aquaflex Standard 　Aquaflex Super Thin 　Aquaflex Permathin	Surfilcon (74%) 　Permaflex	Bufilcon A (45%) 　Hydrocurve II₄₅ 　Soft Mate	Perfilcon (71%) 　Permalens 　Permalens XL 　Permalens Therapeutic
Crofilcon (39%) 　CSI 　Aztech	Lidofilcon A (70%) 　B&L 70 　Genesis 4 　Sauflon 70 　CV 70 　Hydrosight 70 　Q&E 70 　Lubrisof 　PDC 70 　N&N 70	Deltafilcon A (43%) 　Amsoft 　Amsoft Thin 　Aquasoft 　Comfort Flex 　Custom Flex 　Metrosoft 　Soft Form Toric 　Softics 　Softics Super Plus 　Tripol 43 　Sof-form 　Softflow 　Softact	Etafilcon A (58%) 　Vistamarc
Dimefilcon A (36%) 　Gelflex	Ofilcon A (74%) 　DuraSoft 4		Ocufilcon C (55%) 　Ocu-Flex 　O.P.R.-55
Hefilcon A&B (43%) 　B&L Toric 　Flexlens 　Naturvue 　SoftSite 　Miracon 　SoftSite Therapeutic	Xylofilcon A (67%) 　Igel	Droxifilcon A (47%) 　Accugel	Phemfilcon A (55%) 　Durasoft 3 　Durasoft 3 Toric
Phemfilcon A (30%) 　Durasoft 　Durasoft TT	Scafilcon A (71%) 　Scalens	Phemfilcon A (38%) 　Durasoft 2 　Durasoft TT 　Durasoft 2 Toric	Tetrafilcon B (58%) 　Aquaflex 58
Isofilcon (36%) 　AL-47		Ocufilcon (44%) 　Tresoft 　Tresoft Thin	Methafilcon (55%) 　Hydracon 　Metro 55 　Hydracon Toric
Mafilcon (33%) 　N&N Menicon			Vifilcon A (55%) 　Softcon 　Softcon EW
Polymacon (38%) 　CustomEyes 38 　Vesoft 　PDC 　Softics 　Synsoft 　Cellusoft 　Hydron 　Hydron Zero 　Hydron Toric 　Hydron Zero T 　Sof-Form II 　Soflens 　Omega 　Nuview 　SoftView 　Cooper 30 　Metrosoft II			

systems are not continuous disinfection systems; that is, if the patient disinfects the lens; opens the case and handles the lens, thereby contaminating it; then places the lens back in the case, the organisms introduced may thrive. With chemical systems the chemicals would still be present to counteract the contamination after the lens handling. Transportation of the disinfection unit, and the availability of electricity when camping and of appropriate current when traveling overseas, can also be problems with heat-disinfection systems. Lenses can be heat disinfected by placing the lens and case in a pan of boiling water for 15 to 20 minutes. However, one must be careful that the water does not boil away, allowing the case to rest against the bottom of the pan and melt. The case must be tightly closed and should be removed from the water when the boiling is complete so that water from the pan is not drawn into the case on cooling.

Many of the present heat-disinfecting units are easy to use, reliable, and small enough to transport easily. Since the units automatically turn off following the disinfection cycle, the patient can place the lens in the unit, activate it, and leave it until the next morning, when the lenses are ready to be worn again. The patient should occasionally check the unit to be sure that it is heating. Most of the units are low-temperature systems with the temperature reaching only 80° to 90°C. This kills the organisms but minimizes lens damage.

SALT TABLET SYSTEMS

Preparing saline solution by dissolving a salt tablet in distilled water represents an inexpensive system that eliminates all the chemicals to which a patient may be sensitive. Usually a 135 mg salt tablet is dissolved in 15 ml distilled water, or a 250 mg salt tablet is dissolved in 27.7 ml distilled water, to make the solution. Some tablets contain buffers in addition to salt. Only salt tablets formulated for hydrogel lenses should be used, since others may contain binders that can damage the lenses, or iodine, which might cause corneal insult. If the patient follows the proper procedures, salt tablet systems are safe and effective. However, patient compliance is a major problem.[24] For this reason the use of salt tablets is strongly discouraged, since *Pseudomonas* is common in distilled water and a majority of *Acanthamoeba* infections have been attributed to the use of saline prepared from salt tablets.[25–27]

To prevent the possibility of introducing pathogenic organisms into the eye with the salt tablet system, the patient must not place such saline into the eye unless it has been disinfected. This means that when the patient removes the lenses from the eyes, the lenses should be cleaned, rinsed, and placed in the case with the saline solution. Once the lenses and solution are disinfected, the patient should not open the case until the lenses are to be worn. In preparation for wearing the lenses, the hands should be washed and the soap rinsed off. The lenses are removed from the case and placed directly on the eye, using only the solution in the storage case. The patient should not use the solution in the bottle to rinse the lenses before placement because the distilled water used to prepare the solution is probably contaminated.[28] In addition, the salt tablets are handled before being placed in the bottle, which introduces organisms into the system. For the same reasons the saline from the bottle should not be used as an eyedrop.

To minimize the problem of contamination, the solution should be prepared fresh daily, and any remaining solution should be discarded. The bottle should be disinfected periodically, such as weekly, by placing the bottle in a pan of boiling water for 15 to 20 minutes.

Another problem with salt tablet systems is that the patient may not use distilled water. If minerals such as calcium carbonate are present, they will crystallize on and in the lens, causing white deposits (Fig. 14.5). This will damage the lens due to invasion of the deposit (Fig. 14.6) and affect comfort and vision. Often distilled water, mineral water, artesian water, and drinking water are commercially packaged in identical containers except for some small print on the label. Initially, the patient usually reads the label but may later inadvertently obtain the incorrect water. After a few heat disinfection cycles the crystalline deposits appear, and the lenses must be replaced. This can also occur if tap water or water from a dehumidifier or other sources is used.

UNPRESERVED SALINE

To overcome the problems with salt tablets, different methods of packaging prepared saline have been used (Table 14.9). One method is unit-dose packages that contain only enough solution in each package for 1 use. The top of the container is broken off or the package torn open, the solution is used, and the package is discarded. Another method is to use saline in a can under positive pressure. By depressing the top, the desired amount is dispensed. The advantages of such systems are that the solution is sterile, it can be used as an eyedrop to rewet lenses, and it does not contain minerals to damage the lens. Buffers are added to some of these solutions to maintain the proper pH. One manufacturer has even added a surfactant.

The main problem with the unit-dose or limited-dose prepared saline is cost. For this reason some patients will attempt to retain the opened container for later use, with the potential problem of contamination. This practice must be discouraged.

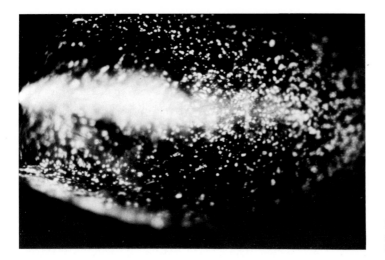

FIGURE 14.5 **White crystalline deposits on the surface of a hydrogel lens due to heat disinfection in water containing minerals.**

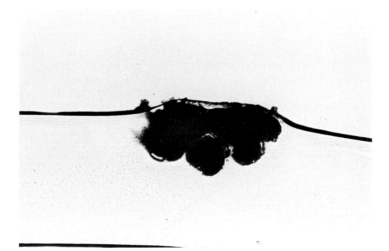

FIGURE 14.6 **A mineral deposit that has invaded the matrix of a hydrogel lens.**

TABLE 14.9
Unpreserved Saline for Hydrogel Lenses

Trade Name	Manufacturer	Formulation	Other Ingredients
Lens Plus Preservative Free	Allergan	240 ml aerosol	
Hypo-Clear	Bausch & Lomb	118 ml aerosol	
Saline, Unpreserved	Bausch & Lomb	10 ml single-dose packets	
Unisol	CooperVision	15 ml	Boric acid, sodium borate
Unisol 4	CooperVision	120 ml	Boric acid, sodium borate
Soft Mate Saline Preservative-Free	Barnes-Hind	15 ml	Borate buffer

Some practitioners and patients will use prepared saline in 1 liter bottles obtained from a hospital supply outlet. This is discouraged because these solutions can become contaminated after opening. Also, saline packaged in such containers is sometimes preserved, which could cause hypersensitivity reactions.

PRESERVED SALINE

To overcome many of the potential problems with salt tablet systems and unpreserved saline, as well as with patient inconvenience with these systems, preserved saline is commonly used, generally in a preservative concentration that is bacteriostatic but not bactericidal (Table 14.10).

The first preservatives used were thimerosal (0.001%) and EDTA (0.1%). Although many patients find this to be very satisfactory, some patients develop an allergic or toxic reaction to the thimerosal.[29-36] The signs and symptoms as well as the time course of such reactions vary with each patient. If patients have previously been sensitized to thimerosal, they can develop a very injected and irritated eye within minutes after the lens, soaked in the solution, is placed on the eye. A relatively severe reaction can also occur in these patients by irrigating the eye with a thimerosal-preserved irrigating solution. A more common history is that the patient seems to do well with the lenses for weeks to months, and then the eyes become injected and irritated immediately on lens placement. These patients had not been previously sensitized to the thimerosal but develop the delayed hypersensitivity during use. Skin patch tests will often be positive to thimerosal[37,38,96] (Color Plate III). The other type of reaction is characterized by the signs and symptoms progressively worsening. The clinical appearance is often very similar. In addition to the conjunctival inflammation, there may be corneal subepithelial infiltrates, limbal infil-

TABLE 14.10
Preserved Saline for Hydrogel Lenses

Trade Name	Manufacturer	Preservative	Other Ingredients
Boil 'n' Soak	Alcon	Thimerosal (0.001%), disodium edetate (0.1%)	Boric acid, sodium borate, NaCl (0.7%)
Opti-Soft	Alcon	Polyquad (0.001%), edetate disodium (0.1%)	Borate buffer, NaCl
Saline Solution for Sensitive Eyes	Alcon	Sorbic acid (0.125%), edetate disodium (0.1%)	Borate buffer, NaCl
Hydrocare Preserved Saline	Allergan	Thimerosal (0.001%), disodium edetate (0.01%)	Boric acid, sodium borate, sequestering agent, sodium hexametaphosphate, NaCl
Lensrins	Allergan	Thimerosal (0.001%), edetate disodium (0.1%)	Sodium phosphate, NaCl (0.85%)
Sorbi-Care	Allergan	Sorbic acid (0.1%)	Boric acid, sodium borate, sequestering agent, NaCl, sodium hydroxide
Soft Mate ps	Barnes-Hind	Potassium sorbate (0.13%), disodium edetate (0.025%)	Borate buffer, NaCl
ReNu	Bausch & Lomb	Dymed (0.00003%), edetate disodium	Boric acid, NaCl
Sensitive Eyes	Bausch & Lomb	Sorbic acid (0.1%), disodium edetate	Borate buffer, NaCl
Sensitive Eyes Saline/Cleaning	Bausch & Lomb	Sorbic acid (0.1%), edetate disodium (0.1%)	Borate buffer, NaCl, surfactant
Sterile, Preserved Saline	Bausch & Lomb	Thimerosal (0.001%), disodium edetate (0.1%)	Boric acid, sodium borate, NaCl
Saline Sensitive Eyes	Charter	Sorbic acid (0.1%), EDTA (0.1%)	Borate buffer, NaCl
Murine Preserved All Purpose Saline	Ross Labs	Sorbic acid (0.1%), edetate disodium	Borate buffer, NaCl
Mirasol	CooperVision	Thimerosal (0.001%), disodium edetate (0.1%), sorbic acid (0.1%)	Poloxamer 407, sodium borate, NaCl, KCl

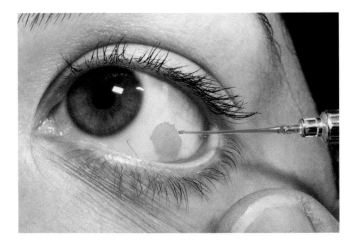

PLATE I A drop of sodium fluorescein 2 μl in volume (1/25 the volume of a standard drop) is administered by touching the conjunctiva with a flexible plastic tube. In the laboratory such dosing is simple, reproducible, and effective in delivering medications to the eye. This method was developed from an unpublished technique of Maurice.

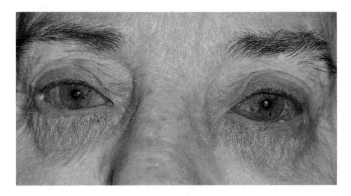

PLATE II Bacterial blepharoconjunctivitis complicated by hypersensitivity to neomycin. Patient was treated with gramicidin–neomycin–polymyxin B (Neosporin). There is erythema and edema of eyelids, as well as intense itching. (Courtesy Debra Bezan, O.D.)

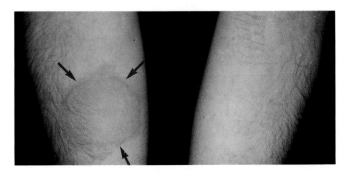

PLATE III Results of positive occlusive patch test performed for 48 hours by taping a cotton pad soaked in thimerosal-preserved saline to the inner surface of the right forearm. The left arm serves as a control by taping a nonmedicated cotton pad to its inner surface. Arrows indicate the well-circumscribed area of redness reflecting thimerosal sensitivity. (Courtesy Joseph F. Molinari, O.D.)

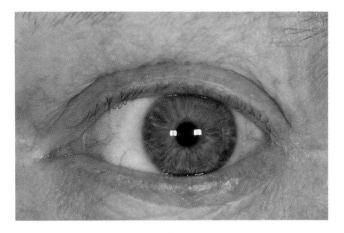

PLATE IV Madarosis and hyperemia of eyelid margins characteristic of staphylococcal blepharitis.

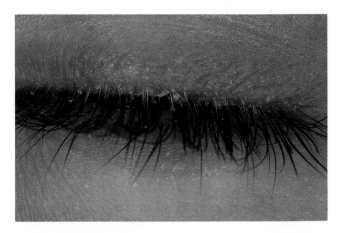

PLATE V Seborrheic blepharitis, characterized by greasy crusts and minimal hyperemia of the eyelid margin.

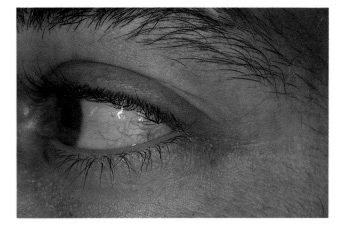

PLATE VI Inflammation of temporal bulbar conjunctiva and excoriation of outer canthus, characteristic of angular blepharoconjunctivitis.

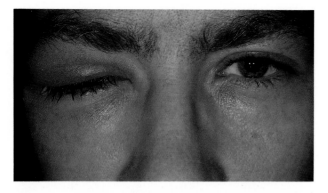

PLATE VII Preseptal cellulitis of right upper eyelid. Note generalized swelling and erythema of eyelid. There were no pupillary abnormalities and no proptosis, and visual acuity was 20/25.

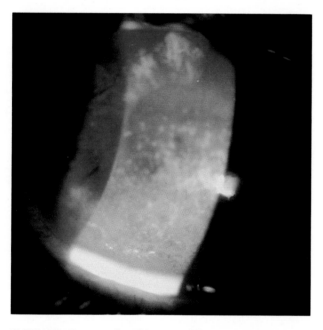

PLATE VIII Exposure keratitis. Note diffuse superficial punctate staining of central and inferior cornea using sodium fluorescein.

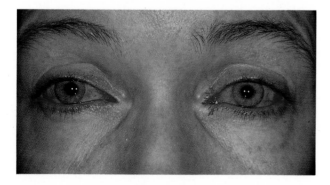

PLATE IX Keratoconjunctivitis sicca with characteristic interpalpebral rose bengal staining of bulbar conjunctiva. (Courtesy Jimmy D. Bartlett, O.D.)

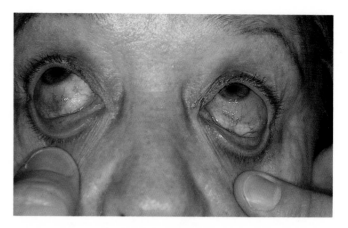

PLATE X Mucus fishing syndrome. Note characteristic rose bengal staining pattern on inferior bulbar conjunctiva secondary to mechanical irritation. (Courtesy Jimmy D. Bartlett, O.D.)

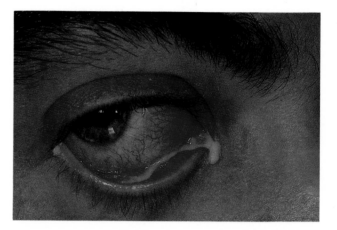

PLATE XI Acute conjunctivitis secondary to *Staphylococcus aureus*. Mucopurulent discharge is stained with sodium fluorescein. (Courtesy Jimmy D. Bartlett, O.D.)

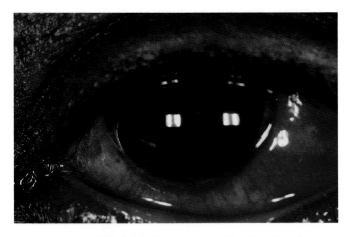

PLATE XII **Allergic blepharoconjunctivitis. There is redness and swelling of both the conjunctiva and eyelids, along with pronounced itching and watery discharge. (Courtesy Jimmy D. Bartlett, O.D.)**

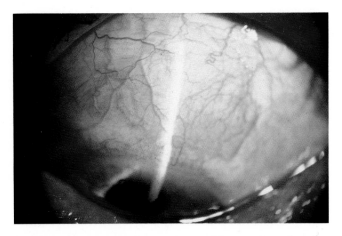

PLATE XIV **Superior bulbar conjunctival hyperemia and rose bengal staining in superior limbic keratoconjunctivitis.**

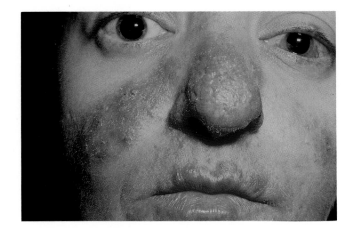

PLATE XIII **Ocular rosacea with typical dermatologic involvement and rhinophyma.**

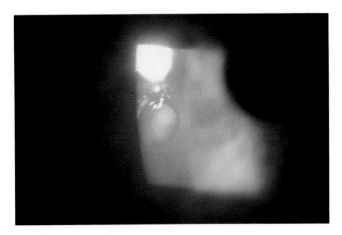

PLATE XV **Central corneal ulcer due to *Streptococcus pneumoniae.***

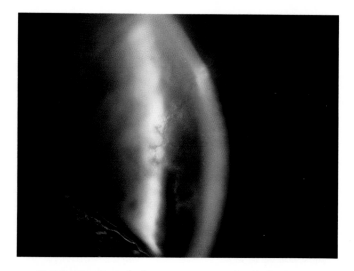

PLATE XVI   **Central arborescent pattern of epithelial herpes simplex virus keratitis stained with rose bengal.**

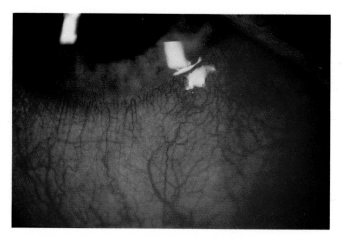

PLATE XIX   **Diffuse scleritis with deep vessel injection and associated episcleritis.**

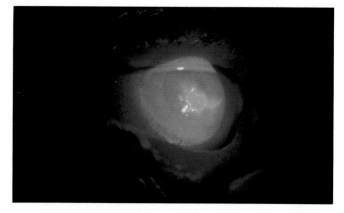

PLATE XVII   **Geographic (ameboid) epithelial herpes simplex virus keratitis stained with sodium fluorescein.**

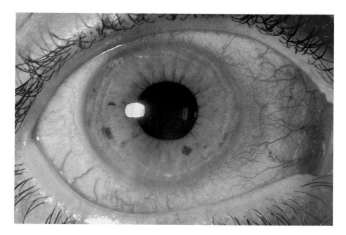

PLATE XX   **Circumcorneal ciliary flush in anterior uveitis. (Courtesy Jimmy D. Bartlett, O.D.)**

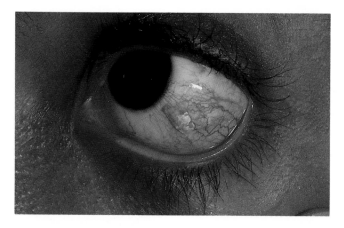

PLATE XVIII   **Episcleritis in sectorial configuration. (Courtesy Jimmy D. Bartlett, O.D.)**

trates (Fig. 14.7), punctate epithelial keratitis, or swollen lids. With long-term use neovascularization can occur. The patient may complain of itching, burning, dryness, photophobia, pain, and decreased visual acuity. When any of these signs or symptoms occurs with a well-fitted lens, the patient's care system should be changed to unpreserved saline or to a solution without thimerosal, such as sorbic acid–preserved saline or hydrogen peroxide.

With the introduction of sorbate– and sorbic acid–preserved salines, many of these adverse reactions can be alleviated or avoided. Patients sensitive to thimerosal-preserved saline do not appear to be sensitive to solutions containing sorbic acid. A small number of patients will report mild discomfort or stinging with sorbic acid– or sorbate–preserved solutions. With high-water-content lenses it may cause a slight lens yellowing or discoloration. If a higher concentration (0.3% or greater) of sorbate or sorbic acid than in present solutions is used, discoloration is very common. The discoloration apparently results from the breakdown of sorbic acid to aldehydes, which in turn react with amino acids from proteins coating the lens.[39] The use of sorbic acid–preserved saline has greatly reduced the need for unpreserved saline and the use of salt tablets. It must be emphasized that sorbate and sorbic acid are weaker preservatives than is thimerosal. If the microbial contamination level is high, these preservatives may not prevent microbial growth.

When changing from a preserved saline or chemical disinfection system to another system, it may be necessary to purge the lenses of the chemicals.[40] This is especially helpful if the patient has exhibited an allergic reaction or if a chemical system containing polymers was used. Purging is accomplished by thoroughly cleaning the lens with a surfactant cleaner not containing the offending chemical and rinsing the lens well with distilled water or unpreserved saline. The lenses should be soaked in several changes of the water or saline and then heat disinfected 2 or 3 times before being worn.

An advantage of heat disinfection is that it will kill all organisms including *Acanthamoeba,* which is not killed with present chemical methods. Other heat disinfection systems have been evaluated, such as the use of microwave sterilization, but these have not as yet proved clinically useful.[41]

Chemical (Cold) Disinfection

Some of the problems and inconveniences of heat disinfection can be overcome with the use of chemical (nonthermal) disinfection systems (Table 14.11). Since no heat or electricity is required, this method is more convenient for travel. It minimizes the problem of deposits and lens deterioration. Disinfection occurs constantly as long as the lens is in the disinfecting solution.

As with preserved saline solutions, a major problem with some chemical disinfection systems is hypersensitivity to the solutions. Patient compliance with disinfection systems requiring multiple steps can also be a problem.[42]

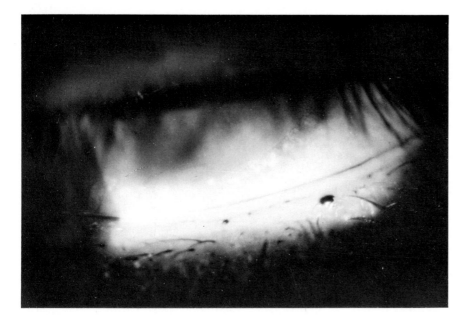

FIGURE 14.7 **Limbal staining and infiltrates resulting from sensitivity to thimerosal-preserved saline.**

TABLE 14.11
Chemical Disinfecting Solutions for Hydrogel Lenses

Trade Name	Manufacturer	Preservative	Other Ingredients
Flex-Care for Sensitive Eyes	Alcon	Chlorhexidine (0.005%), disodium edetate (0.1%)	Sodium borate, boric acid, NaCl
Opti-Free	Alcon	Polyquad (0.001%), edetate disodium (0.05%)	Citrate buffer, NaCl
Opti-Soft	Alcon	Polyquad (0.001%), edetate disodium (0.1%)	Borate buffer, NaCl
Hydrocare Cleaning & Disinfection	Allergan	Thimerosal (0.002%), tris and bis (2-hydroxyethyl) tallow ammonium chloride	Sodium bicarbonate, sodium phosphate, propylene glycol, polysorbate 80, soluble poly-HEMA, hydrochloric acid, buffers
ReNu	Bausch & Lomb	Dymed (0.00005%), edetate disodium	Sodium borate, poloxamine, NaCl
Sterile Disinfecting Solution	Bausch & Lomb	Thimerosal (0.001%), disodium edetate (0.1%), chlorhexidine (0.005%)	Sodium borate, boric acid, NaCl
Soft Mate Disinfection (Thimerosal free)	Barnes-Hind	Chlorhexidine (0.005%), edetate disodium (0.1%)	Povidone, octylphenoxyl (oxyethylene), ethanol, borate buffer, NaCl

THIMEROSAL-CHLORHEXIDINE SYSTEMS

The first chemical disinfecting systems employed thimerosal (0.001%), chlorhexidine gluconate (0.005%), and EDTA (0.1%) as preservatives in saline with appropriate buffers. In some cases agents that increase viscosity were added. These solutions disinfect the lenses after soaking for several hours.

The sensitivity reactions that occur are the same as with the thimerosal-preserved salines.[43,44] In addition, reactions to the chlorhexidine can also occur. The chlorhexidine may bind to tear film components on the lens surface and become a source of irritation. Chlorhexidine may also make the lens surface hydrophobic, which increases adherence of lipids to the lens surface.[45] Decomposition may turn the lens yellow to yellow-green.[45]

The incidence of reactions to the thimerosal-chlorhexidine solutions varies in different studies.[46,47] The specific solutions used, lens material, methods by which patients handle them, and individual patient susceptibility can be factors. If the solution is viscous and a large quantity is introduced into the eye with each lens placement, the symptoms tend to be greater. If deposits develop on the lens surface, the hypersensitivity problem is often worse. Some practitioners instruct patients to rinse the lenses with a preserved or unit-dose unpreserved saline after removing them from the chemical disinfection solution.

Many of the symptoms are mild, and most patients are still able to wear the lenses but are not as comfortable as they might be with other systems. Varying degrees of burning, irritation, tearing, dryness, or pain can occur in up to 50% of patients.[46]

ALKYLTRIETHANOL AMMONIUM CHLORIDE–THIMEROSAL SOLUTION

This disinfecting system, introduced by Allergan, contains Tris (2-hydroxyethyl) tallow ammonium chloride (0.013%), bis (2-hydroxyethyl) tallow ammonium chloride, thimerosal (0.002%), polymers, and surfactants including a soluble HEMA, propylene glycol, and polysorbate 80 as well as buffers and salts to adjust tonicity. It is thought that micelles (grouping or clumping of molecules) are formed with the tallow ammonium preservative and the surfactant polysorbate 80 to minimize sensitivity to the solution. Greenberger[48] and Stein and associates[49] suggest that some patients do better with this system than with thimerosal-chlorhexidine systems. However, these studies were performed with patients previously using thimerosal solutions. Thus, those patients sensitive to thimerosal would not have been entered into the studies. Since this solution does contain thimerosal, some thimerosal-sensitive patients may have difficulty.

POLYQUAD-PRESERVED SOLUTION

This large quaternary ammonium molecule (molecular weight about 5000) does not significantly invade the lens polymer and therefore does not cause toxic reactions. The first formulation of this solution resulted in a fairly high reaction rate with high-water, ionic lenses

(Group IV lenses) but little to no reactions with other materials. A revised formulation appears to have solved the reaction problem with the Group IV lenses. Patients who have sensitivities to thimerosal solutions normally do not have problems with this solution. This is used in the Alcon OptiSoft and Opti-Free solutions and can be used as a preserved saline for heat as well as for chemical disinfection.

POLYHEXAMETHYLENE BIGUANIDE (DYMED)

This is another new preservative developed to overcome the problems of preservative sensitivity and toxic reactions. This compound is a relatively large molecule (molecular weight about 2000) and has had few reported reactions. It is used in the Bausch and Lomb ReNu Disinfecting solution.

HYDROGEN PEROXIDE

Hydrogen peroxide (H_2O_2) is an oxidizing agent that has been used for many years to disinfect hydrogel lenses.[50,51] It is relatively effective in killing most bacteria and does not appear to result in clinically significant sensitivity problems because it is broken down into water and oxygen. Since it is an oxidizing agent, it may have some small effect in keeping the lenses clean but does not eliminate the need for cleaners. The primary disadvantages are patient compliance and instability of the hydrogen peroxide, since it can decompose in the bottle. New formulations of hydrogen peroxide are stable if kept out of sunlight and if fresh solution is regularly obtained. Numerous systems have been devised to make patient compliance easier (Table 14.12).

The lenses must soak in the 3% hydrogen peroxide solution for at least 10 minutes (see Chapter 13 for a discussion of microbial effectiveness). Since hydrogen peroxide causes considerable discomfort if placed on the eye, it must be neutralized. Several methods of neutralization have been devised (see Chapter 13).

The first neutralization procedure consisted of rinsing and soaking the lenses in a 0.5% sodium bicarbon-

TABLE 14.12
Hydrogen Peroxide Disinfection Systems

Trade Name	Manufacturer	Disinfection	Neutralization
Lens Plus Oxysept	Allergan	Oxysept I: 3% hydrogen peroxide, sodium stannate, sodium nitrate, phosphate buffer (10 minutes minimum)	Oxysept II: Catalase, edetate disodium, mono and dibasic sodium phosphate, NaCl (10 minutes minimum)
Quik-Sept	Bausch & Lomb	Quik-Sept: 3% hydrogen peroxide, sodium stannate, sodium nitrate, phosphate buffer (20 minutes minimum)	Saline dilution (10 minutes minimum)
Consept	Barnes-Hind	Consept 1, 3% hydrogen peroxide, polyoxyl 40 stearate, sodium stannate, sodium nitrate, phosphate buffer (10 minute minimum)	Consept 2, sodium thiosulfate (0.5%), borate buffers, NaCl
Charter Hydrogen Peroxide	Charter Labs	3% hydrogen peroxide, sodium stannate, sodium nitrate, phosphate buffer	No neutralization available
AOSept	Ciba	3% hydrogen peroxide, sodium stannate, sodium nitrate, phosphate buffer, 0.85% NaCl	Catalytic disc (6 hours total)
Lensept	Ciba	3% hydrogen peroxide, sodium stannate, sodium nitrate, phosphate buffer	Catalase, borate buffer, sorbic acid, edetate disodium, NaCl (5 minutes minimum)
Septicon	Ciba	3% hydrogen peroxide, sodium stannate, sodium nitrate, phosphate buffer (10 minutes minimum)	Catalytic disc, saline solution (6 hours minimum)
MiraSept	CooperVision	MiraSept Disinfection: 3% hydrogen peroxide, sodium stannate, sodium nitrate, phosphoric acid (10 minutes minimum)	MiraSept Rinsing & Neutralization: 0.5% sodium pyruvate, boric acid, sodium borate, edetate disodium, sorbic acid (0.1%) (10 minutes minimum)
Murine PureSept	Ross Labs	3% hydrogen peroxide, sodium stannate, sodium nitrate, phosphate buffer	Saline dilution

ate neutralizing solution followed by placing them in preserved saline. This was too time consuming for daily use by the patient. Next a platinum catalytic disk was introduced to break down any residual hydrogen peroxide. With this Septicon system the lens is again placed in the hydrogen peroxide for 10 minutes, then transferred to the case with the catalyst and filled with preserved saline. The lens is allowed to soak in this case for at least 3 to 4 hours, at which time the residual hydrogen peroxide should be broken down. This is still a 2-step procedure and requires that a preserved saline be used as the last solution, which introduces potential preservative reactions. Unpreserved saline should not be used for lens storage after the hydrogen peroxide soak because the saline could be contaminated, and no further disinfection occurs.

A further refinement of this system eliminates the step of removing the lens from the hydrogen peroxide and placing it in the second case with saline. In the AOSept system the hydrogen peroxide is placed in the case with the catalytic disk and the lens. The disk immediately begins to break down the hydrogen peroxide to water and oxygen. After 6 hours the lens can be removed and worn. The only difference between the hydrogen peroxide used in this system (AOSept) and the Lensept hydrogen peroxide (Septicon System) is that the former solution contains NaCl and phosphate buffer so the lens ends up in normal saline instead of distilled water. Since oxygen is given off as the hydrogen peroxide is decomposed, the case has vent holes to allow the gas to escape. If the patient uses a surfactant cleaner before disinfecting with AOSept and does not properly rinse the cleaner off, there may be excessive foaming of the solution, resulting in foam exuding from the case. The surfactant is a soap and will form bubbles. The catalytic disk must be replaced periodically to prevent complaints of burning or stinging on lens placement in the morning. This should be done after a hundred or so uses of the system.

Another method of neutralizing the hydrogen peroxide is to use a chemical neutralizer (sodium pyruvate or sodium thiosulfate) or an enzyme (catalase). These systems result in rapid neutralization, less than 5 minutes. One advantage of such systems is that the patient can clean and disinfect lenses in less than 30 minutes. This may be important for patients using extended wear lenses who want to disinfect the lenses without leaving them out overnight. Most companies recommend that the lenses be placed in the 3% hydrogen peroxide for 10 to 20 minutes before neutralization. Another way to use such a system is to allow the lenses to soak overnight in the hydrogen peroxide and neutralize them before wearing in the morning. This system has 2 advantages: (1) the patient does not have to

wait 10 to 20 minutes following lens removal to change the solution before going to bed, and (2) there is a longer disinfection time (overnight), which has been shown to be more effective against some organisms than are shorter disinfection times (see Chapter 13). The disadvantage is that some polymers (the high-water lenses) may change shape and take an hour or longer to return to prehydrogen peroxide soak dimensions.[52]

Another way to eliminate the hydrogen peroxide after disinfection is to simply rinse and dilute it. Rinsing once or twice with preserved saline and then allowing the lenses to soak in saline so that the residual hydrogen peroxide will diffuse out will result in a low enough level of hydrogen peroxide for many patients. However, there will be enough residual hydrogen peroxide that many patients will complain of burning and stinging on lens placement.[97]

Hydrogen peroxide systems can discolor some tinted hydrogel lenses over time.[53] Where possible it is best to use another chemical system. However, if necessary, hydrogen peroxide can continue to be used, since it will fade most tints only slightly.

IODINE SYSTEMS

Iodine is a disinfecting compound that has been used to disinfect hydrogel lenses.[54,55] Polyvinylpyrrolidone iodine (also termed povidone-iodine) (0.1%) systems are marketed outside the United States.[56] This method is an effective disinfectant and apparently does not cause many sensitivity reactions.

To use the system the patient cleans the lenses in the normal fashion, places the lenses in the case, and adds 2 or 3 drops of the iodine compound. The case is then filled with a neutralizing solution. The lens soaks in this solution, and after about 15 minutes the iodine decolors, indicating completion of disinfection. It is best to allow the lens to soak for 2 to 4 hours before wearing to allow complete neutralization of the iodine. Heat accelerates neutralization of the iodine.

If the patient inadvertently places the lens on the eye before the solution decolors, discomfort and corneal damage could occur. Iodine systems may cause lens yellowing.

OTHER DISINFECTION SYSTEMS

A number of other agents and systems have been studied or have found limited use in disinfecting hydrogel lenses. One compound is sodium dichloroisocyanurate.[57] It is supplied in a tablet that is dissolved in unpreserved saline. The lenses are soaked in the solution overnight, removed, and rinsed with saline before placement. The disinfection is completed in less than 2 hours.

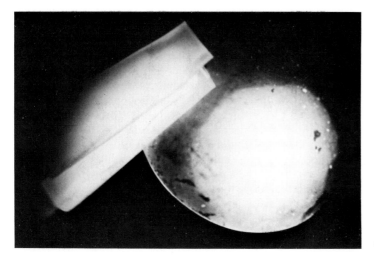

FIGURE 14.8 **Surface coating of tear film components on a hydrogel lens.**

Nipastat (0.01%) with EDTA (0.1%) is also used as an alternative disinfecting compound in the same manner as the thimerosal-chlorhexidine solutions.

Ozone has been suggested as a disinfecting method,[58] but because of numerous problems it has not been used clinically. Ultrasound, refrigeration, and brine solutions have also been explored, but all have major problems in providing adequate bactericidal properties or convenience in use.

Cleaning of Hydrogel Lenses

A variety of surface coatings and deposits develop on hydrogel lenses as a result of surface drying during wear, heat disinfection, lens handling, and exposure to the environment.[20,21,59–64] The most common deposit is a relatively uniform surface coating (Fig. 14.8) of tear film components, mainly proteins. These coatings are limited to the surface or surface layers of the polymer.[60] Soft silicone lenses can also develop surface coatings that appear similar to hydrogel coatings but that develop cracks in the deposits due to the elasticity of the material. Lipids can coat the surfaces of both types of lenses. If ions or minerals are present in the solution used with heat disinfection, crystalline formation will occur on and in the hydrogel lens.[20,60–62] These usually consist of calcium carbonate or calcium phosphate along with other tear film components. In some cases lenses will turn brown, possibly due to the formation of a melanin-like pigment from aromatic compounds in the tears.[65,66]

Discrete spots, probably lipids and calcium salts, can develop on extended-wear lenses (Fig. 14.9). These

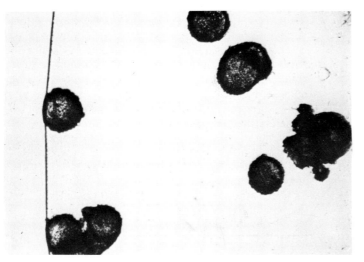

FIGURE 14.9 **Deposits on a high-water-content extended wear lens.**

invade the polymer and will leave a surface defect if removed.

MECHANICAL CLEANING

Hydrogel lenses can be cleaned of many substances by simply rubbing the lens surface between the fingers or in the palm of the hand using only saline. However, denatured or crystallized material is not removed. The use of lens rubbing is important in conjunction with most of the cleaning solutions and systems.

Polishing the lens surface using XPAL in water and a soft pad will also remove some deposits.[67,68]

SURFACTANT CLEANERS

Many surfactant cleaners are available for use with hydrogel lenses (Table 14.13). Surfactants lower surface tension and emulsify lipids, oils, and other materials. In addition to nonionic surfactants, these cleaners contain salts, buffers, and preservatives. Most of the surfactants are prophylactic cleaners that must be used daily to prevent deposits. Once material is denatured on the surface, these cleaners will not remove it. There are some exceptions, notably Soft Mate Weekly Cleaning Solution (also called Hexaclean), Opti-Clean, and Restore. Opti-Clean contains abrasive particles (Fig. 14.10), and Restore contains finely milled salt supplied in powder form. All the surfactants depend on mechanical rubbing of the surface for cleaning. Since various cleaners employ different surfactants and formulations, they may have varying effectiveness against different contaminants. Some contain other cleaners, such as isopropyl alcohol (e.g., MiraFlow), to dissolve lipids.

OXIDIZING CLEANERS

These cleaners act by breaking down proteins and other contaminants into small molecules that can be removed. Some can be strong oxidizing agents and with prolonged or repeated use can damage lens polymers. Because of the possibility of ocular damage if the cleaner is not neutralized or properly rinsed, these cleaners are not generally available in the United States.

Liprofin is an oxidizing cleaner consisting primarily of sodium perborate. It is used by heating to 50° to 60°C for 2 to 4 hours.[69] Constant stirring during this time with a magnetic stirrer aids the cleaning. The lens must be rinsed and neutralized in saline after cleaning.

Monoclens consists of ethylene oxide and propylene oxide as a copolymer and sodium perborate as the oxidizing agent. It is supplied as a powder that is mixed with water. The lens can be soaked for 2 hours or longer in this solution. A more effective method is to boil the lens in the solution for 10 minutes and then maintain it at 70° to 80°C for 2 hours.[69] Following use the lens must be thoroughly rinsed and neutralized by boiling in saline.

Hydrogen peroxide is also a useful oxidizing agent for cleaning as well as disinfecting lenses. As previously described, 3% hydrogen peroxide is used by the patient but has only limited cleaning ability. Some practitioners have used 10% to 30% hydrogen peroxide with low heat and stirring with a magnetic stirrer, but this is an in-office procedure not intended for patient use.

Duragel tablet system is an oxidizing system for patient use. A tablet containing dichloroisocyanurate dihydrate, sodium chloride, citric acid, and sodium bicarbonate is dissolved in water.[69] As the tablet effervesces, chlorine is released and serves as the oxidizing compound. The cleaning lasts about 10 minutes; the lens is then removed, rinsed, and boiled in saline.

The oxidizing cleaners are reasonably effective in cleaning the lenses but can cause lens damage, change lens parameters, and result in possible severe ocular damage if not properly neutralized. Therefore, if these systems are used, the practitioner or patient must be extremely careful to follow precisely all the appropriate procedures.

ENZYMATIC CLEANERS

Enzymatic cleaners (Table 14.14) are effective for removing proteinaceous coatings from hydrogel lenses. They act by breaking up the attached proteins into small molecules. Papain, the first proteolytic enzyme used, still is widely used. It is derived from the papaya and has been used in meat tenderizers.[70] It is active against a wide range of proteins by breaking the peptide bonds. The enzyme cleaners are provided in tablet form and are dissolved in water for use. Preserved saline or sterile unpreserved saline should be used to dissolve the tablets rather than using tap or distilled water to minimize the possibility of microorganism contamination. The soiled lens is soaked in the solution for a period of time depending on the type of lens. With low-water-content lenses at least 2 hours, and commonly overnight, is recommended. Leaving the lens in the solution more than 8 to 12 hours does not result in additional cleaning, since the enzyme is denatured in the aqueous solution. Since the solution does not disinfect, the lens must be disinfected following the enzyme soak. Heat and hydrogen peroxide disinfection will denature any residual enzyme, but other chemical disinfection systems will not. The tablets have an activator added that causes the papain enzyme tablets to have a characteristic odor.

Since water will slowly deactivate the enzyme, patients should be instructed to discard any tablets of which the foil packages have been opened. Moisture is absorbed from the air. The enzyme is normally quite safe and can be used repeatedly without lens or ocular

TABLE 14.13
Surfactant Cleaning Solutions for Hydrogel Lenses

Trade Name	Manufacturer	Preservative	Other Ingredients
Opti-Clean	Alcon	Thimerosal (0.004%), disodium edetate (0.1%)	Tween 21, polymeric cleaning agents, hydroxyethylcellulose
Opti-Clean II	Alcon	Polyquad (0.01%), edetate disodium (0.1%)	Hydroxyethylcellulose, Tween 21, polymeric cleaning agents
Preflex for Sensitive Eyes	Alcon	Sorbic acid (0.2%), disodium edetate (0.2%)	Hydroxyethylcellulose, polyvinyl alcohol, tyloxapol, phosphate buffer, NaCl
LC-65	Allergan	Thimerosal (0.001%), disodium edetate	Undisclosed cleaner
Lens Clear	Allergan	Sorbic acid (0.1%), edetate disodium	Surfactants
Lens Plus	Allergan	Edetate disodium	Cocoamphocarboxyglycinate, sodium lauryl sulfate, hexylene glycol, sodium phosphate, NaCl
Soft Mate Daily	Barnes-Hind	Thimerosal (0.004%), disodium edetate (0.2%)	Octylphenoxyl, hydroxyethyl cellulose, ethanol, NaCl
Soft Mate Daily II (or ps Daily) (or Hands Off Daily Cleaner)	Barnes-Hind	Potassium sorbate (0.13%), edetate disodium (0.2%)	Octylphenoxyl ethanol, hydroxyethlylcellulose, NaCl
Soft Mate Protein Remover	Barnes-Hind	Edetate disodium	Alkyl carboxylic acid amine, alkyl imidazoline dicarboxylate, polyoxyalkylene dimethylpolysiloxane, borate buffers
Soft Mate Weekly	Barnes-Hind	Thimerosal (0.001%), disodium edetate (0.1%)	Undisclosed cleaner
Sensitive Eyes Daily Cleaner	Bausch & Lomb	Sorbic acid (0.25%), disodium edetate (0.5%)	NaCl, borate buffer, hydropropylmethylcellulose, surfactant
Sensitive Eyes Saline/Cleaning	Bausch & Lomb	Sorbic acid (0.1%), edetate disodium	Borate buffer, NaCl, surfactant
Sterile Daily Cleaner	Bausch & Lomb	Thimerosal (0.004%), disodium edetate (0.2%)	Hydroxyethylcellulose, polyvinyl alcohol, tyloxapol, sodium phosphates, NaCl
DURAcare	Blairex	Thimerosal (0.004%), EDTA (0.1%)	Detergents, salt buffers, NaCl
Charter Cleaning for Sensitive Eyes	Charter Labs	Sorbic acid (0.25%), disodium edetate (0.5%)	Borate buffer, poloxamine, hydroxypropylmethylcellulose, NaCl
Ciba Vision Cleaner	Ciba Vision	Sorbic acid (0.1%), edetate disodium (0.2%)	Cocoamphocarboxyglycinate, sodium lauryl sulfate, hexylene glycol
Mira Flow	CooperVision	None	Isopropyl alcohol (20%), poloxamer 407 (15%), amphoteric 10 (10%)
Pliagel	CooperVision	Sorbic acid (0.25%), trisodium edetate (0.5%)	Poloxamer 407 (15%), KCl, NaCl
Restore	Hayes Marketing	None	NaCl, sodium bicarbonate
Murine Daily Contact Lens Cleaner	Ross Labs	Sorbic acid (0.25%), EDTA (0.5%)	Hydroxypropylmethylcellulose, poloxamine, borate buffer, NaCl
Sof/Pro Clean	Sherman	Thimerosal (0.004%), EDTA (0.1%)	Nonionic detergents, block copolymers of ethylene and propylene oxide, lauryl sulfate salt of imidazoline, octylphenoxypolyethoxyethanol, salt buffers

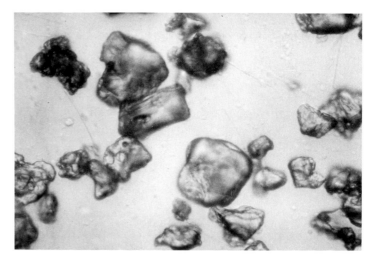

FIGURE 14.10 **Particles found in Opti-Clean as seen under the microscope.**

damage. Although once-weekly soaking will usually keep lenses clean of protein deposits, enzyme cleaners will not remove inorganic deposits.[71,72]

If the enzyme cleaner is not removed or denatured, it may cause a hypersensitivity reaction[73,98] or bind preservatives, causing discomfort.[74] For this reason there has been debate over whether enzyme cleaners should be used with chemical disinfection systems.[75,76] Many patients can use the enzyme with chemical disinfection,[76] but some patients may develop conjunctival injection and discomfort. With high-water-content lenses and extended-wear lenses the soaking time should be decreased to 15 minutes to 1 hour to minimize diffusion of the enzyme into the lens matrix, which might cause a reaction when the lens is worn. In cases where a reaction still occurs, another enzyme must be used or enzyme cleaning must be discontinued.

Pancreatin is another enzyme used to remove deposits from lenses. It is derived from the hog pancreas and has lipase and amylase action as well as protease activity. This enzyme is also effective and is an alternative for patients with sensitivity to papain enzyme. It is used in the same fashion as papain enzyme and has the same limitations.

A newer enzyme for use with contact lenses is subtilisin, which is an extracellular enzyme produced by *B. licheniformis*. It is effective against a wide variety of proteins and over a wide range of temperatures and pH levels. Therefore, it can be used during thermal disinfection (ReNu Thermal) or with hydrogen peroxide (Allergan Ultrazyme). This decreases the patient's time spent cleaning and may thus increase compliance with cleaning. It does not require an activator and thus does not have an odor. It is 90% neu-

TABLE 14.14
Enzymatic Cleaners

Trade Name	Manufacturer	Ingredients
Enzymatic Cleaner for Extended Wear	Alcon	Purified pork pancreatin
Opti-zyme	Alcon	Purified pork pancreatin
Enzymatic Soft Lens Cleaner	Allergan	Stabilized papain, NaCl, sodium carbonate, sodium borate, edetate disodium
Extenzyme Protein Cleaner	Allergan	Same as above
ProFree/GP Weekly Enzymatic Cleaner	Allergan	Same as above
Ultrazyme	Allergan	Subtilisin A
ReNu Effervescent Enzymatic Cleaner	Bausch & Lomb	Stabilized subtilisin, polyethylene glycol, sodium carbonate, tartaric acid, NaCl
ReNu Thermal Enzymatic Cleaner	Bausch & Lomb	Stabilized subtilisin, boric acid, sodium carbonate, NaCl

tralized by an overnight soak in 3% hydrogen peroxide. As an added advantage, the combination of enzyme and hydrogen peroxide is more effective as a disinfectant than is hydrogen peroxide alone. The ReNu thermal enzymatic cleaner should not be used with Sola/Barnes-Hind CSI hydrogel lenses because it will tend to make them stiff and change their shape. An hour or longer may be required for the lens to return to its normal condition and shape once placed back into saline.

Lipases (such as used in Clean-O-Gel) are enzymes used to break down lipid deposits. Other enzyme cleaners (such as Amiclair) use a combination of proteolytic and lipolytic enzymes to remove both lipid and protein deposits.

Most of the tablets are effervescent to shorten the time for the tablet to dissolve and thus decrease cleaning time.

Medications and Contact Lens Wear

Ocular Medications

The use of topical ocular medications with rigid and silicone lenses is permissible in some cases, since the lenses do not absorb the drugs. However, the lens may impede the drug from reaching the cornea, or once under the lens the drug may be held against the cornea for longer than normal. Since contact lenses may compromise the corneal epithelium, reduce the blink rate, and impair tear circulation, topically applied drugs are likely to penetrate the cornea in greater quantity. Ointments will cause blurred vision if instilled with contact lens wear. When possible it is best to instill topical medications without the lenses in place.

Hydrogel lenses, however, present a different situation because they will absorb water-soluble compounds. If a hydrogel lens is placed in a drug solution, the drug will usually concentrate in the lens. This absorption ability of hydrogel lenses has been used to treat various ocular conditions.[77-83] The amount of drug absorbed depends on the lens material, the drug, concentration of the drug in solution, and how long the lens is soaked.[77] The use of hydrogel lenses as drug delivery devices is discussed in Chapter 2.

Because of the exaggerated effect of many drugs when used in conjunction with hydrogel lenses, it is best not to soak lenses in the medication or to use drops while wearing hydrogel lenses, unless such an effect is desired. However, there has been some controversy whether placing a drop of medication on the eye while wearing a lens results in a significant drug absorption or adverse effect.[83-85] Because of the small volume of instilled medication and the rate at which it is washed away by the tears, there appears to be little risk. The same is true for the preservatives in artificial tears and other topically applied solutions.

Soaking lenses in or repeated instillations of epinephrine, phenylephrine, dopa, or related oxidizable adrenergic drugs can stain lenses gray, black, or brown.[83,86,87] Therefore, the wearing of hydrogel lenses by glaucoma patients using topical epinephrine is contraindicated. Once such lens staining has occurred, however, hydrogen peroxide or another oxidizing agent may clear the lens.

Devices for Protecting the Cornea

Hydrogel lenses are sometimes used to protect the cornea following corneal wounds or surgery and to provide comfort for patients with bullous keratopathy. A recently developed product in this regard is the Bio-Cor Fyodorov Collagen Corneal Shield (Bausch & Lomb). It consists of non-cross-linked, homogenized, porcine scleral collagen. It is placed as a bandage on the cornea following surgery or injury, protecting and lubricating the cornea. The shield is applied dry, but it quickly absorbs tears and then gradually dissolves. Early indications are that it accelerates wound healing.

Systemic Medications

A number of systemic medications can affect contact lens wear or discolor hydrogel lenses. Most of the effects on lens wear are the result of changes in the tear film. Some antihistamines, anticholinergic drugs, tricyclic antidepressants, and antianxiety agents may decrease tear production and result in discomfort with lens wear and drying of the lens surface, ultimately causing blurred vision.[88] Propranolol (Inderal), a β-adrenergic blocking agent commonly prescribed to treat hypertension and some cardiovascular diseases, can also cause decreased tearing as well as conjunctival allergic reactions.[89]

Acetylsalicylic acid (aspirin) taken orally is excreted into the tears.[90] This drug might be absorbed into a hydrogel lens and cause corneal epithelial irritation, since aspirin is a known irritant.[91]

Oral contraceptives have been implicated in contact lens–wearing problems.[92] Possible etiologic mechanisms include changes in tear production and in corneal thickness. However, recent evidence[91,93] indicates that the prevalence of contact lens problems associated with this class of drugs is probably less than previously reported.

A number of drugs can be excreted into the tear film and discolor hydrogel lenses. These include phenazopyridine, tetracycline, phenolphthalein, and nitrofurantoin.[89] Rifampin, a drug used to treat meningococcal disease and tuberculosis, is excreted into the tears and may stain hydrogel lenses orange.[94]

Disulfiram (Antabuse), a drug used in the management of chronic alcoholism, has caused a reaction with rigid lens wear similar to that which would occur if alcohol was imbibed. The reaction, reportedly related to the PVA in the wetting solution,[95] consisted of flushing, dry mouth, a prickly sensation, dizziness, nausea, vomiting, and weakness.

For the above reasons, one must carefully question the contact lens patient about the concurrent use of ocular and systemic drugs.

References

1. Petricciani R, Krezanoski JZ. Preservative interaction with contact lenses. Contacto 1977;21:6–10.
2. Feldman GL. Contact lens materials. Int Ophthalmol Clin 1981;21:155–162.
3. Kame R, Asno G, Lee J. Hard lens solutions with the Polycon lens. Contact Lens Forum 1981;6:43–46.
4. Bellows R, Lowther GE. Subepithelial infiltrates. Int Contact Lens Clin 1979;6:73.
5. Hill RM. Escaping the sting. Int Contact Lens Clin 1979;6:27.
6. Hill RM. Aging ophthalmic solutions. Int Contact Lens Clin 1978;5:124.
7. Rosenthal P, Chou MH, Salamone JC, et al. Quantitative analysis of chlorhexidine gluconate and benzalkonium chloride adsorption on silicone/acrylate polymers. CLAO J 1986;12:43–50.
8. Sterling J, Hecht A. BAK adsorption in silicone/acrylates. Contact Lens Forum 1987;12:80.
9. Walters K, Gee H, Meakin B. The interaction of benzalkonium chloride with Boston contact lens material. I. Basic interaction studies. J Br Cont Lens Assoc 1983;6:42–50.
10. Wong MP, Dziabo AJ, Kiral RM. Adsorption of benzalkonium chloride by RGP lenses. Contact Lens Forum 1986;11:25–32.
11. Hoffman W. Ending the BAK-RGP controversy. Int Contact Lens Clin 1987; 14:31–35.
12. Lowther G. Effect of some solutions on HGP contact lens parameters. J Am Optom Assoc 1987;58:188–192.
13. Lasswell LA. Enzymatic cleaning of Polycon II contact lenses. Int Eyecare 1986;2:89–92.
14. Poster MG. Optical efficacy of rewetting and lubricating solutions. Contact Lens Forum 1981;6:25–31.
15. Zand ML. The effect of non-therapeutic ophthalmic preparation on the cornea and tear film. Aust J Optom 1981;64:44–67.
16. Lowther GE. Hydrogel lens classification. Int Eyecare 1986;2:298.
17. Bailey N. Wrong solutions to the cleaning problem. Contact Lens Forum 1976;1:10–15.
18. Jurkus JM, Cedarstaff TH, Nuccio RS. Solution confusion: Photodocumentation of what can happen. Int Contact Lens Clin 1981;8:47–56.
19. Krezanoski JZ. Water and the care of soft contact lenses. Int Contact Lens Clin 1975;2:48–55.
20. Lowther GE, Hilbert J. Deposits on hydrophilic lenses: Differential appearance and clinical causes. Am J Optom Physiol Opt 1975;52:687–692.
21. Hilbert J, Lowther GE, King J. Deposition of substances within hydrophilic lenses. Am J Optom Physiol Opt 1976; 53:51–54.
22. Wilson LA, Schlitzer RL, Aearn DG. Pseudomonas corneal ulcers associated with soft contact lens wear. Am J Ophthalmol 1981;92:546–554.
23. Dada VK, Argarwal LP, Seger KR. Preventable hazard of soft lens wear. Am J Optom Physiol Opt 1976;53:431–432.
24. Gold RM, Melman E. Salt tablets: What price economy? Contact Lens Forum 1981;6:35–39.
25. Moore MB, McCulley JP, Luckenbach M, et al. *Acanthamoeba* keratitis associated with soft contact lenses. Am J Ophthalmol 1985;100:396–403.
26. Centers for Disease Control. *Acanthamoeba* keratitis associated with contact lenses—United States. MMWR 1986; 35:405–408.
27. Dornic DI, Wolf T, Dillon WH, et al. *Acanthamoeba* keratitis in soft contact lens wearers. J Am Optom Assoc 1987;58:482–486.
28. Houlsby RD, Ghajar M, Chavez G. Microbiological quality of water used by pharmaceutical manufacturers and soft lens wearers. Int Contact Lens Clin 1981;8:9–14.
29. Pederson N. Allergy to chemical solutions for soft contact lenses. Lancet 1976;2:1363.
30. Wilson L. Thimerosal hypersensitivity in soft contact lens wearers. Contact Lens J 1981;9:21–24.
31. Neill JC, Hanna JJ. A study of the effect of various media on the radii of microcorneal contact lenses. Contacto 1963;7:10–13.
32. McMonnies CU. Allergic complications in contact lens wear. Int Contact Lens Clin 1978;5:182–189.
33. Josephson JE, Caffery BE. Infiltrative keratitis in hydrogel lens wearers. Int Contact Lens Clin 1979;6:47–71.
34. Rudner EJ. Epidemiology of contact dermatitis in North America, 1972. Arch Dermatol 1973;108:537–540.
35. Rudner EJ, Clendenning WE, Epstein E, et al. The frequency of contact sensitivity in North America, 1972–74. Contact Derm 1975;1:277–280.
36. Lepine EM. Results of routine office patch testing. Contact Derm 1976;2:89–91.
37. Molinari JF, Nash R, Badham D. Severe thimerosal hypersensitivity in soft contact lens wearers. Int Contact Lens Clin 1982;9:323–329.
38. Mondino B, Salamon S, Zaidman G. Allergic and toxic reactions in soft contact lens wearers. Surv Ophthalmol 1982;26:337–344.
39. Sibley M, Chu V. Understanding sorbic acid preserved contact lens solutions. Int Contact Lens Clin 1984;9:531–542.
40. Josephson J. The "Multi-purge Procedure" and its application for hydrophilic lens wearers utilizing preserved solutions. J Am Optom Assoc 1978;49:280–281.

41. Rohrer MD, Terry MA, Bulard RA, et al. Microwave sterilization of hydrophilic contact lenses. Am J Ophthalmol 1986;101:49–57.

42. Sibley MJ. Soft lens cold disinfection solutions: A comparative study. Contact Lens Forum 1981;6:41–49.

43. Wechsler S, George NC. Disinfection of hydrophilic lenses. J Am Optom Assoc 1981;52:179–186.

44. Mondino B, Gorden L. Conjunctival hyperemia and corneal infiltrates with chemically disinfected soft contact lens. Arch Ophthalmol 1980;98:1769–1770.

45. Kleist FD. Appearance and nature of hydrophilic contact lens deposits. II. Inorganic deposits. Int Contact Lens Clin 1979;6:177–186.

46. Kline LN, Deluca TJ. Thermal vs chemical disinfection. Int Contact Lens Clin 1978;5:23–31.

47. Callender M. A comparison of Soflens (polymacon) wearer sensitivity to thermal or cold disinfecting system. Contact Lens J 1978;7:2–3.

48. Greenberger MH. A chlorhexidine-free chemical regimen for hydrophilic contact lenses. Int Contact Lens Clin 1981; 8:13–15.

49. Stein H, Boyaner D, Demers J. Soft contact lens care system alternatives. Int Contact Lens Clin 1981;8:11–16.

50. Gasset A, Ramer R, Katzin D. Hydrogen peroxide sterilization of hydrophilic contact lenses. Arch Ophthalmol 1975;93:412–415.

51. Janoff L. The effective disinfection of soft contact lenses using hydrogen peroxide. Contacto 1979;23:37–40.

52. Janoff LE. The exposure of various polymers to a 24-hour soak in Lensept: The effect on base curve. J Am Optom Assoc 1985;56:222–225.

53. Lowther GE. A review of transparent hydrogel tinted lenses. Contax March 1987;6–9.

54. Siberman HI. An investigation of a method of cold sterilization of hydrogel contact lenses by polyvinylpyrrolidone-iodine complex. J Am Optom Assoc 1973;44:1040–1046.

55. Conn H, Langer R. Iodine disinfection of hydrophilic contact lenses. Ann Ophthalmol 1981;13:361.

56. Josephson JE, Caffery BE. Selecting an appropriate hydrogel lens care system. J Am Optom Assoc 1981;52:227–234.

57. Ganju SN, Cordey P. Evaluation of sodium dichlorisocyanurate as a new soft lens disinfecting preparation. Ophthal Optician 1980;20:774–778.

58. Kamiki T, Kikkawa Y. Ozone sterilization technique of hydrophilic contact lenses, a 20th Congress Paper. Contacto 1976;20:16–18.

59. Hathaway R, Lowther GE. Factors influencing the rate of deposit formation on hydrophilic lens. Aust J Optom 1978;61:92–96.

60. Lowther GE, Hilbert J, King J. Appearance and location of hydrophilic lens deposits. Int Contact Lens Clin 1975;2:30–34.

61. Lowther GE. The relationship between the chemistry of the tear film and hydrophilic lens deposits. In: Soft contact lenses: Second National Research Symposium Proceedings. International Congress Series, 398. Amsterdam: Excerpta Medica, 1977.

62. Gyorffy I. Deposits on contact lenses as a cause of intolerance. Contact Lens 1972;3:19–20.

63. Loran DFC. Surface corrosion of hydrogel contact lenses. Contact Lens 1973;4:3–10.

64. Porter A. Unidentified contaminants of soft contact lens. Rev Optom 1979;116:36.

65. Kleist FD. Appearance and nature of hydrophilic contact lens deposits. I. Protein and organic deposits. Int Contact Lens Clin 1979;6:120–130.

66. Ruben M. Biochemical aspects of soft lenses. Contact Intraocular Lens Med J 1976;2:39–51.

67. Bailey N. Cleaning of coated soft lenses. J Am Optom Assoc 1974;45:1049–1052.

68. Bier N, Lowther GE. Contact lens correction. Boston: Butterworths, 1976;410–424.

69. Phillips AJ. The cleaning of hydrogel contact lenses. Ophthal Optician 1980;20:375–388.

70. Lloyd DJ. Enzyme cleaners: The structure, properties and mode of action of enzymes. Ophthal Optician 1979;19:833–839.

71. Lowther G. Effectiveness of an enzyme in removing deposits from hydrophilic lens. Am J Optom Physiol Opt 1977;54:76–84.

72. Hathaway R, Lowther GE. Soft lens cleaners: Their effectiveness in removing deposits. J Am Optom Assoc 1978;49:259–266.

73. Cumming JS, Karageozian H. Protein conjunctivitis in hydrophilic lens wearers. Contacto 1975;19:8–9.

74. Morris J. Soft lens aftercare. Optician 1974;174:20–26.

75. Fichman S, Baker VV, Horten H. Iatrogenic red eyes in soft contact lens wearers. Int Contact Lens Clin 1978;5:202–206.

76. Bellemare F. Compatibility of enzymatic cleaning with cold contact lens disinfection. Int Contact Lens Clin 1979;6:219–222.

77. Podos SM, Becker B, Assef C, et al. Pilocarpine therapy with soft contact lenses. Arch Ophthalmol 1972;73:336–341.

78. Maddox YT, Bernstein HN. An evaluation of the bionite hydrophilic contact lens for use in a drug delivery system. Ann Ophthalmol 1972;4:789–802.

79. Waltman SR, Kaufman HE. Use of hydrophilic contact lenses to increase ocular penetration of topical drugs. Invest Ophthalmol 1970;9:250–255.

80. Mizutane Y, Miwa Y. On the uptake and release of drugs by soft contact lenses. Contact Intraocular Lens Med J 1975;1:177–183.

81. Marmion VJ. Role of soft contact lenses and delivery of drugs. Trans Ophthalmol Soc UK 1976;96:319–321.

82. Gasset AR. Therapeutic applications. In: Mandell RB, ed. Contact lens practice, ed. 3. Springfield, IL: Charles C Thomas, 1981;607–618.

83. Krezanoski JZ. Topical medications. Int Ophthalmol Clin 1981;21:173–176.

84. Bronson L, Koetting RA, Janoff L, et al. Use of Timoptic with soft lenses. Int Corr Soc Optom 1980;4:2–6.

85. Hales RH. Contact lenses: A clinical approach to fitting. Baltimore: Williams & Wilkins, 1978;32–56.

86. Sugar J. Adrenochrome pigmentation of hydrophilic lenses. Arch Ophthalmol 1974;91:11–12.

87. Miller D, Brooks S, Mobilia E. Adrenochrome staining of soft contact lenses. Ann Ophthalmol 1976;6:65–66.

88. Aucamp A. Drug excretion in human tears and its meaning for contact lens wearers. S Afr Optom 1980;39:128–136.

89. Wartman RH. Contact lens-related side effects of systemic drugs. Contact Lens Forum 1987;12:42–44.

90. Valentic JP, Leopold IH, Dea FJ. Excretion of salicylic acid

into tears following oral administration of aspirin. Ophthalmology 1980;87:815–820.

91. Miller D. Systemic medications. Int Ophthalmol Clin 1981; 21:177–183.

92. Koetting RA. The influence of oral contraceptives on contact lens wear. Am J Optom Physiol Opt 1966;43:268–274.

93. Soni PS. Effects of oral contraceptive steroids on the thickness of human cornea. Am J Optom Physiol Opt 1980;57:825–834.

94. Lyons RW. Orange contact lenses from rifampin. N Engl J Med 1979;300:372–373.

95. Newson SR, Hayer BS. Disulfiram alcohol reactions caused by contact lens wetting solutions. Contact Intraocular Lens Med J 1980;6:407–408.

96. Gordon A. Prospective screening for thimerosal hypersensitivity: A pilot study. Am J Optom Physiol Opt 1988;65:147–150.

97. Paugh JR, Brennan NA, Efron N. Ocular response to hydrogen peroxide. Am J Optom Physiol Opt 1988;65:91–98.

98. Barton BE, James LC, Spencer J, et al. Relative allergenic potential of four proteases used as contact lens cleaners. Am J Optom Physiol Opt 1988;65:70–75.

CHAPTER 15

Topical Anesthesia

Jimmy D. Bartlett

Synthetic local anesthetics enable the practitioner to perform numerous diagnostic or surgical procedures in the office while permitting a comfortable patient and avoiding the relative risk from general anesthesia. The advantages of local anesthesia over general anesthesia include minimal physiologic changes, a relatively pleasant postprocedure period with little or no nausea and hangover, and the potential for prolonged relief of pain when long-acting anesthetics are used for regional nerve block. Since most procedures involving the eye and its adnexa are short and can be accomplished with local anesthesia, there is almost no risk to the patient's general health. In addition, local anesthesia has the advantage of simplicity; no cumbersome equipment is required, and minor in-office diagnostic or surgical procedures can usually be performed with little inconvenience or cost to the patient.

Topical application represents the most common route of administration of local anesthetics for procedures involving the eye. Topically applied anesthetics are surface-acting drugs that produce a reversible inhibition of the sensory nerve endings within the corneal and conjunctival epithelium, producing transient local anesthesia of the corneal and conjunctival surfaces.

Although most of the commonly used topical anesthetics are similar in onset, duration, and depth of anesthesia (see Chapter 4), several important differences exist. Thus, selection of the appropriate topical anesthetic for individual clinical procedures is important to maximize its effectiveness while minimizing undesirable side effects.

Selection of Anesthetic

Most of the commonly employed topical ocular anesthetics provide adequate clinical anesthesia within 10 to 20 seconds following instillation, and their anesthetic action lasts approximately 10 to 20 minutes. Anesthesia can be prolonged, if necessary, by repeated application.

Following the instillation of most topical anesthetics, many patients report a subjective sensation of "heaviness" of the lids that will frequently persist for several minutes following the return of corneal sensation.

Conjunctival hyperemia and mild lacrimation sometimes occur following the application of most topical anesthetics. Even topical cocaine occasionally produces mild hyperemia and lacrimation despite its local vasoconstrictor action.[1] In addition, the reflex action associated with discomfort may cause the fellow eye to become hyperemic when the anesthetic is placed in only 1 eye.

In addition to these direct effects, many topically applied anesthetics produce various indirect effects including increasing the corneal permeability to subsequently applied drugs, occasionally desquamating corneal epithelium, and retarding the mitosis and migration processes associated with corneal epithelial regeneration.[2]

Because the onset, duration of action, and depth of anesthesia of the commonly employed topical anesthetics are quite similar, and since the desirable clinical characteristics of local anesthetics vary only slightly with the ocular procedure to be performed, the clinician should select a single anesthetic that provides effective topical anesthesia for most clinical uses rather than employ different drugs for different purposes.[3] A single topical anesthetic will usually serve this purpose, and the other available drugs can be reserved for specialized uses as discussed in the following sections.

When the clinical usefulness of proparacaine is compared with that of the other commonly employed topical ocular anesthetics, a variety of advantages of proparacaine are evident:

- Rapid onset of surface anesthesia
- Relatively short duration of anesthesia
- Minimal discomfort or pain on instillation
- Absence of associated mydriasis
- Stability at room temperature
- Low incidence of hypersensitivity
- Absence of cross-sensitivity with benoxinate and tetracaine

These advantages make proparacaine the single most useful general-purpose anesthetic for topical use in ophthalmic practice. The other topical anesthetics are usually reserved for specialized uses, as shown in Table 15.1.

Clinical Utilization

The following general guidelines[4-7] should be observed for the safe and effective clinical use of topical anesthetics.

- For routine diagnostic procedures such as applanation tonometry and gonioscopy, topical anesthetics render the eye vulnerable to accidental damage during the period of anesthesia. The protective blink reflex is inhibited, and abnormal drying of the cornea can occur. Since minute foreign bodies can create severe corneal damage if brushed across the hypoesthetic cornea, the patient should be advised against rubbing the eye during the period of anesthesia, usually lasting 20 to 30 minutes following the diagnostic procedure.
- It is beneficial to instill the topical anesthetic into *both* eyes before routine diagnostic procedures such as gonioscopy, applanation tonometry, and fundus contact lens biomicroscopy. This serves to inhibit the blink reflex of the fellow eye, which facilitates the diagnostic procedure on the eye under examination. This practice also reduces examination time, since drug instillation into both eyes is accomplished before beginning the procedure.
- The mild local stinging or burning sensation following instillation of the anesthetic is transient, and treatment requires only patient reassurance.
- Since topically applied anesthetics frequently cause transient irregularity of the surface of the corneal epithelium, this can interfere with subsequent procedures requiring visualization inside the eye, such as ophthalmoscopy and fundus photography. Ideally, these procedures should be performed before application of a topical anesthetic.
- Topical anesthetics are ineffective on skin surfaces and are therefore ineffective for dermatologic procedures such as removal of verrucae.
- Ideally, resumption of contact lens wear should be delayed for at least 60 minutes following application of the anesthetic.[8]
- Epinephrine or other vasoconstrictors have no significant effect on the duration of topical anesthesia and should never be combined with commercially available topical anesthetics. They serve no useful purpose, yet increase the risk of systemic side effects.

Topical ocular anesthetics have many uses in clinical practice. Most commonly they are used to improve patient tolerance of various diagnostic procedures. In addition, these drugs often provide sufficient anes-

TABLE 15.1
Specialized Uses of Topical Anesthetics

Procedure	*Indicated Anesthetic*
Surgery involving the deep conjunctiva	4% lidocaine with 1:1000 epinephrine applied with iontophoresis
Forced duction test	4% cocaine or 4% lidocaine applied with cotton-tipped applicator
Electroretinography	0.5% tetracaine ointment
Goldmann applanation tonometry	0.4% benoxinate-sodium fluorescein or 0.5% proparacaine–sodium fluorescein
Corneal epithelial debridement	4% cocaine

thesia for minor surgical procedures of the cornea and conjunctiva. The following is a discussion of the more commonly employed procedures that are facilitated by topical anesthesia.

Diagnostic Procedures

GONIOSCOPY

One or 2 drops of 0.5% proparacaine allows sufficient topical anesthesia to permit gonioscopy for as long as 15 to 20 minutes. If the anesthetic is instilled into both eyes before beginning the procedure, it need not be reapplied before beginning gonioscopy on the second eye.

APPLANATION TONOMETRY

Two techniques are commonly employed for ensuring topical anesthesia before Goldmann applanation tonometry: (1) the use of a solution of benoxinate-sodium fluorescein or proparacaine–sodium fluorescein, or (2) a 2-step procedure involving the instillation of a topical anesthetic followed by separate application of sodium fluorescein.

Use of a solution of benoxinate–sodium fluorescein (Fluress) or proparacaine–sodium fluorescein allows simultaneous application of the required anesthetic and sodium fluorescein dye. This method increases the efficiency of the procedure by eliminating the need for separate applications of the anesthetic and dye, but it has the disadvantages of irritation from the benoxinate as well as excessive instillation of dye. Sometimes 30 to 60 seconds must elapse to allow the excess dye to dissipate before accurate tonometry can be performed. In addition, solutions of sodium fluorescein have the inherent risk of overflowing and subsequently staining the patient's lids, cheeks, or clothing. Note, however, that differences in the results of tonometry using either benoxinate or proparacaine are not clinically significant.[9]

Also used is a 2-step procedure involving the instillation of a topical anesthetic such as proparacaine followed by the separate application of sodium fluorescein from either a sterile solution or a dye-impregnated paper strip. The application of sodium fluorescein by moistening the impregnated strip with lacrimal fluid and residual anesthetic contained within the inferior conjunctival sac (Fig. 15.1) allows, with experience and practice, a consistent amount of fluorescein to be applied. This technique permits immediate and accurate tonometry by eliminating the excessive dye often associated with sodium fluorescein solutions.

Regardless of which technique is used, the drugs should be applied to both eyes before beginning tonometry. This reduces the blink reflex of the fellow eye and increases the speed and efficiency with which the procedure is performed.

FUNDUS CONTACT LENS BIOMICROSCOPY

Following topical anesthesia the fundus contact lens is applied to the cornea with appropriate gonioscopic bonding solution (see Fig. 16.14). For anesthesia, 1 or 2 drops of 0.5% proparacaine is sufficient. As in gonioscopy and applanation tonometry, applying the anesthetic to both eyes before beginning the procedure serves to increase the speed and efficiency with which the procedure is performed.

EVALUATION OF CORNEAL ABRASIONS

Since repeated applications of a topical anesthetic to an injured cornea may seriously delay or prevent re-

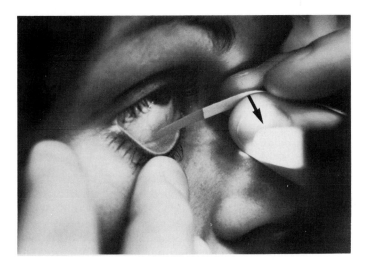

FIGURE 15.1 **Application of sodium fluorescein for applanation tonometry by moistening the dye-impregnated strip with lacrimal fluid and residual anesthetic contained within the inferior conjunctival sac. The sodium fluorescein strip is moistened by placing it within the conjunctival sac, between the bulbar and tarsal conjunctivae. Illumination may be provided by white light on the tonometer prism (arrow).**

generation of the epithelium, the practitioner should refrain from the liberal instillation of topical anesthetics in cases of corneal abrasions, foreign bodies, or other injuries.[10] Often, however, the blepharospasm, lacrimation, and pain accompanying the corneal injury prevent adequate examination of the eye. In such cases, 1 or 2 drops of 0.5% proparacaine will usually relieve the pain and allow slit-lamp evaluation of the injury. The patient, however, should *never* be given a topical anesthetic for self-administration at home. Very serious corneal damage may result[11] (see Chapter 4). Instead, the pain associated with the corneal injury should be treated by cycloplegics, pressure-patching, cold compresses, and aspirin or other systemic analgesics.

FORCED DUCTION TEST

The forced duction test is used to investigate deficient ocular rotations to differentiate between deficiencies due to neurogenic or myogenic weakness and those caused by muscle restrictions such as in Graves' ophthalmopathy.[12] The practitioner is able to detect a mechanical limitation (restrictive myopathy) if, when attempting to actively move the globe, considerable resistance prevents eye movement. On the other hand, a neurogenic cause is isolated if the globe moves freely on forced duction testing. Two methods of performing this test are commonly employed: (1) the traditional technique involving attempted movement of the globe with toothed forceps, or (2) a less traumatic technique involving attempted movement of the globe with a cotton-tipped applicator positioned at the limbus.

In the forceps technique, the practitioner uses the forceps to grasp the insertion of the rectus muscle to be investigated and attempts to move the globe in a direction opposite the field of action of that muscle (Fig. 15.2*A*). Most of the topical anesthetics commercially available fail to completely eliminate the patient's awareness of the forceps. Although this awareness is not particularly painful, the sensation of the eye being touched often increases patient apprehension, provokes blepharospasm, and prevents adequate investigation of the muscle being tested. This problem can be greatly reduced or eliminated by using a 4% solution of lidocaine as the topical anesthetic. A cotton-tipped applicator moistened with this solution should be applied to the surface of the conjunctiva at the site overlying the rectus muscle insertion to be investigated. The applicator should be applied for 1 to 2 minutes. The depth of topical anesthesia achieved using this method has been found to be far more satisfactory than that provided by the more routinely used anesthetics such as tetracaine or proparacaine.[12] Cocaine in a 4% solution applied with a cotton-tipped applicator also provides sufficient local anesthesia to permit traditional forced duction testing.

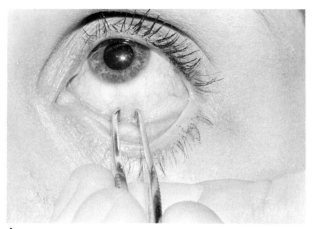

A

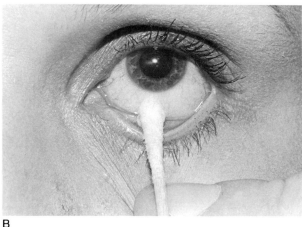

B

FIGURE 15.2   **Forced duction test. (A) Traditional technique involving attempted movement of the globe with toothed forceps. (B) Technique involving attempted movement of the globe with cotton-tipped applicator positioned at limbus.**

A simpler technique for the forced duction test has been described by Smith.[13] Following topical anesthesia with 0.5% proparacaine, movement of the globe is attempted by placing a cotton-tipped applicator at the limbus (Fig. 15.2*B*). This technique allows the practitioner to detect a mechanical limitation of the globe without subjecting the patient to the discomfort associated with toothed forceps.

SCHIRMER NO. 1 TEST

The Schirmer No. 1 test has been used for decades as a quantitative test of aqueous tear production. When performed without topical anesthesia, this test assesses both the basic lacrimal secretion from the lacrimal gland and accessory glands of Kraus and Wolfring, as well as neurogenic lacrimal secretion stimulated by irritation of the conjunctiva and lid tissues with the Schirmer strip. To eliminate the neurogenic component of tear secretion, the Schirmer test can be performed following the application of a topical anesthetic, thus allowing a more accurate assessment of basic lacrimal secretion. The conjunctival sac should be dried with a cotton-tipped applicator following administration of the anesthetic. This will prevent reflex tearing that may result from irritation by the anesthetic and will also prevent false-negative findings from strip wetting by the anesthetic itself. The average Schirmer test result following topical anesthesia in the patient with a normal lacrimal system is approximately 15 mm of strip-wetting at 5 minutes.[14]

ELECTRORETINOGRAPHY

Depending on the specific protocol used for electro-retinography (ERG), the procedure usually lasts any-where from 20 minutes to approximately 1 hour. Placement of the contact lens electrode (Fig. 15.3) is facilitated by the application of 0.5% proparacaine, but the duration of anesthesia does not permit proce-dures exceeding 20 to 30 minutes. When prolonged procedures are anticipated or required, the topical an-esthetic of choice should be 0.5% tetracaine ointment. This preparation allows prolonged patient comfort and thus facilitates determination of the final scotopic val-ues that are so critical in electroretinographic evalua-tions.

LACRIMAL DRAINAGE PROCEDURES

To increase patient comfort during lacrimal dilation and irrigation (see Figs. 20.17 and 20.19), the appli-

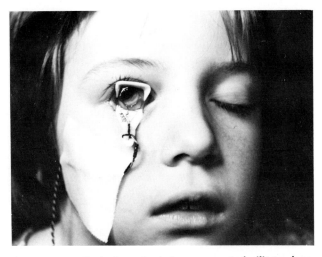

FIGURE 15.3 **Topical anesthesia is necessary to facilitate place-ment of contact lens electrode for electroretinography.**

cation of a topical anesthetic such as 0.5% propara-caine is required. One or 2 drops topically instilled is usually sufficient. Normal blinking following instilla-tion of the anesthetic promotes drainage of the drug through the nasolacrimal drainage system. The dilation and irrigation procedures can begin 1 or 2 minutes following instillation of the anesthetic.

Havener[15] has recommended that, in the probing of an adult's nasolacrimal system, the initial topical an-esthetic be supplemented by irrigation of the lacrimal sac with 0.25 ml of 0.5% tetracaine solution. However, because of the known systemic toxicity of tetracaine, the practitioner should refrain from forcing the tetra-caine into the tissues by manipulating the lacrimal cannula.

One or 2 drops of topically applied 0.5% propara-caine will improve patient comfort for the insertion of collagen implants and other forms of punctal plugs (see Fig. 20.11).

CONTACT LENS FITTING

To evaluate the eye's normal physiologic responses to contact lens wear, contact lenses should be fitted with-out topical anesthesia. However, certain limited cir-cumstances may justify the use of topical anesthetics in contact lens evaluations. These include determining the effect of a rigid contact lens on monocular diplopia when the cornea is suspected to be the etiologic source. Topical anesthesia allows the rigid lens to be easily placed on the eye and to be readily tolerated by the patient during the initial diagnostic evaluation. Topical anesthesia may also be used when fitting infants and very young children with rigid contact lenses. The molding of scleral contact lenses is facilitated by topical anesthesia, as is the fitting of rigid contact lenses to certain mentally retarded patients or other patients whose inability to cooperate prevents necessary eval-uation procedures. The practitioner, however, should avoid the use of topical anesthetics in conjunction with hydrogel lenses. These lenses will absorb the anesthetic and act as a drug reservoir by gradually releasing the drug to the eye, with the potential complications as-sociated with long-term anesthesia.

Therapeutic Procedures

CORNEAL FOREIGN BODY REMOVAL

As with the evaluation of corneal abrasions, the ap-plication of 1 or 2 drops of 0.5% proparacaine is often necessary to allow adequate examination of the eye with a corneal foreign body. Before removal of super-ficial corneal foreign bodies, an additional 1 to 2 drops of topical anesthetic will loosen the epithelium, which, in some cases, may be sufficient to allow removal of the foreign object with a cotton-tipped applicator. The additional topical anesthetic also allows somewhat deeper anesthesia for removal of foreign bodies in the deep epithelium or superficial stroma. The limbal area, however, is often difficult to anesthetize, and a solution of 5% cocaine applied with a cotton-tipped applicator may be useful to achieve adequate anesthesia.[16] Topical anesthetics *must never be prescribed for self-administration by the patient at home.* Following foreign body removal, any associated pain should be treated by cycloplegics, pressure-patching, cold compresses, and aspirin or other systemic analgesics.

MINOR SURGERY OF THE CONJUNCTIVA

The excision of small, superficial conjunctival lesions such as concretions can usually be achieved with topical anesthesia alone (Fig. 15.4). Two or 3 drops instilled at 1-minute intervals allows sufficient anesthesia for this purpose. Alternatively, a cotton pledget or cotton-tipped applicator soaked in the anesthetic solution may be applied for 1 to 2 minutes before surgery. This allows anesthesia of deeper portions of the conjunctiva.

Before routine infiltration anesthesia for chalazion resection, 5% lidocaine ointment can be applied to the tarsal conjunctiva using a cotton-tipped applicator. This procedure effectively reduces the pain of chalazion surgery without side effects.[17]

Iontophoretic local anesthesia for conjunctival surgery has been described in which an iontophoretic unit (Xomed Company), originally designed to deliver local anesthesia to the tympanic membrane, has been adapted for use on the tarsal conjunctiva.[18] Since topical anesthetics, including cocaine, are effective for only superficial conjunctival surgery, iontophoretic anesthesia may be used for lesions such as deeply positioned conjunctival concretions. A solution of 4% lidocaine and 1:1000 epinephrine, in equal parts, is dripped onto a cotton pledget, which touches the tip of the positive electrode overlying the area of the tarsal conjunctiva to be surgically incised. Of the 27 patients on whom this technique was used, no patients reported any discomfort during the induction period. During the surgery that followed, the patients reported no pain except in 3 cases involving chalazions of the deeper portion of the tarsus. This technique has been used successfully for conjunctival surgery involving papillomas, superficial chalazions, and conjunctival concretions.[18]

CORNEAL EPITHELIAL DEBRIDEMENT

At one time mechanical debridement of the corneal epithelium was the only effective treatment for herpetic epithelial keratitis.[19] Although the use of newer antiviral drugs has increased the therapeutic armamentar-

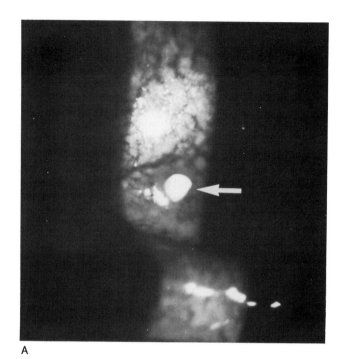

A

B

FIGURE 15.4 **Topical anesthesia permits the removal of symptomatic conjunctival concretion. (A) Concretion (arrow) before removal. (B) Conjunctival depression (arrow) at site of removed concretion. (Courtesy Larry J. Alexander, O.D.)**

ium against herpetic keratitis, debridement remains a safe, effective, and occasionally preferred alternative in the treatment of herpetic corneal infection. The mechanical removal of virus-replicating epithelium abolishes a source of infection for other epithelial cells and eliminates an antigenic stimulus to stromal inflammation.[19]

Debridement is performed at the slit lamp following topical anesthesia with 2 to 3 drops of 4% cocaine applied over several minutes. Not only does the cocaine provide excellent surface anesthesia, it also substantially softens and loosens the corneal epithelium, thereby facilitating its removal with a sterile cotton-tipped applicator (Fig. 15.5). Controlled removal of the epithelium is best achieved by cutting through a margin of healthy epithelium with a semisharp, chisel-ended stick.[19] A sharp knife blade should not be used because of the risk of damaging Bowman's layer and thus creating a portal of virus entry into the corneal stroma.[19] Since simply "wiping off" the herpetic lesion with the applicator may serve to secondarily infect

adjacent, healthy epithelium with virus, a virucidal agent such as phenol or iodine may be applied to the edges of the removed epithelium. This is best achieved by debridement with a chisel-ended stick that has been dipped first in 10% phenol.[19] Care should be taken to remove excessive phenol by blotting before use. If iodine is used, it can be applied with a cotton-tipped applicator. Since cocaine iodide is an insoluble precipitate, the previous application of cocaine protects against stromal damage by the iodine.[15] However, this protection is incomplete, and excessive use of iodine may damage the stroma.

SUTURE BARB REMOVAL

Occasionally suture material may protrude through the surface of the conjunctiva or cornea days, weeks, or even years following cataract surgery or penetrating keratoplasty, giving rise to symptoms such as foreign body sensation, redness, itching, and mucus discharge. Giant papillary conjunctivitis can also occur as a result

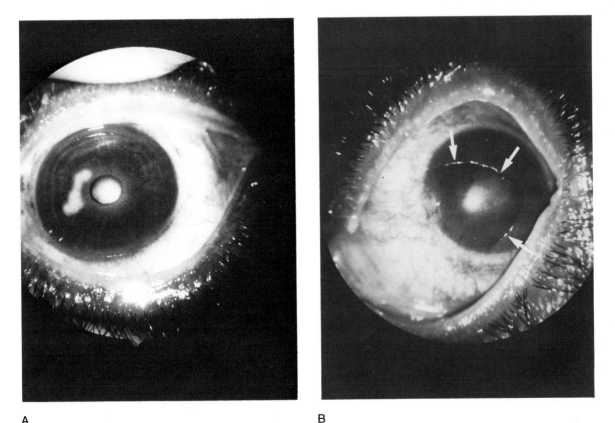

A   B

FIGURE 15.5   **Corneal epithelial debridement. *(A)* Herpetic corneal lesion stained with sodium fluorescein. *(B)* Following the topical application of 4% cocaine, debridement is performed with a sterile cotton-tipped applicator. Edge of debrided area is denoted by arrows. (Courtesy Mark Flora, O.D.)**

of suture-induced irritation.[20] Removal of the offending suture is easily achieved following topical anesthesia using 1 or 2 drops of 0.5% proparacaine.

To ensure adequate healing of the surgical wound, it is prudent to delay suture removal for 3 months following cataract extraction and for as long as 6 to 9 months following penetrating keratoplasty. Furthermore, to reduce the risk of serious complications such as endophthalmitis, a broad-spectrum antibacterial agent such as gentamicin or tobramycin should be used topically several times daily for 2 to 3 days before removal of the offending suture.[21]

The eye should be anesthetized with topically applied 0.5% proparacaine. For deeper anesthesia, 4% lidocaine can be applied with a cotton-tipped applicator held against the suture for 30 to 60 seconds.[22] Broken sutures are removed by firmly grasping the knotted end with jewelers forceps and slowly pulling the suture free. If the suture is intact, the practitioner should grasp the knot with forceps and gently snip the suture using a #11 scalpel or straight blade iris scissors. Following suture removal, the integrity of the surgical wound should be confirmed and the patient given a prophylactic topical antibacterial agent, such as gentamicin or tobramycin, for 3 to 5 days.

Predrug Instillation

Since topical anesthetics increase permeability of the corneal epithelium to subsequently applied drugs,[10] the practitioner may capitalize on this fact to increase the clinical effectiveness of mydriatics and cycloplegics. Moreover, some drugs must be preceded by a topical anesthetic to reduce or eliminate severe stinging or burning associated with those drugs.

MYDRIATICS

The effect of topical anesthetics on phenylephrine-induced mydriasis has been studied by several investigators.[23–25] These studies have shown that when proparacaine precedes phenylephrine, the time required to produce maximum dilation is reduced, the amplitude of maximum dilation is increased, and the duration of dilation is also increased. The enhancement of mydriasis is similar for benoxinate, proparacaine, and tetracaine.[23] Mordi and associates[26] have shown that the prior instillation of 0.5% proparacaine prolongs both the mydriatic as well as the cycloplegic effects of 1% tropicamide. The topically applied anesthetic may increase the mydriatic's bioavailability by inhibiting tear flow and thus increasing corneal absorption of the drug.[23,27] Furthermore, the anesthetic-induced inhibition of tear flow, by increasing the amount of mydriatic

absorbed through the cornea, decreases the quantity of mydriatic available for systemic absorption. This reduces the risk of systemic side effects.[23] This anesthetic-induced enhancement of mydriasis is helpful in eyes difficult to dilate such as in patients with diabetes or those with darkly pigmented irides. The reduced risk of systemic side effects is reassuring in patients with diabetes, cardiovascular disease such as hypertension, and hyperthyroidism.

GLYCERIN

The practitioner should precede the topical instillation of glycerin, a hyperosmotic agent, with a topical anesthetic. Since without topical anesthesia the instillation of glycerin causes severe stinging, burning, or ocular pain, the use of topically applied glycerin is limited to the practitioner's office. Patients should never be permitted to self-administer a topical anesthetic at home in conjunction with the use of topical glycerin as a hyperosmotic agent.

TRICHLOROACETIC ACID

The use of trichloroacetic acid on the cornea as a chemical cauterizing agent should always be preceded by a topical anesthetic. One or 2 drops of 0.5% proparacaine allows sufficient surface anesthesia for such chemical cauterization.

References

1. Jervey JW. Topical anesthetics for the eye. A comparative study. South Med J 1955;48:770–774.
2. Webster RB. Local anesthetics for ophthalmic use. Aust J Optom 1974;57:399–401.
3. Linn JG, Vey EK. Topical anesthesia in ophthalmology. Am J Ophthalmol 1955;40:697–704.
4. Miscellaneous ophthalmic preparations. In AMA drug evaluations. Chicago: American Medical Association, 1980;4:395–407.
5. Allen ED, Elkington AR. Local anaesthesia and the eye. Br J Anaesth 1980;52:689–694.
6. Lyle WM, Page C. Possible adverse effects from local anesthetics and the treatment of these reactions. Am J Optom Physiol Opt 1975;52:736–744.
7. Adriani J, Zepernick R. Clinical effectiveness of drugs used for topical anesthesia. JAMA 1964;188:711–716.
8. Hill RM. Anesthetic impact. Int Cont Lens Clin 1980;7:199–200.
9. Jose JG, Basta M, Cramer KJ, et al. Lack of effects of anesthetic on measurement of intraocular pressure by Goldmann tonometry. Am J Optom Physiol Opt 1983;60:308–310.
10. Bryant JA. Local and topical anesthetics in ophthalmology. Surv Ophthalmol 1969;13:262–283.

11. Duffin RM, Olson RJ. Tetracaine toxicity. Ann Ophthalmol 1984;16:836–837.
12. Raab EL. Traction test (letter). Arch Ophthalmol 1977; 95:1649.
13. Smith JL. The optic nerve. Miami: JL Smith, 1975;49.
14. Ingis TM, Hornblass A. Lacrimal function tests: A comparative study. Surg Forum 1977;28:516–517.
15. Havener WH. Ocular pharmacology. St. Louis: C. V. Mosby Co, 1978;5:72–119.
16. Newell SW. Management of corneal foreign bodies. Am Fam Physician 1985;31:149–156.
17. Gerde LS, Hanson B. Anesthesia in chalazion surgery. South Med J 1983;76:11.
18. Sisler HA. Iontophoretic local anesthesia for conjunctival surgery. Ann Ophthalmol 1978;10:597–598.
19. O'Day DM, Jones BR. Herpes simplex keratitis. In: Duane TD, ed. Clinical ophthalmology, vol. 4. Philadelphia: Harper & Row, 1986; Chap. 19:8.
20. Melore GG. Suture barb syndrome. South J Optom 1987;5:70–73.
21. Gelender H. Bacterial endophthalmitis following cutting of sutures after cataract surgery. Am J Ophthalmol 1982;94:528–533.
22. Dornic DI. How to treat suture barbs. Rev Optom 1987; 124:67–68.
23. Lyle WM, Bobier WR. Effects of topical anesthetics on phenylephrine-induced mydriasis. Am J Optom Physiol Opt 1977;54:276–281.
24. Jauregui MJ, Polse KA. Mydriatic effect using phenylephrine and proparacaine. Am J Optom Physiol Opt 1974;51:545–549.
25. Kubo DJ, Wing TW, Polse KA, et al. Mydriatic effects using low concentrations of phenylephrine hydrochloride. J Am Optom Assoc 1975;46:817–822.
26. Mordi JA, Lyle WM, Mousa GY. Does prior instillation of a topical anesthetic enhance the effect of tropicamide? Am J Optom Physiol Opt 1986;63:290–293.
27. Patton TF, Robinson JR. Influence of topical anesthetics on tear dynamics and ocular drug bioavailability in albino rabbits. J Pharm Sci 1976;64:267–271.

CHAPTER 16

Dilation of the Pupil

Jimmy D. Bartlett

Since the invention of the direct ophthalmoscope in the 19th century, mydriatic drugs have been used to facilitate examination of the crystalline lens, vitreous, retina, and optic nerve. With the advent of the binocular indirect ophthalmoscope, 3-mirror fundus contact lenses, and other diagnostic instrumentation, a panoramic and stereoscopic view of the fundus from ciliary body to optic nerve has been made available to the ophthalmic practitioner. Much of this view, however, is accessible only with the use of mydriatics. The proper use of mydriatics enables the practitioner to more accurately identify and diagnose various abnormalities of the eye that might otherwise go undetected. This chapter considers the incorporation of routine pupillary dilation into office practice, anterior angle evaluation before dilation, dilation drug regimens, clinical procedures facilitated by the use of mydriatics, and pupillary dilation as a therapeutic procedure.

Incorporation of Pupillary Dilation into Examination Routine

The successful incorporation of pupillary dilation procedures into the examination routine improves the clinical effectiveness of mydriatics by allowing the drugs to be used in patients for whom they are indicated without disrupting normal patient flow in the office. Such use requires attention to certain patient management aspects, the examination routine itself, and the selection of patients for dilation.

Patient Management Aspects

Some practitioners acquiesce to the wishes of their patients who decline to be dilated. Although this is acceptable in some cases, the ability to communicate to patients the desirability of pupillary dilation is largely a matter of practitioner-patient rapport. Many older adult patients may remember being dilated as a child when the standard drug regimen was atropine or scopolamine, the effects of which lasted 1 or 2 weeks. These patients can be reassured that contemporary mydriatics are rapid acting with little or no debilitating effect on vision. Other patients sometimes have unrealistic conceptions of "dilation" procedures. Thus, to prevent or minimize dilation-related patient apprehension, the effects of the drugs should be explained before dilation, and the benefits of their use should be emphasized. With this approach, most patients are not only willing to be dilated, but they actually desire the procedure once they understand the reasons for it.

The reasons most commonly cited by practitioners for not routinely using mydriatics relate to time constraints, patient inconvenience, concern for systemic drug reactions, or fear of angle-closure glaucoma.[1,2] Some practitioners consider the routine use of mydriatics unnecessary, while other clinicians contend that the use of mydriatics is not cost effective because it takes too long.

Regarding the problem of patient inconvenience, most patients desire the most current diagnostic procedures even though they may cause transient ocular irritation or blurred vision. Patients seem to agree that a few hours of inconvenience is much more acceptable than a lifetime of blindness. Since many patients equate *dilation* with *complete eye examination*, they are attracted to ophthalmic practices in which mydriatics are routinely used.

When mydriatic drugs and associated diagnostic procedures are appropriately used, the incidence of adverse ocular or systemic drug reactions is extremely low. The prevalence and significance of these complications are discussed later in this chapter. Likewise, the risks of angle-closure glaucoma are extremely low and are considered elsewhere in this chapter. Concern for angle-closure glaucoma should not prevent the practitioner from routinely using mydriatics when appropriate precautions are taken.

Some practitioners may contend that effective diagnosis of cataracts as well as vitreal, retinal, or optic nerve disease can be rendered with an undilated pupil. Most astute clinicians, however, would argue that even the *detection* of posterior segment disease is handicapped by the undilated pupil. Furthermore, the *definitive diagnosis* of posterior segment disease is in many instances impossible without the appropriate use of mydriatics.

The routine use of mydriatics requires little, if any, additional time for the practitioner. However, depending on the diagnostic procedure to be performed, additional time requirements for the patient may range from 20 to 45 minutes. Most of this additional time requirement is consumed in dilation of the pupil. The routine use of mydriatics allows a much greater wealth of diagnostic information to be obtained in the same amount of time that would otherwise be consumed by frustration at the inability to visualize the affected area through the undilated pupil.

Examination Routine

Most clinicians dilate patients only after most other examination procedures have been performed. Complete histories, visual acuities, external examination, pupillary examination, ocular motility, refraction, biomicroscopy, Goldmann tonometry, and other routine evaluation procedures are performed before instilling the mydriatic(s) (Fig. 16.1). This ensures that dilation does not interfere with the refraction, assessment of accommodation or binocularity, or any other refractive finding. In most routine cases, ophthalmoscopy is the only procedure remaining to be performed following dilation. After the drops have been instilled for dilation, the patient may proceed to the reception area or to the dispensary for spectacle frame selection while the pupils dilate. Frame selection can usually be completed without interference from the mydriatic, and the patient not requiring frame selection can relax in the reception area or "dilation room."[3] While this

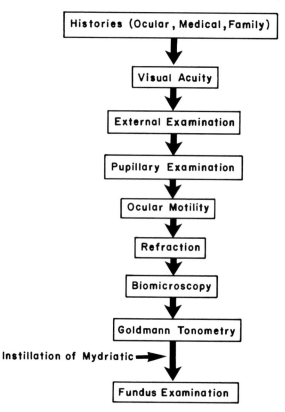

FIGURE 16.1   **Example of examination routine in which the mydriatic is instilled near the conclusion of the examination.**

patient's pupils dilate, the next scheduled patient is examined. In 20 to 30 minutes, after all procedures except dilation have been performed on the second patient and the pupils of the first patient have dilated, the second patient then proceeds to frame selection or to the dilation room while the first patient returns for ophthalmoscopy and any other procedures that may be indicated. This "round robin" or "leap frog" approach (Table 16.1) is used by most practitioners who incorporate pupillary dilation as a routine part of their service.[1] Note, however, that patient appointment schedules will vary depending on the number and responsibilities of staff personnel and of practitioners in the office.[4]

The placement of dilation procedures toward the conclusion of the routine examination enables the practitioner to perform all the mydriatic preinstillation examination as a standard routine. All the procedures that should be accomplished before instilling the mydriatic—visual acuity, tonometry, anterior angle evaluation, drug sensitivity history—are permitted in a natural and logical sequence. Thus, the patient may immediately undergo pupillary dilation if warranted.

TABLE 16.1
Illustration of "Round Robin" Procedure for Incorporating Dilation into Examination Routine[a]

Time (AM)	Patient A	Patient B	Patient C
8:00	(8:00) Arrives for appointment		
	(8:05–8:10) Preliminary work-up by technician		
8:15	(8:10–8:30) Examination by optometrist	(8:15) Arrives for appointment	
8:30	(8:30) Drops instilled for pupillary dilation	(8:20–8:30) Preliminary work-up by technician	
8:45	(8:30–8:50) Frame selection or "dilation room"	(8:30–8:50) Examination by optometrist	(8:45) Arrives for appointment
9:00	(8:50–9:00) Ophthalmoscopy and other indicated procedures, patient consultation	(8:50) Drops instilled for pupillary dilation	(8:50–8:55) Preliminary work-up by technician
		(8:50–9:10) Frame selection or "dilation room"	(8:55–9:10) Examination by optometrist
9:15		(9:10–9:20) Ophthalmoscopy and other indicated procedures, patient consultation	(9:10) Drops instilled for pupillary dilation
			(9:10–9:30) Frame selection or "dilation room"
9:30			(9:30–9:40) Ophthalmoscopy and other indicated procedures, patient consultation

[a]Time allotments represent approximations and may vary according to practitioner requirements, patient punctuality for appointment, and other factors. These suggestions are for illustration purposes only.

If the practitioner does not wish to dilate the pupils, direct ophthalmoscopy or monocular indirect ophthalmoscopy can then be performed in the usual manner.

Indications and Contraindications

When the various clinical and legal factors governing patient care are considered, a standard of care (see Chapter 34) appears to be emerging that requires that virtually all "new" patients presenting for comprehensive eye examination undergo dilated fundus examination using binocular indirect ophthalmoscopy. The fact that pupillary dilation allows a substantially more thorough evaluation of the ocular media, fundus including peripheral retina, and optic disc than is permitted without dilation suggests that careful indirect ophthalmoscopy with or without fundus biomicroscopy be performed through a dilated pupil in a variety of clinical circumstances (Table 16.2).[5]

In rare clinical situations dilation of the pupil may be contraindicated (Table 16.3), but if patient history, signs, or symptoms seem to indicate that dilation is necessary, the practitioner should proceed by following the guidelines given later in this chapter. Legal issues of negligence (failure to dilate) and patient informed consent are extremely important and can play a pivotal role in the selection of patients whose pupils should be dilated (see Chapters 33 and 34).

Anterior Angle Evaluation

Acute angle-closure glaucoma is a well-recognized complication of mydriatic drug use. Since the risk of such a complication is greatest in eyes with shallow chambers and narrow anterior angles, the anterior angle must be evaluated before instilling the mydriatic. The anterior angle can be assessed by employing the shadow test, slit-lamp method, or gonioscopy.

Shadow Test

The easiest and most rapid method of evaluating the anterior angle is by employing a penlight to illuminate the iris (Fig. 16.2). This method is less accurate than

TABLE 16.2
Indications for Pupillary Dilation

- Symptoms of floaters or flashes of light
- Visual acuity not correctable to 20/20
- Visual field loss
- Presence of cataract or other media opacities
- Myopia exceeding 6 D
- Episodes of intermittent blurred vision or blackouts
- Ocular contusion injury
- History of diabetes
- Unexplained ocular pain or redness
- History of lattice degeneration, retinal holes, or retinal detachment
- Afferent pupillary defect (Marcus Gunn pupil)
- History of metastatic tumors
- Miotic pupils
- Nystagmus or unsteady fixation
- Unexplained headaches
- History of use of drugs with known toxicity to lens, retina, or optic nerve
- Any symptom suggesting posterior segment involvement

TABLE 16.3
Contraindications to Pupillary Dilation

- Iris-supported intraocular lens (IOL)
- Subluxated crystalline lens
- Subluxated IOL
- Extremely narrow or closed anterior chamber angles[a]
- History suggesting angle-closure glaucoma, with or without surgical or laser intervention[a]

[a]Dilate with caution.
Adapted from Alexander LJ, Scholles J. Clinical and legal aspects of pupillary dilation. J Am Optom Assoc 1987; 58:432–437.

are the slit-lamp or gonioscopic procedures to be discussed; nevertheless, it is reliable and satisfactory for identifying critically narrow angles that might be predisposed to angle closure. Furthermore, it is useful in the pediatric age group, when slit-lamp examination or gonioscopy may not be permitted.

This method involves directing the penlight beam from the temporal side at the level of the pupil. The entire iris will be illuminated if the iris lies in a flat plane (Fig. 16.2*A*). This is characteristically observed in eyes with deep anterior chambers, such as those in myopia and aphakia, in which the open angle (grade

4) makes a 45° angle between the iris and the cornea.[6] When the angle between the iris and cornea is 20° or less (grade 2 to 0), the lens-iris diaphragm is displaced anteriorly. As a result, the penlight beam will illuminate the temporal iris, but a shadow will be observed on the nasal aspect of the iris in proportion to the convexity of the lens-iris diaphragm.

Although this method of evaluating the anterior angle is reliable in most patients, the practitioner must avoid misinterpretation. It is possible to estimate the angle as being narrower than it actually is because of central shallowing of the anterior chamber. This is especially common in older patients with enlarged lenses. In such eyes, the peripheral iris often recedes from the trabecular meshwork, leaving the angle incapable of closure.[6] The accuracy of this method can be enhanced by properly positioning the penlight exactly perpendicular to the visual axis.[7] If the penlight is positioned too far anteriorly, or if the eye is deviated

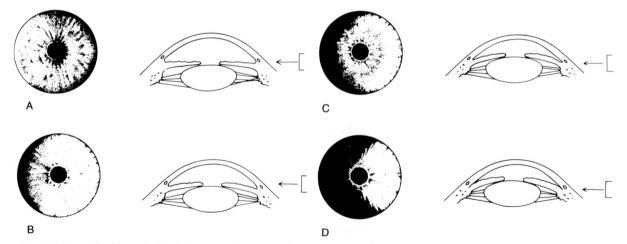

FIGURE 16.2   **Shadow test. The light source illuminates the nasal aspect of the iris to varying degrees depending on the depth of the anterior chamber. *(A)* Wide open angle (grade 4). *(B)* Open angle (grade 3). *(C)* Moderately narrow angle (grade 2). *(D)* Extremely narrow angle (grade 1).**

temporally, the nasal aspect of the iris may be illuminated directly, thus giving a false-negative result.

Slit-Lamp Method

A more accurate method for anterior angle evaluation is provided by the slit-lamp method described by van Herick, Shaffer, and Schwartz.[6] With the patient at the slit lamp, the vertical slit-lamp beam is placed at the temporal limbus just inside the corneoscleral junction. The slit lamp beam should be as narrow as possible, and should be directed toward the eye at an angle of about 60° from the direction of the observation microscope (Fig. 16.3). The depth of the anterior chamber at the temporal limbus is compared with the thickness of the cornea through which the beam travels. In the case of a wide open, or grade 4, angle, the depth of the anterior chamber is equal to or greater than the thickness of the cornea. If the depth of the anterior chamber is equal to approximately half the thickness of the cornea, the angle is classified as grade 3. An anterior chamber depth equal to one-fourth the corneal thickness is classified as a grade 2 angle, and an anterior chamber depth less than one-fourth the corneal thickness is classified as grade 1. The implications of such a classification in terms of the risk for angle closure are shown in Table 16.4.

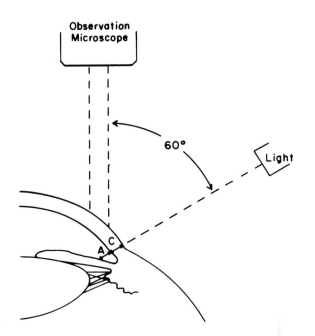

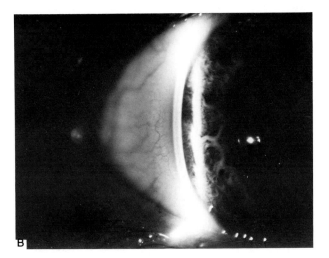

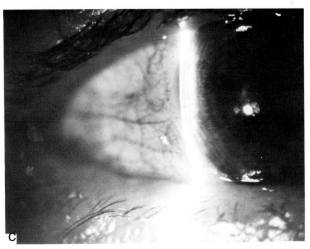

FIGURE 16.3 **Slit-lamp method for anterior angle evaluation.** *(A)* **The slit lamp beam should be as narrow as possible and should be directed toward the eye at an angle of approximately 60° from the direction of the observation microscope. The depth of the anterior chamber (A) is compared with the thickness of the cornea (C) through which the beam travels.** *(B)* **Slit-lamp view of a wide open (grade 4) angle in which the depth of the anterior chamber is greater than the thickness of the cornea.** *(C)* **Slit-lamp view of a grade 2 angle in which the depth of the anterior chamber is one-fourth the thickness of the cornea.**

TABLE 16.4
Classification and Implications of Slit-Lamp Assessment of Anterior Angle

Ratio of Anterior Chamber Depth to Corneal Thickness	Grade (van Herick)	Implication
1	4	Angle incapable of closure
0.5	3	Angle incapable of closure
0.25	2	Narrow angle—perform gonioscopy
Less than 0.25	1	Dangerously narrow angle—perform gonioscopy

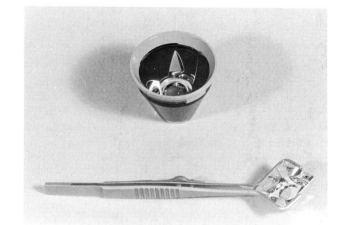

FIGURE 16.4 **Goldmann (top) and Zeiss gonioprisms.**

This method is an extremely rapid (requiring only seconds) and accurate technique for estimating the depth of the anterior chamber angle and tends to correlate well with gonioscopic findings.[6,8] Such slit-lamp grading is based on the findings at the temporal and sometimes nasal limbus and serves as a reliable average of the entire angle.[6]

Using this technique, van Herick and associates[6] found grade 1 narrow angles to have a prevalence of only 0.64% and grade 2 a prevalence of 1%. The prevalence of grades 1 and 2 angles increases with age, but this is an expected finding considering the normal increase of lens thickness with age.[6] The practical implication of the slit-lamp method is that assessments of 0.25 or less indicate a risk of angle closure and merit gonioscopic confirmation before dilation of the pupil.[8]

Gonioscopy

Gonioscopy provides the most definitive method for evaluating the anterior angle. This procedure allows direct or indirect visualization of the anterior angle structures and thus serves to indicate with greater accuracy the risk of angle closure associated with pupillary dilation. The most commonly employed techniques involve use of the Goldmann or Zeiss gonioprisms (Fig. 16.4). Each of these gonioprisms allows an indirect view of the anterior chamber angle by reflection through a mirror.

When viewed gonioscopically, the normal anterior angle is most often narrower superiorly, is widest inferiorly, and has a depth intermediate between these two extremes at the temporal and nasal aspects.[8] It is important, therefore, to evaluate the major anatomic landmarks of the angle (Fig. 16.5) for the entire 360° and to document the observations by employing a recording system such as the one illustrated in Figure

16.6. The classification and implications of the gonioscopic observations are summarized in Table 16.5.

Since the risk of angle closure is inversely proportional to the extent to which the angle structures are visualized during gonioscopy, a conservative estimate is that anterior angles in which the posterior trabeculum is obscured are at increased risk of closure.[8] Cockburn[9] found 6.0% of eyes in which some or all of the superior trabeculum was obscured and 2.0% in which only the anterior half of the trabeculum was visible. Thus, about 6% of eyes have significantly narrowed angles and 2% have critically narrowed angles. The results of other investigators have been in close agreement using criteria that are generally accepted as defining significantly narrowed anterior angles.

In most instances the slit-lamp method of evaluating the anterior chamber depth correlates well with gonioscopy except when the angle is extremely narrow.[8] For example, patients having a slit-lamp assessment of

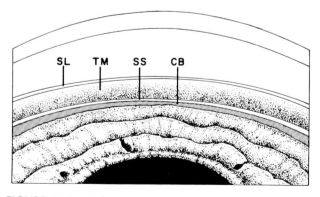

FIGURE 16.5 **Major anatomic landmarks in gonioscopy. Schwalbe's line (SL), trabecular meshwork (TM), scleral spur (SS), and ciliary body (CB).**

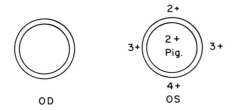

GONIOSCOPY

FIGURE 16.6   **Recording form for gonioscopy. The observations for each of the 4 quadrants of the anterior angle can be quickly and easily recorded by grading each quadrant according to the classification shown in Table 16.5.**

0.3 or less are likely to demonstrate only partial visualization of the trabecular meshwork on gonioscopy.[8] However, it is generally unnecessary to perform gonioscopy on all patients to identify those with significantly narrow angles.[9] The slit-lamp method may be used to select patients in need of gonioscopy—patients having an anterior chamber depth of 0.25 or less should generally undergo gonioscopy. If, during gonioscopy, half or less of the trabeculum is visible in all quadrants, the eye should be considered at risk of angle closure during pupillary dilation.[9] Note, however, that partial angle closure can occur without significant elevation of intraocular pressure or ocular damage.[10] Thus, it is generally the widest quadrant of the anterior chamber angle that is the most critical for evaluation. Furthermore, despite careful gonioscopic analysis of the anterior angle, it is still not possible to predict precisely which eyes will sustain angle closure on pupillary dilation. Methods of dilating pupils of eyes with narrow angles are discussed later in this chapter.

General Considerations and Guidelines

The following general guidelines for the clinical use of mydriatics should enhance the clinical effectiveness of pupillary dilation.

1. Topical anesthesia before instilling the mydriatic enhances pupillary dilation by reducing irritation of the medication and enhancing corneal permeability of the mydriatic.[11,12] By eliminating the stinging sensation produced by the mydriatic, the topical anesthetic diminishes lacrimation and blinking and thus decreases dilution and nasolacrimal drainage of the medication.[11] Benoxinate, proparacaine, and tetracaine produce approximately equal degrees of enhancement of pupillary dilation.[13] If Goldmann applanation tonometry has been performed immediately before dilation, additional topical anesthesia is not required.

2. The goal of dilation should be wide and rapid mydriasis.[1] This is achieved not only by the prior instillation of a topical anesthetic, but also by using a combination of adrenergic and anticholinergic agents. The single instillation of tropicamide or phenylephrine alone may result in some pupillary constriction on intense light stimulation provided by binocular indirect ophthalmoscopy. Furthermore, when tropicamide is used alone for dilation, it may be less effective in the elderly because of decreased sympathetic pupillary tone.[14] Thus, topically administered adrenergic and anticholinergic drugs are frequently used in combination to produce faster and more complete mydriasis. In most cases pupils will obtain maximum mydriasis within 15 to 30 minutes, and virtually all pupils will be maximally dilated within 45 minutes.[15] The combination of phenylephrine and tropicamide is suitable for routine dilation purposes because each drug's duration of action is similar, and tropicamide is less likely to elevate intraocular pressure than are most other anticholinergic drugs.[16]

3. Various combinations of mydriatics have been investigated for their efficacy in pupillary dilation while minimizing side effects.[16-18] The individual agents (usually tropicamide and phenylephrine, or tropicamide and hydroxyamphetamine) can be instilled in any order, and instilling the second drug immediately after the first does not adversely influence the drugs' additive effects.[19] Unfortunately, the commercially avail-

TABLE 16.5
Classification and Implications of Gonioscopic Assessment of Anterior Angle

Visible Angle Anatomy	Grade (Shaffer)	Angular Subtense (°)	Implications
All of ciliary body and trabeculum	4	30–45	Angle incapable of closure
Some ciliary body and all trabeculum	3	20–30	Angle incapable of closure
Most of trabeculum	2	10–20	Narrow angle
Only narrow section of trabeculum	1	10 or less	Dangerously narrow angle
No angle anatomy visible	0	—	Closed angle

able mydriatic combinations, such as 0.2% cyclopentolate combined with 1% phenylephrine (Cyclomydril), or 0.3% scopolamine combined with 10% phenylephrine (Murocoll Phenylephrine), have much too prolonged mydriatic and cycloplegic durations to be conveniently employed for routine pupillary dilation. Use of the cyclopentolate-phenylephrine combination, for example, requires nearly 8 hours for sufficient accommodation to return to allow reading ability.[20]

4. Although mydriatic drug combinations are generally desirable to obtain more rapid and wider dilation, phenylephrine or hydroxyamphetamine may be used alone for dilation when the patient or the practitioner is concerned about the possibility of drug-induced blurred vision. These drugs will spare accommodation but will usually require more than 1 instillation and more time for adequate dilation to occur.[21] Once wide dilation has been achieved, however, pupillary constriction associated with intense light stimulation will usually not occur.[1] The use of these drugs alone for dilation is therefore principally indicated in those patients for whom loss of accommodation might be a significant handicap during the 4 to 6 hours following pupillary dilation.

5. Multiple instillations of mydriatics are rarely required to achieve a wide pupillary dilation. The single instillation of a suitable combination of mydriatic drugs will usually achieve rapid and complete mydriasis while minimizing the risk of side effects associated with drug overdosages.[12,22] Although multiple drops are frequently administered in the belief that this hastens or enhances the mydriatic effect, this is clearly not justified, since a single instillation usually provides clinically effective dilation.

6. A pupillary diameter of 7 mm is usually adequate to permit thorough examination of the fundus, including the peripheral retina.[23] Even smaller pupillary apertures may be adequate in many instances to allow binocular indirect ophthalmoscopy or other stereoscopic examination procedures.

7. The goal of dilation should be a maximally dilated pupil.[1] If pupils are intentionally dilated only minimally, there is a risk of pupillary-block glaucoma that is not present when the pupil is maximally dilated.[24]

8. Unless specifically contraindicated, the pupils of both eyes should be dilated rather than dilating only the pupil of the eye with the suspected lesion.[1] Failure to dilate the pupil of the contralateral eye causes diagnostic errors because lesions considered to be normal variants or benign disease frequently occur bilaterally. Failure to dilate the contralateral eye does not allow comparison with the fellow eye and, thus, may allow errors in diagnostic judgment. In addition, patients can

be disconcerted and annoyed by the Pulfrich phenomenon that is induced by monocular dilation.[1] Patients may experience dizziness, vertigo, or other uncomfortable symptoms, all of which can be prevented or minimized by bilateral pupillary dilation.

9. There may be some variability even in the same patient with regard to the rapidity or degree of dilation obtainable on different occasions.[23]

10. In patients at risk for systemic side effects from topically administered adrenergic mydriatics, manual depression of the puncta (see Fig. 2.5) is a reasonable procedure to minimize nasolacrimal drainage of drug and subsequent absorption into systemic circulation.

11. Although extremely rare, mydriatic-induced angle-closure glaucoma can occur in young patients, and the previous use of mydriatics without adverse effects does not necessarily indicate that angle closure will not develop on subsequent pupillary dilation in patients of any age.[23,25]

Dilation Drug Regimens

Routine Dilation

ADULTS

Rapid and effective mydriasis may be obtained in adult patients by using 1 drop of 0.5% to 1.0% tropicamide.[18] Another effective regimen is 1 drop each of 2.5% phenylephrine and 0.5% to 1.0% tropicamide or 1 drop each of 1% hydroxyamphetamine and 0.5% to 1.0% tropicamide.[1,15,26] These combinations are effective in dilating pupils with senile miosis in which there is decreased sympathetic pupillary tone, where the use of tropicamide alone is less effective.[14]

CHILDREN

Effective dilation in the pediatric age group is accomplished by using no more than 2 drops into each eye of tropicamide 0.5% to 1.0%, cyclopentolate 0.5% to 1.0%, and phenylephrine 2.5%, instilled separately. This combination of agents produces wide mydriasis for fundus examination as well as allowing effective cycloplegia for retinoscopy or subjective refraction.[27]

To minimize ocular irritation and provide mydriasis and cycloplegia with a single-encounter dosage of medication, Caputo and Lingua[28] have recommended a combination mydriatic solution for use in the pediatric age group. The use of such a single-encounter formulation appears to improve the child's trust, comfort, and cooperation during the ophthalmic examination. This combination preparation consists of cyclopentolate 1.3%, tropicamide 0.16%, and phenylephrine

1.6%. By using such minimal effective concentrations of each drug, adverse reactions are avoided.[28] At 1 patient encounter 3 drops of the preparation are instilled, and when the patient is examined 45 to 60 minutes following drug administration, mydriasis is acceptable for binocular indirect ophthalmoscopy. When retinoscopy is compared with atropinization, the resulting cycloplegia approaches the atropine refraction by less than 0.5 D in 80% of eyes.[28]

NEONATES AND INFANTS

Ophthalmoscopic examination of premature infants requires wide pupillary dilation and binocular indirect ophthalmoscopy. Since premature infants treated with oxygen concentrations exceeding room air are at increased risk of developing retinopathy of prematurity, binocular indirect ophthalmoscopy is required to detect early signs of this disease, and safe and effective dilation is necessary.[109] Other neonates or infants may require dilation for evaluation of congenital cataracts or to search for ocular signs of toxoplasmosis, cytomegalovirus, or herpes. Thus, it is important to use mydriatics that are effective and safe in allowing examination of the ocular media, posterior pole, and peripheral retina.

Because of the premature infant's small body mass and less mature cardiovascular and cerebrovascular status, it is prudent to use the lowest concentration yet the most effective combination of mydriatics for pupillary dilation. This will minimize the risk of systemic side effects, which are especially common with topical phenylephrine. Ten percent aqueous or viscous phenylephrine causes innocuous blanching of the skin around the eyes of newborns but, more important, frequently elevates both systolic and diastolic blood pressure.[29] Rosales and associates[30] showed that 80% of low-birth-weight infants who were administered even 2.5% phenylephrine in combination with 0.5% tropicamide had greater than 20% elevation in systolic blood pressure, and 30% of the patients had an elevation of 50% or more. Low-weight infants dilated with cycloplegics alone do not demonstrate a significant elevation in blood pressure.[31] Thus, cycloplegic agents alone—tropicamide alone, cyclopentolate alone, or a combination of tropicamide and cyclopentolate—can be safely used for pupillary dilation in low-birth-weight infants. However, because of possible gastric secretory inhibition and the risk of necrotizing enterocolitis in preterm infants, the concentration of the cyclopentolate should be limited to 0.25%.[32,33] A commercially available combination of phenylephrine 1% and cyclopentolate 0.2%(Cyclomydril) has been found to be even more effective and has minimal risk of cardiovascular or gastrointestinal effects.[31,32]

To facilitate the application of mydriatics in neonates and infants, a single-instillation solution may be prepared by combining 3.75 ml of cyclopentolate 2% with 7.5 ml of tropicamide 1% and 3.75 ml of phenylephrine 10%. The final solution contains cyclopentolate 0.5%, tropicamide 0.5%, and phenylephrine 2.5%.[34] No major side effects have been reported from use of this combination solution, and effective pupillary dilation is obtained.[29,34] In infants with blue irides, 1 drop in each eye is usually adequate, while in other patients a second instillation within 5 to 10 seconds of the first usually provides consistently adequate mydriasis.[34] The solution can also be applied as a spray (see Chapter 2).

Following dilation of the premature infant's eyes, the absolute pupillary diameter may remain somewhat small.[35] The mydriasis, however, is comparable to that of the adult when expressed as a percentage of corneal diameter; that is, the absolute pupillary size of the premature neonate following dilation may remain small simply because of the small size of the infant eye.[35]

During insertion of the lid speculum, binocular indirect ophthalmoscopy, and scleral depression procedures, care should be taken to recognize any stimulation of the oculocardiac reflex and, if necessary, to immediately institute measures for infant resuscitation.[36]

Systemic Disease

Because of the risk of adverse pressor effects from topical phenylephrine, especially the 10% concentration, this drug should generally be avoided for pupillary dilation in patients with cardiac disease, systemic hypertension, aneurysms, and advanced arteriosclerosis.[37] However, mild hypertension not controlled with guanethidine or reserpine is not necessarily a contraindication to the use of phenylephrine.[38] The use of tropicamide alone for dilation of patients with such cardiovascular disease probably represents the safest drug regimen, since tropicamide is virtually free of pressor effect and thus produces little risk of acute hypertensive crisis.[38,39]

Idiopathic orthostatic hypotension is a condition that leads to denervation hypersensitivity.[40] The topical instillation of even 2.5% phenylephrine in patients with this condition often elevates blood pressure dramatically.[40] Thus, because of the increased pressor response to phenylephrine in patients with idiopathic orthostatic hypotension, the practitioner should avoid phenylephrine for dilation in patients with this condition. Instead, hydroxyamphetamine, an indirect-acting adrenergic agent, may provide the desired mydriasis while minimizing the risk for adverse cardiovascular effects.[41]

The addition of tropicamide will improve the mydriasis.

Because of increased sensitivity to circulating catecholamines in patients with hyperthyroidism, patients with this disease may be at increased risk of adverse pressor effects from phenylephrine or hydroxyamphetamine. Thus, these drugs should be avoided or used conservatively in patients with hyperthyroidism.

Sympathetic denervation is common in patients with insulin-dependent diabetes. This sympathetic denervation is caused by autonomic neuropathy, affects the iris and cardiovascular system, and increases the risk of systemic side effects from adrenergic agonists.[42] Smith and Smith[43] have reported that the pupils of patients with diabetes demonstrate hypersensitivity to phenylephrine but show normal reactions to hydroxyamphetamine. This is consistent with a partial postganglionic denervation of the iris dilator muscle.[44] There is a clinical impression,[45] however, that pupillary dilation of patients with diabetes is difficult, presumably because of impairment of the sympathetic innervation to the dilator muscle. This sympathetic autonomic neuropathy may be especially common in female diabetics.[45] An effective mydriatic regimen is tropicamide 0.5% to 1.0% in combination with phenylephrine 2.5%.[43,46] In the insulin-dependent diabetic patient, this regimen usually achieves satisfactory dilation with a minimum of systemic side effects.

Concomitant Drug Therapy

Drug interactions can play an important role in causing systemic side effects following pupillary dilation. Since the tricyclic antidepressants (Table 16.6) and monoamine oxidase (MAO) inhibitors increase the pressor effects of phenylephrine, phenylephrine should be avoided in patients taking these medications.[37] Phenylephrine should be avoided even up to 21 days following termination of MAO inhibitor therapy.[37] Furthermore, the use of topical phenylephrine in atropinized patients can enhance the pressor effects and produce tachycardia.[37] Hydroxyamphetamine should also be avoided in these patients. The use of tropicamide alone will allow effective mydriasis while minimizing the risk of systemic side effects.

Partial sympathetic denervation with resultant hypersensitivity may occur in patients who are taking reserpine, guanethidine, methyldopa, or other α-adrenergic blocking agents.[41,42] Such pharmacologic sympathectomy following the depletion of norepinephrine gives rise to reduced sensitivity to indirect-acting adrenergic agents but also results in increased sensitivity to catecholamines.[41] The resulting denervation hypersensitivity may cause prolonged mydriasis in patients dilated with phenylephrine.[42] More important, however, the risk of adverse pressor effects from phenylephrine is increased. On the other hand, hydroxyamphetamine, an indirect-acting adrenergic, appears to be a safer drug for pupillary dilation in these patients because of a reduced risk of adverse cardiovascular effects in patients with pharmacologic sympathectomy.[41] Depending on the magnitude of the local sympathectomy of the iris dilator muscle, hydroxyamphetamine may have somewhat reduced effectiveness when used alone for dilation in patients taking such drugs. However, adding tropicamide will usually ensure satisfactory mydriasis.

Open-Angle Glaucoma

The management of open-angle glaucoma requires periodic dilation of the pupil for fundus, optic nerve, and visual field examination. This is essential for the following reasons[1]:

- Patients receiving long-term miotic therapy can develop sphincter rigidity and atrophy. Periodic dilation will "rejuvenate" the iris sphincter by allowing it to relax.
- Strong miotics such as the anticholinesterase agents can cause peripheral retinal tears with subsequent rhegmatogenous retinal detachment. Periodic dilation for peripheral retinal examination is thus indicated to identify such patients.[47]
- Stereoscopic examination of the optic nerve head is essential for the proper long-term management of open-angle glaucoma. Critical judgments are often necessary in establishing the initial diagnosis of glaucomatous disc damage, and subtle changes of the nerve head can be easily overlooked with monocular viewing.
- Accurate evaluation of glaucomatous visual fields requires a 3 to 4 mm pupillary aperture so that cataractous changes or miosis do not cause artifactual field loss. Since many glaucoma patients also have progressive lenticular changes, this and other variables may be somewhat better controlled by period-

TABLE 16.6
Commonly Prescribed Tricyclic Antidepressants

Generic Name	Trade Name
Imipramine HCl	Tofranil (Geigy)
Amitriptyline HCl	Elavil, Triavil (Merck)
Doxepin HCl	Sinequan (Roerig)

ically evaluating the visual field with approximately the same pupillary size.

When the pupils of eyes with open-angle glaucoma are dilated with cycloplegics, intraocular pressure can rise significantly.[48–51] This effect is transient and occurs in treated as well as untreated open-angle glaucoma, but is only rarely observed in healthy patients.[48] The incidence of such cycloplegic responsiveness is about 25% in open-angle glaucoma, 33% in miotic-treated open-angle glaucoma, but only 2% in the general population.[48,49] All strong cycloplegics will elevate intraocular pressure, but those with only a minimal effect on accommodation will not produce this response.[49] Tropicamide may elevate intraocular pressure in patients with open-angle glaucoma who are being treated with miotics, but this drug has relatively little effect on intraocular pressure in healthy eyes or in those with untreated open-angle glaucoma.[52] This difference may be caused by competitive inhibition of the miotic at the receptor site in patients treated with miotics.[52] Cyclopentolate, however, causes a 3 to 22 mm Hg elevation of intraocular pressure in most eyes with open-angle glaucoma.[50] As with tropicamide, miotic treatment significantly enhances the incidence of pressure elevation with cyclopentolate but does not, however, significantly influence the magnitude of the response.[48]

Cycloplegic-induced pressure elevations appear to be caused by a decrease of facility of aqueous outflow, but there is no association between the magnitude of pupillary dilation and the intraocular pressure elevation, nor is there any association between pressure elevation and the initial intraocular pressure.[48] Cycloplegic-induced pressure elevations do not appear to be necessarily reproducible in a particular eye or a particular patient.[48] Eyes that are generally responsive may occasionally fail to develop significant elevations of pressure on subsequent dilation. Less commonly, consistently unresponsive eyes may develop significant elevations of pressure. Thus, the use of cycloplegics for dilation of eyes with open-angle glaucoma generally requires some caution.[50,51]

Unlike cycloplegic agents, adrenergic mydriatics have essentially no effect on intraocular pressure in patients with open-angle glaucoma.[49,50,53] Since dilation of the pupil with phenylephrine usually does not elevate the pressure and does not consistently reduce the facility of aqueous outflow, it may be used safely for dilation in patients with open-angle glaucoma.[50] Phenylephrine can also be used to dilate the pupils of patients with primary open-angle glaucoma who are being treated with miotics, even strong miotics such as the anticholinesterase agents.[53] In such cases phenylephrine will partially overcome the miosis but may require up to 60 minutes or longer to obtain a pupillary size adequate for optic disc or fundus examination. Thus, it is possible to dilate the pupils of miotic-treated eyes without altering the intraocular pressure if phenylephrine is used as the mydriatic.

Dilation of eyes with exfoliation or pigmentary glaucoma may liberate pigment into the anterior chamber, which can greatly elevate intraocular pressure.[54,55] Profuse pigment liberation during dilation of such eyes may cause transient blocking of the trabecular meshwork, with obstruction of aqueous outflow and subsequent elevation of intraocular pressure.[55] This elevation of pressure is transient,[54] but it is also possible for pigment to be liberated during pupillary dilation without a concurrent elevation of pressure.[55] Dilation with cycloplegic rather than adrenergic mydriatics is less likely to liberate pigment, but on the other hand it has a greater tendency to raise intraocular pressure because of mechanisms independent of pigment liberation. Thus, no particular mydriatic agent exhibits clear advantages over another for dilation of eyes with exfoliation or pigmentary glaucoma. Note, however, that the pupils of eyes with exfoliation syndrome generally dilate more poorly than do healthy eyes.[56,57] This may be due to bonding of the posterior surface of the iris to the preequatorial lens capsule and anterior zonules by exfoliation material,[58] or to iris infiltration and fibrosis.[59]

In summary, dilation of most eyes with open-angle glaucoma should be accomplished using phenylephrine or hydroxyamphetamine alone[60] or in combination with tropicamide. The combination of phenylephrine and tropicamide generally permits wide mydriasis while minimizing potential elevation of intraocular pressure.[61]

Narrow Angle with Intact Iris

Mydriatic-induced angle-closure glaucoma most commonly occurs in the elderly. It can, however, occur in young patients, and the previous use of mydriatics without adverse sequelae does not necessarily indicate that angle closure will not develop on subsequent dilation.[23,25] Thus, the practitioner should approach the dilation of eyes with narrow anterior angles with the knowledge that there is some risk for angle closure. Unfortunately, gonioscopy is of no value in predicting which narrow angles will close on dilation because it allows only a subjective assessment of the magnitude of the narrow angle.[24] An understanding of the mechanics of pupillary dilation lends support to the various philosophies governing the dilation of eyes with narrow angles.

MECHANICS OF PUPILLARY DILATION AND ANGLE
CLOSURE

Eyes with deep anterior chambers are essentially free
of the risk of pupillary block and iris bombé. However,
in eyes predisposed to angle-closure glaucoma, the lens
is generally displaced anteriorly, which increases the
pressure of the iris against the lens. This situation
favors pupillary block and iris bombé with subsequent
secondary angle closure.[62] When the iris rests on an
anteriorly positioned lens, the forces of pupillary dilation (iris dilator muscle activity) can be resolved into
2 components—a posterior and a lateral. Likewise, the
force of pupillary constriction (iris sphincter muscle
activity) can be resolved into 2 components—a medial
and an anterior[63] (Fig. 16.7A). The total sphincter
pupillary blocking force varies according to size and
position of the pupil.[24] A miotic pupil is generally
associated with a taut iris and small pupillary blocking
force, a mid-dilated pupil is associated with a lax iris
and large pupillary blocking force, and wide dilation
is associated with a compressed iris and small pupillary
blocking force. Thus, the position of greatest risk with
respect to potential angle closure is mid-dilation.[24] With
a mid-dilated pupil, regardless of how it is obtained
pharmacologically, the pupillary blocking force is maximum, and, if the eye is predisposed to angle closure,
some eyes will undergo acute angle closure because of
the increase in pressure in the posterior chamber caused
by pupillary block. The increased pressure produces
iris bombé, which subsequently leads to secondary angle closure[64] (Fig. 16.8).

DILATION PHILOSOPHIES

Routine Dilation.   A valid approach to the dilation
of eyes with extremely narrow angles is to use routine
drug regimens such as the combination of tropicamide
and phenylephrine. If drug-induced angle closure occurs and is promptly recognized and treated, the patient ultimately benefits from the experience, since the
angle-closure attack would occur under controlled conditions in which proper treatment facilities are usually
conveniently available.[65] Thus, the use of routine drug
regimens constitutes essentially a "provocative test."
However, before proceeding with such an approach, it
is best to obtain the patient's informed consent (see
Chapter 33), to dilate only 1 eye at the initial visit,
and to postpone dilation of the fellow eye until the
response of the initial dilation has been ascertained. It
is also prudent to perform the dilation earlier in the
day, when appropriate emergency care is more readily
available. Ideally, the patient should be retained in the
office until the pupil has spontaneously returned to
normal. Before dismissing the patient, intraocular pressure should be determined, and the patient should be
informed of the symptoms of acute angle-closure glaucoma and have specific instructions for emergency
treatment should this become necessary.[39,61]

Anticholinergic Agents Only.   Although dilation of
the pupil with anticholinergic drugs such as tropicamide
can cause angle closure,[64] the risk is generally considered to be much less than from dilation using adrenergic agents. As previously noted, however, reduced

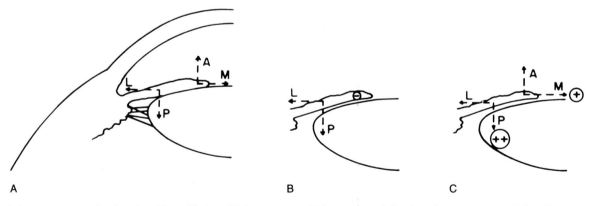

FIGURE 16.7   **Mechanics of pupillary dilation. *(A)* Components of iris muscle activity. Anterior component of iris sphincter
activity (A), medial component of iris sphincter activity (M), lateral component of iris dilator activity (L), and posterior
component of iris dilator activity (P). *(B)* Pupillary dilation with anticholinergic mydriatic. The iris sphincter is inactivated,
and the posterior component of the iris dilator acts peripherally. *(C)* Pupillary dilation with adrenergic mydriatic. The iris
dilator is stimulated and its posterior component is augmented while the medial component of the iris sphincter persists.**

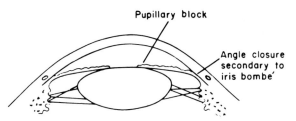

FIGURE 16.8 Pupillary block causes increased pressure in the posterior chamber relative to anterior chamber. This produces iris bombé, which obstructs aqueous outflow and causes secondary angle closure.

aqueous outflow facility may elevate intraocular pressure, but this is unrelated to the angle-closure mechanism.[66]

In eyes with intact irides and shallow anterior chambers, dilation with anticholinergic agents infrequently leads to angle closure because these drugs inhibit the force of iris sphincter contraction, while the force of dilator contraction and the force associated with iris tissue stretching retain their normal values.[62] Consequently, the posterior component of the pupillary dilation force will be located toward the periphery of the iris, where contact between the lens and iris is less than it is near the pupil. The weakened sphincter will have a reduced medial component, resulting in less contact between the iris and lens at the pupillary margin. This allows the aqueous to pass from the posterior to the anterior chambers without obstruction[63] (Fig. 16.7B).

Of the available anticholinergic agents, tropicamide is preferred for routine dilation of eyes with shallow anterior chambers, narrow angles, and intact irides.[63] Homatropine and cyclopentolate are not as rapidly acting as tropicamide and therefore appear to be less safe with regard to precipitating angle closure.[63] However, the disadvantage of using anticholinergic agents is the difficulty in overcoming the dilation with miotics if angle closure occurs.[67] In general, pilocarpine produces little or no miosis following dilation with anticholinergic drugs, and the pupil may remain dilated or partially dilated for a prolonged time.[102]

Angle-closure glaucoma following dilation with tropicamide generally occurs within the first hour following instillation of the medication.[24] If the intraocular pressure has not risen significantly within 1 hour, the probability of angle closure is extremely low, and it is permissible to dismiss the patient without observation. The use of miotics following dilation is discouraged, since it is both unnecessary and may cause angle closure.[24] If angle closure occurs, the intraocular pressure is usually readily brought to normal levels because angle closure following dilation with tropicamide is only rarely complete.[24]

Adrenergic Agents Only. Although Shaffer[61] has recommended the use of phenylephrine for routine dilation of eyes with extremely narrow angles, Mapstone[62] and Lowe[63,68] have advised against the use of such adrenergic agents based on the model of pupillary dilation shown in Figure 16.7. Adrenergic drugs augment the force of dilator contraction while leaving the force of sphincter contraction unaffected. The posterior component of the pupillary dilation force is thus increased at the iris periphery while the medial component of the iris sphincter contraction persists[62,63] (Fig. 16.7C). Consequently, the total force available for causing pupillary block is greater than when an anticholinergic agent is used for dilation, and the contact between iris and lens at the pupillary margin is increased, resulting in pupillary block with subsequent obstruction of aqueous flow from posterior to anterior chamber. This produces iris bombé with secondary angle closure.[63]

Although the risk of pupillary block is greater with the use of phenylephrine compared with tropicamide, dilation with the former is much more easily overcome with the use of miotics such as pilocarpine.[67] The mydriatic effect of most adrenergic agents is rapidly counteracted by pilocarpine in less than 30 minutes.[67] However, pilocarpine-induced miosis following dilation with phenylephrine should generally be avoided because this will lead to angle closure in a significant proportion of eyes by the increased stimulation of the iris sphincter, which enhances the medial component and increases the contact between iris and lens.[24,63]

In contrast to the effects of pilocarpine, the use of adrenergic blocking agents following dilation with phenylephrine leaves the force of sphincter contraction unaffected but decreases the component of dilator contraction toward the lens. By inhibiting the dilator muscle and decreasing the component of the dilator contraction toward the lens, the total pupillary blocking forces are reduced, and iris bombé and secondary angle closure are less probable.[62] Thymoxamine (Opilon), an α-adrenergic blocking agent, can be used to counteract pupillary dilation following phenylephrine administration.[66] The primary advantage of the use of thymoxamine following dilation with phenylephrine is that it rapidly constricts the pupil, usually within 30 minutes, and thus prevents the pupil from remaining in the mid-dilated position.[24,69]

Sector Dilation. As an alternative to full dilation of the pupil, a procedure may be used whereby primarily the inferior aspect of the pupil is dilated. Such sector dilation was first described by Shaffer[61] in 1967. A small, pear-shaped pupillary dilation can be obtained by placing in the inferior conjunctival sac a cotton pledget moistened with 1:1000 epinephrine or 2.5% phenylephrine. The pledget should remain for only 2 to 3 minutes lest too much drug delivery causes complete dilation of the pupil.[61,70] As the drug penetrates into the inferior aspect of the anterior chamber, it dilates the inferior pupillary zone and leaves the remainder of the pupil essentially intact. A vertically oval pupil is produced (Fig. 16.9). Alternatively, 1% epinephrine or 2.5% phenylephrine can be employed by moistening the tip of a thin strip of filter paper (Schirmer strip) and placing it in the inferior conjunctival sac.[70,71] It should be allowed to remain for only 1 minute, since longer contact may dilate the entire pupil. Tropicamide cannot be used for sector dilation because it tends to produce full pupillary dilation even when used in low concentrations.[72]

Before sector dilation, the eye should be anesthetized topically to reduce subsequent lacrimation, which might dilute and spread the mydriatic agent.[71] The sectorially enlarged pupillary aperture obtained from sector dilation usually allows easy access to the posterior segment of the eye by enabling satisfactory binocular indirect ophthalmoscopy or other procedures requiring stereopsis.

Although this technique may not necessarily prevent angle closure, it does seem to reduce the risk of angle closure because of the minimal and brief focal dilation.[1,71]

Narrow Angle Following Surgical Iridectomy or Laser Iridotomy

Lowe[68] has reported that if the pupils of eyes that have undergone peripheral iridectomy for acute angle-clo-

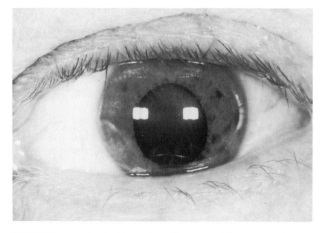

FIGURE 16.9   **Vertically oval pupil produced by sector dilation.**

sure glaucoma are dilated with anticholinergic agents such as cyclopentolate or tropicamide, 50% to 66% of eyes will develop angle closure. Despite the presence of a patent peripheral iridectomy, the anticholinergic agent induces angle closure by causing peripheral crowding of the iris against the trabeculum.[63] In such cases, the degree of angle closure is generally related to the magnitude of pupillary dilation. In contrast, dilation with phenylephrine or other adrenergic agent does not cause peripheral folding of the iris and thus fails to produce angle closure.[63,68,73] In addition, phenylephrine has a relatively brief duration of action and permits rapid pupillary constriction without the need for a miotic.[63] The practitioner should ascertain, however, that the peripheral iridectomy or iridotomy is of full iris thickness because phenylephrine may induce angle closure if only the anterior portion of the iris has been removed or destroyed.[63]

Harris and Galin[74] have challenged the foregoing hypothesis regarding angle closure following dilation of eyes having undergone peripheral iridectomy. Using cyclopentolate, these investigators dilated a number of eyes following iridectomy for angle-closure glaucoma and found no drug-induced episode of angle closure. Since peripheral iridectomy or iridotomy removes the risk of pupillary block, precipitation of angle closure must be primary rather than secondary to pupillary block and iris bombé.[63,74] Eyes with plateau iris undergo angle closure by a mechanism involving crowding of the iris against the trabeculum rather than by a mechanism involving pupillary block.[74] Thus, it has been suggested that mydriatic-induced angle closure despite a patent iridectomy may be associated with the plateau iris syndrome.[75] Wand and associates[75] have reported such cases to be extremely rare. Since the magnitude of pupillary dilation is the crucial factor, one would expect an equal incidence of angle closure with adrenergic and anticholinergic drugs if mydriasis of comparable magnitude is produced.[74] However, until further definitive studies are performed, it is probably wise to use adrenergic rather than anticholinergic agents for routine dilation of eyes having undergone surgical iridectomy or laser iridotomy for acute angle-closure glaucoma.[75]

Ectopia Lentis

Ectopia lentis is commonly found as part of the syndrome of homocystinuria and Marfan's syndrome. Dilation of the pupil is often essential in establishing the initial diagnosis as well as for adequate fundus examination. Because of the risk of precipitating pupillary-block glaucoma, such patients should be dilated in a supine position with the use of a weak mydriatic such as 1% hydroxyamphetamine or 2.5% phenylephrine.[76] Wide pupillary dilation should generally be avoided because there is a risk of subluxation of the lens into the anterior chamber. Following examination of the crystalline lens and fundus, the position of the lens should be inspected to confirm its position behind the iris plane. Gentle tactile pressure may be applied to the lens through the cornea if the lens appears to be in the anterior chamber.[76] Once the lens is placed behind the iris, and with the patient still in a supine position, the mydriasis can be reversed by using a miotic such as 1% pilocarpine.

Effect of Iris Pigmentation

There is a common clinical impression that eyes with greater pigmentation (i.e., darker irides) dilate more poorly than do eyes with less pigmentation (i.e., blue irides). Several investigators[77–79] have demonstrated a greater magnitude of mydriasis in eyes with light irides compared with dark irides. Other investigators,[11,22,80–82] however, have failed to find such differences, reporting equal mydriasis in light and dark irides. Richardson[80] has shown that the pupils in light irides are significantly

larger than in dark irides before pupillary dilation, which may explain the somewhat larger pupillary diameters following dilation of light irides.

Recommended drug regimens for dilation of the pupil in various clinical situations are summarized in Table 16.7.

Clinical Procedures Facilitated by the Use of Mydriatics

Examination of Ocular Media

Dilation of the pupil allows more complete evaluation of the ocular media posterior to the iris plane by permitting detailed biomicroscopy of the crystalline lens and vitreous. The pupil must be dilated to examine the lens for cataract formation, since cortical spoking (Fig. 16.10), off-axis posterior subcapsular opacities (Fig. 16.11), and other opacities of the lens can be entirely overlooked without an adequately dilated pupil.[108] Exfoliation of the lens capsule (see Fig. 29.35) may also be overlooked with the pupil undilated. Posterior vitreous detachment (PVD) (Fig. 16.12) is the

TABLE 16.7
Recommended Drug Regimens for Dilation of the Pupil

Clinical Situation	Drug Regimen
Routine	
Adults	Tropicamide 0.5%–1.0% and phenylephrine 2.5% (hydroxyamphetamine 1%)
Children	Tropicamide 0.5%–1.0%, cyclopentolate 0.5%–1.0%, and phenylephrine 2.5%, instilled separately or as a combination drop or spray
Neonates and infants	Tropicamide 0.5%, phenylephrine 2.5%, and cyclopentolate 0.5%, instilled separately or as a combination drop or spray
Low-birth-weight infants	Phenylephrine 1%–cyclopentolate 0.2% (Cyclomydril)
Systemic disease	
Cardiac disease, systemic hypertension, aneurysms, advanced arteriosclerosis	Tropicamide 0.5%–1.0%
Idiopathic orthostatic hypotension	Tropicamide 0.5%–1.0% and hydroxyamphetamine 1%
Hyperthyroidism	Tropicamide 0.5%–1.0%
Insulin-dependent diabetes	Tropicamide 0.5%–1.0% and phenylephrine 2.5%
Concomitant drug therapy	
Tricyclic antidepressants	Tropicamide 0.5%–1.0%
Atropine	Tropicamide 0.5%–1.0%
β-adrenergic blockers	Tropicamide 0.5%–1.0%
α-adrenergic blockers	Tropicamide 0.5%–1.0% and hydroxyamphetamine 1%
Open-angle glaucoma	Tropicamide 0.5%–1.0% and phenylephrine 2.5% (hydroxyamphetamine 1%)
Narrow angle with intact iris	Tropicamide 0.5%–1.0% and phenylephrine 2.5% (hydroxyamphetamine 1%) as a "provocative test"; tropicamide 0.5%; or sector dilation using phenylephrine 2.5% or hydroxyamphetamine 1%
Narrow angle following peripheral iridectomy	Phenylephrine 2.5% or hydroxyamphetamine 1%
Ectopia lentis	Tropicamide 0.5%, phenylephrine 2.5%, or hydroxyamphetamine 1%

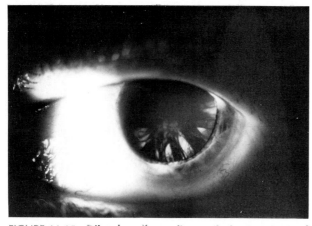

FIGURE 16.10   **Dilated pupil revealing cortical cataract. Visual acuity was 20/20 (6/6).**

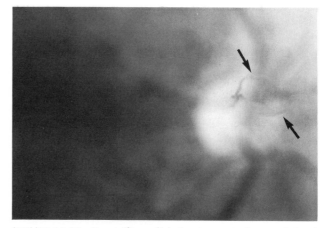

FIGURE 16.12   **Prepapillary glial ring (arrows) characteristic of posterior vitreous detachment.**

most common cause of symptoms of flashes or floaters in patients over 50 years of age, and pupillary dilation is essential for the diagnosis by allowing adequate stereoscopic examination of the vitreous using binocular indirect ophthalmoscopy or fundus biomicroscopy. Furthermore, the dilation of eyes with extremely dense cataract usually permits a satisfactory fundus evaluation, which might otherwise be impossible because of the small pupillary aperture in association with dense nuclear sclerosis or posterior subcapsular opacities.

Once the pupil is dilated, the lens and anterior vitreous can be examined directly with the slit lamp, and use of the Hruby lens, fundus contact lens, or high-power (60 D or 90 D) condensing lens will extend the range of the slit lamp into the mid and posterior vitreous.[83–88] The Hruby lens is attached to the slit lamp

(Fig. 16.13) and does not contact the eye, while the fundus contact lens is placed directly onto the cornea following topical anesthesia (Fig. 16.14). The central contact lens of any gonioscope can also be used as a fundus contact lens. The high-power (60 D or 90 D) condensing lens is positioned near the cornea but without ocular contact (Fig. 16.15). Of the 3 biomicroscopic procedures, the Hruby lens and high-power condensing lens allow more rapid examination of the patient, since they do not require topical anesthesia, the use of gonioscopic bonding solution, or manipulation of the eye for contact lens insertion. The high-power condensing lens, moreover, provides superior stereopsis and permits a larger field of view. All three procedures, however, allow stereopsis and variable magnification according to the capabilities of the slit lamp (Table

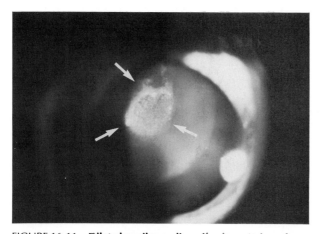

FIGURE 16.11   **Dilated pupil revealing off-axis posterior subcapsular cataract (arrows). Visual acuity was 20/20 (6/6).**

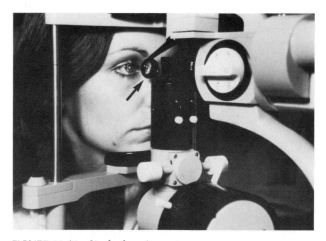

FIGURE 16.13   **Hruby lens (arrow).**

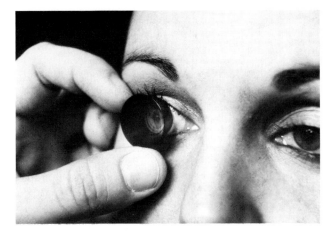

FIGURE 16.14   **Fundus contact lens in situ.**

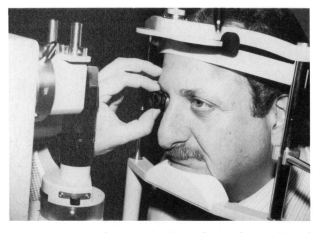

FIGURE 16.15   **High-power (90 D) condensing lens positioned near the cornea.**

16.8). This is particularly advantageous when examining the crystalline lens and vitreous cavity.

With the pupil dilated, the ocular media can also be evaluated by observing the red reflex with the retinoscope, direct ophthalmoscope, or slit lamp. Subtle opacities of the cornea, lens, or vitreous can often be detected more readily than with the pupil undilated. Observation of the red reflex with the direct ophthalmoscope allows rapid and effective comparison of each eye with respect to the density of cataractous changes. Use of the binocular indirect ophthalmoscope, because of its large depth of focus, usually permits rapid detection of subtle vitreal changes, including PVD.

Fundus Examination

Almost without exception, definitive evaluation and diagnosis of diseases of the retina and choroid require dilation of the pupil. Once the pupil is dilated, stereoscopic observation of fundus lesions is permitted,

and various procedures may be used to fully evaluate such lesions. Slit-lamp techniques using the Hruby, fundus contact, or high-power condensing lens are helpful in evaluating lesions of the posterior pole including the macula and optic disc.[83–88] The 3-mirror Goldmann lens or high-power condensing lens may be used to evaluate, using variable magnification and stereopsis, the equatorial and peripheral retina as far anteriorly as the ora serrata and ciliary body processes.[86,89] Unlike the direct or monocular indirect ophthalmoscopes, the binocular indirect ophthalmoscope (Fig. 16.16) allows a broad, panoramic view of the fundus while maintaining stereopsis (Table 16.9). These features enable rapid detection and evaluation of subtle changes in tissue texture, color, depth, or elevation. This significantly improves the evaluation and diagnosis of lesions such as retinal detachment, peripheral retinal disease predisposing to retinal detachment, and extensive disease processes such as presumed ocular histoplasmosis and central retinal vein occlusion. Binocular indirect ophthalmoscopy or fundus biomicros-

TABLE 16.8
Comparison of Fundus Biomicroscopy Techniques

	Hruby Lens	*Fundus Contact Lens*	*90 D Lens*
Field of view	Small	Larger	Largest
Image	Virtual erect	Virtual erect	Real inverted and reversed
Surface reflections	Many	Variable	Variable
Patient tolerance	Good	Variable	Good
Stereopsis	Good	Excellent	Excellent
Photography	Poor	Very good	Excellent

Modified from Gutner R, Cavallerano A, Wong D. Fundus biomicroscopy: A comparison of four methods. J Am Optom Assoc 1988;59:388–390.

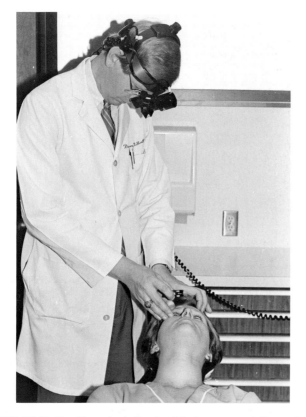

FIGURE 16.16   **Binocular indirect ophthalmoscopy entails use of a hand-held condensing lens and headborne ophthalmoscope. A +20 D condensing lens is generally adequate, but a +28 or +30 D lens may be more satisfactory in patients with only minimal pupillary dilation.**

copy also allows differentiation between significant retinal disease and benign processes such as congenital hypertrophy of the retinal pigment epithelium and retinal pigment epithelial window defects. In some instances serious retinal or choroidal disease has been

overlooked or mismanaged because the pupil was not dilated for fundus examination (Fig. 16.17).[90]

Ophthalmodynamometry (ODM) can be performed with the pupil dilated. This permits the binocular indirect ophthalmoscope to be used and thus facilitates the examination by allowing an assistant to manipulate the plunger while the practitioner directs his or her attention to the central retinal artery (Fig. 16.18). This method of performing ODM is sometimes used in preference to the single-examiner technique because, in the latter method, manipulation of the plunger and simultaneous observation of the central retinal artery with the direct ophthalmoscope can be difficult to coordinate.

Fundus photography, including fluorescein angiography, must generally be performed with the pupil dilated to obtain satisfactory results. Although nonmydriatic cameras are available, these devices do not consider the necessity for pupillary dilation to formulate a definitive diagnosis. Most fundus cameras are essentially monocular indirect ophthalmoscopes that have been adapted for photographic purposes, and dilation of the pupil will therefore increase their effectiveness and use.[89,91]

Dilation before electroretinography (ERG) serves to standardize the results obtained from this electrophysiologic test. Most research and clinical electrophysiologic laboratories therefore incorporate pupillary dilation into the examination protocol.

Examination of Optic Disc

Stereoscopic observation of the optic disc is essential when evaluating abnormalities of the optic nerve head. Following dilation, binocular indirect ophthalmoscopy using the +20 D condensing lens or, for greater magnification the +14 D lens, permits satisfactory evaluation in many instances, but the Hruby, fundus contact,

TABLE 16.9

Comparison of Direct, Monocular Indirect, and Binocular Indirect Ophthalmoscopes

	Direct	Monocular Indirect	Binocular Indirect
Field of view	10° (1½ DD[a])	40° (8 DD[a])	40° (8 DD[a])
Image quality of peripheral fundus	Distorted	Good	Excellent
Stereopsis	Absent	Absent	Present
Image	Erect	Erect	Inverted and reversed
Mydriatic required	No, but helpful	No, but helpful	Yes

[a]DD, Disc diameter.

Modified from Garston MJ. The binocular indirect ophthalmoscope (BIO). J Am Optom Assoc 1977;48:1403–1407.

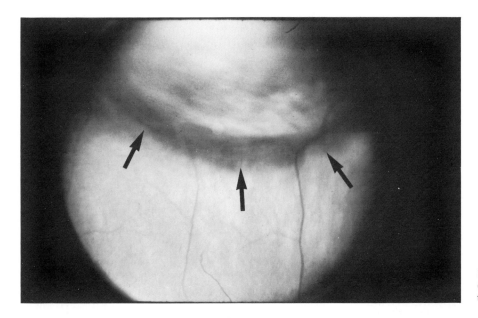

FIGURE 16.17 **Malignant melanoma (arrows) that was overlooked because the pupil was not dilated.**

or high-power condensing lens can be used to enable higher magnification while maintaining stereopsis.[83–88] These procedures allow detailed evaluation of peculiar optic nerve head configurations such as coloboma or tilted disc syndrome. The capability of stereopsis with high magnification is especially important when evaluating subtle abnormalities such as optic disc edema, drusen, optic pits, and various glaucomatous nerve head changes.

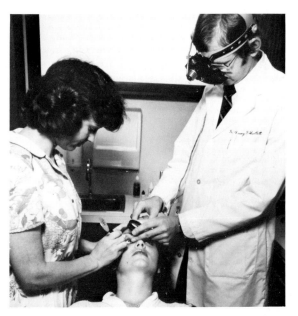

FIGURE 16.18 **Ophthalmodynamometry performed with the binocular indirect ophthalmoscope. An assistant manipulates the plunger while the practitioner scrutinizes the central retinal artery.**

Dilation of Pseudophakic Eyes

When the implantation of intraocular lenses (IOL) became popular during the 1970s, it became clear that eyes with iris-supported lenses (Table 16.10) should not be dilated because of the risk of lens dislocation (Fig. 16.19).[92,93]

Wide dilation is possible with all anterior and posterior chamber lenses (Fig. 16.20).[92,94] However, there may be a slight risk of the IOL becoming entrapped within the pupillary aperture such that the pupil is prevented from returning to its normal size following dilation (Fig. 16.21).[95] If this so-called pupillary capture occurs with an anterior chamber lens, the patient should be placed in a supine position and the pupil should be dilated with phenylephrine or hydroxyamphetamine and then constricted with pilocarpine. The force of gravity should maintain the iris behind the lens. Alternatively, a gonioscope or tonometer prism can be forcibly applied to the cornea after the pupil has been dilated. This maneuver may displace the iris posteriorly, behind the plane of the anterior chamber lens.[96] For an entrapped posterior chamber lens the pupil should be dilated and the patient placed in a prone position, with face downward. Although the force of gravity may

TABLE 16.10
Classification of Intraocular Lenses

- Anterior chamber
- Iris supported
- Posterior chamber

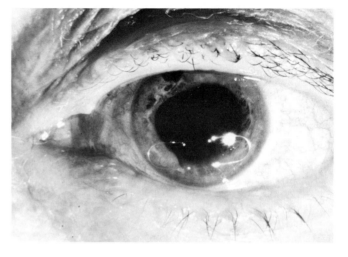

FIGURE 16.19   **Mydriatic-induced dislocation of an intraocular lens. (Copyright 1982, Competency Enhancement Programs. Reprinted with permission from the editors, from the collection of Herbert J. Nevyas, M.D.)**

position the iris in front of the lens, this condition often requires surgical or other noninvasive manipulation for satisfactory correction.[97]

The Plateau Iris

The concept of plateau iris was first proposed and described in the literature by Shaffer[98] in 1960. Wand and associates[75] have subsequently distinguished between *plateau iris configuration* and *plateau iris syndrome.* The former is defined as the preoperative finding of an anterior chamber of normal depth with a flat iris plane as observed directly with the slit lamp, but with an extremely narrow or closed angle by gonioscopy. The latter is defined as the postoperative finding of an anterior chamber of normal depth with a flat iris plane

and patent iridectomy or iridotomy by direct slit-lamp examination, but with gonioscopically confirmed angle closure following dilation of the pupil.

Although the prevalence of plateau iris configuration is unknown, most authors believe it to be rare, and the plateau iris syndrome is considered to be even more uncommon.[75]

Plateau iris configuration results in angle closure by a mechanism independent of pupillary block.[75] Since the anterior chamber is of normal depth and the iris plane is flat, there is little or no pupillary block. Instead, dilation of the pupil causes a peripheral iris roll to approximate and close the angle, thus precipitating an attack of acute angle-closure glaucoma (Fig. 16.22).[75] Since the depth of the anterior chamber in such eyes does not provide a clue to the possible development of angle closure following dilation, gonioscopy is essential for the diagnosis.[75] However, many practitioners

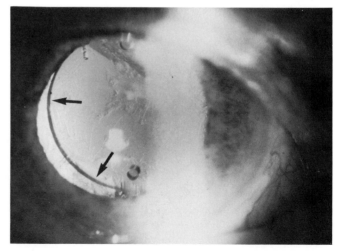

FIGURE 16.20   **Wide pupillary dilation of eye with posterior chamber intraocular lens. Arrows denote edge of lens.**

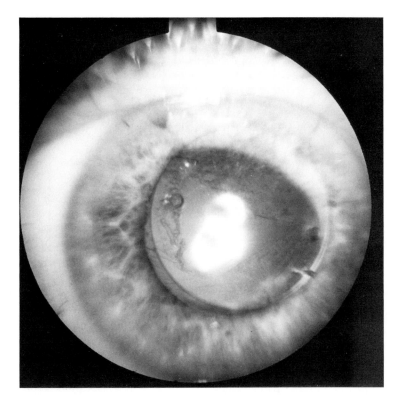

FIGURE 16.21   **Posterior chamber intraocular lens entrapped within the pupillary aperture following dilation. (Courtesy Hernan Benavides, O.D.)**

and investigators believe that plateau iris configuration is difficult to detect even with carefully performed gonioscopy. In many cases, the diagnosis is made only after an apparently open angle has sustained angle closure following pupillary dilation. Once the diagnosis is made, the practitioner should be cautious with dilation, since the existence of plateau iris configuration preoperatively suggests an extremely high risk for mydriatic-induced angle closure postoperatively. These eyes should generally be managed with continuous miotic therapy.[75]

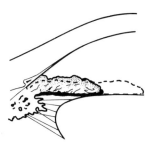

FIGURE 16.22   **Plateau iris. Dilation of the pupil causes the iris to obstruct aqueous outflow, thus causing acute angle-closure glaucoma.**

Postdilation Procedures

Determining Intraocular Pressure

The routine measurement of intraocular pressure following dilation of the pupil is generally unnecessary.[1] In nonglaucomatous patients with open angles, dilation with adrenergic agents, such as phenylephrine, would not be expected to elevate intraocular pressure,[77] while dilation with relatively weak anticholinergic agents such as tropicamide would be expected to elevate intraocular pressure in only about 2% of patients.[49] In glaucomatous patients with open angles, approximately 25% to 33% of patients will demonstrate pressure elevations following dilation with anticholinergic drugs.[48,49] As previously discussed, these pressure elevations are associated with reduced aqueous outflow facility and are unrelated to any angle-closure mechanism.[48] Such pressure elevations are clinically insignificant, decline to normal levels within 4 to 6 hours, and do not require monitoring.[49] Thus, patients with open angles can be dismissed following dilation without regard to the intraocular pressure.

In contrast, the monitoring of intraocular pressure following dilation of eyes with narrow angles is reasonable and prudent.[1] The patient should be retained in the office until the pupils have reached their previous predilation size, and intraocular pressure should be determined before the patient is dismissed. If the patient is dismissed immediately following dilation, he or she should be advised of the symptoms of angle closure and cautioned to return to or telephone the practitioner's office in the event of such an attack. The patient often mistakes the symptoms of angle-closure glaucoma for acute gastrointestinal illness, and these patients have been known to hasten to the hospital only to be met by unwary emergency room physicians.

Use of Miotics

The instillation of miotics such as pilocarpine to counteract the effects of the mydriatic is inadvisable. When pilocarpine is used following dilation with phenylephrine, the relative pupillary block is likely to be increased by the additional stimulation of the iris sphincter, which enhances the medial component of the sphincter force against the lens.[63] In addition, pilocarpine increases aqueous outflow through the trabecular meshwork, which, in the presence of pupillary block, might create a greater differential pressure between the anterior and posterior chambers and lead to iris bombé with secondary angle closure.[69,99] Pilocarpine can also reduce the depth of the anterior chamber, which exacerbates the factors causing angle closure.[100,101] These changes may predispose the eye to angle closure, even in eyes in which closure seems unlikely.[101]

Following dilation with anticholinergic drugs such as tropicamide, pilocarpine will induce little or no miosis, and the pupil will return to its predilation size no more rapidly than without the miotic[67,102] (Fig. 16.23). In addition, the pilocarpine will have no significant beneficial effect on amplitude of accommodation (Fig. 16.24), and the miotic can even have a deleterious effect on distance visual acuity.[102] Thus, the instillation of pilocarpine to counteract the dilation produced by anticholinergic mydriatics is usually nonproductive. It is wise to simply allow the pupils to return spontaneously to their previous size.

Mydriatic Spectacles

Because of increased sensitivity to light and, in some instances, frank photophobia, patients should be given some form of protection while their pupils remain dilated. Commercially available paper sunglasses (U.S. Optical Specialties, Inc., 425 Sycamore Avenue, Mill Valley, California 94941) (Fig. 16.25) are inexpensive and can be discarded after the pupils have returned to normal. If patients are not given such protection, they

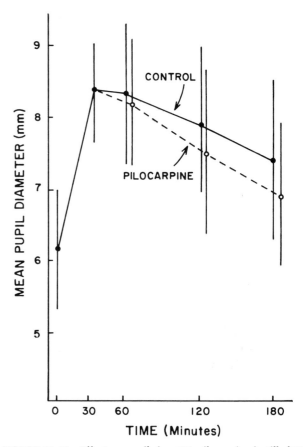

FIGURE 16.23   **Effect on pupil size: 2% pilocarpine instilled 30 minutes after dilation with 0.5% tropicamide has a clinically insignificant effect in returning the pupil to its predilation size. Vertical lines represent 1 standard deviation from mean. (From Nelson ME, Orton HP. Counteracting the effects of mydriatics. Does it benefit the patient? Arch Ophthalmol 1987;105:486–489. Copyright 1987, American Medical Association.)**

can be left significantly incapacitated. Patient objections to dilation frequently relate to a previous experience in which protection from light was not given.[1]

Pupillary Dilation as a Therapeutic Procedure

Nuclear Sclerotic or Posterior Subcapsular Cataract

By increasing the pupillary diameter, patients with central lens opacities such as nuclear sclerotic or posterior subcapsular cataract may experience significant improvement in visual acuity. This can be evaluated in the office by determining visual acuity following pupillary dilation. If significant improvement is obtained, the use of mydriatic therapy on a long-term basis may forestall the need for cataract extraction. This is es-

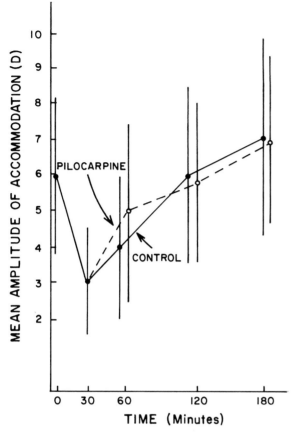

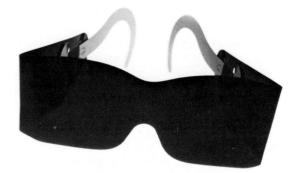

FIGURE 16.25   **Mydriatic spectacles protect the patient from light sensitivity after dilation.**

FIGURE 16.24   **Effect on amplitude of accommodation: 2% pilocarpine instilled 30 minutes after dilation with 0.5% tropicamide has a clinically insignificant effect in returning accommodation to its predilation levels. Vertical lines represent 1 standard deviation from mean. (From Nelson ME, Orton HP. Counteracting the effects of mydriatics. Does it benefit the patient? Arch Ophthalmol 1987;105:486–489. Copyright 1987, American Medical Association.)**

it is wise to avoid cycloplegics for long-term dilation of eyes with open-angle glaucoma.[50] Instead, phenylephrine may be used, since it will overcome the effects of even strong miotics without compromising intraocular pressure.[50,53]

During long-term use of phenylephrine in elderly patients, the pupil may become progressively less responsive to the mydriatic effect.[60] This reduction in mydriasis, which is apparently an age-related phenomenon, may be due to drug-induced damage to the iris dilator muscle[60] or to drug tolerance.

Uveitis

The primary purpose for pupillary dilation of eyes with anterior uveitis is to prevent the formation of posterior synechiae. Any mydriatic can be used for this purpose, but the combination of atropine and phenylephrine acts synergistically to produce strong and wide mydriasis. This combination is also helpful in breaking posterior synechiae that have already developed.[60] Although posterior synechiae are less likely to develop with the iris in this fully dilated position because of less contact between iris and lens, it is nevertheless possible for posterior synechiae to form.[60] Thus, in some cases of severe uveitis it is prudent to use shorter-acting mydriatics such as homatropine or cyclopentolate rather than the longer-acting atropine. The shorter-acting agents allow the pupil to remain somewhat mobile and consequently reduce the risk for development of posterior synechiae.

Complications

Blurred Vision

Patients are likely to encounter some degree of blurred vision following dilation because of spherical aberra-

pecially useful in debilitated elderly patients or in patients otherwise at surgical risk because of systemic illness or having contraindications to general or local anesthesia.

For this purpose, any mydriatic can be used, but agents that are less likely to elevate intraocular pressure are preferred. These include phenylephrine or low concentrations of weak cycloplegic agents such as tropicamide or homatropine. The effect on accommodation is relatively unimportant in elderly patients, but the cycloplegia may be an important consideration in younger patients. It is wise to periodically evaluate intraocular pressure during therapy with cycloplegic mydriatics.

Since cycloplegic mydriatics carry a greater risk of elevating intraocular pressure than do adrenergic agents,

tion associated with the large pupillary aperture and because of accommodative paresis if a cycloplegic has been used. In the latter instance, patients likely to encounter blurred distance vision (driving difficulty) are limited to those with uncorrected nonpresbyopic hyperopia. Most other patients should not encounter significant difficulty with distance vision associated with pupillary dilation.[1]

For reading and other near visual activities following dilation, myopic patients can be advised to simply remove their spectacles, and presbyopic patients may be advised to wear their reading glasses or bifocals. Thus, with proper instructions to the patient, significantly blurred vision following dilation is relatively uncommon.[1] When tropicamide has been used for dilation, most patients will recover the ability to read within 1 to 3 hours, and virtually all patients will completely recover accommodation within 4 to 6 hours.[16,103,104] In many instances, patients never lose the ability to read.[16,81] Patients can therefore be reassured that any postdilation blurred vision will be transient.

Light Sensitivity

The problem of mydriatic-induced light sensitivity has been previously discussed. Patients should be given some form of protection from bright sunlight and other illuminated environments. Commercially available mydriatic spectacles (see Fig. 16.25) are designed specifically for this purpose.

Acute Angle-Closure Glaucoma

Although the prevalence of significantly narrow angles in the general population is from 2% to 6%,[9] Keller[105] estimated the risks of angle-closure glaucoma from the use of mydriatics to be only 1 in 183,000 for the general population and only 1 in 45,000 for the population over 30 years of age. When a practical benefit-risk ratio approach is taken to the problem of potential angle closure following pupillary dilation, the extremely small risk of angle closure should not prevent the practitioner from using mydriatics when necessary.[2] Newell and Ernest[106] suggested that there is a greater danger of overlooking significant retinal disease by failure to dilate than there is of inducing angle closure (see Chapter 34). This statement is supported by Halpern's[107] discovery of peripheral retinal breaks in 6% of 250 patients without symptoms. By evaluating the anterior angle with slit lamp or gonioscopy, eyes predisposed to angle closure are readily identified, and appropriate mydriatics can usually be satisfactorily administered according to the guidelines previously discussed in this chapter.

The signs and symptoms as well as the definitive management of acute angle-closure glaucoma are discussed in Chapter 29.

Systemic Complications

Although adverse systemic reactions to topically administered mydriatic agents have been reported, dilation of the pupil is extremely safe and without adverse sequelae in the vast majority of patients. The risk of adverse systemic reactions is greater in patients with various systemic illnesses or in those taking certain systemic medications such as β-adrenergic blocking drugs or tricyclic antidepressants (see Table 16.6). It should be recognized that there have been very few reports of adverse systemic reactions associated with the use of 2.5% phenylephrine in recommended dosages. The potential for adverse reactions associated with the use of 10% phenylephrine is increased in patients with cardiac disease, systemic hypertension, insulin-dependent diabetes, and idiopathic orthostatic hypotension.[40] In such patients who are predisposed to adverse cardiovascular events, the use of tropicamide either alone or in combination with hydroxyamphetamine should provide satisfactory mydriasis while minimizing the risks of systemic complications.[15] In addition, the use of low concentrations of drug, single applications, and punctum depression will also minimize adverse reactions in susceptible patients.

The diagnosis and management of systemic complications associated with adrenergic mydriatics are considered in Chapter 31.

References

1. Bartlett JD. Pitfalls encountered in the clinical utilization of mydriatic drugs. South J Optom 1980;22:8–14.
2. Steinmann WC, Millstein ME, Sinclair SH. Pupillary dilation with tropicamide 1% for funduscopic screening. A study of duration of action. Ann Intern Med 1987; 107:181–184.
3. Barker A. The logia: Waiting room deluxe. Optom Manage 1979;15:147.
4. Townsend WW. Incorporating ophthalmic pharmaceuticals into your practice. J Am Optom Assoc 1987;58:426–430.
5. Alexander LJ, Scholles J. Clinical and legal aspects of pupillary dilation. J Am Optom Assoc 1987;58:432–437.
6. van Herick W, Shaffer RN, Schwartz A. Estimation of width of angle of anterior chamber. Incidence and significance of the narrow angle. Am J Ophthalmol 1969;68:626–629.
7. Bresler MJ, Hoffman RS. Prevention of iatrogenic acute narrow-angle glaucoma. Ann Emerg Med 1981;10:535–537.
8. Cockburn DM. Slitlamp estimate of anterior chamber depth as a predictor of the gonioscopic visibility of the angle structures. Am J Optom Physiol Opt 1982;59:904–908.

9. Cockburn DM. Prevalence and significance of narrow anterior chamber angles in optometric practice. Am J Optom Physiol Opt 1981;58:171–175.

10. Mapstone R. Outflow changes in positive provocative tests. Br J Ophthalmol 1977;61:634–646.

11. Apt L, Henrick A. Pupillary dilation with single eyedrop mydriatic combinations. Am J Ophthalmol 1980;89:553–559.

12. Caldwell JBH. Use of dilute drug solutions for routine cycloplegia and mydriasis (letter). Am J Ophthalmol 1979;87:727–728.

13. Lyle WM, Bobier WR. Effects of topical anesthetics on phenylephrine-induced mydriasis. Am J Optom Physiol Opt 1977;54:276–281.

14. Borthne A, Davanger M. Mydriatics and age. Acta Ophthalmol 1971;49:380–387.

15. Semes LP, Bartlett JD. Mydriatic effectiveness of hydroxyamphetamine. J Am Optom Assoc 1982;53:899–904.

16. Levine L. Mydriatic effectiveness of dilute combinations of phenylephrine and tropicamide. Am J Optom Physiol Opt 1982;59:580–594.

17. Cable MK, Hendrickson RO, Hanna C. Evaluation of drugs in ointment for mydriasis and cycloplegia. Arch Ophthalmol 1978;96:84–86.

18. Molinari JF. A clinical comparison of mydriatics. J Am Optom Assoc 1983;54:781–784.

19. Geyer O, Godel V, Lazar M. The concurrent application of ophthalmic drops. Aust NZ J Ophthalmol 1985;13:63–66.

20. Levine L. Cyclomydril, a combination mydriatic. Oreg Optom 1981;48:5–7.

21. Doughty MJ, Lyle W, Trevino R, Flanagan J. A study of mydriasis produced by topical phenylephrine 2.5% in young adults. Can J Optom 1988;50:40.

22. Forman AR. A new low-concentration preparation for mydriasis and cycloplegia. Ophthalmology 1980;87:213–215.

23. Feldman JB. Mydriatics. A clinical observation. Arch Ophthalmol 1949;41:42–59.

24. Mapstone R. Dilating dangerous pupils. Br J Ophthalmol 1977;61:517–524.

25. Brooks AMV, West RH, Gillies WE. The risks of precipitating acute angle-closure glaucoma with the clinical use of mydriatic agents. Med J Aust 1986;145:34–36.

26. Levine L. Minimizing risk of adverse reactions to mydriatic agents in binocular indirect ophthalmoscopy. J Am Optom Assoc 1985;56:542–548.

27. Lee PF. Congenital glaucoma. In: Feman SS, Reinecke RD, eds. Handbook of pediatric ophthalmology. New York: Grune & Stratton, 1978;88.

28. Caputo AR, Lingua RW. The problem of cycloplegia in the pediatric age group: A combination formula for refraction. J Pediatr Ophthalmol Strabismus 1980;17:119–128.

29. Caputo AR, Schnitzer RE. Systemic response to mydriatic eyedrops in neonates: mydriatics in neonates. J Pediatr Ophthalmol Strabismus 1978;15:109–122.

30. Rosales T, Isenberg S, Leake R, et al. Systemic effects of mydriatics in low weight infants. J Pediatr Ophthalmol Strabismus 1981;18:42–44.

31. Isenberg S, Everett S, Parelhoff E. A comparison of mydriatic eyedrops in low-weight infants. Ophthalmology 1984;91:278–279.

32. Isenberg SJ, Abrams C, Hyman PE. Effects of cyclopentolate eyedrops on gastric secretory function in pre-term infants. Ophthalmology 1985;92:698–700.

33. Bauer CR, Trottier MCT, Stern L. Systemic cyclopentolate (Cyclogyl) toxicity in the newborn infant. J Pediatr 1973;82:501–505.

34. Caputo AR, Schnitzer RE, Lindquist TD, et al. Dilation in neonates: A protocol. Pediatrics 1982;69:77–79.

35. Carpel EF, Kalina RE. Pupillary responses to mydriatic agents in premature infants. Am J Ophthalmol 1973;75:988–991.

36. Bates JH, Burnstine RA. Consequences of retinopathy of prematurity examinations. Arch Ophthalmol 1987;105:618–619.

37. Fraunfelder FT, Scafidi AF. Possible adverse effects from topical ocular 10% phenylephrine. Am J Ophthalmol 1978;85:447–453.

38. Brown MM, Brown GC, Spaeth GL. Lack of side effects from topically administered 10% phenylephrine eyedrops. A controlled study. Arch Ophthalmol 1980;98:487–489.

39. Chang FW. Pharmacology of mydriasis for modern optometric procedures. J Am Optom Assoc 1977;48:1365–1368.

40. Robertson D. Contraindication to the use of ocular phenylephrine in idiopathic orthostatic hypotension. Am J Ophthalmol 1979;87:819–822.

41. Sneddon JM, Turner P. The interactions of local guanethidine and sympathomimetic amines in the human eye. Arch Ophthalmol 1969;81:622–627.

42. Kim JM, Stevenson CE, Mathewson HS. Hypertensive reactions to phenylephrine eyedrops in patients with sympathetic denervation. Am J Ophthalmol 1978;85:862–868.

43. Smith SA, Smith SE. Evidence for a neuropathic aetiology in the small pupil of diabetes mellitus. Br J Ophthalmol 1983;67:89–93.

44. Thompson HS. 12th pupil colloquium (report). Am J Ophthalmol 1981;92:435–436.

45. Bryant RC. Pupil motility in long-term diabetes (letter). Diabetologia 1980;18:170–171.

46. Huber MJE, Smith SA, Smith SE. Mydriatic drugs for diabetic patients. Br J Ophthalmol 1985;69:425–427.

47. Beasley H. Retinal detachments secondary to miotics. Symposium on drug-induced ocular side effects and ocular toxicology, Little Rock, AR, Sept. 10, 1977.

48. Harris LS, Galin MA. Cycloplegic provocative testing. Effect of miotic therapy. Arch Ophthalmol 1969;81:544–547.

49. Harris LS. Cycloplegic-induced intraocular pressure elevations. A study of normal and open-angle glaucomatous eyes. Arch Ophthalmol 1968;79:242–246.

50. Schimek RA, Lieberman WJ. The influence of Cyclogyl and Neosynephrine on tonographic studies of miotic control in open-angle glaucoma. Am J Ophthalmol 1961;51:781–784.

51. Shaw BR, Lewis RA. Intraocular pressure elevation after pupillary dilation in open angle glaucoma. Arch Ophthalmol 1986;104:1185–1188.

52. Portney GL, Purcell TW. The influence of tropicamide on intraocular pressure. Ann Ophthalmol 1975;7:31–34.

53. Becker B, Gage T, Kolker AE, et al. The effect of phenylephrine hydrochloride on the miotic-treated eye. Am J Ophthalmol 1959;48:313–321.

54. Kristensen P. Mydriasis-induced pigment liberation in the

anterior chamber associated with acute rise in intraocular pressure in open-angle glaucoma. Acta Ophthalmol 1965; 43:714–724.

55. Valle O. The cyclopentolate provocative test in suspected or untreated open-angle glaucoma. III. The significance of pigment for the result of the cyclopentolate provocative test in suspected or untreated open-angle glaucoma. Acta Ophthalmol 1976;54:654–664.

56. Tarkkanen AHA. Exfoliation syndrome. Trans Ophthalmol Soc UK 1986;105:233–236.

57. Carpel EF. Pupillary dilation in eyes with pseudoexfoliation syndrome. Am J Ophthalmol 1988;105:692–694.

58. Dark AJ. Cataract extraction complicated by capsular glaucoma. Br J Ophthalmol 1979;63:465–468.

59. Ghosh M, Speakman JS. The iris in senile exfoliation of the lens. Can J Ophthalmol 1974;9:289.

60. Davidson SI. Mydriatic and cycloplegic drugs. Trans Ophthalmol Soc UK 1976;96:327–329.

61. Shaffer RN. Problems in the use of autonomic drugs in ophthalmology. In: Leopold IH, ed. Ocular therapy: Complications and management. St. Louis: C.V. Mosby Co, 1967;2:18–23.

62. Mapstone R. Mechanics of pupil block. Br J Ophthalmol 1968;52:19–25.

63. Lowe RF. Angle-closure, pupil dilation, and pupil block. Br J Ophthalmol 1966;50:385–389.

64. Mapstone R. The syndrome of closed-angle glaucoma. Br J Ophthalmol 1976;60:120–123.

65. Havener WH. Synopsis of ophthalmology. St. Louis: C.V. Mosby Co, 1975;4:490–494.

66. Mapstone R. Safe mydriasis. Br J Ophthalmol 1970;54:690–692.

67. Anastasi LM, Ogle KN, Kearns TP. Effect of pilocarpine in counteracting mydriasis. Arch Ophthalmol 1968;79:710–715.

68. Lowe RF. Primary angle-closure glaucoma. Investigations using 10% phenylephrine eyedrops. Am J Ophthalmol 1965;60:415–419.

69. Mapstone R. Precipitation of angle closure. Br J Ophthalmol 1974;58:46–54.

70. Chang FW, McCan TA, Hitchcock JR. Sector pupil dilation with phenylephrine and tropicamide. Am J Optom Physiol Opt 1985;62:482–486.

71. Bienfang DC. Sector pupillary dilation with an epinephrine strip. Am J Ophthalmol 1973;75:883–884.

72. Chang FW, Temme BA, Hitchcock JR. Effects of decreasing concentrations of tropicamide on sector pupil dilation. Am J Optom Physiol Opt 1986;63:804–806.

73. Mapstone R. Partial angle closure. Br J Ophthalmol 1977;61:525–530.

74. Harris LS, Galin MA. Cycloplegic provocative testing. Arch Ophthalmol 1969;81:356–358.

75. Wand M, Grant WM, Simmons RJ, et al. Plateau iris syndrome. Trans Am Acad Ophthalmol Otol 1977;83:122–130.

76. Hagee MJ. Homocystinuria and ectopia lentis. J Am Optom Assoc 1984;55:269–276.

77. Haddad NJ, Moyer NJ, Riley FC. Mydriatic effect of phenylephrine hydrochloride. Am J Ophthalmol 1970;70:729–733.

78. Gambill HD, Ogle KN, Kearns TP. Mydriatic effect of four drugs determined with pupillograph. Arch Ophthalmol 1967;77:740–746.

79. Emiru VP. Response to mydriatics in the African. Br J Ophthalmol 1971;55:538–543.

80. Richardson RW. Comparing the mydriatic effect of tropicamide with respect to iris pigmentation. J Am Optom Assoc 1982;53:885–887.

81. Dillon JR, Tyhurst CW, Yolton RL. The mydriatic effect of tropicamide on light and dark irides. J Am Optom Assoc 1977;48:653–658.

82. Levine L. Tropicamide-induced mydriasis in densely pigmented eyes. Am J Optom Physiol Opt 1983;60:673–677.

83. Gutner R, Cavallerano A, Wong D. Fundus biomicroscopy: A comparison of four methods. J Am Optom Assoc 1988;59:388–390.

84. Cavallerano A, Gutner R, Garston M. Indirect biomicroscopy techniques. J Am Optom Assoc 1986;57:755–758.

85. Barker FM. The Volk steady mount holder for the +90 D lens. J Am Optom Assoc 1988;59:558–560.

86. Barker FM. Vitreoretinal biomicroscopy: A comparison of techniques. J Am Optom Assoc 1987;58:985–992.

87. Jackson JE, Fisher M. Evaluation of the posterior pole with a 90 D lens and the slit-lamp biomicroscope. South J Optom 1987;5:80–83.

88. Lundberg C. Biomicroscopic examination of the ocular fundus with a +60-diopter lens. Am J Ophthalmol 1985;99:490–491.

89. Houston G. Peripheral fundus photography using the Volk 90 diopter lens. South J Optom 1988;6:13–15.

90. Semes L, Gold A. Clinical and legal considerations in the diagnosis and management of ocular tumors. J Am Optom Assoc 1987;58:134–139.

91. Houston G. Fundus photography using the Volk 90 D lens. South J Optom 1988;6:23–26.

92. Phillips LJ. Implants (letter). Rev Optom 1981;118:12.

93. Hamburger HA, Lerner L. Surgical treatment of dislocated iris-plane intraocular lenses. Ann Ophthalmol 1985;17:434–436.

94. Devita VJ, Gentile RS. Examination of the pseudophakic patient. J Am Optom Assoc 1985;56:103–107.

95. Nevyas HJ. How to manage the cataract patient. Rev Optom 1986;123:46–52.

96. Wilcox TK. Release of an iris captured IOL following gonioscopy. South J Optom 1987;5:27.

97. Lindstrom RL, Herman WK. Pupil capture: Prevention and management. Am Intra-Ocular Implant Soc J 1983;9:201–204.

98. Shaffer RN. Gonioscopy, ophthalmoscopy, and perimetry. Trans Am Acad Ophthalmol Otol 1960;64:112–127.

99. Gorin G. Angle-closure glaucoma induced by miotics. Am J Ophthalmol 1966;62:1063–1067.

100. Francois J, Goes F. Ultrasonographic study of the effect of different miotics on the eye components. Ophthalmologica 1977;175:328–338.

101. Wilkie J, Drance SM, Schulzer M. The effects of miotics on anterior-chamber depth. Am J Ophthalmol 1969;68:78–83.

102. Nelson ME, Orton HP. Counteracting the effects of mydriatics. Does it benefit the patient? Arch Ophthalmol 1987;105:486–489.

103. Pollack SL, Hunt JS, Polse KA. Dose-response effects of

tropicamide HCl. Am J Optom Physiol Opt 1981;58:361–366.

104. Gettes BC. Tropicamide, a new cycloplegic mydriatic. Arch Ophthalmol 1961;65:48–51.

105. Keller JT. The risk of angle closure from the use of mydriatics. J Am Optom Assoc 1975;46:19–21.

106. Newell FW, Ernest JT. Ophthalmology; principles and concepts. St. Louis: C.V. Mosby Co, 1974;3:150.

107. Halpern JI. Routine screening of the retinal periphery. Am J Ophthalmol 1966;62:99–102.

108. Dziadul J, Teague B, Oshinskie L, et al. A comparison of lens disorders using undilated and dilated biomicroscopy. N Engl J Optom 1988;40:15–17.

109. Sira IB, Nissenkorn I, Kremer I. Retinopathy of prematurity. Surv Ophthalmol 1988;33:1–16.

CHAPTER 17

Cycloplegic Refraction

David M. Amos

Although new methods of refraction have been developed over the years, cycloplegic refraction has remained a time-tested and reliable method for obtaining significant data on difficult refractive patients. Without cycloplegic drugs, determining the true refractive status of patients with accommodative esotropia, pseudomyopia, or latent hyperopia would be fraught with error. In noncommunicative or uncooperative patients, and in patients with aberrations or opacification of the ocular media, cycloplegia is often essential for the proper diagnosis of refractive errors.

This chapter considers the indications, precautions, and contraindications associated with cycloplegics in refraction. Selecting the appropriate cycloplegic agent, techniques of refraction, and principles of spectacle prescribing are also discussed. Recognition and management of adverse reactions to cycloplegics are described in Chapters 3 and 31.

Indications and Advantages

Cycloplegia plays a very important role in the refractive examination of young patients. Although it is certainly not indicated for every child, there are a number of clinical situations in which the practitioner can acquire information that could not otherwise be obtained. As stated by Michaels,[1] "The question is not whether to use cycloplegics, but when."

Cycloplegic refraction is indicated in individuals whose total refractive error does not manifest itself in the course of a subjective noncycloplegic examination. The reasons for determining this latent refractive error are practical ones. In young patients with suspected accommodative esotropia, it is vital to determine the full amount of hyperopia so that plus lenses can be prescribed to relieve the effort placed on the accommodative-convergence system and, in turn, bring the eyes into alignment. As discussed later in this chapter, the full amount of plus lens correction may not be prescribed, especially for children over 4 years of age, but the value derived by the cycloplegic examination serves as an initial starting point that is then molded by clinical judgment and experience.

In a more general sense, cycloplegic refraction is also indicated in young patients who demonstrate any problem with ocular motility. Not only does cycloplegia allow the clinician to diagnose correctly any accompanying refractive error, but it prepares the patient for a dilated fundus examination. All young strabismic patients should have such a thorough evaluation, at least when initially examined. This serves to rule out an occult etiology of the ocular deviation and can conveniently be incorporated into the examination following the cycloplegic refraction, while the pupils are still dilated.

Nonstrabismic children with latent hyperopia are perhaps less obvious in their presentation, but this is another instance in which information gained by cycloplegic examination is essential to the ultimate management plan. When the amount of total hyperopia is considered in conjunction with the patient's signs and symptoms, a successful spectacle prescription can be determined more accurately.

Because patients age 3 years and younger often have unreliable responses during subjective refraction, it is wise to use a cycloplegic-assisted examination in these children. Clearly, as an objective method for determining refractive error in children between the ages of

18 and 48 months, it is superior to noncycloplegic techniques.[2] Not only is cycloplegic retinoscopy of young children and infants more accurate, it is also more easily performed, since the examination does not depend on the patient's position and fixation distance.

It may be worthwhile to use cycloplegics in all children who exhibit myopia for the first time. This is primarily because it allows the practitioner to rule out accommodative spasm (pseudomyopia) as the etiologic source. Once the diagnosis of myopia has been established, future cycloplegic examinations can be excluded if the child is cooperative. A still broader recommendation is made by Duke-Elder and Abrams,[3] who advise that nonmyopic patients up to the age of 16 years have a cycloplegic refraction. Many other clinicians disagree. However, since all children should have a thorough funduscopic evaluation, the use of drugs for pupillary dilation that also allow substantial cycloplegia facilitates both the fundus evaluation and the refraction.

Cycloplegic refraction is also indicated for patients with active accommodative systems whose best-corrected visual acuity in each eye is less than 20/20 (6/6) and for whom there is no apparent reason for the decreased vision. It allows the clinician to be reasonably certain that an uncorrected refractive error is not responsible for the decreased visual acuity.

Patients may benefit from a cycloplegic examination if they demonstrate no known ocular disease but are impaired or handicapped so that they are unresponsive or inconsistent in their responses to subjective refraction. Indeed, this may be the only way the clinician can determine the degree of refractive error, if any. In a similar category are suspected malingering or hysterical patients. The clinician can sidestep the unreliable patient's subjective responses and arrive at objective refractive data through the use of cycloplegics.

Finally, there are patients whose visual signs or symptoms do not correlate with the nature and degree of their manifest refractive error. A cycloplegic refraction will aid in the differential diagnosis in that it can help ensure that the patient's problem is not refractive. The clinician can then concentrate on other aspects of the visual system. Table 17.1 summarizes the indications for cycloplegic refraction.

Disadvantages

Despite the previously mentioned advantages of cycloplegic refraction, it has some disadvantages. Wide dilation of the pupil can create excessive spherical aberration in the ocular media, resulting in difficult retinoscopy and refraction. This is especially true when

TABLE 17.1
Indications for Cycloplegic Refraction

- Accommodative esotropia (any age)
- All children under 3 years of age
- Suspected latent hyperopia
- Suspected pseudomyopia
- Uncooperative patients
- Noncommunicative patients
- Patients whose subjective responses during the manifest refraction are variable and inconsistent
- Suspected malingering
- Suspected hysterical amblyopia
- Visual acuity not corrected to predicted level
- Strabismic children (other than accommodative esotropia)
- Patients whose symptoms seem unrelated to the nature or degree of the manifest refractive error

synergistic agents such as hydroxyamphetamine or phenylephrine are used to permit fundus examination following the retinoscopy. In addition, an allowance for ciliary tonus is usually necessary, and the clinician must consider this to determine the appropriate refractive correction for each patient. The accommodative-convergence relationship must be considered before cycloplegia. Furthermore, since all cycloplegic drugs have potential side effects, caution must be exercised in their use. Cycloplegics may blur vision for 1 to 3 days or longer, and sunlight or any bright light can be extremely annoying even with the use of sunglasses.

Precautions and Contraindications

Before a cycloplegic agent is administered, a preinstillation ocular evaluation should be performed. This not only protects the clinician legally, but also provides valuable information regarding contraindications to the indicated drug(s). Moreover, it furnishes certain baseline clinical information that may be unobtainable after cycloplegia. The following minimum examination is recommended.

- Medical and ocular history, with particular emphasis on present medications, allergies, drug reactions, and previous eye examinations.
- Visual acuity at distance and near.
- Pupillary examination.
- Motility evaluation.
- Manifest ("dry") refraction.
- Accommodative function, if desired.
- Accommodative-convergence relationships, if desired.
- Slit-lamp evaluation with particular attention to the anterior chamber depth, and an estimation of the

anterior angle by van Herick's classification[4] (see Chapter 16).

- Tonometry, if possible.
- Gonioscopy, if a shallow anterior chamber is observed or suspected.[5]

Some of these tests are often not practical or possible with infants or uncooperative children unless performed under general anesthesia. To avoid the need for examination under anesthesia, a penlight estimation of the anterior chamber depth (see Chapter 16) can give the practitioner a reasonable idea regarding the safety of pupillary dilation.

Cycloplegia is contraindicated in patients with a history of angle-closure glaucoma, and atropine, in particular, should be used with caution in patients with Down's syndrome and in patients receiving systemic anticholinergic drugs. Any known sensitivity to a specific cycloplegic agent can be bypassed by substituting another cycloplegic, as discussed below. In addition, some authors recommend that patient or parental consent be obtained before administering cycloplegics[6] (see Chapter 33).

Selection and Use of Specific Cycloplegic Agents

All cycloplegics exhibit anticholinergic properties by blocking the response to acetylcholine at the receptor sites on the smooth ocular muscles innervated by postganglionic cholinergic nerves.[7] This anticholinergic response is observed clinically as some degree of pupillary dilation and cycloplegia.

Cycloplegics, to be clinically useful, should ideally possess the following properties.[8,9]

- Rapid onset of cycloplegia
- Complete paralysis of accommodation
- Adequate duration of maximum cycloplegia
- Rapid recovery of accommodation
- Absence of side effects

Although no cycloplegic meets all these criteria, the more recently developed agents satisfactorily achieve the desired clinical purpose with a minimum of disadvantages. The common cycloplegic agents in current use are listed in Table 17.2.

Atropine

Atropine, a drug from the family Solanaceae, has been known since biblical times. In the Middle Ages, dilated pupils were regarded as a sign of beauty, perhaps associated with the youthful look of innocence, and the term belladonna—"beautiful lady"—was coined for atropine.

TABLE 17.2
Clinical Characteristics of Common Cycloplegic Agents

Cycloplegic Agent	Commonly Used Concentration (%)	Dosage	Onset of Maximum Cycloplegic Effect	Duration of Cycloplegic Effect	Relative Residual Accommodation
Atropine sulfate (ointment or solution)	½[a]	1 gt t.i.d.[b] for 3 days before refraction or	3–6 hours	10–18 days	Negligible
	1	1 gt t.i.d.[b] for 1 day before refraction (see text)			
Scopolamine hydrobromide	0.25	1 gt, repeated in 20 minutes	60 minutes	5–7 days	Negligible
Cyclopentolate hydrochloride	1[c] 2	1 gt, repeated in 10 minutes	20–45 minutes	8–24 hours	Minimal
Tropicamide hydrochloride	1	1 gt, repeated every 5 minutes for 3 instillations	20–30 minutes	4–8 hours	Moderate

[a]Recommended ointment concentration.
[b]Atropine solution; ointment formulation should be instilled b.i.d.
[c]Recommended concentration for most clinical purposes.

The onset of atropine cycloplegia is within 1 hour. Maximum cycloplegia is usually achieved within 6 hours, and accommodation is inhibited for 10 to 18 days. As occurs with most cycloplegics, darkly pigmented irides are often more resistant to atropine than are lightly pigmented irides. In addition, atropine produces mydriasis that may last for 14 to 21 days. The degree of mydriasis is often unreliable in judging the degree of cycloplegia. Atropinized patients often exhibit relatively poor mydriasis while sustaining complete paralysis of accommodation. This seems especially true for patients with darkly pigmented irides.

Atropine is currently available in 0.5% to 3% solution and 0.5% and 1% ointment. The ointment has the advantage of allowing effective cycloplegia while decreasing systemic drug absorption, which minimizes systemic side effects. The traditional dosage for the refraction of patients with accommodative esotropia is 1% atropine solution 3 times daily or 0.5% atropine ointment twice daily for 3 days before examination. This is done at home. The drops or ointment are not instilled on the day of refraction, since no additional cycloplegia is obtained and because the ointment tends to interfere with the refractive procedure by introducing distortions of the optical media. It is important to note that this dosage regimen is excessive, since maximum cycloplegia is usually achieved by the second day. However, it does allow for missed instillations at home. If the parents are reliable, 3 instillations of the atropine solution only 1 day before examination should be adequate.[10] Table 17.3 shows the typical instructions that may be given to the parents for home administration of atropine.

TABLE 17.3
Typical Instructions for Home Administration of Atropine

1. Do not use this medication until _____ (day), _____ (date). This is _____ day(s) before your child's appointment.

2. Place once in each eye as instructed, _____ times a day beginning on the morning of the day noted for the _____ day(s) before the day of appointment. Do not use on the day of appointment.

3. Discontinue medication if child develops a fever or persistent redness of the face.

4. It is normal to notice:
   a. Sensitivity to bright light
   b. Blurred vision
   c. Dilated (enlarged) pupils

5. *Discard medication after the appointment.* This is not "general purpose eye medication."

6. If any problems occur, call our office immediately.

Since atropine provides the most effective cycloplegia of any of the currently available anticholinergic agents, it is the drug of choice for the cycloplegic retinoscopy of infants and children up to age 4 years with suspected accommodative esotropia. The use of atropine allows determination of the maximum amount of hyperopia so that plus lenses can more effectively relieve the effort placed on the accommodative-convergence mechanism. The cycloplegic (atropine) examination should be repeated several months after the patient has worn plus lenses, at which time it is not uncommon to uncover more hyperopia. Refraction of nonstrabismic children and of adults does not require atropine, since complete cycloplegia is not essential in these patients. Furthermore, atropine cycloplegia is usually unnecessary and impractical in adults because of their already reduced amplitude of accommodation and because they are usually intolerant of the prolonged cycloplegia and dilated pupils.[7]

Scopolamine

Scopolamine, or hyoscine, is indicated for cycloplegic retinoscopy only as a substitute for atropine in atropine-sensitive patients. It has an onset of cycloplegia within 1 hour, and maximum cycloplegia is obtained within 1 hour. This allows only negligible residual accommodation and has a duration of cycloplegia from 5 to 7 days.

Scopolamine is available in 0.25% solution. Concentrations greater than 0.5% can cause central nervous system manifestations.[7] A 0.25% solution of scopolamine has approximately the same cycloplegic effect as 1% atropine. The usual dosage for cycloplegic refraction is 1 drop of the 0.25% solution, repeated in 15 to 20 minutes.

Cyclopentolate

The onset of cyclopentolate cycloplegia begins in 5 to 20 minutes and reaches maximum in 20 to 45 minutes. The cycloplegia lasts 8 to 24 hours. Residual accommodation is approximately 1.00 D for white patients but, with the instillation of only 1 drop, can be as high as 5.00 D for black patients.[7]

Cyclopentolate is available in 0.5%, 1%, and 2% solution. One drop of the 0.5% or 1% solution, repeated in 5 or 10 minutes, allows sufficient cycloplegia for most children. However, Miranda[11] found that 1 drop of 1% cyclopentolate alone achieved unsatisfactory cycloplegia in patients with dark brown irides and recommended that a combination of 1% cyclopentolate and 1% tropicamide be used to obtain adequate cycloplegia in such patients. Black children, infants, or children with dark brown irides may require 2 or 3 instillations of the 1% solution to achieve less than 2.00 D residual accommodation. The clinician should avoid use of 2% cyclopentolate because of the increased risk of systemic side effects.

Cyclopentolate has become the drug of choice for the cycloplegic refraction of strabismic patients over age 4 years and nonsquinters of any age. Although atropine is still preferred in patients under age 4 years with suspected accommodative esotropia, there is a definite trend toward the use of cyclopentolate in these patients.

Tropicamide

Tropicamide has a rapid onset of cycloplegia of 5 to 20 minutes, with maximum cycloplegia occurring in 20 to 30 minutes and then quickly diminishing. Residual accommodation has been found to average 3.50 D, which makes tropicamide an unreliable cycloplegic.[12] Another problem with tropicamide is the short duration of maximum cycloplegia. If refraction or retinoscopy is not performed within the few minutes of maximum cycloplegia, residual accommodation will become an unwanted factor and may contribute to errors in refraction. Such timing is often difficult in a busy practice.

Tropicamide is available in 0.5% and 1% solution. One drop of the 1% solution, repeated at least 2 or 3 times at 5-minute intervals, is usually advised for refraction, but even this dosage cannot guarantee adequate cycloplegia. However, Pollack and associates[13] have shown that 1 drop of 1% tropicamide provides effective cycloplegia lasting up to 40 minutes in patients in their twenties and thirties.

Comparison of Cycloplegics

Gettes and Belmont[14] compared the residual accommodation allowed by various cycloplegics relative to 1% atropine. These investigators found cycloplegic efficacies of 92% for 1% cyclopentolate, 80% for 1% tropicamide, and only 54% for 4% homatropine with 1% hydroxyamphetamine. Thus, 1% cyclopentolate produces less residual accommodation than does 1% tropicamide or 4% homatropine and is therefore considered the drug of choice for routine cycloplegic refraction not requiring absolute paralysis of accommodation. Another advantage of cyclopentolate is its shorter duration of action compared with atropine.

Although Havener[7] has reported that 3 drops of 1% cyclopentolate applied at 10-minute intervals will pro-

vide the same cycloplegic effect as the traditional 3-day atropine regimen, Ingram and Barr[15] found that 1% cyclopentolate was significantly less effective than 1% atropine in producing cycloplegia in 1-year-old children.

More recently, Rosenbaum and associates[16] have shown that refraction with 1% atropine is essential to uncover the maximum amount of hyperopia in esotropic children. In this study, which compared the effects of 1% atropine and 1% cyclopentolate, a difference of an additional +1.00 D or more was uncovered with atropine in 22% of the children.

Clinical Procedure

Administration of Cycloplegic Agents

Many clinicians prefer to use a topical anesthetic before instilling the cycloplegic. The anesthetic diminishes the local stinging, irritation, and lacrimation that often accompany cycloplegic drops, but it may also cause desquamation of corneal epithelium, which subsequently interferes with the optical integrity of the refraction. Several authors[17–19] have reported increased corneal drug penetration and therefore increased effectiveness of phenylephrine following topical anesthesia. Increased effectiveness of cycloplegics may also occur following topical anesthesia.[35]

The cycloplegic can be administered alone or as a combination cycloplegic-mydriatic solution to permit adequate binocular indirect ophthalmoscopy in neonates, infants, and young children following cycloplegic retinoscopy. The combination drugs can be administered individually or as a combination solution prepared by mixing certain volumes of each constituent drug as discussed in Chapter 16 and as shown in Figure 17.1.

The cycloplegic or combination cycloplegic-mydriatic solution can be administered to the eye as a drop, a spray (see Chapter 2), or an ointment (atropine). The spray is particularly effective in children who are resistant to drop instillation in the usual manner. To decrease systemic drug absorption and the risk of systemic side effects, many practitioners advocate manual depression of the lower puncta against the nasal bone (see Fig. 2.5).

The practitioner must observe the recommended dosages for cycloplegic refraction. The dosage for all cycloplegic drugs should be the lowest concentration that will satisfactorily achieve the desired cycloplegia. To overmedicate when maximum cycloplegia has been reached increases the probability of systemic drug absorption and the risk of side effects.

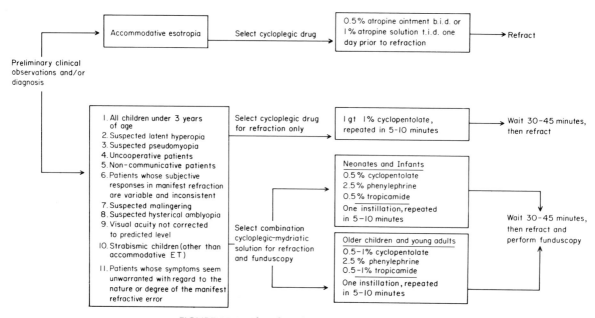

FIGURE 17.1 **Flowchart for cycloplegic refraction.**

Following cycloplegic examination, some clinicians advise the use of a miotic such as pilocarpine to hasten departure of the cycloplegic effect. However, miotic application can cause ciliary spasm, browache, and an increased risk of angle-closure glaucoma by the pupillary-block mechanism. Furthermore, when Nelson and Orton[20] assessed the effects of 2% pilocarpine in countering cycloplegia, they found no significant difference in the decrease of pupil size or the rate of return of accommodation. Distance vision was actually worsened in some subjects. Thus, it is best simply to dispense disposable mydriatic sunglasses to the patient and let the cycloplegic effect run its natural course.[6,21,22] The patient or parent should be advised regarding the expected dilated pupils, increased sensitivity to light, and blurred vision.

Refractive Techniques

After the cycloplegic has been instilled and the time limit for maximum cycloplegia has been reached, the clinician must decide if the degree of cycloplegia is adequate to permit reliable refraction. Reinecke and Herm[23] have described 2 methods of measuring monocular residual accommodation.

1. Lens powers are changed while the patient observes a near accommodative target such as a reading card positioned at a fixed fixation distance. For example, if the eye under cycloplegia cannot read print at 40 cm until a +2.50 D lens is placed over the distance correction, and the print remains clear until the addition of a +4.00 D lens, the residual accommodation is 1.50 D.

2. Another method is to place a +2.50 D lens over the distance correction and then move the print from 40 cm, first away from the eye and then toward the eye, until it blurs in each direction. If the print is clear between 50 cm and 20 cm from the eye, the patient has 3.00 D of residual accommodation.

Of course, these tests are often impossible to perform on the very patients who require cycloplegia, and the experienced clinician quickly learns to use the retinoscope to judge accommodative activity. If residual accommodation exceeds 2.00 D, cycloplegic refraction may be unreliable and inaccurate.[14,24–26]

After the cycloplegia has been determined to be clinically satisfactory, retinoscopy should be performed before the child becomes restless. The best guideline for retinoscopy is to neutralize the central 4 mm of the pupil, ignoring the movement in the periphery, which may be confusing and distracting because of spherical aberration associated with the dilated pupil. A retinoscope light of low to medium intensity will help to reduce such aberrations. The patient should fixate a distant target if the cycloplegia is not completely adequate. However, if the cycloplegia is complete, the patient may fixate directly at the retinoscope light without jeopardizing the retinoscopic result. In addition,

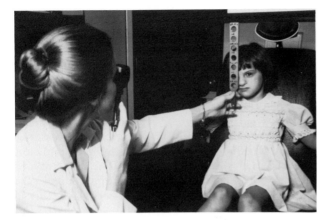

FIGURE 17.2 **Cycloplegic retinoscopy of young child. (Courtesy Jimmy D. Bartlett, O.D.)**

the retinoscope should be as close to the visual axis as possible to avoid errors associated with spherical aberration. It is often difficult to perform retinoscopy on young children through a phoroptor. Instead, loose, hand-held trial lenses or lens bars can be used to facilitate retinoscopy of the young child or infant (Fig. 17.2).

Following retinoscopy, subjective refraction should be attempted. Although a subjective refraction often cannot be performed on many young patients because of lack of maturity and cooperation, it should be attempted when possible. The practitioner should note that spherical aberration can cause errors in the subjective refraction just as it does in retinoscopy.

Spectacle Prescribing

The prescribing of spectacle lenses from cycloplegic findings is truly an art rather than an exact science and thus places great demands on the clinician's judgment, skill, and experience. In many cases determination of the final spectacle prescription is straightforward, but in other cases it requires considerable thought and judgment. Since the ultimate criterion for a satisfactory and successful prescription is relief of patient symptoms, guidelines for spectacle prescribing are necessarily somewhat broad and imprecise. Nevertheless, the following recommendations represent the most widely accepted approaches to spectacle prescribing.

In accommodative esotropia, the full amount of plus lens correction determined by retinoscopy should be prescribed in children younger than 4 years of age. With older children, the plus power can be reduced as long as fusion is maintained. Chapter 28 considers additional guidelines for prescribing spectacles to patients with accommodative esotropia.

Before prescribing lenses for the nonstrabismic patient, the clinician must consider the patient's symptoms. Conservative prescribing, if any, should be the rule in asymptomatic patients. However, for patients with significant symptoms such as asthenopia or reading difficulty, the prescribing of lens powers closer to the cycloplegic amount is indicated. In the vast majority of patients over age 20 years, there is usually very close agreement between the cycloplegic and manifest refractive findings, especially in myopic patients. However, in children the cycloplegic refraction nearly always reveals more plus power in hyperopia than does the manifest refraction, while for myopia the 2 procedures produce more equivalent results.[27] Therefore, for nonstrabismic patients most practitioners usually prescribe the full amount of astigmatic (cylinder power and axis) or myopic correction found by cycloplegic retinoscopy.

In patients with latent hyperopia but no esotropia, a reduced amount of plus lens power should be prescribed to compensate for intrinsic ciliary muscle tonus.[28] A reduction of plus lens power is essential in hyperopic patients who have been accustomed to accommodating 2 to 3 D or more to compensate for their refractive error, because full correcting lenses will result in blurred distance vision and will not be readily accepted. The results from the cycloplegic examination can be used as a guide to a postcycloplegic manifest refraction performed on a different day. This is often helpful to determine, by cyclodamic techniques, the amount of plus lens power actually accepted by the patient.

Since considerable judgment is involved in evaluating and prescribing from cycloplegic findings in patients with latent hyperopia but without accommodative esotropia, it is difficult to give specific guidelines for use in individual clinical circumstances. Mitchell[29] recommends reducing the hyperopic prescription 1.00 D on nonstrabismic atropinized patients, while Reinecke and Herm[23] suggest a 2.00 D subtraction for such patients. As a broad general guideline for use with 1% cyclopentolate, a satisfactory prescription may often be derived by simply reducing the dioptric power according to patient age as shown in Table 17.4.[30] Perhaps a more accurate approach, however, is to prescribe not only according to patient age but also by considering the difference between the manifest and cycloplegic findings, as suggested in Table 17.5. The greater the difference between the manifest and cycloplegic refractions, the greater should be the reduction in plus lens correction.

Regardless of the method used to determine the amount of plus lens correction, a further reduction in power can often be made in accordance with the guidelines ordinarily governing the prescribing of corrections for hyperopia. Prepresbyopic hyperopic patients are

TABLE 17.4
Amount Deducted in Hyperopia Using 1% Cyclopentolate

Age (yr)	Amount Deducted (D)
0–6	1.00
10	0.75
15	0.50
20	0.25
30	0–0.25
40	0

Adapted from Tait EC. Pediatric ophthalmology, Philadelphia: W.B. Saunders Co, 1975.

usually more comfortable with a partial correction than a full correction for their first prescription for the following reasons[29]:

- When some of the plus lens power is subtracted from the cycloplegic refraction, it is easier for accommodation to relax and allow the spectacle lens to compensate for the refractive error. Distance visual acuity is less blurred, and patient cooperation is easier to obtain, especially from the young patient.
- A partial correction does not so violently upset the habitual relationship existing between accommodation and convergence. The abrupt changes made in this relationship by full plus lens correction may give rise to as much discomfort as was associated with the original problem.
- A partial correction forces the patient to accommodate to overcome the uncorrected portion of the refractive error. This may keep the amplitude of

TABLE 17.5
Plus Lens Correction Prescribed for Latent Hyperopia

Manifest Refraction (D)	Cycloplegic Refraction (D)		
	1.00	2.50	5.00
Age 5 years			
Plano	1.00	2.00	4.00
1.00	1.00	2.00	4.00
2.00	a	2.00	4.50
Age 12 years			
Plano	1.00	2.00	3.50
1.00	1.00	2.00	4.00
2.00	a	2.00	4.00
Age 25 years			
Plano	1.00	1.50	3.00
1.00	1.00	2.00	3.50
2.00	a	2.00	4.00

aNot applicable.

accommodation higher and does not allow the patient to become totally dependent on the hyperopic prescription. This can be a significant advantage when the prescription may not be worn, as in sporting events or social functions.

When the final spectacle prescription is dispensed, a mild cycloplegic such as 0.5% cyclopentolate or 0.5% to 1.0% tropicamide may be prescribed if necessary to permit the patient with latent hyperopia to more easily accept the plus lens correction.[31–33] The dosage should gradually be tapered (e.g., 1.0% tropicamide 4 times daily for 1 day, 3 times daily for 1 day, twice daily for 1 day, once daily for 1 day, then discontinued). The clinical procedure for cycloplegic refraction is summarized in Figure 17.1.

Adverse Reactions

Most reactions to cycloplegic agents can be classified as either drug allergy (hypersensitivity) or toxicity. Hypersensitivity reactions to topically applied cycloplegics are usually unexpected responses[34] and are most commonly seen as dermatologic eruptions of the skin of the eyelids. The sequence of toxic drug reactions, however, often follows a predictable pattern. Although the incidence of adverse reactions to cycloplegic agents administered in recommended doses is low, local ocular as well as systemic reactions can occur. These are discussed in detail in Chapters 3 and 31.

References

1. Michaels DD. Visual optics and refraction: A clinical approach. St. Louis: C.V. Mosby Co, 1980;2:523.
2. Maino JH, Cibis GW, Cress P, et al. Noncycloplegic vs cycloplegic retinoscopy in pre-school children. Ann Ophthalmol 1984;16:880–882.
3. Duke-Elder S, Abrams D. System of ophthalmology. Duke-Elder S, ed. St. Louis: C.V. Mosby Co, 1970;5:387.
4. Van Herick W, Shaffer RN, Schwartz A. Estimation of width of angle of anterior chamber. Am J Ophthalmol 1969;68:626–629.
5. Lichter PR. Gonioscopy. In: Duane TD, ed. Clinical ophthalmology. Hagerstown, MD: Harper & Row, 1987;3:Chap. 44:1–19.
6. Milder B, Rubin M. The fine art of prescribing glasses. Gainesville, FL: Triad Scientific, 1980;3:44–51.
7. Havener WH. Ocular pharmacology. St. Louis: C.V. Mosby Co, 1978;4:244–261.
8. Priestly BS, Medine M. A new mydriatic and cycloplegic drug. Compound 75 GT. Am J Ophthalmol 1951;34:572–575.

9. Beitel RJ. Cycloplegic refraction. In: Duane TD, ed. Clinical ophthalmology. Hagerstown, MD: Harper & Row, 1981;1: Chap. 41:2.

10. Michaels DD. Visual optics and refraction. St. Louis: C.V. Mosby Co, 1980;2:318.

11. Miranda MN. Residual accommodation. A comparison between cyclopentolate 1% and a combination of cyclopentolate 1% and tropicamide 1%. Arch Ophthalmol 1972;87:515–517.

12. Gettes BC. Tropicamide, a new cycloplegic mydriatic. Arch Ophthalmol 1961;65:632–635.

13. Pollack SL, Hunt JS, Polse KA. Dose-response effects of tropicamide HCl. Am J Optom Physiol Opt 1981;58:361–366.

14. Gettes BC, Belmont O. Tropicamide: comparative cycloplegic effects. Arch Ophthalmol 1961;66:336–340.

15. Ingram RM, Barr A. Refraction of 1-year-old children after cycloplegia with 1% cyclopentolate: comparison with findings after atropinisation. Br J Ophthalmol 1979;63:348–352.

16. Rosenbaum AL, Bateman JB, Bremer DL, et al. Cycloplegic refraction in esotropic children. Ophthalmology 1981;88:1031–1034.

17. Keller JT, Chang FW. An evaluation of the use of topical anesthetics and low concentrations of phenylephrine HCl for mydriasis. J Am Optom Assoc 1976;47:753.

18. Kubo DJ, Wing TW, Polse KA, Jauregui MJ. Mydriatic effects using low concentrations of phenylephrine hydrochloride. J Am Optom Assoc 1975;46:817–822.

19. Hopkins GA, Lyle WM. Potential systemic side effects of six common ophthalmic drugs. J Am Optom Assoc 1977; 48:1241–1245.

20. Nelson ME, Orton DBO. Counteracting the effects of mydriatics. Arch Ophthalmol 1987;105:486–489.

21. Kolker AE, Heatherington J. Becker-Shaffer's diagnosis and therapy of the glaucomas. St. Louis: C.V. Mosby Co, 1976;4:183–207.

22. Bartlett JD. Administration of and adverse reactions to cycloplegic agents. Am J Optom Physiol Opt 1978;55:229.

23. Reinecke RD, Herm RJ. Refraction. New York: Appleton-Century-Crofts, 1976;2:48–171.

24. Prangen AD. What constitutes satisfactory cycloplegia. Am J Ophthalmol 1931;14:667.

25. Stine GT. Clinical investigation of a new cycloplegic and mydriatic drug. Eye Ear Nose Throat Monthly 1960;22:11–14.

26. Milder B. Tropicamide as a cycloplegic agent. Arch Ophthalmol 1961;66:70–72.

27. Shultz L. Variations in refractive changes induced by Cyclogyl upon children with differing degrees of ametropia. Am J Optom Physiol Opt 1975;52:482–484.

28. Amos DM. Cycloplegics for refraction. Am J Optom Physiol Opt 1978;55:223–226.

29. Mitchell DWA. The use of drugs in refraction. London: The Hereford Times Ltd, 1960;2:57.

30. Tait EC. Pediatric ophthalmology, Philadelphia: W.B. Saunders Co., 1975.

31. Milder B, Rubin M. The fine art of prescribing glasses. Gainesville, FL: Triad Scientific, 1980;2:28–30.

32. Duke-Elder S, Abrams D. System of ophthalmology. Duke-Elder S, ed. St. Louis: C.V. Mosby Co, 1970;5:451–486.

33. Silbert J, Alexander A. Cyclotherapy in the treatment of symptomatic latent hyperopia. J Am Optom Assoc 1987;58:40–46.

34. Ellis PP. Ocular therapeutics and pharmacology. St. Louis: C.V. Mosby Co., 1981:6.

35. Mordi JA, Lyle WM, Mousa GY. Does prior instillation of a topical anesthetic enhance the effect of tropicamide? Am J Optom Physiol Opt 1986;63:290–293.

CHAPTER 18

Abnormalities of the Pupil

Jimmy D. Bartlett

The practitioner can often quickly and easily differentiate the site of impairment in patients with anisocoria by instilling into the eyes various drugs affecting the autonomic nervous system. Since almost all patients with anisocoria have no evidence of significant neurologic disease, these patients can be appropriately evaluated and managed by the optometrist or ophthalmologist without the necessity for neurologic consultation. This chapter considers those diseases or conditions characterized by anisocoria that are most often encountered in ophthalmic practice. The clinical and pharmacologic evaluations of these disorders, as well as appropriate patient management, are discussed.

Clinical Evaluation of Anisocoria

A variety of clinical conditions can exhibit anisocoria as a primary or secondary feature. The most common disorders with unequal pupils as a primary diagnostic sign are listed in Table 18.1. Some of these conditions, such as physiologic (essential) anisocoria, are benign and have an excellent prognosis. Others, such as third-nerve palsy, can indicate significant intracranial disease and may carry a grave prognosis. Although a discussion of all conditions associated with anisocoria is beyond the scope of this chapter, those disorders that most easily lend themselves to evaluation by clinical and pharmacologic methods will be emphasized. These conditions have in common that *only one* pupil is involved and that the basic underlying abnormality manifests itself as an inability of the affected pupil either to *dilate* or to *constrict*. Consequently, either the sympathetic or the parasympathetic nervous system can be

implicated, and various drugs affecting the autonomic nervous system may thus be used to pharmacologically differentiate the site of impairment. The disorders that are most easily evaluated pharmacologically, in which only one pupil is abnormal, are identified in Table 18.1.

The initial clinical evaluation of the patient with unequal pupils will frequently allow diagnosis of the underlying condition without resorting to pharmacologic or other more elaborate methods of examination. Thus, the practitioner must perform the appropriate clinical examination of the patient as the initial phase of the evaluation.

Pupil Size

In addition to the customary evaluation of pupillary function (direct reflexes and evaluation for Marcus Gunn sign), pupil size must be measured accurately. This may be accomplished with flash photography, or it can be accurately estimated using the area of the pupil rather than its diameter.[1] The black semicircles found on rulers and near reading cards are suitable for this purpose and are preferred over simple millimeter rules.

Light Reaction

In testing the response to direct light, if one pupil responds poorly, this clearly indicates the abnormal pupil. Differential diagnosis includes third-nerve palsy, anticholinergic mydriasis, Adie's pupil, or local iris disease. If the light reaction is good in each eye, dif-

TABLE 18.1
Disorders Characterized by Anisocoria

- Physiologic (essential) anisocoria
- Alternating contraction anisocoria
- Claude Bernard syndrome
- Horner's syndrome[a]
- Episodic unilateral mydriasis
- Adie's syndrome[a]
- Third-nerve palsy[a]
- Adrenergic mydriasis
- Anticholinergic mydriasis[a]
- Argyll Robertson pupils
- Local iris disease (sphincter atrophy, posterior synechiae, etc.)
- Hutchinson's pupil
- Angle-closure glaucoma

[a]Disorders that are most easily evaluated pharmacologically, in which usually only one pupil is abnormal.

ferential diagnosis includes Horner's syndrome or physiologic anisocoria.

Nature of Anisocoria in Light versus Dark

A comparison of the anisocoria in bright and dim ambient illuminations may be helpful in reaching a diagnosis by clinical means alone. Although use of a semidarkened room facilitates the clinical evaluation of unequal pupils, this method is often self-defeating when the patient has dark irides, since there is poor contrast between the iris and the pupil. This problem can be overcome by using an ultraviolet light in a completely darkened room.[2,3] The technique employs the principle of lenticular fluorescence from ultraviolet

stimulation and involves instrumentation that is readily available in most ophthalmic and general medical offices. The ultraviolet light source (such as a Burton lamp) should be held 8 to 12 inches from the patient so that the visible emission will not stimulate pupillary activity.[2] If the anisocoria increases in darkness, the differential diagnosis includes Horner's syndrome or physiologic anisocoria (Fig. 18.1). In Horner's syndrome the oculosympathetic paresis does not allow the iris dilator to function properly in darkness; consequently, the anisocoria increases as the normal pupil dilates in response to darkness. Although no autonomic nervous system abnormalities exist in physiologic anisocoria, this benign condition also exhibits increased anisocoria in darkness.

If the anisocoria is greater in the light than in darkness, this generally indicates an abnormal parasympathetic innervation to the iris sphincter (see Fig. 18.1). Differential diagnosis includes Adie's pupil, iris sphincter atrophy (possibly associated with previous anterior segment trauma), or any of the disorders implicated as a "unilateral fixed and dilated" pupil (third-nerve palsy, anticholinergic mydriasis, or Adie's pupil). Since the underlying abnormality is generally associated with the parasympathetic innervation to the iris sphincter, the abnormal (larger) pupil does not appropriately constrict to stimulation by light. The anisocoria is therefore greater in bright light than in dim illumination.

Slit-Lamp Examination

The clinician should carefully examine the physical characteristics of the iris with the biomicroscope for evidence of mechanical restrictions of the pupils. Some

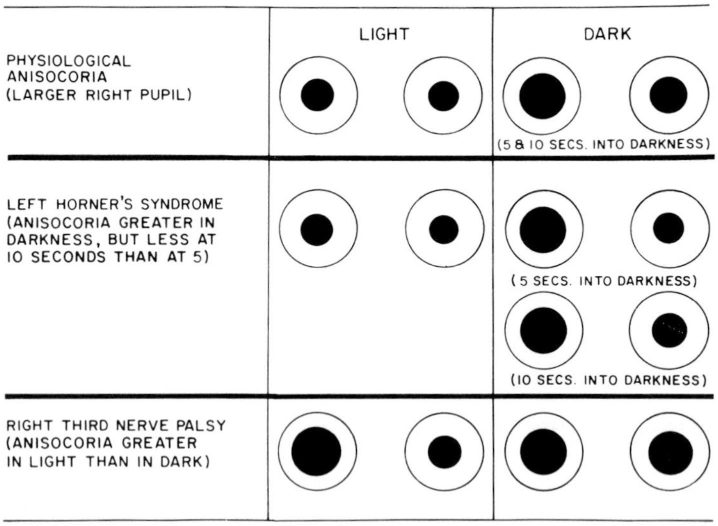

FIGURE 18.1 **Use of light and dark illumination in differentiating the various causes of anisocoria.**

patients have iris damage due to previous ocular inflammation or trauma. Careful evaluation may uncover subtle areas of posterior synechiae that immobilize the pupil. Iris sphincter atrophy can also be detected by careful biomicroscopic examination. Furthermore, careful examination of the iris may reveal sector palsies with associated vermiform movements, indicating Adie's pupil.

Inspection of Photographs

Frequently the question arises whether the anisocoria is recent or long-standing. Patients are often quite insistent that their newly found condition is of recent onset. In such cases, examination of personal photographs (both recent and old) may indicate with some certainty the onset and duration of the condition.

Associated Ocular or Systemic Findings

Diagnostic physical findings are often associated with the observed anisocoria. For example, the existence of ipsilateral ptosis and facial anhydrosis are highly suggestive of Horner's syndrome and allow such a diagnosis without the need for pharmacologic confirmation. In addition, a history of sympathectomy with subsequent unilateral ptosis, anhydrosis, and miosis are all consistent with a diagnosis of Horner's syndrome. On the other hand, the patient with a unilateral sluggish pupil with associated accommodative insufficiency and diminished deep tendon reflexes may be strongly suspected of having Adie's syndrome, especially if these are of recent onset in a healthy young adult female.

Thus, careful pupillary examination, with special attention paid to the patient's history as well as to other ocular or systemic physical findings, may allow the practitioner to establish the diagnosis without resorting to pharmacologic or other more sophisticated methods of examination. When the findings are ambiguous, however, or if insufficient clinical information is available to establish the diagnosis with certainty, pharmacologic evaluations should be performed as discussed in the following sections.

Guidelines for the Pharmacologic Evaluation of Anisocoria

When the patient's history is incomplete or noncontributory, or when the clinical signs and symptoms are too ambiguous to enable a definitive diagnosis, the practitioner should proceed with pharmacologic test-ing. Pharmacologic evaluation of unequal pupils is easily and quickly accomplished in the office and frequently obviates further neuroradiologic or laboratory investigations.

Adherence to the following general guidelines will facilitate pharmacologic evaluation and improve the accuracy with which the drugs allow a definitive diagnosis.[4-6]

- One drop of the indicated drug should be instilled into each eye and repeated after several minutes. This ensures adequate drug application if the first drop is removed by tearing.
- The drops should always be instilled into *both* eyes so that the reaction of the affected pupil can be compared with that of the normal pupil. If the condition is bilateral, as in anticholinergic mydriasis caused by systemic agents, the drop should be placed in only *one* eye so that the response of each pupil can be compared.
- The patient's general status can influence the size of the pupils. A change in alertness, either toward arousal or somnolence, can affect the "before" and "after" comparisons. If the patient becomes uncomfortable or anxious while waiting for the drug to act, both pupils may dilate. If the patient becomes drowsy, both pupils may constrict. In the case of Adie's pupil, drowsiness may constrict the normal pupil more than the Adie's pupil. This fact emphasizes the importance of instilling the drug into both eyes so that one pupil always serves as a control when only one pupil is affected.
- In testing for hypersensitivity to cholinergic or adrenergic drugs, the amount of ambient illumination before and after drug instillation must be constant.
- Accommodation should be carefully controlled during the "before" and "after" evaluations so that it can be eliminated as a factor producing the change in pupil size.
- The use of photography is highly recommended to enable a more accurate evaluation of pupil size both before and after instillation of the indicated drug. Frequently an accuracy of 0.1 mm can be obtained using flash photography.[7] Since appropriate patient management depends on accurate diagnosis, the practitioner should not simply estimate the differences in pupil size because this may lead to an incorrect diagnosis.

Physiologic Anisocoria

Clearly the most common condition characterized by unequal pupils is physiologic (essential) anisocoria. Depending on how it is defined, this condition is found in from 1% to more than 50% of the general population.[8,9] It is seldom greater than 1 mm and can be variable, changing from day to day or even from hour to hour.[9,10] The clinical and pharmacologic features of physiologic anisocoria are listed in Table 18.2.

Horner's Syndrome

In 1869 Johann Friedrich Horner, a Swiss physician, described the findings now associated with the syndrome bearing his name.[11] Although the case reported by Horner was caused by a preganglionic lesion, the term "Horner's syndrome" is now used to refer to any oculosympathetic palsy or paresis.

Etiology

The fibers comprising the oculosympathetic pathway have a long and tortuous course from the hypothalamus to the eye (see Fig. 3.6). Since a variety of vascular, traumatic, or neoplastic lesions can interrupt this pathway and produce the signs characteristic of Horner's syndrome, it is important to understand the clinical anatomy to appropriately evaluate and manage patients with lesions of the oculosympathetic pathway. This sympathetic pathway can be divided into three portions:

1. The central (first-order) neuron originates in the hypothalamus, courses through the brainstem and cervical cord, and terminates at the ciliospinal center of Budge at C8–T2.
2. The preganglionic (second-order) neuron is located in the chest and neck and extends from the cervical cord (C8–T2) through the stellate ganglion at the pulmonary apex to the superior cervical ganglion at the bifurcation of the internal and external carotid arteries.
3. The postganglionic (third-order) neuron originates at the superior cervical ganglion, located at the level

TABLE 18.2
Clinical and Pharmacologic Features of Physiologic Anisocoria

---

- Constricts briskly to light
- No dilation lag in darkness
- No disturbed psychosensory dilation
- Dilates normally with cocaine
- Exhibits greater anisocoria in darkness than in light

---

of the angle of the jaw, and travels through the internal carotid plexus until it penetrates the base of the skull, passes through the cavernous sinus, and accompanies the long ciliary nerves to the dilator muscle of the iris. Postganglionic sympathetic fibers also innervate Mueller's muscle of the upper and lower lids.

The sympathetic fibers for sweating that innervate the face leave the superior cervical ganglion, follow the *external* carotid artery, and are therefore not involved in lesions of the carotid plexus. In some patients, however, a portion of the sympathetic fibers to the sweat glands in the ipsilateral forehead may follow the branches of the *internal* carotid artery, allowing a lesion of the postganglionic oculosympathetic pathway to produce a small area of anhydrosis above the brow.[12]

The most common causes of Horner's syndrome are listed in Table 18.3.[12–19] Maloney and associates[20] retrospectively studied 450 patients with Horner's syndrome and were able to determine the cause for the sympathetic paresis in only 60% of the patients. Of the patients for whom no cause was determined, 35% were reexamined from 6 months to 28 years after the initial finding of Horner's syndrome, and the cause was still not discovered in any patient, indicating that, whatever the cause, the lesion probably was a benign and stable process.

The prevalence of malignant tumors as a cause of Horner's syndrome has been a subject of considerable discussion. The distribution of various tumors causing Horner's syndrome is shown in Table 18.4. In the study reported by Giles and Henderson,[21] the most common cause of Horner's syndrome was neoplasia, which was more often malignant than benign. The most common tumor was bronchogenic carcinoma, usually of the upper lobes (Pancoast's tumor). In contrast, in the series of patients reported by Maloney and associates,[20] fewer than 3% of patients with Horner's syndrome had malignancies.

It has been generally recognized that most lesions causing Horner's syndrome involve the preganglionic neuron.[21] Patients with such lesions may have a lung or breast malignancy that has spread to the thoracic outlet. There may also be a history of surgery or trauma to the neck, chest, or cervical spine. In one study,[21] nonoperative trauma was the etiologic factor in 13% of the cases of preganglionic Horner's syndrome. These included injuries to the brachial plexus due primarily to birth trauma or to automobile accidents.

Only recently has the etiologic significance of the postganglionic Horner's syndrome been clarified.[12,14] As can be seen from Figure 18.2, patients with acute

TABLE 18.3
Etiologies of Horner's Syndrome[12–19,68,74]

Central	Preganglionic	Postganglionic
Basal meningitis	Spinal birth injury	Abnormalities of the internal carotid artery
Pituitary tumor	Tuberculosis	Unilateral vascular headache syndromes
Tumor of third ventricle	Pancoast's tumor	Direct or indirect trauma
Syphilis of midbrain	Aortic aneurysm	Spontaneous or traumatic occlusion
Tumor of pons	Enlarged mediastinal glands	Aneurysms
Syringobulbia	Enlargement of thyroid	Atherosclerosis
Syringomyelia	Lymphadenopathy	Spontaneous dissection
Cervical cord trauma	Thoracic neuroblastoma	Lesions involving the middle cranial fossa and
and tumors	Pulmonary mucormycosis	cavernous sinus
Spinal tabes		Basal skull fractures
Poliomyelitis		Locally invasive neoplasms (meningiomas, etc.)
Stroke		Metastatic neoplasms
Multiple sclerosis		Inflammation of adjacent structures
		Tolosa-Hunt syndrome
		Otitis media
		Trigeminal herpes zoster
		Sinusitis

postganglionic Horner's syndrome can be divided into those without pain and those with pain of the typical cluster headache variety or with pain atypical of cluster headache. The presence of a unilateral headache in a patient with acquired Horner's syndrome therefore helps to localize the lesion to the postganglionic sympathetic pathway, especially if there are no other signs or symptoms of brainstem involvement.[12]

Although most lesions producing postganglionic Horner's syndrome are benign, a variety of potentially serious conditions may interrupt the postganglionic sympathetic pathway (see Table 18.3). Neoplasia as an underlying cause of postganglionic Horner's syndrome is relatively rare. These lesions include nasopharyngeal tumors, meningiomas of the middle cranial fossa, or carcinomas invading from the sphenoid sinus. In one series[12] nearly half the patients with unilateral headache

had typical cluster headache. In these patients the Horner's syndrome is generally believed to result from compromise of the postganglionic oculosympathetic fibers as they course with the sheaths surrounding a swollen internal carotid artery in the bony petrous canal.

The patient's age at the time of onset is an important aid to the clinician investigating a Horner's syndrome of unknown etiology. From birth to age 20 years, trauma is the leading cause in most cases. From 21 to 50 years, almost half the cases result from tumors. In the older age group (51 years of age and older), neoplasia is the most important cause.[21]

Diagnosis

Clinical Evaluation

The primary clinical signs diagnostic of Horner's syndrome are listed in Table 18.5. Although the complete syndrome is quite dramatic, it is only rarely encountered, and diagnosis based on the patient's clinical signs alone can therefore be difficult.

Since Mueller's muscle, which is innervated by oculosympathetic fibers, assists in elevation of the upper lid, interruption of the sympathetic innervation to this muscle results in some degree of ptosis. The degree of ptosis varies. In some patients ptosis may be completely absent, in others it may be substantial, and in some it can worsen with fatigue. If the lesion is located centrally (i.e., in the first-order neuron), the only sign clinically observable may be pupillary constriction,

TABLE 18.4
Tumors Causing Horner's Syndrome[20,21]

Benign	Malignant
Neuroma-neurofibroma	Bronchogenic carcinoma
Thyroid adenoma	Metastatic carcinoma
Meningioma	Sarcoma
Dermal cyst	Hodgkin's lymphoma
Osteoma	Thyroid carcinoma
Pituitary adenoma	Neuroblastoma
	Lacrimal gland
	carcinoma
	Pharyngeal carcinoma

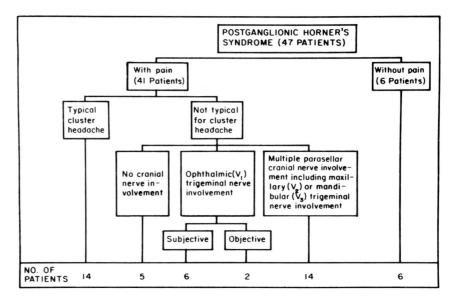

FIGURE 18.2 **Characteristics of patients with the acute onset of postganglionic Horner's syndrome seen at the University of Iowa between 1969 and 1975. Forty-one patients had associated unilateral headache, and 6 patients had no associated pain. Twenty-five patients had no associated parasellar cranial nerve involvement, 8 had involvement of the ophthalmic division of the trigeminal nerve only, and 14 had multiple parasellar cranial nerve involvement. (From Grimson BS, Thompson HS. Raeder's syndrome. A clinical review. Surv Ophthalmol 1980; 24:199–210, with permission of the authors and publisher.)**

without ptosis.[3,22] In contrast, if the lesion is located in the cervical sympathetic region, it is possible that all the signs comprising the syndrome, including ptosis, may be present.[3] However, the clinician should not misinterpret the partial ptosis of Horner's syndrome for retraction of the contralateral lid, since the patient can employ the levator or frontalis muscles to elevate the ptotic lid. The practitioner should simply cover the eye that does not appear to display lid retraction, and, if Horner's syndrome is present, the covered eye will manifest a ptosis.[23]

Since sympathetically innervated smooth muscle fibers also exist in the lower lid, oculosympathetic paresis can produce elevation of the lower lid ("upside-down ptosis"). This is often subtle, but this sign, along with ptosis of the upper lid, contributes to a narrowing of the palpebral fissure, giving the appearance of enophthalmos.[73]

Disruption of the sympathetic innervation to the iris dilator enables the parasympathetically innervated iris sphincter to have the predominant action on the iris,

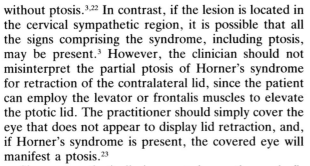

TABLE 18.5
Diagnostic Signs in Horner's Syndrome

- Unilateral ptosis
- Elevation ("upside-down ptosis") of the lower lid
- Narrowed palpebral fissure (apparent enophthalmos)
- Ipsilateral miosis
- Dilation lag
- Absence of dilation to psychosensory stimuli
- Conjunctival hyperemia
- Facial or body anhydrosis
- Heterochromia iridis, if congenital

thus producing miosis. The degree of anisocoria, however, may not be constant in any given patient, since the pupil size can vary with completeness of the syndrome, location of the lesion, patient alertness, ambient illumination, degree of denervation hypersensitivity, patient fixation, and concentration of the neurotransmitter substances.[3]

An extremely helpful sign in the clinical diagnosis of Horner's syndrome is *dilation lag,* in which the pupil fails to redilate quickly to its original size when a bright light is extinguished. This can be easily evaluated by comparing the dilation time in each eye.[22] Following a bright stimulus the normal pupil will return to its original darkness diameter in approximately 12 to 15 seconds, with about 90% of the dilation occurring during the first 5 to 6 seconds. This includes pupils associated with physiologic anisocoria. The Horner's pupil, however, requires approximately 25 seconds to return to its original darkness diameter, reaching about 90% of its final diameter within the first 10 to 15 seconds. The maximum difference between the normal pupil and Horner's pupil on dark dilation occurs after 4 to 5 seconds of darkness. This difference is an expression of the dilation lag that is pathognomonic of Horner's syndrome. Flash Polaroid photographs should first be taken after the patient has been in bright light for a few minutes, then in darkness 4 to 5 seconds after the light has been extinguished, and then finally in darkness 10 to 12 seconds after the light has been extinguished (Fig. 18.3). The criteria for recognizing dilation lag are (1) poor dilation of the more miotic pupil at 4 to 5 seconds compared with the dilation achieved after 10 to 12 seconds of darkness, and (2) increased anisocoria in darkness, more marked at 4 to 5 seconds than at 10 to 12 seconds.

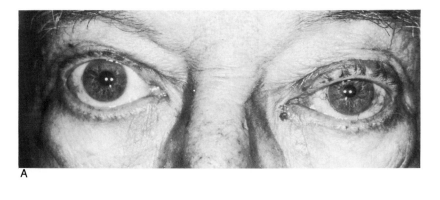

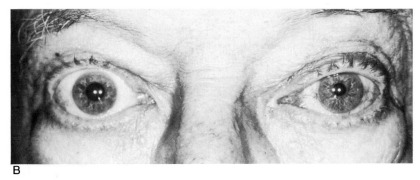

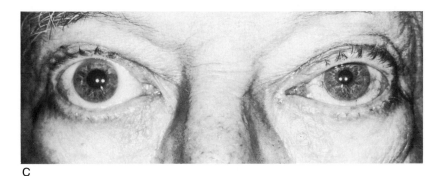

FIGURE 18.3   **Dilation lag in 72-year-old male with left Horner's syndrome.** *(A)* **Obvious anisocoria in bright illumination. Note greater anisocoria at 4 to 5 seconds in darkness** *(B)* **compared with the anisocoria at 10 to 12 seconds in darkness** *(C).*

Conjunctival hyperemia is usually a transient clinical sign and is observed only in the acute phase of Horner's syndrome, usually disappearing after the first several weeks.[24]

Since sweating is mediated by sympathetic innervation, interruption of these fibers results in facial or body anhydrosis, but lesions involving the postganglionic sympathetic pathway generally cause Horner's syndrome without anhydrosis.[22]

The finding of heterochromia iridis indicates congenital or neonatal Horner's syndrome. Normal pigmentation of the iris appears to be associated in some way with the integrity of the cervical sympathetic nervous system. Pigmentation of the iris is not complete until age 2 years. Hypopigmentation of the iris on the

side of the lesion is a characteristic feature of spinal birth injury involving the preganglionic (second-order) neuron.[22] Oculosympathetic paresis occurring after 2 years of age generally does not result in heterochromia. Table 18.6 shows the clinical characteristics of a series of 450 patients with Horner's syndrome studied retrospectively.[20] Of the patients with heterochromia, 77% had Horner's syndrome of congenital origin, and none had disease of recent onset. Thus, heterochromia associated with Horner's syndrome appears to indicate a long-standing sympathetic denervation.[20]

The term *Raeder's syndrome* is used to designate any painful postganglionic Horner's syndrome.[14] The pain may be characterized by a unilateral headache or facial pain in the distribution of the trigeminal nerve.

TABLE 18.6
Clinical Characteristics of 450 Patients with Horner's Syndrome

Sign	Prevalence (%)
Miosis	98[a]
Ptosis	88
Anhydrosis	4
Heterochromia	3

[a]Most authors consider the prevalence of clinically detectable anisocoria to be 100%.

Adapted from Maloney WF, Younge BR, Moyer NJ. Evaluation of the causes and accuracy of pharmacologic localization in Horner's syndrome. Am J Ophthalmol 1980;90:394–402.

Patients with Raeder's syndrome can be divided into 3 major groups[14]: (1) those with either multiple parasellar cranial nerve involvement (III, IV, V, VI) or involvement of the second, third, or all three divisions of the trigeminal nerve; (2) those with a typical history of cluster headache; and (3) those with a pain history that is not typical of cluster headache, who may also have involvement of the first (ophthalmic) division of the trigeminal nerve only. Common to all 3 groups of patients is the association of unilateral headache with the interruption of the postganglionic oculosympathetic fibers along the course of the internal carotid artery. The significance of Raeder's syndrome and its 3 major subclasses becomes apparent with regard to the strategies used in patient management.

Pharmacologic Evaluation

The decision to proceed with pharmacologic testing is based solely on the clinical findings.[3,25] If there is une-

quivocally no ptosis and no dilation lag, the anisocoria can be considered to be physiologic, and the patient need not undergo pharmacologic evaluation. The patient who has minimal anisocoria with minimal ptosis, but without dilation lag, likewise can be considered to have physiologic anisocoria. If there are enough clinical findings, however, to highly suggest the possibility of Horner's syndrome, such as definite ptosis but equivocal dilation lag, then the cocaine test is indicated to confirm the diagnosis.[25] If definite miosis exists in association with definite ptosis, and if there is also an unequivocal dilation lag, the diagnosis of Horner's syndrome can be made on clinical grounds, and the practitioner may proceed directly to the hydroxyamphetamine test. In some cases various clinical signs can have significant localizing value, enabling the clinician to tentatively identify the site of the lesion before proceeding with the pharmacologic testing (Table 18.7). The indications for pharmacologic testing in patients with suspected Horner's syndrome are summarized in Table 18.8.

COCAINE TEST

When topically applied, cocaine produces dilation of the pupil by preventing the reuptake of norepinephrine that has been released into the synaptic junctions of the iris dilator muscle in response to a nerve impulse. If the sympathetic innervation to the eye is interrupted at any level (central, preganglionic, or postganglionic), cocaine should theoretically have no mydriatic effect because in each case the flow of nerve impulses has been impeded and no endogenous norepinephrine is released.[5] However, when the lesion is in the brain stem or spinal cord (first-order neuron), mydriasis with cocaine may be impaired but not entirely abolished.

TABLE 18.7
Clinical Localizing Signs in Horner's Syndrome

Central Neuron Lesions	Preganglionic Neuron Lesions	Postganglionic Neuron Lesions
• Contralateral hypothesia of the body • Loss of sweating on entire half of body • Vertigo • Syringomyelia • Absence of ptosis	• Pain in ipsilateral arm or shoulder • Brachial plexus palsy • Pancoast's syndrome • Anhydrosis of face and neck • Flushing or blanching of face and neck • Thyroidectomy scar and hoarseness • Cervical osteoarthritis • Thoracic surgery	• Facial pain • No loss of sweating, except perhaps in supraorbital area

Modified from Pilley SFJ, Thompson HS. Pupillary "dilation lag" in Horner's syndrome. Br J Ophthalmol 1975;59:731–735.

TABLE 18.8
Indications for Pharmacologic Testing in Suspected Horner's Syndrome

Signs	Presumptive Clinical Diagnosis	Indicated Pharmacologic Testing
No ptosis No dilation lag[a]	Physiologic anisocoria	None
Minimal ptosis No dilation lag[a]	Physiologic anisocoria	None
Definite ptosis Equivocal dilation lag[a]	Horner's syndrome	Cocaine test followed by hydroxyamphetamine test
Definite ptosis Unequivocal dilation lag[a]	Horner's syndrome	Hydroxyamphetamine test

[a]Documented by photography.

This is due to incomplete interruption of the descending sympathetic pathway.[5] Thus, as a rule, *dilation with cocaine will be reduced or absent in any Horner's pupil regardless of the site of impairment.* Consequently, the cocaine test is useful as a screening procedure to confirm the presence or absence of oculosympathetic paresis, but *this test will not indicate the location of the lesion.* Although cocaine cannot be relied on to accurately localize the lesion,[5,12,20,24] it is quite dependable for its usefulness in indicating the existence of a lesion of the oculosympathetic pathway.

Thus, the cocaine test is reliable in most cases in confirming the initial diagnosis of Horner's syndrome.[24] To perform the test, 1 drop of cocaine solution should be instilled into each eye and repeated after several minutes, and the pupils should be evaluated after 30 to 45 minutes[27] (Fig. 18.4). Although 5% or 10% cocaine can be used, the latter is preferred, since weaker concentrations may require several hours before significant dilation is recognized in the normal pupil.[5,27] This is especially true for patients with dark irides, which may dilate very slowly and poorly.[27] The response to cocaine in 12 patients with Horner's syndrome is illustrated in Figure 18.5.

EPINEPHRINE TEST

In 1901 Langley[28] elucidated the physiologic properties of epinephrine, finding that this drug seemed to have the same effect on the eye as did stimulation of the cervical sympathetic nerve, but, unlike cocaine, epinephrine seemed to produce a more marked effect when the sympathetic nerves were interrupted. This observation eventually led to the discovery of the principle of denervation hypersensitivity. In 1910 Cords[29] described a patient with traumatic Horner's syndrome in which the pupil on the affected side dilated to extremely low concentrations of epinephrine. This observation led to the suggestion that it might be possible to pharmacologically distinguish postganglionic lesions from preganglionic lesions. Consequently, the use of epinephrine became a popular adjunct to cocaine in the diagnosis of Horner's syndrome. However, Morone and Andreani[30] and Jaffe[13] demonstrated that the hypersensitivity response to epinephrine is unreliable in differentiating between preganglionic and postganglionic etiologies of Horner's syndrome.

Because there are great individual differences in sensitivity to epinephrine, even repeated instillations

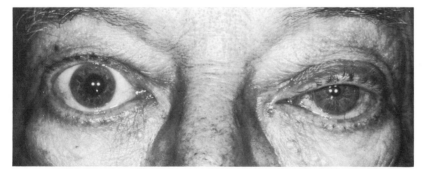

FIGURE 18.4 **Cocaine test for Horner's syndrome (same patient as in Fig. 18.3A). Following instillation of 10% cocaine into each eye, there is dilation of the normal right pupil but absence of dilation of the left Horner's pupil.**

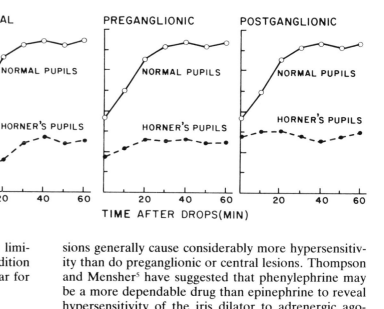

FIGURE 18.5 **Summary of mydriatic responses to 5% cocaine in 12 patients with unilateral Horner's syndrome. The mean dilation curves are shown for each group. The unaffected pupils (12 patients, open circles) dilated normally. All the Horner's pupils (3 central, 6 preganglionic, 3 postganglionic) showed impaired dilation. (Published with permission from The American Journal of Ophthalmology 72:472–480, 1971. Copyright by The Ophthalmic Publishing Company.)**

of this drug may give inconclusive results. This limitation, as well as others discussed in the first edition of this book, make the epinephrine test unpopular for use in clinical practice.[4]

PHENYLEPHRINE TEST

Theoretically, any adrenergic agonist that, in low concentrations, does not dilate the normal pupil can be used to demonstrate the denervation hypersensitivity in Horner's syndrome. Phenylephrine (Neo-Synephrine) is such a drug. When employed in a 1% concentration, phenylephrine will not dilate the normal pupil, but in the presence of sympathetic denervation it may produce mydriasis.[12,23] The 1% concentration is easily prepared by diluting commercially available formulations with extraocular irrigating solution or normal saline (Table 18.9). When phenylephrine is used to demonstrate denervation hypersensitivity, it is subject to the same limitations as is 1:1000 epinephrine. The clinician must judge the degree of hypersensitivity displayed by the iris dilator, since postganglionic le-

sions generally cause considerably more hypersensitivity than do preganglionic or central lesions. Thompson and Mensher[5] have suggested that phenylephrine may be a more dependable drug than epinephrine to reveal hypersensitivity of the iris dilator to adrenergic agonists. However, for correct interpretation of the hypersensitivity response, it must be established that the corneal penetration of phenylephrine has not been altered by tonometry, corneal sensitivity testing, or other clinical procedures that might compromise the corneal epithelium. Furthermore, the corneal epithelium might allow greater drug penetration if trigeminal nerve involvement is associated with a postganglionic Horner's syndrome, thus invalidating the test. Even when higher concentrations of phenylephrine are employed, the hypersensitive iris dilator of the Horner's pupil produces greater dilation than the iris dilator of the normal pupil. Thus, the phenomenon of denervation hypersensitivity can be elicited even without the use of low concentrations of adrenergic drugs. Figure 18.6 summarizes the mydriatic responses to 10% phenylephrine in a series of 12 patients with Horner's syndrome. Although in each instance both pupils of each patient dilated, dilation of the Horner's pupil was most dramatic in those patients with postganglionic lesions.

HYDROXYAMPHETAMINE TEST

In 1971 Thompson and Mensher[5] first suggested that the failure of hydroxyamphetamine (Paredrine) to dilate the postganglionic Horner's pupil could be used to distinguish patients with postganglionic lesions from patients with central or preganglionic lesions. The pharmacologic rationale for this use of hydroxyamphetamine as a localizing drug is sound, and the value of hydroxyamphetamine in localizing the lesion in Horner's syndrome has been established with some certainty.[5,20,31]

The localizing value of hydroxyamphetamine lies in its indirect pharmacologic action.[32] This drug is an

TABLE 18.9
Dilution of Commercially Available Drugs to Obtain Lower Concentrations[a]

Concentration (%) of Commercially Available Drug	Desired Final Concentration (%)			
	0.1	0.125	0.5	1
1[b]	1/9	1/7	1/1	—
2[b]	1/19	1/15	1/3	1/1
2.5[c]	—	—	—	2/3
10[c]	—	—	—	1/9

[a]Dilutions are prepared by mixing the indicated number of drops of commercially available drug (numerator of fraction) with the indicated number of drops of extraocular irrigating solution or normal saline (denominator of fraction). Equal drop sizes should be used.
[b]Pilocarpine.
[c]Phenylephrine.

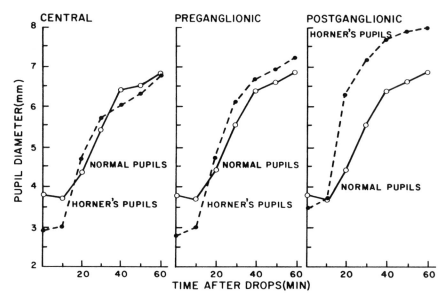

FIGURE 18.6 **Summary of mydriatic responses to 10% phenylephrine in 12 patients with unilateral Horner's syndrome. The data were plotted as in Figure 18.5. Although all pupils dilated well, the Horner's pupil always dilated sooner than the normal pupil. This supersensitivity of the Horner's pupil was most evident in the postganglionic cases. (Published with permission from The American Journal of Ophthalmology 72:472–480, 1971. Copyright by The Ophthalmic Publishing Company).**

indirect acting α-adrenergic agonist that will dilate the pupil only in the presence of endogenous norepinephrine. In the case of postganglionic Horner's syndrome, the postganglionic sympathetic pathway is compromised enough to diminish the normal concentration of norepinephrine contained within the presynaptic vesicles, so that hydroxyamphetamine cannot produce mydriasis or produces incomplete mydriasis[5] (Fig. 18.7). In the case of central or preganglionic lesions, the postganglionic sympathetic pathway is left undisturbed so that the norepinephrine contained within the presynaptic vesicles may be released by the topically instilled hydroxyamphetamine, thus producing normal mydriasis.[5] Hence, hydroxyamphetamine will have a mydriatic effect only when the postganglionic sympathetic pathway to the eye is intact. This drug can be relied on to dilate the Horner's pupil normally in patients with central or preganglionic lesions, but the dilation will be reduced or absent in patients with postganglionic lesions.[5,31]

In contrast to the adrenergic hypersensitivity test using epinephrine or phenylephrine, the response to hydroxyamphetamine is not subject to errors due to interpersonal variations in drug sensitivity or to somewhat uneven administration of the drops.[5] Dilation with topically applied hydroxyamphetamine depends only on the amount of norepinephrine available in the iris for release, and, provided that at least a dose sufficient to dilate the normal pupil is instilled, 1 eye may receive considerably more drug than the other without causing a difference in mydriatic response.[5] One source of error in hydroxyamphetamine testing is its use in infants with acquired preganglionic lesions. Due to the phenomenon of transsynaptic dysgenesis, the pupil may behave pharmacologically as if there were a postganglionic lesion.[72]

The current clinical usefulness of hydroxyamphetamine lies in its ability to distinguish between central or preganglionic and postganglionic lesions. In this regard hydroxyamphetamine provides a clearer dis-

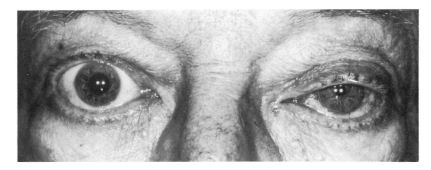

FIGURE 18.7 **Hydroxyamphetamine test in Horner's syndrome (same patient as in Fig. 18.3A). Following instillation of 1% hydroxyamphetamine into each eye, there is dilation of the normal right pupil but absence of dilation of the left Horner's pupil, indicating a postganglionic lesion.**

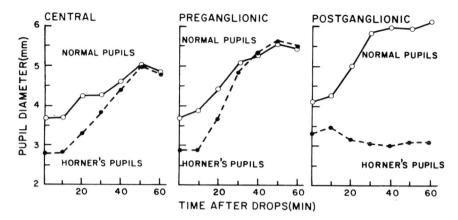

FIGURE 18.8 **Summary of mydriatic responses to 1% hydroxyamphetamine in 12 patients with unilateral Horner's syndrome. The data were plotted as in Figure 18.5. The postganglionic group of Horner's pupils not only failed to dilate but actually became smaller during the test, partly because the patient became progressively bored and sleepy and partly because more light was entering the pupil of the fellow eye, which was dilating normally. (Published with permission from The American Journal of Ophthalmology 72:472–480, 1971. Copyright by The Ophthalmic Publishing Company.)**

tinction between preganglionic and postganglionic defects than is available with any other mydriatic test.[5,31] As previously stated, although the hydroxyamphetamine test is not subject to error due to factors that tend to enhance corneal penetration, the results of this test may be somewhat ambiguous when the Horner's syndrome is incomplete.[23] Furthermore, since pretreatment with cocaine interferes with the action of hydroxyamphetamine,[5] at least 2 days should elapse after cocaine administration before proceeding with the hydroxyamphetamine test. A useful memory device for the hydroxyamphetamine test—"FAIL-SAFE"—has been proposed by Brumberg.[3] This phrase suggests that failure of the pupil to dilate with hydroxyamphetamine indicates a good prognosis (postganglionic lesion). A summary of the mydriatic responses to hydroxyamphetamine in 12 patients with unilateral Horner's syndrome is illustrated in Figure 18.8.

Hydroxyamphetamine has a diagnostic accuracy (accuracy to predict) for postganglionic lesions of 84%, and it has a diagnostic accuracy of 97% for central or preganglionic lesions.[20] The sensitivity (accuracy to confirm) of hydroxyamphetamine for postganglionic lesions is 96%. Van der Wiel and Van Gijn,[31] however, have found that when the pupillary dilation differs more than 1.0 mm between eyes, the predictive value for postganglionic lesions is 100%, but a normal dilation from hydroxyamphetamine provides little diagnostic aid.

Table 18.10 summarizes the expected responses of the Horner's pupil to cocaine and hydroxyamphetamine. This current schema for drug testing in Horner's syndrome applies only to *complete* lesions of the oculosympathetic pathway and should not be relied on in patients with incomplete lesions. Cocaine is used initially to confirm the presence of the Horner's syn-

TABLE 18.10
Current Schema for Mydriatic Drug Tests in Horner's Syndrome

Drug	Normal	Central Lesion	Preganglionic Lesion	Postganglionic Lesion
Cocaine 10% (2 drops)	Mydriasis	Impaired dilation	No dilation	No dilation
Hydroxyamphetamine 1% (2 drops)	Mydriasis	Normal dilation	Normal dilation	No dilation

Modified from Thompson HS. Diagnostic pupillary drug tests. In: Blodi FC, ed. Current concepts in ophthalmology. St Louis: C.V. Mosby Co, 1972; 3:76–90, with permission of the author and publisher.

drome, while hydroxyamphetamine is employed several days later to localize the lesion to the central-preganglionic or postganglionic sympathetic pathway. One should note that *there is presently no pupillary drug test that clearly distinguishes central from preganglionic lesions.*[4,33]

Management

It is crucial to differentiate central or preganglionic lesions from postganglionic lesions, since appropriate patient management depends on accurate localization of the lesion. When the detailed history, clinical examination, and pharmacologic testing indicate a central or preganglionic lesion of unknown etiology, the patient should have cervical spine and chest x-ray films (posteroanterior, lateral, and apical lordotic) and should be referred to a thoracic surgeon or internist because there is some risk of malignancy.[24] When a spinal cord tumor is suspected, myelography should be performed.[21] Routine skull films are also indicated. Neurologic consultation should be considered when central lesions are strongly suspected. If the lesion is postganglionic, however, it is most likely associated with a benign vascular headache syndrome. Such patients with unilateral headache and isolated postganglionic Horner's syndrome usually have a benign course and need no further evaluation. However, if the headaches do not spontaneously resolve within several months, or if objective involvement of the trigeminal nerve or other parasellar cranial nerves is documented, then further investigation should be considered. This decision is facilitated by differentiating the patient with true cluster headache from the patient with no headache or with a vascular headache that is atypical of cluster headache (Table 18.11).[14]

Patients sustaining postganglionic Horner's syndrome with typical cluster headache can be considered to have a benign disorder, whereas patients sustaining postganglionic Horner's syndrome without headache or those with an atypical vascular headache syndrome should be investigated further,[34] preferably by a neurologist. Figure 18.9 summarizes the management of the patient with Horner's syndrome of unknown etiology.

Adie's Syndrome

In 1932, Adie described a syndrome in which usually unilateral defective accommodation and constriction of the pupil were associated with absent or markedly diminished tendon reflexes but without evidence of syphilis.[35] When the association exists between tonic pupils and hyporeflexia, it is known as *Adie's syndrome,* but when the tonic pupil exists alone without associated hyporeflexia, the term *Adie's pupil* is used.

Etiology

Although the etiology of Adie's pupil is usually unknown,[36] it is generally accepted that the lesion is in

TABLE 18.11
Differentiation between Typical and Atypical Cluster Headache

Typical Cluster Headache	*Atypical Cluster Headache*
1. The unilateral headache is very severe. The pain lasts from 30 to 120 minutes and can occur several times daily during the "cluster period," which lasts for several weeks or months. There is a complete absence of pain between the attacks of headaches and also during the months or years separating the "cluster periods."	1. The unilateral headache or facial pain varies from mild to severe, and the degree of pain in each individual varies frequently. The pain occurs in the distribution of the trigeminal nerve, usually lasting for hours or days and may be continuous over several weeks or months.
2. No neurologic signs are found in these patients except for the occurrence of a postganglionic Horner's syndrome in 5% to 22% of the cases. Specifically, no trigeminal nerve involvement is present.	2. Involvement of the first or ophthalmic division of trigeminal nerve is frequently found on the neurologic examination in addition to the postganglionic Horner's syndrome.
3. Other associated systemic conditions are not characteristically present.	3. Common associated conditions include hypertension, arteriosclerosis, past history of vascular headache, head trauma, and recent local infections (viral upper respiratory tract infections, sinusitis).
4. The headache occurs most commonly in middle-aged men and resolves spontaneously over several weeks or months.	4. The headache occurs most commonly in middle-aged men and resolves spontaneously over several weeks or months.

Modified from Grimson BS, Thompson HS. Raeder's syndrome. A clinical review. Surv Ophthalmol 1980;24:199–210, with permission of the authors and publisher.

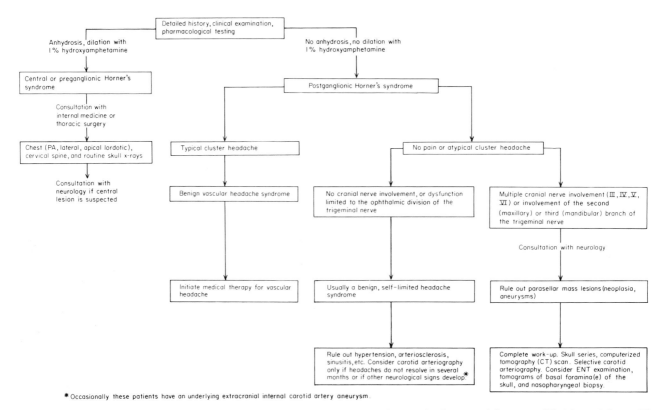

FIGURE 18.9   Flowchart for the management of the patient with Horner's syndrome of unknown etiology. (Modified from Grimson BS, Thompson HS. Raeder's syndrome. A clinical review. Surv Ophthalmol 1980; 24:199–210.)

the ciliary ganglion, with damage to the postganglionic neurons serving the ciliary muscle and iris sphincter.[36,37] Adie's pupil frequently follows a mild upper respiratory infection, and thus in some cases it may be associated with a nonspecific viral illness. In other instances orbital trauma can produce the syndrome. Coppeto and associates[38] have reported Adie's pupils following ipsilateral third-nerve palsy, probably caused by misdirection of injured preganglionic parasympathetic fibers. When Adie's pupil occurs bilaterally, it may be associated with orthostatic hypotension, Riley-Day syndrome, or neurosyphilis.[39]

Perhaps the most widely accepted interpretation of Adie's pupil involves the concept of aberrant regeneration of nerve fibers.[23,37] The parasympathetic accommodative fibers in the ciliary ganglion are believed to be far more numerous than those that supply the iris sphincter. Following destructive ciliary ganglion disease, nerve fiber regeneration may occur with some accommodative fibers becoming misdirected and supplying the iris sphincter. This results in attenuation or loss of the pupillary light response but with preservation of the potential for constriction of the pupil in accommodation, so-called light-near dissociation. Al-

though this hypothesis does not explain the hyporeflexia that often accompanies the ocular findings in Adie's syndrome, it has been proposed that the syndrome may represent a form of mild polyneuropathy,[40] accounting for the diminished deep tendon reflexes. In rare cases Adie's syndrome and a *severe* polyneuropathy can be associated with underlying malignant disease.[41] Perhaps the most noteworthy difference between the clinical signs of Adie's pupil and those of isolated third-nerve pupillary palsy is the presence of light-near dissociation in the former and its absence in the latter.[23]

Diagnosis

Clinical Evaluation

Adie's pupil is a benign disorder.[42] However, because the patient is often alarmed by the presence of a sudden unilateral fixed and dilated pupil, the prompt and accurate diagnosis becomes extremely important. A diagnosis of Adie's pupil will invariably obviate elaborate and expensive neuroradiologic investigations. The pri-

TABLE 18.12
Diagnostic Signs in Adie's Syndrome

• Relative mydriasis in bright illumination
• Absent or poor light reaction
• Slow (tonic) contraction to prolonged near effort
• Slow redilation after near effort
• Vermiform movements of pupillary margin (i.e., sector palsies of iris sphincter)
• Accommodative paresis
• Diminished deep tendon reflexes
• Onset in third to fifth decade
• Females affected in 70% of cases

mary clinical characteristics diagnostic of Adie's syndrome are listed in Table 18.12.

Adie's pupil is unilateral in 80% to 90% of all cases.[6,43] Of the unilateral cases being monitored, approximately 4% become bilateral each year.[6]

In the acute stage, the pupil is usually dilated and reacts very poorly to light. The tonic pupil often changes size in a random manner, possibly being larger in the morning or smaller in the afternoon.[43] Adie's pupils tend to become smaller with time.[6] Some patients have been monitored for several years and have shown a strikingly progressive miosis of the affected pupil. The gradual constriction is more marked than the normal miosis of aging. In an extensive review, Thompson[6] collected data suggesting that Adie's pupils are slightly larger than normal initially and quickly become smaller. In fact, the dilated pupil usually returns to its previous size within a few months, and there is a very slowly progressive additional miosis after approximately 2 years. In darkness most Adie's pupils are smaller than normal, and, if a patient is found with an Adie's pupil larger than the normal pupil in darkness, the condition is most likely of very recent onset.[6] The tendency of Adie's pupils to become progressively miotic and to become bilateral with age suggests that many Adie's pupils eventually become disguised as Argyll Robertson–like pupils or simply become inconspicuous among the smaller pupils of the elderly.[6] Furthermore, the patient learns that the condition is benign and seeks no further medical attention.

The reaction of the Adie's pupil to an accommodative stimulus is very sluggish and poor.[43] The typical slow and tonic near response serves as the mechanism for the most distinguishing clinical feature of this syndrome, namely, tonic and sluggish redilation as the patient changes fixation from near to distance.

Of patients with Adie's pupil, 50% to 90% will demonstrate significantly impaired or absent deep tendon reflexes, and this serves as a helpful clinical confirmation of the diagnosis. In the series of patients reported by Thompson,[6] the majority had tendon re-

flexes that were abnormal throughout the body, but the extent of the impairment was greater in the ankles and triceps than in the knees and biceps. Approximately 33% of patients with Adie's syndrome have entirely normal knee jerks, but about 50% of patients have completely absent ankle jerks. In Thompson's[6] series of patients, only 10% had entirely normal reflexes.

When observed with the biomicroscope, the iris may demonstrate subtle and irregular (vermiform) movements of its sphincter.[6] Segmental palsies of portions of the iris sphincter are present in almost every patient with Adie's pupil. Vermiform movements of the sphincter are nothing more than physiologic pupillary unrest (hippus) of those segments of the sphincter that are intact and still functioning in response to light. Although the affected pupil will show some residual light reaction in most patients, about 10% of patients will have a total palsy of the iris sphincter, and the affected pupil will therefore have no reaction to light.[6,44] Segmental palsies of the iris sphincter are characteristic of Adie's pupil, but they are not pathognomonic.[44,45]

Most patients with Adie's pupil have an accommodative paresis in the involved eye at the onset of the condition, and this is often the primary source of their symptoms.[6] A relative accommodative paresis in the affected eye of 0.50 D or more at initial examination was present in two-thirds of the patients evaluated by Thompson.[6] However, there is clearly a tendency for accommodation to recover, and most of this recovery occurs during the first 2 years.[6]

In summary, the typical patient sustaining Adie's syndrome will be a young (20 to 40 years of age), otherwise healthy female presenting with a unilateral fixed and dilated pupil, with blurred near vision in the affected eye, and with impaired deep tendon reflexes. Clinical evaluation will reveal tonic redilation of the pupil from near to distance. Such a patient can usually be given the diagnosis of Adie's syndrome on clinical grounds alone without the need for pharmacologic, laboratory, or neuroradiologic investigations. In those instances, however, in which the clinical signs are ambiguous or incomplete, pharmacologic testing is indicated.

Pharmacologic Evaluation

METHACHOLINE TEST

Cholinergic hypersensitivity of the denervated iris sphincter in Adie's pupil has been known for many years and is expected according to the principle of denervation hypersensitivity. Although it is clearly helpful in confirming the diagnosis, the diagnosis can be made even when hypersensitivity cannot be demonstrated. Furthermore, the hypersensitivity does not seem to be correlated with the amount of sphincter denervation, the duration of the Adie's pupil, or the amount of light-near dissociation.[6] Occasionally an acute Adie's pupil will show very little hypersensitivity during the first few weeks after onset but will gradually become more hypersensitive several months following the initial episode.[6,43]

In 1940 Scheie[46] showed that most Adie's pupils would constrict to 2.5% methacholine hydrochloride (Mecholyl) but that normal pupils required as strong as 20% methacholine for miosis to occur. Concentrations as high as 15% had no noticeable miotic effect on normal pupils. However, it was soon recognized that many Adie's pupils failed to constrict to 2.5% methacholine because they had not become sufficiently denervated to become hypersensitive. In addition, there were large interindividual variations in sensitivity to methacholine when such low concentrations were used. Although methacholine became popular to elicit the cholinergic denervation hypersensitivity in Adie's pupil, its usefulness was quite limited because less than half of Adie's pupils demonstrated a convincing miosis to the 2.5% solution.[6]

PILOCARPINE TEST

Methacholine has not been commercially available for many years, but pilocarpine, when used in very low concentrations, has been shown to serve as a more useful and more reliable substitute. Various clinicians have demonstrated cholinergic hypersensitivity by using pilocarpine in 0.0625%, 0.1%, 0.125%, or 0.25% solution (see Table 18.9). The usefulness of the pilocarpine test in eliciting cholinergic hypersensitivity depends on the presence of a standardized concentration of drug at the iris. Thus, any clinical procedure that compromises the corneal epithelium, the use of wetting agents, or other factors that enhance corneal penetration may result in false-positive findings. Although not clinically practical, the pilocarpine should ideally be administered in a vehicle that is not preserved with benzalkonium chloride or other preservative that may enhance corneal penetration of the drug.[23]

Younge and Buski[10] have recommended that pilocarpine be used as a 0.1% solution. These investigators report that too many false-positive reactions occur when pilocarpine is used in a concentration of 0.2%, and when 0.05% pilocarpine solution is used, too many insufficient responses (false negative) of the Adie's pupil result. These authors found that a 0.1% concentration of pilocarpine performed the best clinically to confirm the Adie's pupil. This concentration of pilocarpine will not usually constrict the normal pupil but will constrict the tonic pupil.

Thompson[6] and Pilley and Thompson,[47] however, have recommended that pilocarpine be used as a 0.125% solution. When used in this concentration, pilocarpine will slightly constrict most normal pupils, with the degree of miosis differing among individuals from just noticeable to several millimeters.[6] The advantage of using a concentration that slightly constricts the normal pupil is that it allows the clinician to ascertain whether or not an adequate amount of drug has been instilled into each eye. In the typical patient with Adie's pupil, 0.125% pilocarpine will cause a slight constriction of the normal pupil, while the affected pupil becomes even more miotic[4] (Fig. 18.10).

When the 0.125% pilocarpine test is compared with the 2.5% methacholine test, the former is clearly the most clinically useful and reliable pharmacologic test to confirm the diagnosis of Adie's pupil. If the strict definition of cholinergic hypersensitivity is followed (i.e., the Adie's pupil constricts to a cholinergic stimulus more than the fellow normal pupil does to the same stimulus), and if 0.2 mm of excessive constriction of the Adie's pupil is required before it can be considered to be hypersensitive, then the methacholine test is positive in only about 64% of patients with Adie's pupil, whereas the pilocarpine test is positive in about 80%.[6]

Management

Since Adie's syndrome is a benign disorder, the most important aspect in patient management is reassurance. The associated accommodative paresis will tend to recover during the first several years, and any visual impairment will thus improve. The patient should be advised that the second eye may become involved but that the other changes associated with the syndrome (decreased light reaction and diminished deep tendon reflexes) do not represent significant functional impairments. For many patients the chief concern is for the cosmetic appearance of the unequal pupils. Most patients can be reassured that, with time, this should become less noticeable.

In most cases the clinician should *not* prescribe pilocarpine for the affected pupil because the intermittent drug-induced accommodative spasm, which is aggravated by the hypersensitivity of the ciliary muscle, will not usually be tolerated. Symptomatic patients, however, may benefit from the instillation of 0.1% to 0.125% pilocarpine into the affected eye 3 or 4 times daily.[48,49] Because of individual variability, various low concentrations of pilocarpine should be attempted to determine the optimum concentration of miotic that alleviates symptoms such as periocular discomfort, headache, photophobia, or blurred vision.[49] If a miotic is used in this fashion, the patient should be carefully

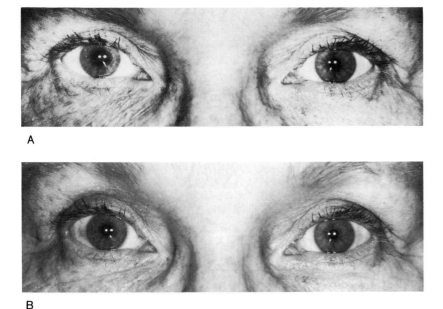

A

B

FIGURE 18.10   **Pilocarpine test in 57-year-old woman with right Adie's pupil. (A) Before drug instillation. (B) Following instillation of 0.125% pilocarpine into each eye, the normal left pupil constricts slightly while the right Adie's pupil constricts significantly.**

monitored in anticipation of modifying the drug regimen if the degree of cholinergic hypersensitivity changes with time.

The practitioner can also prescribe tinted lenses, which not only shield the cosmetic appearance of the unequal pupils but also alleviate perception of the Pulfrich phenomenon produced by the anisocoria. Furthermore, when affected patients are presbyopic, unequal bifocal powers are clearly justified and frequently serve to alleviate the asthenopia associated with near vision. Reading lenses may be indicated for patients who are prepresbyopic.

Unilateral Fixed and Dilated Pupil

A unilateral fixed and dilated pupil in an ambulatory and otherwise healthy patient is seldom associated with significant neurologic disease, yet, historically, the practitioner has been cautioned to consider this a sign of potentially grave intracranial disease. Although the possible causes of a fixed and dilated pupil are numerous and include potentially destructive vascular and neoplastic processes (Table 18.13), the clinician is usually able, by a careful history and physical examination, to narrow the possible diagnoses to three:[50] (1) involvement of the intracranial third nerve, (2) Adie's pupil, or (3) anticholinergic mydriasis.

Since the fixed and dilated pupil is clearly the abnormal pupil, the pharmacologic evaluation involves instillation of a miotic, usually pilocarpine, to assess the degree to which the iris sphincter or its parasympathetic innervation has been impaired. In the majority

of cases only one pupil is dilated and fixed, and false-positive or false-negative drug tests can be avoided by instilling the drug into both eyes. Constriction of the normal pupil thus indicates that enough pilocarpine was instilled. When both pupils are dilated and fixed, the drops should be placed in only one eye so that any constriction can be attributed solely to the drug.[50]

In the following sections the most common disorders associated with a unilateral fixed and dilated pupil will be considered, including third-nerve palsy, anticholinergic mydriasis, iris sphincter atrophy, and adrenergic mydriasis. Since Adie's syndrome is not always characterized by a dilated pupil, this disorder has been discussed separately.

Third-Nerve Palsy

The patient presenting with the classic signs of a complete third-nerve palsy (Fig. 18.11) need not undergo pharmacologic testing; the diagnosis can be made on clinical grounds alone, and the patient should be referred to a neurologist, since a complete third-nerve palsy of recent onset is of neurologic significance. The most common cause of a sudden unilateral third-nerve palsy in an adult with a dilated and fixed pupil and with headache is an aneurysm at the junction of the ipsilateral internal carotid artery and the posterior communicating arteries.[69] The practitioner should recall, however, that the most common cause of a sudden unilateral third-nerve palsy in an adult with headache but with *spared* pupil is diabetes mellitus.[43,51] The pupillary findings, therefore, are extremely important in the

TABLE 18.13
Possible Causes of a Fixed and Dilated Pupil

1. Midbrain damage
   Vascular accidents, tumors, degenerative and infectious diseases, etc.
   Dorsal (Edinger-Westphal nucleus and its connections)
      Relatively rare
      Usually involves both pupils
      Pupillary near vision reaction often retained
      Often associated with supranuclear vertical gaze palsy
   Ventral (fascicular part of third nerve)
      Often associated with other neurologic deficits (e.g., Nothnagel's, Benedikt's, Weber's syndromes)
      Unlikely to spare the extraocular components of the third nerve

2. Damage to the third nerve (from interpeduncular fossa to ciliary ganglion)
   Basal aneurysms
   Supratentorial space-occupying masses, causing displacement of the brain stem or transtentorial herniation of the uncus
      These patients are usually stuporous or comatose
   Basal meningitis
      Often causes bilateral internal ophthalmoplegia
   Ischemic oculomotor palsy ("diabetic ophthalmoplegia")
      Usually spares the pupillary fibers
   Parasellar tumor (e.g., pituitary adenoma, meningioma, craniopharyngioma, nasopharyngeal carcinoma, or distant metastases)
   Parasellar inflammation (e.g., "Tolosa-Hunt," temporal arteritis, herpes zoster)

3. Damage to the ciliary ganglion or short ciliary nerves results in Adie's pupil
   Viral ciliary ganglionitis or involvement of the ciliary nerves (e.g., herpes zoster)
   Orbital trauma or tumor
   Choroidal trauma or tumor
   Blunt trauma to the globe may injure the ciliary plexus at the iris root (traumatic iridoplegia)

4. Damage to the iris
   Degenerative or inflammatory diseases of the iris
   Posterior synechiae
   Mechanical influences from intraocular lenses
   Acute rise of intraocular pressure (hypoxia of sphincter)
   Blunt injury to the globe with sphincter damage (traumatic iridoplegia)
   Pharmacologic blockade by atropinic substances

Modified from Thompson HS, Newsome DA, Loewenfeld IE. The fixed dilated pupil. Sudden iridoplegia or mydriatic drops? A simple diagnostic test. Arch Ophthalmol 1971;86:21–27. Copyright 1971, American Medical Association.

evaluation and differential diagnosis of an acute third-nerve palsy.

If, however, the patient exhibits only a unilateral fixed and dilated pupil without evidence of ptosis or extraocular muscle involvement, the clinician should perform the pilocarpine test, first using a 0.125% solution to reveal any cholinergic hypersensitivity as evidence for Adie's pupil. If there is no local iris damage by slit-lamp examination, no sector palsy of the iris sphincter, and no cholinergic hypersensitivity demonstrated by the 0.125% pilocarpine, then the condition might be associated with interruption of the preganglionic innervation to the iris sphincter (i.e., third-nerve palsy). If the patient has incurred a third-nerve palsy, the muscarinic receptor sites on the iris sphincter will be activated by topically instilled pilocarpine in moderate concentrations. Therefore, if no cholinergic hypersensitivity is revealed with 0.125% pilocarpine, the practitioner should subsequently instill pilocarpine in a concentration of 0.5% or 1.0%. This should

promptly constrict the affected pupil (Fig. 18.12).[7,52] Slamovits and associates [70] have shown, however, that some patients with intracranial third-nerve palsy may manifest hypersensitivity to low concentrations of pilocarpine. Thus, the clinician should carefully evaluate all clinical signs and symptoms before reaching a final diagnosis.

Anticholinergic Mydriasis

ETIOLOGY

Anticholinergic mydriasis, also known as pharmacologic blockade or "atropinic" mydriasis, refers to the fixed and dilated pupil resulting from the accidental inoculation into the eye of drugs or substances with anticholinergic properties. Medical personnel such as doctors, nurses, and pharmacists are particularly susceptible to this condition, since they frequently handle such medications. Often some medication spills over

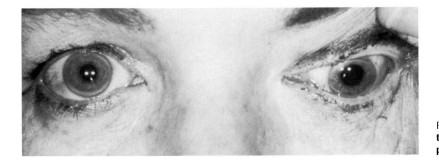

FIGURE 18.11   **Complete third-nerve palsy.** Note the left ptosis, exotropia, hypotropia, and dilated pupil.

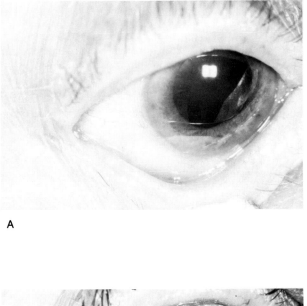

A

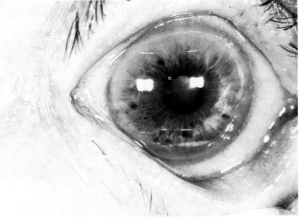

B

FIGURE 18.12   **Pilocarpine test in third-nerve palsy.** *(A)* Before drug instillation. *(B)* Following instillation of 1.0% pilocarpine, the pupil promptly constricts.

the side of the bottle container, and the practitioner or nurse who next handles the bottle comes into contact with the dried medication. The drug is then easily transferred to the eye by simple rubbing. Although such medications commonly include cyclopentolate, homatropine, and atropine, other drugs or substances with anticholinergic properties have been implicated. On occasion, the patient will admit to having placed some drops into the affected eye but will often not be able to recall the name of the medication. In these cases the practitioner should inquire about the color of the medication cap, since most cycloplegics are commercially packaged with red caps, while miotics have green caps. It is not uncommon for these patients to have instilled into their mildly irritated eye atropine drops that had previously been prescribed for an episode of iritis.

Other substances have also been implicated in anticholinergic mydriasis. Jimson weed (*Datura stramonium*) is found in many parts of the United States, and the entire plant from root to flower contains significant concentrations of belladonna alkaloids including atropine, scopolamine, hyoscine, and hyoscyamine.[53] A farmer working in a dusty field often sustains relatively insignificant ocular foreign bodies, and a particle of jimson weed dust may be no more irritating to the eye than any other particle of plant origin. The drug-induced dilated pupil and blurred vision may not be noticed until the following day, and the patient often does not associate the onset of the condition with an ocular foreign body. Numerous cases of jimson weed mydriasis have been reported.[54-56] Hence, the practitioner should entertain a suspicion of jimson weed mydriasis in farmers, or in children who have been "picking flowers," if these patients present with an acute onset of unilateral mydriasis. Moreover, the dried pods of the plant are often used in floral arrangements for indoor decoration during the winter, and this may contribute to an increased risk of systemic toxicity in the pediatric age group, since children have been known to consume such "berries." In fact, fatal cases have been reported in children in whom the seeds were recovered from the stomach contents at autopsy.[53] In addition to *bilaterally* dilated pupils, the early symptoms of systemic toxicity when the weed is consumed orally are those typical of anticholinergic drugs: blurred vision, dryness of the mouth, extreme thirst, constipation, urinary retention, convulsions, dry and flushed skin, diffuse erythematous rash, tachycardia, and elevated temperature.

The practitioner should be alert to the possible inoculation into the eye of *any* drug or substance with anticholinergic properties, including plants, cosmetics, perfumes, or medicines. Two women have been reported to have sustained unilateral fixed and dilated pupils following the use of propantheline bromide lotion (Ercoril) as an antiperspirant.[57] In several patients the use of transdermal scopolamine (Transderm Scōp) for the treatment of motion sickness has been associated with the development of unilateral fixed and dilated pupils.[58–61] Scopolamine from the disk placed behind the ear can be inadvertently inoculated into the eye, producing the typical signs of anticholinergic mydriasis. Fixed and dilated pupils have also resulted from direct droplet contamination associated with the use of anticholinergic aerosols for treatment of acute asthma and other airflow obstructions.[62,71]

DIAGNOSIS

Since the pupillary paralysis of neurogenic origin (i.e., third-nerve palsy) is clinically indistinguishable from anticholinergic mydriasis, many practitioners have unnecessarily subjected patients to extensive neurologic, radiologic, and laboratory investigations for possible intracranial disease. Clearly, the diagnostic procedure of choice in such instances is 1 or 2 drops of 0.5% or 1.0% pilocarpine instilled into each eye (Fig. 18.13). If the muscarinic receptor sites on the affected iris sphincter have been occupied by an anticholinergic drug, the pilocarpine will be unable to activate the receptors and constrict the pupil. Thus, this simple test will quickly and easily differentiate between anticholinergic mydriasis and pupillary paralysis associated with third-nerve palsy; the former will not react to the pilocarpine, while the latter will constrict.[7,52,55]

Thompson and associates[50] have recommended that pilocarpine be initially used in a 0.5% rather than 1.0% concentration because a pupil that is only weakly dilated with an anticholinergic drug might be constricted by the stronger pilocarpine solution, resulting in a

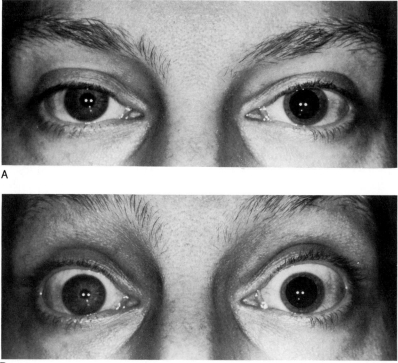

FIGURE 18.13 **Pilocarpine test in anticholinergic mydriasis.** *(A)* 27-year-old man with fixed and dilated left pupil. *(B)* Following instillation of 1.0% pilocarpine into each eye, the right pupil constricts while the left pupil does not.

false-positive finding. If neither the normal nor the affected pupil constricts when the 0.5% pilocarpine is instilled, the stronger solution should then be used.

MANAGEMENT

Once the diagnosis of anticholinergic mydriasis has been made, the patient should be reassured that with time, usually a few days to a few weeks, the pupil will spontaneously return to its original size, and vision (accommodation) will improve as the effects of the inoculated substance subside.

Damage to the Iris

Damage to the iris sphincter muscle by high intraocular pressure, trauma, or inflammation may impair pilocarpine's ability to constrict the pupil. Clinically, these conditions can usually be ruled out by careful history and physical (biomicroscopic) examination. Mechanical factors associated with malpositioned intraocular lenses[63] or posterior synechiae may also limit movement of the iris. Depending on the extent of iris damage, the pupil may demonstrate constriction ranging from complete to nonexistent.[7,50,52]

Keratoconic Mydriasis

In some patients following uncomplicated penetrating keratoplasty for keratoconus, the pupil becomes irreversibly dilated a few days after surgery and will not react to various miotics including pilocarpine, carbachol, physostigmine, or echothiophate.[64] In 1 series of patients, 2 pupils failed to respond to acetylcholine injected into the anterior chamber 3 to 4 weeks following keratoplasty.[65] In the less severe cases, however, a sudden reduction of the mydriasis may be observed during the months following the corneal transplantation. This spontaneous postoperative dilation of the pupil has never been observed in eyes that have been

grafted for other corneal diseases, even if the identical surgical techniques were employed.[64]

The etiology of keratoconic mydriasis remains obscure. Bertelsen and Seim[64] have observed that patients with keratoconus very often have hypoplasia of the iris stroma. These investigators have proposed that the hypoplasia may be the etiology for the postoperative mydriasis. Uribe,[65] on the other hand, believes that the iris abnormality is a consequence rather than a cause of the postoperative mydriasis. Since these pupils fail to respond to topically administered anticholinesterase drugs, the mechanism may have a neurochemical origin. Uribe[65] has postulated that the cause for irreversible mydriasis may be related to a paralysis of the local parasympathetic nervous system by disturbance of the normal liberation of acetylcholine.

Adrenergic Mydriasis

Although the pupil that has become dilated in response to topically instilled adrenergic drugs is often not completely immobile, this condition is included here for the sake of completeness. A patient who is unusually sensitive to adrenergic agonists may sustain a dilated pupil as a consequence of the accidental inoculation into the eye of nose drops, nasal sprays, or other substances with adrenergic properties.[66] In addition, some patients with minor corneal epithelial compromise may sustain a dilated pupil following the instillation of decongestant eyedrops. In these instances, however, the adrenergic mydriasis can usually be distinguished from the dilated pupil of third-nerve palsy or anticholinergic mydriasis by the blanched conjunctiva, the residual light reaction, and the occasional retracted upper eyelid[23,50] (Fig. 18.14). Although dilation associated with adrenergic agonists is usually incomplete and short-lived, the concomitant use of topical epinephrine and timolol for the treatment of glaucoma may occasionally result in the development of long-standing fixed and dilated pupils.[67] A careful history

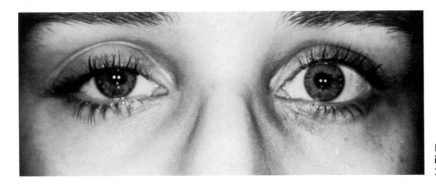

FIGURE 18.14 **Retracted left upper lid following instillation of 0.012% naphazoline (Degest 2) as a decongestant.**

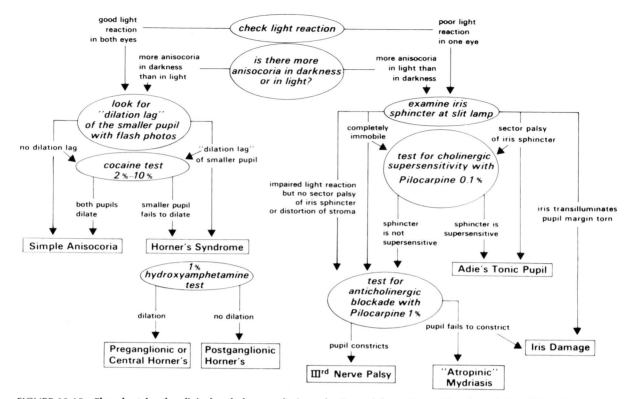

FIGURE 18.15   **Flowchart for the clinical and pharmacologic evaluations of the patient with anisocoria in which only one pupil is affected. (Modified from Thompson HS, Pilley SFJ. Unequal pupils. A flow chart for sorting out the anisocorias. Surv Ophthalmol 1976;21(1):45–48, with permission of the authors and publisher.)**

and clinical evaluation of the patient will usually eliminate the need for pharmacologic testing.

Figure 18.15 summarizes the clinical and pharmacologic evaluations of the patient with anisocoria in which only one pupil is affected.

References

1. Gray LG. The five-step pupil evaluation. Rev Optom 1981;118:38–44.

2. Alexander LJ. Use of "black light" in assessing pupillary responses. Am J Optom Physiol Opt 1977;54:792–796.

3. Brumberg JB. Horner's syndrome and the ultraviolet light as an aid in its detection. J Am Optom Assoc 1981;52:641–646.

4. Thompson HS. Diagnostic pupillary drug tests. In: Blodi FC, ed. Current concepts in ophthalmology. St Louis: C.V. Mosby Co, 1972;3:76–90.

5. Thompson HS, Mensher JH. Adrenergic mydriasis in Horner's syndrome. Hydroxyamphetamine test for diagnosis of postganglionic defects. Am J Ophthalmol 1971;72:472–480.

6. Thompson HS. Adie's syndrome: Some new observations. Trans Am Ophthalmol Soc 1977;75:587–626.

7. Czarnecki JSC, Pilley SFJ, Thompson HS. The analysis of anisocoria. The use of photography in the clinical evaluation of unequal pupils. Can J Ophthalmol 1979;14:297–302.

8. Loewenfeld IE. "Simple, central" anisocoria: A common condition, seldom recognized. Trans Am Acad Ophthalmol Otolaryngol 1977;83:832–839.

9. Lam BL, Thompson HS, Corbett JJ. The prevalence of simple anisocoria. Am J Ophthalmol 1987;104:69–73.

10. Younge BR, Buski ZJ. Tonic pupil: A simple screening test. Can J Ophthalmol 1976;11:295–299.

11. Horner F. Uber eine form von ptosis. Klin Monatsbl Augenheilkd 1869;7:193–201.

12. Grimson BS, Thompson HS. Postganglionic Horner syndrome. In: Glaser JS, ed. Neuro-ophthalmology. St. Louis: C.V. Mosby Co, 1977;9:190–197.

13. Jaffe NS. Localization of lesions causing Horner's syndrome. Arch Ophthalmol 1950;44:710–728.

14. Grimson BS, Thompson HS. Raeder's syndrome. A clinical review. Surv Ophthalmol 1980;24:199–210.

15. Swann PG, Johnson LB. Horner's syndrome: An unusual precursor of occlusive disease of the carotid arterial system. J Am Optom Assoc 1985;56:131–132.

16. Musarella MA, Chan HSL, DeBoer G, et al. Ocular involvement in neuroblastoma: Prognostic implications. Ophthalmology 1984;91:936–940.

17. Kline LB, Vitek JJ, Raymon BC. Painful Horner's syndrome

due to spontaneous carotid artery dissection. Ophthalmology 1987;94:226–230.

18. Levy H, Sacho H, Feldman C, et al. Pulmonary mucormycosis presenting with Horner's syndrome. S Afr Med J 1986;70:363–365.

19. Smith PG, Dyches TJ, Burde RM. Topographic analysis of Horner's syndrome. Otolaryngol Head Neck Surg 1986;94:451–457.

20. Maloney WF, Younge BR, Moyer NJ. Evaluation of the causes and accuracy of pharmacologic localization in Horner's syndrome. Am J Ophthalmol 1980;90:394–402.

21. Giles CL, Henderson JW. Horner's syndrome: An analysis of 216 cases. Am J Ophthalmol 1958;46:289–296.

22. Pilley SFJ, Thompson HS. Pupillary "dilatation lag" in Horner's syndrome. Br J Ophthalmol 1975;59:731–735.

23. Carter JH. Diagnosis of pupillary anomalies. J Am Optom Assoc 1979;50:671–680.

24. Thompson HS. Diagnosing Horner's syndrome. Trans Am Acad Ophthalmol Otolaryngol 1977;83:840–842.

25. Thompson BM, Corbett JJ, Kline LB, et al. Pseudo-Horner's syndrome. Arch Neurol 1982;39:108–111.

26. Thompson HS, Mensher JH. Horner's syndrome (letter). Am J Ophthalmol 1974;78:739–740.

27. Friedman JR, Whiting DW, Kosmorsky GS, et al. The cocaine test in normal patients. Am J Ophthalmol 1984;98:808–810.

28. Langley JN. Observations on the physiological action of extracts of the supra-renal bodies. J Physiol 1901;27:237–256.

29. Cords R. Ein fall von schlafenschuss mit lahmung des augen sympathicus. Arch Klin Exp Ophthalmol 1910;75:113–128.

30. Morone G, Andreani F. Richerche pupillografiche nella sindrome di Bernard-Horner sotto l'azione di alcuni medicamenti. Riv Oto-neuro-oftal 1949;24:180–194.

31. Van der Wiel HL, Van Gijn J. Localization of Horner's syndrome. Use and limitations of the hydroxyamphetamine test. J Neurol Sci 1983;59:229–235.

32. Heitman K, Bode' DD. The Paredrine test in normal eyes. A controlled study. J Clin Neuro-ophthalmol 1986;6:228–231.

33. Lepore FE. Diagnostic pharmacology of the pupil. Clin Neuropharmacol 1985;8:27–37.

34. Journal Club Ophthalmology. New York: Medical Information Systems, 1975.

35. Adie WJ. Tonic pupils and absent tendon reflexes: A benign disorder sui generis; its complete and incomplete forms. Brain 1932;55:98–113.

36. Purcell JJ, Krachmer JH, Thompson HS. Corneal sensation in Adie's syndrome. Am J Ophthalmol 1977;84:496–500.

37. Czarnecki JSC, Thompson HS. Spontaneous cyclic segmental sphincter spasms in an Adie's tonic pupil. Am J Ophthalmol 1976;82:636–637.

38. Coppeto JR, Monteiro MLR, Young D. Tonic pupils following oculomotor nerve palsies. Ann Ophthalmol 1985;17:585–588.

39. Fletcher WA, Sharpe JA. Tonic pupils in neurosyphilis. Neurology 1986;36:188.

40. Fite JD, Walker HK. The pupil. In: Walker HK, Hall WD, Hurst JW, eds. Clinical methods: The history, physical and laboratory examinations. Boston: Butterworths, 1980;2:577–585.

41. Bell TAG. Adie's tonic pupil in a patient with carcinomatous neuromyopathy. Arch Ophthalmol 1986;104:331–332.

42. Scheinberg IH, Adler RI. Adie's syndrome: Case report. Ann Ophthalmol 1979;11:247–248.

43. Smith JL. The pupil. Miami: Smith, 1975.

44. Thompson HS. Segmental palsy of the iris sphincter in Adie's syndrome. Arch Ophthalmol 1978;96:1615–1620.

45. Cox TA. Spontaneous contractions of the pupillary sphincter in traumatic ophthalmoplegia. Am J Ophthalmol 1986;102:543–544.

46. Scheie HG. Site of disturbance in Adie's syndrome. Arch Ophthalmol 1940;24:225–237.

47. Pilley SFJ, Thompson HS. Cholinergic supersensitivity in Adie's syndrome: Pilocarpine vs. Mecholyl (abstr.). Am J Ophthalmol 1975;80:955.

48. Flach AJ, Dolan BJ. The therapy of Adie's syndrome with dilute pilocarpine hydrochloride solutions. J Ocular Pharmacol 1985;1:353.

49. Flach AJ, Dolan BJ. Adie's syndrome: A medical treatment for symptomatic patients. Ann Ophthalmol 1984;16:1151–1154.

50. Thompson HS, Newsome DA, Loewenfeld IE. The fixed dilated pupil. Sudden iridoplegia or mydriatic drops? A simple diagnostic test. Arch Ophthalmol 1971;86:27.

51. Nadeau SE, Trobe JD. Pupil sparing in oculomotor palsy: A brief review. Ann Neurol 1983;13:143–148.

52. Thompson HS, Pilley SFJ. Unequal pupils. A flow chart for sorting out the anisocorias. Surv Ophthalmol 1976;21:45–48.

53. Blattner RJ. Jimson weed poisoning: Stramonium intoxication. J Pediatr 1962;61:941–943.

54. Reader AL. Mydriasis from *Datura wrightii*. Am J Ophthalmol 1977;84:263–264.

55. Thompson HS. Cornpicker's pupil: Jimson weed mydriasis. J Iowa Med Soc 1971;61:475–478.

56. Simmons FH. Jimson weed mydriasis in farmers. Am J Ophthalmol 1957;44:109–110.

57. Nissen SH, Nielsen PG. Unilateral mydriasis after use of propantheline bromide in an antiperspirant (letter). Lancet 1977;2:1134.

58. McCrary JA, Webb NR. Anisocoria from scopolamine patches. JAMA 1982;248:353–354.

59. Verdier DD, Kennerdell JS. Fixed dilated pupil resulting from transdermal scopolamine (letter). Am J Ophthalmol 1982;93:803–804.

60. Rosen NB. Accidental mydriasis from scopolamine patches. J Am Optom Assoc 1986;57:541–542.

61. Bienia RA, Smith M, Pellegrino T. Scopolamine skin-disks and anisocoria. Ann Intern Med 1983;99:572–573.

62. Jannum DR, Mickel SF. Anisocoria and aerosolized anticholinergics. Chest 1986;90:148–149.

63. Lippman JI. Pupillary abnormalities associated with posterior chamber lens implantation. Ophthalmic Surg 1982;13:197–200.

64. Bertelsen TI, Seim V. The cause of irreversible mydriasis following keratoplasty in keratoconus: A preliminary report. Ophthalmic Surg 1974;5:56–58.

65. Uribe LE. Fixed pupil following keratoplasty. Evaluation of six cases. Am J Ophthalmol 1967;63:1682–1686.

66. Stirt JA, Shuptrine JR, Sternick CS, et al. Anisocoria after anaesthesia. Can Anaesth Soc J 1985;32:422–424.

67. Laibovitz RA. The fixed, dilated pupil: A new cause. Tex Med 1980;76:59.

68. Wimalaratna HS, Capildeo R, Lee HY. Herpes zoster of second and third segments causing ipsilateral Horner's syndrome. Br Med J 1987;294:1463.

69. Brodsky MC, Frenkel REP, Spoor TC. Familial intracranial aneurysm presenting as a subtle stable third nerve palsy. Arch Ophthalmol 1988;106:173.

70. Slamovits TL, Miller NR, Burde RM. Intracranial oculomotor nerve paresis with anisocoria and pupillary parasympathetic hypersensitivity. Am J Ophthalmol 1987;104:401–406.

71. Helprin GA, Clarke GM. Unilateral fixed dilated pupil associated with nebulised ipratropium bromide. Lancet 1986;2:1469.

72. Weinstein JM, Cutler JI. Observations on transsynaptic changes in acquired Horner's syndrome. Am J Ophthalmol 1983;95:837–838.

73. Nielsen PJ. Upside down ptosis in patients with Horner's syndrome. Acta Ophthalmol 1983;61:952–957.

74. Monteiro MLR, Coppeto JR. Horner's syndrome associated with carotid artery atherosclerosis. Am J Ophthalmol 1988;105:93–94.

CHAPTER 19

Diseases of the Eyelids

Jimmy D. Bartlett

Disorders of the eyelids are among the most common ocular abnormalities encountered by the optometrist and other primary care practitioners. Because of their widespread prevalence and the fact that eyelid diseases are often associated with conjunctival, corneal, or systemic involvement, the practitioner must be able to recognize and manage specific diseases affecting the eyelids. This chapter considers the pharmacologic management of the most common and clinically significant disorders affecting the eyelids.

Clinical Anatomy and Physiology

A meaningful discussion of eyelid disease requires knowledge of the important anatomic structures and functions of the lids. The important anatomic features are shown in Figure 19.1. The eyelid is limited anteriorly by the dermis, which often plays an important role in allergic eyelid manifestations. The orbicularis muscle is innervated by the seventh cranial nerve and is primarily responsible for normal involuntary blinking as well as tight eyelid closure. The eyelashes (cilia) emerge from individual follicles, surrounding which are the glands of Zeis and Moll. Posterior to the lash line is the row of meibomian glands. The meibomian glands and glands of Zeis are sebaceous glands, which secrete oil, while the glands of Moll are modified sweat glands. The meibomian glands serve an important function in tear physiology, since they supply the lipid layer of the tear film, which prevents evaporation of the underlying aqueous component. Meibomian gland abnormalities may thus play an important role in dry eye syndrome.

The levator muscle is innervated by the third cranial nerve and is responsible for elevation of the upper eyelid. Mueller's muscle, innervated by the sympathetic division of the autonomic nervous system, augments the action of the levator muscle in elevating the upper lid.

Congenital Abnormalities

Coloboma

Congenital eyelid coloboma is a rare clinical entity characterized by absence of a portion of the eyelid. In 90% of cases the upper lid is involved,[1] and the most common position of the coloboma is at the junction of the medial and middle third of the lid.[2] A variety of other orbital, facial, or ocular abnormalities may be associated, including limbal dermoids, strabismus, and corneal opacities.[3]

The primary problem caused by congenital eyelid coloboma is exposure keratopathy, which occurs when 30% or more of the upper lid is absent.[4] Management is thus dictated by the severity of the individual situation. Surgical correction is generally indicated for cosmesis, but this can be delayed until the child is 3 to 6 months old, at which time general anesthesia is a less serious risk. In the meantime, the cornea should be protected by use of topically applied lubricating ointments as well as antibiotic ointments if infection is a significant risk. If four-fifths of the upper lid is absent, corneal exposure and scarring are quite likely, and surgery may be necessary within the first 48 hours

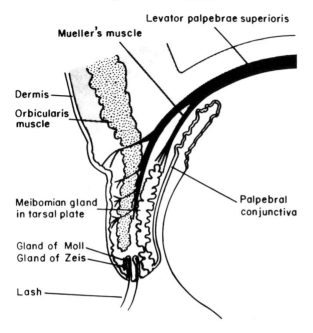

FIGURE 19.1 **Major anatomic features of the eyelids.**

of life.[1] Even topical antibiotics or lubricating ointments are often unsatisfactory in such cases.

Distichiasis

Congenital distichiasis is a rare condition in which an accessory row of eyelashes lies posterior to the normal lashes (Fig. 19.2). The accessory row of lashes arises from the meibomian gland orifices.[5] The meibomian glands themselves may be rudimentary, atrophic, or normal.[6] This disorder occurs sporadically or as an autosomal dominant trait.[6,7] There is often wide variation in the number of eyelids involved; the number of abnormal lashes; the diameter, length, or pigmentation of the lashes; and the direction of their shafts. Associated findings can include corneal hypoesthesia and corneal epithelial staining with sodium fluorescein.[7] In rare instances distichiasis can be associated with skeletal abnormalities and may occur along with congenital heart disease and peripheral vascular anomalies.[8]

Distichiasis requires no treatment if the patient is asymptomatic, but when the lashes cause corneal irritation, they should be removed. If only a few lashes are involved, they can be removed by epilation or electrolysis. When the condition is extensive, however, surgical correction[9,10] or cryotherapy[6,11] is indicated. The application of artificial tear solutions or lubricating ointments or, in severe cases, antibiotics may be indicated before surgical intervention.

Abnormalities Associated with Trauma

Thermal Burns

Flame, flash, and scald burns are the most common causes of eyelid burns.[12–14] It is vital to exclude the possibility of ocular damage by exposing and examining the globe for penetrating injury or thermal burns of the cornea and conjunctiva. Once ocular injury has been excluded, first- or second-degree burns of the lids usually result only in temporary loss of lashes and

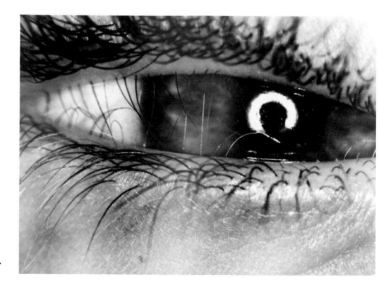

FIGURE 19.2 **Congenital distichiasis. (Courtesy Jerry R. Pederson, O.D.)**

require no more than general supportive care.[12] Initial therapy should include careful lid and lash hygiene with gauze and saline to keep crusting of the lids to a minimum.[15] Topically applied burn creams should be avoided because they can irritate the conjunctiva and impair lid motion.[13] Antibiotic ointments should be applied to the lids 2 to 4 times daily to prevent secondary infection. If applied soon after the injury, the use of cold compresses or iced-saline gauze over the eyelids has been found to be effective in reducing edema.[14] Healing is generally uncomplicated (Fig. 19.3).Immediately following the injury trichiasis may occur due to charring, distortion of the lashes, or lid edema. Since corneal abrasion can result from the trichiasis, the offending lashes should be epilated, or the cornea and globe should be protected with soft contact lenses or scleral shells.[15]

In cases of severe, third-degree burns of the lids, the cornea should be protected with any combination of artificial tears, bland lubricating ointment, or soft contact lenses. Since structural deformities resulting from extensive lid scarring are likely, immediate consultation with an oculoplastic surgeon is indicated.[12,13]

Chemical Burns

The accidental inoculation of foreign chemicals into the eye may result in only minor irritation or serious, destructive burns depending on the chemical involved. Acid burns are generally self-limited, and the resultant injury is usually superficial unless the acid is in contact with the tissues for a prolonged time. On the other hand, alkaline fluids typically cause more extensive tissue damage because they can penetrate eyelid or ocular tissue.[14]

Regardless of the type of chemical injury, speed is essential in the initial first-aid of the chemical burn. The eye(s) should be irrigated with copious amounts of clean water or irrigating solution. The irrigation will be more comfortable if a topical anesthetic is first instilled. In most cases only 1 to 2 minutes of irrigation is required, except in the instance of acid or alkali burns, which should receive prolonged irrigation.[16] In addition, if the contaminant is chemically reactive or has an oily or viscous base, the irrigation should also be extended. Every 5 to 10 minutes during the course of irrigation the conjunctival sac should be tested with

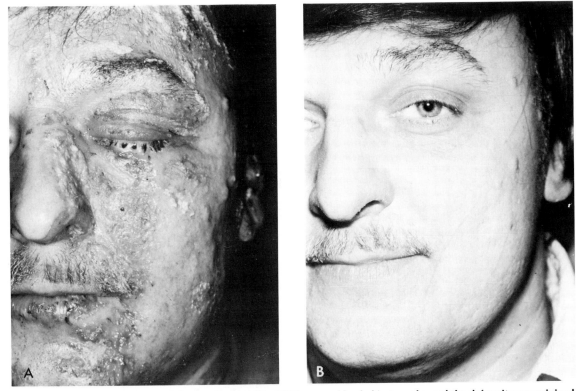

FIGURE 19.3   *(A)* **Burn injuries of the face and eyelid.** *(B)* **The wound healed in 2 weeks, and the deformity was minimal. (From Huang TT, Blackwell SJ, Lewis SR. Burn injuries of the eyelids. Clin Plast Surg 1978; 5:571–581, with permission of the authors and publisher).**

a pH test paper. Once the pH has returned to normal, it is unnecessary to continue irrigation. The sticky paste and powder of lime (calcium hydroxide) can be removed from the lids and conjunctival sac by using cotton-tipped applicators that have been soaked in ethylenediaminetetraacetic acid (EDTA), 0.01 M.[17] Following irrigation, the cornea and conjunctiva should be carefully examined for damage, and whenever it is possible that the eye is contaminated with solid particles, the entire conjunctival sac must be inspected for any residual particles.

In the case of an alkali burn,[16] the eye or eyelids should be treated with a topical antibiotic, which may include gentamicin solution 4 times daily or erythromycin or bacitracin ointment 4 times daily. Cycloplegia with cyclopentolate 1%, homatropine 5%, or atropine 1%, 1 to several times daily, should be instituted according to the severity of the chemical burn. Elevated intraocular pressure can be treated with acetazolamide, 250 mg 4 times daily, or a topical β blocker twice daily. For several days following the alkali burn, topical steroids such as dexamethasone 0.1% or prednisolone 1% can be used several times daily along with the topical antibiotic to reduce the severity of any anterior uveitis. However, steroids should not be used for more than 5 to 7 days, since they tend to suppress tissue repair processes.[16,17] If the chemical injury is serious enough to cause potential eyelid, conjunctival, or corneal deformities, immediate consultation with an oculoplastic surgeon is warranted.[17]

Cyanoacrylate Tarsorraphy

Cyanoacrylate adhesives (e.g., Krazy Glue, Super Glue) are widely used in both industrial and household settings. Occasionally the adhesive can be inadvertently spilled onto the ocular tissues, and in some instances the similarity of containers can lead to accidental instillation into the eye.[18,19] Although chemically induced tarsorraphy or even total ankyloblepharon can result, the condition is temporary and does not cause permanent injury.[20,21] However, the patient will often experience extreme anxiety and functional vision impairment as long as the eyelids are apposed.

Unless there are other complicating factors, surgical lysis of the adhesion should not be undertaken. This is unnecessary, since most of the adhesion is between the lashes of the upper and lower lids.[22] Because the glue can be irritative, the involved lashes can be cut, allowing the lids to be quickly and easily separated with only mild pressure.[22] A more conservative approach consisting of the application of tap water–or mineral oil–soaked eyepads has been shown to be effective and results in less eyelid morbidity.[20,23] The

moistened eyepads may need to be applied for at least 24 hours. Another approach is to instill antibiotic ointment into the conjunctival sac and onto the adhesion, covering the eye with a light pressure dressing. This conservative management often allows the glue to be easily removed with forceps 24 hours later.[21] Oral analgesics may be needed for patient discomfort or pain.

Although cyanoacrylate adhesives generally cause no permanent ocular damage, some patients have residual epithelial keratopathy or corneal abrasion.[18,19,21] This should be treated in the usual fashion, using topical antibacterial ointment and pressure-patching, if necessary.

Inflammatory Diseases

External Hordeolum

External hordeolum (common stye) is one of the most common eyelid disorders encountered in clinical practice. It is often self-treated by the patient using various home remedies, but the optometrist or other primary care clinician is often consulted because of its painful and cosmetically displeasing course.

ETIOLOGY

An external hordeolum is an acute staphylococcal infection of the glands of Zeis and Moll. This is usually a localized area of inflammation, but it may be associated with staphylococcal blepharitis. The lesions are often associated with fatigue, poor diet, and stress and can be recurrent.[24]

DIAGNOSIS

The lesion usually presents as a localized area of redness, tenderness, and swelling near the lid margin (Fig. 19.4). The primary symptom is localized pain of recent onset. Within a few days of onset of redness and tenderness, the localized area develops a yellow point. In most cases the abscess will spontaneously drain within 3 or 4 days following pointing.

MANAGEMENT

The application of hot compresses several times daily will serve to hasten pointing and drainage. Generally this is all that is necessary for resolution. Topically applied antibiotic solutions or ointments several times daily may be used to prevent infection of surrounding lash follicles, but this will not affect the course of the external hordeolum itself.[25] One of the best methods to hasten drainage of the lesion is simply to epilate 1

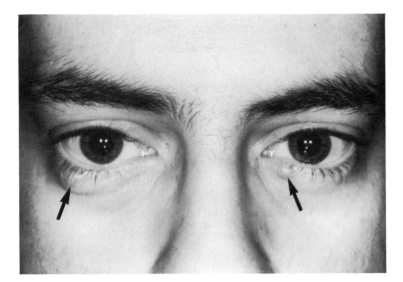

FIGURE 19.4 **Bilateral external hordeola (arrows), presenting as localized areas of redness, tenderness, and swelling near the lid margin.**

or 2 involved lashes, which creates an effective drainage channel.[26]

For lesions resistant to the usual therapy, an incision can be made with a sterile needle or blade into the area of pointing, without using a topical anesthetic.[24,26,27] This will allow the abscess cavity to drain. Following the stab incision, topical antibiotic ointment such as gentamicin or bacitracin–polymyxin B should be applied to the lid margin and conjunctival sac.[26]

Fraunfelder[27] recommends gentamicin solution or ointment applied 4 times daily during the acute phase and continued twice daily for 1 week thereafter. Topical steroids are indicated only if inflammation is severe.[27] If staphylococcal infection exists elsewhere in the body, or if there is preauricular lymphadenopathy, systemic antibiotics may be necessary. Erythromycin 250 mg or dicloxacillin 125 to 250 mg can be administered orally 4 times daily for up to 2 weeks.[27] If recurrence is likely, long-term prophylactic therapy may consist of tetracycline 250 mg administered twice daily 1 hour before meals for several months.[27] If the

hordeolum is recurrent despite such antibiotic therapy, a lid culture should be obtained to identify the organism so that specific antibiotic therapy can be instituted.[24]

Internal Hordeolum

ETIOLOGY

An internal hordeolum is a localized staphylococcal infection of the meibomian gland.[24] The infection usually results from blockage of the gland and is found more frequently in the upper lid.

DIAGNOSIS

Palpation of the affected lid area will reveal a localized area of swelling, inflammation, and tenderness within the tarsus (Fig. 19.5). The onset and course of the internal hordeolum are usually more prolonged than that of the external hordeolum.[24]

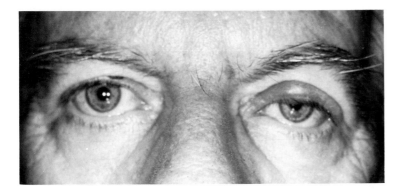

FIGURE 19.5 **Internal hordeolum of left upper lid, characterized by swelling, inflammation, and tenderness within a localized area of tarsus. The swelling has caused pseudoptosis.**

MANAGEMENT

Because the infection is deep within the lid tissue, the topical application of antibiotics is usually ineffective. In mild cases the application of hot compresses several times daily is sufficient for resolution. However, in moderate to severe cases oral antibiotic therapy is indicated. Erythromycin 250 mg 4 times daily or tetracycline 250 mg 4 times daily will usually allow resolution within 1 to 2 weeks. In cases resistant to such therapy, puncture and drainage using a sterile needle or blade may be necessary. Topically applied antibiotic solution or ointment following drainage will serve to prevent secondary infection.

Chalazion

ETIOLOGY

A chalazion is a chronic, sterile, lipogranulomatous inflammation of the meibomian gland due to retention of normal secretions.[24,28] Such duct obstruction and granuloma formation may occur during *Demodex brevis* invasion of the meibomian glands, but the precise role of this organism in the formation of chalazia has not been established.[29,30] Chalazia occur spontaneously or may follow an episode of acute internal hordeolum.

DIAGNOSIS

The lesion usually develops over several weeks and is more common in the upper lid, appearing as a hard, immobile lump[31] (Fig. 19.6). The lesion can be as small as 2 mm to as large as 7 or 8 mm in diameter.[31] It is often associated with seborrhea, including seborrheic blepharitis, and rosacea.[31–33] Palpation of the lesion produces no pain or tenderness, an important feature differentiating it from internal hordeolum. If the chalazion enlarges, it may produce mild discomfort, be cosmetically displeasing, or induce corneal astigmatism.[34,35] Cottrell and associates[36] have reported that at least 25% of chalazia will resolve spontaneously within 6 months of onset, but most will require treatment.

MANAGEMENT

In most cases chalazia can be treated successfully by the simple application of physical therapy. Topically or systemically administered antibiotics are ineffective and are not justified, because the lesion is sterile.[32] The application of hot compresses followed by vigorous digital massage to the chalazion several times daily for 2 to 4 weeks often leads to resolution, especially when the mass is small.[37] Bohigian[32] found no significant difference in improvement of chalazia using hot moist compresses 4 times daily as compared with topical

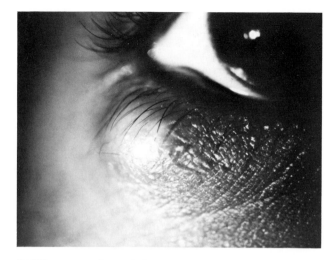

FIGURE 19.6 **A large chalazion located at the lateral aspect of the lower eyelid.**

sulfonamide 4 times daily following the hot compress therapy. In each group approximately half the patients improved after 1 month, and the cure rate after 1 month was about 40% with this conservative therapy. Perry and Serniuk[38] employed a different form of conservative therapy that resolved the chalazia in almost 80% of patients. Patients were instructed to apply warm saline soaks to the eyelids a few times daily and to use a moistened cotton-tipped applicator to the base of the eyelashes (Table 19.1). This therapy reportedly resolves the condition in about 3 weeks, ranging from 2 days to 4 weeks.

Chalazia that fail to respond to such conservative management may be treated with intralesional steroids.[39–43] Ten milligrams per milliliter of triamcinolone acetonide (Kenalog-10)) is diluted with normal saline to a concentration of 5 mg/ml.[44] Some clinicians, however, use triamcinolone in a concentration of 10 mg/ml.[40,41] A volume of 0.05 to 0.3 ml of this steroid suspension is injected into the lesion after topical anesthesia, using a 1 ml tuberculin syringe fitted with a 27- or 30-gauge 5/8 inch needle.[44,45] For lesions of the upper lid, a chalazion clamp can be gently placed around the lesion, allowing the full thickness of the eyelid to be everted to accommodate the injection. Although Jacobs and associates[39] have shown poor results with intralesional steroids compared with conventional incision and curettage, most other investigators[40–43,206] have demonstrated good to excellent results. Chalazia typically resolve within 1 or 2 weeks following a single injection of steroid, but larger lesions (≥ 6 mm in diameter) often require a second injection 2 to 4 weeks after the first.[41,42] Following the initial treatment, the chalazion should be reevaluated after 1 week, at which

TABLE 19.1
Instructions for Lid Hygiene

A. Warm Saline Soaks
  1. Prepare a saline solution using ½ teaspoon of table salt in 1 quart of warm water.
  2. Place 1 saline-soaked, sterile cotton ball on each eye with the lids closed until the cotton ball cools.
  3. Replace the cotton balls with fresh ones as they cool, and continue the soak for 10 minutes.
B. Cleaning the Lashes
  1. Gently brush the lashes using a cotton-tipped applicator moistened with the warm salt water.
  2. Clean the lashes twice daily.

Adapted from Perry HD, Serniuk RA. Conservative treatment of chalazia. Ophthalmology 1980;87:218–221.

time the need for additional intralesional steroid can be reassessed. The overall success rate has been reported to be 77% to 93% after 1 or 2 injections,[40,41,43,45] thus making intralesional steroids a viable treatment alternative in the management of chalazia. It is effective in all age groups and for lesions of both short and long duration.[41] This treatment modality is particularly suitable for use in children and for lesions located near the lid margin or lacrimal drainage apparatus. It is also useful for patients who are allergic to local anesthetics.[43]

The rationale for the use of locally injected steroid is that chalazia are composed chiefly of steroid-sensitive histiocytes, multinucleated giant cells, lymphocytes, plasma cells, polymorphonuclear leukocytes, and eosinophils.[44] The injected steroid serves to suppress additional inflammatory cells and impedes chronic fibrosis. The advantages of intralesional steroid therapy over conventional surgery are as follows:[45] (1) the in-office time required is usually less than 5 minutes; (2) since patching the eye is unnecessary, multiple chalazia in eyelids of both sides can be treated at one sitting; (3) bleeding and pain are minimal; (4) surgical damage to the lacrimal drainage apparatus is avoided in the treatment of chalazia near the medial canthus; and (5) this treatment has a high patient acceptance and reduces the cost of therapy.

Complications from intralesional steroid therapy are usually minimal (Table 19.2) and include depigmentation of the eyelid at the injection site.[46] This depigmentation can be avoided by using a transconjunctival rather than a transepidermal injection in darkly pigmented patients.[47] When depigmentation occurs, it is usually reversible. Thomas and Laborde[48] reported a single case of retinal and choroidal vascular occlusion in an 8-year-old boy that immediately followed steroid injection into a chalazion.

TABLE 19.2
Complications of Intralesional Steroids for Treatment of Chalazia

- Pain on injection
- Subcutaneous white (steroid) deposits
- Depigmentation of eyelid
- Retinal and choroidal vascular occlusion

If, after 1 or 2 months of conservative therapy or 2 to 4 weeks of intralesional steroid therapy, the chalazion has not resolved, surgical resection can be recommended.[49] For cases that are atypical or that recur following surgical removal, the chalazion should be submitted for pathologic examination to exclude the possibility of sebaceous gland carcinoma.[50]

Blepharitis

The term *blepharitis* refers to a variety of inflammatory conditions of the eyelid margin. Although some authors have maintained that *Demodex folliculorum,* the hair follicle mite, or *Demodex brevis,* found in sebaceous glands including the meibomian glands, are important factors in the development of chronic blepharitis,[29] most investigators[28,51–55] still believe there is no evidence, either histopathologic or pathogenetic, that confirms a role for these organisms in blepharitis. McCulley and associates[51] have developed a classification of chronic blepharitis (Table 19.3) that takes into consideration recent data on the significance of infectious, seborrheic, as well as meibomian gland factors in the production of this disease.

STAPHYLOCOCCAL BLEPHARITIS

Etiology. Bacterial infection of the lid margin is caused almost exclusively by *Staphylococcus aureus* and *S. epidermidis.*[28,56] Since these bacteria have been found on the bodies of *Demodex* organisms, these mites may serve as vectors of the staphylococcal organisms.[57] In

TABLE 19.3
Classification of Chronic Blepharitis

Staphylococcal
Seborrheic
  Alone
  Mixed seborrheic/staphylococcal
  Seborrheic with meibomian seborrhea
  Seborrheic with secondary meibomianitis
Primary meibomianitis

Adapted from McCulley JP, Dougherty JM, Deneau DG. Classification of chronic blepharitis. Ophthalmology 1982;89:1173–1180.

addition, although most retail eye mascaras appear to be initially free of microbial contamination, the cosmetics are subject to contamination during use and may therefore be an important source of bacterial infection.[58] Hypersensitivity to *S. aureus* may also play a role in the pathogenesis of this condition.[59]

Diagnosis.   The more common, squamous, type of staphylococcal blepharitis is characterized by the presence of hard, brittle, fibrinous scales surrounding the lashes and on the lid margin.[57] These scales are less greasy than those observed in seborrheic blepharitis.[51] There is also a characteristic hyperemia of the lid margin (Color Plate IV). Symptoms include foreign body sensation, mattering of the lids on awakening, itching, tearing, and burning. The less common, ulcerative type is characterized by matted, hard crusts surrounding the individual lashes.[57] When these crusts are removed, small ulcers can often be observed, and bleeding may occur. When staphylococcal blepharitis is chronic, associated findings may include loss of lashes (madarosis), trichiasis, or thickened lid margins (tylosis ciliaris).[57]

A chronic, papillary conjunctivitis is almost invariably associated, and the minimal mucopurulent discharge contains a preponderance of polymorphonuclear leukocytes.[57] An epithelial keratitis, due to the liberation of exotoxins from the lid margin, is often observed as a superficial punctate keratitis affecting predominantly the inferior quadrant of the cornea (see Fig. 22.2).

Management.   Since staphylococcal blepharitis can become chronic and more difficult to treat, it must be treated aggressively to be successful. It is important to stress to the patient that treatment is usually intended to *control* the condition rather than to *cure* it. The first phase of therapy, lasting 2 to 8 weeks, consists of vigorous treatment to bring the condition under control, while the chronic phase of therapy is directed at keeping the signs and symptoms in check. However, in contrast to treatment of other forms of blepharitis, staphylococcal blepharitis can sometimes be completely irradicated without the need for long-term maintenance therapy.[60]

The mainstay of therapy should be careful lid hygiene. This is accomplished at home by the patient, who is instructed to use hot compresses (15 or 20 minutes 2 to 4 times daily), each application followed by lid scrubs using a mild detergent cleanser compatible with ocular tissues. Although use of baby shampoo has been popular, recent experience has shown other commercially available cleansers (Table 19.4) to be as effective with potentially less ocular stinging and toxicity.[61,62] Polack and Goodman[61] and Leibowitz and

TABLE 19.4
Commercially Available Eyelid Cleansers

Trade Name	Manufacturer
EV Lid-Cleanser	Eagle Vision
I-Scrub	Spectra Pharmaceutical Services
SIS (Sterile I-Scrub Solution)	Spectra Pharmaceutical Services
OcuSoft Lid Scrub	Ocusoft
OcuSoft Lid Scrub Pads	Ocusoft
Ultra-Mild Eyelid Cleanser	Medmoor

Capino[62] have shown I-Scrub to be effective and well tolerated when applied with a cotton-tipped applicator.

Following each session of hot compresses and hygienic scrubs, antibiotics should be applied in the form of a lid scrub directly to the lid margin. Although use of sulfonamides has been popular for many years, McCulley and associates[51] have shown that only about 30% of *S. aureus* strains cultured from the lids are sensitive to sulfonamides. These investigators have further shown that 56% of *S. epidermidis* strains are sensitive to tetracycline, 90% to erythromycin, but only 33% to sulfonamides. Since bacitracin and erythromycin ointment are each effective against both *S. aureus* and *S. epidermidis,* these antibiotics have become the treatment of choice.[55,60] Aminoglycosides such as gentamicin and tobramycin are also effective and can be administered in solution or ointment form as a lid scrub.[55,60] Note, however, that long-term treatment with an aminoglycoside can lead to chemical blepharitis, necessitating withdrawal of the drug.[63] Several investigators[64,65] have reported the combination of trimethoprim–polymyxin B to be effective in the treatment of staphylococcal blepharitis. Whichever antibacterial agent is chosen as initial therapy, it is important to alternate treatment using a different antibiotic on consecutive weeks to avoid or minimize the development of resistant organisms.[60]

Yellow mercuric oxide ointment (Stye) can be applied to the lids when there is only minimal involvement or when the condition has already been brought under control. Nightly application of this ointment may prevent exacerbation of the condition.[25] Kastl and associates,[66] moreover, have shown 1% yellow mercuric oxide ointment to be effective in reducing bacterial lid counts in 87% of patients with blepharitis who used the medication twice daily.

Since locally applied steroids may be useful for the hypersensitivity component that is often present and will serve to reduce the congestion and irritation that often provoke the patient to rub the eyelids and aggravate the blepharitis, a combination steroid-antibacterial agent may provide the most effective treatment in some cases.[25] Donshik and associates[67] have shown the combination of gentamicin-betamethasone to be more effective than either of its components alone in relieving the signs and symptoms of staphylococcal blepharitis. Topical steroids are generally not required, however, and, indeed, can lead to serious ocular complications if used indiscriminantly by the patient.

In cases that are resistant to the initial antibiotic therapy, discontinuation of contaminated cosmetics sometimes results in marked improvement.[58] Silver nitrate 1% may be effective when applied to the lid margins.[68] The topical application of rifampin, a drug known to kill intraleukocytic staphylococci, may also be considered, although this route of administration has not been approved by the Food and Drug Administration (FDA).[57,69] Systemic antibiotic therapy may also be helpful. Oral erythromycin or tetracycline, 1 g initially then 250 mg daily, can be administered.[70] Tetracycline, however, should not be used in the treatment of children or pregnant women and the estylate form of erythromycin should be avoided.[57] If the blepharitis is unilateral, the lacrimal drainage system should be carefully examined as the etiologic factor.

If culture and sensitivity studies show the blepharitis to be caused by methicillin-resistant *S. epidermidis*, a trial of topical vancomycin should be considered.[56,71] A 50 mg/ml solution can be prepared by mixing a single ampule (500 mg) of vancomycin hydrochloride with 10 ml of phosphate-buffered artificial tears. The patient should shake the bottle vigorously before instilling the medication 4 times daily. This solution will retain its antibacterial activity for at least 2 weeks without refrigeration.[71]

It is important to impress upon the patient the importance of complying with the recommended therapy. Because of complications associated with chronic staphylococcal blepharitis, the importance of early and effective treatment cannot be overemphasized. The practitioner should observe the patient perform lid scrubs to be sure that the patient is able to properly administer the therapy at home.

Since the incidence of associated keratoconjunctivitis sicca is significantly higher in patients with chronic blepharitis than in healthy patients,[51,60] it is important that symptoms of dry eye be adequately treated with artificial tears and lubricants. Otherwise, symptoms may persist despite adequate treatment of the obvious infection.

Since any associated toxic epithelial keratitis should respond to treatment of the lid infection, the use of topical steroids for the keratitis is unnecessary.[57] However, if symptoms are severe, steroid drops such as prednisolone 0.12% may be used 2 or 3 times daily for a few days. If a hypersensitivity corneal infiltrate occurs, prednisolone drops should be added to the treatment regimen in doses ranging from 0.12% 2 or 3 times daily to 1.0% 4 or more times daily.[57]

SEBORRHEIC BLEPHARITIS

Etiology. Seborrheic blepharitis is nearly always associated with a more generalized seborrheic dermatitis and probably represents a localized form of a more generalized disorder.[51]

Diagnosis. As in staphylococcal blepharitis, seborrheic blepharitis is characterized by lid and lash crusting, but in the latter the crusts are more greasy and the lid margins are less inflamed (Color Plate V).[51]

Management. The treatment of seborrheic blepharitis involves careful lid hygiene. This can be performed by softening the crusts with warm compresses and then gently cleaning the lid margin with a cotton-tipped applicator moistened with an eyelid cleanser such as I-Scrub.[24,61,62] This should be done at home by the patient 2 to 4 times daily. In addition, the hair and scalp should be vigorously cleaned by the patient, using a shampoo containing selenium sulfide (Selsun). In cases resistant to such therapy, antibiotic lid scrubs may be employed using bacitracin or erythromycin ointment twice daily for 3 weeks to discourage staphylococcal infection.[60] Any associated keratoconjunctivitis sicca should be treated using an appropriate regimen of artificial tears and lubricants.

MIXED SEBORRHEIC-STAPHYLOCOCCAL BLEPHARITIS

Most cases of blepharitis involve a combination of staphylococcal and seborrheic changes.[24] Thus, the patient should be instructed carefully in adequate lid hygiene techniques, and the application of antibiotics as previously described should be instituted. In addition, the patient should shampoo the scalp and eyebrows with an antiseborrheic product such as selenium sulfide (Selsun). If not treated properly, this form of blepharitis can lead to chronic conjunctivitis, permanent thickening of the lid margin, and madarosis.[60]

SEBORRHEIC BLEPHARITIS WITH MEIBOMIAN SEBORRHEA

Etiology. Meibomian seborrhea is characterized by an increase of normal meibomian secretions without associated solidification of the secretions or surrounding inflammation.[51,55,60]

Diagnosis. Patients are often relatively asymptomatic but more often complain of burning, itching, or tearing. The marked symptoms are typically out of proportion to the observed signs, since there are frequently no signs of inflammation.[51,72] The diagnostic signs, when present, are moderate foam in the tear meniscus and occasionally minimal bulbar conjunctival injection.[51] A thickened oily layer of the precorneal tear film may be observed with the slit lamp as an increased interface phenomenon manifested by multiple colors of the spectrum.[72] Contact lens wearers may develop buildup of this material on the lenses, which can lead to reduced visual acuity, allergic manifestations, or vague, nonspecific symptomatology associated with lens wear.

Management. The management of meibomian seborrhea in symptomatic patients is extremely difficult because of the relative inability to reduce normal meibomian secretions. Symptoms can sometimes be reduced but not eliminated entirely by treating the seborrheic component of the blepharitis as previously described. Digital meibomian gland massage and expression can be performed in the office by the practitioner, and the patient can be instructed in these techniques to be performed twice daily at home. These procedures are designed to "milk" the meibomian glands of their excessive secretions and thus should be performed immediately after the use of hot compresses but before lid scrubs.[60]

SEBORRHEIC BLEPHARITIS WITH SECONDARY
MEIBOMIANITIS

Etiology. A meibomianitis (meibomitis) secondary to the seborrheic blepharitis may be manifest as stagnation or solidification of meibomian secretions. This occurs in a spotty pattern involving scattered clusters of meibomian glands.[51]

Diagnosis. The typical findings of seborrheic blepharitis are observed along with scattered clusters of inflamed meibomian glands whose orifices are observed to be plugged with white, stagnant secretions. Digital massage over these isolated areas results in expression of a thick, creamy-white material from the glands.

Management. Treatment involves attention to lid hygiene and the use of antibiotics as previously described. In addition, the meibomianitis is treated with hot compresses 2 to 4 times daily followed by digital expression of the meibomian glands.

These procedures will usually bring the condition under control within 2 to 8 weeks. If, however, the condition seems to be resistant, a trial of oral tetracycline, 250 mg 4 times daily, should be considered.[60] Once sufficient improvement has occurred, the dosage of tetracycline can be tapered and discontinued. Rarely is oral drug therapy required beyond 8 weeks.[60]

PRIMARY MEIBOMIANITIS

Etiology. Primary meibomianitis (meibomitis) appears to represent a form of generalized sebaceous

gland dysfunction and is therefore frequently found in association with seborrheic dermatitis or rosacea.[33,51] Both clinical as well as cytologic studies indicate that the condition is due to obstruction of the meibomian gland orifices by desquamated epithelial cells that tend to aggregate in keratotic clusters.[73] This results in stagnation of the sebaceous secretion, which causes an alteration in the contribution of the meibomian gland to the tear film.[74] *Demodex brevis* organisms have been implicated,[29] but cultures have failed to yield *S. aureus*, which implies that this disease is not a primary bacterial disorder.[51,75]

Diagnosis. In contrast to secondary meibomianitis, primary meibomianitis tends to involve all meibomian glands to a similar degree.[51] The meibomian gland changes are not always accompanied by significant inflammatory signs, and the condition may be easily overlooked.[74] Although the clinical findings can vary considerably, symptoms usually consist of complaints of irritation, chronic burning, stinging, foreign body sensation, or mild conjunctival hyperemia. Signs include inspissated plugs at the orifices of the meibomian glands, hyperemia and mild papillary hypertrophy of the palpebral conjunctiva, and thickened, rounded eyelid margins (Fig. 19.7). Special examination techniques, such as transilluminated biomicroscopy and infrared photography, may document morphologic abnormalities of the meibomian glands themselves.[76] Superficial punctate keratopathy, with rose bengal staining of the cornea and conjunctiva in the interpalpebral space, contributes to an unstable tear film.[51,77] Stagnation of the meibomian glands, which produce the lipid layer of the tear film, may also account for the tear film instability, which is clinically evident by a markedly reduced tear breakup time (TBUT).

Management. The most effective treatment for primary meibomianitis involves relieving the obstruction of the meibomian ducts and orifices by applying digital massage and gland expression 2 to 4 times daily.[74] This can be performed in the office, and the patient can be instructed in the proper technique for meibomian expression at home. The application of hot compresses before gland expression is usually more effective in promoting return of normal meibomian gland flow.

In addition to the use of hot compresses and meibomian gland expression several times daily, antibiotic ointment can be applied to the lid margin twice daily. Although no pathogen is implicated in primary meibomianitis, the use of lid scrubs to deliver bacitracin or erythromycin ointment to the lid margin is recommended and often allows significant improvement in the condition within 2 to 4 weeks.[60,72]

In cases that are resistant to therapy 1% silver

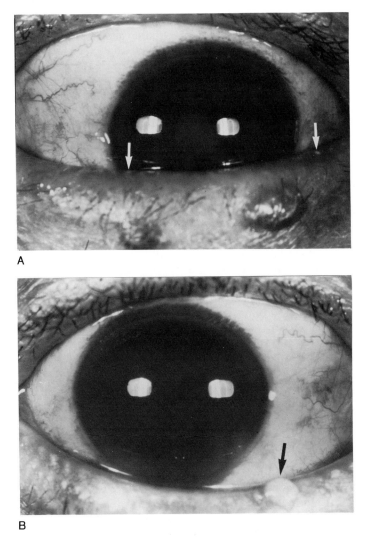

A

B

FIGURE 19.7 *(A)* Primary meibomianitis, characterized by inspissated plugs at orifices of the meibomian glands (arrows), and thickened, rounded lid margin. *(B)* Digital massage expresses thick, white, creamy material from the meibomian glands (arrow).

nitrate applied to the lid margins is sometimes effective.[68] A trial of oral tetracycline may be worthwhile.[52,60,70] Although its mechanism of action is unknown, tetracycline may reduce the quantity of lipolytic enzymes elaborated by bacteria residing on the lid margin,[78] reducing free fatty acids in the sebum[79] and thus stabilizing the tear film.[52,70] This can be accomplished even without killing the organisms.[60] Sometimes low maintenance doses of oral tetracycline (250 mg daily) are required to ensure long-term control.[60]

Since there is only a minimal increase of inflammatory cells in affected meibomian glands, the use of local steroids is unlikely to be of any benefit.[52]

During the course of therapy attention should be given to the keratoconjunctivitis sicca that is present in nearly every case of primary meibomianitis.[51] The use of artificial tears or lubricating ointments is indicated to ensure improvement in symptoms.

ANGULAR BLEPHARITIS

Etiology. Angular blepharitis is caused by infection with *Moraxella* species, but this condition can also represent a form of eczematoid blepharitis caused by staphylococci.[28] Glasser[80] has described a case apparently caused by Gram negative bacillus DF-2.

Diagnosis. The characteristic signs of angular blepharitis include chronic hyperemia, desquamation, and ulceration of the lateral, and sometimes medial, canthal regions (Color Plate VI).[28] There is often simultaneous involvement of the conjunctiva. Symptoms include irritation and tenderness of the involved area.

Management. Angular blepharitis secondary to *Moraxella* responds well to zinc sulfate 0.25% solution applied with a cotton-tipped applicator several times daily. If this is ineffective, the condition is probably caused by staphylococcal organisms, and therapy should be changed to erythromycin or bacitracin ointment.

Preseptal (Periorbital) Cellulitis

ETIOLOGY

Preseptal, or periorbital, cellulitis involves inflammation of the lid structures anterior to the orbital septum. It is often caused by direct inoculation of a pathogenic organism following penetrating trauma or spread of infection from the skin of the lids or face. One of the most common presentations is caused by extension of an internal or external hordeolum, which spreads to involve most of the lid.[81] Jackson and Baker[82] found sinusitis to be a common predisposing factor, with *Haemophilus influenzae* the most frequently isolated pathogenic organism. Other authors,[81] however, have reported *S. aureus* to be the most common pathogen, while streptococci and anaerobic bacteria play a secondary role or occasionally serve as primary pathogens. In rare cases preseptal cellulitis may be associated with a toxic shock syndrome,[83] ectopic lashes,[84] or can follow eyebrow tweezing.[85] Occasionally preseptal cellulitis may invade the postseptal region and cause orbital cellulitis, but orbital cellulitis more commonly occurs as a result of a sinus infection.[81]

DIAGNOSIS

It is important to differentiate preseptal cellulitis from the more serious orbital cellulitis (Table 19.5). Preseptal cellulitis occurs with greater frequency in the pediatric population[82] and is characterized by generalized swelling, erythema, and mild tenderness of the eyelid (Color Plate VII). Pain is minimal, and there is no proptosis nor limitation of motility.[81,86] Orbital cellulitis, on the other hand, is a potentially lethal disease characterized by marked lid swelling, erythema, chemosis, proptosis, limitation of motility, pain, decreased vision, and leukocytosis in a febrile patient.[81,86-88]

H. influenzae can cause a distinctive preseptal cellulitis in children 6 to 36 months of age. This is manifested by elevated temperature, irritability, and upper respiratory infection (URI). The lids and cheek are often sharply demarcated with a purple area of involvement.[81] Chemosis and a mucopurulent discharge are present. *H. influenzae* can produce paranasal sinusitis with secondary orbital cellulitis.[89]

MANAGEMENT

Preseptal cellulitis secondary to hordeolum should be treated with hot compresses (15 to 20 minutes, 2 to 4 times daily) along with oral tetracycline or erythromycin, 250 mg 4 times daily.[81] Marked chemosis and other severe inflammatory signs can be treated with topical steroids such as prednisolone acetate 1.0%, 4 to 8 times daily. Concomitant antibacterial therapy, such as topical gentamicin or tobramycin, will reduce the risk of secondary infection of the external ocular tissues. If an abscess forms, incision and drainage become necessary, with microbiologic investigation of the drainage material and provision of appropriate antibiotic therapy.

Other antibiotics reported to be effective in treatment of preseptal cellulitis include ampicillin[85] and intravenous oxacillin.[84,85] If a conjunctival scraping for Gram staining and culture suggests the pathogenic organism to be *H. influenzae*, the drugs of choice are ampicillin and chloramphenicol. It is prudent to begin

---

TABLE 19.5
Differential Diagnosis between Preseptal Cellulitis and Orbital Cellulitis

Clinical Finding	Bacterial Preseptal Cellulitis	Orbital Cellulitis
Lid edema	Moderate to marked	Marked
Proptosis	Absent or slight	Marked
Chemosis	Moderate	Marked
Vision	Normal	Often reduced
Pupils	Normal	May be afferent defect
Motility	Usually normal	Usually restricted
Pain on motion	Absent	Present
Intraocular pressure	Normal	May be elevated
Temperature	Normal or slightly elevated	Elevated (102° to 104°F)

Modified from Jones DB. Microbial preseptal and orbital cellulitis. In: Duane TD, Jaeger EA, eds. Clinical ophthalmology. Hagerstown, MD: Harper & Row, 1987; vol. 4, Chap. 25, 1–19.

therapy with both drugs initially until results of sensitivity testing are complete.[89]

Therapy should generally be continued for at least 5 to 7 days or until the suppuration subsides. However, cases due to streptococci require 10 days of treatment to prevent the complication of glomerulonephritis.[89] If intravenous antibiotics have been used initially, oral therapy may be substituted after 48 to 72 hours if there has been sufficient clinical improvement.

Patients who have sustained penetrating injuries with potentially contaminated wounds should have their tetanus immunization status reviewed to prevent serious sequelae.[90]

Herpes Simplex Blepharoconjunctivitis

ETIOLOGY

Blepharoconjunctivitis secondary to herpes simplex virus (HSV) usually occurs as a primary infection in children, but can also occur in adults.[91,92] It is usually caused by HSV type 1 (HSV-1), but cases of HSV type 2 (HSV-2) involvement have been reported. Primary infection occurs, with or without skin involvement, in the totally nonimmune host,[93] but cases of recurrent HSV blepharitis have been reported as a distinct clinical entity occurring in a previously exposed host.[91]

DIAGNOSIS

Two forms of clinical involvement have been described. Classically, HSV lesions of the eyelids are characterized by the presence of vesicles along the base of the eyelashes. The vesicles are pinhead in size, have erythematous bases, and may involve the lid margins

as well as the periocular skin.[94] These vesicles break and ulcerate, the eyelid margins become edematous, and dermatitis of the eyelids results.[91]

Egerer and Stary[94] have described an erosive-ulcerative form of HSV blepharitis that is much more prevalent than the vesicular herpetic lid lesions. This is characterized by erosions of the mucocutaneous junction of the lid, skin ulcers located at the lid margins, or a combination of both features (Fig. 19.8). This occurs in the absence of typical vesicular eruptions. The erosions are readily visualized by staining with sodium fluorescein. The involved portion of the lid usually demonstrates mild swelling and tenderness on palpation. There may be pronounced conjunctival injection adjacent to the lid lesion, and the regional lymph nodes are swollen. Both forms of HSV blepharoconjunctivitis are characterized by the presence of follicular conjunctivitis, occasionally associated with symptoms of a viral illness.

MANAGEMENT

Since topically administered antiviral agents have little or no effect on skin lesions,[95,96] treatment of HSV infection of the eyelid is nonspecific. In the immunologically competent host, the vesicular lesions from primary herpetic infection of the lids remain localized, are generally self-limited, and resolve without scarring, usually within 10 to 14 days.[97,98] In the absence of corneal involvement, it is prudent to use antiviral therapy such as trifluridine prophylactically in both eyes several times daily until the skin lesions resolve.[93,96,99] Simon and associates,[98] however, have suggested that even prophylactic therapy may be unnecessary, since the risk of corneal involvement in the child with normal immune mechanisms is remote. Affected children

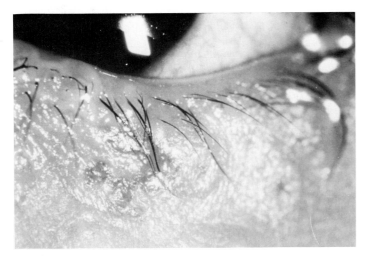

FIGURE 19.8 **Herpes simplex blepharitis with erosions and ulceration along the lid margin. (Courtesy William Wallace, O.D.)**

should be restrained from handling the lid lesions. If corneal involvement occurs, vigorous antiviral therapy should be instituted as described in Chapter 22.

Treatment of the skin lesions themselves requires only warm saline compresses and maintenance of good hygiene.[97] Drying agents can be applied to skin lesions other than those on the lid margins. These agents include Cetaphil lotion, calamine lotion, Unibase, spirits of camphor, or 70% alcohol.[68,95] If the lesions become secondarily infected, topical antibiotic ointment should be applied.[68] Steroids are contraindicated because they may predispose to a serious corneal involvement.

Varicella Zoster Blepharoconjunctivitis

ETIOLOGY

The varicella, or chickenpox, virus and the herpes zoster virus are the same organism.[100] The term varicella zoster refers to recurrent infection of the partially immune patient who had previous exposure to chickenpox but who failed to develop an adequate immune system.[101] In recent years the incidence and severity of varicella zoster infection have increased because of the growing number of immunosuppressed patients, including those with Hodgkin's disease, chronic lymphocytic leukemia, and acquired immunodeficiency syndrome (AIDS).[102–104]

The cranial nerves are frequently affected, but the thoracic dermatomes are most commonly involved, with vesicular skin lesions occurring over the sensory dermatome innervated by the affected dorsal root ganglion.[100] When the first, or ophthalmic, division of the fifth cranial nerve is affected, the resultant disease is referred to as herpes zoster ophthalmicus. One or all nerves of the first division may be involved. The frontal nerve is the most frequently affected, involving the upper lid, forehead, and some superior conjunctiva. The primary sensory nerve to the globe is the nasociliary branch. Its nasal branch innervates the sclera, cornea, iris, ciliary body, and choroid as well as the side and tip of the nose. Involvement of the nasociliary branch thus allows the virus direct access to the intraocular tissues.[105]

DIAGNOSIS

The disorder is initially characterized by headache, malaise, fever, and chills, followed in 1 or 2 days by neuralgic pain and 2 or 3 days later by hot, flushed hyperesthesia and edema of the dermatome(s). The skin overlying the affected dermatome then erupts with a single crop of clear vesicles from which virus can be cultured for only about 3 days.[100,106] The vesicles are distributed on only 1 side of the face and almost never cross more than 1 to 2 mm beyond the midline (Fig. 19.9).[100] These vesicles then become yellow and turbid and form deep eschars, which may leave permanent, pitted scars over the affected dermatome.

Occasionally the pain is represented by relatively minor tingling and numbness, but the disease is often accompanied by excruciating neuralgic pain.[100] In most cases the severe pain will subside during the first several weeks, but many patients will develop postherpetic neuralgia, a chronic condition caused by scarring of the nerves. Thus, one of the most important aspects of therapy is to prevent such scarring and subsequent neuralgia.[100] Although the acute inflammatory stage lasts only 8 to 14 days, the skin ulceration may require many weeks to heal and can result in the equivalent of third-degree burns. As a result, sometimes serious complications arise, including total lid retraction, ptosis, or madarosis.

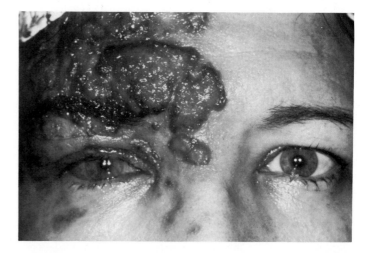

FIGURE 19.9 **Herpes zoster ophthalmicus. Note unilateral nature of vesicular eruptions.**

MANAGEMENT

In most cases the skin and lid lesions of varicella zoster are self-limited and benign.[95] The primary therapeutic concern should be for any coincident keratitis, and the swollen lids must therefore be carefully separated so that the cornea can be examined. The treatment of corneal lesions is discussed in Chapter 22. The following regimen is recommended as the general approach to varicella zoster infection.[25,93,95,103,105,107,108]

- For patients who have little or no pain or mild or no ocular involvement, no therapy is required.
- Topical steroids, such as prednisolone acetate 1.0%, should be administered up to every 3 hours for corneal edema and anterior uveitis.
- Vidarabine ointment or trifluridine solution may be administered 4 times daily along with the topical steroid as prophylaxis against potential HSV infection.
- Ulcerative keratitis should be treated with topical antibiotics.
- During the first 10 days nonnarcotic or narcotic analgesics may be administered for neuralgic pain. If there is no relief from pain, a chest x-ray film, complete blood count (CBC), and evaluation of immune status should be obtained, followed by prednisone, 20 mg orally 4 times daily for 7 days, decreasing to 15 mg orally twice daily for 7 days, then decreasing to 15 mg orally every day for 7 days, with continuation of topical steroids and cycloplegics. The patient should be monitored frequently, in consultation with an internist, for dissemination of virus.
- Postherpetic neuralgic pain can be treated with narcotic and nonnarcotic analgesics, tricyclic antidepressants and antianxiety agents, or anticonvulsants.[108] It is often necessary to use several different drugs within a group before an effective agent is found. Some patients experience pain relief from a phenothiazine, sometimes in combination with antidepressants. A useful combination is amitriptyline 25 to 50 mg orally at bedtime with fluphenazine 1 mg orally twice daily.[108] Other treatment modalities include sympathetic nerve block and subcutaneous infiltration of a steroid-anesthetic combination.[108] It should be recognized that postherpetic neuralgia associated with herpes zoster ophthalmicus is extremely difficult to treat successfully.

In recent years considerable attention has been given to the use of acyclovir to prevent complications arising from severe inflammatory changes often associated with varicella zoster infection. This drug has been employed intravenously and orally, and the oral route of administration has been shown to be effective in hastening resolution of signs and symptoms, reducing viral shedding and formation of new skin lesions, and decreasing both the incidence and severity of ocular complications.[106,109] The beneficial effect of oral acyclovir, however, is most pronounced when the drug is given within 72 hours of initial onset of skin lesions. If administered later, there is little or no alteration of the natural course of the disease. In the nonimmunocompromised patient, dosage should be 600 to 800 mg 5 times daily for 10 days.[106,109,110] This dosage regimen is well tolerated by most patients, the most common side effect being gastrointestinal disturbances (nausea and vomiting). Perhaps the most significant factor in favor of acyclovir use is the fact that most of the common complications of the disease are minimized, including dendriform keratopathy, stromal keratitis, and anterior uveitis.[106] Cobo and associates[106] have shown, moreover, that acyclovir reduces zoster-related pain during the acute phase of the infection, but the drug is of no benefit for the postherpetic neuralgia.

Topically applied steroid ointment may expedite healing of lid lesions, and antibiotics can be used prophylactically against secondary bacterial infection. Thus, the application of an antibiotic-steroid ointment for the skin and lids is beneficial.[107] This regimen appears to adequately prevent the development of large crusts and severe secondary infection. The antibiotic-steroid ointment should be applied 2 or 3 times daily and continued until all the crusts have separated. This usually occurs within 3 weeks following onset of the disease.[107] Drying lotions should not be used, since they may increase scarring.[95] For the child or adult in whom the skin lesions itch or are irritating, an oral antihistamine such as chlorpheniramine or diphenhydramine (Benadryl) may be useful in preventing scratching, which can predispose to a secondary infection and scarring.[95] In some cases a solution of aluminum acetate (Burrow's solution) is effective when applied to the skin and lid lesions as supportive therapy.[68] If there is severe lid involvement, lubricating ointments should be instilled into the eye to prevent complications arising from exposure or trichiasis. Scarring and contraction of lid tissue that creates cicatricial ectropion, lid retraction, lid margin deformity, or severe corneal complications should be managed by an oculoplastic surgeon.

In the management of lid involvement it must be recognized that the acute lid edema that occurs soon after onset of the disorder is not due to bacterial cellulitis, and this condition will resolve within a few days without antibiotic therapy.[107]

Steroids have a well-established role in the therapy of herpes zoster ophthalmicus. They act to suppress destructive inflammation while permitting the infection to run its natural course. Their use is entirely justified if the disease is sufficiently severe with regard to ocular involvement or pain. The use of systemic steroids, however, is still controversial.[103] Steroid-induced dissemination of virus is possible in patients who are immunologically compromised, such as in lymphoma, AIDS, or leukemia. Elderly patients who have debilitating systemic disease may also respond less satisfactorily. For nonimmunocompromised patients older than 60 years, Liesegang[103] has recommended that oral prednisone be given in a dosage of 60 mg daily for 5 days, tapered over a 2-week period. Oral steroids should probably be withheld in immunosuppressed individuals, patients with an underlying medical disorder, and younger patients.

Phthiriasis Palpebrarum

Phthiriasis palpebrarum is an uncommon eyelid infestation by *Phthirus pubis* (crab louse) and, less commonly, by *Pediculus humanus* species.[111,112] The term pediculosis refers to infestation by *Pediculus corporis* (body louse) or *Pediculus capitis* (head louse) and should not generally be used when referring to eyelid manifestations.

ETIOLOGY

Phthiriasis or pediculosis usually occur when sanitary conditions are inadequate. Phthiriasis palpebrarum is caused by lid infestation by the pubic louse, whose habitat is normally the pubic and inguinal areas.[113] The eyelashes and eyebrows are special sites of predilection for phthiriasis in children.[111] Phthiriasis is usually transmitted by sexual contact, but in children infestation occurs from contact with an infested parent, usually the mother.[111] The lice may also be transferred from bedding and towels contaminated with lice eggs.[113]

The fecal material and saliva excreted by the parasites can be both toxic and antigenic, resulting in an inflammatory response manifested by conjunctivitis, marginal keratitis, and preauricular lymphadenopathy.[114,115]

Pediculosis palpebrarum, on the other hand, occurs only when there is florid infestation of the scalp with the head louse.[113] This condition is also transmitted by close contact with an infested individual or by contaminated bedding or clothing.[111]

DIAGNOSIS

Diagnosis is easily accomplished by careful slit-lamp examination, by which the adult lice and eggs (nits) are readily detected. The adult lice vary from 1 to 1.5 mm.[113] The translucent lice can be more easily visualized by epilating 1 or more infested lashes for examination under low power of a light microscope.[28]

Phthiriasis palpebrarum is characterized by itching and irritation, and there may be blepharoconjunctivi-

tis, blood-stained thickened discharge on the lid margins, and the presence of nits and adult parasites on the eyelashes (Fig. 19.10). The presence of parasites and their nits, along with tiny, granular, reddish black fecal material matted to the lids and lashes, leads to a dark crusty discoloration of the lid margins.[112] A preauricular lymphadenopathy may also be present.[113]

MANAGEMENT

Treatment is essentially the same for all varieties of lid infestation, whether caused by *Pediculus* or *Phthirus*.[111] The scalp, body, or pubic areas should be treated as well as the lid condition. In addition, for treatment to be effective, thorough investigation and treatment of contacts should be performed, including family members, clothing, and bedding.

In cooperative patients it is possible to remove the adult parasites with forceps or cotton-tipped applicators using the slit lamp, but this procedure is somewhat uncomfortable, especially in children. Cilia bearing eggs should be epilated. Cryotherapy has been recommended as providing rapid cure.[111] Pharmacologically, a variety of treatment modalities can be employed and have been shown to be effective.[68,111–113] Treatment involving yellow mercuric oxide 1% ophthalmic ointment applied twice daily for 1 week is effective. In addition, bland petrolatum ointment can be thickly applied twice daily for 8 days to smother the parasites. Anticholinesterase agents, such as 0.25% physostigmine ointment, may be applied to the lid margins. These agents, however, have little effect on the nits, and therapy should therefore be continued twice daily for about 10 to 14 days to ensure that all eggs have hatched and that the emerging parasites have been adequately treated. The use of such anticholinesterase treatment is limited by annoying ocular side effects (e.g., miosis, browache). The use of gamma benzene hexachloride (Kwell) for the lid condition should be avoided because of potential ocular irritation and chemical conjunctivitis.[112,113] Similarly, pyrethrin gel (A-200 Pyrinate) and other pediculocides should not be used near the eye.[113]

Scalp, body, and pubic hair must be treated with an appropriate pediculocidal agent (Table 19.6) in combination with careful nit removal. Although gamma benzene hexachloride (Kwell) is generally considered the drug of choice for the treatment of head and pubic lice, a pyrethrin-based pediculocide, RID, has been shown to be equally effective and safe and is available over the counter, without prescription.[116] A single application to the affected areas is usually adequate to eradicate the lice.[113] The application should be repeated in 1 week if viable nits persist or if new nits appear. Translucent, empty nits are signs of inactive infestation and require no further treatment.[112] Because gamma

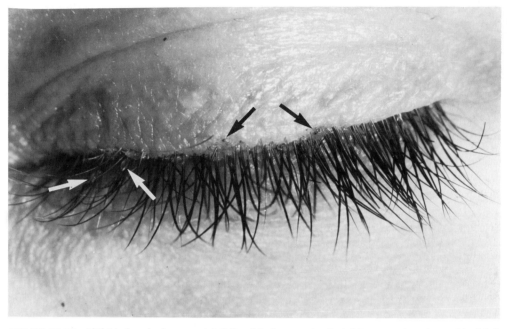

FIGURE 19.10   **Phthiriasis palpebrarum. Adult lice (black arrows), nits (white arrows), and parasitic debris are matted to the base of the lashes. (Courtesy Rodney Nowakowski, O.D.)**

benzene hexachloride may lead to central nervous system (CNS) toxicity, it must be used cautiously in infants, children, and pregnant women, and excessive application should be avoided.[113] Pubic lice are not resistant to gamma benzene hexachloride.[112] If treatment appears to be ineffective, there is either patient noncompliance or reinfestation has occurred.

In addition to treating the lids and body hair, family members or sexual contacts should be examined and treated if infested. This is important because of the high risk of concurrent sexually transmitted disease in patients with *Phthirus pubis* infestation.[117] Clothing, linens, and grooming instruments should be laundered

or sterilized by exposing to dry heat at 140°F (50°C) for 20 to 30 minutes.[112,113] This can usually be accomplished at the highest temperature settings of most household dryers. Contaminated cosmetics should be discarded.

Allergic Diseases

The eyelid is one of the most common sites of ocular allergy. The intimate relationship of the palpebral conjunctiva and skin at the eyelid margin predisposes to simultaneous allergic involvement of both the conjunc-

TABLE 19.6
Pediculocidal Agents[a]

Trade Name	Formulation	Manufacturer
A-200 Pyrinate	Gel, shampoo	Norcliff Thayer
Barc	Gel, liquid	Commerce Drug
Kwell[b]	Cream, lotion, shampoo	Reed & Carnrick
Licetrol	Liquid	Republic
R & C	Shampoo	Reed & Carnrick
RID	Liquid	Leeming/Pacquin
Triple X	Shampoo	Carter Products

[a]Not for use on or near the eye.
[b]Prescription product. All others are available over the counter.

tiva and the eyelid. The extreme thinness of its skin and its loose arrangement of connective tissue make the eyelid particularly susceptible to allergic involvement.[118]

URTICARIA AND ANGIONEUROTIC EDEMA

Urticaria (hives) refers to localized patches of edema in the superficial layers of the skin, whereas angioneurotic edema involves primarily the deeper subcutaneous tissues.[119]

Etiology. Most cases of urticaria or angioneurotic edema are thought to represent anaphylactoid (type I) hypersensitivities[119,120] and usually result from ingestion of a food or drug to which the patient is sensitive. Bites or stings of insects can also cause the reaction, and less commonly topical drugs may produce acute wheals or eyelid edema.[119] Clinically, the reaction may appear within seconds or minutes following the initiating episode, and the reaction can manifest itself independently in the eyelid or can occur in association with acute allergic reactions elsewhere in the body.

The histopathologic changes of angioneurotic edema and urticaria are identical except for the predilection of the former for the deep cutaneous tissues and predilection of the latter for the superficial tissues.[119] Thus, both conditions are treated in similar fashion.

Diagnosis. The history and clinical findings usually provide an immediate diagnosis. Urticaria is characterized by one or more circumscribed plaques of edema with an erythematous margin and a blanched center.[119] Angioneurotic edema, on the other hand, demonstrates localized dermal edema with an essentially normal epidermis (Fig. 19.11). Depending on the severity

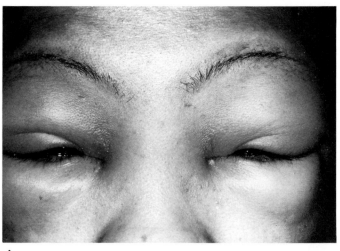

A

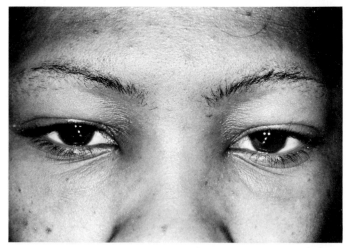

FIGURE 19.11 *(A)* **Angioneurotic edema secondary to hair dressing solution.** *(B)* **Complete resolution after 3 days of oral antihistamines and application of warm compresses.**

B

TABLE 19.7
Characteristics of Contact Dermatitis

Characteristic	Primary Irritant Dermatitis	Allergic Contact Dermatitis
Incidence	Common	Uncommon
Occurrence	Occurs upon first exposure	Occurs with previous sensitizing exposure
Onset	1–24 hours	12–72 hours
Immunity	None	Cell mediated
Clinical appearance	Flat, dry, scaly	Papular, vesicular
Exposure required	Concentration dependent	Minimal exposure

Modified from Rich LF, Hanifin JM. Ocular complications of atopic dermatitis and other eczemas. Int Ophthalmol Clin 1985;25:61–76.

of the condition, there may be mild to moderate discomfort and itching.

The intradermal skin test is sometimes used to confirm the diagnosis. A small amount of the suspected allergen can be applied to a superficial epidermal scratch or can be injected intradermally. The rapid appearance, within seconds or minutes, of a wheal and flare indicates a positive reaction.[119] As an alternative, a small amount of the substance may be instilled topically into the conjunctival sac, and the nearly immediate onset of eyelid swelling, chemosis, conjunctival hyperemia, and itching indicates a positive response. It must be emphasized, however, that these skin and conjunctival tests are not necessarily innocuous in that they can cause anaphylaxis in highly susceptible individuals.[119] Thus, when performing the conjunctival test, it is prudent to use relatively low concentrations of drug or to instill relatively small amounts. Unfortunately, a negative skin or conjunctival test does not ensure that the drug can be administered safely. Severe, even fatal reactions have been reported following negative skin testing.[121]

Management.   Since complications rarely arise following such acute episodes, prudent management involves the administration of systemic antihistamines such as oral chlorpheniramine maleate, 4 mg every 4 hours, cold compresses during the first 24 to 48 hours, then warm compresses, and reassurance.[68,119,120] If the condition is severe, immediate therapy may include the subcutaneous administration of 0.3 to 0.5 ml of epinephrine 1:1000.[68] Systemically or topically administered steroids can be used for general discomfort and itching, but they should be used only when the condition is severe or debilitating. Orally administered aspirin has been reported to be a valuable antipruritic agent in such cases.[68]

It is important to eliminate the cause of the reaction, and if continued exposure cannot be prevented, the patient should be desensitized by serial administration of small amounts of the offending allergen. This should be performed by an allergist.

CONTACT DERMATITIS

Etiology.   Contact dermatitis is often classified as either primary irritant (nonallergic) or allergic (Table 19.7).[122] Primary irritant dermatitis is more common but less often seen in practice because it occurs within minutes to hours and thus allows a self-diagnosis and avoidance of the offending irritant. Allergic contact dermatitis, however, is a delayed, cell-mediated (type IV) hypersensitivity that involves the eyelid skin and may secondarily involve the conjunctiva.[119] Sensitization usually requires at least 5 to 10 days for strongly sensitizing allergens[123] but can require months or even years when less potent sensitizers are involved. After the patient has been sensitized, the time interval between subsequent exposure to the allergen and the appearance of the reaction is usually 12 to 72 hours.

Although virtually any medication can cause allergic contact dermatitis, certain drugs or substances are particularly potent sensitizers (Table 19.8).[118–120,122,124–128] Facial creams and cosmetics are especially common causes of contact dermatitis in women.[129] Interestingly, erythromycin has never been reported to cause allergic

TABLE 19.8
Drugs or Substances Known to Cause Allergic Contact Dermatitis or Dermatoconjunctivitis

- Cosmetics (including nail polish)
- Local anesthetics
- Neomycin
- Tobramycin
- Gentamicin
- Bacitracin
- Benzalkonium chloride
- Thimerosal
- Parabens
- Atropine
- Timolol
- Phenylephrine
- Lanolin
- Rubber or nickel (eyelash curler)
- EDTA

contact dermatitis, nor has it ever been associated with positive patch test reactions.[130,131]

Allergic contact dermatitis of the lids associated with topically administered ocular medications usually occurs following contact conjunctivitis. On the other hand, allergic contact dermatitis without conjunctivitis is usually caused by a drug or substance coming in contact with the eyelids without having been instilled into the conjunctival sac.[132]

Diagnosis. As with urticaria and angioneurotic edema, diagnosis of contact dermatitis is usually made by a careful history and physical examination. However, identification of the specific causative agent is sometimes difficult because of the myriad of possible irritants and allergens.

The primary cutaneous signs of irritant dermatitis are mild scaly eruptions with slight eyelid edema and faint erythema.[122] It is often localized to the skin of the eyelid, whereas allergic contact dermatitis frequently spreads to involve periorbital skin. Allergic contact dermatitis is manifest as erythema, vesiculation, oozing, crusting, scaling, or thickening (Fig. 19.12). Eyelid edema is often present, and a linear fold of skin beneath the lower lid (Dennie-Morgan fold) may be observed.[118,133] The primary symptom is itching. The conjunctiva may also manifest signs of allergic involvement, including a papillary reaction, hyperemia, chemosis, and watery discharge.

It should be recognized that once the patient is sensitized, the offending allergen can cause allergic reactions in the skin virtually anywhere in the body.[122,134,135] This can account, for example, for the eyelid manifestations of allergic reactions to nail polish, which can be confined entirely to the lids.

A skin patch test can be used to confirm the diagnosis. This should be performed on a relatively hairless area of skin such as the inner aspect of the forearm or the back.[119] The drug or substance to be tested is applied to the skin and covered by a small piece of impermeable material such as Saran Wrap or aluminum foil, and fixed with tape. Alternatively, the substance can be applied under a Band-Aid or cotton ball if the edges are sealed with tape.[122] The adhesive eye patches that are used for amblyopia therapy may also be used. The skin to which the medication or substance has been applied for 48 hours should be observed 24 to 48 hours after the dressing has been removed to allow time for the pressure-induced effects to subside (Color Plate III). It is possible for false-negative results to occur because the skin to which the substance has been applied is relatively resistant to the development of allergic contact dermatitis. Similarly, false-positive results may occur from the application of a substance that is too concentrated and that therefore produces an eczematous reaction by irritation rather than by immunologic hypersensitivity.[119] Since asymptomatic individuals can demonstrate positive skin patch tests, a positive result does not necessarily indicate the specific cause of the dermatitis. Thus, a careful history is probably more important than skin patch-testing in delineating the specific cause.

Another important test that can be employed to make a positive diagnosis of allergic contact dermatitis is to simply instruct the patient to use the suspected allergen (such as a cosmetic). By employing such a usage test either alone or in combination with skin patch-testing, the accuracy of diagnosis increases significantly.[122,129]

Management. The most effective treatment for contact dermatitis is to eliminate the offending substance. In many cases no other therapy is required, but in persistent or severe cases the application of soothing compresses saturated with water and Burow's solution (aluminum acetate) 1:16, or Domeboro tablets (alu-

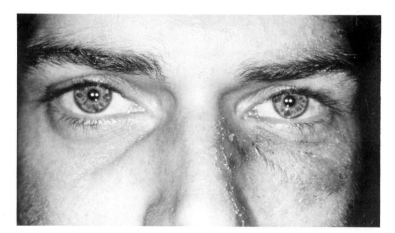

FIGURE 19.12 **Eczematoid reaction characteristic of allergic contact dermatitis.**

minum sulfate and calcium acetate) dissolved in water is effective for the acute, weeping stages of the disorder and will often cause drying of the dermatitis within a few days.[68,119] The application of steroid cream or ointment, such as 0.5 to 1% hydrocortisone, is helpful in the dry, subacute, and chronic stages and can be applied to the eyelids several times daily until the reaction subsides. Use of steroids, however, must be strictly supervised because of the risk of serious complications, including glaucoma.[136] Topically applied antihistamines have no effect on this type IV hypersensitivity and may even be sensitizing.[119] However, when orally administered, antihistamines can provide relief from the associated itching. Desensitization to offending substances has largely been ineffective.[130]

It should be emphasized that allergic contact dermatitis may worsen even with steroid therapy if contact with the offending substance continues. Thus, the use of combination preparations such as neomycin-hydrocortisone can lead to continued irritation if neomycin is the sensitizer. Moreover, topically applied fluorinated steroids have been reported to cause persistent periocular dermatitis.[137] Successful management requires withdrawal of the steroid and treatment with oral tetracycline, 250 mg 4 times daily, along with 0.5% to 1% hydrocortisone ointment.

Abnormalities of Motility

Ptosis

ETIOLOGY

Although establishing the initial diagnosis of ptosis is not difficult, determining the specific etiology can be challenging. Before the ptosis can be properly managed, it is therefore imperative that the underlying etiology be identified.

There are both congenital as well as acquired forms of ptosis (Table 19.9).[138] In addition, various ocular diseases or abnormalities may simulate ptosis (pseudoptosis). Congenital ptosis can vary from complete closure to only slight asymmetry between sides. It is usually autosomal dominant and is caused by incomplete differentiation of the levator muscle.[25] Acquired ptosis, on the other hand, is usually caused by abnormality of the levator muscle or its innervation. This may be associated with neurogenic lesions, myogenic problems such as myasthenia gravis, trauma, or mechanical effects. Thiamine deficiency in childhood has also been reported to be a cause of ptosis.[139,140] Involutional (senile) ptosis is common and thought to be caused by disinsertion of the levator aponeurosis.[141–143]

TABLE 19.9
Classification of Ptosis

Congenital ptosis
　With normal superior rectus function
　With superior rectus weakness
　Blepharophimosis
　Synkinetic ptosis
　　Marcus Gunn
　　Misdirected third nerve
Acquired ptosis
　Neurogenic
　Myogenic
　Traumatic
　Mechanical
Pseudoptosis
　Microphthalmia, phthisis bulbi, anophthalmia, or
　　enophthalmos
　Hypotropia
　Dermatochalasis
　Lid cellulitis

Adapted from Beard C, Sullivan JH. Ptosis—current concepts. Int Ophthalmol Clin 1978;18:53–73.

DIAGNOSIS

The following examination should be performed for the evaluation of ptosis.[138,144]

- The lid level should be measured by instructing the patient to fixate a distant object while the practitioner measures the vertical height of the affected palpebral aperture. The vertical height of the normal palpebral aperture is about 10 mm, and in unilateral cases, the fellow eye serves as a control.
- Action of the levator muscle can be assessed by instructing the patient to look up and down while the practitioner's hand stabilizes the frontalis muscle. The prognosis for a successful surgical result is better if the levator function is good. Levator function can also be assessed by observing the presence of a lid fold. The presence of a fold at the upper margin of the tarsal plate indicates levator function.
- Congenital ptosis can often be distinguished from acquired ptosis by observing the position of the lids in full downgaze. The inelasticity of the lid in congenital ptosis results in lid lag, whereas in acquired myogenic ptosis, the affected lid usually assumes a lower position on downgaze.
- Orbicularis muscle function should be assessed by observing closure of the lids.
- When the history reveals generalized muscular weakness, the patient should be evaluated for myasthenia gravis, preferably in consultation with a neurologist. A tuberculin syringe containing 10 mg of edrophonium chloride (Tensilon) should be prepared with an intravenous needle, and 2 mg is injected intravenously within 15 to 30 seconds. The needle should

be left in place, and if there is prompt elevation of the ptotic lid, a diagnosis of myasthenia gravis is indicated. If no reaction occurs after 45 seconds, the remaining 8 mg should be injected. If a cholinergic reaction consisting of muscarinic side effects, skeletal muscle fasciculations, and increased muscle weakness occurs after injection of 2 mg, the test should be discontinued and atropine sulfate 0.4 to 0.5 mg should be administered intravenously.

If Horner's syndrome is suspected, 1 drop of 2.5% phenylephrine can be instilled into each eye and the lid positions compared after 5 minutes. The lid on the affected side will be observed to elevate when compared with the noninvolved side (Fig. 19.13).[145] This lid retraction is caused by denervation hypersensitivity of Mueller's muscle to the adrenergic agonist. This test must be performed before pupillary dilation with adrenergic mydriatics, because instilling the drops for dilation may cause lid retraction on the noninvolved side.

MANAGEMENT

Surgery represents the most effective treatment modality for most forms of ptosis. In some instances,

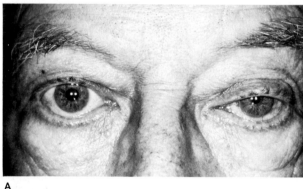

A

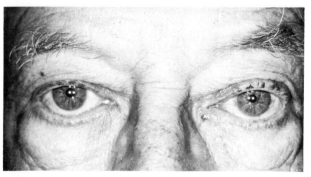

B

FIGURE 19.13   *(A)* **Ptosis of left upper lid associated with Horner's syndrome.** *(B)* **Marked left upper lid retraction 5 minutes after instillation of 2.5% phenylephrine.**

however, topically applied or systemically administered medications may be of value.

Surgery for congenital ptosis is usually indicated for cosmetic reasons and can thus be deferred until the child is of school age, at which time the degree of ultimate ptosis is most easily assessed.[25] However, if the ptosis interferes with vision or if compensatory head tilt or furrowed brow become established, surgical correction should be performed earlier.

The treatment of acquired ptosis should necessarily be determined from its cause. Any residual ptosis can be managed by surgical correction.[207] However, if the ptosis is minimal or if surgery is contraindicated or refused, a ptosis crutch attached to the spectacle frame can be employed.[146] Many conventional ptosis crutches do not permit full lid closure, thus necessitating that the patient slide the spectacles down the nose once every 5 minutes to allow lid closure and normal ocular wetting. Failure to do this often results in severe complications from corneal exposure. As an alternative, an ocular prosthesis has been described that permits full lid closure and thus prevents corneal exposure.[147] This prosthetic device is particularly useful for patients with chronic progressive external ophthalmoplegia (CPEO), in which there is often loss of normal corneal protective mechanisms and, consequently, a high risk of postoperative corneal exposure.[148]

The treatment of ptosis associated with myasthenia gravis involves the use of orally administered anticholinesterase agents. Therapy is usually begun with neostigmine bromide (Prostigmin) 15 mg 3 to 5 times daily.[25] If neostigmine is unsatisfactory in controlling the systemic manifestations as well as the lid signs, therapy can be changed to pyridostigmine bromide (Mestinon).[149] In addition, thymectomy may be beneficial.[25] Although anticholinesterase therapy frequently controls the systemic manifestations of myasthenia gravis, it is less effective for the lid signs and extraocular muscle palsies.[150] Therefore, for cases that do not adequately respond to such therapy, systemically administered steroids may be required. Following initiation of steroid therapy, the ocular signs may begin to improve within a few days, but substantial improvement may not be observed for as long as 3 months.[149] The goal of long-term steroid therapy is a maintenance dosage of prednisone 15 or 20 mg every other day.[149] If the ptosis remains refractory to steroid and anticholinesterase therapy, corrective lid surgery may be considered if the ptosis has remained stable for at least 3 to 4 years.[151]

When there is minimal ptosis, a trial of topical ocular phenylephrine 2.5% or 10% every 4 hours can be used to intermittently elevate the lid for social occasions.[152] The phenylephrine acts on Mueller's muscle to elevate the lid, and the effect may be dramatic within 5 to 10 minutes, especially in patients with Horner's syndrome, where there is denervation hypersensitivity (see Fig. 19.13).

Ptosis associated with thiamine deficiency often responds rapidly to corrective therapy, sometimes within 2 to 48 hours.[140]

Myokymia

Lid myokymia is a common condition in which mild to moderate fasciculations of the orbicularis muscle cause annoying symptoms, often with no observable eyelid signs.

ETIOLOGY

Etiologic factors include fatigue, stress, tension, anxiety, lack of sleep, irradiated corneal or conjunctival lesions, and occasionally excessive use of alcohol or smoking.[153] The topical ocular use of anticholinesterase agents can also produce lid myokymia,[153] and cases of lid myokymia associated with use of fluphenazine[154] and haloperidol[155] have been reported.

DIAGNOSIS

The patient often complains that the eye "jumps" or "quivers." However, gross external as well as slit-lamp examination fail to uncover any ocular movement abnormality, and the astute clinician soon learns to interpret such complaints to be related to eyelid fasciculations. Rarely, the patient may report associated oscillopsia, correlating with "pseudonystagmus" observed on slit-lamp examination.[156] The lower lid is more commonly involved, and the condition is usually unilateral.

MANAGEMENT

In cases that are not drug induced, management involves patient reassurance, since in most cases the myokymia spontaneously resolves. Occasionally, however, the condition is persistent or severe, and more specific treatment is indicated. Topically administered antihistamines, such as antazoline or pheniramine, are often effective and may give significant relief within 15 to 20 minutes. Antihistaminic therapy relaxes the spasming orbicularis muscle by prolonging its refractory time. The topical medication should be used every 4 hours as needed to abolish symptoms. If this is ineffective, 12.5 to 25 mg of promethazine (Phenergan) can be administered orally 1 to 3 times daily, or 75 mg of tripelennamine can be administered orally 4 times daily.[153] For recalcitrant cases oral quinine, 200 to 300 mg, may be administered 1 to 3 times daily either

alone or in combination with antihistaminic therapy.[153] Quinine relaxes the orbicularis muscle by a curari-like action, but it must be avoided in pregnant women because of its abortifacient properties.

Essential Blepharospasm

Essential blepharospasm is a chronic and progressive disorder in which bilateral, almost symmetric eyelid closure occurs involuntarily. It can occur alone or be associated with dyskinetic disorders of other facial muscles.

ETIOLOGY

The blepharospasm is a result of abnormal involuntary contraction of the orbicularis muscles, but other muscles innervated by the seventh cranial nerve can also be involved.[157] Although the precise pathophysiology of the disorder remains unknown, a dopaminergic imbalance in the central nervous system has been proposed.[158]

DIAGNOSIS

The condition is found more often in women and usually begins in the fifth or sixth decade.[159] The severity of the spasms slowly progresses over 6 months to 3 years, and the condition nearly always becomes bilateral. The severe, involuntary muscle contractions can cause profound functional impairment and may preclude many routine daily activities such as reading or driving. The spasms, however, do not occur during sleep, but emotional stress or fatigue will often increase their intensity.

Gladstone and Putterman[160] have described a repetitive forced closure test that can be used to elicit symptomatic spasms in the patient with only mild facial or lid signs. The patient is instructed to close the lids maximally for about 5 seconds and then to open them fully. This cycle is repeated at least 3 to 10 times, during which severe blepharospasm, with or without facial spasm, will often become apparent.

MANAGEMENT

Since patients are often self-conscious and depressed, reassurance is required and psychologic counseling may sometimes be needed. Although numerous medications have been used to suppress the spasms, the response to treatment has generally been variable, unpredictable, and usually transient. The pharmacologic approach has included trials of anticholinergics, anticonvulsants, antidopaminergics, antianxiety agents, antipsychotics, and monoamine depletors.[158] The results of various surgical interventions, including seventh-nerve resection and myectomy, have likewise been variable.[161] The effectiveness of biofeedback training has also been explored.[162]

The therapeutic approach receiving the greatest attention in recent years has been the use of botulinum toxin. Although still an experimental procedure, treatment with this agent has shown impressive results in numerous series of patients.[163–175] Botulinum toxin (type A) is derived from the bacterium *Clostridium botulinum* and is supplied in a purified crystalline form (Oculinum) for ophthalmic use.[169] When injected into striated muscle, this neurotoxin blocks the release of acetylcholine from nerve terminals, thus preventing transmission of the nerve impulse and temporarily paralyzing the injected muscle.[159] Limited histologic studies have failed to detect any pathologic lesions induced by the toxin.[165]

Although the specific technique for injection of botulinum-A toxin varies,[159,163,166,169,172] most investigators use a procedure similar to the following: a 1½ inch 27- or 30-gauge needle on a tuberculin syringe is used to infiltrate the pretarsal orbicularis muscle at multiple sites in the upper and lower lids, without using a local anesthetic. A total of 25 units (10 ng) of toxin in 10 separate injection sites is commonly administered.

Use of botulinum-A toxin appears to be effective in reducing or eliminating spasms in almost all patients (Fig. 19.14). The beneficial effects of treatment occur within 2 or 3 days, but the duration of the therapeutic response is only about 10 to 12 weeks, necessitating retreatment.[159,166,169,171,172] Although some authors have reported no evidence of increasing duration of clinical improvement after multiple injections,[164] Engstrom and associates[159] have demonstrated a progressive increase in response time after repeated treatments from the first to fourth injection, after which the duration of improvement seems to stabilize. This finding, along with the work of others,[166,167] appears to indicate that tolerance to the toxin does not develop.

Side effects and complications of botulinum-A toxin injection are not uncommon but tend to be minimal and well tolerated. All reported effects have been local (Table 19.10), and no systemic side effects have been observed.[166,169,170] The most common complication is ptosis, caused by toxin infiltration of the levator muscle.[168,172,174] The development of ptosis cannot be predicted nor controlled, and it usually occurs within 2 or 3 days after injection and gradually subsides in 4 to 8 weeks. Diplopia is most commonly caused by toxin-induced paresis of the inferior oblique muscle, and this complication may be reduced by avoiding injection of toxin in the medial two-thirds of the lower lid.[163,171]

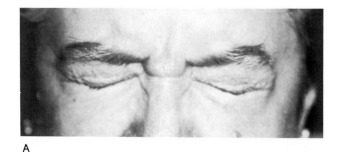

A

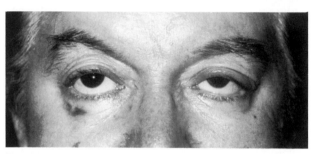

B

FIGURE 19.14 **Elimination of blepharospasm with injection of botulinum-A toxin.** *(A)* **Before treatment, blepharospasm occurred 75% of the time.** *(B)* **Appearance 2 weeks after treatment. Note ptosis of left upper lid and small subcutaneous hemorrhage beneath right lower lid at one of the injection sites. (From Malinovsky V. Benign essential blepharospasm. J Am Optom Assoc 1987; 58:646–651, with permission of the author and publisher.)**

Lagophthalmos

Lagophthalmos is a condition in which there is an inability to fully close the eyelids.

ETIOLOGY

Lagophthalmos can be classified as:[176–178]

- Physiologic or nocturnal. This occurs during sleep, and symptoms arising from the condition occur more often in adults than in children, probably because of a reduction of tears in the former group.
- Orbital. This is usually associated with severe proptosis (see Fig. 27.6).
- Mechanical. Scarring of the lid muscles or lids may prevent closure.
- Paralytic. Seventh-nerve palsy is the most common type of paralytic lagophthalmos.

DIAGNOSIS

Symptoms include ocular irritation, especially on awaking. This symptom is accompanied by punctate keratitis of the central or inferior cornea, often in the shape of

TABLE 19.10
Side Effects of Botulinum Toxin Injection

- Ptosis
- Lacrimation or epiphora
- Dry eye
- Lagophthalmos
- Exposure keratopathy
- Ectropion
- Entropion
- Diplopia
- Subcutaneous hemorrhage

a horizontal band (Color Plate VIII). If the exposure is severe enough, melting of the inferior cornea can occur.[176] In addition, the conjunctiva is often injected, and the affected portion of the cornea may be hypoesthetic.[176]

The physical examination should confirm the presence of lagophthalmos. This is usually demonstrated easily by instructing the patient to gently close the eyes. In cases of nocturnal lagophthalmos, the presence of lagophthalmos may not be noted until the patient is in a supine position and the closed eyelids are examined carefully with a penlight (Fig. 19.15). Another simple way to determine if nocturnal lagophthalmos is occurring is to query the spouse or parent if the patient sleeps with his or her eyes open. The presence or absence of a Bell's reflex is immaterial, since this phenomenon is unrelated to the position of the globe during gentle lid closure or during sleep.[176]

MANAGEMENT

When the degree of corneal exposure is mild, bland ocular lubricating ointment applied at bedtime will be sufficient to eliminate symptoms. Artificial tears instilled every 2 to 4 hours during the day may also be required according to the severity of the exposure. In addition, the eyelids can be taped closed at bedtime by applying the tape first to the cheek, then pulling the lower lid upward as the tape is attached to the brow and forehead.[176] This form of treatment is usually well tolerated. In cases of severe lagophthalmos, a moisture chamber can be formed of Saran Wrap and placed over the eye at bedtime. Antibiotic ointment may also be indicated if infection seems imminent. Extended wear bandage contact lenses may also be employed along with antibiotic or lubricant therapy. When these conservative measures fail, or if the condition is long-standing, surgical correction may be necessary.[179–181]

Incomplete Blink

Abelson and Holly[182] have described a condition in which incomplete blinking contributes to inferior punctate keratopathy. Impaired blinking may cause the corneal lesions by producing exposure and inadequate tear film. The condition is treated by blink training,[183] the application of artificial tears or bland lubricating ointment, or bandage soft contact lenses.

Lid Retraction

Lid retraction is most commonly associated with thyroid disease and is considered in Chapter 27.

Abnormalities of Lid Margin Position

Ectropion

Ectropion is a condition in which usually the lower, but sometimes the upper, lid becomes everted, expos-

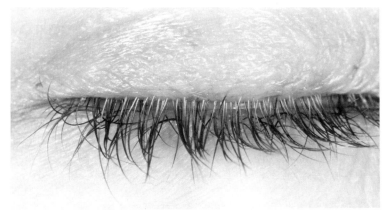

FIGURE 19.15 **Nocturnal lagophthalmos.**

ing the conjunctiva and cornea and causing irritation and occasionally secondary infection.

ETIOLOGY

Ectropion is classified as involutional (senile), cicatricial, and paralytic.[141] By far the most common type is involutional, which is caused by horizontal laxity of the eyelid tissue components.[184,185] This allows gravity to evert the lower lid and expose the conjunctiva and inferior cornea.

Scarring of the skin of the lids produces cicatricial ectropion. This can be caused by chemical or thermal burns or chronic dermatoses, or it can be secondary to trauma or previous surgery.

Paralytic ectropion is caused by prolonged paralysis of the orbicularis muscle of the lower lid, most often from Bell's palsy. Failure of the upper lid to protect the cornea aggravates this condition.

DIAGNOSIS

In mild cases of involutional ectropion, there may be no obvious signs of lower eyelid eversion. The lid margin is often in its normal position against the globe, but, if pulled away, it will return slowly rather than briskly. As the ectropion becomes advanced, the patient often complains of tearing or epiphora, since the lower punctum will not be in its normal position to drain the lacrimal lake. The diagnosis is further confirmed by excluding a history of trauma, previous surgery, and burns. There will be absence of ectropion accentuation on opening the mouth widely, an inability to palpate scar tissue within the eyelid, and the ability to pinch the horizontally redundant, full-thickness eyelid together.[185]

The diagnosis of lower eyelid cicatricial ectropion is made by palpating scar tissue within the eyelid. In addition, when the patient opens the mouth widely, the ectropion will be accentuated because this places a stretch on the facial skin.[185] In the case of upper eyelid cicatricial ectropion, there is usually evidence of lid lag on downgaze, lid retraction, and lagophthalmos.

MANAGEMENT

In addition to cosmesis, the primary clinical significance of ectropion is resultant exposure of the conjunctiva and cornea, which leads to irritation, secondary infection, and, in some cases, serious complications such as corneal ulceration. Appropriate treatment is therefore indicated.

If the ectropion is mild to moderate, lubricants can be employed for corneal protection. Bland lubricating ointment should be used at bedtime, and artificial tears during the day as needed. In more severe cases extended wear soft contact lenses can be applied for corneal protection, either alone or in combination with a lateral tarsorrhaphy. If epiphora is a major problem, the lower lid can be brought into apposition with the globe by simple lid-taping at the medial canthus.[186]

With failure of such conservative therapy to adequately protect the eye, surgical correction is indicated.[187,188] If the everted palpebral conjunctiva has become keratinized (Fig. 19.16), this does not require treatment.[187] Moreover, if the lid is returned to its proper position surgically, this will not damage the cornea, and the conjunctiva will revert to its normal character.

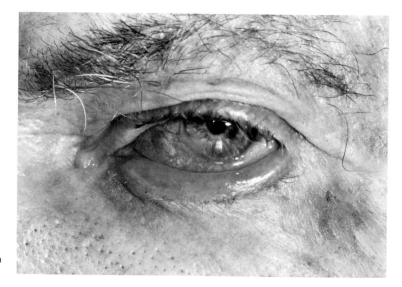

FIGURE 19.16 **Severe involutional (senile) ectropion with keratinized palpebral conjunctiva.**

Floppy Eyelid Syndrome

First reported in 1981 by Culbertson and Ostler,[189] the floppy eyelid syndrome refers to the clinical findings of chronic papillary conjunctivitis associated with nonspecific irritative symptoms, along with a soft, rubbery, "floppy," and easily everted upper eyelid. It is usually seen in middle-aged, obese men who may complain of chronic, thick, mucoid discharge and spontaneous eversion of the eyelids during sleep. The condition is usually bilateral but tends to be worse on the side on which the patient sleeps. The mechanism is thought to relate to loss of tarsal integrity, causing eyelid eversion during sleep, which creates mechanical irritation to the lids and conjunctiva.[190,191]

Diagnosis is made by careful history, including sleeping patterns, and the observation of a rubbery upper lid that easily everts on elevation. A mucoid discharge with papillary conjunctivitis may also be seen.

Treatment consists of discontinuing all previously prescribed medications except those required for concurrent conditions. Symptoms or signs of dry eye, lagophthalmos, and medicamentosa should be managed appropriately. Symptoms of floppy eyelid syndrome cannot usually be controlled with topical steroids or lubricants alone, and lid taping or use of a shield at bedtime is generally required to prevent lid eversion. The definitive treatment, however, is surgical, employing a lid-shortening procedure.[190,191]

Entropion

Entropion is a condition in which the lower or upper lid is inverted toward the globe. The primary complication is trichiasis, which can lead to irritation or corneal ulceration.

ETIOLOGY

Entropion is classified as congenital, involutional (senile), cicatricial, and spastic.[25,141,192] The most common type of entropion is involutional, or senile. There is a reduction in tone of the orbicularis muscle, elongation of the lid structures, influence by gravity on these structures, relaxation of the tarsus, and weakness of the inferior lid retractors.[141] Atrophy of the orbital tissues creates slight enophthalmos, which enhances the possibility of entropion. Because of the lack of passive resistance provided by the retractors of the lower lid, and the combination of horizontal lid laxity, the lower tarsal border moves outward while the upper tarsal border moves inward, resulting in frank entropion.[193] This form of entropion never occurs in the upper lid.[141]

The cicatricial form of entropion occurs as a result of conjunctival scarring. This is sometimes seen in the upper lid as a complication of trachoma.

True spastic entropion occurs only in cases of severe conjunctival and corneal disease, in which irritation of the lid structures provokes lid spasm, resulting in entropion.[141]

DIAGNOSIS

In moderate to severe cases, the diagnosis is straightforward by observing the inverted lid border, with or without trichiasis. Frequently, however, the entropion is not observable early in the course of its development, and pressure from the upper lid on the lower lid margin during tight lid closure is necessary to produce the clinical signs (Fig. 19.17).

MANAGEMENT

Since the primary problem associated with entropion is irritation resulting from trichiasis, the in-turned lashes must be epilated. This often must be repeated every few weeks or months. The eye can be protected with lubricating ointment or artificial tears, and, in cases of severe irritation, prophylactic antibiotic ointment may be indicated. Electrolysis can produce a more permanent cure by destroying the affected lash follicles.

The outer layers of the lower lid can be nonsurgically tightened by applying collodion. As the collodion contracts, it causes mild cicatricial ectropion.[194] Cyanoacrylate adhesive (Krazy Glue) is even more effective in the correction of involutional entropion.[194] The glue can be used to attach a horizontal fold of excess skin of the lower lid to the cheek. Since fumes from the glue may be irritating to the eye, the eyelids must be closed during the application. This form of correction may last from several hours to several weeks, but cleaning the skin well and applying benzoin compound may prolong the adhesion.

If these conservative measures fail, surgical procedures can be undertaken.[141,193,195]

Trichiasis

Trichiasis is a common clinical problem characterized by the presence of one or more inturning lashes of the upper or lower lid. When severe, the condition may lead to blindness, especially in areas of the world where trachoma is endemic.

ETIOLOGY

In most cases trichiasis is the result of aging changes of the lid, and there is no underlying disease process.

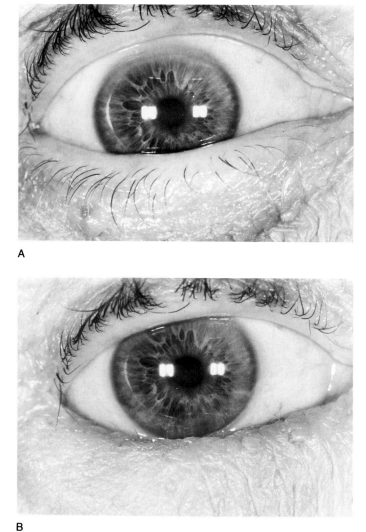

A

B

FIGURE 19.17 **Involutional (senile) entropion.** *(A)* **Lower lid margin in normal position between blinks.** *(B)* **Entropion evident immediately after tight lid closure.**

Other causes include conditions such as trachoma, Stevens-Johnson syndrome, ocular pemphigoid, and trauma, all of which can produce deformity of the lid and conjunctiva.

DIAGNOSIS

Diagnosis is made by careful physical examination, especially with the slit lamp. One or more inturned lashes is observed (Fig. 19.18), and conjunctival hyperemia or corneal staining in the area of the inturned lash may be evident.

MANAGEMENT

Management involves removal of the offending lash as well as attention to the compromised conjunctiva or cornea. When only a few lashes are involved, manual epilation is effective but usually must be repeated every few weeks or months, since it fails to destroy the lash follicle.

Electrolysis can be employed to destroy the lash follicle when only a few lashes are involved. The Perma Tweez unit (General Medical Company, Department OA 145, 1935 Armacost Avenue, West Los Angeles, California 90025) is effective for this purpose. Topical anesthesia with an agent such as proparacaine 0.5% usually permits the procedure to be tolerated well with little discomfort. Sisler,[196] however, has described a procedure that combines anesthesia and cautery in a single unit. The unit consists of an ordinary syringe to which a short, disposable 30-gauge hypodermic needle is attached. An anesthetic mixture consisting of lido-

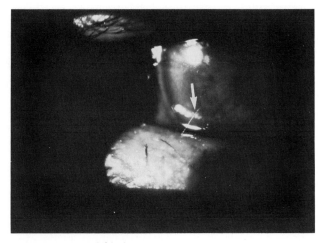

FIGURE 19.18   **Trichiasis (arrow).**

caine, hyaluronidase (1 ampule of 150 units/30 ml of solution), and epinephrine 1:1000 is placed in the syringe. The offending lash is inserted into the needle, and the needle is then inserted into the eyelid margin with the base of the lash guiding the needle toward its own follicle. Without withdrawing the needle, the clinician allows about 20 seconds for anesthesia to become effective and then touches the needle with the electrocautery source. Advantages of the technique include minimal anesthesia that is optimumly placed, and reliability of perfectly positioned cautery. Following electrolysis it is wise to use a broad-spectrum antibiotic ointment for several days to prevent infection.

When one-third or more of the eyelid margin is involved, simple epilation or electrolysis is impractical. In such cases surgical procedures are indicated, including conventional techniques,[197] cryosurgery,[198] and argon laser thermal ablation.[199,208]

Benign Tumors

Verrucae (Papillomata)

Verrucae, commonly known as warts, are benign skin tumors that can affect any part of the body, including the eyelids.

ETIOLOGY

Verrucae are caused by viral infection of localized areas of epidermis.[200] Human wart virus has also been found in a papilloma of the eyelid.[201] The virus stimulates, by an unknown mechanism, the infected cells to proliferate, causing thickened and keratotic epider-

mis. Whether the various types of warts are caused by the same virus or a group of closely related viruses is unknown. Verrucae are more common in children, patients with diabetes, and patients who are immunosuppressed.[200]

DIAGNOSIS

The most common type of wart to occur on the face and lid area is the flat wart (verrucae planae).[200] These are flat-topped, round, slightly raised, 2 to 6 mm in diameter, tan to yellow pink, and have a granular surface. They may be quite numerous and even confluent (Fig. 19.19A).

MANAGEMENT

Treatment of verrucae is indicated primarily for cosmetic reasons but also to prevent further dissemination. Since most verrucae will resolve spontaneously after several years, therapy should be conservative so that it does not result in scarring. The lesions are limited entirely to the epidermis, and treatment limited to this level should not result in scarring.[200] Specific antiviral therapy is not available, and systemic treatment, including vaccines, is ineffective. Thus, treatment is limited to the topical application of various keratolytic agents or removal by excision.

Dichloroacetic acid (Bichloracetic Acid), a chemical cauterizing agent, is easily employed by applying small amounts to each lesion with a wooden applicator.[202] The lesion will immediately turn white (Fig. 19.19B), then gray-white after several days (Fig. 19.19C), and within 7 to 10 days the wart will desquamate. Usually only one application is necessary. This treatment modality is limited to lesions on the surface of the lid and must not be used for verrucae on the lid margin because of potential injury to the conjunctiva or cornea.

Sudoriferous Cysts

Sudoriferous cysts are small, round, translucent, elevated masses caused by blockage of the ducts of the gland of Moll. One or more lesions ranging from 1 to 2 mm in diameter may be observed on the eyelid margin. They are always painless but occasionally can cause irritation or interfere with successful contact lens wear.

They tend to reform following puncture but will rarely reappear if the dome of the cyst is excised.[25] After cleaning the eyelid margin with an antiseptic such as benzalkonium chloride, and after anesthetizing the surface of the cyst with a drop of local anesthetic, the thin overlying membrane should be dissected with the sterile tip of a 25- or 27-gauge needle.[37] Material

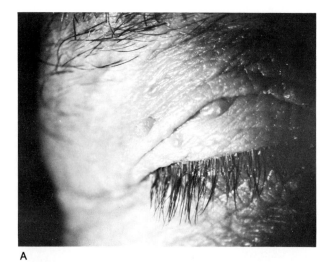

A

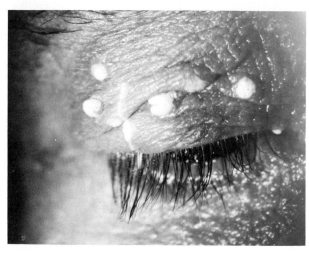

B

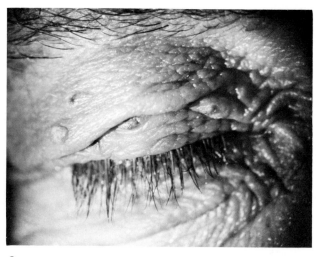

C

FIGURE 19.19   *(A)* **Verrucae planae of eyelids.** *(B)* **White phase following application of dichloroacetic acid.** *(C)* **Gray-white phase several days following application of dichloroacetic acid. (Courtesy Gerald G. Melore, O.D., M.P.H.)**

from the cyst can then be expressed with 2 sterile cotton-tipped applicators placed on each side of the base of the cyst. Application of an antibiotic ointment such as bacitracin or bacitracin–polymyxin B (Polysporin) will prevent infection.

Xanthoma Palpebrarum

Xanthoma palpebrarum (xanthelasma, xanthoma) is an elevated, yellowish discoloration that occurs most commonly in women during the fourth and fifth decades of life. The lesions usually occur bilaterally on the medial aspect of the upper eyelids. The plaque-like character of xanthoma is caused by infiltration of the dermis by xanthoma cells, which are benign histiocytes that imbibe fat.[203] The condition usually occurs inde-

pendently without associated systemic disease, but in some patients a hypercholesterolemia or other associated disturbance of lipid metabolism may be found.[203–205]

The patient should undergo general medical and serum lipid evaluations to exclude the possibility of hyperlipemic syndromes or other medical problems such as diabetes, arteriosclerosis, and cirrhosis.

Removal is indicated for cosmetic reasons only. The lesions can be concealed with a spectacle frame or tinted lenses, or they can be removed surgically, by electrocoagulation, by CO_2 laser, or by chemical cauterization.[68,204] A solution of dichloroacetic acid (Bichloracetic Acid) can be carefully applied to the lesion with a wooden applicator. If necessary this may be repeated after several weeks.

References

1. Casey TA. Congenital colobomata of the eyelids. Trans Ophthalmol Soc UK 1976;96:65–68.
2. Patipa M, Wilkins RB, Guelzow KWL. Surgical management of congenital eyelid coloboma. Ophthalmic Surg 1982;13:212–216.
3. Miller MT, Deutsch TA, Cronin C, Keys CL. Amniotic bands as a cause of ocular anomalies. Am J Ophthalmol 1987;104:270–279.
4. Bullock JD, Fleishman JA. Eyelid coloboma. In: Fraun-

felder FT, Roy GH, eds. Current ocular therapy. Philadelphia: W.B. Saunders Co, 1985;362–363.

5. Anderson RL. Surgical repair for distichiasis (letter). Arch Ophthalmol 1977;95:169.

6. Frueh BR. Treatment of distichiasis with cryotherapy. Ophthalmic Surg 1981;12:100–103.

7. Kremer I, Weinberger D, Cohen S, Sira IB. Corneal hypoaesthesia in asymptomatic familial distichiasis. Br J Ophthalmol 1986;70:132–134.

8. Goldstein S, Qazi QH, Fitzgerald J, et al. Distichiasis, congenital heart defects and mixed peripheral vascular anomalies. Am J Med Genet 1985;20:283–294.

9. White JH. Correction of distichiasis by tarsal resection and mucous membrane grafting. Am J Ophthalmol 1975;80:507–508.

10. Anderson RL, Harvey JT. Lid splitting and posterior lamella cryosurgery for congenital and acquired distichiasis. Arch Ophthalmol 1981;99:631–634.

11. Delaney MR, Rogers PA. A simplified cryotherapy technique for trichiasis and distichiasis. Aust J Ophthalmol 1984;12:163–166.

12. Frank DH, Wachtel T, Frank HA. The early treatment and reconstruction of eyelid burns. J Trauma 1983;23:874–877.

13. Edlich RF, Nichter LS, Morgan RF, et al. Burns of the head and neck. Otolaryngol Clin North Am 1984;17:361–388.

14. Huang TT, Blackwell SJ, Lewis SR. Burn injuries of the eyelids. Clin Plast Surg 1978;5:571–581.

15. Burns CL, Chylack LT. Thermal burns: The management of thermal burns of the lids and globes. Ann Ophthalmol 1979;11:1358–1368.

16. Rost KM, Jaeger RW, deCastro FJ. Eye contamination: A poison center protocol for management. Clin Toxicol 1979;14:295–300.

17. Pfister RR. Chemical injuries of the eye. Ophthalmology 1983;90:1246–1253.

18. Morgan SJ, Astbury NJ. Inadvertent self administration of superglue: A consumer hazard. Br Med J 1984;289:226–227.

19. Silverman CM. Corneal abrasion from accidental instillation of cyanoacrylate into the eye. Arch Ophthalmol 1988;106:1029–1030.

20. Bock GW. Skin exposure to cyanoacrylate adhesive. Ann Emerg Med 1984;13:486.

21. Kimbrough RL, Okereke PC, Stewart RH. Conservative management of cyanoacrylate ankyloblepharon: A case report. Ophthalmic Surg 1986;17:176–177.

22. Donnenfeld ED, Perry HD, Nelson DB. More of the conservative management of cyanoacrylate ankyloblepharon. Ophthalmic Surg 1987;18:74–75.

23. Raynor LA. Treatment for inadvertent cyanoacrylate tarsorrhaphy. Arch Ophthalmol 1988;106:1033.

24. Alexander KL. Some inflammations of the external eye and adnexa. J Am Optom Assoc 1980;51:142–146.

25. Trevor-Roper PD. Diseases of the eyelids. Int Ophthalmol Clin 1974;14:362–393.

26. Hudson RL. Treatment of styes and meibomian cysts. Practical procedures. Aust Fam Phys 1981;10:714–717.

27. Fraunfelder FT. Hordeolum. In: Fraunfelder FT, Roy FH, eds. Current ocular therapy. Philadelphia: W.B. Saunders Co, 1985;363–364.

28. Jones DB, Liesegang TJ, Robinson NM. Laboratory diagnosis of ocular infections. Washington, DC: American Society for Microbiology,1981;9–10.

29. English FP, Nutting WB. Demodicosis of ophthalmic concern. Am J Ophthalmol 1981;91:362–372.

30. English FP, Cohn D, Groeneveld ER. Demodectic mites and chalazion. Am J Ophthalmol 1985;100:482–483.

31. Gershen HJ. Chalazion. In: Fraunfelder FT, Roy FH, eds. Current ocular therapy. Philadelphia: W.B. Saunders Co, 1985,354–355.

32. Bohigian GM. Chalazion: A clinical evaluation. Ann Ophthalmol 1979;11:1397–1398.

33. Browning DJ, Proia AD. Ocular rosacea. Surv Ophthalmol 1986;31:145–158.

34. Nisted M, Hofstetter HW. Effect of chalazion on astigmatism. Am J Optom Physiol Optics 1974;51:579–582.

35. Bogan S, Simon JW, Krohel GB, Nelson LB. Astigmatism associated with adnexal masses in infancy. Arch Ophthalmol 1987;105:1368–1370.

36. Cottrell DG, Bosanquet RC, Fawcett IM. Chalazions: The frequency of spontaneous resolution. Br Med J 1983; 6405:1595.

37. Catania LJ. Lumps and bumps of the eyelids or "what is that thing?" South J Optom 1979;21:16–19.

38. Perry HD, Serniuk RA. Conservative treatment of chalazia. Ophthalmology 1980;87:218–221.

39. Jacobs PM, Thaller VT, Wong D. Intralesional corticosteroid therapy of chalazia: A comparison with incision and curettage. Br J Ophthalmol 1984;68:836–837.

40. Watson AP, Austin DJ. Treatment of chalazions with injection of a steroid suspension. Br J Ophthalmol 1984;68:833–835.

41. King RA, Ellis PP. Treatment of chalazia with corticosteroid injections. Ophthalmic Surg 1986;17:351–353.

42. Palva J, Pohjanpelto PEJ. Intralesional corticosteroid injection for the treatment of chalazia. Acta Ophthalmol 1983;61:933–937.

43. Castren J, Stenborg T. Corticosteroid injection of chalazia. Acta Ophthalmol 1983;61:938–942.

44. Pizzarello LD, Jakobiec FA, Hofeldt AJ, et al. Intralesional corticosteroid therapy of chalazia. Am J Ophthalmol 1978;85:818–821.

45. Dua HS, Nilawar DV. Nonsurgical therapy of chalazion (letter). Am J Ophthalmol 1982;94:424–425.

46. Cohen BZ, Tripathi RC. Eyelid depigmentation after intralesional injection of a fluorinated corticosteroid for chalazion (letter). Am J Ophthalmol 1979;88:269–270.

47. Jakobeic FA, Silvers D. Eyelid depigmentation after intralesional injection of a fluorinated corticosteroid for chalazion—reply (letter). Am J Ophthalmol 1979;88:270.

48. Thomas EL, Laborde RP. Retinal and choroidal vascular occlusion following intralesional corticosteroid injection of a chalazion. Ophthalmology 1986;93:405–407.

49. Gershen HJ. Chalazion excision. Ophthalmic Surg 1974;5:75–76.

50. Tesluk GC. Should all chalazia be sent to pathology? Ann Ophthalmol 1985;17:621.

51. McCulley JP, Dougherty JM, Deneau DG. Classification of chronic blepharitis. Ophthalmology 1982;89:1173–1180.

52. Gutgesell VJ, Stern GA, Hood CI. Histopathology of mei-

bomian gland dysfunction. Am J Ophthalmol 1982;94:383–387.

53. Roth AM. Demodex folliculorum in hair follicles of eyelid skin. Ann Ophthalmol 1979;11:37–40.

54. Heacock CE. Clinical manifestations of demodicosis. J Am Optom Assoc 1986;57:914–919.

55. McCulley JP, Dougherty JM. Blepharitis associated with acne rosacea and seborrheic dermatitis. Int Ophthalmol Clin 1985;25:159–172.

56. Khan J, Hoover D, Ide CH. Methicillin-resistant *Staphylococcus epidermidis* blepharitis. Am J Ophthalmol 1984;98:562–565.

57. Smolin G, Okumoto M. Staphylococcal blepharitis. Arch Ophthalmol 1977;95:812–816.

58. Wilson LA, Julian AJ, Ahearn DG. The survival and growth of microorganisms in mascara during use. Am J Ophthalmol 1975;79:596–601.

59. Mondino BJ, Caster AI, Dethlefs B. A rabbit model of staphylococcal blepharitis. Arch Ophthalmol 1987;105:409–412.

60. McCulley JP. Blepharoconjunctivitis. Int Ophthalmol Clin 1984;24:65–77.

61. Polack FM, Goodman DF. Experience with a new detergent lid scrub in the management of chronic blepharitis. Arch Ophthalmol 1988;106:719–720.

62. Leibowitz HM, Capino D. Treatment of chronic blepharitis. Arch Ophthalmol 1988;106:720.

63. Kaufman HE. Chemical blepharitis following drug treatment. Am J Ophthalmol 1983;95:703.

64. Lamberts DW, Buka T, Knowlton GM. Clinical evaluation of trimethoprim-containing ophthalmic solutions in humans. Am J Ophthalmol 1984;98:11–16.

65. Nozik RA, Smolin G, Knowlton G, Austin R. Trimethoprim-polymyxin B ophthalmic solution in treatment of surface ocular bacterial infections. Ann Ophthalmol 1985;17:746–748.

66. Kastl PR, Ali Z, Mather F. Placebo-controlled, double-blind evaluation of the efficacy and safety of yellow mercuric oxide in suppression of eyelid infections. Ann Ophthalmol 1987;19:376–379.

67. Donshik P, Kulvin SM, McKinley P, Skowron R. Treatment of chronic staphylococcal blepharoconjunctivitis with a new topical steroid anti-infective ophthalmic solution. Ann Ophthalmol 1983;15:162–167.

68. Ellis PP. Ocular therapeutics and pharmacology. St Louis: C.V. Mosby Co, 1985;7:105–120.

69. Smolin G. Staphylococcal blepharitis. In: Fraunfelder FT, Roy FH, eds. Current ocular therapy. Philadelphia: W.B. Saunders Co, 1980;434–435.

70. Salamon SM. Tetracyclines in ophthalmology. Surv Ophthalmol 1985;29:265–275.

71. Fleischer AB, Hoover DL, Khan JA, et al. Topical vancomycin formulation for methicillin-resistant *Staphylococcus epidermidis* blepharoconjunctivitis. Am J Ophthalmol 1986;101:283–287.

72. Flora MR. Meibomianitis and meibomian hypersecretion. South J Optom 1979;21:46–48.

73. Lambert R, Smith RE. Hyperkeratinization in a rabbit model of meibomian gland dysfunction. Am J Ophthalmol 1988;105:703–705.

74. Korb DR, Henriquez AS. Meibomian gland dysfunction and contact lens intolerance. J Am Optom Assoc 1980;51:243–251.

75. Seal DV, McGill JI, Jacobs P, et al. Microbial and immunological investigations of chronic non-ulcerative blepharitis and meibomianitis. Br J Ophthalmol 1985;69:604–611.

76. Robin JB, Jester JV, Nobe J, et al. In vivo transillumination biomicroscopy and photography of meibomian gland dysfunction. Ophthalmology 1985;92:1423–1426.

77. McCulley JP, Sciallis GF. Meibomian keratoconjunctivitis. Am J Ophthalmol 1977;84:788–793.

78. Dougherty JM, McCulley JP. Bacterial lipases and chronic blepharitis. Invest Ophthalmol Vis Sci 1986;27:486–491.

79. Dougherty JM, McCulley JP. Analysis of the free fatty acid component of meibomian secretions in chronic blepharitis. Invest Ophthalmol Vis Sci 1986;27:52–56.

80. Glasser DB. Angular blepharitis caused by gram-negative bacillus DF-2. Am J Ophthalmol 1986;102:119–120.

81. Barad RF. Differential diagnosis and treatment of periorbital cellulitis. Intern Med Special 1986;7:209–215.

82. Jackson K, Baker SR. Periorbital cellulitis. Head Neck Surg 1987;9:227–234.

83. Brower MF, Levine RA, Boyer KM. Preseptal cellulitis complicated by toxic shock syndrome. Arch Ophthalmol 1987;105:1631–1632.

84. Riffle JE. Ectopic cilia and preseptal orbital cellulitis. Am J Ophthalmol 1984;98:119–120.

85. Insler MS, Zatzkis S. Periorbital cellulitis after eyebrow tweezing. Am J Ophthalmol 1986;102:534–535.

86. Lawless M, Martin F. Orbital cellulitis and preseptal cellulitis in childhood. Aust NZ J Ophthalmol 1986;14:211–219.

87. Bergin DJ, Wright JE. Orbital cellulitis. Br J Ophthalmol 1986;70:174–178.

88. Jackson K, Baker SR. Clinical implications of orbital cellulitis. Laryngoscope 1986;96:568–574.

89. Jones DB. Microbial preseptal and orbital cellulitis. In: Duane TD, Jaeger EA, eds. Clinical ophthalmology. Hagerstown, MD: Harper & Row, 1987;vol.4, Chap. 25,1–19.

90. Searl SS. Minor trauma, disastrous results. Surv Ophthalmol 1987;31:337–342.

91. Jakobiec FA, Srinivasan BD, Gamboa ET. Recurrent herpetic angular blepharitis in an adult. Am J Ophthalmol 1979;88:744–747.

92. Darougar S, Wishart MS, Viswalingam ND. Epidemiological and clinical features of primary herpes simplex virus ocular infection. Br J Ophthalmol 1985;69:2–6.

93. Pavan-Langston D. Ocular antiviral therapy. Int Ophthalmol Clin 1980;20:149–161.

94. Egerer I, Stary A. Erosive-ulcerative herpes simplex blepharitis. Arch Ophthalmol 1980;98:1760–1763.

95. Ostler HB. The management of ocular herpesvirus infections. Surv Ophthalmol 1976;21:136–147.

96. Wander AH. Herpes simplex and recurrent corneal disease. Int Ophthalmol Clin 1984;24:27–38.

97. Chu W, Pavan-Langston D. Ocular surface manifestations of the major viruses. Int Ophthalmol Clin 1979;19:135–167.

98. Simon JW, Longo F, Smith RS. Spontaneous resolution of herpes simplex blepharoconjunctivitis in children. Am J Ophthalmol 1986;102:598–600.

99. Cykiert RC. Spontaneous resolution of herpes simplex blepharoconjunctivitis in children (letter). Am J Ophthalmol 1987;103:340.

100. Pavan-Langston D. Varicella-zoster ophthalmicus. Int Ophthalmol Clin 1975;15:171–185.

101. Tanaka Y, Harino S, Danjo S, et al. Skin test with varicella-zoster virus antigen for ophthalmic herpes zoster. Am J Ophthalmol 1984;98:7–10.

102. Bucci FA, Savia PV, Mauriello JA. Herpes zoster ophthalmicus. Am Fam Physician 1987;35:121–128.

103. Liesegang TJ. Herpes zoster ophthalmicus. Int Ophthalmol Clin 1985;25:77–96.

104. Cole EL, Meisler DM, Calabrese LH, et al. Herpes zoster ophthalmicus and acquired immune deficiency syndrome. Arch Ophthalmol 1984;102:1027–1029.

105. Pavan-Langston D. Diagnosis and therapy of common eye infections: bacterial, viral, fungal. Compr Ther 1983;9:33–42.

106. Cobo LM, Foulks GN, Liesegang T, et al. Oral acyclovir in the treatment of acute herpes zoster ophthalmicus. Ophthalmology 1986;93:763–770.

107. Marsh RJ. Current management of ophthalmic herpes zoster. Trans Ophthalmol Soc UK 1976;96:334–337.

108. Mayne GE, Moya F. Herpes zoster/postherpetic neuralgia. Intern Med Special 1987;8:198–212.

109. Cobo LM, Foulks GN, Liesegang T, et al. Oral arclovir in the therapy of acute herpes zoster ophthalmicus. An interim report. Ophthalmology 1985;92:1574–1583.

110. Büchi ER, Herbort CP, Ruffieux C. Oral acyclovir in the treatment of acute herpes zoster ophthalmicus. Am J Ophthalmol 1986;102:531–532.

111. Awan KJ. Cryotherapy in phthiriasis palpebrarum. Am J Ophthalmol 1977;83:906–907.

112. Chin GN, Denslow GT. Pediculosis ciliaris. J Pediatr Ophthalmol Strabismus 1978;15:173–175.

113. Couch JM, Green WR, Hirst LW, et al. Diagnosing and treating phthirus pubis palpebrarum. Surv Ophthalmol 1982;26:219–225.

114. Kairys DJ, Webster HJ, Terry JE. Pediatric ocular phthiriasis infestation. J Am Optom Assoc 1988;59:128–130.

115. Dornic DI. Ectoparasitic infestation of the lashes. J Am Optom Assoc 1985;56:716–719.

116. Smith DE, Walsh J. Treatment of pubic lice infestation: A comparison of two agents. Cutis 1980;26:618–619.

117. Chapel TA, Katta T, Kuszmar T, et al. Pediculosis pubis in a clinic for treatment of sexually transmitted disease. Sex Transm Dis 1979;6:257–260.

118. Friedlander MH. Ocular allergy. J Allergy Clin Immunol 1985;76:645–657.

119. Wilson FM. Adverse external ocular effects of topical ophthalmic medications. Surv Ophthalmol 1979;24:57–88.

120. Bloomfield SE. Clinical allergy and immunology of the external eye. In: Duane TD, Jaeger EA, eds. Clinical ophthalmology. Hagerstown, MD: Harper & Row, 1987;Vol.4, Chap.2,1–25.

121. Zimmerman MC. The prophylaxis and treatment of penicillin reactions with penicillinase. Clin Med 1958;5:305–311.

122. Rich LF, Hanifin JM. Ocular complications of atopic dermatitis and other eczemas. Int Ophthalmol Clin 1985;25:61–76.

123. de Weck AL. Contact eczematous dermatitis. In: Fitzpatrick TB, Arndt KA, Clark WH, et al, eds. Dermatology in general medicine. New York: McGraw-Hill, 1971;669–679.

124. Hätinen A, Teräsvirta M, Fräki JE. Contact allergy to components in topical ophthalmologic preparations. Acta Ophthalmol 1985;63:424–426.

125. Richmond PP, Allansmith MR. Allergic disorders of the anterior segment. Int Ophthalmol Clin 1983;23:43–61.

126. Fernandez-Vozmediano JM, Blasi NA, Romero-Cabrera MA, et al. Allergic contact dermatitis to timolol. Contact Dermatitis 1986;14:252.

127. Romaguera C, Grimalt F, Vilaplana J. Contact dermatitis by timolol. Contact Dermatitis 1986;14:248.

128. Ducombs G, de Casamayor J, Verin P, Maleville J. Allergic contact dermatitis to phenylephrine. Contact Dermatitis 1986;15:107–108.

129. Sher MA. Contact dermatitis of the eyelids. S Afr Med J 1979;55:511–513.

130. Fisher AA. Contact dermatitis. Philadelphia: Lea & Febiger, 1973;2:39–70.

131. Fisher AA. Erythromycin: A nonsensitizing topical antibiotic. Arch Dermatol 1976;112:732.

132. Theodore FH, Schlossman A. Ocular allergy. Baltimore: Williams & Wilkins, 1958;64–77.

133. Uehara M. Infraorbital fold in atopic dermatitis. Arch Dermatol 1981;117:627–629.

134. Jennings BJ. Allergic contact dermatitis. J Am Optom Assoc 1985;56:474–478.

135. Whittington CV. Elicitation of contact lens allergy to thimerosal by eye cream. Contact Dermatitis 1985;13:186–203.

136. Eisenlohr JE. Glaucoma following the prolonged use of topical steroid medication to the eyelids. J Am Acad Dermatol 1983;8:878–881.

137. Fisher AA. Periocular dermatitis akin to the perioral variety. J Am Acad Dermatol 1986; 15:642–644.

138. Beard C, Sullivan JH. Ptosis—current concepts. Int Ophthalmol Clin 1978;18:53–73.

139. Cogan DG, Witt ED, Goldman-Rakic PS. Ocular signs in thiamine-deficient monkeys and in Wernicke's disease in humans. Arch Ophthalmol 1985;103:1212–1220.

140. Varavithya W, Dhanamitta S, Valyasevi A. Bilateral ptosis as a sign of thiamine deficiency in childhood. Clin Pediatr 1975;14:1063–1065.

141. Beyer CK. Repair of entropion and ectropion. Int Ophthalmol Clin 1978;18:19–52.

142. Martin PA, Rogers PA. Involutional ptosis: Recognition and management. Aust NZ J Ophthalmol 1985;13:185–187.

143. Shore JW, McCord CD. Anatomic changes in involutional blepharoptosis. Am J Ophthalmol 1984;98:21–27.

144. Werb A. Ptosis. Trans Ophthalmol Soc NZ 1976;28:29–32.

145. Laibovitz RA, Cain R. Lost lid signs in topical neuro-ophthalmic diagnosis. Tex Med 1977;73:68–69.

146. Cohen MB. Case history: Use of a bilateral ptosis crutch. N Engl J Optom 1987;40:26–27.

147. Moss HL. Prosthesis for blepharoptosis and blepharospasm. J Am Optom Assoc 1982;53:661–667.

148. Lane CM, Collins JRO. Treatment of ptosis in chronic progressive external ophthalmoplegia. Br J Ophthalmol 1987;71:290–294.

149. Anderson FG. Treatment of myasthenia gravis ptosis and extraocular muscle palsies. Tex Med 1976;72:84–86.

150. Walsh FB, Hoyt WF. Clinical neuro-ophthalmology. Baltimore: Williams & Wilkins, 1969;3:1292.

151. Castronuovo S, Krohel GB, Kristan RW. Blepharoptosis in myasthenia gravis. Ann Ophthalmol 1983;15:751–754.

152. Beasley H. Ptosis. In: Fraunfelder FT, Roy FH, eds. Current ocular therapy. Philadelphia: W.B. Saunders Co., 1980;432–433.

153. Jaffe NS, Shults WT. Lid myokymia. In: Fraunfelder FT, Roy FH, eds. Current ocular therapy, ed 2. Philadelphia: W.B. Saunders Co., 1985;366.

154. Freed EDD. Rapid tremor of the eyelids after overdose of fluphenazine. Br J Psychiatr 1983;143:525–526.

155. Barbaro AC. Tremor of the eyelids. Br J Psychiatr 1984;144:437–438.

156. Krohel GB, Rosenberg PN. Oscillopsia associated with eyelid myokymia. Am J Ophthalmol 1986;102:662–663.

157. Casey DE. Essential blepharospasm. In: Fraunfelder FT, Roy FH, eds. Current ocular therapy, ed. 2. Philadelphia: W.B. Saunders Co, 1985;360–362.

158. Jankovic J, Ford J. Blepharospasm and orofacial-cervical dystonia. Clinical and pharmacological findings in 100 patients. Ann Neurol 1983;13:402–411.

159. Engstrom PF, Arnoult JB, Mazow ML, et al. Effectiveness of botulinum toxin therapy for essential blepharospasm. Ophthalmology 1987;94:971–975.

160. Gladstone GJ, Putterman AM. A repetitive forced closure test. Arch Ophthalmol 1985;103:477–480.

161. Waller RR, Kennedy RH, Henderson JW, Kesty KR. Management of blepharospasm. Trans Am Ophthalmol Soc 1985;83:367–386.

162. Halperin E, Yolton RL. Ophthalmic applications of biofeedback. Am J Optom Physiol Optics 1986;63:985–998.

163. Frueh BR, Nelson CC, Kapustiak JF, Musch DC. The effect of omitting botulinum toxin from the lower eyelid in blepharospasm treatment. Am J Ophthalmol 1988;106:45–47.

164. Elston JS. Long-term results of treatment of idiopathic blepharospasm with botulinum toxin injection. Br J Ophthalmol 1987;71:664–668.

165. Spector JG, Burde RM. Botulinum-A toxin for ocular muscle disorders. Lancet 1986;1:855.

166. Mauriella JA, Coniaris H, Haupt EJ. Use of botulinum toxin in the treatment of one hundred patients with facial dyskinesias. Ophthalmology 1987;94:976–979.

167. Biglan AW, Gonnering R, Lockhart B, et al. Absence of antibody production in patients treated with botulinum A toxin. Am J Ophthalmol 1986;101:232–235.

168. Burns CL, Gammon A, Gemmill MC. Ptosis associated with botulinum toxin treatment of strabismus and blepharospasm. Ophthalmology 1986;93:1621–1627.

169. Biglan AW, May M. Treatment of facial spasm with Oculinum *(C. botulinum* toxin). J Pediatr Ophthalmol Strabismus 1986;23:216–221.

170. Perman KI, Baylis HI, Rosenbaum AL, Kirschen DG. The use of botulinum toxin in the medical management of benign essential blepharospasm. Ophthalmology 1986;93:1–3.

171. Frueh BR, Musch DC. Treatment of facial spasm with botulinum toxin. An interim report. Ophthalmology 1986;93:917–923.

172. Scott AB, Kennedy RA, Stubbs HA. Botulinum A toxin injection as a treatment for blepharospasm. Arch Ophthalmol 1985;103:347–350.

173. Shorr N, Seiff SR, Kopelman J. The use of botulinum toxin in blepharospasm. Am J Ophthalmol 1985;99:542–546.

174. Lingua RW. Sequelae of botulinum toxin injection. Am J Ophthalmol 1985;100:305–307.

175. Frueh BR, Felt DP, Wojno TH, Musch DC. Treatment of blepharospasm with botulinum toxin. A preliminary report. Arch Ophthalmol 1984;102:1464–1468.

176. Katz J, Kaufman HE. Corneal exposure during sleep (nocturnal lagophthalmos). Arch Ophthalmol 1977;95:449–453.

177. Harvey JT, Anderson RL. Lid lag and lagophthalmos: A clarification of terminology. Ophthalmic Surg 1981;12:338–340.

178. Jobe RP. Lagophthalmos. In: Fraunfelder FT, Roy FH, eds. Current ocular therapy, ed. 2. Philadelphia: W.B. Saunders Co, 1985;364–366.

179. Hinzpeter EN, Riehm E. Preliminary experience with lid magnets for paralytic lagophthalmos. Trans Ophthalmol Soc UK 1976;96:73–78.

180. D'Hooghe PJ, Hendrick EM. Upper lid loading with dermis graft and levator weakening. Management of lagophthalmos due to facial palsy. Ophthalmologica 1975;171:419–424.

181. Smith MFW, Goode RL. Eye protection in the paralyzed face. Laryngoscope 1979;89:435–442.

182. Abelson MB, Holly FJ. A tentative mechanism for inferior punctate keratopathy. Am J Ophthalmol 1977;83:866–869.

183. Collins M, Heron H, Larsen R, Lindner R. Blinking patterns in soft contact lens wearers can be altered with training. Am J Optom Physiol Optics 1987;64:100–103.

184. Stefanyszyn MA, Hidayat AA, Flanagan JC. The histopathology of involutional ectropion. Ophthalmology 1985;92:120–127.

185. Putterman AM. Combined z-plasty and horizontal shortening procedure for ectropion. Am J Ophthalmol 1980;89:525–530.

186. Miller GR, Tenzel RR, Buffam FV. Lid taping in the preoperative management of tearing or asthenopia. Arch Ophthalmol 1976;94:1289–1290.

187. Frueh BR, Schoengarth LD. Evaluation and treatment of the patient with ectropion. Ophthalmology 1982;89:1049–1054.

188. Lisman RD, Smith B, Baker D, Arthurs B. Efficacy of surgical treatment for paralytic ectropion. Ophthalmology 1987;94:671–681.

189. Culbertson WW, Ostler HB. The floppy eyelid syndrome. Am J Ophthalmol 1981;92:568–575.

190. Dutton JJ. Surgical management of floppy eyelid syndrome. Am J Ophthalmol 1985;99:557–560.

191. Moore MB, Harrington J, McCulley JP. Floppy eyelid syndrome. Management including surgery. Ophthalmology 1986;93:184–188.

192. Tse DT, Anderson RL, Fratkin JD. Aponeurosis disinsertion in congenital entropion. Arch Ophthalmol 1983;101:436–440.

193. Rainin EA. Senile entropion. Arch Ophthalmol 1979;97:928–930.

194. Baylis HI, Hamako C. Office and bedside techniques for treatment of involutional entropion. Trans Am Acad Ophthalmol Otolaryngol 1977;83:663–668.

195. Baylis HI, Hamako C. Tarsal grafting for correction of cicatricial entropion. Ophthalmic Surg 1979;10:42–48.

196. Sisler HA. Trichiasis combined anesthesia-cautery unit. Trans Am Acad Ophthalmol Otolaryngol 1977;83:881–882.

197. Fein W. Surgical repair for distichiasis, trichiasis, and entropion. Arch Ophthalmol 1976;94:809–810.

198. Johnson RLC, Collin JRO. Treatment of trichiasis with a lid cryoprobe. Br J Ophthalmol 1985;69:267–270.

199. Awan KJ. Argon laser treatment of trichiasis. Ophthalmic Surg 1986;17:658–660.

200. Schmidt LM. Warts: Their diagnosis and treatment. Pediatr Ann 1976;5:782–790.

201. Angevine DM, Norback DH, Dortzbach RK. Virus in papilloma (letter). JAMA 1981;246:1087–1088.

202. Melore GG. Verrucae and their treatment. South J Optom 1985;2:20–25.

203. Depot MJ, Jakobiec FA, Dodick JM, Iwamoto T. Bilateral and extensive xanthelasma palpebrarum in a young man. Ophthalmology 1984;91:522–527.

204. Gladstone GJ, Beckman H, Elson LM. CO_2 laser excision of xanthelasma lesions. Arch Ophthalmol 1985;103:440–442.

205. Parkes ML, Waller TS. Xanthelasma palpebrarum. Laryngoscope 1984;94:1238–1240.

206. Epstein GA, Putterman AM. Combined excision and drainage with intralesional corticosteroid injection in the treatment of chronic chalazia. Arch Ophthalmol 1988;106:514–516.

207. Linberg JV, Vasquez RJ, Chao GM. Aponeurotic ptosis repair under local anesthesia. Prediction of results from operative lid height. Ophthalmology 1988;95:1046–1052.

208. Bartley GB, Bullock JD, Olsen TG, et al. An experimental study to compare methods of eyelash ablation. Ophthalmology 1987;94:1286–1289.

CHAPTER 20

Diseases of the Lacrimal System

Leo Semes
Richard J. Clompus

Tearing is a common complaint among ophthalmic patients.[1] To pinpoint the offending site within the lacrimal system and to institute appropriate management for these patients, a logical approach is necessary.

Since tears are continually produced and drained, any alteration of this equilibrium can result in tearing. Temporary overproduction of aqueous tears by stimulation of the ophthalmic (first) division of the trigeminal nerve is known as hypersecretion. An example is the reflex tearing resulting from superficial foreign-body irritation. True hypersecretion, resulting from lacrimal nerve stimulation secondary to a mass or lacrimal gland enlargement, is extremely rare.

More frequently encountered is pseudoepiphora. A chronic aqueous deficiency associated with keratoconjunctivitis sicca and Sjögren's syndrome results in an increased production of reflex (aqueous) tears.

All reflex tears are produced by the lacrimal gland on signals from the lacrimal nucleus. Distinct from continuous (or basic) lacrimal secretions, reflex tears are of a solely aqueous composition. Any imbalance in the constituency of the tears can result in an unstable tear film. Some authors[2] believe that such an instability is the major source of tearing complaints.

Obstruction of the lacrimal drainage passageways can result in tearing. A normal tear production rate is too much for a malfunctioning or blocked excretory system to handle. Tearing is usually seen near the medial canthus.

Management of each patient follows from accurate diagnosis. A careful case history combined with logical testing of the entire lacrimal system, based on its anatomy, will usually allow the practitioner to provide effective treatment.

Clinical Anatomy and Physiology

A convenient conceptual separation of the lacrimal system can be made based on function. The secretory system produces sufficient quality and quantity of tear film to allow the ocular surface to function normally. A smooth refractive surface, ocular comfort, and resistance to disease and exposure all depend on a healthy tear film.

The lids serve as the distribution system for the tear film. Lid irregularities or disorders can interfere with lid function, resulting in ocular discomfort or compromise.

The excretory system must effectively drain a proper quantity of tears. Deficient access to the lacrimal lake or a blockage within the drainage passageways will result in epiphora—classically, tearing secondary to obstruction. The delicate balance among these components of the lacrimal system will determine both the comfort and health of the ocular surface (Fig. 20.1).

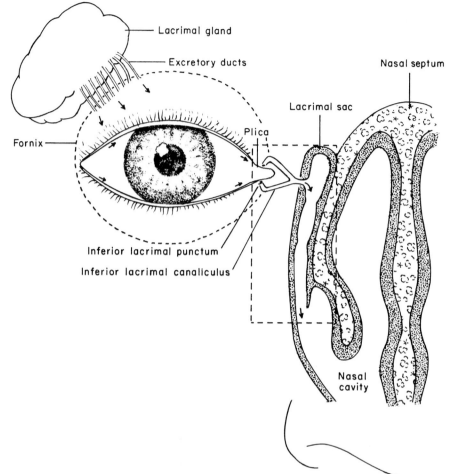

FIGURE 20.1   **Schematic view of the lacrimal system. The lacrimal gland supplies only aqueous (reflex) secretions. Arrows indicate the pathway that tears follow to drainage beginning at the punctum. The area enclosed by dashed lines represents the drainage apparatus. (Adapted from Botelho SY. Tears and the lacrimal gland. Sci Am 1964; 211:78–85. Copyright 1964 by Scientific American, Inc. All rights reserved.)**

Secretory System

The secretory portion of the lacrimal system is composed of 2 sets of glands. Reflex (aqueous) secretion comes from the lacrimal gland. About the size and shape of a shelled almond, the lacrimal gland consists of main and accessory portions separated by the aponeurosis of the levator muscle.[1,3] The efferent nerve supply to the lacrimal gland is cholinergic through the anastomosis of the lacrimal and zygomatic nerves. Impulses travel with the seventh cranial nerve from the lacrimal nucleus in the pons through the sphenopalatine ganglion to eventually reach the lacrimal gland (see Fig. 3.31).[1,3–5] Drugs that inhibit cholinergic activity therefore inhibit aqueous secretion and often cause dry eye signs or symptoms.

Input to the lacrimal nucleus is from several sources. The "emotional" center of the frontal cortex, basal ganglion, thalamus, and hypothalamus are all thought to contribute.[4] Reflex tearing is also stimulated by

irritation of trigeminal nerve endings located in the cornea, conjunctiva, and surface of the face.[1,5] In addition, stimulation of the retina by bright light can cause reflex tearing.[5]

Perhaps more important to maintenance of the tear film and ocular surface integrity are the basic secretors. The 3-layer tear film has numerous contributors (Fig. 20.2). The outermost, oily or lipid, layer is produced primarily by the sebaceous meibomian glands of the lids. They are located in the tarsus of both the upper and lower eyelids. Also contributing to this layer are the glands of Zeis, at the palpebral margin of each eyelid, and the glands of Moll, found at the roots of the eyelashes. The oily secretions function to thicken, stabilize, and prevent premature evaporation of the underlying aqueous layer of the tear film.[1,2,5]

The accessory lacrimal glands of Krause and Wolfring are primarily responsible for producing the intermediate, or middle, layer of the tear film. Most of the glands of Krause are located in the superior conjunc-

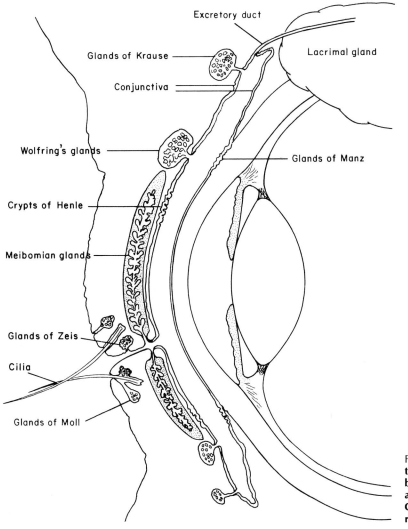

Excretory duct

Glands of Krause

Conjunctiva

Lacrimal gland

Wolfring's glands

Glands of Manz

Crypts of Henle

Meibomian glands

Glands of Zeis

Cilia

Glands of Moll

FIGURE 20.2 **Cross-section of the lacrimal secretory system. See text for products of the labelled basal secretors. (Adapted from Botelho SY. Tears and the lacrimal gland. Sci Am 1964; 211:78–85. Copyright 1964 by Scientific American, Inc. All rights reserved.)**

tival fornix, but a few can be found in the lower fornix. The accessory glands of Wolfring are located posterior to the upper margin of the tarsal plate superiorly and inferiorly.[1,3] These exocrine glands form the bulk of the continuous tear film.

Gillette and associates[6] have pointed out the histologic and immunohistologic similarity of main and accessory lacrimal gland tissue. Combined with their finding of myoepithelial cells among accessory lacrimal gland material, these authors believe that some form of autonomic innervation exists to this tissue.[6] These findings may point to a common source of stimulated (reflex) and unstimulated (continuous) tears. For practical purposes, continuous tears can be thought of as available on an unstimulated (basal) basis.

The inner layer of the tear film contributes greatly to lubrication of the lids and provides an adsorbing site for the aqueous layer of the tear film to the normally hydrophobic corneal epithelium. The inner layer of tear film is a mucoid layer of polysaccharide composition (sialomucus)[7] derived primarily from the conjunctival goblet cells located in the fornices. Also contributing to this layer are the tarsal crypts of Henle and limbal glands of Manz[1,3] (see Fig. 20.2).

The basic secretors together produce the continuous flow of tears that bathe the globe. They have no confirmed afferent nerve supply, and their output has been shown to decrease with age. A basic secretory deficit is responsible for hyposecretion disorders but has never been implicated in true hypersecretion.[1,5]

Distribution System

The distribution system for the tear film consists of the lids and the tear meniscus along the lid margins in the open eye.[7] The need for renewal of the tear film caused by its breakup is the stimulus for the blink reflex.[2] Each blink compresses the superficial lipid layer. The mucus layer acts as a scavenger to pick up any lipid-containing debris and carry it to the fornices. As the eyelid reopens, a new tear-film layer is spread across the ocular surface. Inadequacies of any layer of the tear film will increase its instability and accelerate tear breakup time (TBUT).

The distribution system of the lids also acts as a pumping mechanism to draw tears into the excretory system (see Fig. 20.1). Controversy exists over the exact mechanism for tear fluid dynamics.[2,8–10] It is agreed, however, that the lids act to direct the lacrimal fluid toward the inner canthi for drainage into the puncta. Whether this is an active or passive process and whether tears are propelled by positive or negative conjunctival pressure remain unanswered.[1,3,8–10]

Excretory System

Blinking is an important factor in tear distribution. It also plays a pivotal role in tear drainage.[3,8,10,11] Crucial to proper lacrimal excretory function is the punctum, entry point for lacrimal drainage. Each punctum is located on the posterior eyelid margin at the nasal end of the tarsus about 6 mm from the nasal canthus. Each punctum is 0.2 to 0.3 mm in diameter and points toward the globe.[3] Proper tear elimination requires that the punctum be apposed to the globe. If it is visible without everting the lid, it is out of position. Should a patient's lower punctum become exposed on upgaze, tear drainage may be adversely affected.

Anatomically the lacrimal drainage system, except for the punctum, is hidden from direct observation. Understanding its physical characteristics and dimensions is extremely important. Following entry of tears into the punctum, they flow through a 2 mm vertical segment of each canaliculus. Each canaliculus then turns nasalward and runs a horizontal course of approximately 8 mm to reach the lacrimal sac. The lacrimal sac is about 12 mm vertically, ballooning above the junction of the superior and inferior canaliculi to form their entrance to the sac (internal punctum), the common canaliculus (Fig. 20.3). The nasolacrimal duct is continuous with the lacrimal sac inferiorly, extends 15 to 20 mm caudalward, narrows, and finally opens into the inferior meatus. Tears are then drained over the nasopharynx and oropharynx to be swallowed.

The drainage pathway is traditionally thought to

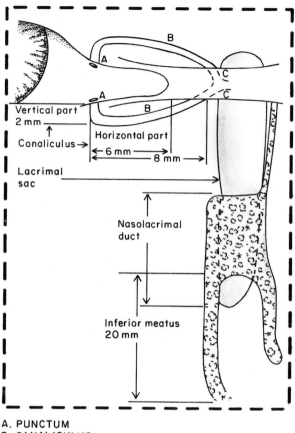

A. PUNCTUM
B. CANALICULUS
C. COMMON CANALICULUS

FIGURE 20.3 **Cut-away view showing the lacrimal excretory system. Tears drain through the punctum and eventually under the inferior turbinate bone of the nose. Dimensions of the canaliculi serve as references for probing and irrigation. (Redrawn with permission from Jones LT. Ophthalmic anatomy: A manual with some clinical applications. I. The orbital adnexa. American Academy of Ophthalmology 1970, 70.)**

account for about 90% of the fate of tears. The remainder is lost by evaporation. The importance of the punctum to proper physiologic drainage of tears has been stressed.[3,11] Gravitational attraction suggests that the inferior (lower) punctum is the more important in each pair, but the superior punctum may allow compensatory drainage if the lower punctum becomes nonfunctional.[12,13,99]

General Examination Procedures

Specific examination routines may vary, but the following strategy, with its basis in the anatomic logic of the lacrimal system, can serve as an outline for any patient with a complaint of tearing (Fig. 20.4).

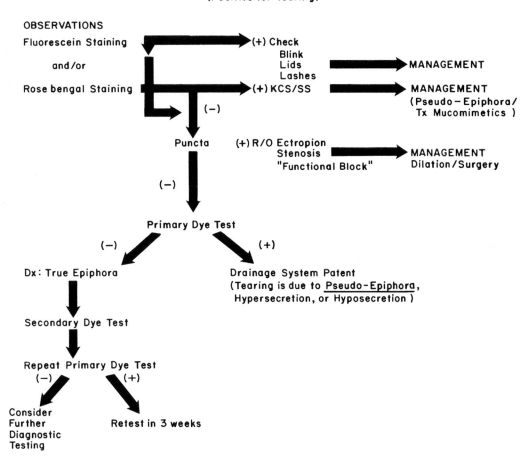

FIGURE 20.4   **Flowchart outlining authors' approach to lacrimal function testing.**

History

A careful patient interview often assists greatly in the diagnosis of lacrimal system disorders before any clinical tests are performed (Table 20.1). McMonnies[14] has proposed a sensitive and specific dry eye questionnaire. His approach is to discern information regarding the risk or presence of dry eye conditions based on gender, as well as other information cited in Table 20.1.

Factors such as the patient's sex, age, occupation, and environment may influence differential diagnostic considerations between secretory and excretory abnormalities. For example, infants who present with tearing are more likely to suffer from a drainage problem, while such a "wet" eye in an adult patient whose occupation includes exposure to noxious fumes is likely to be the result of lacrimal gland stimulation.

Pseudoepiphora, resulting from an aqueous deficiency, is most common among postmenopausal women.

TABLE 20.1
Subjective Assessment of Lacrimal System Disorders

- Duration and severity (acute, chronic, progressive; seasonal; previous medical or surgical treatment)
- Ocular and visual history
- Systemic health history
- Medication history
- Allergy history
- Occupational or environmental exposures
- Location of tearing (medial/lateral)

The dry eye of contact lens wearers may remain subclinical and, therefore, asymptomatic for tearing until environmental factors, for example, upset the aqueous equilibrium.

Medications such as anticholinergic agents, antianxiety drugs, and antihistamines can decrease aqueous production and cause a dry eye (see Chapter 30).

Patients whose drainage system is obstructed may have adapted to carrying a handkerchief or tissue to accommodate the epiphora.

Objective Examination of the Tear Film

Following a comprehensive health and medication history, the clinician can focus on objective examination of the patient. Physical findings should include fluorescein and rose bengal staining patterns. The presence of fluorescein staining of the cornea or conjunctiva is an indication to examine the blink function, lids, and lashes. Abnormal (devitalized or dead) epithelial cells of the cornea and conjunctiva will stain positively with rose bengal dye[15] (Color Plate IX). The presence of staining in the interpalpebral region is generally diagnostic of an aqueous deficiency.

The diagnosis of lacrimal system disorders may begin by observing any staining with sodium fluorescein viewed with cobalt blue light. The presence of fluorescein staining indicates a disrupted corneal epithelium.[15] The dye is also useful in evaluating tear-film stability by performing the TBUT test.[16] Fluorescein also enhances observation of the tear meniscus, which is reduced in aqueous deficiencies.

The TBUT test quantifies the stability of the precorneal tear film using sodium fluorescein as an indicator dye. It must be performed on a cornea that has not been manipulated by earlier tests, including the instillation of a topical anesthetic. A drop of sodium fluorescein is instilled into each inferior cul-de-sac. If a fluorescein strip is used, it should be moistened with saline or irrigating solution rather than rigid contact lens wetting solution. The increased viscosity of contact lens wetting solutions will artificially prolong the TBUT and yield misleading results.

The cornea should be scanned under low slit-lamp magnification using cobalt blue light. The patient is instructed to blink once or twice and then stare straight ahead without blinking. Without holding the lids, the practitioner should note the time it takes for the first randomly formed dry spot to appear (Fig. 20.5). A clinical measurement of 10 seconds or less is consistent with the diagnosis of dry eye.[16] It is important to note that a decreased TBUT finding indicates only tear film instability, not whether the deficiency is mucin or aqueous.[17]

Absent from our approach to the evaluation of the lacrimal system is the Schirmer test. Because there is confusion regarding its reliability,[18–22] a review of the components of Schirmer's[23] original strategy will be given with a perspective on its current clinical use.

The Schirmer I or "routine" Schirmer test is performed without topical anesthesia. A piece of What-

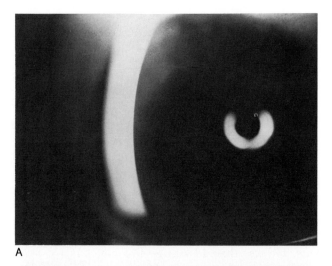

A

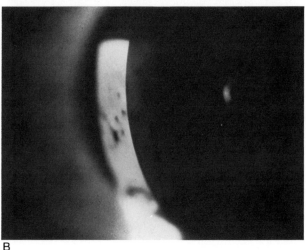

B

FIGURE 20.5 **Tear breakup time (TBUT) test. (A) Immediately following several complete blinks, there is homogeneous tear film stained with sodium fluorescein. (B) Randomly formed dry spot signals conclusion of the test and indicates instability of the tear film.**

man No. 41 filter paper is cut into a strip 5 mm × 50 mm, folded, and inserted into the inferior conjunctival fornix about one-third of the way from the lateral canthus. The patient is instructed to look slightly above the horizon at a distance. After 5 minutes, the strip is removed, and the extent of wetting from the fold is measured (Fig. 20.6). Some observers obtain useful results when consistently applied conditions are followed. In 1972, a 1-minute variation was shown to be equivalent to the 5-minute test when the amount of wetting was multiplied by 3.[13] Milder[24] suggests that the test be performed simultaneously in both eyes.

The practical clinical information obtained from the Schirmer I test appears to be the confirmation of hy-

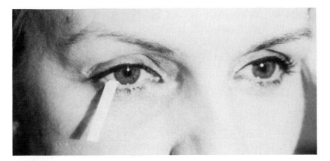

FIGURE 20.6   Position of filter-paper strip for Schirmer testing. Note that the strip is placed over the lid near the lateral canthus and away from the more sensitive cornea.

posecretion when less than 5 mm of strip wetting occurs. Greater than 15 mm wetting could indicate decreased, normal, or increased compensatory (reflex) secretion.

When more than 15 mm wetting occurs, it is useful to differentiate the "basic" from "reflex" contributions to the tear film. Since reflex secretion can occur secondary to a variety of stimuli, its contribution is sought to be eliminated by use of a topical anesthetic before performing the basic secretion test. Any residual anesthetic should be wiped from the conjunctival sac using a dry sterile cotton-tipped applicator. When a fresh Schirmer strip is inserted following application of topical anesthetic, the difference between the Schirmer I value and basic secretion test value represents the reflex portion of the tear film.

Less than 5 mm of wetting on the basic secretion test ensures a diagnosis of hyposecretion. Whether this is due to an actual deficiency of basic tear-film secretion or to "peripheral sensory fatigue block" can be determined using the Schirmer II test. Jones [1,3] proposed that decreased sensory input to the lacrimal nucleus results in the absence of reflex secretion. The Schirmer II test is qualitative and is performed immediately following a low value on the basic secretion test. With the same strip in place, mechanical or chemical irritation of the nasal mucosa is carried out. Increased wetting is testimony to integrity of the efferent reflex pathway (peripheral sensory fatigue block[1,3]), while no increase in wetting implies a fault of the reflex secretors.[1,3,24,25] The Schirmer test sequence is summarized in Figure 20.7. The objective of Schirmer's tests is the evaluation of tear secretion, but this function probably can be evaluated more reliably by using dye tests (sodium fluorescein and rose bengal).

Another test available to the clinician is quantitative lysozyme assay.[26] Tear lysozyme level is a useful measure of aqueous tear secretion, since lysozyme constitutes nearly one-fourth of total tear protein. Lysozyme levels will be reduced by dilution in hypersecretion and are known to be reduced in such aqueous-deficient conditions as Sjögren's syndrome. The basis for the test is inhibition of bacterial growth. The bacterium used is *Micrococcus lysodeikticus*.

Lysozyme concentration in tears has been measured clinically by spectrophotometric[26] and microdiffusion[27] methods. Of these techniques, the immunologic micro-

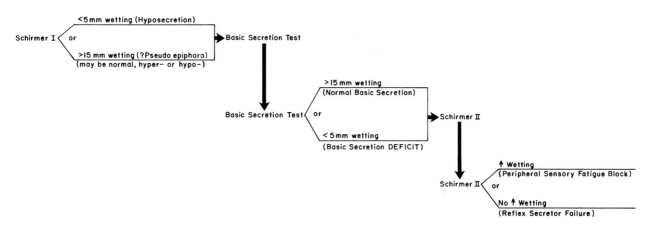

FIGURE 20.7   **Flowchart for Schirmer tests. Exhaustive Schirmer testing includes performing the Schirmer I, basic secretion, and Schirmer II tests sequentially. A small amount of wetting on the Schirmer I test confirms [HYPOSECRETION]; greater than 15 mm wetting is inconclusive. [NORMAL BASIC SECRETION] is indicated by > 15 mm wetting in the basic secretion test (BST). When fewer than 5 mm of the strip is wet on the BST, [BASIC SECRETION DEFICIT] is indicated. The Schirmer II test is now performed to differentiate between [PERIPHERAL SENSORY FATIGUE BLOCK] and [REFLEX SECRETOR FAILURE].**

diffusion procedure appears to be more applicable to office use.

An alternative to lysozyme assay (which may require sophisticated laboratory facilities) for lacrimal gland function is the measurement of lactoferrin concentration in tears. In a clinical comparison between lysozyme and lactoferrin assays among both control and dry eye patients, consistent results were found.[28] The strength of lactoferrin measurement lies in its ease of use in the office environment. The commercial version of the test is marketed as Lactoplate (Eagle Vision, Inc., 6485 Poplar Avenue, Memphis, TN 38119) (Fig. 20.8), and the procedure appears to be a reliable marker in the diagnosis of keratoconjunctivitis sicca.[28] The results are read after 2 to 3 days.

Another sophisticated diagnostic strategy for confirming dry eye is the use of cellulose acetate impressions to investigate ocular surface integrity. Conjunctival impression "cytology" is performed to determine goblet-cell density of the bulbar or palpebral conjunctival surface. A strip of commercially available filter paper (MF Millipore Filter VS) is gently pressed against the bulbar or palpebral conjunctiva with a glass rod.[29] Nelson and associates[29] prefer the rougher (versus smooth) side of the paper as the more useful in obtaining specimens. Following staining with Schiff's reagent and counterstaining with hematoxylin, the specimens are graded using a microscope. The results of studies of normal and "dry" eyes (keratoconjunctivitis sicca, ocular pemphigoid, Stevens-Johnson syndrome) have reflected normal or decreased goblet-cell counts, respectively.[29,30] Impression cytology has also been applied in monitoring vitamin A deficiency.[31]

Blink, Lid, and Lash Disorders

Since the lids represent the distribution system for lacrimal fluids, their neural, muscular, and structural components must be intact for proper maintenance of the tear film. Incomplete or twitch blinking may pose a problem to contact lens wearers or patients with marginal (subclinical) dry eye. Nocturnal lagophthalmos can result in exposure keratitis with characteristic inferior corneal staining observable with sodium fluorescein.

The seventh cranial nerve is responsible for lid closure during the blink reflex. Bell's palsy can interrupt these impulses, resulting in exposure keratitis. Loss of muscular tone can lead to ectropion, disrupt the "lacrimal pump," and result in impaired tear drainage.

Lid margins normally are smooth and regular. Inflammatory conditions and trauma can distort the lid margins, with potential for disrupted flow of tear film. An inturned lash (trichiasis) or blepharitis can disturb the tear film or irritate the cornea to cause physical signs of fluorescein staining and tearing along with symptoms of irritation. Chapter 19 considers lid abnormalities in further detail.

Dacryoadenitis

Etiology

Acute inflammation of the lacrimal gland may accompany local or systemic viral or bacterial infection or be secondary to trauma.[32]

Diagnosis

Pathologic enlargement of the lacrimal gland is characterized by swelling in the temporal one-third to one-half of the upper lid. Milder[32] calls attention to the S curve of the upper lid in lacrimal gland disorders, since it is diagnostic for lacrimal gland disease and is unique

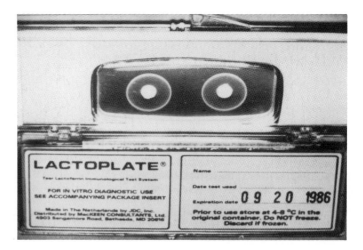

FIGURE 20.8 **Lactoferrin immunologic test system (Lactoplate). A tear sample is collected on a filter paper disc and transferred to reagent gel (shown). The results are read after 3 days of incubation (diffusion) at room temperature.** (Courtesy Eagle Vision, Inc., Memphis, TN.)

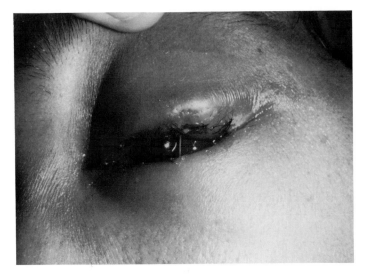

FIGURE 20.9   **Dacryoadenitis. Inflammation of the lacrimal gland is characterized by swelling of the superolateral lid and adnexal tissue and the diagnostic S curve of the upper lid. (Courtesy Michael A. Callahan, M.D.)**

among lid abnormalities (Fig. 20.9). Tumors of the lacrimal gland are relatively rare but should be differentiated histopathologically and distinguished clinically from inflammatory disorders of the lacrimal gland.[33–35]

A painless swelling without inflammatory signs in the region should suggest benign mixed tumor (pleomorphic adenoma), while acute onset and pain suggest malignant tumors (carcinoma). Computed tomography following plain x-ray films can be useful in the differential diagnosis of lacrimal gland lesions.[32,36] The role of magnetic resonance imaging (MRI) studies in preoperative differentiation of benign mixed tumors from carcinoma has yet to be established.[36] Pain or tenderness suggests an acute inflammatory process. Table 20.2 summarizes clinical signs in dacryoadenitis.

Acute dacryoadenitis is an inflammatory process of the lacrimal gland generally seen in infants or children.[36] Aside from age, clinical characteristics include unilateral local tenderness, redness, lid swelling, conjunctival chemosis, discharge or suppuration, and enlarged preauricular nodes.[35,36]

Management

Acute dacryoadenitis usually responds rapidly to systemic corticosteroids.[36] Viral dacryoadenitis associated with acute epidemic parotitis (mumps), infectious mononucleosis, or herpes zoster infection should receive supportive therapy.[33,35] Supportive therapy for mumps should be continued for its typical 2- to 4-week self-limiting course[32] and may take the form of rest, local application of ice, and use of oral analgesics such as acetaminophen.

Bacterial dacryoadenitis should be treated with specific antibiotics following culture and sensitivity test-

ing.[32,33] Broad-spectrum coverage is offered by a combination of gentamicin, 4 mg/kg body weight daily intramuscularly in 3 divided doses, and a cephalosporin, such as cefazolin, 1 g every 4 hours intravenously with probenecid, 0.5 g orally 4 times daily.[32] This regimen should be followed for 7 days. Gonorrheal dacryoadenitis is treated with penicillin administered intramuscularly or tetracycline taken orally.[32]

Persistent enlargement of the lacrimal gland, when tumor has been ruled out, generally represents chronic dacryoadenitis.[32,33] Biopsy may be necessary when the episode does not follow sarcoidosis, tuberculosis, Graves' ophthalmopathy, Mikulicz's syndrome, "sclerosing pseudotumors," or Wegener's granulomatosis.[36] Table 20.3 lists systemic conditions that have been associated with chronic dacryoadenitis. Histopathology studies appear to be useful in the differential diagnosis (Table 20.4).[32,36]

Disorders of the Tear Film

Holly and Lemp[2] have arranged tear film abnormalities into 5 different categories according to physiologic con-

TABLE 20.2
Clinical Signs in Dacryoadenitis[32–36]

Consistent in All	Associated with Acute Cases or Suggestive of Tumor
• Superolateral swelling • S curve of upper lid	• Local tenderness • Discharge • Proptosis • Diplopia

TABLE 20.3
Systemic Conditions Associated with Chronic Dacryoadenitis[32,33,36]

- Sarcoidosis
- Tuberculosis
- Thyroid ophthalmopathy
- Sclerosing pseudotumors
- Wegener's granulomatosis

TABLE 20.5
Tear Film Abnormalities

Disorder	Example
Aqueous deficiency	Keratoconjunctivitis sicca
Mucin deficiency	Cicatricial pemphigoid
Lipid abnormality	Secondary to chronic blepharitis
Impaired lid function	Exposure keratitis secondary to Bell's palsy
Epitheliopathy	Microepithelial irregularity

Adapted from Holly FJ, Lemp MA. Tear physiology and dry eyes. Surv Ophthalmol 1977;22:69–87.

siderations (Table 20.5). This classification is useful for patient management once appropriate examination procedures have led to an accurate diagnosis.

Aqueous Deficiency

ETIOLOGY

A decrease in aqueous production by the basic secretors is known to occur with advancing age. Thinning of this, the thickest, segment of the precorneal tear film results in premature contamination of the mucin layer of the tear film and is observed clinically as a rapid TBUT.[16]

Lack of aqueous production at birth is a disorder termed congenital alacrima.[37] This rare condition may be due to hypoplasia of lacrimal gland tissue or congenital paresis of cranial nerves.[2] Another congenital and equally rare cause of aqueous deficiency is familial dysautonomia (Riley-Day syndrome).[38] This disorder is associated with a short lifespan.

Considerably more common is the aqueous deficiency seen among adults during the fifth and sixth decades of life. Keratoconjunctivitis sicca occurs in a disproportionate ratio of women to men (9:1). It has a gradual onset with periods of exacerbation that may be heightened by decreases in ambient humidity. The following discussion will consider only the acquired aqueous deficiencies.

DIAGNOSIS

Symptoms of keratoconjunctivitis sicca may include burning, foreign-body sensation, and scratchiness. These

TABLE 20.4
Differential Diagnosis in Dacryoadenitis[32,33,36]

- Dermoids, dermoid cysts
- Congenital cysts
- Dacryops (lacrimal gland cysts)
- Pseudotumor of lacrimal gland
- Tumor
  - Benign mixed (pleomorphic adenoma)
  - Malignant (carcinoma)

symptoms tend to increase in severity during the course of the day. Due to the thinned aqueous, lipid-contaminated mucus strands collect in the fornices.[2] Patients may also complain of increased "mattering" associated with the presence of dried mucus at the nasal canthus on arising. The irritation accompanying the disorder itself combined with excess mucus may prompt the patient to manually attempt to remove the strands. The resulting mechanical irritation can cause further irritation and tearing. This vicious cycle has been termed the *mucus-fishing syndrome* and is characterized by rose bengal staining of the affected bulbar conjunctiva and cornea[39] (Color Plate X).

Clinical signs can include the observation of increased debris in the tear film (due to an increased desquamation rate of the epithelial cells),[2] reduced marginal tear strip, increased mucus strands, rose bengal staining of bulbar conjunctiva or cornea (see Color Plate IX),[15] filamentary keratitis, reduced TBUT, and corneal staining with sodium fluorescein.[40]

Simple clinical observation and physical findings combined with the history generally confirm the diagnosis. Sophisticated procedures such as tear protein determination are rarely necessary to begin treatment but may be helpful in the early identification of the patient with keratoconjunctivitis sicca.[40]

MANAGEMENT

Tear substitutes have been the mainstay of treatment for aqueous-deficient dry eye. It is generally most useful to begin the patient on a regimen of artificial tear solutions 4 to 8 times per day along with the application of a bland ophthalmic ointment at bedtime. Although rare, some artificial tear solutions may contain viscosity-enhancing components (substituted cellulose ethers) that tend to precipitate out of solution and cause crust to form on the eyelids.[41] An alternative approach to the formulation of tear replacements is to substitute polymers (e.g., polyvinyl alcohol) for the cellulose compounds. The treatment strategy, in either case, is to enhance contact time to preserve the scanty aqueous secretion. Clinicians should also be aware that the preservative benzalkonium chloride has been reported to reduce TBUT.[42]

One novel formulation in the artificial tear armamentarium is the incorporation of a solubilized lipid component.[43] Since this solution (Tear Gard, Med Tech) has been designed to supplement each component of the tear film—lipid, aqueous, and mucin—it is thought by some to be the ideal physiologic tear replacement. LaMotte and Lesher,[43] however, have reported a slightly negative response by patients due to the increased viscosity the lipid imparts. The transient blurring of vision is often seen as a trade-off for subjective benefits.

The use of a soft contact lens with frequent instillation of saline or artificial tear solution has been advocated as another level of dry eye treatment. A low-water contact lens is preferred.[44,45] Although agreement is not uniform, such a strategy may be most useful in treating abnormalities of the tear film, especially those resulting in recurrent corneal erosion.[46]

Another approach to the management of patients with aqueous deficiency and excessive mucus filaments is the topical application of mucolytic agents such as n-acetylcysteine (Mucomyst, Mead Johnson). Initially intended for asthmatics, n-acetylcysteine can be diluted with artificial tears to 2% to 10% concentration for lysing mucus strands in the fornices.[47] However, because this agent has not been FDA-approved for use in the eye, it is not widely employed.

Preservation of existing tears is another treatment strategy sometimes used for patients with aqueous deficiency. Both thermal and laser cauterization of the punctal openings have been attempted,[48] and removable silicone plugs (Figs. 20.10 and 20.11) currently offer a reversible method of punctoplasty.[49] In addition, dissolvable collagen implants (Fig. 20.12) can be used diagnostically by insertion into the inferior canaliculus to determine whether permanent punctoplasty may be effective.[50]

Nonpharmacologic methods of treatment of dry eyes may include the use of home humidifiers or local means of decreasing evaporation of tears. Conservation of tears by punctal occlusion has been discussed. Osmotic infusion pumps and constant flow devices have been proposed and prototypes developed. These, however, remain unpopular. Methylcellulose inserts to provide a constant reservoir of artificial tears have met with resistance from most patients.[51]

Severe dry eye states have been managed with vitamin A ointment, and results appear encouraging for a spectrum of dry eye syndromes, including goblet-cell and surface ocular abnormalities.[52]

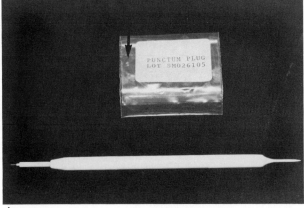

A

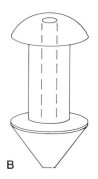

B

FIGURE 20.10 **Punctum plugs and dilator/inserter instrument.** *(A)* **Silicone removable punctum plugs are packaged in a sterile envelope. Each end of the supplied instrument serves as dilator or inserter, respectively.** *(B)* **Enlarged drawing of plug to illustrate detail. (Adapted from product information, Eagle Vision, Inc., Memphis, TN.)**

Mucin Deficiency

ETIOLOGY

The conjunctival mucin made by the goblet cells is needed to produce and maintain wettability of the corneal epithelium. Instability of the tear film due to mucin deficiency results from goblet-cell dysfunction. The causes of goblet-cell destruction vary from vitamin A deficiency to direct conjunctival trauma (chemical burns, radiation) or disease. Etiologies of mucin deficiency are listed in Table 20.6.[53,54]

Traumatic destruction of conjunctival architecture is generalized; fibrous tissue replaces normal conjunctiva. In contrast, destruction in cases of avitaminosis A appears to be more specific. The microcirculation supporting the goblet cells is lost in this vitamin deficiency, resulting in keratinization.[52,53]

Ocular cicatricial pemphigoid (OCP), a chronic inflammatory disease that can affect the conjunctiva, is

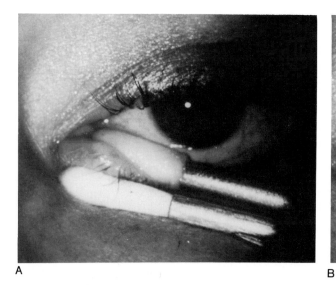

A

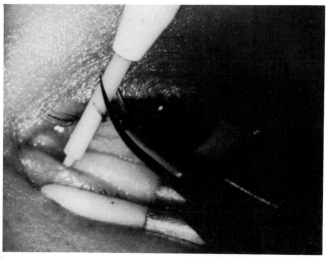

B

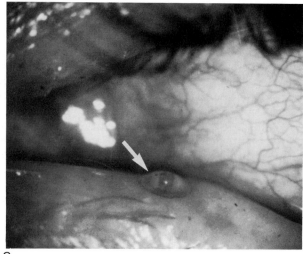

C

FIGURE 20.11 **Method of inserting removable punctum plugs.** *(A)* **After topical anesthesia is obtained, the punctal opening is exposed.** *(B)* **The plug is buried into punctum with the inserting instrument. Forceps grasp the movable sleeve of the inserting end, forcing the plug from the shaft into the punctum.** *(C)* **Close-up showing plug in place in the inferior punctum (arrow). (Courtesy Eagle Vision, Inc., Memphis, TN.)**

presumed to have an autoimmune etiology. Support for this concept comes from a report of 10 patients with pseudopemphigoid[55] (OCP associated with ocular drug administration). All patients had clinically proven OCP that responded positively to immunosuppressive therapy.[55] Stevens-Johnson syndrome (erythema multiforme major) manifests similar clinical signs but occurs as acute recurrent episodes without the chronic relentless progression of OCP.[56] Thoft[57] argues that ocular surface disorders such as OCP and Stevens-Johnson syndrome manifest aqueous *and* mucin deficiencies secondary to pathologic changes of the corneal and conjunctival surface epithelium. For this reason, OCP represents the diagnostic and treatment prototype

for the mechanical forms of mucin deficiency secondary to conjunctival shrinkage.

DIAGNOSIS

Cicatricial pemphigoid (benign mucosal pemphigoid) is a subepithelial bullous disease of the aged. It affects the skin and mucous membranes, leading to shrinkage, scarring, and adhesions. In the conjunctiva, normal tissue is replaced by scar tissue (cicatrization). The incidence is low (1 in 20,000 ophthalmic patients), and women are affected in a 7:3 ratio to men. The average age at presentation is over 60 years, and there is no racial predilection.[58]

History of trauma combined with the observation of persistent dry spots on the cornea should alert the clinician to consider the possibility of early mucus deficiency. Persistent dry spots are observed as areas of nonwetting or areas of recurrent tear-film breakup. The loss of corneal surfacing by mucus is responsible for this clinical picture.

OCP may begin with typical dry eye complaints in an elderly patient. The progressive submucosal shrinkage can also involve the lacrimal and accessory lacrimal gland ducts, contributing to aqueous deficiency.[59]

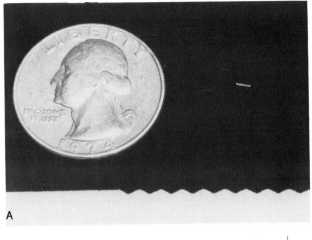

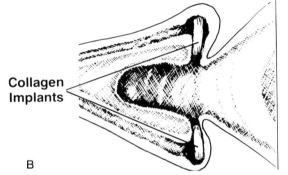

Collagen
Implants

B

FIGURE 20.12 **Temporary intracanalicular collagen implants.** *(A)* **Photograph illustrating a single implant compared with a U.S. quarter dollar. The serrated structure at the bottom of the photograph is the foam insert for packaging.** *(B)* **Temporary intracanalicular insert in place. (Fig.** *B* **courtesy Eagle Vision, Inc., Memphis, TN.)**

Continued progression of conjunctival shrinkage and scarring can lead to symblepharon formation with entropion and trichiasis, lagophthalmos and exposure keratitis, and inability to elevate the eyes. Keratinization involving the cornea (see Fig. 21.23) will result in decreased visual acuity. Other ocular complications include corneal erosion, corneal neovascularization, and pseudopterygia.[59]

The differential diagnoses of OCP are few. Conjunctival shrinkage and scarring secondary to membranous conjunctivitis of viral etiology (adenovirus types 8 and 9, primary herpetic keratoconjunctivitis) or infection with β-hemolytic *Streptococcus* are acute and self-limiting, in contrast to the chronic and progressive nature of the conjunctival shrinkage in OCP.

MANAGEMENT

As in any tear-film deficiency, treatment of mucin-deficient dry eye with artificial tears plays a major

TABLE 20.6
Etiology of Mucin Deficiency[53,54]

Conjunctival destruction (mechanical)
   Ocular cicatricial pemphigoid (OCP); benign mucosal
      pemphigoid
   Erythema multiforme (EM)
   Toxic etiologies
      Chemical burns, irradiation
      Drug-induced (pseudopemphigoid)
         Echothiophate iodide
         Pilocarpine
         Epinephrine
         Systemic practolol
Avitaminosis A

therapeutic role. The strategy is to keep the patient comfortable rather than attempting to arrest progression of the disorder. Frequent application of artificial tears during the waking hours combined with bland ointment at bedtime may be useful in early stages or in mild cases. If only clinical signs are present (persistent dry spots) but the patient is asymptomatic, artificial tears can be applied 4 times daily in addition to bland ointment at bedtime. This approach is often effective in mild cases. The ointment apparently has a salubrious effect on the corneal epithelium during sleep, and with continuation of the regimen some patients may show reversal of the clinical signs of corneal drying.

In addition to the basic disease process, secondary bacterial infections can complicate the clinical condition. Eyelid scrubs followed by antibiotic ointments are effective for any associated blepharitis (see Chapter 19).

A recent report[60] calls attention to the observation that timolol can induce and exacerbate OCP. The authors[60] recommend that elevated intraocular pressure be treated, alternatively, with carbonic anhydrase inhibitors.

Entropion with trichiasis may be corrected in the early stages of the disease by oculoplastic surgical techniques, but care must be taken not to further shorten the already shrunken conjunctiva.[59] Traditional approaches to the trichiasis may also be used: electrolysis, epilation, and cryoablation.[56,59]

Systemic steroids are useful in the acute stages of OCP.[61] Gardner and associates[59] have suggested that immunosuppressive agents may be promising for selected cases. Mucous membrane transplantation has been shown to have only limited success.[54]

The treatment of other forms of mucin deficiency is similar to that for OCP. Alkali burns are an emergency, and the conjunctival fornices should be copiously flushed with water immediately. Testing the tears in the fornices following lavage can be carried out with pH paper to determine whether all the alkaline material has been flushed. Management of subsequent scarring should follow the same course as treatment of OCP. Table 20.7 summarizes the approach to treatment of mucin-deficient dry eyes.

A recent approach to the mucin-deficient eye that shows promise is the local application of 0.1% or 0.01% all-trans retinoic acid (vitamin A). Vitamin A is locally deficient when cicatricial tissue replaces normally vascularized tissue. Since vitamin A is one of the essential factors for epithelial growth and differentiation, its local application is thought to stimulate goblet-cell activity.[52] A series of selected cases was studied by Tseng and associates.[52] Of 16 patients (27 eyes) with Stevens-Johnson syndrome, OCP, or traumatic goblet-cell loss, all showed improvement in clinical signs and symptoms when treated with local vitamin A. Concentrations used were either 0.01% or 0.1% (weight/weight) of all-trans retinoic acid in ointment form. Spectacular improvements were recorded over a relatively short follow-up period (all less than 12 months), but this report[52] may represent the first nonsurgical attempt at treating mucin deficiencies by reversing changes in the diseased ocular surface epithelium.

The clinical response to vitamin A in histologically proven goblet-cell loss has been documented by Sullivan and associates.[62] Systemic administration of vitamin A contributed to reversal of corneal and conjunctival keratinization as well as to some restoration of goblet cells after 3 weeks of treatment. This report suggested that vitamin A may be helpful for patients with goblet-cell loss due to dietary deficiency.[62] Recently, vitamin A ointment has been shown to be effective for some surface ocular abnormalities characterized by metaplasia of the surface epithelium.[100]

Lipid Deficiency

ETIOLOGY

Lipid deficiency is extremely rare. Complete absence of meibomian secretion has been described in cases of congenital anhidrotic ectodermal dysplasia.[54] Sebum from the skin of the eyelid then contaminates the aqueous layer. Because of the higher polarity and lower molecular weight of sebum, complete "dewetting" of the ocular surface can result.[54,63]

A milder degree of lipid deficiency occurs secondary to chronic blepharitis. The inflammatory process of the eyelids alters the polarity of the meibomian secretion. This alteration takes the form of free fatty acid formation associated with the lipase activity of staphylococcal organisms.[62] Often, however, this is offset by a proportional increase in the rate of meibomian secretion.[54]

TABLE 20.7
Treatment Strategies for Mucin Deficiencies

Ocular cicatricial pemphigoid, Stevens-Johnson syndrome
  Tear substitutes
  Consider systemic steroids and immunosuppressive agents
  Abort bacterial infections with lid prophylaxis
  Manage complications of entropion, trichiasis on an
    individual basis
Chemical burns (acid, alkali, solvents)
  Flush with water or sterile saline *immediately* (first aid)
  Tear substitutes once acute phase has cleared
  Manage complications on an individual basis
Drug-induced (pseudopemphigoid)
  Consider alternative ocular medications
  Consult concerning use of immunosuppressive agents

DIAGNOSIS

Both staphylococcal and seborrheic blepharitis have distinctive clinical signs. The former is characterized by collarettes at the base of the lashes. The eyelids show a fibrinous scale and significant inflammation but occasionally can exhibit an ulcerative appearance.[64]

Patients with seborrheic blepharitis generally have eyelids with less inflammation combined with more oily or greasy scaling.[64] Clinical symptoms are similar between the two and may be indistinguishable from keratoconjunctivitis sicca, which may be an associated condition. Chief among the clinical signs of either tear-film disorder is a reduced TBUT.

The lipase activity of staphylococcal organisms gives rise to the formation of free fatty acids.[62] Clinically this may be associated with "foam" or "soap bubble" accumulation at the outer canthi when viewed with the biomicroscope.

MANAGEMENT

The treatment of lipid deficiency associated with blepharitis consists of a combination of eyelid hygiene, topical antibiotic therapy, and occasionally systemic antibiotic therapy[64] (see Chapter 19). The strategies are designed to reverse the destabilizing effects on the tear film. Typical palliative treatment with tear substitutes during the day and ocular lubricating ointments at bedtime will help to keep the patient comfortable while the supervening blepharitis is controlled.

Both Jones'[53] and Holly's[54] classifications of tear dysfunction states or lacrimal abnormalities include mechanisms related to disorders of the eyelids. Since the eyelids serve as distributors of the tear film, this is a logical inclusion. Chapter 19 considers in greater detail the diagnosis and treatment of eyelid abnormalities.

Disorders of Lacrimal Drainage

Congenital Epiphora

ETIOLOGY

The lacrimal drainage system is generally completely canalized by term. It is generally agreed that the last portion to become patent is the most distal.[65–67] A vestigial remnant of epithelialization of the canal (Hasner's membrane) may occlude this most distal opening, and this is the most frequent cause of congenital epiphora.

DIAGNOSIS

Any obstruction of lacrimal drainage will cause tearing. The clinical characteristics of congenital epiphora include an infant with tearing and possibly a secondary dacryocystitis. The condition may have a prevalence as high as 6%.[68] Congenital epiphora generally appears within the first month of life,[65] and, when accompanied by dacryocystitis, the purulent discharge must be differentiated from neonatal conjunctivitis. The diagnosis of dacryocystitis can be confirmed in many cases by gently pressing over the nasolacrimal sac and observing mucopurulent reflux from either punctum.[69]

MANAGEMENT

Conservative treatment appears to be a consistent feature of large studies.[65,68–71] However, the exact timing for more aggressive intervention is controversial. Jones[65] has suggested that patients over 1 year of age with epiphora be examined for inflammation and presence of purulent discharge. Topical antibiotics and decongestants are indicated in the presence of inflammatory signs, but in the absence of inflammation, the parents should be instructed in the technique of hydrostatic nasolacrimal massage.[69]

The hydrostatic technique was described originally by Crigler.[72] It consists of placing the index finger over the common canaliculus to prevent reflux of material through either punctum. With a firm downward "stroking" motion, an attempt is made to increase hydrostatic pressure within the nasolacrimal duct (Fig. 20.13). The objective is to catalyze rupture of membranous obstruction (Hasner's membrane) at the distal end of the nasolacrimal duct. This maneuver should be repeated 5 times twice a day. Treatment should be continued until epiphora stops or until the child is 3 months old. Use of antibiotic (erythromycin) ointment several times daily is recommended if mucopurulent discharge is present.[69]

Another conservative strategy is to allow time for a spontaneous cure. Suckling[70] projected that 94% of

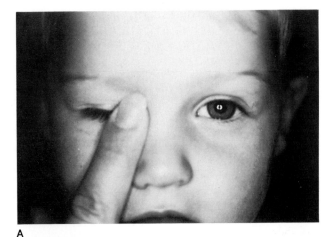

A

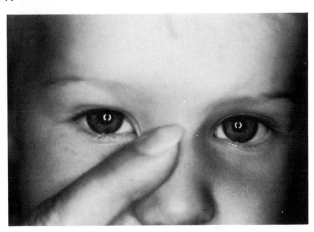

B

FIGURE 20.13 **Sequence illustrating the method for applying digital pressure in congenital dacryocystitis secondary to incomplete distal lacrimal drainage system canalization (see text).**

infants with obstruction at age 7.5 months will cure themselves if left untreated until 21 months of age. The efficacy of delayed intervention beyond 13 months of age has been confirmed in a large series of patients.[71] In fact, 93.5% were cured following a single probing performed under general anesthesia.[71] An alternative approach to probing is high-pressure irrigation.[67]

If irrigation procedures are unsuccessful, careful probing can be performed. This procedure[73] is best performed in a hospital operating room. General anesthesia is obtained by inhalation administered by an anesthesiologist. The ophthalmic surgeon uses a Bowman probe of small diameter (usually #1 or #2) (Fig. 20.14). The probe's tip can be lightly coated with a sterile ophthalmic ointment. Once general anesthesia is induced, the Bowman probe is inserted in the superior punctum of the involved eye. It is then directed downward so that the probe is parallel to the nose. A

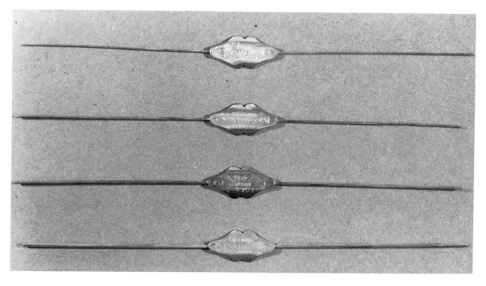

FIGURE 20.14 **Bowman probes.**

gentle insertion technique is needed until the tip of the probe is seen exiting the ipsilateral nare. In some cases, a cracking sound can be heard as the probe is pushed through the structures of the nose. Extreme care should be taken to respect the anatomic structures of the nasolacrimal system.

To test the integrity of the lacrimal system after probing, a few drops of 1% sodium fluorescein are instilled into the cul-de-sac of the involved eye. A small clear plastic tube is inserted immediately into the area of the inferior meatus to aspirate the fluorescein. If the nasolacrimal system is patent, the surgeon will observe fluorescein in the clear plastic aspiration tube. With the inherent risk using general anesthesia on an infant, the procedure should be practiced and performed in less than 3 to 4 minutes. The child can recover from the anesthesia in a few more minutes and be back in the mother's arms for recovery. More time is spent in preoperative preparation and postoperative recovery than performing the actual procedure.

Failures of probing pose a management dilemma. Bony malformations appear to be the cause of nearly all failures.[67,73–78] The inability to pass a probe through the nose or to irrigate saline through the nasolacrimal duct indicate nasal pathology.[74–78]

Regardless of age, the infant should be observed carefully for the presence of true epiphora, and the prospect of parent compliance should play a role in the management decision. Following conservative treatment, lack of spontaneous cure much beyond 1 year of age significantly increases the likelihood of 2 events: nasal pathology is more likely to be present, and more complex procedures probably will be needed to resolve the tearing problem.[71,77,78]

Acquired Epiphora

The lacrimal drainage apparatus serves to channel tears from the eye. It plays a vital role in the equilibrium established between tear production and excretion. Except for observation of the punctum, the clinician must rely largely on patient symptoms and evidence from indirect evaluation to arrive at a diagnosis of a lacrimal drainage disorder. Tests for acquired lacrimal drainage dysfunction are based on anatomy of the lacrimal drainage system.

ACQUIRED PUNCTUM OCCLUSION

Etiology. Occlusion of the lacrimal puncta is called atresia when congenital and stenosis when it is acquired. Each will produce true epiphora.

Weil[79] has divided the lacrimal excretory system into upper and lower components conceptually. This separation appears to violate the embryologic, histologic, and anatomic continuity of the system, but it allows consideration of problems of the puncta and canaliculi separate from the more distal portions of the system.

Diseases of the eyelids and lid margins can result in malposition of the punctum. These include blepharitis; seborrheic, atopic, or neurodermatitis; and collagen diseases such as scleroderma.[79] Stenosis (occlusion by flattening) of the punctum can be secondary to lid dermatoses or simply be the result of age. The latter is the most frequent cause of acquired epiphora.

Diagnosis. The diagnosis of true epiphora is often accomplished before the clinician begins formal examination procedures. A history of persistent tearing and the presence of a handkerchief or tissue in the patient's hand will virtually secure the diagnosis.

Apart from direct observation, the clinician may wish to perform the diagnostic dye tests. Controversy exists, however, over the approach to interpretation of fluorescein as a marker for tear drainage. Jones[80] has suggested instilling fluorescein into the inferior cul-de-sac and awaiting its appearance in the nose after 5 minutes. He favored direct exploration of the inferior meatus of the nose using a cotton-tipped wire applicator. Alternatively, direct observation for fluorescein can be performed with a cobalt-filtered light source (Burton lamp or angioscopy filter in place on a binocular indirect ophthalmoscope headset). Perhaps the most effective method of detecting the fluorescein-stained tears is to incline the patient forward and have the patient clear the nose into a white tissue. This test is performed on one side at a time and reveals evidence that is particularly dramatic whether the test is positive or negative.[81]

Other authors[82] have correlated the *dis*appearance of fluorescein from the cul-de-sac with the Jones fluorescein test. The conclusion is that rapid excretion of the fluorescein-stained tears from the marginal tear strip observed with the slit lamp indicates normal physiologic lacrimal drainage.

Whichever interpretive strategy is used, blockage of the lacrimal drainage system will not allow fluorescein to be detected in the nose. This is the Jones No. 1 test, or primary dye test.[80] When fluorescein is present, the test is considered positive (normal lacrimal drainage) and implies physiologic patency of the system. Should the dye remain in the eye or not be detected further along the drainage passageways, then a negative test result is recorded and further diagnostic evaluation is indicated (see Fig. 20.4).

Punctal dilation is the next indicated diagnostic test. Enlargement with a dilator (Fig. 20.15) may open a stenotic punctum, although only, perhaps, temporarily.[79] If a repeated fluorescein dye test then reveals a positive result, the punctal dilation procedure will have solved the patient's problem, even if only temporarily.[79] The patient should be monitored within 2 to 3 weeks.

Punctal dilation can be accomplished easily with little or no patient discomfort. Topical anesthesia can be obtained with the instillation of 1 or 2 drops of 0.5% proparacaine. Deeper anesthesia can also be obtained with the following procedure.

A 6 inch sterile cotton-tipped applicator can be broken in half and the cotton tip saturated with a few drops of 0.5% proparacaine. The patient should look straight ahead with lids opened as wide as possible. The cotton tip, containing the proparacaine, is then held over the punctum. The patient then closes the lids securely to hold the shortened applicator for about 15 to 30 seconds. The proparacaine can now remain in contact longer with the lid margin and puncta and provide deeper anesthesia (Fig. 20.16). This method also provides the practitioner with a "patient anxiety index" by observing how much the wooden tip of the applicator wiggles due to lid tension. A rapidly wiggling applicator informs the clinician that the patient may require more support or empathy.

To dilate the inferior punctum, the lower lid is gently pulled away from the globe and the dilator is inserted vertically into the opening of the punctum. The dilator should be rolled slowly between the practitioner's finger and thumb to ease insertion. After traveling about 2 mm inferiorly, the dilator must be lowered to a horizontal position with continued gentle forward motion (Fig. 20.17). Excessive pressure should not be exerted with the dilator. As the dilator is in-

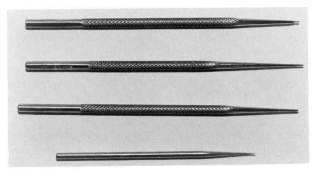

FIGURE 20.15 **Lacrimal dilators. Top dilator is Muldoon instrument; note the medium tip and rapid expansion. The next two are different sizes of the Wilder dilator. The bottom dilator is the Reudemann. It has a very fine tip and narrow taper, making it perhaps the most useful of the group.**

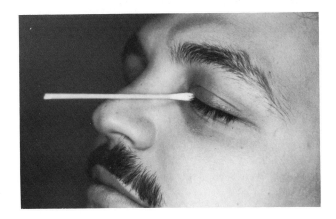

FIGURE 20.16 **Method of obtaining deeper anesthesia for punctum procedures. The cotton-tipped applicator is saturated with topical anesthetic and placed between the superior and inferior puncta. The patient then closes the lids.**

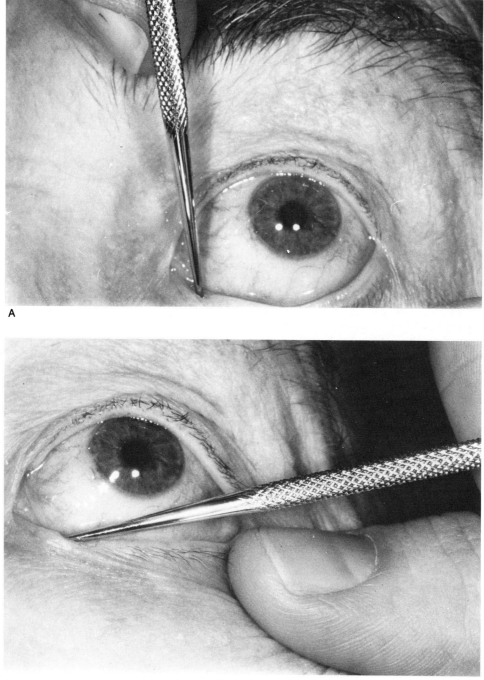

A

B

FIGURE 20.17   **Procedure for lower punctum dilation. (A) The dilator is inserted vertically about 2 mm. (B) It is then brought near the horizontal plane of the lower lid. The lower lid can be gently pulled laterally to straighten the canaliculus.**

serted further into the canaliculus and the punctal opening dilates, the ring of elastic tissue surrounding the punctum (punctal ring) will blanch. If further pressure is exerted against the punctum by the dilator, the punctum and lower lid will begin to turn inward and outward with the turning of the dilator. This indicates to the practitioner that sufficient pressure is being exerted and temporary dilation of the punctum is taking place. If the punctal opening is occluded with a thin layer of epithelial cells, it can still be opened with the needle-tipped dilator (see Fig. 20.15) or a sterilized safety pin. Most dilation procedures are directed to the lower lid, but the superior punctum can be dilated as well.

If the dye test following punctal dilation still proves

negative, then the secondary dye test, or Jones No. 2 test, is indicated. Some preparation is needed before the test is performed. Any remaining fluorescein should be rinsed from the cul-de-sac, and the patient should be administered a topical anesthetic. A 2 ml syringe is filled with sterile saline or extraocular irrigating solution and attached to a 23-gauge lacrimal cannula (Fig. 20.18). With the patient inclined forward and holding an emesis basin beneath the nose, the cannula is inserted through the lower punctum into the vertical and horizontal portions of the lower canaliculus (Fig. 20.19).

A reinforced 23-gauge straight cannula is the instrument preferred by some clinicians for this procedure. The base of the cannula is reinforced by a metal sleeve to prevent the cannula from breaking and lodging in the canaliculus following repeated use. This thickened shaft also serves the important function of punctal occluder during forced irrigation to prevent saline from regurgitating through the ipsilateral punctum. Other cannulas are available. The 23-gauge West cannula with blunt end and the side opening offers the advantages of easy advancement through the canaliculus and alignment with the nasolacrimal duct, respectively.

Once a hard stop is reached, a distance of approximately 13 mm from the punctum has been traversed.

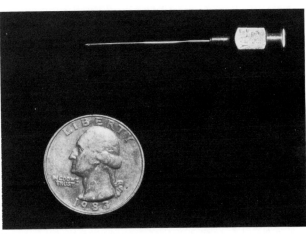

A

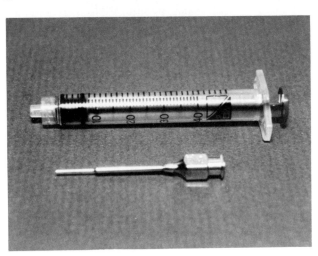

B

FIGURE 20.18 **Lacrimal cannulas. *(A)* The 23-gauge West cannula. The shaft is straight and approximately 25 mm long. The tip is blunt with needle hole in the side. *(B)* Reinforced 23-gauge cannula and syringe.**

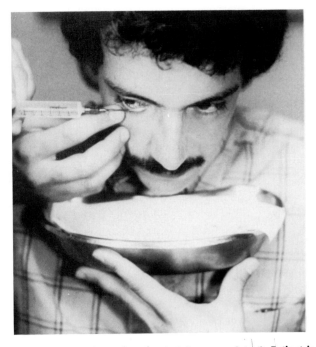

FIGURE 20.19 **Secondary dye test (Jones no. 2 test). Patient is seated and inclined forward for irrigation. Note basin to catch effluent. (From Semes L, Melore GG. Dilation and diagnostic irrigation of the lacrimal drainage system. J Am Optom Assoc 1986; 57:518–525. Reprinted with permission of the authors and publisher.)**

At this point, at least 0.5 ml of solution should be expressed from the syringe. One of 4 possible outcomes can occur[84]:

1. No fluid appears, indicating complete obstruction of the nasolacrimal duct.
2. Fluorescein-stained fluid appears, indicating partial distal obstruction of the nasolacrimal duct.
3. Clear fluid appears, indicating a negative Jones No. 2 (secondary) dye test. No fluorescein entered the drainage system, and an ectropion or stenosis of the punctum should be ruled out.
4. Regurgitation of saline or discharge appears at the superior punctum. This could indicate an inflammatory or neoplastic process. Table 20.8 summarizes the localizing value of regurgitation by type and site.

An alternative to the classic Jones No. 2 technique places the patient in a reclined position. The patient is requested to signal when he or she tastes the salty solution. The clinician can also be alert to observe the swallow reflex. It is important to use only a few milliliters of saline, since the patient will experience an overwhelming gag response if more is irrigated.

Management.   Effective management of minor cases of punctal occlusion may require only periodic (or in some cases single) dilation of the stenotic punctum. Some clinicians disdain the transient effects of punctal dilation and favor snip procedures or punch punctumplasty.[79] Most patients, however, prefer repeated dilation to surgical intervention.

If the punctum is involuted such that it cannot be identified or opened, then a dacryocystorhinostomy is required.[79] This surgical procedure shunts the tears directly from the lacrimal lake to the nasolacrimal duct.

CANALICULAR DISORDERS

Etiology.   Canaliculitis is a relatively rare disorder. In one study[85] only 2% of patients with tearing problems had a final diagnosis of canaliculitis. Actinomycotic and herpetic infections appear to be the most likely causative agents.[86,87] Recently, however, an allergic etiology has been reported.[88]

Diagnosis.   The patient complains of a smoldering, usually unilateral, red eye that has been resistant to antibiotic therapy.[85,86] Epiphora has a variable association.[88] Diagnostic irrigation may be met with resistance ("soft stop") before reaching the hard stop of the lacrimal bone. An important clinical sign in the diagnosis of obstructed canaliculus has been termed the *wrinkle sign.*[89] When a soft stop is encountered during probing or irrigation, the clinician can observe compression of the medial canthal skin (wrinkling) in the presence of internal obstruction. The visualization of smooth skin and advancement of the instrument to the lacrimal bone indicates a patent proximal drainage system. The secondary dye test may be negative.[88]

The initial diagnostic suspicion of canaliculitis may be aided by considering the patient's age. Actinomycotic infections are more likely to appear among patients over age 50 years,[85,86] while primary herpetic infections (herpes simplex, herpes zoster, varicella, and vaccinia) have a distinctly higher prevalence among patients under 20 years of age and will present with cutaneous manifestations of the infectious disease.[87]

Diagnostic testing beyond Gram-stained smears or cultures employs sophisticated means. Dacryoscopy (Dyonics, Inc., 71 Pine St., Woburn, MA 01801) allows direct visualization of lacrimal drainage passages through a needlescope.[90] Patients who are patent to irrigation may have incomplete anatomic obstruction that can be demonstrated by intubation dacryocystography with subtraction.[91] Advances in digital subtraction imaging now allow instantaneous high-resolution, magnified, bone-free radiographs of the lacrimal drainage system.[92] A contrast medium is injected before the x-ray film. The greatest advantage of this technique is its dynamic nature, allowing the clinician to interpret the flow of tears as it occurs.

Another diagnostic view of the lacrimal drainage pathways is possible using lacrimal scintigraphy.[93] In this procedure a radioisotope is instilled into the conjunctival sac and serves as the marker for tear drainage. Some authors[94] believe that this noninvasive imaging medium, when coupled with digital subtraction macrodacryocystography, provides the ultimate in anatomic and physiologic views of the lacrimal drainage system.

Canalicular disorders can also be secondary to trauma.[95] Standard primary diagnostic testing should reveal impatencies or lacerations of this nature. Failure to reach a conclusion in the presence of a history of trauma or previous unsuccessful surgery should prompt consideration of higher-level investigations of the lacrimal drainage system.

TABLE 20.8
Localization of Obstruction by Regurgitation of Irrigating Solution

Site/Type of Regurgitation	Site of Obstruction
Ipsilateral	Ipsilateral canaliculus
Contralateral	Common canaliculus or lacrimal sac
Mucoid	Lacrimal sac
Mucopurulent	Nasolacrimal duct inflammation (dacryocystitis)
Delayed reflux	Nasolacrimal duct

Management. Infectious disorders causing canaliculitis should be treated at the direction of the microbiologic tests. Although these tests generally suggest the presence of *Actinomyces,* topical and systemic antibacterial therapy appear to be beneficial. Some authors favor chloramphenicol, while others recommend neomycin, polymyxin B, and bacitracin in combination with systemic penicillin or ampicillin.[85,86] Success in eradicating the infection depends on removal of concretions and purulent material from the involved canaliculi.[85,86]

Herpetic canaliculitis may be the result of ocular viral infection or be secondary to its treatment with antiviral agents. Following the recognition of viral blepharoconjunctivitis, especially in the presence of lid vesicles, persistent epiphora should not be ignored. Harley and associates[87] have recommended irrigation of the involved lacrimal drainage apparatus on a biweekly schedule. Failure to maintain patency, due to cicatrization, may require a shunt or external dacryocystorhinostomy.[87]

Relief of allergic canalicular obstruction has been reported with use of cromolyn sodium.[88] This report indexed the resolution of intermittent epiphora and eye rubbing to symptomatic relief and lacrimal patency.

Acquired Dacryocystitis

Etiology

When a patient over 1 year of age is observed to have swelling over the lacrimal sac, it is most often due to acquired dacryocystitis. Culture studies usually find the offending organism to be *Staphylococcus aureus,* with *Haemophilus influenzae* a common pathogen in children.[96]

Diagnosis

The swelling characteristic of dacryocystitis is limited in its upward extent by the medial canthal tendon. Mucoceles and solid tumor masses may extend above the tendon and masquerade as dacryocystitis. Although pain and hyperemia are consistent features of acquired dacryocystitis, a mucocele is nontender.[96] More sophisticated analysis by percutaneous aspiration biopsy is also possible.[96]

Lacrimal passageway inflammation can be assessed by thermography, in which subtle temperature differences can be detected by infrared scanning devices.[97] A rudimentary comparison between the affected and normal sides can be made at the primary care level simply by judging the symmetry of temperature on each side.

Management

Hurwitz and Rodgers[96] have emphasized the importance of recognizing the stage of acquired dacryocystitis. The presence of a pyocele (pus-filled sac) with orbital cellulitis is a life-threatening condition. Since penicillin-resistant *Staphylococcus* is the most common pathogen, cloxacillin is the antibiotic of choice. Application of hot compresses will minimize the cellulitis and localize the infection to the lacrimal sac.[96,97] If the sac enlarges or if cellulitis is absent, hot compresses should be avoided because the risk of spontaneous sac perforation is too great. An initial administration of oral ampicillin (a semisynthetic penicillin) can be attempted while awaiting the results of culture and sensitivity studies.[96] An alternative that provides interim coverage would be use of a cephalosporin.[98] In children, it is appropriate to treat for *Haemophilus,* but since reports of ampicillin-resistant *Haemophilus* are common, third-generation cephalosporins (e.g., cefotaxime, Claforan) may be more effective.[98]

After the inflammation resolves, diagnostic irrigation should be carried out. The symptomatic patient deserves the very highest level of lacrimal investigation,[96] since any decision concerning surgery should be based on this information.

References

1. Jones LT. The lacrimal secretory system and its treatment. Am J Ophthalmol 1966;62:47–60.
2. Holly FJ, Lemp MA. Tear physiology and dry eyes. Surv Ophthalmol 1977;22:69–87.
3. Jones LT. An anatomical approach to problems of the eyelids and lacrimal apparatus. Arch Ophthalmol 1961;66:111–124.
4. Botehlo SY. Tears and the lacrimal gland. Sci Am 1964; 211:78–85.
5. McEwen WK, Goodner EK. Secretion of the tears and blinking. In: Davson H, ed. The eye, ed. 2, vol. 3. New York: Academic Press, 1969:357–359.
6. Gillette TE, Allansmith MR, Greiner JV, et al. Histologic and immunohistologic comparison of main and accessory lacrimal tissue. Am J Ophthalmol 1980;89:724–730.
7. Holly FW, Lamberts DW, Buessler JA. The human lacrimal apparatus: Anatomy, physiology, pathology and surgical aspects. Plast Reconstr Surg 1984;74:438–445.
8. Hill JC, Bethell W, Smirmaul HJ. Lacrimal drainage—a dynamic evaluation. I. Mechanics of tear transport. Can J Ophthalmol 1974;9:411–424.
9. Ahl N, Hill JC. Horner's muscle and the lacrimal system. Arch Ophthalmol 1982;100:488–493.
10. Doane MG. Blinking and the mechanics of the lacrimal drainage system. Ophthalmology 1981;88:844–851.

11. Milder B. Physiology of lacrimal excretion. In: Milder B, Weil BA, eds. The lacrimal system. Norwalk, CT: Appleton-Century-Crofts, 1983;56.

12. Canavan YM, Archer DB. Long-term review of injuries to the lacrimal drainage apparatus. Trans Ophthalmol Soc UK 1979;99:201–204.

13. Jones LT, Marquis MM, Vincent NT. Lacrimal function. Am J Ophthalmol 1972;73:658–659.

14. McMonnies CW, Ho A. Patient history in screening for dry eye conditions. J Am Optom Assoc 1987;58:296–301.

15. Norn MS. Vital staining of the cornea and conjunctiva. Acta Ophthalmol 1972; Suppl 13:9–65.

16. Lemp MA, Hamill JR. Factors affecting tear film breakup in normal eyes. Arch Ophthalmol 1973;89:103–105.

17. Vanley GT, Leopold IH, Gregg TH. Interpretation of tear film breakup. Arch Ophthalmol 1977;95:445–448.

18. Wiggins HE, Karian BK. Evaluation of the lacrimal system: The Schirmer tests and fluorescein dye tests. J Oral Surg 1974;32:622–625.

19. Feldman F, Wood MM. Evaluation of the Schirmer tear test. Can J Ophthalmol 1979;14:257–259.

20. Patton TF. Reliability of the Schirmer tear test (letter). Can J Ophthalmol 1979;15:101.

21. Hornblass A, Ingis TM. Lacrimal function tests. Arch Ophthalmol 1979;97:1654–1655.

22. Shapiro A, Merrin S. Schirmer test and breakup time of the tear film in normal subjects. Am J Ophthalmol 1979;88:752–757.

23. Schirmer O. Studien zur physiologie and pathologie der tränenabsonderung und tranenabfuhr. Arch Klin Ophthalmol 1903;56:197–291.

24. Milder B. Diagnostic tests of lacrimal function. In: Milder B, Weil BA, eds. The lacrimal system. Norwalk, CT: Appleton-Century-Crofts, 1983;71–78.

25. van Bijsterveld OP. Diagnostic tests in the sicca syndrome. Arch Ophthalmol 1969;82:10–14.

26. de Luise VP, Tabbara KF. Quantitation of tear lysozyme levels in dry-eye disorders. Arch Ophthalmol 1983;101:634–635.

27. Velos P, Cherry PMH, Miller D. An improved method for measuring human tear lysozyme concentration. Arch Ophthalmol 1985;103:31–33.

28. Boersma HGM, van Bijsterveld OP. The lactoferrin test for the diagnosis of keratoconjunctivitis sicca in clinical practice. Ann Ophthalmol 1987;19:152–154.

29. Nelson JD, Havener VR, Cameron JD. Cellulose acetate impressions of the ocular surface. Arch Ophthalmol 1983;101:1869–1872.

30. Nelson JD, Wright JC. Conjunctival goblet cell densities in ocular surface disease. Arch Ophthalmol 1984;102:1049–1051.

31. Natadisastra G, Wittpenn JR, West KP Jr, et al. Impression cytology for detection of vitamin A deficiency. Arch Ophthalmol 1987;105:1224–1228.

32. Milder B. Diseases of the lacrimal gland. In: Milder B, Weil BA, eds. The lacrimal system. Norwalk, CT: Appleton-Century-Crofts, 1983;105–110.

33. Wright JE, Steward WB, Krohel GB. Clinical presentation of lacrimal gland tumors. Br J Ophthalmol 1979;63:600.

34. Henderson JW, Farrow GM. Primary malignant mixed tumors of the lacrimal gland. Report of 10 cases. Ophthalmology 1979;87:466–475.

35. Wright JE. Lacrimal gland tumors. Trans Ophthalmol Soc NZ 1983;35:101–106.

36. Mafee MF, Haik BG. Lacrimal gland and fossa lesions: Role of computed tomography. Radiol Clin North Am 1987;25:767–779.

37. Mondino BJ, Brown SI. Hereditary congenital alacrima. Arch Ophthalmol 1976;94:1478–80.

38. Riley CM, Day CL, Greely DM, et al. Central autonomic dysfunction with defective lacrimation. Report of five cases. Pediatrics 1949,3:468–478.

39. McCulley JP, Moore MB, Matoba AY. Mucus fishing syndrome. Ophthalmology 1985;92:1262–1265.

40. Baum J. Clinical manifestations of dry eye states. Trans Ophthalmol Soc UK 1985;104:415–423.

41. Lemp MA. Artificial tear solutions. Int Ophthalmol Clin 1973;13:221–229.

42. Norn M. The effects of drugs on tear flow. Trans Ophthalmol Soc UK 1985;104:410–414.

43. LaMotte J, Lesher G. Relief of dry eye complaints by a lipid-containing tear substitute. Int Eye Care 1986;2:582–585.

44. Baldone JA, Kaufman HE. Soft contact lenses and clinical diseases. Am J Ophthalmol 1983;95:851–852.

45. Mackie IA. Contact lenses in dry eyes. Trans Ophthalmol Soc UK 1985;104:477–483.

46. Farris RL. Contact lens wear in the management of the dry eye. Int Ophthalmol Clin 1987;27:54–60.

47. Messner K, Leibowitz HM. Acetylcystine treatment of keratitis sicca. Arch Ophthalmol 1971;86:357–359.

48. Dohlman CH. Punctal occlusion in keratoconjunctivitis sicca. Trans Am Acad Ophthalmol Otolaryngol 1978;85:1277–1281.

49. Freeman JM. The punctum plug: Evaluation of a new treatment for dry eyes. Trans Am Acad Ophthalmol Otolaryngol 1975;79:874–879.

50. Lemp MA. Recent developments in dry eye management. Ophthalmology 1987;94:1299–1304.

51. Wright P. Other forms of treatment of dry eyes. Trans Ophthalmol Soc UK 1985;104:497–498.

52. Tseng SCG, Maumenee AE, Stark WJ, et al. Topical retinoid treatment for various dry-eye disorders. Ophthalmology 1985;92:717–727.

53. Jones DB. Prospects in the management of tear-deficiency states. Trans Am Acad Ophthalmol Otolaryngol 1977;83:693–700.

54. Holly FJ. Tear film physiology. Int Ophthalmol Clin 1987;27:2–6.

55. Pouliquen Y, Patey A, Foster CS, et al. Drug-induced cicatricial pemphigoid affecting the conjunctiva: light and electron microscopic features. Ophthalmology 1986;93:775–783.

56. Mondino BJ. Cicatricial pemphigoid and erythema multiforme. In: Foulks GN, ed. Noninfectious inflammation of the anterior segment, vol. 23. Boston: Little, Brown, 1983;63–78.

57. Thoft RA. Relationship of the dry eye to primary ocular surface disease. Trans Ophthalmol Soc UK 1985;104:452–457.

58. Beyer CK. The management of special problems associated with Stevens-Johnson syndrome and ocular pemphigoid. Trans Am Acad Ophthalmol Otolaryngol 1977;83:701–704.

59. Gardner KM, Rajacich GM, Mondino BJ. Ophthalmological manifestations of adult rheumatoid arthritis and cicatricial

pemphigoid. In: Callen JP, Eiferman RA, eds. Oculocutaneous diseases, vol. 25. Boston: Little, Brown, 1985;1–34.

60. Fiore PM, Jacobs IH, Goldberg DB. Drug-induced pemphigoid: A spectrum of diseases. Arch Ophthalmol 1987;105: 1660–1663.

61. Mondino BJ, Brown SI, Lempert S, et al. The acute manifestations of ocular cicatricial pemphigoid: Diagnosis and treatment. Ophthalmology 1979;86:543–552.

62. Sullivan WR, McCulley JP, Dohlman CH. Return of goblet cells after vitamin A therapy in xerosis of the conjunctiva. Am J Ophthalmol 1973;75:720–725.

63. McCulley JP, Sciallis GF. Meibomian keratoconjunctivitis. Am J Ophthalmol 1977;84:788–793.

64. Bowman RW, Dougherty JM, McCulley JP. Chronic blepharitis and dry eyes. Int Ophthalmol Clin 1987;27:27–35.

65. Jones LT. Treatment of lacrimal duct obstructions in the infant. J Pediatr Ophthalmol 1966;3:42–45.

66. Sevel D. Development and congenital abnormalities of the nasolacrimal apparatus. J Pediatr Ophthalmol Strabismus 1981;18:13–19.

67. Busse H, Müller KM, Kroll P. Radiological and histological findings of the lacrimal passages in newborns. Arch Ophthalmol 1980;98:528–532.

68. Baker JD. Treatment of congenital nasolacrimal system obstruction. J Pediatr Ophthalmol Strabismus 1985;22:34–35.

69. Nelson LB, Calhoun JH, Menduke H. Medical management of congenital nasolacrimal duct obstruction. Ophthalmology 1985;92:1187–1190.

70. Suckling RD. The natural history of congenital epiphora. NZ Med J 1981;93:74–75.

71. El-Mansoury J, Calhoun JH, Nelson LB, et al. Results of late probing for congenital nasolacrimal duct obstruction. Ophthalmology 1986;93:1052–1054.

72. Crigler LW. The treatment of congenital dacryocystitis. JAMA 1923;81:23–24.

73. Robb RM. Probing and irrigation for congenital nasolacrimal duct obstruction. Arch Ophthalmol 1986;104:378–379.

74. Cibis GW, Jazbi BU. Nasolacrimal duct probing in infants. Trans Am Acad Ophthalmol Otolaryngol 1979;86:1488–1491.

75. Sterk CC. Probing in congenital dacryocystitis or atresia. Doc Ophthalmol 1981;50:321–325.

76. Mittleman D. Probing for congenital nasolacrimal duct obstruction (letter). Arch Ophthalmol 1986;104:1125.

77. Wesley RE. Inferior turbinate fracture in the treatment of congenital nasolacrimal duct obstruction and congenital nasolacrimal duct anomaly. Ophthalmic Surg 1985;16:368–371.

78. Katowitz JA, Welsh MG. Timing of initial probing and irrigation in congenital nasolacrimal duct obstruction. Ophthalmology 1987;94:698–705.

79. Weil BA. Diseases of the upper excretory system. In: Milder B, ed. The lacrimal system. Norwalk, CT: Appleton-Century-Crofts, 1983;125–132.

80. Jones LT, Linn ML. The diagnosis and causes of epiphora. Am J Ophthalmol 1969;67:751–754.

81. Campbell HS, Smith JL, Richman DW, et al. A simple test for lacrimal obstruction. Am J Ophthalmol 1962;53:611–613.

82. Zappia RJ, Milder B. Lacrimal drainage function. I: The Jones fluorescein test. Am J Ophthalmol 1972;74:154–159.

83. Hecht SD. Evaluation of the lacrimal drainage system. Am Acad Ophthalmol Otolaryngol 1978;85:1250–1258.

84. Jones BR. Syndromes of lacrimal obstruction and their management. Trans Ophthalmol Soc UK 1973;93:581–588.

85. Demant E, Hurwitz JJ. Canaliculitis: Review of 12 cases. Can J Ophthalmol 1980;15:73–75.

86. Smith RL, Henderson PN. Actinomycotic canaliculitis. Aust J Ophthalmol 1980;8:75–79.

87. Harley RD, Stefanyszyn MA, Apt L, et al. Herpetic canalicular obstruction. Ophthalmic Surg 1987;18:367–370.

88. Wojno TH. Allergic lacrimal obstruction. Am J Ophthalmol 1988;106:48–52.

89. Burns JB, Penland WR, Cahill KV. The wrinkle sign in tear duct obstruction. Ophthalmic Surg 1984;15:930–931.

90. Cohen SW, Prescott R, Sherman M, et al. Dacryoscopy. Ophthalmic Surg 1979;10:57–63.

91. Rosenstock T, Hurwitz JJ. Functional obstruction of the lacrimal drainage passages. Can J Ophthalmol 1982;17:249–255.

92. Galloway JE, Kavic TA, Raflo GT. Digital subtraction macrodacryocystography. Ophthalmology 1984;91:956–962.

93. Amanat LA, Hilditch TE, Kwok CS. Lacrimal scintigraphy. II. Its role in the diagnosis of epiphora. Br J Ophthalmol 1983;67:720–728.

94. Millman A, Liebeskind A, Putterman AM. Dacryocystography: The technique and its role in the practice of ophthalmology. Radiol Clin North Am 1987;25:781–786.

95. Jones LT. The cure of epiphora due to canalicular disorders: Trauma and surgical failures on the lacrimal passages. Trans Am Acad Ophthalmol Otolaryngol 1962;66:506–524.

96. Hurwitz JJ, Rodgers KJA. Management of acquired dacryocystitis. Can J Ophthalmol 1983;18:213–216.

97. Rosenstock T, Chart P, Hurwitz JJ. Inflammation of the lacrimal drainage system—assessment by thermography. Ophthalmic Surg 1983;14:229–237.

98. Linberg JV. Disorders of the lower excretory system. In: Milder B, Weil BA, eds. The lacrimal system. Norwalk, CT: Appleton-Century-Crofts, 1983;133–143.

99. Linberg JV, Moore CA. Symptoms of canalicular obstruction. Ophthalmology 1988;95:1077–1079.

100. Soong HK, Martin NF, Wagoner MD, et al. Topical retinoid therapy for squamous metaplasia of various ocular surface disorders. A multicenter, placebo-controlled, double-masked study. Ophthalmology 1988;95:1442–1446.

CHAPTER 21

Diseases of the Conjunctiva

William Wallace IV

Infections and inflammations of the conjunctiva are second only to refractive errors as the cause of the majority of patient visits to the eyecare practitioner. Because of its exposed nature, the conjunctiva is the part of the eye most frequently affected by toxic, allergic, and infective agents. Thus, it is imperative for the practitioner to understand the many clinical presentations of conjunctival disease and the pharmacologic agents used to manage these conditions. This chapter considers the more frequently encountered disorders of the conjunctiva in the context of a clinically oriented discussion of therapeutic management.

Histology of the Conjunctiva

The conjunctiva develops from tissue that is embryologically derived from the surface ectoderm.[1] This ectoderm also forms the corneal epithelium, the epithelium of the lens, and the epidermis of the skin.[2] This common embryologic origin predisposes the simultaneous involvement of the conjunctiva in a number of dermatologic disorders and forms an important basis in understanding the participation of the conjunctiva in a variety of systemic diseases.

A thin mucous membrane, the conjunctiva derives its name from the fact that it joins the eyelids to the globe.[3] It is divided anatomically into three portions[4] (Fig. 21.1): (1) palpebral or tarsal conjunctiva, (2) fornix conjunctiva, and (3) bulbar conjunctiva.

Palpebral Conjunctiva

At the posterior lid margin, which is actually a transition zone between the skin of the lid and the con-

junctiva proper, the keratinized lid epidermis gradually transforms into the moist mucous membrane known as the palpebral conjunctiva.[5]

The palpebral conjunctiva is nonkeratinized stratified squamous epithelium that decreases in thickness as it proceeds from the lid margin.[6] Beneath this epithelium is an underlying stroma, or substantia propria, composed of connective tissue and vessels with scattered collections of lymphocytes, lymphoid follicles, and plasma cells.[6] It is these cellular elements that may undergo extensive proliferation in many pathologic processes, such as vernal conjunctivitis.

The palpebral conjunctiva adheres tightly to the superior tarsus over its whole extent, but it is much less adherent to the inferior tarsus.[5] This anatomic difference between the superior and the inferior palpebral conjunctiva is the basis for the different clinical appearance of papillary conjunctivitis affecting the superior palpebral conjunctiva versus the inferior palpebral conjunctiva.[5]

Fornix Conjunctiva

The conjunctival fornix is a continuous cul-de-sac that is broken medially only by the plica semilunaris and caruncle.[5] The tissue of the fornix loosely adheres to the underlying fibrous tissue, which allows free motion during eye movements. Lymphoid follicles and inflammatory cells are prominent here, and the accessory lacrimal glands of Krause are located in the upper fornix.[6]

Bulbar Conjunctiva

From the fornix the conjunctiva continues onto the globe, forming the bulbar conjunctiva. It lies in loose

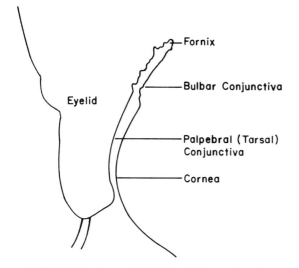

FIGURE 21.1   **Anatomic division of the conjunctiva.**

connection with the underlying Tenon's capsule and contains numerous unmyelinated nerve fibers and free nerve endings. A highly developed network of perilimbal vessels is present within the substantia propria.[6] Goblet cells are numerous and resemble the goblet cells of the large intestine but differ in that they degenerate after discharging their contents.[7] These goblet cells are actually unicellular mucous glands that moisten and protect the conjunctiva and cornea.[7] Their loss in the cicatricial and xerotic disorders of the conjunctiva can lead to profound deterioration of ocular function. The population of goblet cells may be greatly increased in inflammatory conditions of the conjunctiva.[8]

Langerhans cells are members of a family of dendritic cells found in skin, lymphoid tissue, thymus, spleen, and stratified squamous epithelium such as the conjunctiva. There is growing evidence that conjunctival Langerhans cells, which are in greatest concentration at the limbus, play a primary role in initiating the ocular immune response through antigen recognition.[9]

Conjunctival Inflammation

Two important clinical manifestations of acute and chronic conjunctival inflammation are follicles and papillae. These entities are distinct both clinically and histopathologically (Table 21.1).

Papillae represent a nonspecific response of conjunctival tissue to many acute and chronic inflammatory disorders. Their clinical appearance is due to a diffuse infiltration of various types of inflammatory cells such as lymphocytes, plasma cells, eosinophils, or polymorphonuclear leukocytes into the conjunctival stroma, with the papillary projections of the epithelium and stroma forming a delineating margin (see Fig. 21.8). Centered in the papillae is a small vessel that is the origin of this focal exudation of cells.[10] This papillary reaction gives the conjunctiva a velvet appearance in bacterial and allergic conjunctivitis.

Follicles are a focal hyperplasia of lymphoid tissue and appear clinically as milky, translucent, lobular projections (see Fig. 21. 18). They are derived from preexisting lymphoid tissue in the conjunctival stroma, which is particularly abundant in the fornices. The central avascular portion contains immature lymphocytes and macrophages, with the periphery made up of the more mature cells. Follicles are particularly common reactions to viral infections, which tend to produce a prominent lymphocytic response.[10]

Laboratory Evaluation of Conjunctival Disease

Although many pathologic states of the conjunctiva, such as vernal conjunctivitis, are readily identifiable by clinical appearance alone, the use of relatively simple laboratory procedures, such as conjunctival cultures or cytologic smears, can often yield valuable information that aids the clinician in establishing a definitive diagnosis.

It is often helpful for the relatively inexperienced clinician to use such laboratory studies to reinforce clinical judgment in diagnosis. The more experienced

TABLE 21.1
Clinical and Histopathologic Comparison of Follicles and Papillae

Condition	Clinical Appearance	Histopathology
Follicle	White to yellow, translucent, avascular elevation of conjunctiva	Central core of germinal cells (immature lymphocytes and macrophages) with surrounding mature lymphocytes
Papilla	Vascularized clear conjunctival elevation, often giving velvety appearance to affected surface	Diffuse infiltration of acute (neutrophils) and chronic (lymphocytes, plasma cells) inflammatory cells surrounding a central conjunctival vessel

TABLE 21.2
**Conjunctivitis Requiring Mandatory
Laboratory Investigation**

* Hyperacute conjunctivitis
* Membranous conjunctivitis
* Moderately severe chronic conjunctivitis
* Ophthalmia neonatorum
* Parinaud's oculoglandular syndrome

Adapted from Hyndiuk RA, Seideman S. Clinical and laboratory techniques in external ocular disease and endophthalmitis. In: Fedukowicz HB. External infections of the eye. New York: Appleton-Century-Crofts, 1978; 2:258.

clinician can usually defer use of these laboratory studies in the diagnosis of obvious clinical entities.

It is important, however, to realize that laboratory investigation is mandatory for proper patient management in several disorders, such as hyperacute conjunctivitis (Table 21.2). In addition, there are conditions, such as chronic unilateral conjunctivitis, in which bacterial cultures and cytologic smears are not only helpful but may provide the etiology of a diagnostically elusive disorder (Table 21.3).

Conjunctival Cultures

Routine cultures of the conjunctiva require the use of bacteriologic media capable of supporting the growth of a number of fastidious organisms that may be present in relatively small quantities in the eye specimen.

Solid media are advantageous because of the morphologic and quantitative information they provide. The two solid media most commonly used for conjunctival cultures (and nonocular cultures as well) are blood agar and chocolate agar.

Blood agar is a general-purpose culture medium composed of a trypticase-soy agar combined with 5% or 10% defibrinated sheep blood.[11] It can isolate most common bacterial pathogens of the conjunctiva, except for *Neisseria* and *Haemophilus*.

Chocolate agar is essentially an agar base, such as beef infusion agar, to which 5% or 10% defibrinated

TABLE 21.3
Conjunctivitis Suggesting Laboratory Investigation

* Chronic conjunctivitis
* Allergic conjunctivitis
* Infectious eczematoid conjunctivitis

Adapted from Hyndiuk RA, Seideman S. Clinical and laboratory techniques in external ocular disease and endophthalmitis. In: Fedukowicz HB. External infections of the eye. New York: Appleton-Century-Crofts, 1978; 2:259.

sheep or rabbit blood has been added. The mixture is then heated to 80°C until hemolysis of the blood occurs, resulting in the chocolate color.[12] The presence of free hemin and nicotinamide adenine dinucleotide (NAD) in the chocolate agar allows the cultivation of such fastidious conjunctival pathogens as *Neisseria* and *Haemophilus*.[13] Although all bacteria that can be cultured on blood agar can also be isolated on chocolate agar, the converse is not true. Thus, both media must be used to ensure recovery of potential pathogens.

Mannitol-salt agar is a selective solid medium useful in the isolation and differentiation of pathogenic from nonpathogenic *Staphylococcus*. The agar contains an indicator (phenol red) that changes from red to yellow to signify fermentation of the mannitol. *Staphylococcus aureus* (80% of strains) is capable of fermenting mannitol, while *Staphylococcus epidermidis* is not. The salt concentration allows for a selective inhibition of nonstaphylococcal species.[14]

Thayer-Martin medium is a selective chocolate agar that contains antibiotics (vancomycin, colistimethate, and nystatin) to allow for better recovery of *Neisseria* in patients with suspected gonococcal conjunctivitis.[15]

Sabouraud's agar is one of the most commonly employed media used for the cultivation of fungi from ocular infection.

Although maintenance of viral culture media is generally prohibitive for smaller laboratories, most state health department laboratories are equipped to perform viral studies. Viral transport solution such as Earle's balanced salt solution can be used to hold the conjunctival material until it can be used to inoculate the viral culture media.[16] Fortunately, the two most commonly encountered viral infections of the conjunctiva, herpes simplex and adenovirus, can usually be diagnosed by clinical findings alone or by cytologic smears without the need for such sophisticated laboratory procedures.

Specimens for conjunctival culture should be obtained without the use of topical anesthesia, since the anesthetic and preservatives can greatly reduce the recovery of some pathogenic bacteria.[17] This is especially true if the anesthetic is transferred with the specimen into the culture medium. The conjunctival specimen itself is obtained by everting the lower lid and wiping a sterile cotton-tipped applicator moistened with sterile broth or unpreserved normal saline along the lower cul-de-sac. The applicator should be wiped rather than rolled in the lower cul-de-sac because wiping gives higher bacterial yields. The applicator is then swabbed directly onto the appropriate culture medium. For plating, the streaking method described originally by Thygeson[18] and now widely used in ocular microbiology allows contaminants to be differentiated from actual growth of conjunctival organisms. Both eyes

TABLE 21.4
Antibiotics for Sensitivity Testing in Conjunctivitis

- Bacitracin
- Chloramphenicol
- Colistin (Polymyxin)
- Erythromycin
- Gentamicin
- Neomycin
- Sodium sulfacetamide
- Sulfisoxazole
- Tetracycline
- Tobramycin

should always be cultured, as well as both upper and lower lid margins. Use of the commercially available cotton-tipped applicator–transport media combinations should be avoided, since the transport solution further dilutes the often already low concentration of bacterial pathogens in the conjunctival specimen, making recovery all the more difficult.

Antibiotic sensitivity testing (Table 21.4) should be obtained routinely on culture specimens. Sensitivity is determined at the laboratory by the size of the zone of growth inhibition surrounding an antibiotic disk on the agar plate on which the ocular pathogen has been isolated. The clinician should be familiar with antibiotic sensitivity patterns of the various microbial pathogens to better guide initial therapy (Table 21.5).

Conjunctival Scrapings and Smears

Conjunctival exudate may be swabbed directly onto a clean glass slide and studied by the use of bacterial (Gram) or cytologic (Giemsa or Diff-Quik) stains. In most cases of conjunctival infection, recognizable organisms will not be seen in a smear of the exudate. A conjunctival scraping, however, will often demonstrate the pathogenic bacteria or at least a cytologic response indicating a particular disease process. That such a scraping can often provide an early diagnosis is well known in such entities as gonococcal conjunctivitis, in which the intracellular gram-negative diplococci are essentially pathognomonic.

In general, the Giemsa (or Diff-Quik) stain will provide more information about a conjunctivitis of unknown etiology than will a Gram stain. When collecting material for a cytologic staining, a scraping of the conjunctiva should be obtained from the site of maximum involvement. After topical anesthesia the conjunctiva is scraped with a platinum spatula (Kimura spatula, Storz) that has been flamed and cooled. The conjunctiva should be only mildly blanched by the spatula, since a scraping containing excessive blood will contain peripheral blood elements and will be misleading. The material obtained should be spread evenly on a clean glass slide. Slides prepared for Giemsa staining must be placed immediately in methanol to preserve cellular features, while slides prepared for the Gram stain should be fixed in methanol or flamed lightly.[19]

TABLE 21.5
Antibiotic Sensitivity Patterns of Important Conjunctival Pathogens

Pathogen	*Principal Effective Antibiotics*
	Gram-positive cocci
Staphylococcus aureus	Bacitracin, gentamicin, erythromycin,[a] chloramphenicol,[a] sulfonamides[a]
S. pneumoniae	Bacitracin, chloramphenicol, gentamicin,[a] erythromycin[a]
S. pyogenes	Bacitracin, chloramphenicol, gentamicin[a]
S. viridans	Bacitracin, chloramphenicol, gentamicin
	Gram-negative cocci
Neisseria gonorrhoeae	Bacitracin, gentamicin, penicillin G[a]
N. meningitidis	Bacitracin, gentamicin, penicillin G[a]
	Gram-negative rods
Haemophilus	Polymyxin B, gentamicin, chloramphenicol
Moraxella	Polymyxin B, neomycin, sulfonamides, tetracycline
Proteus mirabilis	Gentamicin, neomycin, chloramphenicol
Pseudomonas aeruginosa	Polymyxin B, gentamicin, tobramycin
Enteric rods (*Enterobacter, Escherichia coli, Serratia*)	Gentamicin, polymyxin B, chloramphenicol[a]

[a]Significant resistance may be encountered.

Recently, direct immunofluorescent monoclonal antibody tests have become available for a variety of ocular pathogens, such as *Chlamydia*.[18] These direct tests offer distinct advantages over the traditional methods of virus and chlamydia isolation and identification using human cell cultures.

Microbiology of the Conjunctiva

Normal Microbial Flora

The healthy conjunctiva may harbor a number of indigenous microbial organisms. Serial cultures from normal conjunctiva generally yield *S. epidermidis* as well as aerobic diphtheroids. In one study[20] involving repetitive cultures from the conjunctival sacs of 92 healthy eyes, almost 61% of specimens contained at least one organism. Obligate anaerobes, predominantly *Propioni-bacterium acnes,* were recovered from over half the eyes cultured. Aerobic and facultatively anaerobic bacteria, which were present in 32.6% of the eyes cultured, were less common than obligate anaerobes. Coagulase-negative *S. epidermidis* was the most common isolate. The origin of such bacteria is probably the skin of the eyelids.[21] On occasion a few colony-forming units (CFUs) of potential pathogens such as *Streptococcus pneumoniae, S. aureus, Haemophilus,* and even gram-negative enteric bacteria may be recovered from the healthy conjunctiva. In such cases these organisms are thought to be transient rather than indigenous flora. Many references are made in the literature about isolation of indigenous fungi from the conjunctiva. Although *Candida albicans* and other yeasts are occasional isolates from normal conjunctiva, serial cultures tend to indicate a transient seeding from an exogenous source rather than an indigenous ocular fungal flora.[18]

Microbial Pathogens

Although many causes of conjunctivitis are not infectious, the list of infectious causes is substantial and includes bacteria, *Chlamydia, Rickettsia,* fungi, and viruses. Among the bacterial causes of conjunctivitis, *S. aureus, Streptococcus pneumoniae,* and *Haemophilus* probably account for over 90% of infections. Less frequently encountered are *Streptococcus* species, *Neisseria gonorrhoeae,* and the gram-negative rods, such as *Pseudomonas aeruginosa* and *Proteus.*[21]

Numerous mechanisms protect the conjunctiva from infection. Establishment of infection requires more than the introduction of an infective agent. The innoculum must be of sufficient quantity and quality such that it is not washed out by the normal flow of tears or inactivated by lysozyme, antibodies, or other tear components. The severity of the infection largely depends on the pathogen's ability to cause disease as well as the infected tissue's immunologic and structural competency. The various diseases and disorders affecting the conjunctiva are classified in Table 21.6.

Papillary Conjunctivitis

Hyperacute Bacterial Conjunctivitis

ETIOLOGY

The most common cause of this infrequently seen papillary conjunctivitis is one of the pathogenic *Neisseria* species, with *N. gonorrhoeae* being by far the most common.[22] Although it can occur at any age, hypera-

TABLE 21.6
Classification of Diseases of the Conjunctiva

Papillary conjunctivitis
 Hyperacute bacterial conjunctivitis
 Acute bacterial conjunctivitis
 Chronic bacterial conjunctivitis
 Ophthalmia neonatorum
 Simple allergic conjunctivitis
 Giant papillary conjunctivitis
 Vernal conjunctivitis
Follicular conjunctivitis
 Viral conjunctivitis
 Chlamydial conjunctivitis
 Toxic conjunctivitis
 Miscellaneous follicular conjunctivitis
Toxic and mechanical conjunctivitis
Conjunctivitis associated with dermatologic disorders
 Acne rosacea
 Psoriasis
 Atopic dermatitis
Conjunctivitis associated with mucous membrane disorders
 Benign mucous membrane pemphigoid (BMMP)
 Erythema multiforme (Stevens-Johnson syndrome)
Conjunctivitis associated with collagen disorders
 Reiter's syndrome
 Relapsing polychondritis
 Polyarteritis nodosa
 Systemic lupus erythematosus (SLE)
Miscellaneous conjunctival disorders
 Phlyctenular conjunctivitis
 Pinguecula
 Pterygium
 Superior limbic keratoconjunctivitis (SLK)
 Subconjunctival hemorrhage
 Conjunctival abrasions and lacerations

cute papillary conjunctivitis is most frequently a disease of the neonate, adolescent, or young adult. Gonococcal conjunctivitis is generally acquired by the adolescent through fomite spread, while the adult tends to suffer from autoinfection from the infected genitalia.

Although gonorrhea is the most common reportable infection in this country, with over 800,000 cases reported in 1985, ocular involvement is rare.[23] National figures for adult gonococcal conjunctivitis are not maintained, but 1 recent series involving 700 cases of acute conjunctivitis disclosed only 4 cases of hyperacute conjunctivitis by *N. gonorrhoeae*.[23] A seasonal peak in incidence was also reported in this series, with a preponderance of cases in spring and summer, despite the temperate climate of the study location.

DIAGNOSIS

The initial signs and symptoms of gonococcal conjunctivitis are similar to those of acute mucopurulent conjunctivitis. The affected individual often complains of a mild to moderate foreign body sensation as well as intermittent blurring of vision secondary to the copious purulent exudate (Fig. 21.2). The conjunctivitis, however, demonstrates rapid progression with tenderness of the globe, throbbing pain, and swelling of the eyelids. Preauricular swelling may be prominent and tender. Because the infection is severe, the patient normally will seek medical attention before it involves both eyes.

More than 50% of patients in 1 series of 21 cases of adult gonococcal conjunctivitis had signs and symptoms of genitourinary gonorrhea, 9 of whom had genital cultures positive for *N. gonorrhoeae*.[23]

The gonococcus is the only ocular pathogen of major importance capable of penetrating intact epithelium. The sequence of events leading to gonococcal infection can be understood from electron microscopy of tissue cultures challenged with gonococci. The gonococci first adhere to the epithelial cells, after which microvillae from the host cell make initial contact with the gonococci. The bacteria are then engulfed by the cell membrane, which forms a phagocytic vacuole within the cell. Intracellular multiplication then occurs, with subsequent bacterial penetration of the subepithelial connective tissue, which gives rise to the marked local inflammatory response typical of the disease.[24] Thus, if not treated promptly and aggressively, gonococcal conjunctivitis will progress to corneal ulceration with subsequent perforation and panophthalmitis.

Neisseria meningitidis can cause a hyperacute conjunctivitis that is clinically indistinguishable from gonococcal conjunctivitis. This condition usually occurs in younger individuals than does gonococcal conjunctivitis, but it is potentially more serious due to the possible development of metastatic meningitis.

In all cases of hyperacute papillary conjunctivitis, laboratory investigation is mandatory due to the potentially vision- and even life-threatening nature of this

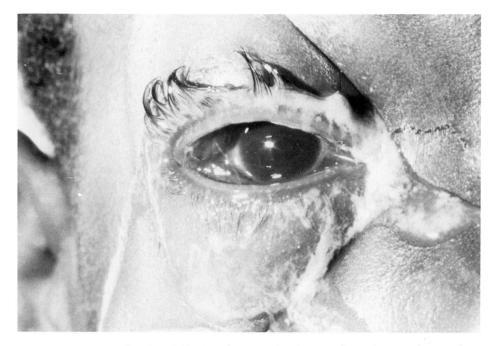

FIGURE 21.2 **Neonatal conjunctivitis secondary to *Neisseria*. Note the copious purulent exudate and pronounced chemosis of the conjunctiva.**

type of conjunctivitis. Conjunctival scrapings are preferred for both Giemsa and Gram stains. Examination of such smears will demonstrate an overwhelming polymorphonuclear leukocyte response with gram-negative intracellular diplococci (Fig. 21.3) observed in many cases. This observation by direct smear is diagnostic for *Neisseria* conjunctivitis. Thayer-Martin and chocolate agar are required media for cases of suspected hyperacute conjunctivitis and should be streaked directly from the infected eye to ensure viability of the infective organism.

MANAGEMENT

Hyperacute conjunctivitis must be treated aggressively and promptly. Inadequate therapy, especially of gonococcal conjunctivitis, may only mask the infection and allow progression to more severe ocular involvement, including panophthalmitis. During the course of antibiotic treatment lavage with sterile saline or other irrigating solution is useful, since the accumulation of purulent discharge leads to maceration of the corneal epithelium. Full doses of systemic antibiotics should be used in addition to topical antibiotics.

Penicillin is still the drug of choice for treatment of nonsensitive patients. Before 1955 few strains of gonococcus required more than 0.05 unit/ml of penicillin for in vitro inhibition.[25] By 1965 over 15% of strains were resistant to this same level of antibiotic.[25] Currently, even though penicillinase-producing strains of *N. gonorrhoeae* currently represent less than 1% of all

gonococcal infections, strains introduced from southeast Asia are so resistant that bactericidal plasma concentrations cannot be achieved. This demonstrates the importance of bacterial cultures and sensitivities in the management of hyperacute bacterial conjunctivitis.

Suggested parenteral therapy consists of 5.0 million units of aqueous procaine penicillin delivered intramuscularly in 2 divided doses daily for 10 days plus 1 g of probenecid daily orally. Probenecid is a derivative of benzoic acid that causes increased plasma concentrations of penicillin by blocking penicillin secretion by the renal tubules.[25]

Ampicillin, a broad-spectrum semisynthetic penicillin, may be given in an oral dose of 3.5 g simultaneously with 1 g of probenecid. This is a highly effective regimen.[25] Alternative treatment in the case of penicillin allergy includes 4 g of spectinomycin given daily in 2 divided doses or tetracycline hydrochloride with a loading dose of 1.5 g followed by 0.5 g 4 times a day for 4 days.[25] The usual contraindications to tetracycline therapy in children should be observed.

The third-generation cephalosporins, such as ceftriaxone, have long half-lives (>8 hours) and exceptionally low minimum inhibitory concentrations (MICs) for both penicillin-susceptible and penicillinase-producing strains, which make them attractive therapy for gonococcal disease. Current treatment recommendations for penicillinase-producing *N. gonorrhoeae* conjunctivitis include 1.0 g of cefoxitin or 500 mg of cefotaxime intravenously 4 times daily or 1.0 g of ceftriaxone intramuscularly daily for 5 days.[26] Although some reports have supported the

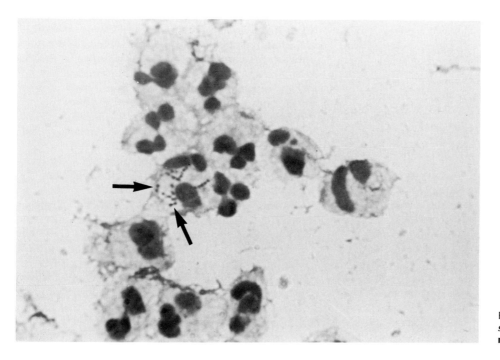

FIGURE 21.3 **Intracellular *Neisseria gonorrhoeae* (arrows) from neonatal conjunctivitis.**

use of single-dose cephalosporin therapy,[27] particularly in mild or early cases, any attempt at single-dose treatment should be undertaken only with careful observation and microbiologic monitoring.[135]

Preliminary topical therapy based on the clinical appearance of hyperacute papillary conjunctivitis may consist of an antibiotic such as gentamicin (Garamycin) solution (0.3%) instilled hourly, alternated with bacitracin ointment (500 units/g) every 2 hours.[28] The aminoglycoside gentamicin, together with the cell membrane destabilization of bacitracin, provide synergistic bactericidal effect against a variety of gram-positive cocci and *Neisseria* species. Once gonococci have been identified by culture or from conjunctival scrapings, it is useful to substitute a "fortified" topical bacitracin solution that contains 10,000 units/ml.[28] This can be prepared by using commercially packaged vials of bacitracin for injection and adding them to a volume of tear substitute (see Chapter 22).

Appropriate therapy of hyperacute bacterial conjunctivitis usually eliminates the purulent discharge within 48 hours. Conjunctival hyperemia and chemosis, as well as lid edema, may take 1 to 2 weeks to resolve. If the inflammatory reaction was severe enough, subconjunctival fibrosis may occur with scarring and secondary entropion leading to corneal injury. This is particularly common in inadequately treated cases in which inflammatory membranes have been allowed to develop on the tarsal conjunctiva.[29]

Acute Bacterial Conjunctivitis

ETIOLOGY

Acute bacterial conjunctivitis is caused by a number of microbial agents. The primary causative organisms include *S. aureus*, *S. pneumoniae*, and *Haemophilus*. More rarely isolated bacteria include *Moraxella*, *Serratia marcescens*, and even *P. aeruginosa*.

DIAGNOSIS

Acute bacterial conjunctivitis is less severe than gonococcal conjunctivitis and is accompanied by a relatively mild mucopurulent discharge, the accumulation of which often causes the lids to stick together in the morning on awakening. Initial complaints of tearing and irritation of one eye, followed by redness, usually signal onset of the infection. The fellow eye is often involved 2 to 3 days after the first. Initially a diffuse superficial punctate keratitis may be present, but this usually disappears within a few days.

In contrast to hyperacute bacterial conjunctivitis, acute bacterial conjunctivitis tends to be a self-limiting infection. Important exceptions to this include conversion of acute staphylococcal conjunctivitis to a chronic blepharoconjunctivitis and acute *Haemophilus* conjunctivitis progressing to orbital cellulitis in infants.

Staphylococci are gram-positive extracellular organisms that are constant inhabitants of the skin. They are pyogenic organisms and elaborate numerous toxins and enzymes, which enhance their virulence and pathogenicity. *S. aureus* is the most common cause of bacterial conjunctivitis.[18] Acute conjunctivitis is less common than is chronic staphylococcal conjunctivitis and has a fairly typical appearance. The conjunctivitis involves the lower palpebral conjunctiva predominantly, and a mucopurulent discharge is a relatively constant feature (Color Plate XI). Marginal corneal infiltrates are not uncommon (see Fig. 22.8). If improperly treated, the infection may become chronic and lead to substantial conjunctival and corneal disease.

S. pneumoniae organisms are gram-positive diplococci. They are quite invasive, and the pathogenic varieties elaborate a polysaccharide capsule that delays or prevents phagocytosis by leukocytes. It is a frequent cause of acute bacterial conjunctivitis that may even take on epidemic proportions, especially among schoolchildren. Pneumococcal conjunctivitis tends to be more prevalent in the colder months and northern climates. Children are especially susceptible, and a concomitant upper respiratory tract infection is characteristic. Pneumococcal infection tends to produce a moderately severe conjunctivitis with only a mild mucopurulent discharge (Fig. 21.4). Follicle formation is not infrequent in children, but the disease is generally purely papillary in adults. The conjunctivitis is basically self-limiting and subsides in 7 to 10 days even without antibiotic therapy. A common finding in pneumococcal conjunctivitis is the formation of petechial hemorrhages, especially in the upper fornix, which probably result from damage to conjunctival capillary beds by inflammatory cells attracted to bacterial antibody-antigen complexes.[30] Corneal involvement generally takes the form of marginal infiltrates that clear as the conjunctivitis subsides. Chronic pneumococcal dacryocystitis may serve as a reservoir for recurrent conjunctivitis.

Haemophilus aegyptius, or Koch-Weeks bacillus, is a small gram-negative bacillus that can be quite pleomorphic. *Haemophilus* is often a cause of acute bacterial conjunctivitis in the southeast, especially in young children, and has a peak incidence in the early fall. The conjunctivitis is quite similar to that seen with *S. pneumoniae,* with the occurrence of petechial hemorrhages (Fig. 21.5). However, the involvement tends to be more severe and last longer than pneumococcal conjunctivitis, and the organism may cause marginal

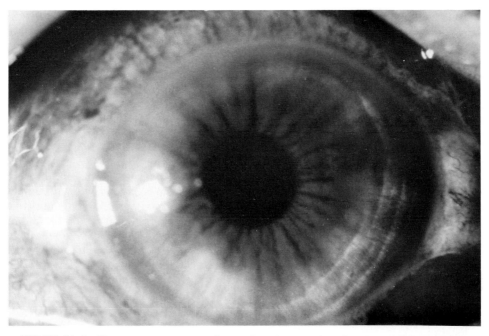

FIGURE 21.4 *Streptococcus pneumoniae* conjunctivitis with subconjunctival hemorrhage.

corneal infiltrates more commonly than staphylococci or *S. pneumoniae*.[31] If improperly treated, the infection may progress to preseptal cellulitis or even metastatic meningitis, especially in children between 6 months and 3 years of age. This is probably due to a lack of immunologic competency, and transplacental antibodies are no longer present in quantities sufficient for protection.

Conjunctival scrapings reveal a predominantly polymorphonuclear response when stained by the Giemsa

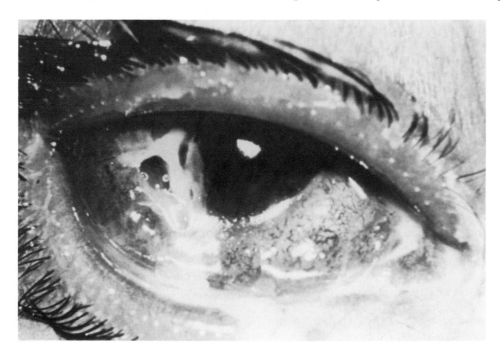

FIGURE 21.5 *Haemophilus* conjunctivitis.

or Diff-Quik method. Gram stain of the material may provide presumptive diagnosis, while bacterial cultures obtained with blood and chocolate agar provide confirmational and antibiotic sensitivity information. Most practitioners, however, do not employ laboratory studies routinely for most cases of acute bacterial conjunctivitis. Familiarity with clinical features of the various etiologic organisms is usually sufficient for empiric management, but laboratory investigation and consideration of a nonbacterial etiologic agent are indicated if the condition does not respond to accepted treatment.

MANAGEMENT

Topical antibiotic therapy is generally sufficient to adequately manage most cases of acute bacterial conjunctivitis.[32] Culture and antibiotic sensitivities will provide information for definitive therapy, but the history and clinical findings are all that are usually required.

The sulfonamides (sodium sulfacetamide and sulfisoxazole) have a range of activity against both gram-positive and gram-negative organisms. They generally exert only a bacteriostatic effect in vivo, and the patient's humoral and cellular immunologic mechanisms are required for final elimination of the infection. This is particularly important in patients with compromised immune systems and in eyes in which immune responses may themselves mediate considerable damage to ocular tissue. S. pneumoniae and Haemophilus tend to be highly susceptible, but acquired resistance to sulfonamides may be significant in infections due to Staphylococcus. The antibacterial action of the sulfonamides is inhibited by purulent exudation, which contains para-aminobenzoic acid (PABA), a finding that further lowers their use in acute bacterial conjunctivitis. Not infrequently, the use of sulfonamides will convert an acute staphylococcal conjunctivitis into a chronic blepharoconjunctivitis rather than eradicate the organism. As with all antibiotics, the sulfonamides can produce potentially serious allergic reactions. Although the administration of systemic sulfonamides has been known to cause erythema multiforme in rare cases, this potentially fatal syndrome has apparently been precipitated by the topical administration of 10% sulfacetamide.[33] For these reasons, use of the topical sulfonamides is not strongly recommended.

Erythromycin may be either bacteriostatic or bactericidal and is most effective against gram-positive cocci such as S. aureus and S. pneumoniae. Neisseria and Haemophilus are inhibited as well. Erythromycin has one of the lowest incidences of toxic or allergic side effects of any antibiotic applied topically to the eye. However, other antibiotics may be more effective when topically administered, and the emergence of appreciable numbers of erythromycin-resistant strains of S. aureus in some geographic areas precludes the drug as a first choice in the treatment of acute bacterial conjunctivitis.

Although chloramphenicol has a relatively broad spectrum of activity among the gram-negative rods and S. pneumoniae, resistance of Staphylococcus, through an inducible acetyltransferase, approaches 50% in some geographic areas. One study, for example, compared the efficacy of chloramphenicol to that of a trimethoprim–polymyxin B ophthalmic solution in the treatment of acute bacterial conjunctivitis. The latter solution was found to be significantly better than chloramphenicol in reducing the signs and symptoms of infection.[34]

Although the drug has been widely used to treat serious ocular infections, it is being replaced by other topical agents that are more effective and have less potential for inducing severe adverse reactions. A number of cases of aplastic anemia have been reported with use of topical chloramphenicol.[35] Although these cases are extremely rare, the availability of other agents negates justifying the use of chloramphenicol in acute bacterial conjunctivitis.

The tetracyclines, although valuable in chlamydial infections, suffer from widespread bacterial resistance that make the group generally unreliable as initial therapy for acute bacterial conjunctivitis.

Bacitracin is bactericidal for many gram-positive organisms, and Haemophilus species are inhibited as well. Because of its severe nephrotoxicity, the drug is rarely used systemically. When topically administered, however, its polar structure makes it quite safe, and it only rarely causes hypersensitivity. This drug is one of the most effective topical antibiotics available for treatment of staphylococcal blepharoconjunctivitis. It can be prepared as a fortified drop using the dry powder (50,000 units/vial) reconstituted with an artificial tear preparation.

Polymyxin B exerts a bactericidal effect against a variety of gram-negative bacteria (except Neisseria and Proteus). Because of significant nephrotoxicity, as well as occasional neurologic blockade, the drug is not used systemically. Polymyxin B is not absorbed from denuded skin or mucous membranes, and hypersensitivity is rare. Bacterial resistance is infrequent, and the drug is especially active against Haemophilus and Pseudomonas species. A combination of polymyxin B and bacitracin (Polysporin) provides excellent coverage of the common causes of acute bacterial conjunctivitis and can be conveniently applied at bedtime as an ointment to supplement topical drop therapy during the day. Polymyxin B has been used in combination with trimethoprim, a potent antimicrobial with a wide range of activity against both gram-positive and gram-negative organisms. In one study this combination was shown to be as safe and effective as a preparation of polymyxin B–neomycin-gramicidin in the treatment of acute bacterial conjunctivitis.[36]

Gentamicin sulfate is a broad-spectrum aminoglycoside that has become a mainstay as the initial drug of choice in a wide range of ocular infections, especially those caused by *Pseudomonas. Pseudomonas* and the gram-negative enteric rods are quite sensitive, as are practically all strains of *S. aureus. Haemophilus* species are moderately sensitive while *Neisseria* species may be relatively resistant. Rare instances have been reported of gentamicin-induced pupillary mydriasis and conjunctival paresthesia.[37] The neuromuscular blocking activity of various antibiotics, such as gentamicin, have been proven by in vivo and in vitro studies. Great caution should be used in administering the aminoglycosides, along with the tetracyclines and polymyxins, to patients with myasthenia gravis, because myasthenia gravis further sensitizes patients to these antibiotics' neuromuscular blocking action, possibly resulting in respiratory failure in susceptible patients.[37] Hypersensitivity reactions occasionally occur but are less frequent than with neomycin.

Tobramycin (Tobrex) is similar to gentamicin in antibacterial spectrum but is less active than gentamicin for most gram-negative bacteria, except *Pseudomonas* species, against which it is 2 to 4 times more active by concentration than is gentamicin.[38] It is available as a topical ophthalmic solution and ointment.

Neomycin is quite similar to gentamicin in antibacterial spectrum, except that *Pseudomonas* and *Streptococcus pyogenes* are not very sensitive. Neomycin is available in over a hundred different brands of dermatologic creams, ointments, and sprays and in combination with bacitracin and polymyxin B, other antibiotics, and a number of corticosteroids for ophthalmic use. Hypersensitivity reactions occur with topical use of neomycin in 6% to 8% of patients.[39]

Recent studies have demonstrated the efficacy of fusidic acid (Fucithalmic) in the management of acute bacterial conjunctivitis.[40] Fusidic acid is a potent antistaphylococcal antibiotic that is moderately active against streptococci, diplococci, gonococci, some *Haemophilus* species, and *Moraxella*. Fusidic acid acts by inhibiting bacterial protein synthesis. It is not inactivated by β lactamases, and it has not demonstrated cross-resistance with any other antibiotic in clinical use. The drug can be used on a convenient twice-a-day dosage schedule and is devoid of known severe toxic effects.[41] Fusidic acid promises to be a valuable new preparation for the treatment of bacterial conjunctivitis.

From the above discussion of available topical ocular antibiotics, one rational empiric choice for initial treatment of acute bacterial conjunctivitis would be gentamicin 0.3% solution instilled initially every 3 to 4 hours and tapered over 7 to 10 days, with bacitracin–polymyxin B ointment (Polysporin) applied in the lower cul-de-sac at bedtime.[136–138] Especially with staphylococcal infections, it is important to eradicate the organism from the lid margins to ensure against recurrent or chronic infections. Polysporin ointment applied twice a day with a cotton-tipped applicator as a lid scrub is valuable for this purpose. An advantage of this approach is the probable synergism against gram-positive organisms by the combination of bacitracin and gentamicin, with definitely increased activity against gram-negative bacteria by gentamicin and polymyxin B.

Topical steroids are contraindicated in routine cases of acute bacterial conjunctivitis because their inherent risks outweigh almost any possible benefit. The widespread use of such agents has led to an increased incidence of fungal infections, exacerbation of herpetic keratitis, and other complications. Their use is strongly discouraged except in bacterial conjunctivitides with marked chemosis and severe conjunctival hyperemia or those associated with extreme discomfort. In such cases a 3- to 5-day course of a topical antibiotic-steroid combination permits a more rapid recovery from the severe inflammatory changes.

Chronic Bacterial Conjunctivitis

ETIOLOGY

Chronic papillary conjunctivitis can be caused by a number of agents, both bacterial and toxic. *S. aureus* is not only the most frequently encountered cause of acute papillary conjunctivitis, but it is also a common cause of chronic papillary conjunctivitis. The pathogenic staphylococci tend to establish themselves on the patient's lid margins, either following an inadequately treated acute conjunctivitis or, as in many cases, simply because of their ubiquitous presence on the skin. Their presence leads to a variable presentation of ocular signs and symptoms depending on a complex balance of host immune responses and changing local conditions. The pathogenic staphylococci elaborate a variety of exotoxins, including coagulase and hemolysins that are directly toxic to the ocular tissues. This is responsible for many of the manifestations of chronic staphylococcal conjunctivitis, such as inferior superficial punctate keratitis and marginal corneal infiltrates.

Rarely, gram-negative enteric bacteria such as *Escherichia coli, Klebsiella pneumoniae,* and *S. marcescens* can produce a chronic bacterial conjunctivitis. A number of patients, all of whom wore soft contact lenses, have been encountered with chronic papillary conjunctivitis secondary to *Proteus mirabilis* cultured from their contact lenses and storage cases.[a] The infection may be quite recalcitrant to therapy and has required permanent discontinuation of contact lens wear due to recurrent infection.

In older individuals, especially those debilitated by alcoholism or chronic disease, *Moraxella* species (*lacunata* and its subspecies *liquefaciens*) can cause a chronic mixed papillary-follicular conjunctivitis. The nose appears to be the usual habitat of the organism. The conjunctivitis may be endemic in institutional settings, and mild epidemics may occur in the southwest during hot, dusty seasons. *Moraxella* often occurs in a mixed infection with *Staphylococcus*.

DIAGNOSIS

The clinical findings of patients with chronic bacterial conjunctivitis are often quite nonsuggestive and can be easily overlooked in a cursory examination. Thickening of the conjunctiva with obscuration of normal meibomian architecture in the lid, along with hyperemia and a fine micropapillary response, are common. Minimal discharge is usually present, but the patient may complain of mild mattering of the lids on awakening. There is often associated blepharitis that may serve as a reservoir for continued infection. Madarosis and recurrent hordeola are common with mild to moderate foreign body sensation, more prominent in the morning. Concretions and retention cysts in the palpebral conjunctiva are seen in a large percentage of affected individuals.

Chronic papillary conjunctivitis with associated signs and symptoms—lid margin hyperemia, madarosis, recurrent hordeola, and mattering of the eyelids, which is worse in the mornings—is highly indicative of chronic staphylococcal infection. A crusty, yellow exudate is often observed to encase the base of the lashes. Small ulcerations may be observed at the lid margin, which represent small abscesses of the lash follicles. This is quite different from the greasy scales observed in seborrheic blepharitis, in which dermatitis involving the scalp and eyebrow is a constant finding.

Chronic staphylococcal infection may result in both madarosis and trichiasis with subsequent mechanical damage to the conjunctiva and cornea. Internal hordeola (infected meibomian gland) and external hordeola (infected lash follicle) may be recurrent.

Maceration of lateral canthal skin is not uncommon in chronic staphylococcal infection, with staphylococci being a more common cause than *Moraxella*. Other cutaneous manifestations include infectious (eczematoid) dermatitis consisting of superficial excoriation of

the skin of the eyelids. The findings may be confused with contact dermatitis.

Production of exotoxins is probably responsible for the fine micropapillary reaction observed. A superficial punctate keratitis affecting the inferior cornea is common and is thought to be due to a dermonecrotic toxin. The accumulation of this toxin during sleep is responsible for the increased symptomatology in the morning hours compared with later in the day. This presentation is in contrast to that seen in the tear deficiency state of keratoconjunctivitis sicca, in which the patient's symptoms are more intense later in the day.

Frequently both diseases are present simultaneously, and the signs and symptoms are difficult to differentiate. Not uncommonly, patients with chronic staphylococcal conjunctivitis will demonstrate multiple marginal corneal infiltrates, which are separated from the limbus by clear zones (see Fig. 22.8). They are thought to be secondary to infiltration of inflammatory cells into the corneal epithelium and superficial stroma, probably in response to an antibody-antigen complex involving bacterial cell wall components. Multiple recurrences may result in superficial corneal neovascularization.

Phlyctenular conjunctivitis may be a result of chronic staphylococcal infection. Corneal involvement is not unusual, and the condition is generally bilateral. This disorder is discussed in more detail later in this chapter.

Laboratory investigation is especially beneficial in cases of chronic papillary conjunctivitis. Because of the relatively low level of bacteria often present in chronic versus acute bacterial conjunctivitis, bacterial cultures are usually of greater value than is cytologic examination of conjunctival scrapings. Smears may demonstrate occasional gram-positive cocci, but a nonspecific polymorphonuclear response without demonstration of bacteria is not uncommon. Culture media should include both blood and chocolate agar as well as a suitable broth medium, such as thioglycolate, to ensure recovery of organisms present in small quantities in the innoculum. *S. aureus* is a common isolate, with many strains exhibiting resistance to numerous antibiotics, especially the sulfonamides. In such cases antimicrobial sensitivities using antibiotics available in topical form (see Table 21.4) are exceedingly valuable.

MANAGEMENT

In the majority of patients with chronic bacterial conjunctivitis, *Staphylococcus* species are the predominant organism. Because of their propensity to colonize the lid margin, therapy must be directed at this area as well as at the conjunctiva proper. The patient must be instructed in the performance of daily lid margin hygiene using antibiotic ointment applied with a sterile

---

[a]Personal observation of the author.

cotton-tipped applicator. Bacitracin or a bacitracin–polymyxin B combination ointment (Polysporin) is excellent for this purpose and will significantly reduce the bacterial population if performed at bedtime for 2 to 3 weeks. Once the condition is reduced to a level where the patient is asymptomatic, a regimen of hygienic lid scrubs can be effectively substituted for antibiotic use. In addition to lid hygiene, topical gentamicin is especially effective due to its broad gram-positive and gram-negative spectrum.

Although this empiric approach is often effective, sensitivity patterns of bacterial cultures are still of obvious importance, especially in the case of gram-negative organisms. Fleischer and associates[42] have described cases of chronic *S. epidermidis* blepharoconjunctivitis unresponsive to empiric therapy that were successfully treated only with topical vancomycin, now considered the drug of choice for treating methicillin-resistant *S. epidermidis* infections. Recurrences may require periodic bacterial cultures and reinstitution of antibiotic therapy. Recurrent acute internal hordeola may be managed by warm compresses and topical antibiotics such as gentamicin, but severe involvement may require the use of oral penicillinase-resistant antibiotics such as dicloxacillin (Dynapen).

Only in cases of infectious (eczematoid) dermatitis occurring in chronic staphylococcal eye disease is the use of an antibiotic-corticosteroid preparation indicated. The sodium sulfacetamide–prednisolone acetate combinations (Blephamide) are quite effective and are available in ointment and suspension form. Used 4 to 5 times daily for 1 week, they will usually eliminate the patient's symptoms and significantly resolve the hypersensitivity component of the disease, especially marginal corneal infiltrates. Once the eczematoid component of the disease resolves, steroid use should be suspended but antibiotic therapy should be continued as needed.

A tendency toward the production of recurrent and recalcitrant bacterial lid disease, as well as the elaboration of multiple exotoxins and immunologically active substances, makes *Staphylococcus* an often difficult organism to treat in cases of chronic bacterial conjunctivitis. Some patients are never really free of the disorder and progress through periods of exacerbation and remission but with ever increasing permanent structural changes (conjunctival hypertrophy and corneal neovascularization). It is therefore important to recognize that selective immunoglobulin deficiencies, especially in the IgG subclasses, can be associated with an increased susceptibility to chronic bacterial infection.[43] Since gamma globulin replacement may greatly benefit these patients, it is not unreasonable for any patient, particularly a child, with a history of recurrent bacterial blepharoconjunctivitis to undergo a thorough evaluation for immunodeficiencies. Attempted desensitization to bacterial toxins has been attempted using intracutaneous staphylococcal toxoid, but without significant benefit.

Ophthalmia Neonatorum

ETIOLOGY

Infection of the neonatal conjunctiva occurs by essentially 3 routes of inoculation: (1) ascending infection from the cervix and vagina due to premature membrane rupture, (2) inoculation from passage through the infected birth canal, or (3) contact with infected individuals or material during the early postpartum period.

Infants are normally exposed to a number of potential pathogens during passage through the birth canal. In fact, conjunctivitis is the most frequently seen ophthalmic disorder occurring in the newborn, with an incidence rate varying between 1.6% and 12% in some institutions.[44] In one study[45] aerobic and anaerobic cultures were obtained from cervical swabs of mothers and their newborns' conjunctival sacs. An average of 6 bacterial isolates was obtained per eye, with the predominant aerobes isolated being *Staphylococcus*, *Haemophilus vaginalis*, and *Streptococcus viridans*. Anaerobes included *Bacteroides fragilis* and *Peptostreptococcus*.

A variety of factors can lead to the development of neonatal conjunctivitis. These include susceptibility of the infant's conjunctiva to infection, which reflects local immunity and mechanical integrity. Equally important is the mother's infective status and the organisms present in the genitourinary tract as well as the infant's duration of exposure to the pathogenic agent. Prolonged delivery or premature rupture of membranes can allow infectious agents, such as gonococci, to have prolonged exposure to the conjunctiva, increasing the likelihood of penetration of conjunctival epithelium. This will significantly decrease the efficacy of surface prophylaxis using irrigation with silver nitrate. Prolonged delivery or premature membrane rupture can significantly alter the apparent time of onset of the neonatal conjunctivitis and can lead to erroneous conclusions regarding the etiologic agent (Table 21.7). The form and adequacy of prophylaxis, such as with silver nitrate, as well as proper treatment of the mother during pregnancy are important considerations that decrease the risk of ophthalmia neonatorum.

DIAGNOSIS

Unlike conjunctivitis in the adult, the clinical signs of neonatal conjunctivitis do not provide clues to the

TABLE 21.7
Differential Diagnosis of Ophthalmia Neonatorum, by Time of Onset

Causative Agent	Onset after Exposure
Chemical (silver nitrate)	24 hours
Bacterial (*Neisseria* species)	3–4 days
Chlamydial	5+ days
Viral (rare)	5+ days

Adapted from Ostler B. Oculogenital disease. Surv Ophthalmol 1976; 20:334.

responsible agent. However, the time of onset following exposure to the etiologic agent is often helpful in formulating an initial diagnosis (see Table 21.7).

Bacterial.   The principal causes of bacterial neonatal conjunctivitis include *S. aureus*, *S. pneumoniae*, and *S. pyogenes*. Gram-negative organisms are not uncommon and consist of the enteric rods, *Haemophilus*, *P. aeruginosa*, and *N. gonorrhoeae*. As noted previously, numerous species of bacteria can be found in the birth canal and on the cervix during labor, and a significant number of these are transient inhabitants of the neonate's conjunctiva. Inoculation from delivery room personnel is not unusual.

Although classically described as occurring within 3 to 5 days postpartum, bacterial neonatal conjunctivitis can manifest itself at any time. In 1 series [46] of 100 infants with neonatal conjunctivitis, patients with bacterial conjunctivitis presented at an average of 21 days versus 13 days for patients with chlamydial conjunctivitis. Clinical signs are nonspecific and not of particular benefit in the differential diagnosis. Evaluation should include appraisal of the cornea and conjunctiva for evidence of mechanical trauma. Nasolacrimal duct obstruction, which occurs in 2% to 4% of newborns, can result in secondary infection. Systemic involvement is not unusual, especially in cases of *N. gonorrhoeae* and *P. aeruginosa*, and can result in septicemia and death, making rapid diagnosis and aggressive treatment mandatory.

Although clinical signs are variable, the typical gonococcal conjunctivitis in the neonate is similar to that in the adult. A hyperacute conjunctivitis with marked exudation and lid swelling begins 2 to 5 days after birth. Delayed or inadequate treatment may lead to corneal ulceration and perforation because the organism can penetrate intact epithelium.

Diagnosis is based on the recognition of intracellular gram-negative diplococci on the Gram stain of conjunctival scrapings. Cultures using Thayer-Martin or chocolate agar incubated at 37°C under 2% to 10% CO_2 are mandatory. Because of the rising number of penicillinase-producing strains, antibiotic sensitivities are essential. Since *Neisseria meningitidis* causes neonatal conjunctivitis indistinguishable from that caused by *N. gonorrhoeae*, biochemical differentiation is vital due to the danger of metastatic meningitis. The infant should be monitored carefully for central nervous system (CNS) signs, and a spinal tap should be obtained if necessary.

Chlamydial.   Chlamydiae replicate within the cytoplasm of infected cells and form characteristic intracellular inclusions that are visible by light microscopy (Fig. 21.6). They are the leading infective agent responsible for neonatal conjunctivitis in the United States, affecting 2% to 6% of all newborns. [47] One study [47] revealed that almost 13% of women shed *Chlamydia* from the urogenital tract during the third trimester of pregnancy. The high incidence of this agent in neonatal conjunctivitis is undoubtedly due to the newborn's frequent exposure to it during birth as well as to the ineffectiveness of silver nitrate prophylaxis on *Chlamydia*.

The clinical involvement may be quite variable but is often that of a bilateral mucopurulent conjunctivitis (Fig. 21.7). Lid edema and conjunctival chemosis are mild relative to those of gonococcal infection, but a hyperacute conjunctivitis is not unusual. Unilateral cases are not infrequent, and onset may vary from 24 hours to several weeks postpartum. [48] Because lymphoid follicles are absent in the neonate until 4 or 5 months of age, the conjunctival reaction is a nonspecific papillary reaction rather than follicular as seen in adult chlamydial inclusion disease. The conjunctivitis may be severe with inflammatory membrane formation in the palpebral conjunctiva and even corneal pannus formation and corneal infiltration. Systemic involvement is common, with pneumonitis, rhinitis, and otitis media as the major manifestations.

Conjunctival scrapings reveal intracytoplasmic inclusions with polymorphonuclear leukocytes, conjunctival epithelial cells, and lymphocytes. The inclusions are basophilic staining with Giemsa preparations. A direct immunofluorescent monoclonal antibody test for *Chlamydia* is available (Syva Co., Palo Alto, CA), and has been shown to be superior to both the Papanicolaou and Giemsa stains in the diagnosis of chlamydial neonatal conjunctivitis. [49]

Viral.   Cutaneous or disseminated herpes simplex virus (HSV) is an uncommon agent of neonatal conjunctivitis, but ocular damage is potentially severe. The infant acquires the infection in most cases by contact

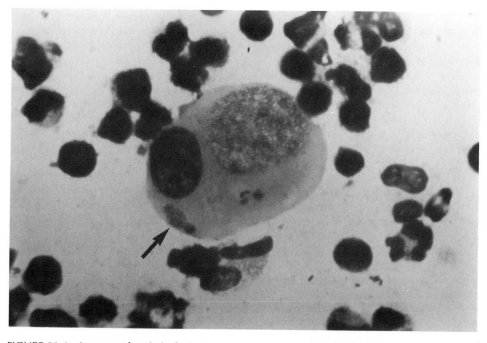

FIGURE 21.6   **Intracytoplasmic inclusions (arrow) associated with neonatal inclusion conjunctivitis.**

with herpetic lesions in the infected mother's birth canal. Severe infection generally occurs in premature infants in particular, possibly due to low titers of protective maternal antibodies. Viremia may result with subsequent meningitis or an acute necrotizing enceph-

alitis. Of the two serotypes (types 1 and 2) of HSV, type 2, or venereal herpes, is the most common cause of HSV ophthalmia neonatorum (70%). Normally within 2 weeks of birth a nonspecific chemosis, hyperemic conjunctiva with mucoid discharge, and lid edema

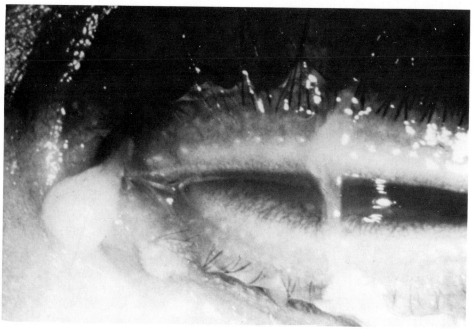

FIGURE 21.7   **Neonatal inclusion conjunctivitis.**

develop. Within days the typical epithelial or stromal keratitis may develop. As stated, viremia may ensue with chorioretinitis, CNS involvement, mucocutaneous vesicles, and even death. Conjunctival scrapings reveal multinucleated cells or eosinophilic intranuclear inclusions in conjunctival epithelial cells. Inflammatory cells are few, especially in premature infants.

An increasing number of women shed HSV-2 during pregnancy, even in the absence of demonstrable genital lesions.[50] Women with a history of recurrent genital herpes have been urged to deliver their children by cesarean section in an attempt to reduce the infant's risk of exposure to HSV-2 during delivery. However, the efficacy of this procedure is questionable, since infants delivered in this manner have gone on to develop HSV-2 neonatal conjunctivitis. Abraded or traumatized mucous membrane is more susceptible to infection than is intact mucous membrane, a point that may be important in surgical or complicated delivery.

Other viruses, such as cytomegalovirus (CMV), can cause ophthalmia neonatorum. CMV infection has been detected in 0.5% to 2.5% of newborns and is the most commonly identified cause of congenital systemic viral infection.[50] Approximately 8% of women have been shown to shed CMV from the cervix during pregnancy. Only 10% of infants born with CMV infection will be clinically symptomatic, but when complete the syndrome includes mental retardation, jaundice, petechieae, hepatomegaly, cerebral calcifications, and chorioretinitis. Conjunctivitis is exceedingly rare.

Chemical. The majority of infants who receive topical 1% silver nitrate at birth develop chemical conjunctivitis. A similar conjunctivitis may occur after instillation of other topical antibiotics for prophylaxis of ophthalmia neonatorum. Chemical conjunctivitis typically begins with conjunctival hyperemia and watery discharge and lasts 1 or 2 days. The common use of single-dose 1% buffered silver nitrate solution in wax ampules has largely eliminated the more severe pseudomembrane and corneal scar formation observed with the more concentrated solutions used in the past. Superinfection with staphylococci is not uncommon and superimposes an acute purulent process on the initial chemical conjunctivitis. Silver nitrate denatures protein in the conjunctival epithelium, which disrupts the protective epithelial barrier and greatly increases the risk of infection. Credé's prophylaxis remains the most common cause of ophthalmia neonatorum.

LABORATORY STUDIES

Prompt and appropriate treatment is the key to successful management of all forms of ophthalmia neonatorum. A complete maternal history with special emphasis on previous venereal infection or exposure is vital. Evidence of cervicitis as well as duration of membrane rupture and length of labor should be thoroughly detailed. Gram and Giemsa stains should be performed on conjunctival scrapings obtained with a Kimura spatula.

Conjunctival culture specimens should be obtained using a sterile, cotton-tipped applicator moistened with liquid culture broth. Blood, chocolate, and Thayer-Martin agar should be inoculated. Antibiotic sensitivities are often useful. Specimens can be obtained for both viral and chlamydial cultures. Virus isolation and the demonstration of viral antigen cells are the methods of choice in confirming the diagnosis of viral ophthalmia neonatorum. Inoculation of human embryonic fibroblasts with HSV-containing specimens will demonstrate typical cytopathic effects (CPE) within 12 to 24 hours. Immunologic methods include immunoperoxidase assays, solid-phase radioimmunoassay, and immunofluorescence. Of these, immunofluorescence is the most widely used.

A rapid serodiagnostic test has been developed for neonatal inclusion conjunctivitis.[51] The technique is based on a modified microimmunofluorescence test for detecting antichlamydial IgG and IgM in blood and IgG and IgA in tears. In patients with acute chlamydial infections, it has similar sensitivity to chlamydial culture with irradiated McCoy cells but is more rapid and less expensive than cultures.

PREVENTION

In 1881 Credé introduced the use of topical 1% silver nitrate solution as prophylaxis against gonococcal ophthalmia neonatorum.[52] This procedure has played a major role in significantly reducing the incidence of blindness due to neonatal gonococcal eye infections. Before the widespread use of silver nitrate prophylaxis, the incidence of ophthalmia neonatorum was around 10%. Within 2 years of its introduction, the Credé method reduced the incidence to around 0.5%. Although silver nitrate is quite toxic to sensitive bacteria, even when diluted to 10^{-5} M, its antibacterial spectrum is relatively narrow. Its mechanism of action is by denaturation of proteins, bacterial as well as human epithelial. Thus, repeated instillation of silver nitrate solution is contraindicated because of conjunctival and corneal toxicity. Disruption of the epithelium reduces an important barrier to ocular infection and predisposes the development of bacterial conjunctivitis, especially that due to *S. aureus*.

The original Credé's procedure consisted of 2 parts[53]: (1) mechanical cleaning of the infant's eyelids as soon as the head was visible and before the eyes opened; and (2) the instillation of 1% silver nitrate into the conjunctival sac. Although the technique was very successful in reducing the incidence of gonococcal ophthalmia, gonococcal neonatal conjunctivitis still occurs. This is probably due to inadequate instillation or the fact that the tissue fluid chlorides precipitate silver from solution, which prevents deep penetration of the agent and thus spares more deeply established gonococcal infection.[53] Careful observation of the newborn's eyes is necessary to identify early signs of infection due to inadequate prophylaxis.

Even with the success of silver nitrate prophylaxis, it has several shortcomings[53]: (1) it does not provide certain protection against gonococcal neonatal conjunctivitis; (2) it has no effect against the more common chlamydial agents; and (3) it causes a chemical conjunctivitis. Nevertheless, the use of silver nitrate remains the major form of prophylaxis for ophthalmia neonatorum in the United States, and a majority of states[32] require or recommend its use.

Although the prevention of gonococcal ophthalmia neonatorum has never been evaluated by a controlled clinical study, various series support the efficacy of a number of antibiotic regimens. Although bacitracin has an excellent bactericidal effect on most all strains of *Neisseria* and can be safely applied to the eye in a 10,000 unit/ml solution, its results have been less satisfactory than those obtained with silver nitrate.[53] Some authors[54] have recommended the use of topical aqueous penicillin (2,500 units/ml) applied once daily for 3 days. This therapy is well tolerated, easily administered, and nontoxic. The disadvantages, however, are those of potential sensitization, thus preventing systemic use; the emergence of penicillin-resistant *N. gonorrhoeae* strains; and the lack of activity against *Chlamydia*. Tetracycline solutions and ointments have been widely used to prevent ophthalmia neonatorum, and Laga and associates[139] have recently reported that effective prophylaxis against both chlamydial and gonococcal conjunctivitis is provided by 1% tetracycline ointment given as a single application immediately after delivery.

The Centers for Disease Control (CDC) recommend 0.5% erythromycin ointment as an alternative to silver nitrate for the prophylaxis of gonococcal ophthalmia neonatorum. Erythromycin has the additional advantages of activity against *Chlamydia* and a low incidence of conjunctival toxicity. For these reasons erythromycin ointment is currently a prophylactic antibiotic of choice for the prevention of both gonococcal and chlamydial ophthalmia neonatorum.

MANAGEMENT

Systemic treatment of gonococcal ophthalmia neonatorum, either alone or in conjunction with topical ther-

apy, is now preferred to topical therapy alone. This is due to the relatively high level of treatment failures (over 19% in 1 study[55]) observed with topical treatment alone, the fact that systemic treatment of the neonate is often simpler and less demanding than topical therapy, and, most important, the high risk of systemic spread.

The CDC recommend that an infant with gonococcal conjunctivitis be hospitalized and isolated for 24 hours. Aqueous benzylpenicillin, 50,000 units/kg body weight daily, should be given intravenously in 2 doses for 7 days. Topical antibiotics alone are considered inadequate. Irrigation of the cul-de-sac to remove purulent exudate is beneficial. Both parents of an infant with gonococcal disease must be treated. Simultaneous systemic or topical use of penicillin and tetracycline must be avoided because the bacteriostatic tetracycline will block penicillin's bactericidal effect.

In 1976, a completely penicillin-resistant variety of *N. gonorrhoeae* was first encountered, the resistance being due to acquisition of a plasmid coding for penicillinase production through conjugation of gonococci with *H. influenzae*.[55] In some areas of the world, penicillinase-producing *N. gonorrhoeae* (PPNG) represent over 60% of gonococcal strains isolated from cases of ophthalmia neonatorum.[55] Excellent treatment results have been obtained with a single intramuscular injection of kanamycin combined with topical gentamicin ointment.[56] More recently, an intramuscular dose of 125 mg of ceftriaxone has been shown to be extremely effective against PPNG ophthalmia neonatorum, without the need for concomitant topical antibiotic therapy.[57]

Bacterial neonatal conjunctivitis of nongonococcal origin is usually managed by topical therapy alone. Initial therapy should include a combination of bacitracin ointment instilled 4 to 6 times daily alternated with gentamicin solution every 3 to 4 hours, then tapered as the condition responds. This is especially valuable when a bacterial agent is suspected but the Gram stain reveals no organism. Erythromycin is effective against many gram-positive organisms as well as *Haemophilus* species and is well tolerated by the eye when instilled as a 0.5% ointment 4 to 6 times daily. Gram-negative organisms, especially *P. aeurginosa*, are best treated by topical gentamicin or tobramycin 5 to 6 times daily for 10 to 14 days. Gentamicin-resistant isolates have been reported.[58] The practitioner should be alert for evidence of systemic infection.

In most developed countries the incidence of chlamydial ophthalmia neonatorum far exceeds that caused by *N. gonorrhoeae*. At one time it was thought possible to cure chlamydial ophthalmia neonatorum with topical applications of tetracycline ointment. It is now known that topical treatment alone is inadequate, since *C.*

trachomatis can be isolated in up to 50% of infants after such therapy.[53] Current recommended therapy is oral erythromycin, 50 mg/kg body weight daily, in 4 divided doses for at least 2 weeks.

Viral ophthalmia neonatorum due to HSV-2 frequently responds well to trifluridine (Viroptic) but is often resistant to idoxuridine (IDU) and vidarabine (Vira-A). Trifluridine has been shown to be more potent, both in vivo and in vitro, than is IDU. It is considerably more soluble and better tolerated as well. It is available as a 1% solution and is instilled every 2 hours for a total of 9 times daily for 3 weeks. Acyclovir (Zovirax) is well tolerated in the eye and is considerably more potent against HSV-1 and -2 than is either IDU or vidarabine. Although systemic vidarabine may be used to treat viremia from HSV, acyclovir is less toxic than vidarabine when administered systemically. Recurrent conjunctivitis in neonatal herpes infection has been reported.[59]

Simple Allergic Conjunctivitis

ETIOLOGY

Immunologic responses to antigens of exogenous agents can be important causes of conjunctival inflammation. These responses are known as hypersensitivity reactions and result from humoral or cell-mediated immunologic interaction, with resulting release of vasoactive amines and lymphokines. Most hypersensitivity reactions are classified clinically into 2 types based on the time between exposure to the antigen and the appearance of the immune response: (1) immediate or type I hypersensitivity is mediated by serum immunoglobulins (antibodies) and produces a predominantly eosinophilic cellular response, and (2) delayed or type IV hypersensitivity is mediated by cells (lymphocytes) sensitized to antigen and produces a predominantly mononuclear cellular response. Although not completely understood, the physiology of allergic conjunctivitis is clearly linked to the cascade of events triggered by mast cell degranulation. Human conjunctiva has a mast cell density averaging 5000 cells/mm³, with the limbus having the highest concentration.[60] Each mast cell contains hundreds of granules filled with preformed chemical mediators such as histamine, as well as precursors of biologically potent prostaglandins, thromboxanes, and leukotrienes. On the cell membrane surface are thousands of IgE receptors, which react with antigen-specific IgE antibodies synthesized from mature plasma cells.[60] The resulting mast cell degranulation is responsible for the itching, tearing, hyperemia, and swelling that are the typical signs and symptoms of allergic conjunctivitis (see Chapter 11).

The immediate, antibody-mediated response develops within minutes after exposure to the offending antigen and is characterized by conjunctival hyperemia and chemosis secondary to vascular dilatation and serous exudation. Histopathologically, there is a pattern of eosinophil infiltration, goblet cell discharge, and epithelial damage similar to that produced by histamine alone.[61] Conjunctival itching is a prominent symptom in most patients, and micropapillary reaction of the palpebral conjunctiva (Fig. 21.8) is often seen in more chronic antigen exposure states. Seasonal allergic (hay fever) conjunctivitis is the prototype type I allergic eye disease. It is the only allergic disorder of the eye for which the specific antibody has been isolated from the serum and tears of affected individuals.[62]

The delayed, cell-mediated response develops within hours or days after introduction of the antigen and is characterized by the same general conjunctival signs of chemosis and hyperemia as in the immediate reaction, but in many cases a mild follicular reaction may be superimposed. Type IV, or cell-mediated, hypersensitivity often plays a major role in many forms of allergic conjunctivitis, especially in those associated with hypersensitivity to topical antibiotics and preservatives.

Allergic conjunctivitis, in its various forms, is especially common in persons aged 20 to 30 years. A history of atopic conditions, such as hay fever or atopic dermatitis, is often present. Determination of an etiologic agent is often quite difficult because multiple antigenic involvement is common. One study[63] of 5000

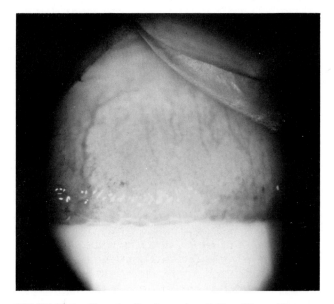

FIGURE 21.8 **Chronic allergic conjunctivitis with papillary reaction of superior palpebral conjunctiva.**

children undergoing treatment for allergy found ocular involvement in 3.5%. In those with eye signs, 94% demonstrated anterior segment signs, with 80% of those having conjunctivitis. Respiratory or dermatologic involvement was present in 66% of patients, while in 32% ocular involvement was the only sign of the allergic disorder. Conjunctival allergy to airborne dust and pollens is common in the spring and summer, while allergic states secondary to topical drug use and cosmetics show no seasonal variation.

Airborne pollens, dust, and other environmental contaminants probably constitute the largest single group of agents responsible for allergic conjunctivitis. The allergens responsible are mainly graminaceae pollen, along with house dust, animal hair, and yeasts. Cosmetics, perfumes, soaps, detergents, aftershave lotions, and hair dressing are also frequent causes. Ophthalmic drugs are not uncommon causes of allergic conjunctivitis. Neomycin, sulfonamide preparations, proparacaine, and cyclopentolate are commonly encountered etiologic agents along with atropine, timolol, and thimerosal.[64,65]

Patients with allergic conjunctivitis will often demonstrate eosinophils in Giemsa (or Diff-Quik) stains of conjunctival scrapings. Increased tear fluid concentrations of histamine and IgE, along with cyclic AMP, is a common finding. Tada and associates[66] reported 175 patients with atopic asthma, allergic rhinitis, and dermatitis, 61% of whom exhibited conjunctival signs. Of those, 52% demonstrated a positive skin test for house dust, 35% for *Candida* species, and 12% for pollen. This illustrates the value of antigen testing in recalcitrant cases of allergic conjunctivitis and emphasizes the relationship of allergic conjunctivitis to general allergy.

DIAGNOSIS

Thorough history and the typical appearance of conjunctival and eyelid chemosis and hyperemia, along with itching and tearing, are necessary for the correct diagnosis and determination of the responsible agent. The symptoms of itching and tearing are frequently more prominent than are the signs of chemosis and hyperemia (Color Plate XII).

MANAGEMENT

The general approach to the management of allergic conjunctivitis includes desensitization, pharmacologic agents, and avoidance of offending allergens. The latter is obviously the ideal situation but may be impossible, as in the case of dust allergy, or impractical, as in the case of hay fever. However, management by avoiding allergens is quite successful in cases of allergic conjunctivitis secondary to ophthalmic drug preparations and facial cosmetics. Desensitization may be of value in cases associated with pollen or other airborne allergens. Tada and associates[66] desensitized 120 children to graminaceae pollen, alone or in combination with dust. The results were encouraging, since 47% were cured and 24% demonstrated considerable improvement. Most of the failures involved children with multiple allergies, including vernal conjunctivitis.

Pharmacologic management of allergic conjunctivitis includes the use of topical vasoconstrictors, antihistamines, corticosteroids, and inhibitors of vasoactive substances (cromolyn sodium).

Topical preparations containing naphazoline, phenylephrine, or oxymetazoline are valuable aids in the treatment of allergic conjunctivitis. The vasoconstriction produced by these drugs reduces conjunctival congestion and edema and can greatly relieve the patient's symptoms. Dosage is typically 4 to 6 times daily. However, long-term or frequent use of phenylephrine or combinations containing phenylephrine may be accompanied by reactive (rebound) hyperemia that may be a greater problem to the patient than the allergic condition being treated.

Mild allergic conjunctivitis can be treated with an over-the-counter (OTC) preparation, Estivin, which contains a dilute rose petal extract and provides a nonspecific soothing action on the conjunctiva.

Release of histamine and other vasoactive substances from tissue is responsible for the hyperemia, tearing, and itching occurring in conjunctivitis due to hay fever and other forms of immediate-response, antibody-mediated allergy. Drugs that inhibit histamine are usually effective in the relief of these symptoms. Although antihistamines are often more effective when used systemically than topically, topical 0.5% antazoline used in conjunction with a vasoconstrictor, such as 0.05% naphazoline (Vasocon-A), has been shown to be quite effective in reducing the signs and symptoms of allergic conjunctivitis.[67] The usual dosage is 1 drop every 3 to 4 hours as required to relieve symptoms, but these preparations are well tolerated and may be instilled as often as every 1 to 2 hours for particularly severe cases. Promethazine hydrochloride (Phenergan) and chlorpheniramine maleate (Chlor-Trimeton) are commonly used oral preparations and should be titrated to the smallest dosage needed to provide symptomatic relief. The most common side effect of systemic antihistamine use is sedation, but gastrointestinal upset and dizziness are often encountered as well. Terfenadine (Seldane) has been shown to be as effective as chlorpheniramine in relieving symptoms of seasonal allergic conjunctivitis, but with significantly less sedation.[68] The recommended dosage regimen is 60 mg twice daily. Since sedatives and narcotics are greatly potentiated by systemically administered antihistamines, proper care must be exercised in their use.

Contact allergies to cosmetics and topical drugs are predominantly cell mediated (type IV) and thus do not respond well to antihistaminic preparations. In such cases, topical steroids, with their more generalized effect in reducing inflammation, are of particular value. A pulse of topical steroid, such as 1 drop of 1% prednisolone acetate (Pred Forte) every 2 hours for 1 to 2 days, can often reduce the allergic reaction enough that topical vasoconstrictors and cool compresses can be used until the condition subsides. Prolonged use of topical steroids is not recommended because they may lead to ocular infection and glaucoma.

In the past few years increased interest has centered around the use of drugs that inhibit the release of histamine and other vasoactive substances in the treatment of allergic conjunctivitis. The drug receiving the most investigation in this regard is cromolyn sodium (disodium cromoglycate). Lindsay-Miller[69] and Vakil and associates[70] have shown a topical solution of 2% cromolyn (Opticrom) to be more effective in the treatment of allergic conjunctivitis than are antihistamine-vasoconstrictor preparations, and it is without significant side effects. When used every 4 to 6 hours it is reasonably well tolerated by the eye and, in many individuals, is as effective as topical steroids in controlling the signs and symptoms of allergic conjunctivitis, but without the danger of chronic steroid use. In more severe cases of seasonal allergic conjunctivitis, a topical solution of 4% cromolyn is superior to the 2% solution in controlling symptoms.[70] Cromolyn sodium has thus proved to be a major advancement in the management of allergic conjunctivitis.

Giant Papillary Conjunctivitis

ETIOLOGY

Giant papillary conjunctivitis (GPC) is a specific conjunctival inflammatory reaction to both soft and rigid contact lens wear and has been reported even in patients using methylmethacrylate ocular prostheses.[71] It is characterized by a papillary hypertrophy primarily affecting the superior tarsal conjunctiva. Eosinophils and basophils, as well as mast cells, characterize the cellular infiltrate.

Analysis of soft contact lenses from individuals with contact lens–associated GPC has failed to reveal differences between lens surface deposits in those patients and deposits on soft contact lenses of asymptomatic individuals. Studies of bacterial attachment to soft contact lenses in patients with GPC and asymptomatic soft contact lens wearers have also failed to show any sig-

nificant differences between the two groups. These findings tend to support the concept that the development of GPC is a reflection of individual immunologic response rather than individual differences in lens deposits or bacterial contamination.[72]

Ballow and associates[73] have identified greatly reduced levels of lactoferrin in the tears of patients with GPC. These reduced levels returned to normal as the GPC subsided after discontinuing contact lens wear. Lactoferrin, an iron-complexing protein found in normal tears, has both bacteriostatic and bactericidal properties that make it an important component of the nonspecific defense system of the external eye. Lactoferrin has also been shown to have a strong inhibitory effect on the complement system by blocking the formation of C3 convertase.[73] Thus, the reduced levels of tear lactoferrin observed in patients with GPC, the cause of which is unknown, could further contribute to the inflammation and tissue damage observed in the disorder.

GPC probably represents a chronic conjunctival inflammatory response to denatured proteins adherent to the anterior lens surface. The more intimate association between the contact lens and the upper palpebral conjunctiva probably explains the location of the giant papillary hypertrophy. Biopsy specimens of the upper palpebral conjunctiva in soft contact lens–associated GPC demonstrate plasma cells, with 20% of these cells exhibiting Russell bodies.[74] The plasma cell is seen in various forms of ocular inflammation and is a major producer of antibodies. As the plasma cell degenerates, the nucleus eventually leaves a hyaline mass called a Russell body. Thus, the presence of Russell bodies in tissue signifies a long-standing, chronic inflammatory process.[74]

DIAGNOSIS

The upper lids of patients wearing contact lenses, especially soft lenses, should be everted for careful inspection of the upper palpebral conjunctiva. Variable amounts of papillary hypertrophy (Fig. 21.9) will generally correspond to symptoms of itching, burning, stinging, loose lenses, fluctuating vision, mucoid discharge, and general contact lens intolerance. These symptoms are frequently relieved when the lenses are removed.

MANAGEMENT

In the early stages of GPC, with only mild symptoms, discontinuation of soft lens wear may resolve the process relatively promptly. More advanced GPC, however, may require use of topical antihistaminic-vasoconstrictor preparations for symptomatic relief. Increased mucin production may be a prominent component of GPC.

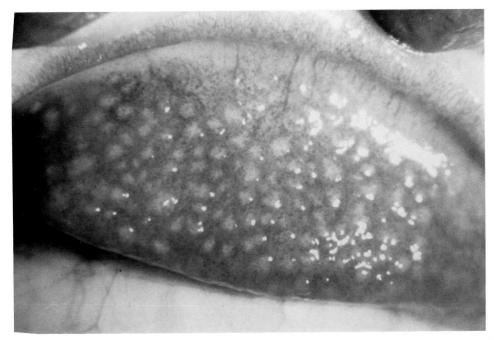

FIGURE 21.9 **Giant papillary conjunctivitis in a 27-year-old soft contact lens wearer.**

Mucolytic agents such as N-acetyl-L-cysteine (Mucomyst) applied topically in 1% to 2% solution in artificial tears 4 to 6 times daily can be quite effective in reducing this problem. Once the patient has been rendered asymptomatic, it may be possible to reinstitute contact lens wear using a more vigorous schedule of enzymatic and surfactant cleaning in an attempt to prevent recurrence of GPC, or at least to keep it at an asymptomatic level. The use of disposable extended-wear soft contact lenses may also be beneficial in keeping signs and symptoms of GPC to a minimum.[140] Cromolyn sodium has been advocated as treatment for severe GPC. Donshik and associates[75] found that by using a 2% cromolyn solution in combination with frequent contact lens replacement, 82% of the patients with GPC were able to continue wearing contact lenses. Although the risk of significant ocular morbidity due to GPC is slight, the chronic use of cromolyn, suprofen,[141] or other mast cell inhibitors in the management of contact lens wearers with GPC may be of questionable clinical practice.

Vernal Conjunctivitis

ETIOLOGY

Vernal conjunctivitis is a bilateral inflammation affecting primarily the upper palpebral conjunctiva and not infrequently the limbal conjunctiva. The disease is seasonal in occurrence, having peak activity during the warm months. It is typified by formation of so-called cobblestone papillae on the upper palpebral conjunctiva (Fig. 21.10), which represent new blood vessel formation with surrounding accumulations of inflammatory cells, especially eosinophils and plasma cells. Papillary hypertrophy can occur at the limbus and is characterized by a gelatinous thickening of the superior limbus, which can actually override the cornea. Within the limbal papillae, whitish chalky dots may occur (Horner-Trantas' dots, Fig. 21.11), which represent calcification of eosinophils. Histologically, patients with vernal conjunctivitis demonstrate basophils, eosinophils, and mast cells in the conjunctival epithelium. Normally few if any mast cells are found in the upper palpebral conjunctiva; however, in patients with vernal conjunctivitis the density of mast cells in this area can exceed $15,000/mm^3$.[76] Tear histamine levels are significantly higher than in healthy eyes. Conjunctival scrapings show many eosinophils as well as eosinophilic granules on Giemsa (or Diff-Quik) staining.[77]

Although vernal conjunctivitis is worldwide in prevalence, it occurs more commonly in warm climates. This disease rarely occurs before age 3 years or after the mid-20s. Males are affected more than twice as often as females.[78] Vernal conjunctivitis usually runs a course lasting 4 to 10 years, although cases can last longer, with periods of remission. Family history of atopic disease is a common finding, as is atopic involvement in affected patients themselves. In a series reported by Allansmith,[78] almost 50% of patients with vernal conjunctivitis had asthma, eczema, allergic rhin-

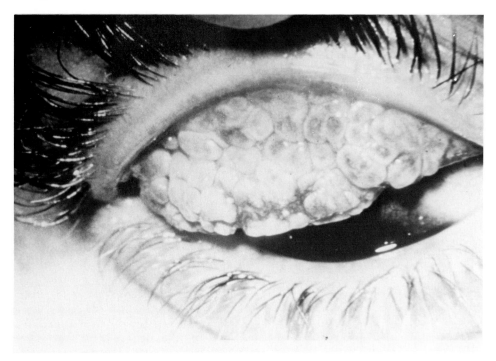

FIGURE 21.10   **Vernal conjunctivitis with cobblestone papillae on upper palpebral conjunctiva.**

itis, hay fever, or a combination of the disorders. Although the name of the disorder is derived from the fact that the patient's symptoms are worse in the spring and summer, many patients are affected year round. Of the 2 forms of vernal conjunctivitis, the palpebral form tends to predominate in whites, while the limbal variety tends to be more common in blacks and American Indians. Both forms of vernal conjunctivitis, however, tend to occur together, with one form usually being the more conspicuous.

DIAGNOSIS

Patients with vernal conjunctivitis demonstrate giant papillae and mast cells in the upper palpebral conjunctiva along with eosinophils and basophils in the conjunctival epithelium and substantia propria. Essentially all affected individuals complain of intense itching during warm months, with some relief during colder weather. A thick, ropy discharge is characteristic. The lids do not stick together, however, unless the patient develops a secondary bacterial infection. With corneal involvement photophobia may be marked. Hypertrophy of the upper tarsus may result in slight ptosis, which is usually bilateral.

MANAGEMENT

Patients with vernal conjunctivitis may derive considerable symptomatic relief from the use of topical an-

tihistamine-vasoconstrictor combinations. Especially in individuals with mild forms of the disease, these preparations, in combination with cold compresses several times daily, may be all that is required for symptomatic control.

In comparison to the topical antihistamine-vasoconstrictor preparations, topical steroids provide superior symptomatic relief from vernal conjunctivitis. Unfortunately, the duration of the disease makes the long-term use of topical steroids, with the risk of glaucoma,

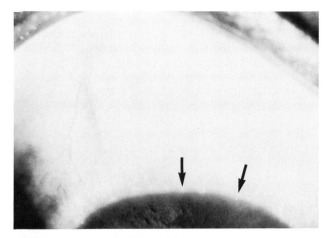

FIGURE 21.11   **Horner-Trantas' dots (arrows) in limbal vernal conjunctivitis.**

cataract, and infection, unacceptable. For individuals with severe vernal conjunctivitis, a pulse of topical steroids may reduce the symptoms to the point where nonsteroidal preparations may become effective in managing the disease. A regimen of topical 1% prednisolone acetate (Pred Forte) every 1 to 2 hours (while awake) for 3 days and then tapered results in substantial relief of symptoms. The patient can then receive topical antihistamine-vasoconstrictors and use cold compresses. The patient must be encouraged to tolerate mild levels of discomfort and not to become dependent on continuous use of corticosteroids. In severe cases pulses of topical steroid several times a year may be beneficial. When the long-term continuous use of topical steroids is required, fluorometholone (FML) should be used, since this preparation has a reduced risk of steroid-induced glaucoma.

Cromolyn sodium in a 4% solution applied 4 times daily is as effective in some cases as topical steroids in controlling the disease.[69] The drug is well tolerated and has demonstrated no significant toxicity in long-term use. Many patients, especially after an initial pulse of topical steroids, require no drug other than cromolyn to remain essentially asymptomatic.

Abelson and associates[76] have described patients with vernal conjunctivitis recalcitrant to cromolyn who have been successfully managed by adding oral aspirin to their therapy. Aspirin prevents the formation of prostaglandin D_2, a secondary mast cell mediator that may play a key role in allergic ocular disease, and thus would be expected to diminish the signs and symptoms of vernal conjunctivitis. The experience of other investigators[79] using adjunctive aspirin therapy for severe vernal conjunctivitis has been disappointing, but a therapeutic trial may still be warranted in severe cases. Recommended dosage is 650 mg 3 times daily, with careful attention to the potential side effects of aspirin, such as gastritis and increased bleeding time.

Dramatic clinical improvement in patients with severe chronic vernal conjunctivitis has been described after topical treatment with a 2% solution of cyclosporine.[79] The therapeutic effect of cyclosporine may result from either a direct stablizing effect on conjunctival mast cells or the drug's inhibitory effect on both the release of interleukins and the clonal expansion of T helper-inducer lymphocytes.[79] Although the drug was well tolerated, most patients in the study demonstrated recurrence of disease after discontinuing the cyclosporine.

Patients with atopic disease often derive benefit from desensitization. Unfortunately, however, the relief of symptoms in atopic patients with concomitant hay fever conjunctivitis is not shared by atopic individuals with vernal conjunctivitis, and desensitization thus represents a last-resort therapy. Although not gener-

ally practical, moving to a cooler climate often reduces symptoms. This is probably the result of not only the lower concentration of pollens in the air, but of the vasoconstrictive effect of the cool air itself. Table 21.8 summarizes the important differential diagnostic and management criteria for the various forms of papillary conjunctivitis.

Follicular Conjunctivitis

Follicular conjunctivitis is a nonspecific response to a variety of exogenous substances and agents. Specific characteristics depend on the type of agent and interaction with the host. Follicular conjunctivitis may present a diagnostic and management dilemma because it is caused by a number of noninfective processes as well as by viral and bacterial organisms. Although often presenting as an acute episode, such as seen in epidemic keratoconjunctivitis, follicular conjunctivitis may run a prolonged course with secondary corneal involvement. In some instances cytologic examination of conjunctival scrapings, along with bacterial cultures, may be necessary to determine the causative agent.

Follicular conjunctivitis is characterized by the prominent formation of conjunctival follicles during some point in the disease. Lymphoid follicles are elevated, avascular lesions primarily involving the palpebral conjunctiva. They are 0.1 to 2 mm and represent lymphoid germinal centers. Usually yellowish-white and translucent, they should not be confused with papillae.

Marked conjunctival follicular hypertrophy occurs with relative frequency in young children. In such cases other signs of ocular inflammation are generally absent unless the patient also has a superimposed bacterial infection. A specific agent has not been identified in chronic folliculosis in young children, and this form of mild lymphoid hyperplasia may represent a condition related to the tonsillar lymphoid hyperplasia also seen in many children. A chronic viral infection of the conjunctiva may be the causative agent in conjunctival folliculosis, but treatment is usually not necessary, since these individuals tend to be asymptomatic and the condition resolves as the child approaches adolescence.

Herpes Simplex Conjunctivitis

ETIOLOGY

Herpetic conjunctivitis occurs as a manifestation of primary infection with HSV. More common in children than in adults, herpetic conjunctivitis presents typically as a follicular conjunctivitis with prior or simultaneous appearance of vesicular lesions on the eyelids and lid

TABLE 21.8
Summary of Differential Diagnosis and Management of Papillary Conjunctivitis

Condition	Symptoms	Signs	Cytology	Management
Hyperacute bacterial conjunctivitis	Globe tenderness, throbbing pain, often foreign body sensation	Acute conjunctival hyperemia with purulent discharge. Often marked lid swelling and even preauricular lymphadenopathy	Significant polymorphonuclear (PMN) leukocyte response	Laboratory studies, gentamicin 0.3% q1h alternated with bacitracin–polymyxin B ointment
Acute bacterial conjunctivitis	Mild tearing and foreign body sensation	Mild mucopurulent discharge with moderate hyperemia	Predominant polymorphonuclear (PMN) leukocyte response	Gentamicin q3h–q4h with bacitracin–polymyxin B ointment at bedtime
Chronic bacterial conjunctivitis	Mild foreign body sensation	Mild hyperemia, often with blepharitis	Nonspecific PMN response	Laboratory studies, bacitracin–polymyxin B ointment at bedtime
Ophthalmia neonatorum	Marked photophobia and irritability	Purulent discharge with prominent lid swelling	Nonspecific PMN, lymphocytes, and intracytoplasmic inclusions (with chlamydia)	Laboratory studies mandatory; fortified bacitracin q2h alternated with gentamicin q4h for bacterial; tetracycline ointment q3h for chlamydial; 1% trifluridine q2h for 9 administrations daily for 3 weeks for viral
Allergic conjunctivitis	Itching, dryness, general irritation	Conjunctival chemosis and hyperemia without watery discharge	Eosinophils	Avoidance of allergen; topical antihistaminic-decongestant q4h; pulse of corticosteroid q2h × 2d; 4% cromolyn q4h
Giant papillary conjunctivitis	Itching, excessive contact lens movement, mild foreign body sensation	Superior tarsal papillary hypertrophy, mucus discharge (mild)	Eosinophils, basophils, mast cells	Discontinue lens wear in mild cases; topical antihistaminic-vasoconstrictor q4h; mucolytic agents such as Mucomyst 1% q4h (in artificial tears)
Vernal conjunctivitis	Extreme itching and photophobia	Cobblestone papillae; many with superior keratitis or pannus, limbal involvement not uncommon; mucus discharge	Diffuse eosinophils	Topical antihistaminic-vasoconstrictor q2h–q4h; cool compresses; steroid pulse if severe (prednisolone acetate 1% q1h–q2h × 3d); 4% cromolyn q4h

margins. These vesicles eventually break down into superficial ulcerations. Even without the typical lid lesions, herpetic blepharoconjunctivitis must be considered in any case of follicular conjunctivitis. Primary HSV infection generally occurs in children between 6 months and 5 years of age.[80] This is related to the fact that maternal neutralizing antibodies specific for HSV, which are acquired by the infant transplacentally, tend

to disappear by the time the child is 6 months of age. From that time until about 2 years of age the child is most susceptible to infection with the virus. However, about 90% of primary HSV infections are asymptomatic and do not result in ocular involvement.

Although most cases of herpetic ocular infection are due to the nonvenereal form of the virus (HSV-1), ocular infection with venereal HSV-2 is often seen in newborns and adults. It is thought to result from contact with the virus in the infected birth canal (neonatal) or by autoinoculation after sexual contact with an infected partner (adults). The ocular manifestations of HSV-1 and -2 infection do not differ clinically.

DIAGNOSIS

HSV conjunctivitis can last for 3 to 4 weeks and may present with pseudomembrane formation and, rarely, conjunctival ulceration. Although the cornea may be spared during the primary episode, herpetic corneal involvement in the form of punctate keratitis or even typical dendritic ulceration is not uncommon. The patient should be monitored closely for this development. Herpetic conjunctivitis tends to occur unilaterally, and the fellow eye, if involved, becomes affected within a week of onset.

The differential diagnosis in HSV conjunctivitis includes a number of agents producing acute follicular conjunctivitis. In particular, the syndromes to be considered are chlamydial inclusion conjunctivitis and follicular conjunctivitis secondary to adenovirus, either epidemic keratoconjunctivitis or pharyngoconjunctival fever. Of particular consideration is accompanying upper respiratory infection (adenovirus), skin lesions (HSV), or type of discharge (mucopurulent in adult inclusion conjunctivitis).

All these disorders are usually unilateral at onset, with a mild, nontender preauricular node on the side of the affected eye. HSV and *Chlamydia* often involve one eye alone, but the fellow eye may develop the disease 7 to 10 days after onset. The discharge is watery (Fig. 21.12) in all cases except adult inclusion conjunctivitis, which tends to be mucopurulent. Cytologic examination of conjunctival scrapings during follicular conjunctivitis reveals many lymphocytes, except for adult inclusion disease, in which equal numbers of polymorphonuclear leukocytes and lymphocytes are usually noted.

MANAGEMENT

Infection with HSV may lead to prolonged disease, necessitating lifelong treatment. Recurrence is a hallmark of herpetic eye disease, with 50% of patients having a second ocular involvement within 2 years of their initial episode.[80] The patient must be aware of the possible complications of the infection as well as the chronic nature of the disease. Any "trigger" mechanism, such as fever or emotional upset, that can be identified in various patients must be avoided.

Several topical preparations are available for the treatment of HSV conjunctivitis and keratitis. IDU (Herplex, Stoxil) dosage is 1 drop of the 0.1% solution in the conjunctival sac every hour during the day and

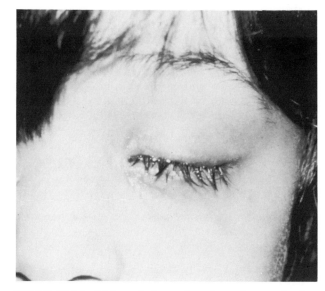

FIGURE 21.12 **Watery discharge in primary herpes simplex blepharoconjunctivitis.**

every 2 hours at night until the condition begins to respond. At that time the dosage is halved (every 2 hours during the day, every 4 hours during the night), and therapy should be continued for 3 to 5 days after healing is complete. The 0.5% ointment should be applied 4 times a day and once before bedtime. Although IDU is a relatively stable compound, older solutions may produce irritation and punctate keratitis. This is thought to be due to breakdown of IDU into iodouracil. Iodouracil may also antagonize the antiviral activity of IDU when present in quite low (0.00001%) concentration and is toxic to conjunctival epithelium. IDU is generally well tolerated in the eye, but cases of IDU allergy, some of which can be moderately severe, are not uncommon. IDU-induced conjunctival cicatrization similar to ocular pemphigoid has been described in several patients receiving chronic topical IDU treatment of from 1 to 3 years' duration.[81] Lack of response to IDU in suspected HSV conjunctivitis should always suggest resistance to the drug.

Vidarabine is less toxic and perhaps more effective, in terms of healing time, than is IDU. It is useful in individuals sensitive to IDU and is available in a 3% ointment. The dosage is 5 times daily, continued until 3 to 5 days after the infection has resolved.

Trifluridine (Viroptic) is well tolerated by the eye and is effective against many IDU-resistant strains of HSV. Dosage is 1 drop of the 1.0% solution every 2 hours for a maximum of 9 drops daily, with the dosage reduced to 1 drop every 4 hours as the conjunctivitis responds. Treatment should be continued for 3 to 5 days after clinical elimination of the infection.

Acyclovir is a relatively nontoxic, highly specific antiherpetic drug that may be administered topically, orally, or intravenously. More potent in vitro than the other antiherpetic agents, acyclovir is well tolerated in the eye and, unlike the other antivirals, does not appear to interfere with corneal wound healing. Treatment consists of topical application of the 3% ointment 5 times daily for 1 week, tapering as the infection subsides.

Corticosteroids are absolutely contraindicated in active herpetic epithelial infections, since they increase the activity of virus replication.[82]

Pharyngoconjunctival Fever

ETIOLOGY

Adenoviruses typically cause diseases confined to the respiratory tract. They are spherical DNA viruses that have been subdivided into seven subgenera (A to G) and over 40 species that are infective for humans. Pharyngoconjunctival fever (PCF) is a common manifestation of adenoviral ocular infection and, as its name implies, is characterized by a syndrome of pharyngitis, follicular conjunctivitis, and fever.

Although adenovirus 3 is the most frequently isolated cause of PCF, the syndrome may be associated with essentially all the 40 adenovirus species.[83,84] Even adenovirus 19, usually a cause of epidemic keratoconjunctivitis (EKC), has been documented to cause PCF.[85]

Although the virus is typically not able to be cultured from the throat and conjunctiva after 14 days, viral excretion may continue for 30 days in the feces, which serves as an important vector for spread of the virus.

Outbreaks of PCF can be epidemic and, in such instances, may be associated with contaminated public swimming pools.

DIAGNOSIS

Following an incubation period of 2 to 10 days, PCF presents with the classic triad of mild pharyngitis, often with submaxillary adenopathy, follicular conjunctivitis, and fever that can reach 104°F. The conjunctivitis can be unilateral and involves essentially the lower fornix conjunctiva. The fellow eye may be involved, usually with less severity, 2 to 5 days after onset. Corneal findings tend to be transient.

Although the epidemic presentation of the PCF triad is essentially pathognomonic for adenoviral infection, sporadic cases, which can occur without systemic symptoms, may be easily confused with herpetic or other causes of follicular conjunctivitis. In these cases virus

isolation is of obvious importance, as is the presence of acute blepharitis or skin eruptions seen in HSV infections.

MANAGEMENT

Although corneal involvement, typically superficial keratitis, may occur in some cases of PCF, it is rarely severe. The disease may last from 1 to 3 weeks and is self-limiting. Thus, management is entirely supportive and consists of topical vasoconstrictors, lubricants, and cool compresses. Cycloplegic agents, such as 5% homatropine twice a day, may be indicated to prevent anterior uveitis when there is severe corneal involvement. There is no evidence that the currently available antiviral drugs alter the natural course of this disease. Topical steroids are also of unproved value and present a significant risk if the etiologic agent is in doubt. Steroid use may even prolong the infection and exacerbate the disease.

Topical antibiotics are indicated only in cases of secondary bacterial infection. Proper diet and rest may be encouraged to increase the patient's resistance. Live adenovirus vaccine may be of value in preventing epidemics, but its use is questionable.

Epidemic Keratoconjunctivitis

ETIOLOGY

In 1955 Jawetz and associates[86] first isolated adenovirus type 8 from a well-documented outbreak of epidemic keratoconjunctivitis (EKC). Previous epidemics among shipyard workers had established EKC, or "shipyard disease," as a distinct entity. Although adenovirus type 8 was the predominant causative agent for EKC before 1973,[87] since then types 19 and 21 have been documented to cause EKC.[88] Currently, type 37 is the predominant virus recovered from persons with EKC in the United States and Europe.[89] Although the relationship between serologic type and clinical disease is not always constant, in epidemics the relationship tends to be relatively stable.

Outbreaks of EKC may occur frequently in outpatient clinics and factory dispensaries.[90] The source of the epidemic is often unrecognized but is frequently associated with applanation tonometry, slit-lamp examination, instillation of eyedrops, and, in some cases, the practitioner. The simple procedures of washing the hands between patients and mechanical wiping and drying of instruments are usually effective in preventing spread of this disease.

Since infected individuals continue to shed virus in both the tears and the nasopharynx for 2 weeks, they should be considered infective during this period and encouraged to have limited contact with other individuals during that time.[87] The prevalence of neutralizing antibodies to adenovirus type 37 in the general population is probably less than 5%, which means that most individuals exposed to the virus are susceptible to infection. Humans appear to be the only hosts for the important adenoviruses, including type 37, but the role and duration of immunity have not been determined.

DIAGNOSIS

EKC presents classically as an acute follicular conjunctivitis in the lower fornix. Conjunctival petechiae and chemosis, as well as edema of the caruncle and semilunar fold, are a constant feature. EKC is usually unilateral at onset and is associated with preauricular lymphadenopathy. Systemic involvement is usually lacking, but a case has been described of acute bilateral retrobulbar optic neuropathy associated with EKC in a patient with drug-suppressed cellular immunity.[91] A low-grade fever may accompany the infection. The patient complains of a foreign body sensation that can be moderately severe. Pseudomembrane formation is not uncommon in severe cases.

Corneal involvement, however, distinguishes EKC from the other forms of adenoviral conjunctivitis. Frequently in the first week of the disease the patient will manifest a diffuse superficial punctate keratitis. At this point the corneal appearance is quite nonspecific, and the patient is relatively asymptomatic. However, after about 7 days, the cornea frequently develops discrete elevated epithelial lesions that stain with fluorescein and are associated with moderate to marked foreign body sensation. From 10 to 14 days after onset, subepithelial opacities begin to form beneath the existing epithelial lesions (see Fig. 22.7) and may produce transient visual loss. The epithelial lesions gradually disappear by the end of 4 weeks, and the subepithelial opacities normally disappear within 3 to 4 months.

The acute follicular conjunctivitis observed with EKC is indistinguishable from the other viral conjunctivitides. Twenty-five patients presenting with the clinical features of moderate to severe follicular conjunctivitis, superficial punctate keratitis with subepithelial opacities, and no systemic involvement were found by cultural or serologic testing to have herpes simplex keratoconjunctivitis.[92] No adenovirus was isolated. Of these 25 patients, only 5 developed typical herpetic lesions of the lids or cornea.[92] The remainder could be easily confused with EKC, which underscores the importance of herpes simplex in the differential diagnosis of follicular conjunctivitis.

Marked lid swelling may be present as well as prominent subconjunctival hemorrhage involving the bulbar conjunctiva (Fig. 21.13). In severe cases membranous conjunctivitis must be differentiated from that caused by beta *Streptococcus* or, rarely, *Corynebacterium diphtheriae* or even erythema multiforme (Stevens-Johnson syndrome).

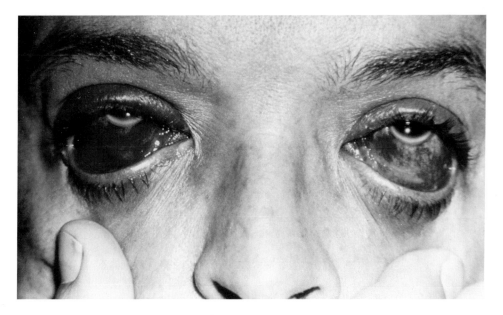

FIGURE 21.13 **Subconjunctival hemorrhages in a 38-year-old man with epidemic keratoconjunctivitis.**

MANAGEMENT

In most cases, EKC is a self-limiting, although aggravating and at times debilitating, ocular disease with excellent prognosis for complete recovery. Although the follicular conjunctivitis generally runs a self-limiting course over 7 to 14 days, with the corneal involvement (subepithelial opacities) subsiding within 3 months, the opacities may persist for over 2 years. The conjunctival membrane formation that may be seen in severe cases of EKC can be followed by conjunctival scar formation that, when extensive, can lead to cicatricial entropion. Secondary bacterial infection is common, especially by *Staphylococcus,* and can lead to severe disease if not recognized. Therefore, affected patients should be monitored closely to minimize potential complications. During the acute phase of EKC, supportive therapy such as cold compresses and topical astringents, decongestants, or lubricants are often effective in relieving symptoms. Prophylactic topical antibiotics are justified due to the frequency of secondary bacterial infection.

Much controversy has surrounded the role of corticosteroids in the management of EKC. In patients with markedly reduced visual acuity from the subepithelial opacities, topical steroid therapy will reduce the opacities and improve vision. However, since the subepithelial opacities probably represent a local immune response to viral protein, suppressing such an immune response with steroids may only interfere with clearing of the viral antigen and ultimately prolong the corneal disease. Indeed, patients have been observed to be steroid dependent many months after their initial EKC infection; discontinuing the topical steroid resulted in recurrence of the subepithelial opacities sufficient to decrease visual acuity.[93] The existence of an EKC-like variant of HSV keratoconjunctivitis should only further discourage the use of topical steroids.

Although IDU is ineffective in the management of EKC, vidarabine is of mild benefit on the severity of the disease, especially the formation of subepithelial infiltrates. In addition, Hiti and associates[94] have shown that trifluridine (Viroptic) may be effective against some adenovirus serotypes known to cause EKC. Virus production in vitro was reduced ten-fold for type 7 and 1000-fold for type 19 in trifluridine-treated cell cultures.[94] Although this drug's clinical use in EKC has not been fully investigated, preliminary results are promising.

Topical interferon has been evaluated as a treatment for EKC,[95] and although the results were disappointing in terms of treatment of the affected eye, the interferon was effective in protecting the second eye from developing significant conjunctivitis.[95]

The importance of proper office procedures for the prevention of EKC transmission cannot be overemphasized.

Acute Hemorrhagic Conjunctivitis

ETIOLOGY

The first reports of acute hemorrhagic conjunctivitis (AHC) came from western Africa in 1969.[96] Since that time major pandemics have occurred throughout Africa and Asia. Before 1981 AHC had not been reported outside of southeast Asia and the Indian subcontinent. In 1981 AHC was introduced into the western hemisphere and caused outbreaks in South America, Central America, and Florida. AHC is associated with two viral pathogens, enterovirus 70 and coxsackievirus A24, which are antigenically unrelated.[96]

DIAGNOSIS

AHC is an acute follicular conjunctivitis whose hallmark is the formation of prominent subconjunctival hemorrhages. Following an incubation period of 18 to 48 hours, AHC is typically bilateral at onset with symptoms persisting for 3 to 5 days. Systemic involvement is usually lacking, but a low-grade fever may occur. Corneal involvement is rare.

The prominent hemorrhagic character and lack of systemic symptoms set AHC apart from PCF, while the lack of corneal involvement in AHC is in distinct contrast with EKC. Hemorrhagic conjunctivitis due to bacterial agents, such as *Haemophilis* species, is papillary rather than follicular, with a mucopurulent rather than watery discharge.

MANAGEMENT

Most patients with AHC recover uneventfully in less than 1 week. Only in cases of secondary bacterial infection is there danger of significant ocular morbidity. The course of AHC, although explosive in onset, resolves rapidly compared with EKC. As in EKC and PCF, treatment is supportive with topical vasoconstrictors, lubricants, and cool compresses. Since the disease is highly contagious, proper patient education is important. Topical antibiotics may be useful in preventing secondary bacterial infection.

General Viral Conjunctivitis

General viral conjunctivitis is defined in this discussion as those conjunctivitides associated with generalized viral syndromes. Although the major clinical significance of these diseases is not ocular, conjunctivitis may nevertheless be a frequent and even relatively important part of the clinical picture of the infection. Examples include varicella zoster virus, measles, mumps, Newcastle disease, and, rarely, rubella.

ETIOLOGY

Herpes zoster (shingles) results from reactivation of the dormant varicella zoster virus, usually acquired during childhood chickenpox. It is characterized by dorsal root ganglia inflammation, often with associated neuralgic pain, and clustered vesicles localized to the distribution (dermatomes) innervated by the affected ganglia. The involvement is nearly always unilateral (Fig. 21.14). Transmission appears to occur from direct contact with infected vesicles. The incidence and severity of herpes zoster increase with age and immunosuppression. Peak incidence is between 50 and 75 years, with only about 7% of cases occurring in children.[97] An increased incidence of herpes zoster

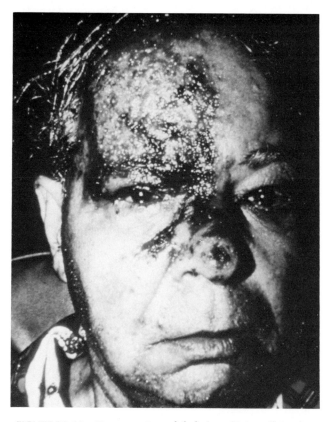

FIGURE 21.14 **Herpes zoster ophthalmicus. Note unilateral nature of the dermatologic involvement.**

ophthalmicus has also been identified among patients at risk for acquired immunodeficiency syndrome (AIDS). Ocular lesions occur in about one-third of patients with zoster, involving the ophthalmic division of the trigeminal nerve. Conjunctivitis is the most common ocular manifestation, although keratitis, anterior uveitis, and cranial nerve palsies are not infrequent. Pustules and follicles appear on the superior palpebral conjunctiva, with similar lesions at the limbus.[98]

Measles is one of the most contagious of the childhood viral diseases. Brief contact can be followed by infection, but intimate exposure results in infection in over 90% of susceptible individuals. The upper respiratory tract is probably the primary entry site, although the conjunctiva may be an important secondary site. Measles is worldwide in distribution, with no racial or sex predilection. Conjunctivitis is a classic feature of the prodromal and early eruptive period of the measles. It is typically of a mild catarrhal character, although occasionally marked chemosis can occur. A mild punctate keratitis may persist for several months.[99]

Mumps is an acute, general infection caused by a member of the RNA paramyxovirus group. It is primarily a disease of childhood, and over 85% of cases occur in children under 14 years of age. Transmission occurs through direct contact with saliva, infected aerosol droplets, or contaminated fomites. Conjunctivitis is not infrequent and is generally mild, often without discharge. Interstitial keratitis, dacryoadenitis, and optic neuritis are more dramatic presentations.[100]

Newcastle disease is due to another member of the paramyxovirus group. A serious and typically fatal disease of poultry, it may occasionally produce a mild conjunctivitis in exposed individuals, such as poultry workers. There is follicular conjunctivitis, often swelling of the preauricular glands, and mild upper respiratory symptoms.[100]

The rubella virus, although classified as a member of the togavirus group, is similar in terms of clinical features and epidemiology to those of the paramyxoviruses. The virus appears to be spread by infected droplet inhalation. It is only moderately contagious, with its greatest communicability within 3 to 4 days preceding and following the appearance of the rash. After an incubation period of 1 to 5 days, a mild prodrome of anorexia, headache, low-grade fever, and conjunctivitis occurs. The conjunctivitis is mild, bilateral, and follicular, with minimal discharge. Subconjunctival hemorrhage is not frequent but does occur.

DIAGNOSIS

Knowledge of the systemic manifestations of the general disease state allows relatively straightforward diagnosis. Secondary bacterial infection is not uncommon and may convert a mild follicular conjunctivitis to a purulent condition.

MANAGEMENT

Most patients with conjunctival involvement secondary to these general viral syndromes recover totally without complication. However, corneal involvement in zoster or mumps can be serious and lead to permanent visual and ocular disability. Bacterial infection is an important and potentially devastating complication.

Management of most types of general viral conjunctivitis is essentially supportive. Cold compresses, vasoconstrictors, and ocular lubricants are helpful during acute stages. Early and accurate diagnosis of herpes zoster ophthalmicus is extremely important, however, since acyclovir will have its greatest effect on the disease when administered within 72 hours of the cutaneous eruption.[97] Data from a recent multicenter study[97] indicate that the acute ocular complications of herpes zoster ophthalmicus can be significantly reduced or even avoided by the use of oral acyclovir. A rising creatinine level, one of the more common complications of systemic acyclovir therapy, is avoided with oral administration.[97]

The role of systemic steroid therapy in herpes zoster remains controversial, especially in immunocompromised patients. Bucci and associates[97] have shown that in immunocompetent elderly patients with herpes zoster ophthalmicus, systemic steroids can decrease the incidence of postherpetic neuralgia without affecting the healing rate or increasing the risk of systemic dissemination. Systemic steroids, however, should generally not be used in young patients, immunosuppressed patients, or patients with serious underlying disease. Topical steroids are quite effective in treating the ocular inflammation associated with herpes zoster, but the condition tends to relapse if the steroid is tapered too quickly. Topical antibiotics are of benefit as prophylaxis against potentially serious bacterial infections. Artificial tear preparations are often useful as well.

Chlamydial Conjunctivitis

ETIOLOGY

The *Chlamydia* are obligate intracellular parasites that depend on the host cell for high-energy compounds to carry out metabolic-biosynthetic processes. Two species are recognized, *Chlamydia trachomatis* and *Chlamydia psittaci*, with numerous serotypes within each species.

In humans, *Chlamydia* species produce a variety of oculogenital diseases, such as inclusion conjunctivitis, trachoma, lymphogranuloma venereum, and nonspecific urethritis. In 1963, the Congress of Microbiology assigned the name TRIC to the causative agent of trachoma and inclusion conjunctivitis.

Chlamydia species are the most commonly encountered group of organisms producing chronic follicular conjunctivitis, with trachoma being a prototype for the other forms of chronic conjunctivitis. Trachoma and its complications still represent serious public health problems in many underdeveloped areas of the world, especially Asia, Africa, and South America. Trachoma is thought to affect almost one-tenth of the world's population, although antibiotic therapy and public health programs have made substantial progress in decreasing its incidence. In the United States, trachoma is still seen mainly among the American Indian population of the Southwest.[101]

Spread of trachoma is essentially from eye to eye or by contact with infected material. Shedding of *C. trachomatis* in tears of patients with moderate to severe hyperendemic trachoma is a major factor in transmission by flies, hands, and towels. These patients are thought to be the main reservoir of infection. In areas where the disease is sporadic, such as the United States, extraocular infection is essentially genital. The newborn may become infected when the agent localizes in the mother's cervix and produces inclusion conjunctivitis.

The chlamydial agent of inclusion conjunctivitis is the most common cause of acute follicular conjunctivitis, which tends to become chronic. Asymptomatic *C. trachomatis* eye infections are thought to represent an important epidemiologic problem.[102] Outbreaks of the disease tend to be sporadic and to occur almost invariably from sexual exposure. The disease is often relatively asymptomatic in terms of urogenital symptoms, although non-specific urethritis and chronic vaginal discharge are not uncommon.

Although the risk of transmission in infected women is poorly defined, infected women constitute an important reservoir of infection. Women infected with *C. trachomatis* have neither signs nor symptoms, and infection can last for many months.

DIAGNOSIS

Although *C. trachomatis* appears to be the agent of both trachoma and inclusion conjunctivitis, the clinical presentations, as well as the epidemiologic characteristics, of the two diseases are quite different.

Trachoma, in its early stages, presents as a chronic follicular conjunctivitis that is essentially limited to the upper palpebral conjunctiva. With the development of papillary hypertrophy and inflammatory infiltration, the follicular character may be obscured. Symptoms of photophobia and lacrimation may be accompanied by a mucoid or purulent exudate. Secondary bacterial infection with *Haemophilus* or *Moraxella* is not uncommon and is probably responsible for the frank purulent exudation in some patients.

As the disease progresses, conjunctival scarring (Fig. 21.15) with resultant cicatricial entropion or trichiasis occurs, leading to corneal ulceration and scarring. Patients with pronounced conjunctival scarring develop severe dry eye syndrome secondary to goblet cell destruction. Stenosis of the puncta can also occur, but it is of little value in ameliorating the tear deficiency. Corneal involvement is typically a superiorly located epithelial keratitis, although marginal infiltration, superficial vascularization (pannus), and limbal edema are also common. The pannus is usually more marked superiorly. Limbal follicles occur in severe cases, and their eventual cicatrization produces whitish depressions known as Herbert's pits.[103]

The various stages of trachoma are usually described according to the MacCallen classification, which is based purely on conjunctivial findings (Table 21.9). In areas where it is endemic, the presence of two of the typical signs—upper tarsal follicles, pannus, or limbal follicles (Herbert's pits)—is sufficient for diagnosis. Milder cases, such as those often seen in the southwest United States, may require careful slit-lamp examination for diagnosis.

Laboratory studies may be quite useful in mild cases, either by isolation of *C. trachomatis* in tissue culture or detection of chlamydial antibodies in serum or tears by immunofluorescent techniques.

Trachoma, especially in nonendemic populations, must be differentiated from other causes of chronic follicular conjunctivitis such as *Moraxella,* adenovirus, molluscum contagiosum virus, and chemical conjunctivitis. Conjunctival scarring is not uncommon in these cases, but Herbert's pits are absent. The presence of angular conjunctivitis should make *Moraxella* suspect, while clinical history is important in cases of chemical conjunctivitis, sometimes seen with chronic administration of topical physostigmine. The predilection of trachoma to affect the upper palpebral conjunctiva as well as the superior cornea (pannus) is of great value in the differential diagnosis.

Inclusion conjunctivitis presents in adults as an acute follicular conjunctivitis with a mucopurulent discharge. Upper respiratory symptoms and fever are lacking, in contrast to the acute follicular conjunctivitis due to adenovirus (PCF). The disease typically occurs in sexually active young adults who have acquired a new sexual partner in the past 1 or 2 months. After an incubation period of 5 to 12 days a relatively sudden onset of conjunctival injection, mixed follicular-papillary hypertrophy (Fig. 21.16), and foreign body sensation develop. The disease is usually unilateral, with a small, slightly tender, preauricular node on the affected side. During the second week keratitis may develop along with marginal or central infiltrates, superficial pannus, and even EKC-like opacities. Iritis, as well as Reiter's syndrome, can occur in late stages, with the keratitis being a more prominent feature as the disease progresses. Typical cytoplasmic inclusions may occasionally be demonstrated by Giemsa stain, but they are seen with much less frequency than in neonatal inclusion disease. In contrast to trachoma, inclusion conjunctivitis affects predominately the lower fornix and palpebral conjunctiva. The cellular response is typically monocytic and neutrophilic, an important differentiation from viral disease. Clinical and social history are crucial. Rapid serologic tests are available

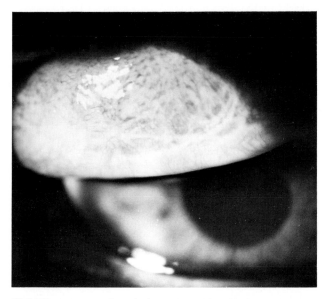

FIGURE 21.15 **Conjunctival scarring with Arlt's line in stage IV trachoma.**

TABLE 21.9
MacCallen Classification of Trachoma

Stage I	Upper tarsal plate demonstrates immature follicles without conjunctival scarring
Stage IIA	Upper tarsal plate demonstrates mature follicles with moderate papillary hypertrophy
Stage IIB	Papillary hypertrophy obscures follicular hypertrophy
Stage III	Conjunctival scarring develops with continued follicular hypertrophy
Stage IV	Follicular hypertrophy on upper tarsal plate replaced by cicatricial scarring

Adapted from Apple DJ, Rabb MF. Clinicopathologic correlation of ocular disease. St Louis: C.V. Mosby Co, 1978;2:467.

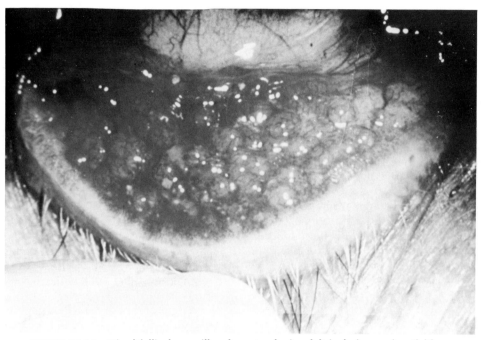

FIGURE 21.16 **Mixed follicular-papillary hypertrophy in adult inclusion conjunctivitis.**

using modified microimmunofluorescence for detection of antichlamydial IgG and IgM in blood and IgG and IgA in tears.[51]

MANAGEMENT

Trachoma usually responds to a 3-week course of oral tetracycline (1 g daily in 4 divided doses) or oral erythromycin (2 g daily in 4 divided doses).[104] The clinical response itself is relatively slow and may not be significant until 3 to 4 months after starting therapy. In pregnant patients and children under 8 years of age, tetracycline is contraindicated because it can discolor the teeth and depress bone growth in premature infants. Long-acting sulfonamide preparations are of value, but toxic and allergic reactions must be considered.

Topical treatment with tetracycline or erythromycin ointment, 2 to 3 times daily for 60 days, has been advocated for mass treatment campaigns in hyperendemic areas. Darougar and associates[105] evaluated the efficacy of topical drugs on hyperendemic trachoma in preschool children. Using examination of the upper tarsus alone as the criterion for cure, 1% rifampicin, 1% oxytetracycline, or 1% spiramycin ointment was instilled twice daily for a 6-week period. Examination 1 week after the trial period revealed only moderate clinical success (54% to 67%) for all 3 antibiotics. Chlamydial cultures performed 7 months later revealed

moderately low recovery rates in patients treated with rifampicin and oxytetracycline, but not in the spiramycin-treated group. This study suggests that although topical preparations are effective in reducing trachomatous inflammation, incomplete cure and subsequent transmission are significant, especially in hyperendemic populations. This supports the need for concomitant systemic treatment in areas of hyperendemic trachoma. Ozawa and associates,[106] however, have indicated that sustained-release ocular inserts using erythromycin estolate may offer much improved treatment of trachoma over current topical regimens without the increased possibility of side effects seen with parenteral drug administration.

Topical therapy alone is relatively ineffective in the treatment of adult inclusion conjunctivitis. Although oral tetracycline, 1 g daily in divided doses for 3 weeks, has traditionally been regarded as appropriate systemic therapy for adult inclusion disease, recent work has shown that minocycline, rifampicin, and doxycycline are markedly more active against in vitro *C. trachomatis*. Of these 3 agents, doxycycline (Vibramycin) has been used systemically to treat adult inclusion conjunctivitis and has been reported to be the most effective antibiotic yet investigated.[107] The advantages of doxycycline over other tetracyclines are that it requires a minimum daily dosage schedule; it is better absorbed from the intestine; and its absorption is not affected by diet. Usual dosage is 100 mg every 12 hours for 1 day, followed by 100 mg daily for 2 to 3 weeks. Gastrointestinal irritation can occur but can be controlled by taking the drug with food (not milk or milk products) or antacids that are free of calcium, magnesium, or aluminum. Phototoxicity with summer sun exposure can also occur with doxycycline administration, and proper precautions should be taken. Resistant organisms have not been a clinical problem, and the in vitro susceptibility closely corresponds to the clinical results of antimicrobial therapy. Tetracycline therapy should be avoided in pregnant and lactating women as well as in children under 8 years of age.

Toxic Follicular Conjunctivitis

ETIOLOGY

Toxic conjunctivitis is a condition resulting from chronic exposure of the conjunctiva to injurious substances. The more common causes include chronic use of eye medications, eye makeup, and molluscum contagiosum.

Chronic follicular conjunctivitis is not uncommon in glaucoma patients receiving long-term therapy with the strong miotics such as echothiophate (Fig. 21.17). In addition, pilocarpine and phenylephrine have been described as causes of toxic follicular conjunctivitis.[108] A marked follicular response is not unusual in women using excessive amounts of eye makeup. Cosmetic granules are frequently observed within individual follicles. Molluscum contagiosum, produced by a DNA virus of the poxvirus group, has never been cultured outside the human body. Transmission is by direct contact with the umbilicated papules or by fomite spread. Veneral spread can occur.

DIAGNOSIS

The follicular conjunctivitis observed in patients with molluscum lesions of the lid margin or palpebral conjunctiva is thought to be due to toxic viral protein or to hypersensitivity to the virus itself. This is because the virus itself does not generally infect the conjunctiva, although conjunctival lesions have been reported. Diagnosis is relatively easy when multiple papules are present, but the lesions are often hidden among the cilia and may be overlooked during cursory examination. In contrast to the other causes of toxic follicular conjunctivitis, molluscum contagiosum is generally unilateral. The disease may produce considerable thickening of the upper palpebral conjunctiva, which can resemble trachoma. Epithelial, punctate, marginal, or pannus types of keratitis may develop. The presence of typical molluscum lesions on the lid margins and the absence of cytoplasmic inclusions are helpful diagnostic signs.

Toxic follicular conjunctivitis secondary to chronic eye medication can appear indistinguishable from trachoma. Tarsal follicles, papillary hypertrophy, con-

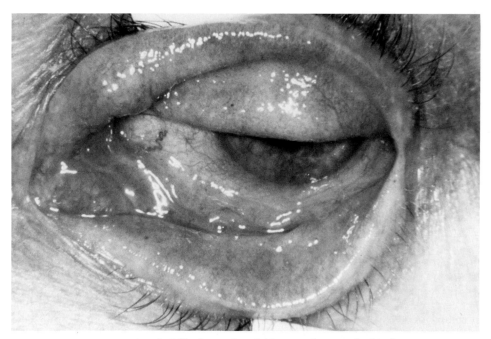

FIGURE 21.17 **Chronic follicular conjunctivitis secondary to echothiophate.**

junctival scarring, keratitis, and pannus are all seen, but not Herbert's pits.[109] Laterality depends, of course, on the laterality of drug administration. Detailed history of topical medication use is essential for diagnosis.

Toxic follicular conjunctivitis due to use of eye makeup is generally asymptomatic, and patients normally exhibit dark granules, presumably cosmetic or breakdown products, within the follicles.

MANAGEMENT

Management of toxic follicular conjunctivitis involves eliminating the injurious agent. Surgical excision of lid margin lesions in molluscum contagiosum is curative. Changing patients receiving long-term miotic therapy, as for glaucoma, to newer preparations, such as β blockers, is often effective. Discontinuation of eye cosmetics is not usually necessary, but secondary bacterial infection may be managed with topical antibiotics.

Miscellaneous Follicular Conjunctivitis

Less frequently encountered causes of follicular conjunctivitis include the large gram-negative diplobacillus *Moraxella lacunata,* a number of agents responsible for the oculoglandular involvement of Parinaud's syndrome, and the chronic follicular conjunctivitis of Axenfeld. These entities comprise an important group of clinical syndromes that must be differentiated from the other agents producing follicular conjunctivitis.

ETIOLOGY

Moraxella species (*M. osloensis* and *M. nonliquefaciens*) are members of the normal flora of humans. *M. lacunata* was once relatively common among children in orphanages and other institutions as well as in American Indian children. Although once considered the principal cause of chronic angular blepharoconjunctivitis, *M. lacunata* is now probably less frequently the cause of this infection than is *S. aureus.* Epidemics have occurred, especially among schoolgirls sharing eye cosmetics. The disease is not uncommon in the southwest United States.[110,111]

Parinaud's oculoglandular conjunctivitis is associated with ipsilateral regional lymphadenitis. A variety of etiologic agents have been implicated, including the fungus *Sporotrichum;* the agent of tularemia, *Francisella tularensis;* and the agent of cat-scratch disease. Young children exposed to cats, farmers with traumatic exposure to *Actinomyces israelii,* and hunters coming in contact with infected rabbit and squirrel (tularemia) are typically affected. Tuberculosis, coccidiomycosis, and syphilis are occasionally implicated causes of Parinaud's oculoglandular syndrome.

Axenfeld's chronic follicular conjunctivitis, a mild asymptomatic follicular conjunctivitis involving the upper palpebral conjunctiva, has been described as occuring in orphanages and boarding schools. The disease is self-limiting and is similar in many respects to the mild form of trachoma seen among American Indians.[112]

DIAGNOSIS

A history of borrowed eye makeup in a young girl with moderate bilateral follicular conjunctivitis, often with mild mucopurulent discharge, should prompt suspicion of *M. lacunata* infection. Conjunctival scrapings may reveal the large gram-negative bacillus (often as diplobacilli) but are devoid of chlamydial inclusions. Bacterial cultures reveal *M. lacunata,* often mixed with *S. aureus.* The clinical differentiation of viral from *Moraxella* chronic follicular conjunctivitis may be difficult, particularly in the presence of preauricular adenopathy, punctate keratitis, or the appearance of subepithelial infiltrates. The misdiagnosis of *Moraxella*-induced follicular conjunctivitis as a chlamydial infection can have severe social repercussions.

Parinaud's oculoglandular syndrome is characterized by a unilateral follicular conjunctivitis associated with deep yellowish lesions (granulomas) and prominently enlarged preauricular, submaxillary, or cervical nodes on the affected side. Fever and general malaise are usually present (vomiting in tularemia), and there is a frequent history of exposure to an animal, especially a cat. Laboratory studies should include Gram and Giemsa staining of smears, bacterial cultures, complete blood count (CBC) and erythrocyte sedimentation rate (ESR), chest x-ray study (tuberculosis, sarcoidosis, and coccidiomycosis), specific skin tests (Hanger-Rose test, PPD and Frie test), and conjunctival biopsy.

Axenfeld's chronic follicular conjunctivitis is insidious in onset, generally asymptomatic, and accompanied by a minimal discharge. The follicles involve the upper tarsus as well as the palpebral and fornix conjunctiva (Fig. 21.18). The cornea is typically not involved.

MANAGEMENT

Moraxella species are generally susceptible to topical sulfonamides, erythromycin, and tetracycline. Incidence of toxic or hypersensitivity reactions is low with erythromycin and tetracycline when topically administered, but use of sulfonamides increases the risk of allergic reactions. Zinc salts have been traditionally used in *Moraxella* infection, especially to treat keratitis in the preantibiotic era, and have an almost specific effect on the infection. Application of 0.25% or 0.5%

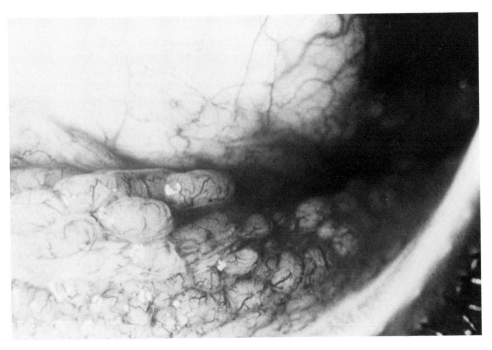

FIGURE 21.18   **Axenfeld's chronic follicular conjunctivitis.**

zinc sulfate solution (Zincfrin), although effective against the bacteria, is not as effective as the previously mentioned antibiotics. Neomycin and gentamicin are usually effective, but sensitivity is variable. *Moraxella* is sensitive to the penicillins, but their use is normally not indicated either topically or systemically.

Systemic involvement occurs in the majority of cases of Parinaud's oculoglandular syndrome. Antibiotics should be selected only after thorough consideration of the nature of the causative agent. The affected lymph node may be treated with local heat. Oral and topical antibiotics are indicated. Initial therapy should include gentamicin sulfate 0.3% ointment, bacitracin ointment (500 units/g), or 1% tetracycline ointment (Achromycin) instilled into the involved eye every 2 or 3 hours for 2 days, then 4 or 5 times daily until the condition resolves. Cycloplegics often provide symptomatic relief, and frequent lavage of mucopurulent discharge is beneficial. Topical or oral corticosteroids should be avoided. Cat-scratch disease is best treated with analgesics and antipyretics such as aspirin. Systemic or topical antibiotics do not shorten the natural course of the disease. Some investigators believe the disease may be shortened by excising the conjunctival lesion. In general, however, a conservative approach is warranted because of the self-limited nature of the disease, which resolves without sequelae. Sporotrichosis responds well to oral potassium iodide, 1 ml in a glass of water 3 times daily, gradually increasing the daily dose by 1 ml for a total daily dose of 8 to 10

ml. Therapy must be continued for 1 to 2 months for complete cure.

Oculoglandular syndrome due to *Francisella tularensis* (tularemia) is most effectively treated by streptomycin, 1 g daily delivered intramuscularly for 1 week. Prompt results may be obtained with the use of oral tetracycline or chloramphenicol, but these bacteriostatic agents often fail to eradicate the organism, and relapses occur. Resistance apparently does not develop, since reinstitution of therapy with the initial antibiotic regimen brings about prompt clinical recovery. Without treatment, tularemia has a fatality rate of approximately 5%. Mortality increases to 30% when pneumonia is associated.

Specific therapy for Axenfeld's conjunctivitis is generally not required, but its possible relationship to mild trachoma may warrant a course of oral tetracycline or a sulfonamide.

Table 21.10 summarizes the important differential diagnostic and management criteria for the various forms of follicular conjunctivitis.

Mechanical and Toxic Conjunctivitis

ETIOLOGY

Various antibiotics and other medications can cause conjunctivitis. Overtreatment of acute or chronic in-

TABLE 21.10
Summary of Differential Diagnosis and Management of Follicular Conjunctivitis

Condition	Symptoms	Signs	Cytology	Management
Herpes simplex conjunctivitis	Rubbing eye, foreign body complaint	Conjunctival hyperemia, often lid vesicles, possible dendritic keratitis, watery discharge	Lymphocytes	Vidarabine (Vira-A) 3% ointment q3h for 5 instillations daily until 3–5 days after resolution
Pharyngoconjunctival fever (PCF)	Sore throat, irritability, mild foreign body complaints	Pharyngitis, fever, watery discharge, submaxillary adenopathy	Lymphocytes	Supportive therapy (cool compresses, vasoconstrictors, antipyretics)
Epidemic keratoconjunctivitis (EKC)	Moderate to severe foreign body complaint	Marked chemosis and petechiae, preauricular lymphadenopathy, keratitis with subepithelial infiltrates (10–14 days from onset)	Lymphocytes	Supportive therapy (topical antibiotic to prevent bacterial infection; consider trifluridine 1% q2h if severe)
Adult inclusion conjunctivitis	Foreign body sensation, photophobia, burning on urination (with urethritis)	Mucopurulent discharge, preauricular node, urethral discharge, mixed follicular-papillary hypertrophy, corneal infiltrates (often)	Intracytoplasmic inclusions, PMN, lymphocytes	Tetracycline 250 mg qid PO for 3 weeks
Toxic follicular conjunctivitis	Mild to moderate irritation	Cosmetic granules from excessive eye makeup; molluscum lesions on lid margin	Nonspecific	Elimination of injurious agent
Moraxella conjunctivitis	Mild irritation	Mild mucopurulent discharge	Large gram-negative bacillus	Topical sodium sulfacetamide 10% q4h for 10 days; or erythromycin (Ilotycin) ointment q6h for 10 days
Parinaud's syndrome	Tender lymph nodes (preauricular, cervical, submaxillary), malaise, vomiting	Deep, yellowish conjunctival granulomas	Variable, depending on etiology	Laboratory studies with selection of appropriate oral antibiotic
Chronic follicular conjunctivitis of Axenfeld	Generally asymptomatic	Minimal discharge, uninvolved cornea	Lymphocytes	No treatment indicated

fectious conjunctivitis may produce conjunctival hyperemia and irritation, termed medicamentosa; it is often indistinguishable from the original infection and is relieved only after the medication is withdrawn.

The abuse of OTC eye preparations containing vasoconstrictors, especially phenylephrine, often leads to a chronic conjunctivitis characterized by marked hyperemia and even chemosis. Not infrequently the disease was first treated as bacterial. As noted in Chapter 19, mechanical conjunctival and corneal trauma associated with the various forms of entropion comprise an important source of ocular morbidity. Mechanical trauma of a similar nature occurs in trachoma.

DIAGNOSIS

In the patient presenting with chronic conjunctivitis in which a multitude of antibiotics and other topical preparations have been used without success, it is often rewarding to totally withdraw all topical medications. Often the conjunctivitis will begin to resolve in 1 to 2 days, and the diagnosis of medicamentosa is easily made. The patient's medication history is vital. It is particularly important to recognize that many patients do not consider OTC eye preparations to be "medicine." Thus, the patient should be specifically questioned about the use of these preparations, since such medications constitute a major cause of mild, "nonspecific" conjunctivitis.

Streeten and Streeten[113] have described the appearance of intensely basophilic inclusions in Giemsa-stained conjunctival scrapings of patients who used various topical antibiotics to treat conjunctivitis. These "blue-bodies" differed in morphology from bacterial, chlamydial, and other more frequently encountered cytoplasmic inclusions. Electron microscopy showed these inclusions to consist of a variety of dense bodies as well as phagolysomal vacuoles containing complex lipids, indicating epithelial cell injury. The existence of more than a few random "blue-bodies" in a conjunctival scraping may indicate drug toxicity.[113]

The diagnosis of mechanical conjunctivitis is based on the concomitant lid involvement (entropion) that is produced by a variety of cicatricial and senile entropion processes.

MANAGEMENT

The management of toxic conjunctivitis can be as simple as eliminating a chronically administered topically applied antibiotic or as difficult as attempting to isolate the offending agent from a multitude of aerosols, eye rinses, and skin preparations. In any case, the condition improves once the offending agent is withdrawn, although complete resolution is often prolonged.

In some forms of toxic conjunctivitis, such as that seen in chemotherapy patients receiving methotrexate followed by leucovorin rescue, topical cromolyn sodium (Opticrom) is highly effective.[114]

The management of mechanical conjunctivitis secondary to trichiasis, entropion, or distichiasis takes a variety of forms. Surgical intervention includes entropion repair and lysing of cicatricial conjunctival bands. Epilation of offending cilia, either mechanically or by electrolysis, is effective but is often only temporary in relieving mechanical conjunctival irritation. Bandage soft contact lenses and ocular lubricants for treatment of tear deficiencies due to loss of conjunctival goblet cells are effective both in relieving symptoms and preventing further conjunctival trauma.

The management of trachoma and other cicatricial disorders is discussed elsewhere in this chapter.

The Conjunctiva in Systemic Diseases and Syndromes

Oculodermatologic Disorders

ETIOLOGY

These disorders are often characterized by conjunctival inflammation associated with a generalized dermatologic disease. Examples include rosacea, psoriasis, and atopic dermatitis.

Rosacea is a chronic condition characterized by acneform papular-pustular eruptions with cutaneous erythema. Histologically, the disease is typified by sebaceous gland hypertrophy. Females are more susceptible to the disease than are males, and the peak onset is between 30 and 50 years of age. Once thought to be a disease associated with alcoholism, this relationship is now considered to be somewhat circumstantial.[115]

Psoriasis, a chronic papulosquamous disorder, is characterized by sharply demarcated erythematous patches with overlying gray scales. Onset is typically between the ages of 10 and 35 years, with females significantly more susceptible to develop the disease than males. Psoriasis is more common in whites than in blacks. Ocular involvement occurs in approximately 10% of patients with psoriasis and may be the only sign of the disease. In contrast to the systemic disorder, ocular involvement occurs almost twice as frequently in males than in females.

Atopic dermatitis represents a hypersensitivity state caused by predispositional, constitutional, or hereditary factors rather than by acquired hypersensitivity to specific allergens, as in contact dermatitis. Patients usually have a personal or family history of allergy, particularly asthma or hay fever. The disorder is found in an estimated 3% of the population, affects all races, and is more common in males. The condition usually appears in the late teens and lasts until the fourth or fifth decade of life.[116]

DIAGNOSIS

Rosacea is a chronic acneform process that is also characterized by multiple facial telangiectasia and the typical rhinophyma in advanced cases (Color Plate XIII). Ocular involvement can be significant, even in conjunction with only mild dermatologic disease, but typically parallels the generalized disease. Conjunctival hyperemia, often with actual conjunctival telangiectasia and chronic blepharitis, is the most common ocular manifestation.

Ocular rosacea typically presents with symptoms of foreign body sensation, burning, and complaints of recurrent chalazia. Less commonly encountered signs are corneal thinning, vascularization, and infiltration. Unless the conjunctivitis is recognized as part of the generalized dermatitis, proper diagnosis and thus proper treatment are often delayed.

Psoriasis typically involves the scalp and extensor surfaces of the knees and elbows. Itching and burning sensations are characteristic symptoms, and psoriatic arthritis may be severe and mutilating. Conjunctival involvement is in the form of granulated lesions affecting both the palpebral and bulbar conjunctiva. Corneal neovascularization causes the development of marked photophobia. There is often marked scaling along the base of the lashes. Inflammatory ectropion, entropion with trichiasis, or madarosis are not uncommon in severe cases.

Atopic dermatitis is characterized by patches, often multiple, of thickened, excoriated, lichenified skin very similar to that of chronic contact dermatitis (Fig. 21.19). The skin is typically dry and itchy and is sensitive to heat, external irritants, and even perspiration. Ocular involvement takes the form of hyperemia and chemosis, particularly affecting the superior palpebral and bulbar conjunctiva. Corneal involvement is not uncommon, even to the point of development of the classic shield ulcer (Fig. 21.20), which is sterile, or pannus (Fig. 21.21). Various types of cataract (anterior capsular shield cataract) are also noted. As mentioned previously, other forms of allergy, such as asthma or hay fever, are often observed in patients with atopic ocular disease as well as a strong hereditary predisposition.

MANAGEMENT

Oral tetracycline, 250 mg 4 times daily and tapered over several weeks, is effective for the treatment of rosacea.[115] The mechanism of action is thought to be due to the lipase-inhibiting action of tetracycline, thus

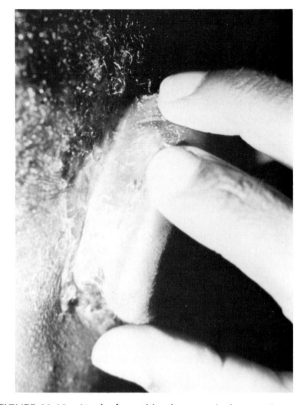

FIGURE 21.19 **Atopic dermatitis of retroauricular area in a 9-year-old black boy.**

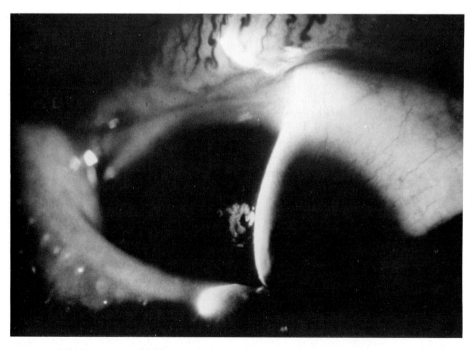

FIGURE 21.20 **Shield corneal ulcer associated with atopic conjunctivitis.**

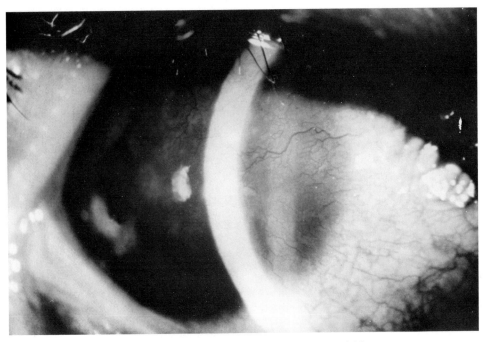

FIGURE 21.21   **Pannus in atopic keratoconjunctivitis.**

preventing the conversion of lipids present in sebaceous gland secretions into free fatty acids, which irritate the conjunctiva and facial skin. Patients with
ocular rosacea often have concomitant staphylococcal
blepharitis, which is best treated by antibacterial (bacitracin–polymyxin B) lid scrubs before bedtime. Most
patients can taper and discontinue oral tetracycline
therapy without recurrence of symptoms, although patients with severe disease often require prolonged
maintenance therapy (such as 250 mg daily) or pulses
of therapy to remain free of symptoms.[115]

Isotretinoin (13-*cis*-retinoic acid) has been used successfully in the treatment of severe rosacea for a number of years. In severe, recalcitrant cases therapeutic
success with isotretinoin has been much greater than
with the standard remedies such as oral tetracycline or
metronidazole.[117] Side effects frequently encountered
include cheilitis, dermatitis, conjunctivitis, and pruritus.

Psoriasis has been treated with variable success by
a number of agents. Anthralin is a mild irritant with
weak antimicrobial activity. Available in ointment form,
it is often very effective in treating psoriasis not responsive to other treatment. It can be irritating, however, and should not be used around the eyes. Azaribine
(Triazure), an oral agent, is used to treat severe psoriasis, and resolution typically occurs within 8 weeks,
often with a remission of several months. Its use may
result in significant but reversible suppression of eryth-
ropoiesis. Striking improvement has been seen in
patients with severe psoriasis treated with the anti-

metabolite methotrexate. Twenty percent zinc oxide
ointment and 6% resorcinol ointment are both commonly used to treat typical cases of psoriasis, but these
agents are not designed for ocular use. Fortunately,
treatment of generalized psoriasis often reduces the
ocular involvement.

The management of atopic ocular disease includes
treatment of the generalized dermatitis as well as local
ocular therapy including topical corticosteroids and antihistamines. Topical steroids should be used judiciously, and special attempts should be exerted to avoid
making the patient dependent on their use. Topical
antihistamines can provide considerable relief, along
with topical vasoconstrictors and cool compresses.
Topical cromolyn sodium 2% has been shown to be
less effective than 1% medrysone,[116] but a higher concentration of cromolyn (4%) has been found to be
quite effective in some cases and may allow for a
significant reduction in topical steroid use during treatment with cromolyn.[118] Patients with severe atopic keratoconjunctivitis may benefit from treatment with
plasmapheresis if the condition is resistant to more
conservative therapy.[142]

Mucous Membrane Disorders

ETIOLOGY

Mucous membrane disorders that often involve the
conjunctiva include benign mucous membrane pem-

phigoid (BMMP) and erythema multiforme (Stevens-Johnson syndrome). Cicatricial pemphigoid is a bullous disease of the skin and mucous membranes that affects women with almost twice the frequency of men. There is no apparent racial or geographic predilection, and the average age of onset is about 60 years. The disorder is relatively rare, accounting for approximately 1 in 30,000 ophthalmic cases.[119]

Erythema multiforme is an acute but generally self-limiting bullous disorder of the skin and mucous membranes. Males are more often affected than females. Although the highest incidence is before 30 years of age, the disorder may occur at any age. Although there appears to be no racial or geographic predilection, an increased incidence of the disease exists during the winter and spring. A number of factors appear to precipitate the disease in susceptible individuals. Toxic or allergic reactions to drugs such as penicillin, barbiturates, sulfonamides, salicylates, and phenylbutazone have been implicated, as well as radiation exposure, neoplasia, and certain infections (e.g., HSV). In significant numbers of cases no precipitating factor can be identified.[120]

DIAGNOSIS

Chronic and progressive conjunctival shrinkage and symblepharon formation characterize the ocular involvement in BMMP (Fig. 21.22.) The differential di-

agnosis includes a number of conditions associated with such conjunctival changes, making the clinical diagnosis of BMMP one of exclusion. Chronic topical administration of pilocarpine, epinephrine, or echothiophate may in some cases produce a clinical picture very similar to BMMP. Symblepharon has been described in sarcoidosis and even in severe dry eye states. Severe alkali burns and radiation may produce a similar clinical condition. The acute membranous conjunctivitis that can occur in EKC, HSV, group A streptococci, and in rare cases of diphtherial conjunctivitis may cause conjunctival scarring. Their acute presentation and generally self-limiting course is quite different from the chronic, progressive conjunctival shrinkage and symblepharon formation observed in BMMP.

BMMP generally begins with involvement of one eye and becomes bilateral within 1 or 2 years. The course of the disease involves slowly progressive conjunctival shrinkage that is often interrupted by periods of acute disease activity with intense conjunctival hyperemia and chemosis. As the disease progresses, subconjunctival fibrosis produces symblepharon, which may eventually impair ocular motility. Severe dry eye syndrome, secondary to fibrotic occlusion of the ducts of the lacrimal and accessory lacrimal glands, can lead to actual keratinization of the conjunctiva and cornea (Fig. 21.23).

Stevens-Johnson syndrome—the major form of erythema multiforme—is characterized by cutaneous le-

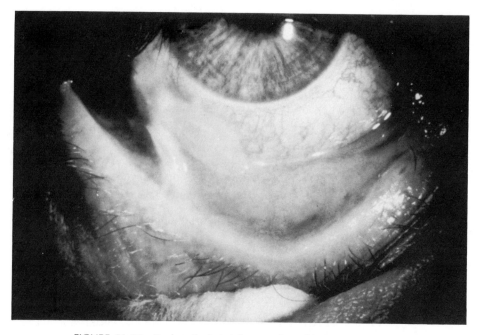

FIGURE 21.22 **Conjunctival shrinkage and symblepharon formation in benign mucous membrane pemphigoid.**

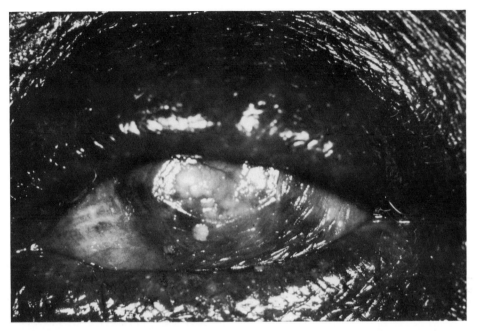

FIGURE 21.23   **Keratinization of conjunctiva and cornea in benign mucous membrane pemphigoid.**

sions as well as by frequently severe ocular involvement and can be confused with toxic epidermal necrolysis. However, the mucous membrane lesions are more severe in Stevens-Johnson syndrome than in toxic epidermal necrolysis. Of particular value is the fact that the Nikolsky sign (spreading of the epidermal bullae by sliding pressure with the finger) is demonstrable in toxic epidermal necrolysis but not in Stevens-Johnson syndrome. The associated fever of Stevens-Johnson syndrome typically persists after appearance of the skin eruptions, unlike that observed in toxic epidermal necrolysis, which disappears at that point in the disease. The ocular involvement in Stevens-Johnson syndrome characteristically results in conjunctival scarring and symblepharon, while toxic epidermal necrolysis does not normally produce significant permanent conjunctival changes.

The acute phase of ocular involvement observed in erythema multiforme generally lasts 2 to 4 weeks. Conjunctival involvement runs the spectrum from mild catarrhal conjunctivitis, which resolves without sequelae, to severe membranous conjunctivitis, which resolves with conjunctival scarring, symblepharon formation, and entropion with trichiasis in a clinical picture similar to that of BMMP. Severity of late ocular complications depends on the severity of the systemic disease rather than on the localized ocular treatment. The condition is self-limited, so that any conjunctival shrinkage and symblepharon produced by the disorder is static, unlike the chronic progressive course of BMMP.[120]

MANAGEMENT

Intensive use of artificial tear preparations is of particular value in controlling the symptoms produced by the severe dry eye condition seen in BMMP. Drops must frequently be used hourly to be of benefit. Lubricating ointments (e.g., Lacri-Lube, Duratears) may be instilled at bedtime or continuously during the day according to the severity of ocular involvement. Systems for prolonged delivery of tear substitutes (Lacrisert) appear to be effective in the treatment of severe keratitis sicca. Because of the high incidence of concomitant staphylococcal lid disease, patients with BMMP often have the basic disease process aggravated by acute or chronic bacterial infections. Thus, frequent use of antibiotic (bacitracin or bacitracin–polymyxin B) lid scrubs is of definite benefit in reducing the general ocular morbidity. Surgical procedures may be valuable in correcting entropion and trichiasis, and electrolysis and even cryotherapy may be valuable in treating trichiasis. Therapeutic soft contact lenses can protect the cornea from both desiccation and trichiasis. However, their use becomes increasingly difficult with obliteration of the fornices. Frequent lysis of symblepharon with a glass rod, using topical anesthesia, is useful but probably serves only as a temporizing measure. Therapy with topical, subconjunctival, and oral corticosteroids has been generally disappointing. Topical therapy alone is ineffective, and subconjunctival injection is only temporarily effective. Oral steroids are of definite value in treatment of the acute periods of disease activity. Mondino and associates[119] have shown oral immunosuppressive agents to be beneficial in some patients, and these may become a major treatment modality. Keratoprostheses may restore useful vision in patients with endstage disease characterized by ankyloblepharon and sclerocornea. Penetrating keratoplasty has been universally unsuccessful.

Management of the ocular complications of erythema multiforme is similar to that in BMMP. Local treatment with steroids does not appear to influence the severity of the ocular disease. Treatment of secondary bacterial infection, ocular lubricants, early lysis of symblepharon, and bandage soft contact lenses may provide symptomatic relief and reduce the severity of secondary complications.[120]

Collagen Disorders

ETIOLOGY

The collagen disorders include various systemic diseases that are characterized as primary disturbances of the connective tissue of the body. Since lesions of blood vessels accompany the connective tissue changes, the term collagen-vascular disease is widely used. Much evidence supports autoimmunity or hypersensitivity as an underlying process in the pathogenesis of these disorders.[121]

In collagen-vascular disorders, connective tissues demonstrate differing degrees of fibroblastic proliferation and degeneration. Collagen fibers are swollen and fragmented, and the ground substance increases both in prominence and actual quantity. The previous architecture is lost.[121]

Commonly included within the collagen disorders are rheumatoid arthritis, systemic lupus erythematosus (SLE), polyarteritis nodosa, scleroderma, dermatomyositis, rheumatic fever, and thrombotic thrombocytopenic purpura. Other less common entities, often with ocular manifestations, are Reiter's syndrome and relapsing polychondritis. Only the latter two entities, along with polyarteritis nodosa and SLE, involve the conjunctiva as a primary ocular involvement.

SLE has a peak onset in the third and fourth decades of life and is 5 to 10 times more frequent in women than in men.[121] The disease may last for weeks to years, and the prognosis is generally poor. SLE-like manifestations can occur in patients receiving certain drugs, such as isoniazid, phenytoin (Dilantin), sulfonamide preparations, and even penicillin.

Polyarteritis nodosa represents a widespread arteritis of small and medium vessels. Its onset is typically in the second to fifth decades, and it affects men at 2 to 3 times the rate observed in women. Its etiology has been linked to allergy, rheumatic fever, infection with streptococci, and even a virus-related antigen. Asthma and other allergic states are frequently associated, suggesting that the disease may indeed be a severe manifestation of hypersensitivity.[121]

Relapsing polychondritis is a recurrent inflammation of cartilage, with involvement of the pinnae of the ears the most common clinical feature. Onset is typically in the third to sixth decades, and men and women are equally affected.[121]

Reiter's syndrome is a nongonococcal triad of conjunctivitis, urethritis, and arthritis. The disease is usually limited to young adults, with over 90% of those being male. Conjunctivitis occurs in approximately one-third of affected patients. Although the pathogenesis is uncertain, much evidence supports an infective basis for the disorder. Chlamydial infection, in particular, seems to be an important preexisting finding, and the disease may represent an altered host response rather than a primary infective process. A postdysenteric form has been noted in several major epidemics of bacillary dysentery.[121] The disease is rare in children.[121]

DIAGNOSIS

The conjunctivitis observed in SLE tends to be nonspecific and is characterized by hyperemia of the bulbar conjunctiva with a micropapillary reaction of the palpebral conjunctiva. Such a presentation, with evidence of systemic symptoms of migratory polyarthritis and polyarthralgias, suggests a collagen disorder as the underlying entity. Various cutaneous lesions often occur as well. These are frequently symmetric erythematous and maculopapular lesions involving the face, neck, and extremities. Although not universally observed, a characteristic "butterfly" malar erythematous rash is sometimes seen. The LE cell test, based on a factor present in the gamma globulin fraction of plasma of affected patients, is typically positive in patients with active SLE. A variety of antinuclear antibodies has also been described. Gastrointestinal symptoms may mimic acute surgical abdomen, and acute nephritis is seen in 50% of affected patients.

In polyarteritis nodosa the ocular signs are typically those of conjunctival hyperemia with occasional subconjunctival hemorrhages. Other ocular findings include Cogan's syndrome (nonluetic interstitial keratitis and deafness), papilledema in up to 10% of affected patients, third and sixth cranial nerve palsies, Horner's syndrome, and even homonymous hemianopsia. Systemic symptoms are those generally associated with the various collagen-vascular diseases, such as fever, malaise, polyarthralgia, myalgia, and weight loss. Renal disease develops in 70% to 80% of affected patients, with systemic hypertension a secondary finding. Bladder involvement is characterized by hemorrhagic cystitis, and cardiopulmonary complications include endocarditis and myocarditis. Gastrointestinal findings include nausea, vomiting, hemorrhage, and jaundice.[122]

The diagnosis of relapsing polychondritis is based on inflammation of cartilage of the ear, nose, trachea, and peripheral joints. Ocular complications occur in up to two-thirds of affected patients and include conjunctivitis, episcleritis, anterior uveitis, optic neuritis, and extraocular muscle paresis. The conjunctivitis is nonspecific and is generally mild with little exudation. It is seen in approximately one-fourth of affected patients, while episcleritis is the most common ocular manifestation.

The diagnosis of Reiter's syndrome is based on a history of urethritis with evidence of chronic vesiculitis or prostatitis, polyarthritis, and conjunctivitis. Elevated ESR, leukocytosis, and chronic low-grade fever are additional findings. The arthritis seen in rheumatoid disease usually involves the hands, while the feet and heels are more often involved in Reiter's syndrome. Hyperkeratosis of the plantar surfaces (keratodermia blenorrhagica) occurs in 5% to 8% of affected patients and is pathognomonic[123] (Fig. 21.24).

MANAGEMENT

In all the collagen disorders described in this section, the conjunctival involvement tends to be mild and self-limiting and is generally a minor problem in relation to the overall morbidity and even mortality associated with the underlying disease process.

Management of the concomitant conjunctivitis observed in the collagen disorders essentially takes the form of supportive therapy such as topical vasoconstrictors and prophylactic antibiotics according to the severity of ocular involvement. The primary therapy should be aimed at treating the underlying systemic disorder.

Aspirin, chloroquine, and corticosteroids are usually effective in the management of SLE. Clinical remission has occurred in patients with polyarteritis nodosa with use of systemic steroids. Relapsing polychondritis also responds to adequate early treatment with steroids. Patients with Reiter's syndrome do well with steroids, while some patients respond to oxytetracycline, which lends credence to the evidence supporting a chlamydial agent as an underlying etiology. Reiter's syndrome is self-limiting, usually lasting only

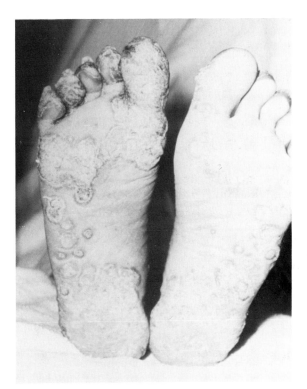

FIGURE 21.24   **Keratodermia blenorrhagica in Reiter's syndrome.**

1 to 6 months, and only rarely results in serious complications.

Table 21.11 summarizes the important differential diagnostic and management criteria for the various conjunctival disorders associated with systemic diseases and syndromes.

Miscellaneous Conjunctival Disorders

Tear Deficiencies

The etiology, diagnosis, and management of the various tear deficiency states are discussed in Chapter 20.

Phlyctenular Conjunctivitis

ETIOLOGY

Phlyctenular conjunctivitis is an inflammatory condition characterized by the development of conjunctival or corneal nodules (Fig. 21.25). Long associated with a delayed hypersensitivity response to tubercular protein, it is now thought that the condition represents a

TABLE 21.11
Summary of Differential Diagnosis and Management of Conjunctival Disorders Associated with Systemic Diseases and Syndromes

Condition	Symptoms	Signs	Cytology	Management
Rosacea conjunctivitis	Mild to moderate irritation	Mild hyperemia to frank telangiectasia, chronic blepharitis, multiple facial telangiectasia and rhinophyma in advanced cases	Nonspecific	Tetracycline 250 mg qid PO for 1 week, then tapering dose 250 mg daily each week until control of condition, lid scrubs (antibiotic ointment if severe) 2–3 times a week
Psoriasis conjunctivitis	Burning, itching; marked photophobia with corneal involvement	Conjunctival granulations; inflammatory ectropion, entropion, madarosis	Nonspecific	Oral agents (methotrexate); topical nonocular preparations (Anthralin, zinc oxide 20%)
Atopic conjunctivitis	Itching, burning, and photophobia	Hyperemia and chemosis; superior keratitis (shield ulcer and pannus formation not common); anterior capsular cataract	Nonspecific	Topical antihistaminic-vasoconstrictor q2h–q4h; 4% cromolyn q4h; topical corticosteroid use (prednisolone acetate 1% q3h–q4h) if severe
Benign mucous membrane pemphigoid (BMMP)	Chronic irritation	Progressive conjunctival shrinkage with symblepharon formation and secondary dry eye	Nonspecific	Intensive artificial tear therapy q1h; ocular lubricant (LacriLube, Duratears) q6h; prophylactic antibiotic (bacitracin–polymyxin B, bacitracin); lysis of symblepharon; oral corticosteroids (20–60 mg daily) during acute episodes
Erythema multiforme (Stevens-Johnson syndrome)	Same as BMMP except disease is not progressive and thus carries better prognosis	Same as BMMP except disease is not progressive and thus carries better prognosis		
Collagen-vascular disorders (Reiter's syndrome, relapsing polychondritis, polyarteritis nodosa, systemic lupus erythematosus)	Mild to moderate irritation	Nonspecific hyperemia and chemosis with micropapillary hypertrophy	Nonspecific	Topical vasoconstrictors/ antibiotics in prophylactic doses (e.g., sodium sulfacetamide 10% q6h); treatment of underlying disorder

nonspecific delayed hypersensitivity to foreign (bacterial) protein.[124]

Histologically, the cellular reaction of the phlyctenule is a typical delayed hypersensitivity reaction with focal epithelial infiltration of round cells and macrophages. Only when the central epithelium of the phlyctenule undergoes necrosis does a large number of polymorphonuclear leukocytes invade the area. Langerhans cells and T lymphocytes are observed in far greater numbers in scrapings from phlyctenules than from normal conjunctiva. Langerhans cells can function as antigen presenting and activating cells for T lymphocytes, which in turn amplify the initial cellular response by the recruitment of other lymphocytes. Normally, antibody-producing B lymphocytes are absent from normal conjunctival scrapings. Their pres-

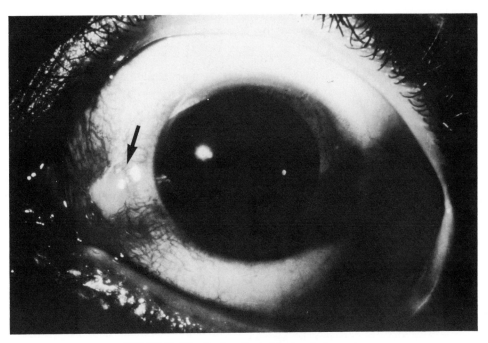

FIGURE 21.25 **Conjunctival phlyctenule (arrow).**

ence in phlyctenule scrapings can be explained by recruitment of B lymphocytes following activation of helper T lymphocytes. These findings indicate that phlyctenular conjunctivitis can be more accurately characterized as an initial cell-mediated immune response to bacterial antigens, such as the teichoic acid polysaccharide of the *Staphylococcus* cell wall, followed by an antibody-mediated reaction.[125]

Phlyctenular conjunctivitis (or keratoconjunctivitis) occurs worldwide, typically affecting children. A higher incidence is still reported in females than in males. There remains an association between the disorder and tuberculosis, with phlyctenulosis being uncommon in areas where the rate of tuberculosis is low. In the United States, phlyctenulosis is usually associated with hypersensitivity to *Staphylococcus* antigens.[126]

DIAGNOSIS

Vernal conjunctivitis, primarily with limbal involvement, may be confused with phlyctenulosis, but the presence of cobblestone papillae, marked itching, and moderate conjunctival inflammation distinguishes vernal disease from phlyctenulosis.

The corneal involvement observed in acne rosacea is probably based on the same type of allergic mechanism as is phlyctenulosis. Although sometimes observed as a primary ocular finding without dermatologic manifestations, acne rosacea typically presents in association with characteristic facial telangiectasia, which provides a valuable diagnostic clue in most cases.

Inflamed pingueculae can be distinguished from a limbal phlyctenule by the lack of microabscess formation in the former and absence of conjunctival hypertrophy in the latter.

MANAGEMENT

Phlyctenular keratoconjunctivitis can be a severe and potentially blinding disorder. However, conjunctival phlyctenules are typically transient, resolving without sequelae, although corneal involvement may lead to ulceration, scarring, and even perforation. If mildly symptomatic, conjunctival phlyctenulosis can be treated with topical decongestants or astringents. A pulsed dose of topical steroid, such as 1% prednisolone acetate (Pred Forte) every 2 hours for 3 to 4 days, then tapered, is reserved for more severe cases.

Although topical steroids have long been the treatment of choice for phlyctenulosis, oral tetracycline in cases of recalcitrant or recurrent nontuberculosis phlyctenular keratoconjunctivitis has provided often dramatic relief of symptoms and arrested the disease. Patients may receive 500 mg to 1 g of tetracycline daily, tapered to maintenance doses of 250 to 500 mg daily.[125] This therapy is not recommended for children younger than 8 years because tetracycline may permanently discolor the teeth.

Patients with phlyctenulosis should be evaluated for tuberculosis, and children or young adults with a positive tuberculin test, or adults demonstrating recent conversion, should be treated for tuberculosis. The patient's family should be examined for active tuberculosis.

Pinguecula

ETIOLOGY

A pinguecula represents a hyperplasia of conjunctival tissue, probably in response to environmental irritation. Occurring on the exposed bulbar conjunctiva within the palpebral fissure, it may become inflamed (pingueculitis) or be associated with overlying exposure keratosis.

DIAGNOSIS

Inflamed pingueculae can be confused with conjunctival phlyctenulosis. Conjunctival hypertrophy is not present in the latter, and the pingueculitis is not as painful as typical phlyctenulosis. Precancerous and cancerous lesions may mimic pingueculae.

MANAGEMENT

Other than intermittent inflammation or development of dellen adjacent to a partially elevated pinguecula, the patient with pingueculae is very rarely symptomatic and typically requires no therapy. However, intermittent inflammation of pingueculae is greatly aided by the use of topical decongestants or ocular lubricants. More severe inflammations respond to a short course of topical steroid therapy, such as 1% prednisolone acetate 4 times daily for 5 to 7 days. Surgical removal by conjunctival resection may be necessary if the lesion becomes a cosmetic problem or is chronically inflamed. Triethylenethiophosphoramide (Thiotepa), an antimitotic agent related to the nitrogen mustards, has been successfully used to prevent recurrence of both pingueculae and pterygia after surgical resection.[127]

Pterygium

Pterygium formation represents a basophilic degeneration of the bulbar conjunctival stroma that may even demonstrate secondary calcification. Histologically, pterygium is identical to pinguecula, with corneal involvement characterizing the former (Fig. 21.26). Neither condition is premalignant, and the epithelium of pterygia demonstrates only alternate atrophy and reactive hyperplasia.[128,143]

Recurrence after excision varies from 20% to 40%. Beta irradiation and Thiotepa have been used to reduce the recurrence rate.[127,144]

Thiotepa is as effective in reducing the recurrence

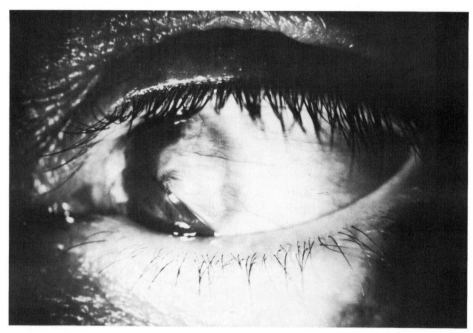

FIGURE 21.26 **Pterygium.**

of pterygium as is beta radiation, and complications of irritation, skin depigmentation, and hypersensitivity reactions are less than those of beta radiation, which include conjunctival and corneal scarring, radiation cataract, and iritis. A typical regimen for Thiotepa is 1 drop of a 1:2000 dilution (Ringer's solution) every 3 hours while awake for 6 to 8 weeks beginning 2 days postoperatively. Optimum potency requires a fresh solution biweekly. Recurrence rates vary from 3.3% to 16.1% compared with 31.3% in controls.[127]

Superior Limbic Keratoconjunctivitis

ETIOLOGY

Superior limbic keratoconjunctivitis (SLK) is a chronic and recurrent inflammation of unknown etiology affecting the superior palpebral and bulbar conjunctiva. Histologic studies demonstrate acanthosis, dyskeratosis, keratinization, nuclear degeneration, and intracellular accumulation of glycogen. There is a great increase in the number of superior palpebral conjunctival goblet cells, while the superior bulbar conjunctiva is devoid of these cells.[129]

Viral, fungal, and specific bacterial cultures have not been productive, and conjunctival scrapings reveal a polymorphonuclear leukocyte response.

DIAGNOSIS

The disease characteristically demonstrates rose bengal staining of the superior cornea and limbal area. The disorder is typically bilateral, although often asymmetric. The superior bulbar and palpebral conjunctiva are markedly hyperemic (Color Plate XIV), and the patient complains of moderate to severe foreign body sensation, photophobia, and often sharp pain. A filamentary keratitis involving the superior cornea occurs in approximately one-third of cases and is the cause of particularly severe irritation.[130]

SLK must be differentiated from limbal vernal conjunctivitis, marginal ulcers, phlyctenulosis, and some presentations of atopic conjunctivitis. The eosinophilic response and extreme itching of vernal disease are absent in SLK, and phlyctenulosis and marginal corneal ulcer secondary to microbial hypersensitivity characteristically do not involve the palpebral conjunctiva. Atopic disease typically involves various areas of the scalp and face along with the ocular manifestations.

MANAGEMENT

SLK is usually a chronic disorder exhibiting periods of exacerbation and remission. The disorder tends to run a course of several months to years, and although often quite annoying, rarely does it result in significant sequelae. Pannus formation, however, is not uncommon in severe cases. Management is aimed at making the patient as comfortable as possible.

Although the condition is relatively unresponsive to topical corticosteroids, an immune mechanism is suggested because of the lack of recoverable infective organisms. Artificial tear preparations often improve the patient's comfort, and a pulse of topical steroids may reduce inflammation.

Application of 0.5% silver nitrate solution on a cotton swab results in keratinization and eventual sloughing of the treated conjunctival area. This procedure may provide relief from symptoms lasting from 6 to 8 weeks after treatment. Bandage soft contact lenses can be effective in relieving symptoms. Thermal cautery of the superior bulbar conjunctiva has been shown to be highly effective and represents a simple, low-risk procedure that should be considered before conjunctival resection.[131] Surgical resection of the superior bulbar conjunctiva, however, has produced permanent remission in many patients and now appears to be the treatment of choice in severe cases or in cases unresponsive to medical therapy.

Subconjunctival Hemorrhage

Subconjunctival hemorrhage (see Fig. 21.14) is commonly encountered in a variety of traumatic and infectious conditions. Hemorrhagic conjunctivitis due to adenovirus (EKC) is common in clinical practice and is easily recognized by the associated follicular hypertrophy, preauricular lymphadenopathy, and absence of trauma.[132] *S. pneumoniae* and *Haemophilus* species also commonly produce conjunctival petechiae that often progress to frank subconjunctival hemorrhage.

Typical Valsalva's maneuvers, such as lifting weights or straining at stool, raise the episcleral venous pressure to the point of rupture of conjunctival vessels, especially in adults over 50 years of age, in whom the blood vessels are particularly friable due to generalized vascular disease. Anemia and conjunctival microvascular anomalies are also common causative agents. Recurrent subconjunctival hemorrhages without explainable cause should be investigated for underlying systemic abnormalities.[132]

Initial treatment includes cool compresses to reduce the typically mild inflammation induced by the hemorrhage, followed by warm compresses to speed reabsorption of the hemorrhage. Reassurance is beneficial, since many patients are initially alarmed by the striking cosmetic appearance of the hemorrhage.

TABLE 21.12
Summary of Differential Diagnosis and Management of Miscellaneous Conjunctival Disorders

Condition	Symptoms	Signs	Cytology	Management
Phlyctenular conjunctivitis	Mild to moderately severe burning and foreign body sensation	Elevated conjunctival nodule with intense hyperemia	Epithelial cells	Topical steroid (prednisolone acetate 1%) q1h–q2h on a tapering dose; oral tetracycline (1 g daily, decreasing over 2–4 weeks) in patients more than 8 years old. Evaluate for tuberculosis.
Pinguecula	Cosmetic to mild irritation	Elevated vascularized hyperplastic conjunctiva	Nonspecific epithelial degeneration	Intermittent topical decongestants or artificial tears; pulse of topical steroid if inflamed. Surgical resection with recurrent inflammation.
Pterygium	Cosmetic to mild irritation; decreased visual acuity if visual axis is involved	Vascularized conjunctival hyperplasia encroaching onto cornea, typically in interpalpebral distribution	Same as pinguecula	Surgical excision followed by beta radiation or Thiotepa (1:2000 q3h for 6–8 weeks)
Superior limbic keratoconjunctivitis	Moderate to severe foreign body sensation; photophobia, sharp pain	Superior bulbar and palpebral conjunctival hyperemia with superior filamentary keratitis in ⅓ of cases	PMN response	Artificial tears (q2h–q4h); 0.5% silver nitrate cautery to involved area; bandage soft contact lenses; surgical resection of superior bulbar conjunctiva in severe cases.
Subconjunctival hemorrhage	Cosmetic	Purple to red subconjunctival lesion with irregular margin	Nonspecific	Cool compresses q4h for 1–2 days followed by warm compresses
Conjunctival abrasion or laceration	Ocular pain; foreign body sensation	Localized conjunctival hyperemia, chemosis, and subconjunctival hemorrhage		Topical gentamicin ointment prophylactically; pressure-patch; warm compresses; oral analgesics

Conjunctival Abrasions and Lacerations

ETIOLOGY

Conjunctival abrasions, although not encountered as frequently as conjunctival infection or inflammation, are nevertheless a relatively common entity in clinical practice. Conjunctival lacerations are much less commonly seen and are often associated with more generalized trauma to the globe and adnexa. They are significant because they may conceal a penetrating or even perforating injury to the underlying sclera.[133]

Conjunctival abrasions most often involve the exposed bulbar conjunctiva and consist of mechanical removal of the superficial conjunctival epithelium, often without damage to the underlying substantia propria. Conjunctival lacerations represent an injury to the conjunctiva caused by a sharp object penetrating conjunctival epithelium, stroma, Tenon's capsule, and episclera.

DIAGNOSIS

A conjunctival abrasion exhibits prominent staining with sodium fluorescein. Localized conjunctival hyperemia, chemosis, and subconjunctival hemorrhage are common. The patient typically reports mild to moderate ocular pain and foreign body sensation. On cursory examination a conjunctival laceration may appear somewhat similar to a conjunctival abrasion, but movement of the eye away from the side of the injury will often make the edges of the laceration more visible.

MANAGEMENT

The eye with a conjunctival abrasion should be thoroughly irrigated with sterile saline solution to remove any retained foreign material. A topical broad-spectrum antibiotic, such as gentamicin, should be used prophylactically, especially in large abrasions in which pressure-patching may aid the healing process and reduce patient discomfort. Warm compresses can be applied several times a day to aid in resorption of subconjunctival hemorrhage. Oral analgesics may be necessary to control pain.[133]

Lacerating or perforating injuries of the bulbar conjunctiva may conceal a penetrating or perforating injury of the underlying sclera. The associated chemosis and hemorrhage often make it difficult to rule out the presence of underlying prolapsed uvea, retina, or vitreous. Thus, every conjunctival laceration should be initially treated as though the globe has been perforated.[133] Careful slit-lamp examination should be performed using topical anesthesia, since exploration with forceps may be necessary to properly visualize the area of sclera in question. Pressure on the globe should be minimized to avoid potential prolapse of intraocular tissue. Dissection of the conjunctiva under the operating microscope may be required in the presence of significant conjunctival chemosis and hemorrhage. Indirect ophthalmoscopy through a widely dilated pupil should always be undertaken to further rule out the possibility of perforating injury. Although small perforations of the globe are often self-sealing, low intraocular pressure may provide evidence of perforation.[134]

Conjunctival lacerations typically heal rapidly without complications, although treatment with topical antibiotics is recommended to prevent infection. Only in cases of significant tissue loss is primary surgical repair necessary, since normal healing is usually cosmetically acceptable. Surgical repair of medial lacerations often requires mobilization of adjacent conjunctiva to prevent traction on the caruncle or plica, leading to a poor cosmetic result.[134]

Table 21.12 summarizes the important differential diagnostic and management criteria for the miscellaneous conjunctival disorders.

References

1. Wolff E. Anatomy of the eye and orbit. Philadelphia: W.B. Saunders Co, 1976;7:451.
2. Wolff E. Anatomy of the eye and orbit. Philadelphia: W.B. Saunders Co, 1976;7:438–441.
3. Wolff E. Anatomy of the eye and orbit. Philadelphia: W.B. Saunders Co, 1976;7:205.
4. Apple DJ, Rabb MF. Clinicopathologic correlation of ocular disease. St Louis: C.V. Mosby Co, 1978;2:457.
5. Wolff E. Anatomy of the eye and orbit. Philadelphia: W.B. Saunders Co, 1976;7:206.
6. Apple DJ, Rabb MF. Clinicopathologic correlation of ocular disease. St Louis: C.V. Mosby Co, 1978;2:458.
7. Wolff E. Anatomy of the eye and orbit. Philadelphia: W.B. Saunders Co, 1976;7:210.
8. Wolff E. Anatomy of the eye and orbit. Philadelphia: W.B. Saunders Co, 1976;7:211.
9. Bron AJ, Mengher LS, Davey CC. The normal conjunctiva and its response to inflammation. Trans Ophthalmol Soc UK 1985;104:424–435.
10. Apple DJ, Rabb MF. Clinicopathologic correlation of ocular disease. St. Louis: C.V. Mosby Co, 1978;2:465.
11. Lennett EH, Balows A, Hausler WJ, Truant JP. Manual of clinical microbiology. Washington, DC: American Society of Microbiology, 1980;3:974.
12. Lennette EH, Balows A, Hausler WJ, Truant JP. Manual of clinical microbiology. Washington, DC: American Society of Microbiology, 1980;3:978.
13. Lennette EH, Balows A, Hausler WJ, Truant JP. Manual of clinical microbiology. Washington, DC: American Society of Microbiology, 1980;3:125,332.
14. Lennette EH, Balows A, Hausler WJ, Truant JP. Manual of clinical microbiology. Washington, DC: American Society of Microbiology, 1980;3:84.
15. Lennette EH, Balows A, Hausler WJ, Truant JP. Manual of clinical microbiology. Washington, DC: American Society of Microbiology, 1980;3:994.
16. Lennette EH, Balows A, Hausler WJ, Truant JP. Manual of clinical microbiology. Washington, DC: American Society of Microbiology, 1980;3:760.
17. Kleinfeld J, Ellis PP. Effects of topical anesthetics on growth of microorganisms. Arch Ophthalmol 1966;76:712–715.
18. Wilson LA. Bacterial conjunctivitis. In: Duane TD, Jaeger EA, eds. Clinical ophthalmology. Hagerstown,MD: Harper & Row, 1987;vol 4; Chap. 5:1–16.
19. Rapoza PA, Johnson S, Taylor HR. Platinum spatula vs Dacron swab in the preparation of conjunctival smears. Am J Ophthalmol 1986;102:400–401.
20. McNutt J, Allen SD, Wilson LA, et al. Anaerobic flora of the normal human conjunctival sac. Arch Ophthalmol 1978:96:1448.
21. Meek ES, Golden B. Conjunctivitis and scleritis. In: Hoeprich PD, ed. Infectious diseases. Hagerstown,MD: Harper & Row, 1977;2:1172.
22. Wilson LA. Bacterial conjunctivitis. In: Duane TD, Jaeger EA, eds. Clinical ophthalmology. Hagerstown,MD: Harper & Row, 1987;vol 4; Chap. 5:9.
23. Wan WL, Farkas GC, May WN, et al. The clinical char-

acteristics and course of adult gonococcal conjunctivitis. Am J Ophthalmol 1986;102:575–583.

24. Watt PJ. Pathogenic mechanisms of organisms virulent to the eye. Trans Ophthalmol Soc UK 1986;105:26–31.

25. Havener WH. Ocular pharmacology. St Louis: C.V. Mosby Co, 1978;4:647.

26. Kestelyn P, Meheus A. Gonococcal conjunctivitis (letter). Br J Ophthalmol 1986;70:875–876.

27. Zajdowicz TR, Kerbs SB, Berg SW, et al. Laboratory-acquired gonococcal conjunctivitis: Successful treatment with single-dose ceftriazone. Sex Transm Dis 1984;11:28–29.

28. Havener WH. Ocular pharmacology. St Louis: C.V. Mosby Co, 1978;4:648.

29. Havener WH. Ocular pharmacology. St. Louis: C.V. Mosby Co, 1978;4:557–583.

30. Fedukowicz HB. External infections of the eye. New York: Appleton-Century-Crofts, 1978;2:126.

31. Fedukowicz HB. External infections of the eye. New York: Appleton-Century-Crofts, 1978;2:160.

32. Baum JL. Antibotic use in ophthalmology. In: Duane TD, Jaeger EA, eds. Clinical ophthalmology. Hagerstown,MD: Harper & Row, 1987;vol 4; Chap. 26:1–20.

33. Genvert GI, Cohen EJ, Donnenfeld ED, et al. Erythema multiforme after use of topical sulfacetamide. Am J Ophthalmol 1985;99:465–468.

34. Gibson JR. Trimethoprim-polymyxin B ophthalmic solution in the treatment of presumptive bacterial conjunctivitis—a multicentre trial of its efficacy versus neomycin–polymyxin B–gramicidin and chloramphenicol ophthalmic solutions. J Antimicrob Chemother 1983;11:217–221.

35. Fraunfelder FT, Bagby GC, Kelly DJ. Fatal aplastic anemia following topical administration of ophthalmic chloramphenicol. Am J Ophthalmol 1982;93:356–360.

36. Nozik RA, Smolin G, Knowlton G, et al. Trimethoprim-polymyxin B ophthalmic solution in treatment of surface ocular bacterial infections. Ann Ophthalmol 1985;17:746–748.

37. Awan KJ. Mydriasis and conjunctival paresthesia from local gentamicin (letter). Am J Ophthalmol 1985;99:723–724.

38. Annable WI. Therapy for ocular infections. Pediatr Clin North Am 1983;30:389–396.

39. McGill JI. Bacterial conjunctivitis. Trans Ophthalmol Soc UK 1986;105:37–40.

40. Hvidberg J. Fusidic acid in acute conjunctivitis. Acta Ophthalmologica 1987;65:43–47.

41. Van Bijsterveld OP, el Batawi Y, Sobhi FS, et al. Fusidic acid in infections of the external eye. Infection 1987;15:16–19.

42. Fleischer AB, Hoover DL, Khan JA, et al. Topical vancomycin formulation for methicillin-resistant staphylococcus epidermidis blepharoconjunctivitis. Am J Ophthalmol 1986;101:283–287.

43. Insler MS, Gordon RA. Absolute IgG4 deficiency and recurrent bacterial blepharokeratoconjunctivitis (letter). Am J Ophthalmol 1984;98:243–244.

44. Sandstrom KI, Bell TA, Chandler JW, et al. Microbial causes of neonatal conjunctivitis. J Pediatr 1984;105:706–711.

45. Brook I, Barrett CT, Brinkman CR, et al. Aerobic and anaerobic bacterial flora of the maternal cervix and newborn gastric fluid and conjunctiva: A prospective study. Pediatrics 1979;63:451–455.

46. Rapoza PA, Quinn TC, Kiessling LA, et al. Epidemiology of neonatal conjunctivitis. Ophthalmology 1986;93:456–461.

47. Chandler JW, Alexander ER, Pheiffer TA, et al. Ophthalmia neonatorum associated with maternal chlamydial infections. Ophthalmology 1977;83:302–308.

48. Stenberg K, Mardh PA. Persistent neonatal chlamydial infection in a 6 year old girl (letter). Lancet 1986;2:1278–1279.

49. Duggan MA, Pomponi C, Kay D, et al. Infantile chlamydial conjunctivitis. A comparison of Papanicolaou, Giemsa and immunoperoxidase staining methods. Acta Cytol 1986;30:341–346.

50. Hanshaw JB, Dudgeon JA. Viral diseases of the fetus and newborn. Maj Prob Clin Pediatr 1978;17:356.

51. Darougar S, Trehavne JD, Minassian D, et al. Rapid serological test for diagnosis of chlamydial ocular infections. Br J Ophthalmol 1978;62:503.

52. Havener WH. Ocular pharmacology. St Louis: C.V. Mosby Co, 1978;4:645.

53. Oriel JD. Ophthalmia neonatorum: Relative efficacy of current prophylactic practices and treatment. J Antimicrob Chemother 1984;14:209–219.

54. Havener WH. Ocular pharmacology. St Louis: C.V. Mosby Co, 1978;4:646–647.

55. Lockie P, Leong LK, Louis A. Penicillinase-producing *Neisseria gonorrhoea* as a cause of neonatal and adult ophthalmia. Aust NZ J Ophthhalmol 1986;14:49–53.

56. Fransen L, Nsanze H, D'Costa L, et al. Single-dose kanamycin therapy of gonococcal ophthalmia neonatorum. Lancet 1984 Dec 1;2:1234–1237.

57. Laga M, Naamara W, Brunham RC, et al. Single dose therapy of gonococcal ophthalmia neonatorum with ceftriaxone. N Engl J Med 1986;315:1382–1385.

58. Traboulsi EI, Shammas IV, Ratl HE, et al. Pseudomonas aeruginosa ophthalmia neonatorum (letter). Am J Ophthalmol 1984;98:801–802.

59. Alpert G, Plotkin SA. Recurrent conjunctivitis in neonatal herpes infection. Pediatr Infect Dis 1983;2:311–312.

60. Allansmith MR, Ross RN. Ocular allergy and mast cell stabilizers. Surv Ophthalmol 1986;30:229–244.

61. Woodward DF, Spada CS, Hawley SB, et al. Conjunctival eosinophil infiltration evoked by histamine and immediate hypersensitivity. Modification by H_1- and H_2-receptor blockade. Invest Ophthalmol Vis Sci 1986;27:1495–1503.

62. Dart JK, Buckley RJ, Monnickendan M, et al. Perennial allergic conjunctivitis: Definition, clinical characteristics and prevalence. A comparison with seasonal allergic conjunctivitis. Trans Ophthalmol Soc UK 1986;105:513–520.

63. Marrache F, Brunet D, Frandeboeuf J, et al. The role of ocular manifestations in childhood allergy syndromes. Rev Fr Allergol Immunol Clin 1978;18:151–155.

64. Fernandez-Vozmediano JM, Blasi NA, Romero-Cabrera MA, et al. Allergic contact dermatitis to timolol. Contact Derm 1986;14:252.

65. Fisher AA. Allergic reactions to contact lens solutions. Cutis 1985;36:209–211.

66. Tada R, Yuasa T, Shimomura Y. Response of the con-

junctiva in atopic diseases. Acta Soc Ophthalmol Jpn 1979;83:921.

67. Duzman E, Warman A, Warman R. Efficacy and safety of topical oxymetazoline in treating allergic and environmental conjunctivitis. Ann Ophthalmol 1986;18:28–31.

68. Kemp JP, Buckley CE, Gershwin ME, et al. Multi-center, double-blind, placebo-controlled trial of terfenadine in seasonal allergic rhinitis and conjunctivitis. Ann Allergy 1985; 54:502–509.

69. Lindsay-Miller ACM. Group comparative trial of 2% sodium cromoglycate (Opticrom) with placebo in the treatment of seasonal allergic conjunctivitis. Clin Allergy 1979;9:271.

70. Vakil DV, Ayiomamitis A, Nizami RM. Treatment of seasonal conjunctivitis: Comparison of 2% and 4% sodium cromoglycate ophthalmic solutions. Can J Ophthalmol 1984;19:207–211.

71. Srinivasan RD, Jakobiec FA, Iwamoto T, et al. Giant papillary conjunctivitis with ocular prostheses. Arch Ophthalmol 1979;97:892.

72. Fowler SA, Greiner JV, Allansmith MR. Soft contact lenses from patients with giant papillary conjunctivitis. Am J Ophthalmol 1979;88:1056.

73. Ballow M, Donshik PC, Rapaca P, et al. Tear lactoferrin levels in patients with external inflammatory ocular disease. Invest Ophthalmol Vis Sci 1987;28:543–545.

74. Henriquez AS, Allansmith MR. Russell bodies in contact lens associated giant papillary conjunctivitis. Arch Ophthalmol 1979;97:473.

75. Donshik PC, Ballow M, Luistro A, et al. Treatment of contact lens-induced giant papillary conjunctivitis. CLAO. 1984;10:346–350.

76. Abelson MB, Butrus SI, Weston JH. Aspirin therapy in vernal conjunctivitis. Am J Ophthalmol 1983;95:502–505.

77. Allansmith MR, Baird RS, Greiner JV. Vernal conjunctivitis and contact lenses-associated papillary conjunctivitis compared and contrasted. Am J Ophthalmol 1979;87:544–555.

78. Allansmith MR. Vernal conjunctivitis. In: Duane TD, Jaeger EA, eds. Clinical ophthalmology. Hagerstown,MD: Harper & Row, 1987;vol. 4; Chap. 9:1–8.

79. BenEzra D, Pe'er J, Brodsky M, et al. Cyclosporine eyedrops for the treatment of severe vernal keratoconjunctivitis. Am J Ophthalmol 1986;101:278–282.

80. Nahmias AJ, Starr SE. Infections caused by herpes simplex viruses. In: Hoeprich PD, ed. Infectious diseases. Hagerstown, MD: Harper & Row, 1977;2:727.

81. Lass JH, Thoft RA, Dohlman CH. Idoxuridine-induced conjunctival cicatrization. Arch Ophthalmol 1983;101:747–750.

82. Havener WH. Ocular pharmacology. St Louis: C.V. Mosby Co, 1978;4:382–383.

83. Fedukowicz HB. External infections of the eye. New York: Appleton-Century-Crofts, 1978;2:211–214.

84. O'Donnell B, Bell E, Payne SB, et al. Genome analysis of species 3 adenoviruses isolated during summer out-breaks conjunctivitis and pharyngoconjunctival fever in the Glasgow and London areas in 1981. J Med Virol 1986;18:213–227.

85. Taylor JW, Chandler JW, Cooney MK. Conjunctivitis due to adenovirus type 19. J Clin Microbiol 1978;8:209–213.

86. Jawetz E, Kimura S, Nicholas AW, et al. New type of apc virus from epidemic keratoconjunctivitis. Science 1955; 122:1190.

87. Dawson C, Hanna L, Wood TR, et al. Adenovirus type 8 keratoconjunctivitis in the United States. Epidemic, clinical and microbiologic features. Am J Ophthalmol 1970;69:473.

88. Kemp MC, Hierholzer JC, Cabradilla CP, et al. The changing etiology of epidemic keratoconjunctivitis: Antigenic and restriction enzyme analyses of adenovirus types 19 and 37 isolated over a 10-year period. J Infect Dis 1983;148:24–33.

89. Aoki K, Kawana R, Matsumoto I, et al. Viral conjunctivitis with special reference to adenovirus type 37 and enterovirus 70 infection. Jpn J Ophthalmol 1986;30:158–164.

90. Thygeson P. Office and dispensary transmissions of epidemic keratoconjunctivitis. Am J Ophthalmol 1957;43:98.

91. Manor RS, Cohen S, Ben-Sira T. Bilateral acute retrobulbar optic neuropathy associated with epidemic keratoconjunctivitis in a compromised host (letter). Arch Ophthalmol 1986;104:1271–1272.

92. Darougar S, Hunter PA, Viwalingam M, et al. Acute follicular conjunctivitis and keratoconjunctivitis due to herpes simplex virus in London. Br J Ophthalmol 1978;62:843–849.

93. Laibson PR, Dhiri S, Oconer J, et al. Corneal infiltrates in epidemic keratoconjunctivitis. Arch Ophthalmol 1970;84:36–40.

94. Hiti H, Hanselmayer H, Hofmann H. Experience in therapy and prophylaxis of epidemic keratoconjunctivitis (abstr.). Klin Monatsbl Augenheikd 1979;174:456–461.

95. Adams CP Jr, Cohen EJ, Albrecht J, et al. Interferon treatment of adenoviral conjunctivitis. Am J Ophthalmol 1984;98:429–432.

96. Doug-Deen R, Paul R, Watson B, et al. Acute hemorrhagic conjunctivitis caused by coxsackievirus A24-caribbean. MMWR 1987;36:245–251.

97. Bucci FA Jr, Savia PV Jr, Mauriello JA Jr. Herpes zoster ophthalmicus. Am Fam Phys 1987;35:121–128.

98. Fedukowicz HB. External infections of the eye. New York: Appleton-Century-Crofts, 1978;2:208–211.

99. Fedukowicz HB. External infections of the eye. New York: Appleton-Century-Crofts, 1978;2:214–216.

100. Fedukowicz HB. External infections of the eye. New York: Appleton-Century-Crofts, 1978;2:217–218.

101. Fourth WHO Scientific Group on Trachoma Research: Report WHO Tech Rep series no. 330, 1966.

102. Insler MS, Anderson AB, Murray M. Latent oculogenital infection with *Chlamydia trachomatis*. Ophthalmology 1987;94:27–29.

103. Fedukowicz HB. External infections of the eye. New York: Appleton-Century-Crofts, 1978;2:177.

104. Dawson CR. Follicular conjunctivitis. In: Duane TD, Jaeger EA, eds. Clinical ophthalmology. Hagerstown, MD: Harper & Row, 1987;vol. 4; Chap. 7:1–19.

105. Darougar S, Jones BR, Viswalingam N, et al. Topical therapy of hyperendemic trachoma with rifampicin, oxytetracycline, or spiramycin eye ointments. Br J Ophthalmol 1980;64:37–42.

106. Ozawa H, Hosaka S, Kunitomo T, et al. Ocular inserts for

controlled release of antibiotics. Biomaterials 1983;4:170–174.

107. Viswalingam ND, Darougar S, Yearsley P. Oral doxycycline in the treatment of adult chlamydial ophthalmia. Br J Ophthalmol 1986;70:301–304.

108. Mathias CGT, Maibach HI, Irvine A, et al. Allergic contact dermatitis to echothiophate iodide and phenylephrine. Arch Ophthalmol 1979;97:286–287.

109. Dawson CR. Follicular conjunctivitis. In: Duane TD, Jaeger EA, eds. Clinical ophthalmology. Hagerstown, MD: Harper & Row, 1987;vol. 4; Chap. 7:16.

110. Fedukowicz HB. External infections of the eye. New York: Appleton-Century-Crofts, 1978;2:153.

111. Kowalski RP, Harwick JC. Incidence of *Moraxella* conjunctival infection. Am J Ophthalmol 1986;101:437–440.

112. Dawson CR. Follicular conjunctivitis. In: Duane TD, Jaeger EA, eds. Clinical ophthalmology. Hagerstown, MD: Harper & Row, 1987;vol. 4; Chap. 7:17–18.

113. Streeten BW, Streeten EA. "Blue-body" epithelial cell inclusions in conjunctivitis. Ophthalmology 1985;92:575–579.

114. Cohen JM. Cromolyn for chemotherapy conjunctivitis (letter). J Clin Oncol 1985;3:1690.

115. Jenkins MS, Brown SI, Lempert SL, et al. Ocular rosacea. Am J Ophthalmol 1979;88:618–622.

116. Vajpayee RB, Gupta SK, Uppal RK. Evaluation of sodium cromoglycate and medrysone in the management of atopic keratoconjunctivitis: A double masked clinical study. Aust NZ J Ophthalmol 1986;14:251–253.

117. Hoting E, Paul E, Plewig G. Treatment of rosacea with isotretinoin. Int J Dermatol 1986;25:660–663.

118. Leino M, Touvinen E. Clinical trial of the topical use of disodium cromoglycate in vernal, allergic, and chronic conjunctivitis. Acta Ophthalmol 1980;58:121–124.

119. Mondino BJ, Brown SI, Lempert S, et al. Acute manifestations of ocular cicatricial pemphigoid: Diagnosis and treatment. Ophthalmology 1979;89:543–552.

120. Dohlman CH, Doughamm DJ. The Stevens-Johnson syndrome. In: Symposium on cornea. Trans New Orleans Acad Ophthalmol. St Louis: C.V. Mosby Co, 1972;236–252.

121. Robbins SL, Angell M. Basic pathology. Philadelphia: W.B. Saunders Co, 1976;2:182–201.

122. Rose GA. The natural history of polyarteritis. Br Med J 1957;2:1148.

123. Miehle W. Reiter's syndrome. Fortsehr Med 1979;97:182–186.

124. Sorsby A. The aetiology of phlyctenular ophthalmia. Br J Ophthalmol 1942;26:159–179, 189–215.

125. Abu el Asrar AM, Geboes K, Maudgal PC, et al. Immunocytological study of phlyctenular eye disease. Int Ophthalmol 1987;10:33–39.

126. Thygeson P. Observations of nontuberculosis phlyctenular keratoconjunctivitis. Trans Am Acad Ophthalmol Otolaryngol 1954;58:128.

127. Orlander K, Haik KG, Haik GM. Management of pterygia: Should Thiotepa be used? Ann Ophthalmol 1978;7:853–861.

128. Apple DJ, Rabb MF. Clinicopathologic correlation of ocular disease. St Louis: C.V. Mosby Co, 1978;2:474–475.

129. Wilson FM, Ostler HB. Superior limbic keratoconjunctivitis. Int Ophthalmol Clin 1986;26:99–112.

130. Eifevman RA, Wilkins EL. Immunological aspects of superior limbic keratoconjunctivitis. Can J Ophthalmol 1979;14:85–87.

131. Udell IJ, Kenyon KR, Sawa M, et al. Treatment of superior limbic keratoconjunctivitis by thermocauterization of the superior bulbar conjunctiva. Ophthalmology 1986;93:162–166.

132. Wilson RJ. Subconjunctival hemorrhage: Overview and management. J Am Optom Assoc 1986;57:376–380.

133. Locke LC. Conjunctival abrasions and lacerations. J Am Optom Assoc 1987;58:488–493.

134. Goldberg MF, Paton D. Management of ocular injuries. Philadelphia: W.B. Saunders Co, 1976;214–235.

135. Ullman S, Roussel TJ, Forster RK. Gonoccocal keratoconjunctivitis. Surv Ophthalmol 1987;32:199–208.

136. Timewell RM, Rosenthal AL, Smith JP, et al. Safety and efficacy of tobramycin and gentamicin sulfate in the treatment of external ocular infections of children. J Pediatr Ophthalmol Strabismus 1983;20:22–26.

137. Gigliotti F, Hendley O, Morgan J, et al. Efficacy of topical antibiotic therapy for acute conjunctivitis in children. J Pediatr 1984;104:623–626.

138. Baum J. Therapy for ocular bacterial infection. Trans Ophthalmol Soc UK 1986;105:69–77.

139. Laga M, Plummer FA, Piot P, et al. Prophylaxis of gonococcal and chlamydial ophthalmia neonatorum. N Engl J Med 1988;318:653.

140. Cho MH, Norden LC, Chang FW. Disposable extended-wear soft contact lenses for the treatment of giant papillary conjunctivitis. South J Optom 1988;6:9–12.

141. Wood TS, Stewart RH, Bowman RW, et al. Suprofen treatment of contact lens-associated giant papillary conjunctivitis. Ophthalmology 1988;95:822–826.

142. Aswad MI, Tauber J, Baum J. Plasmapheresis treatment in patients with severe atopic keratoconjunctivitis. Ophthalmology 1988;95:444–447.

143. Jaros PA, DeLuise VP. Pingueculae and pterygia. Surv Ophthalmol 1988;33:41–49.

144. Aswad MI, Baum J. Optimal time for postoperative irradiation of pterygia. Ophthalmology 1987;94:1450–1451.

CHAPTER 22

Diseases of the Cornea

Jack E. Terry

The cornea is one of the most important ocular structures, considering the prevalence and clinical significance of disorders that affect it.[1] The maintenance of normal corneal integrity is crucial in sustaining normal visual acuity. The possible sequelae of corneal disease include ulceration, corneal pannus and scarring, secondary uveitis, and endophthalmitis. This chapter considers the diagnosis and management of the most common corneal diseases encountered in clinical practice.

Examination

The examination of patients with corneal disease is facilitated by many of the same basic techniques that are performed routinely on any eyecare patient; these include case history, visual acuities, gross external and corneal observations, corneal sensitivity, and biomicroscopy including vital staining.

History

The initial aspect of the history of a patient with a corneal disorder is the specific complaint. This can range from the more subtle intermittent blur experienced by patients with corneal edema to the severe pain of those with bacterial corneal ulcers. Since many corneal disorders are due to trauma, the exact nature and circumstances of the injury must be obtained. A number of corneal disorders become activated or exaggerated in response to various trigger mechanisms. These include seasonal variations, changes in humidity,

exposure to ultraviolet light, or fever. Any daily fluctuation of symptoms should be noted.

The medication history of the patient also must be determined. The preservatives in many ophthalmic medications can cause, with long-term use, a toxic superficial punctate keratitis. The phenylmercuric and thimerosal agents also have been associated with calcific band keratopathy. Various anti-infective agents such as idoxuridine (IDU) and gentamicin can cause a keratitis.

The family history is often helpful, since a number of corneal disorders have a genetic basis. In addition, knowledge of the patient's systemic disease history is mandatory.

Visual Acuity

The cornea is normally transparent because of its fibril uniformity, avascularity, and deturgescence. However, in numerous corneal diseases, visual acuity decreases. Hence, the accurate determination of best correctable or pinhole visual acuity is essential for the detection, diagnosis, and subsequent follow-up of the diseased cornea.

Gross Observation

As the practitioner begins to evaluate the patient with suspected corneal disease, any gross abnormalities of the skin, face, eyelids, conjunctiva, and pupils should be noted. Conditions affecting the periorbital area or conjunctiva, such as rosacea, herpes labialis, or herpes zoster, may be associated with corneal disease.

Biomicroscopy

Examination of the cornea is facilitated by use of the slit lamp because it provides variable magnification with stereopsis. The cornea can be evaluated using almost every slit-lamp evaluation technique.[2] When using the direct technique and its subtypes, the practitioner should frequently look to the side of the illuminated area to gain an indirect view. In this way many minor and subtle changes can be detected. Also, use of specular reflection, sclerotic scatter, and retroillumination techniques can frequently assist the practitioner in evaluating an abnormal cornea.

It is crucial to augment slit-lamp examination of the cornea with the use of vital stains, including sodium fluorescein and rose bengal.

General Forms of Superficial Keratitis

Since critical information is obtained by direct observation of the cornea, the clinician can often either greatly simplify the diagnostic possibilities or make the diagnosis outright by carefully scrutinizing the pattern and location of the keratitis. Several types of superficial keratitis are shown in Figure 22.1 and include punctate epithelial erosions, punctate epithelial keratitis, punctate subepithelial infiltrates, and filamentary keratitis.

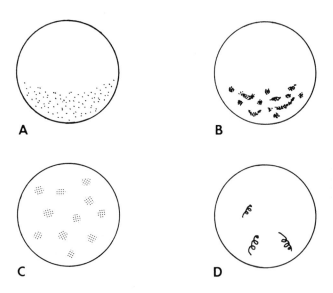

FIGURE 22.1   **Various types of superficial corneal involvement diagrammatically represented. (A) Punctate epithelial erosions (PEE). (B) Punctate epithelial keratitis (PEK). (C) Punctate subepithelial infiltrates. (D) Filamentary keratitis (keratopathy).**

Punctate Epithelial Erosions

Punctate epithelial erosions (PEE) are fine depressions or pits extending through or partially through the epithelium (see Fig. 22.1A). These can be detected when viewed under high magnification with the slit-lamp biomicroscope. Although quite common clinically, PEE may be very difficult to see with direct illumination due to their transparency; however, the tiny pits stain brightly with sodium fluorescein[3] (Fig. 22.2). Photophobia, foreign body sensation, and tearing often accompany these erosions, whose specific location on the cornea may give a clue about their etiology.

Punctate Epithelial Keratitis

In contrast to punctate epithelial erosions, punctate epithelial keratitis (PEK) presents as an area of white or gray opaque spots that are easily seen with direct slit-lamp illumination (see Fig. 22.1B). They can vary in size, shape, and location. Rose bengal stains these areas more prominently than does sodium fluorescein.[4] PEK is often seen in conjunction with PEE, and, as with PEE, location may help determine etiology.

Punctate Subepithelial Infiltrates

Punctate subepithelial infiltrates appear as clusters of gray-white to yellow spots in the superficial stroma, just beneath Bowman's layer (see Fig. 22.1C). These lesions are often sequelae to PEE or PEK, producing a more intense epithelial-subepithelial involvement. Often the epithelium will heal, leaving punctate subepithelial infiltrative involvement.[3]

Filamentary Keratitis (Keratopathy)

Once thought to be idiopathic, filamentary keratitis is now known to be caused by specific entities. The most common etiologies are listed in Table 22.1. Filamentary keratitis is usually a chronic disease characterized by short stalks or strands of proliferative hyperplastic epithelial cells protruding anterior to the corneal surface (Figs. 22.1D and 22.3). Most likely, these coiled epithelial cells are produced by aberrant epithelial healing.[5] Therefore, any condition causing localized epithelial erosions may produce filamentary keratitis. Mucus strands are often seen attached to the filaments, aggravating the condition.[3] Beneath the attachment site, there may be a gray subepithelial granular opacity. The patient with filamentary keratitis frequently has symptoms that include foreign body sensation, photo-

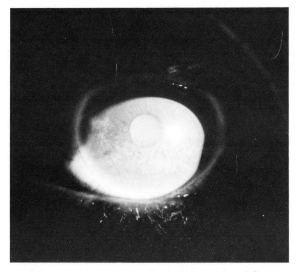

FIGURE 22.2   **Inferior punctate epithelial erosions of the cornea associated with staphylococcal blepharitis.**

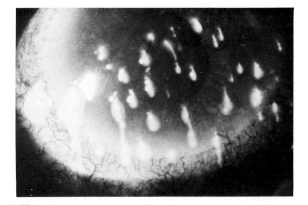

FIGURE 22.3   **Strands of corneal epithelium in filamentary keratitis associated with Sjögren's syndrome. (Courtesy William Wallace, O.D.)**

phobia, blepharospasm, increased blink reflex, and epiphora.[6]

Treatment usually involves identifying the specific etiology so that proper therapy can be administered. However, the use of 5% sodium chloride drops 3 to 4 times daily has been shown to be highly effective[6] regardless of the cause. The filaments can be removed with forceps if their number is small.[3] If a dry eye is suspected, use of ocular lubricants may prevent further filament formation. Topical steroids may be used in severe cases, as can a thin soft contact lens, which usually allows adequate epithelial growth and inhibits further filament proliferation.[7]

TABLE 22.1
Common Etiologies of Filamentary Keratitis

Sjögren's syndrome
Keratitis sicca
Stevens-Johnson syndrome
Pemphigoid
Superior limbic keratoconjunctivitis
Prolonged patching
Radiation or chemical keratitis
Herpes simplex keratitis
Thygeson's keratitis
Recurrent corneal erosion
Trachoma
Retained foreign body of upper lid
Ectodermal dysplasias
Diabetes
Psoriasis

Conditions Affecting the Inferior Cornea

Staphylococcal Blepharitis

ETIOLOGY

In the Western world, *Staphylococcus aureus* is probably the single most common cause of bacterial conjunctivitis and blepharoconjunctivitis. The presence of *S. aureus* in the conjunctival sac and on the lid margins varies among countries, apparently according to climate.[3] It is an important feature of the pathogenesis of staphylococcal infection that phagocytosed staphylococci can remain viable for significant intervals and are likely to produce chronic, latent, or smoldering infections of long duration, often characterized by remissions and exacerbations.[8]

DIAGNOSIS

Staphylococcal blepharitis is an infection of the lid margins and glands of the lids by pathogenic staphylococci. It can be classified as two different types.[9] In the common squamous type, hard, brittle, fibrinous scales are evident. The less common ulcerative type is characterized by matted, hard crusts surrounding the cilia. Small ulcers of the hair follicles are found along the lid margins, and bleeding may occur.

Characteristic of both types of staphylococcal blepharitis are dilated blood vessels (rosettes) on the lid margins, white lashes (poliosis), lash loss (madarosis), trichiasis (misdirected lashes), and scales around the cilia.[10]

The principal mechanism of attack by *S. aureus* is the secretion of necrotizing exotoxins. There is almost invariably an associated chronic papillary conjunctivitis due to the liberation of these toxins. Although usually not aggressively invasive, the organism is very toxigenic and can provoke corneal involvement. When this takes place, a broad, amorphous epithelial keratitis of the inferior quadrant of the cornea usually occurs, and inferior punctate epithelial erosions are frequently seen[10] (see Fig. 22.2). Corneal limbal infiltration, which represents an antigen-antibody reaction, and phlyctenulosis, which represents a delayed hypersensitivity reaction to *S. aureus,* are among the other ocular complications due to staphylococcal infection.[11] Conjunctival staining with rose bengal will usually accompany the corneal lesions.

Patients with rosacea have an increased predisposition to develop a staphylococcal blepharoconjunctivitis. It is important, therefore, in the management of rosacea to treat the blepharoconjunctivitis if it is present.[7]

Laboratory findings in *S. aureus* infection include complete hemolysis on blood agar, mannitol fermentation, and coagulase production, with coagulase production being the most conclusive for pathogenicity of the organism.[12]

Staphylococcus epidermidis, which usually exists in low to moderate population density in the normal flora of the outer eye, may, if present in greater numbers, produce the symptoms and signs of staphylococcal blepharitis. These strains have been known to sometimes secrete a necrotizing toxin similar to that of *S. aureus.*[13] Also, *S. epidermidis* is a common contaminant in eye cosmetics and can establish replicating colonies of pathogenic strains.[14]

MANAGEMENT

The first line of defense against staphylococcal blepharitis consists of proper local measures including careful lid hygiene and warm compresses. The patient should be instructed to cleanse the lid margins thoroughly of flakes and debris twice daily, using baby shampoo or eyelid cleanser applied with a cotton-tipped applicator. Warm compresses will help improve circulation, mobilize meibomian gland secretions, and help cleanse crusting deposits on the lashes.[5]

When the above procedures fail to improve the condition, the staphylococcal blepharitis may need to be treated with an antibiotic ointment or solution.[15] In long-standing cases, a culture and antibiotic sensitivity tests are highly recommended to isolate the causative organism and to plan rational therapy. Mild cases can be controlled with 1 daily application of an antibiotic ointment (e.g., erythromycin, bacitracin, or bacitracin-polymyxin B) at bedtime as a lid scrub. Severe cases may require that the ointment be applied 3 or 4 times daily as a lid scrub. Treatment for 7 to 10 days should, in most cases, shorten the course of the disease, al-

though intermittent treatment for many months or years is commonly required to control this chronic condition.

The integrity of the lacrimal drainage system should be evaluated in cases of chronic unilateral staphylococcal infection. Chronic, long-standing blepharitis is due to the inability to eradicate the staphylococcal organism (resistance) or to a hypersensitivity reaction to the staphylococcal exotoxins.[7] In addition to careful lid hygiene, hot compresses, and intermittent topical antibiotics, lash base debridement and oral tetracycline (250 mg 4 times daily for 7 to 10 days) may be necessary to adequately control the condition.[15]

The management of staphylococcal blepharitis is considered in further detail in Chapter 19.

Adult Inclusion Conjunctivitis

ETIOLOGY

Chlamydia trachomatis, a trachoma inclusion conjunctivitis (TRIC) agent, causes adult inclusion conjunctivitis. Morphologically, *Chlamydia* resemble both viruses and bacteria. They probably most resemble rickettsiae, which, like viruses, simulate obligate intracellular parasites.[16] However, some studies suggest that they are most similar to gram-negative bacteria because of the presence of a muramic acid coat containing both RNA and DNA and a susceptibility to antibiotics. Both *Chlamydia* and rickettsiae are cell-wall-defective microbes whose small "bacterial" forms have lost the ability to reproduce as bacteria during evolution.[17]

C. trachomatis organisms infect the superficial mucosal linings of the genitourinary tract and other mucous membranes of the body.[16] Adult inclusion conjunctivitis involves the conjunctiva of one or both eyes, along with the genital or urinary tract infection, and is therefore classified as an oculogenital disease.

DIAGNOSIS

Adult inclusion conjunctivitis presents as an acute follicular conjunctivitis with moderate mucopurulent discharge (see Fig. 21.16). The follicles are seen primarily in the inferior fornix, but occasionally the caruncle and plica will be involved. Papillary hypertrophy may occur, especially in the upper fornix and tarsus. The bulbar conjunctiva displays mild to moderate hyperemia, whereas the palpebral conjunctiva is severely hyperemic.[18]

Corneal involvement usually occurs late in the disease process, but a fine to coarse punctate epithelial keratitis may develop during the second week after onset. The keratitis usually occurs in the inferior half of the cornea (Fig. 22.4) but is not limited to this area.[18] It is occasionally accompanied by marginal or

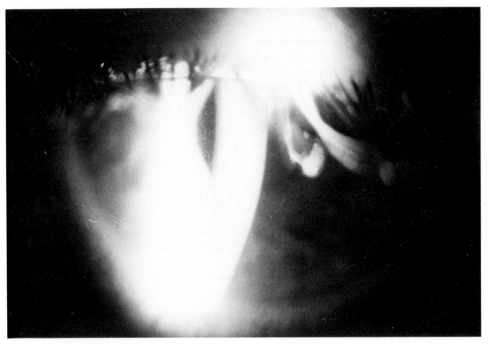

FIGURE 22.4   **Fine epithelial keratitis associated with adult inclusion conjunctivitis.**

central subepithelial infiltrates resembling epidemic keratoconjunctivitis (EKC).[19] The disease usually runs a chronic, remittent course, and in long-standing infections, micropannus, in the form of superficial neovascularization, limbal swelling, and conjunctival involvement resembling trachoma, may be noted. This can be differentiated from trachoma by the absence of Herbert's pits in the cornea, by the flat and sheet-like conjunctival cicatrization as opposed to stellate cicatrization that is seen in trachoma, and by the presence of an accompanying genital or urinary tract infection.[19] Generally, the preauricular lymph node will be swollen on the same side as the affected eye.[18] The disease is rarely accompanied by Reiter's syndrome or an upper respiratory tract infection.[20]

Common symptoms include lid swelling, redness, moderate lacrimation, photophobia, and occasionally a foreign body sensation.[18] The patient may not describe vaginal discharge (female) or urethritis (male), since the genitourinary infection is often asymptomatic and is demonstrable only by cervical or urethral smears.[21]

Inclusion conjunctivitis is most common in young adults, age 18 to 35 years, who have acquired a new sexual partner in the preceding 2 or 3 months.[5] However, there have been reports of infections in young children and adults over age 60 years.[22] *Chlamydia* can form chronic, often quiescent infections in the human genital tract that may be reactivated by urethritis in the male and by gonorrhea or oral contraceptives in the female.[21] *Chlamydia* can be difficult to demonstrate in chronic infections of the eye, and a provocative administration of steroids has occasionally been successful in reactivating the infection.[23]

Before proper chlorination, swimming pools were a major source of transmission of inclusion conjunctivitis. The disease is now known to be transmitted almost exclusively by sexual contact, with subsequent passage by hand from the genital tract to the eye.[24] Once thought to affect both eyes, inclusion conjunctivitis is now known to be unilateral in approximately 70% of cases. The incubation period for the disease is 4 to 12 days.[5] Although the disease affects all social classes, it is slightly more prevalent in groups unable to practice proper hygiene.

Normal bacterial culture techniques will not isolate *Chlamydia,* but they can provide useful information for differential diagnosis, since growth of any significant bacteria in the culture would not be expected. Probably the most common method of diagnosis is the use of cytology smears for morphologic identification, which show Prowazek's intracytoplasmic inclusion bodies in the epithelial cells. These inclusion bodies are indistinguishable from those found in conjunctival samples taken from patients with trachoma, and laboratory findings must be well supported by clinical evidence in making the final diagnosis. *Chlamydia* is isolated more easily by swabbing rather than scraping the conjunctiva, and this is less traumatic to the patient.[25] Inclusions are frequent in very active, acute, severe infections, but they are rare in chronic infections. Predominant neutrophilic and monocytic cellular responses will occur and will aid in the diagnosis of adult inclusion conjunctivitis.[26]

MANAGEMENT

Oral tetracyclines have been accepted as the treatment of choice for adult nongonococcal genital infections attributable to *Chlamydia* as well as for adult inclusion conjunctivitis.[27] Topical antibiotics are relatively ineffective in treating adult inclusion conjunctivitis.[28] There are 3 different tetracycline congeners: short acting, intermediate acting, and long acting (see Table 6.11). The short-acting agents include oxytetracycline and tetracycline, while the intermediate-acting group includes methacycline and demeclocycline. Long-acting tetracycline agents include doxycycline and minocycline.

Milk products and antacids should generally be avoided by the patient, since they decrease blood levels of the tetracycline by as much as 50%. However, the effect of dietary intake is much less significant for doxycycline and minocycline. Hence, if the patient's lifestyle does not permit him or her to take the tetracycline approximately 2 hours before eating, then one of these agents would be the preferred alternative. In addition, patient compliance is often better with either doxycycline or minocycline because they are both taken only twice daily. Minocycline can cause vestibular symptoms, especially in women, that require discontinuation of the antibiotic. However, this is minimized if the dosage is 50 mg 4 times daily. Systemic tetracycline should be avoided during pregnancy because it can cause skeletal and dental abnormalities in the fetus.

The most accepted therapy for adult inclusion conjunctivitis, especially when medication cost is taken into consideration, is oral tetracycline, 250 mg 4 times daily for 21 days, or 500 mg 4 times daily for 14 days. If the clinical situation warrants (e.g., poor patient compliance, incompatible eating schedules), doxycycline 100 mg daily may be the most appropriate choice.[29] During pregnancy and lactation, erythromycin, 500 mg 4 times daily for 14 days, should be substituted. Systemic tetracyclines are also contraindicated for use in young children (8 years or younger) and therefore cannot be used against neonatal inclusion conjunctivitis. Topical erythromycin 0.5% ointment and oral erythromycin ethylsuccinate, 25 mg/kg body weight, should be prescribed every 12 hours for 14 days.[30] It is important to note that milk increases the systemic absorption of systemic erythromycin succinate.[30]

Exposure Keratitis (Keratopathy)

ETIOLOGY

Any condition causing incomplete lid closure or inadequate corneal coverage by the lids may lead to exposure keratitis. Although many etiologies exist, the most common causes are Bell's palsy, proptosis (especially in Graves' disease), nocturnal lagophthalmos, and extreme ectropion.[5]

DIAGNOSIS

Clinically, slit-lamp examination reveals punctate corneal staining with sodium fluorescein in the inferior interpalpebral area of the cornea and conjunctiva (Color Plate VIII). The desiccation is due to inadequate corneal moistening and can produce a very painful, injected eye. Although the keratitis is usually sterile, secondary infection is always a constant threat. Corneal ulceration may follow, especially in severe cases.[7]

MANAGEMENT

Management usually begins with treating the underlying cause(s) of the corneal drying, if possible. Treatment depends on the severity of the condition. Mild cases can be treated simply by frequent instillation of lubricating drops during the day and application of a bland lubricating ointment at bedtime. Taping the eyelids shut at bedtime, as in nocturnal exposure, may also be helpful. In more moderate cases, a soft contact lens along with lubricating drops will aid in keeping the cornea covered and moist.[5] In extreme cases, such as severe proptosis or Bell's palsy, a tarsorrhaphy may be required.[15]

Rosacea Keratitis

ETIOLOGY

Rosacea is primarily a disease of the sebaceous glands of the skin, which can lead to ocular rosacea.[5] Although of unknown etiology, the disease is thought to be triggered or exacerbated in affected individuals by certain dietary factors, such as the intake of carbohydrates, alcohol, and other foods.[3]

DIAGNOSIS

The disease usually presents as a rash consisting of small macular, slightly scaling lesions on an erythematous base, usually around the nose and cheeks (Color Plate XIII). Being chronic, with periods of exacerbation and remission, the disease can lead to a permanent telangiectasia. Ocular manifestations are rather common, and corneal involvement not infrequently leads to visual impairment.[31] The cutaneous lesions need not always precede the ocular involvement, and the converse is always a possibility.[3]

The ocular findings usually begin with a mild non-ulcerative blepharitis, associated with marked plugging of the meibomian glands. The glands may be expressed by pressure applied to the lids. Scaling of the lid margins will occur along with a diffuse, nonspecific, low-grade conjunctival hyperemia.[5]

When the cornea becomes involved, it usually exhibits a peripheral marginal punctate keratitis with subepithelial opacities and infiltrates. Vascular infiltration may follow, and ulceration of the cornea can occur, usually at the limbus, but it can move progressively inward. Inferior corneal involvement is most common. Progressive epithelial erosion may occur, leading to corneal thinning and irregularity.[3] Although the activity of the inflammation may fluctuate, the corneal ulceration can move centrally, eventually affecting the entire cornea, with resulting perforation of the cornea and possible iris prolapse.[5] Often a secondary staphylococcal infection will occur due to the cornea's compromised condition.[12] The end result may be chronic corneal scarring and a circumferential wedge-shaped pannus formation.

MANAGEMENT

Management is difficult, since there is no specific etiology. Elimination of possible dietary factors along with treatment of the skin lesions is usually pursued.[3] Ocular treatment should begin with careful lid hygiene including warm compresses, lid margin scrubs with baby shampoo or other lid cleanser, and mechanical removal of any crusts from the lashes.

Topical antibiotics such as bacitracin or erythromycin may be used as a preventative measure to control any secondary infection. Ocular lubricants may aid in alleviating corneal surface irregularities or tear film instability.[5] Topical steroids may reduce the inflammatory and vascular reactions to the keratitis, and low doses are usually effective. However, steroids should be used cautiously, since with prolonged therapy ulceration can lead to perforation. Dosage should be limited to no more than 1.0% prednisolone acetate twice daily; however, 0.12% prednisolone acetate is much safer.[3] Oral tetracycline has been shown to be highly effective in the treatment of rosacea.[32] Patients with ocular signs and symptoms of rosacea should be treated with 250 mg of tetracycline 4 times daily for 4 to 6 weeks. Assuming no drug intolerance, the tetracycline dosage frequency should be reduced to 3 times

daily for 2 to 4 weeks. The dosage can be reduced further if the clinical situation warrants. The medication can ultimately be discontinued in some patients or the patient can receive a maintenance dose of 250 mg daily or every other day.[33]

Conditions Affecting the Central Cornea

Superficial Punctate Keratitis of Thygeson

ETIOLOGY

The etiology of Thygeson's superficial punctate keratitis (TSPK) is unknown. It was once thought to be viral based on its clinical similarity to adenovirus infection.[34] A hyperimmune mechanism has been suggested, although this has not been proved. No evidence suggests that the disease is communicable.[3]

DIAGNOSIS

Thygeson's superficial punctate keratitis is a specific clinical entity seen as a coarse punctate epithelial keratitis affecting the central cornea.[34] Characteristic clinical findings include symptoms of photophobia, foreign body sensation, and tearing.[3] The corneal lesions are faint gray and appear as coarse punctate epithelial defects (Fig. 22.5). They are usually round to oval and under high magnification are seen to be made up of many tiny gray opacities.[3] They stain with rose bengal and appear slightly elevated.[5] When microerosions occur, fluorescein will stain these spots. The tiny lesions

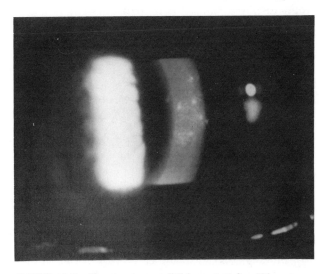

FIGURE 22.5 **Thygeson's superficial punctate keratitis, appearing coarse and gray. (Courtesy Jimmy D. Bartlett, O.D.)**

act as convex lenses and will converge the beam of a penlight into tiny bright spots on the iris.[3] The defects can range from as few as 2 up to as many as 50 lesions. The disease process almost always affects only the epithelium without any stromal involvement. It is usually bilateral but can be asymmetric, and it is not associated with inflammation elsewhere in the eye.[35] There is usually no accompanying conjunctival or anterior chamber involvement. Corneal sensitivity is normal, and a significant increase in the wetting of the filter paper has been noted in the Schirmer's test.[36]

An uncommon entity, it can affect any age group. However, most females with TSPK are 21 years of age or younger, while affected males are 28 years or younger.[36] The inflammation usually runs a chronic course involving remissions and exacerbations, with the Schirmer values returning to normal during periods of remission. The disease can last from 6 months to 30 or more years, with intermittent, transient attacks. No residual findings are seen between attacks.[36]

MANAGEMENT

Weak topical steroids are usually effective in treating the disease.[3] Frequent instillations of 0.12% prednisolone acetate should be used for the first 3 or 4 days, then quickly tapered. However, the keratitis can recur quite readily. One drop of 0.12% prednisolone acetate instilled weekly may keep the patient asymptomatic. Any corneal trauma or abrasion may reactivate the disease.[37] Antibacterial agents have no effect on the disease.[3]

Soft bandage contact lenses may be used in the management of TSPK to allow discontinuation or reduction of the topical steroid.[38] In addition, symptomatic relief can be achieved after pressure-patching for 24 hours.[39]

Conditions Affecting the Superior Cornea

Trachoma

ETIOLOGY

The causative organism of trachoma is *C. trachomatis.*

DIAGNOSIS

Trachoma presents as a chronic follicular conjunctivitis that usually initially affects the upper tarsal plate.[40] The insidious onset of trachoma can aid in the differential diagnosis from adult inclusion conjunctivitis, which usually presents with an acute onset. Initial symptoms typically include tearing, photophobia, dis-

charge, pain, lid edema, chemosis, and hyperemia, often imitating a bacterial conjunctivitis.[3]

Papillary hypertrophy and conjunctival inflammatory infiltration may become so prominent that they mask the follicular response.[3] As the disease progresses, conjunctival scarring seen as fine, white, linear scars on the tarsal plate (Arlt's lines) will occur (see Fig. 21.15).[41]

Corneal involvement (Fig. 22.6) includes epithelial keratitis, marginal and central infiltrates, superficial vascularization, shallow ulcers, pannus, limbal swelling, limbal follicles and their sequelae, and Herbert's pits. All the signs of trachoma most often affect the upper half of the cornea and conjunctiva, but they are not limited to this area.[3]

MacCallen has classified trachoma into 4 stages based on conjunctival findings only (see Table 21.9), although corneal signs must be present to establish the diagnosis.[42]

The epithelial and subepithelial keratitis presents as a keratitis of the superior cornea. The marginal and central infiltrates range from being so small that biomicroscopic examination is necessary for detection to being large pustules that are actually small ulcers at the site of the infiltrate.[3] The trachomatous pannus consists of a fibrovascular membrane with infiltrates and scarring.[5] The limbal follicles appear as gelatinous, semiopaque, dome-shaped elevations, and their sequelae (Herbert's pits) appear as small depressions of the connective tissue at the limbus. Both the limbal follicles and Herbert's pits are pathognomonic of trachoma. Vascular loops usually extend from these pits and expand onto the cornea.[20]

Sequelae of long-standing trachoma include severe scarring, tear deficiency syndromes, dacryostenosis, trichiasis, and entropion. The latter two are the most common causes of blindness associated with trachoma, since they cause corneal ulceration and scarring.[24] Populations with trachoma usually have a high incidence of other corneal disease such as bacterial ulcers, due to the vulnerability of the compromised cornea. The final tragic result seen in trachoma is xerophthalmia, a cicatricial degeneration of the entire cornea and conjunctiva. The eye appears dry, thick, and lusterless, resembling skin.[42]

Giemsa staining of conjunctival scrapings taken from the upper tarsal plate shows predominantly a polymorphonuclear reaction, but plasma cells, Leber cells (giant histiocytic macrophages containing phagocytosed debris), follicle cells, lymphocytes, and lymphoblasts may also be seen. Inclusion bodies, known as Halberstraedter-Prowazek bodies, may not always be isolated. These are identical to those seen in adult inclusion conjunctivitis, appearing as dark purple, purplish blue, or blue inclusions that cap the nucleus of

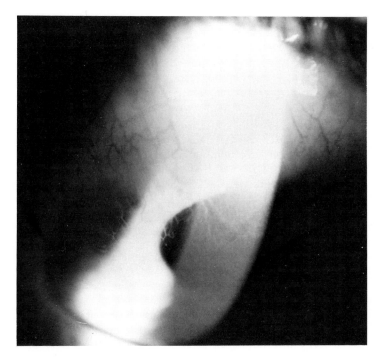

FIGURE 22.6   **Corneal involvement in trachoma. Note the superficial pannus.**

the epithelial cell.[14] Microimmunofluorescence studies are needed to differentiate serologically the agents of trachoma and inclusion conjunctivitis.[43]

MANAGEMENT

The treatment of choice is systemic tetracycline or erythromycin. Oral administration of 1 g daily (250 mg 4 times daily) for 21 days or 500 mg twice daily for 14 days is usually effective.[44] The usual contraindications to tetracycline use should be observed. Topical ointments or drops have had some success, but they are not the treatment of choice.[45] Sulfonamides, tetracycline, or erythromycin ointment applied topically twice daily for 10 weeks may be successful.[4] It may require 10 to 12 weeks from commencement of therapy to achieve maximum effect. Therefore, a lingering follicular reaction following discontinuation of therapy should not be construed as therapeutic failure.[44]

Vernal Conjunctivitis

ETIOLOGY

Vernal conjunctivitis is an uncommon, seasonally recurrent, bilateral allergic inflammation of the conjunctiva. The disease is mediated by an immediate (humoral) hypersensitivity reaction.[46]

Vernal conjunctivitis occurs worldwide but is much more common in warm climates. The disease has a seasonal predilection for the spring, early summer, and fall.[47] It is a disease of youth, usually occurring in the prepubertal years. It is very rarely seen in children under 3 years of age or in adults over age 25 years. It is much more common in males than in females (3:1).[48] When the disease strikes, it has an average duration of 4 to 10 years. There is usually a family history of atopic allergies (hay fever, eczema), and the atopic disease may be present in the patient.

DIAGNOSIS

Symptoms include extreme itching, burning, foreign body sensation, photophobia, and a ropy discharge. Itching is the most constant and prominent feature. The patient commonly refers to the eyes as "irritated" to describe the uncomfortable, hot, tight, sensitive feeling. Bloodshot eyes are commonly reported by the patient, who is usually able to pull a thick strand of whitish yellow material from the lower fornix. The lids are not matted together unless a secondary bacterial conjunctivitis is present. Ptosis may be a sign, due to the thickened upper lid, but it is usually present only slightly.[3]

The palpebral form of vernal conjunctivitis primarily affects the upper tarsal plate. The superior border of the tarsal plate is the most severely affected area. Mild papillary hypertrophy may occur first, but this usually progresses to form large papillae resembling cobblestones (see Fig. 21.10). The papillae are distinctive, with tiny twigs of vessels pushing up through the center. The papillae accumulate and crowd together, and a milky veil forms over the area.[49]

The limbal form presents with gelatinous swelling of the upper limbal conjunctiva. These limbal nodules (papillae) have vessels in the center of the lesions and must be differentiated from limbal follicles, which have vessels coming up the sides of the mounds. The limbal mass usually overrides the cornea as a semiopaque hood, typically with no more than 3 mm of corneal encroachment.[49] Associated with these masses are white, chalky concretions called Horner-Trantas' dots (see Fig. 21.11). These are composed of eosinophilic concretions and are pathognomonic for the disease.[3]

The two forms of vernal conjunctivitis usually occur together, but one may predominate over the other at any particular stage of the disease. Corneal findings are common and usually are the most distressful to the patient.[3] Characteristic superficial epithelial keratitis can occur, with punctate stippling of the superior cornea. Keratitis epithelialis vernalis of Tobgy may be an additional finding, presenting as small gray patches of necrosing epithelium in a syncytium of superficial disease involving the upper one- to two-thirds of the cornea.[3] If the disease is allowed to progress further, the cornea may stain with fluorescein in a diffuse punctate fashion, appearing as if it had been dusted with flour.[50]

A less common corneal finding is the vernal or shield ulcer of the superior cornea.[5] The ulcer is usually oval and somewhat shallow. The edges are composed of grayish white, dead epithelial cells leading into a shallow center containing necrotic debris. Infiltrates invade the superficial stroma. The ulcerative lesion tends not to spread, but secondary scarring and opacification are possible. Although micropannus may occur, total corneal pannus is quite rare.[3]

Giemsa staining of conjunctival scrapings shows a prominent eosinophilic response and is of great diagnostic value. Many of the eosinophils will be fractured, with release of eosinophilic granules. Lymphocytes and plasma cells may also be present.[49] These findings, combined with the seasonal predilection of the disease and patient's allergic history, should provide useful information for the differential diagnosis of vernal conjunctivitis.[3]

MANAGEMENT

Historically, the treatment of vernal conjunctivitis has entailed the use of topical steroids, but their side effects (glaucoma, cataract formation, and the aggravation of corneal ulcers) have raised concern about their long-term use.

Cromolyn sodium is an anti-allergy agent that tra-ditionally has been used in the medical management of bronchial asthma. It is known to alter the mast cell membrane permeability to the influx of calcium from the extracellular fluid. By preventing calcium entry, cromolyn inhibits contraction of the peripheral microfilaments and extrusion of the histamine-loaded granules. Hence, cromolyn sodium interrupts the release of histamine, leukotrienes, and eosinophil chemotactic factor (ECF-A).[51] The overall effect is to secondarily block the inflammatory effect that occurs in vernal, giant papillary, and ragweed conjunctivitis and atopic keratoconjunctivitis.[52] Cromolyn sodium also increases the tear-film breakup time (TBUT)[53] and allows a reduced steroid dosage in patients with severe symptoms in whom cromolyn therapy alone is not adequate.[54] The use of cromolyn sodium 4% (Opticrom) on a schedule of 1 to 2 drops 4 times daily normally reduces symptoms after 1 to 2 weeks of therapy. It also decreases the number of Trantas' dots as well as the degree of limbal infiltration and punctate keratitis.

It must be emphasized that cromolyn sodium is ineffective in the management of type IV hypersensitivity disorders such as contact dermatitis and hypersensitivity to preservatives in contact lens solutions.

Side effects from the use of cromolyn sodium are minor and transient. The most commonly reported side effects include stinging and watering on instillation of the medication.[55] On rare occasions patients may develop acute chemotic reactions of the conjunctiva.[56]

Topical steroids are useful for quickly relieving patient symptoms, but this may lead to indiscriminant long-term use. Therefore, steroid therapy must be carefully monitored by the practitioner.[3] A "pulse" regimen of steroid therapy may be used if patients with severe vernal keratoconjunctivitis cannot be treated with cromolyn sodium. For severely afflicted patients, 1.0% prednisolone acetate can be instilled topically, 1 drop every 2 hours for 4 days. This usually reduces the symptoms, and other less potent forms of therapy can be used between pulses. When the symptoms become severe again, another pulse of steroid can be administered. During the vernal season, this usually can be accomplished with only 1 to 3 periods of steroid therapy.[3] In milder cases in which cromolyn cannot be used, an anti-inflammatory agent such as medrysone (HMS) can be employed. For the most severe cases that do not otherwise respond to topical treatment, the use of systemic steroid therapy for 1 or 2 weeks, several times a year, may provide relief.

Other useful forms of therapy include cold compresses (10 minutes several times daily) and topical decongestants (with or without antihistamines). Since aspirin prevents the synthesis of prostaglandins that are released in vernal keratoconjunctivitis, the use of aspirin may be advantageous in some recalcitrant cases of vernal conjunctivitis. Depending on the patients' age and the severity of the condition, the dosage can range from 500 mg to 2.5 g daily.[57]

Sleeping and working in a cool, air-conditioned environment can keep the patient relatively comfortable. The best remedy is to remove the offending antigen or to reduce its presence. Relocation of the patient from a warm climate to a cool, moist environment often relieves symptoms.[37]

Superior Limbic Keratoconjunctivitis

ETIOLOGY

Superior limbic keratoconjunctivitis (SLK) is a bilateral inflammation of the upper tarsus and superior limbus.[58] The etiology is unknown, but it was once thought to be viral. It is speculated that the disease is thyroid related, but no conclusive evidence for this has been found. Nevertheless, patients presenting with SLK should undergo thyroid function studies.[1]

DIAGNOSIS

Clinical features include inflammation of the tarsal conjunctiva of the upper lid with mild papillary hypertrophy. The superior bulbar conjunctiva is hyperemic and chemotic (Color Plate XIV). Thickening and keratinization of the superior limbus along with epithelial keratitis of the superior cornea are observed.[3] Filamentary keratopathy of the superior cornea is also associated with the disease.[5] Usually, one-third to one-half of patients with SLK will have filaments. Superior micropannus may occur in some cases.

Fluorescein dye will stain the superior bulbar conjunctiva, and fine punctate corneal staining at the upper limbus will be seen. Decreased tear stability will be observed in about one-half the cases.[58]

Symptoms include photophobia, severe foreign body sensation, and tearing. These symptoms may come and go, since the disease runs a chronic course (1 to 10 years) with exacerbations and remissions. During a period of remission, the patient may not exhibit any residual signs. Although bilateral, the signs and symptoms of SLK may be more predominant in one eye.[3]

Laboratory findings are usually negative, since no causative organism has ever been conclusively linked to SLK.[5]

MANAGEMENT

Topical ocular lubricants and topical steroids provide some relief, but this therapy rarely completely alleviates the problem.[5] The standard treatment, although often unsatisfactory, has consisted of use of a silver nitrate solution. The instillation of 0.5% to 1.0% silver nitrate solution followed by irrigation causes chemical debridement of the degenerate, keratinized epithelial cells. It has been suggested that SLK may be better managed by using a pressure-patch to eliminate the lid's mechanical effect on the globe and by protecting the cornea with a soft contact lens.[59] Surgical intervention may be required in patients who do not respond to the above therapy.[3]

Conditions Causing Diffuse Superficial Keratitis

Keratitis Secondary to Bacterial Conjunctivitis

ETIOLOGY

Bacterial keratitis (keratoconjunctivitis) is defined as an active invasion of the cornea by proliferating bacteria with varying pathogenicity and virulence.[60] The invasion leads to stromal abscess formation and is accompanied by inflammatory findings of variable intensity. Only 4 pathogens can invade a healthy, intact cornea: *Corynebacterium diphtheriae*, *Neisseria gonorrhoeae*, *Streptococcus pneumoniae*, and *Haemophilus influenzae*.[60,61] Active invasion by any other pathogen must be secondary to an already compromised cornea.

The entire cornea may become infected in undiagnosed or undertreated cases, causing severe visual impairment or even corneal perforation and loss of the globe. Therefore, a bacterial keratitis should be considered a serious ocular infection requiring immediate and proper management to avoid corneal destruction.[62] This should be accomplished by identifying and eliminating the invasive organism, minimizing the accompanying inflammation, and aiding in rapid corneal reepithelialization.

Staphylococcus aureus, *Streptococcus pneumoniae*, *Moraxella* species, and *Pseudomonas aeruginosa* are by far the most common causes of bacterial keratitis in the United States.[60] *Pseudomonas* predominates in the southeastern states, *S. aureus* and *S. pneumoniae* are common in the other areas, and *Moraxella* is fairly uniform in all areas of the country, although the geographic distribution can be quite variable.[3]

The normal flora of the eyelid margins and periorbital skin includes *Staphylococcus epidermidis*. Aerobic diphtheroids are found in conjunctival tissue, as are occasional low numbers of *Haemophilus* species, *S. pneumoniae*, *S. aureus*, *Moraxella* species, and a few gram-negative rods.[14] All these organisms can cause conjunctivitis. The most common causes of bacterial conjunctivitis are listed in Table 22.2.[7]

Bacterial conjunctivitis is the most frequently encountered conjunctivitis and the most common of all

TABLE 22.2
Most Common Causes of Bacterial Conjunctivitis

Purulent
    Neisseria gonorrhoeae
    Neisseria meningitidis
Acute catarrhal
    Streptococcus pneumoniae (pneumococcus)—temperate
        climates
    Haemophilis aegyptius (Koch-Weeks bacillus)—tropical
        climates
Subacute catarrhae
    Haemophilus influenzae—temperate climates
Chronic
    Staphylococcus aureus
    Moraxella lacunata (diplobacillus of Morax-Axenfeld)
Rare (acute, subacute, chronic)
    Streptococci
    Neisseria catarrhalis
    Coliforms
    Proteus species
    Corynebacterium diphtheriae

eye diseases in the Western hemisphere.[8] It is usually characterized by a history of a red eye of short duration (2 or 3 days), without pain or photophobia, and with a mucopurulent discharge causing sticky lids.[60] If the cornea becomes involved (keratoconjunctivitis), the patient will usually complain of pain and photophobia. The pain is usually expressed as a foreign body sensation, as if something is lodged under the upper lid.[5] The matted lids are due to the incubating effect of the closed eye during sleep, which causes a temperature increase and promotes the growth of bacteria under the lids. Liberation of bacterial exotoxins causes the mucopurulent discharge. When the lids are open, exposure to air limits growth of the organisms.[5]

GRAM-POSITIVE BACTERIAL ORGANISMS

S. Aureus. *S. aureus* is colonized in the human within a few days after birth and remains a continuous or intermittent inhabitant throughout life. *S. aureus,* an aerobic gram-positive coccus, is harbored in the conjunctiva, skin, upper respiratory tract, and colon as part of the normal flora, although it is rarely cultured from the healthy outer eye.[3] On microscopic examination, *S. aureus* appears as a gram-positive coccus occuring singly, in pairs, or in clusters. Other characteristics include the production of the enzyme coagulase, complete hemolysis on blood agar, and the fermentation of mannitol.[14]

The conjunctivitis due to *S. aureus* is normally of the diffuse papillary type. This papillary response may be caused by the liberation of toxins rather than by direct invasion of the conjunctival or corneal epithelium by the organism itself.[9] This response differs from the chronic follicular hypertrophy characteristic of diplobacillary conjunctivitis.

Although not usually aggressively invasive, *S. aureus* is very toxigenic and can provoke corneal infiltrates, eczematous blepharitis, phlyctenular keratitis, and angular blepharitis.[5] When *S. aureus* invades a compromised cornea, it tends to remain localized but can eventually involve the entire cornea. Since most of the bacteria are harbored in the lower cul-de-sac,[7] exotoxins produce a superficial keratitis of the inferior cornea. If left untreated, the keratitis may advance to a corneal ulcer. The ulcer is usually grayish white and round to oval with distinct borders. The margins of the ulcer are often blurred by stromal infiltrates and epithelial edema. Further destruction of the cornea can occur, with corneal perforation within 7 days, if the ulcer is left untreated or is undertreated.[49]

S. pneumoniae (Pneumococcus). Pneumococci are aerobic, encapsulated, gram-positive diplococci. They are a part of the normal flora of the upper respiratory tract in up to 70% of healthy human adults.[60] The frequency of acute conjunctivitis, keratitis, and corneal ulceration caused by *S. pneumoniae* is evidence of its presence in close proximity to the eye.

Pneumococcus most commonly produces a moderately severe acute conjunctivitis. Corneal involvement is rather rare in the United States. If corneal complications do occur, a diffuse punctate keratitis is seen along with marginal infiltrates that may later form corneal ulcers. The borders of the ulcer are usually obscured by replicating bacteria. *Pneumococcus* is considered to be a common cause of central corneal ulcers (Color Plate XV) in some countries, and many authorities believe it is the major causative organism in central hypopyon and serpiginous ulcers. Chronic dacryocystitis can occur secondary to pneumococcal infection.[37]

Pneumococci are lancet shaped and are distinct enough morphologically to be identified by Gram staining. They are readily cultured on blood or chocolate agar, appearing as small, glistening, nonpigmented colonies. Surrounded by a zone of incomplete hemolysis, they are optochin-sensitive.[14] These organisms are more common in children and in the northern United States during the colder months.

Streptococcus pyogenes. *Streptococcus pyogenes,* an aerobic gram-positive coccus, is an infrequent cause of outer eye infection. However, the organism is a serious pathogen in other organ systems and can invade the eye in compromised individuals.[3] Invasive and toxigenic, the organism can cause a pseudomembranous conjunctivitis. The pseudomembrane is a fibrinous layer entrapping inflammatory cells and is attached to the conjunctival surface. It can be easily removed with minimal bleeding of the underlying tissue.[5] *S. pyogenes* most commonly causes lid cellulitis. Corneal involvement is rarely seen, but a severe purulent or primary hypopyon keratitis can occur in some cases. Uveitis, iritis, iridocyclitis, orbital cellulitis, and panophthalmitis may occur in severe, long-standing cases.

S. pyogenes organisms usually grow in chains, are round or elongated, and exhibit complete beta hemolysis on blood agar.[14]

Streptococcus viridans.   Although not usually a part of the normal flora, it is not uncommon to find *S. viridans* within the ocular normal flora. *S. viridans* can cause chronic focal infection and usually does so to a greater degree than does *S. pyogenes*. *S. viridans* can produce infections manifested as acute catarrhal conjunctivitis, hypopyon keratitis, chronic dacryocystitis, and postoperative infections similar to those caused by *Pneumococcus*.[13]

Morphologically, *S. viridans* appears similar to pneumococci on culture media except that the latter is encapsulated. *S. viridans* is alpha-hemolytic and can therefore be differentiated from the beta hemolysis of *S. pyogenes*.[13]

GRAM-NEGATIVE BACTERIAL ORGANISMS

Moraxella lacunata (Morax-Axenfeld).   *M. lacunata,* an aerobic gram-negative diplobacillus, is a common cause of angular blepharoconjunctivitis. *Moraxella* species can cause an acute conjunctivitis that may proceed to one of chronicity, with follicular reaction.[5]

The cornea may become involved in the form of a marginal keratitis and central or paracentral ulceration with or without hypopyon. Ulcers are usually found only in previously debilitated elderly patients (e.g., chronic alcoholics or cancer patients).[6] The ulcer may form a posterior abscess late in the disease. Sequelae such as persistent sterile stromal inflammation, diffuse endothelial degeneration with corneal edema, posterior synechiae, and secondary glaucoma have been reported.[3]

Conjunctival or corneal scrapings show *M. lacunata* to be a nonmotile, uncapsulated, paired gram-negative rod. It may be cultured on blood and chocolate agar and is oxidase-positive. Some strains of *Moraxella* species retain crystal violet stain and may be misinterpreted as gram-positive organisms.[14]

Neisseria gonorrhoeae.   The gonococcal organism is usually introduced into the conjunctival sac by direct transfer from the genitalia, through contact with infected articles (in adults), or by passage through an infected cervix during delivery (in newborns). The organism may cause a rampant acute purulent conjunctivitis with potential corneal ulceration occurring secondarily. The infection quickly progresses to severe edema of both lids of the involved eye, excessive mattering, aching pain, and ocular tenderness. The cornea appears lusterless, and without proper diagnosis and treatment, corneal ulceration will occur. Pus production and mucopurulent discharge are usually profuse (see Fig. 21.2).[3]

Gonorrheal conjunctivitis is the most common form of hyperacute conjunctivitis, and it occurs concomitantly with infection of other body parts. The gonorrheal organisms produce a soluble toxin that, when present in the anterior chamber, can cause a toxic iritis. In gonococcal ophthalmia, corneal ulceration progresses rapidly to corneal perforation and blindness.[14] The seriousness of the disease is accentuated by the rapid progress from conjunctivitis to corneal scarring or perforation within 24 hours if treatment is not prompt and effective.

Haemophilus influenzae.   *H. influenzae* is a fastidious, aerobic, gram-negative pleomorphic organism often seen as a slender rod or in coccobacillary form.[14] It is carried in the upper respiratory tract in healthy adults, but more often it causes an acute conjunctivitis in younger children during warm weather in warmer climates. In the United States, it is more prevalent in the southern states, with a peak incidence from May to October.[3] *H. influenzae* is a toxigenic organism and can cause patchy conjunctival hemorrhages during the infection. Untreated, it is usually self-limiting and resolves in 9 to 12 days, but can progress to periorbital cellulitis associated with respiratory infection.[3] In young children, the infection may lead to a bacteremia.[37] Symptoms include mucopurulent discharge with characteristic watering and irritation. The infection is usually unilateral initially but typically transfers to the other eye within 1 or 2 days. The eyelids are commonly matted together, and corneal limbal infiltrates are associated with the acute infection.[14]

DIAGNOSIS

It is imperative to diagnosis as quickly and as specifically as possible the cause of keratitis secondary to a bacterial conjunctivitis. Even though numerous clinical situations arise in which a smear or culture is not required (e.g., acute bacterial conjunctivitis without corneal involvement), if the cornea is affected, as shown by keratitis, a smear or culture is advisable. This microbiologic data will most accurately specify the diagnosis. Once the diagnosis is established, treatment options can be approached more logically.

The specific diagnostic criteria for acute, hyperacute, and chronic bacterial conjunctivitis are discussed in Chapter 21.

MANAGEMENT

The management of diffuse superficial keratitis caused by a bacterial conjunctivitis depends on the etiologic agent. In general, when managing the keratitis, the primary attack is to control the conjunctivitis; thereafter, the keratitis will normally begin to resolve spontaneously. Therefore, treatment consists of careful lid hygiene if exudate and debris are present. Gentamicin or tobramycin ophthalmic solution should be instilled, 1 drop every 3 to 4 hours, and an ointment such as bacitracin–polymyxin B (Polysporin), bacitracin, or erythromycin can be applied at bedtime. After the infection begins to improve, the therapy should be tapered.[15]

In the management of hyperacute bacterial conjunctivitis, the conjunctiva must be frequently irrigated with normal saline or physiologic irrigating solution, and proper lid hygiene must be initiated to wash away the purulent exudate and lid crusting. Cycloplegics, such as homatropine 5%, atropine 1%, or cyclopentolate 1%, can be used twice daily to prevent uveal involvement. Topical antibiotic solutions such as tobramycin or gentamicin should be used, 1 drop every 2 hours for the first 48 hours, then tapered to 1 drop 5 times daily. These antibiotics may also be used in ointment form.[61] Bacitracin ointment can also be used every 2 hours for 48 hours, then tapered to 5 times daily. Systemic amoxicillin is used against *N. gonorrhoeae* in a dose of 3 g orally along with probenecid 0.5 to 1.0 g daily.

The keratitis associated with a chronic bacterial conjunctivitis should be managed by including meticulous attention to eyelid hygiene for a minimum of 3 to 4 weeks. The topical antibiotics that normally produce the best results are erythromycin, bacitracin, tetracycline, or the combination agents such as bacitracin–polymyxin B. These can be instilled directly into the cul-de-sac 2 to 4 times daily and can be used as a lid scrub twice daily. The clinician should keep in mind that keratitis sicca may contribute to the chronicity of the infective process, especially in the elderly.

Epidemic Keratoconjunctivitis

ETIOLOGY

Epidemic keratoconjunctivitis (EKC) is an acute inflammatory disease caused by adenovirus types 8 and 19[63] and most predominantly by type 37.[64] Several sporadic cases of EKC due to adenovirus types 3 and 7 and herpesvirus were included among typical cases studied by O'Day and associates.[65] This experience illustrates the potential for error that exists in making an etiologic diagnosis without the benefit of laboratory investigation.

DIAGNOSIS

EKC differs from other adenoviral infections of the conjunctiva in that it is a source of considerable morbidity and may cause visual impairment.[66–68] It is usually characterized by an acute onset of a watery discharge, follicular conjunctivitis, focal corneal epithelial lesions, and preauricular lymphadenopathy. The conjunctivitis subsides after approximately 10 to 15 days, and discrete subepithelial opacities appear in the superficial layers of the corneal stroma at the site of the epithelial lesions (Fig. 22.7).[63] These diagnostic lesions usually regress over several months, without loss of visual function, but they may persist for up to 2 years.

Three predisposing factors to clinical adenovirus type 8 infection have been described. Infection can follow direct inoculation of the virus into the eye, or it can occur secondary to ocular trauma. Adenovirus type 8 also has been associated with concurrent bacterial infection.[69] Direct inoculation and trauma can be caused by ocular instrumentation, and in epidemics involving eyecare facilities, applanation tonometry, minor surgical procedures,[70,71] and finger-to-eye contact[72] have been regularly associated with increased risk of infection.

It has been postulated that the corneal opacities result from the proliferation of virus in the epithelium

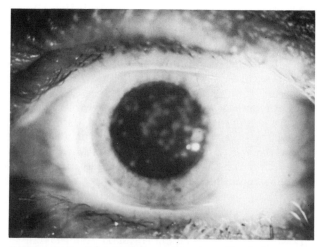

FIGURE 22.7 **Subepithelial opacities in epidemic keratoconjunctivitis. (Courtesy Jimmy D. Bartlett, O.D.)**

with local deposition of viral antigens in the anterior stroma. The host's immune response results in the discrete, persistent opacities.[73] The corneal lesions are round and punctate and may increase in number and size, often becoming as large as 0.5 mm in diameter.[74] Outbreaks of EKC have been associated with the bacterial conjunctivitis of the Koch-Weeks bacillus (*Haemophilus aegyptius*). The relatively large amounts of exudate present with bacterial disease may serve as a mechanical medium to spread the infection.

Adenovirus types 8 and 19 can be cultivated on HeLa cells and identified by neutralization tests. Giemsa staining of conjunctival scrapings shows primarily a mononuclear inflammatory reaction.[7]

MANAGEMENT

As with most viral infections, chemotherapy is not particularly effective in treating EKC. However, topical antibiotics should be routinely used to prevent secondary bacterial infection. IDU, which is useful in the treatment of herpesvirus keratitis, is ineffective in infections due to adenovirus.[75] Steroid therapy may delay the appearance of the corneal opacities, but it will not completely prevent their formation. Topical steroids have caused opacities to resolve up to 1 year after the acute infection, but on withdrawal of therapy the infiltrates usually reappear. The steroids probably act by suppressing the edema that results from the minimal but continuing antigen-antibody reaction in the stroma.[74]

Eyes afflicted with adenovirus type 8 or 19 should not be treated with topical steroids unless photophobia and lacrimation become extremely severe and incapacitating or the infiltrates and opacities deeply involve the stroma over the pupillary area with concomitant iridocyclitis or reduced vision.[74] The basis for this recommendation, in addition to the usual side effects of steroids, is that once steroids are discontinued, the subepithelial opacities often return. This could require the patient to take steroids for years. In those situations in which the patient must take steroids, the mildest agent and lowest dosage that are effective should be prescribed.

Cyloplegics, such as homatropine 5%, decrease ocular pain and help manage the iridocyclitis. Aspirin or ibuprofen may be used to aid patient comfort, and topical decongestants or ocular lubricants can also help decrease the inflammation and improve patient comfort. Cold compresses can be used to control conjunctival hyperemia and swelling.

Epidemic keratoconjunctivitis is extremely contagious. Care must be taken to wash hands and instrumentation after each patient to prevent further spread of the infection.

Pharyngoconjunctival Fever

ETIOLOGY

Pharyngoconjunctival fever (PCF) is caused by adenoviral serotypes 3 and 7.

DIAGNOSIS

PCF is an acute and highly infectious disease characterized by fever of 101° to 104°F (38.5° to 40°C), sore throat, and follicular conjunctivitis in one or both eyes. However, the syndrome may be incomplete, with only one or two of the cardinal signs of the triad (fever, pharyngitis, and conjunctivitis) being present. The follicles are often very prominent on both the conjunctiva and pharyngeal mucosa.[7] In the early stages, the condition can be confused with herpes conjunctivitis, acute inclusion conjunctivitis, or acute hemorrhagic conjunctivitis. Symptoms include injection and tearing, usually bilateral, and there may be transient superficial epithelial keratitis and occasionally some subepithelial opacities, although the cornea is rarely severely affected. The disease is also at times associated with preauricular lymphadenopathy as well as with nonspecific systemic complaints including malaise, myalgia, headache, abdominal discomfort, and diarrhea.

Adenovirus type 3 can be grown in HeLa cells, and neutralization tests will help identify the organism. As the disease progresses, a rising titer of the antibody that neutralizes the virus is seen.

MANAGEMENT

The disease is usually self-limiting, lasting from 5 to 14 days. Therapy should be directed toward preventing complications, preventing secondary bacterial infection, and relieving symptoms.[7] The patient may experience considerable discomfort, which is best treated with cold compresses and other supportive measures, including the use of topical decongestants and ocular lubricants.

PCF is milder and resolves more quickly than the conjunctivitis seen in EKC. EKC causes a much more severe keratitis and is more likely to result in visual disturbances.

Atopic Keratitis (Keratoconjunctivitis)

ETIOLOGY

Patients with atopic dermatitis (eczema) often have an accompanying atopic keratoconjunctivitis. Symptoms are much the same as in hay fever but demonstrate no seasonal incidence. Atopic individuals—those who exhibit a higher than normal incidence of bronchial asthma and reactions to intracutaneous skin testing with protein allergens—are most often affected.

DIAGNOSIS

Atopic keratoconjunctivitis is manifested by chemosis of the palpebral and bulbar conjunctivae, conjunctival vascular engorgement, and a papillary conjunctival reaction. Corneal involvement may occur as a superficial peripheral keratitis, with or without peripheral superficial corneal infiltrates. Rarely, in severe cases, the entire cornea becomes hazy and vascularized, and vision is reduced.

Giemsa staining of conjunctival smears shows a mild eosinophilic reaction.

MANAGEMENT

Since the underlying cause of the ocular problem is cutaneous, the patient usually is concurrently under a dermatologist's care. The most effective management is removal of the offending allergen, although its identity is often difficult to establish. The most effective pharmacologic treatment consists of topical cromolyn sodium 4%, 1 or 2 drops 4 times daily.[76] Some forms of palliative treatment, such as topical decongestants, may give some relief. Short-term intensive steroid therapy may be instituted in more severe cases, but side effects must be carefully monitored. Since topical ocular cromolyn was introduced, the need for topical steroids has lessened. Topical ocular antihistamines seem to have little effect, but cold compresses may help in acute cases.

Topical Medications (Medicamentosa)

ETIOLOGY

Medicamentosa is caused by a toxic reaction to topical medications. A chronic keratoconjunctivitis is not uncommonly encountered after long-term topical antibiotic treatment of a surface ocular infection. The inflammation can be regarded mistakenly as a continuation of the previous infection.

DIAGNOSIS

The keratoconjunctivitis results from direct contact of the chemical irritant, and it develops minutes to hours after exposure to the toxic agent. Symptoms worsen as encounters with the irritant continue and can vary from mild to severe irritation and hyperemia depending on the offending irritant's potency and degree of toxicity. The skin of the eyelid can be involved. The conjunctiva

is injected, and diffuse papillae and follicles may develop later. If the toxic agent is not discontinued, the conjunctivitis can become chronic and may progress to involve the cornea, manifested as a superficial punctate keratitis. In severe cases a secondary iritis may also occur.

MANAGEMENT

Treatment consists of removing the toxic agent. However, this may prove difficult, especially in the case of topical therapeutic agents, since patients may question discontinuing medication when their symptoms temporarily persist. Removal of all medications is indicated, replacing them with cold compresses. A latent period of several days may precede improvement. Topical decongestant agents can provide a soothing effect but can mask symptoms of a continuing toxic reaction. Topical ocular antihistamines appear to be of little benefit. Topical ocular lubricants may offer some relief but should be provided without preservative to reduce the risk of preservative toxicity.

Conditions Causing Superficial Keratitis of Random Distribution

Molluscum Contagiosum

ETIOLOGY

The molluscum contagiosum virus is a member of the poxvirus (DNA, double-stranded) group, which causes tumor-like epithelial eruptions involving the skin.

DIAGNOSIS

Although children are most frequently affected, adults are not immune to the molluscum contagiosum virus. Ocular involvement presents as a nodule affecting the skin of the eyelids (particularly the lid margins) and, rarely, the conjunctiva. It is characterized by the production of a slowly progressive, enlarging nodule, the center of which usually undergoes necrosis and becomes umbilicated. The pale nodules can become multiple, ranging up to 2 mm in diameter. A cheesy material may be expressed from the lesion. When the pearly nodules affect the lid margin, a follicular conjunctivitis and epithelial keratitis may be produced, presumably due to toxicity to products released from the lesions into the cul-de-sac. The conjunctivitis tends to be of the chronic follicular type, with the keratitis presenting as a diffuse or focal epithelial keratitis. The keratitis may become chronic and, if left untreated, can lead to subepithelial infiltration and peripheral corneal vascularization. The lid lesion must be differentiated from other eyelid tumors, including sebaceous cysts, verrucae, chalazia, keratoacanthomas, and small fibromas.

Cultivation of the virus is difficult if not impossible. Humans are the only known hosts, since animal inoculation experiments have failed.

MANAGEMENT

The most successful method of treatment is surgical excision of the lesions, especially when the conjunctiva and cornea are involved. The conjunctivitis and keratitis usually spontaneously resolve following surgical eradication of the lesion. Additionally, electrocoagulation or cryotherapy may be attempted.

Trichiasis

ETIOLOGY

Trichiasis is a condition in which the lashes are directed toward the globe and irritate the cornea and conjunctiva (see Fig. 19.18). The condition often follows diseases that cause scarring of the lid margin and an inward turning of the lid. Causes of trichiasis are primary entropion or entropion due to trachoma, Stevens-Johnson syndrome, cicatricial pemphigoid, blepharitis, chronic blepharoconjunctivitis, and chemical burns. Primary trichiasis is thought to be acquired, with distortion and misdirection of the cilia.

DIAGNOSIS

The in-turned eyelashes are readily diagnosed by direct visualization with the slit lamp. In some patients with spastic entropion, the trichiasis will be intermittent rather than constant. When the patient is actually examined, the eyelid often will not be in a state of spasm and the eyelashes will not be turned inward, onto the globe. The examiner can often induce the condition by having the patient tightly close the eyelids. In addition, staining the cornea with fluorescein will demonstrate eyelash track marks across its surface.

MANAGEMENT

Removal of the aberrant lashes is only a temporary solution, since the lashes tend to regrow. Destroying the hair follicles by electrolysis is a more permanent treatment but is usually effective only if a few lashes are involved. If many lashes are affected, surgical reconstruction of the lid margin, producing lid eversion, may be necessary.

Entropion

ETIOLOGY

Entropion is a condition in which the eyelid is turned in toward the globe (see Fig. 19.17).[77] It is classified into 4 forms: congenital, spastic, involutional (senile), and cicatricial.

DIAGNOSIS

Congenital entropion is rare and is usually associated with other congenital abnormalities. The spastic form arises from excessive contraction of the orbicularis oculi muscle (blepharospasm). The involutional type follows loss of tone of the orbicularis muscle combined with loss of skin elasticity and is usually seen in the elderly. Cicatricial entropion follows scarring of the palpebral conjunctiva and can be caused by many factors, such as chemical burns, lacerations, surgical procedures, and certain ocular diseases. The lower lid is usually affected, although the cicatricial form can also affect the upper lid.

Corneal involvement usually accompanies entropion and can complicate chronic conjunctivitis, keratitis, and ocular surgery. Secondary trichiasis can occur, causing corneal irritation and encouraging corneal ulceration. Secondary bacterial infection is a constant threat when the cornea is compromised.

MANAGEMENT

The best treatment is surgical intervention, since many surgical procedures have been devised to evert the lid margin and the lashes. Scarred conjunctival tissue can be replaced with mucous membrane tissue transplanted from the mouth.

The best procedures are those that restore the action of attenuated eyelid retractors and those that tighten a lax lower lid. Nonsurgical alternatives include taping or gluing the lower lid to the cheek, although this provides only temporary relief.

Conditions Affecting the Limbus

Marginal Infiltrates (Ulcers)

ETIOLOGY

Marginal corneal ulcers and infiltrates are caused by a hypersensitivity reaction to the exotoxin of *S. aureus*.[11] They are the result of sensitization to bacterial products, with antibodies from the limbal vessels reacting with antigens that have diffused through the corneal epithelium.[154] They are almost invariably associated with an acute or chronic bacterial conjunctivitis.

DIAGNOSIS

The lesions usually begin as oval or linear infiltrates separated from the limbus by an interval of clear cornea (Fig. 22.8). Later, ulceration and vascularization occur. They are usually self-limited and resolve in 7 to 10 days. If left untreated, however, the primary bacterial blepharoconjunctivitis is likely to recur. The ulceration and infiltration are *not* infectious processes, and corneal scrapings are usually void of the causative organisms unless a concomitant bacterial infection is present. The ulcers are typically benign, although the patient often presents with extreme pain and photophobia.

MANAGEMENT

Topical steroids relieve the painful symptoms and usually shorten the course of the disease. However, these ulcers must be differentiated from marginal herpetic keratitis, for which steroid therapy is contraindicated. This can usually be easily accomplished by observing the corneal anesthesia of herpetic involvement as contrasted to the pain seen with the hypersensitivity-type marginal ulcer. If steroid therapy is to be initiated, it should be done with concomitant topical antibiotic administration to prevent the reproliferation of the underlying bacterium. Tobramycin drops and erythromycin ointment are generally effective, as discussed later in this chapter.

Phlyctenular Keratoconjunctivitis

ETIOLOGY

Phlyctenular keratoconjunctivitis is characterized by a nodule of lymphocytes that results from a delayed hypersensitivity to reexposure to an antigen.[154] The antigens most often implicated in phlyctenular keratoconjunctivitis are *S. aureus* and *Mycobacterium tuberculosis*.[78,79]

DIAGNOSIS

Phlyctenules appear as pinkish white, avascular mounds of varying size (pinpoint to several millimeters), typically occurring at or near the limbus (see Fig. 21.25). They migrate toward the center of the cornea in a pie-shaped section. The untreated phlyctenule can develop a central ulcer over several days. This area may scar through the depth of the cornea, with pannus formation.

The usual patient symptomatology includes mild irritation, tearing, and pruritis, which become more intense when the cornea is involved. Photophobia invariably occurs as the cornea becomes affected.

MANAGEMENT

Treatment of phlyctenular keratitis is primarily aimed at reducing the hypersensitivity inflammatory response with prednisolone acetate 1% administered every 2 to 4 hours.[76] The steroid should be carefully tapered to decrease the possibility of a recurrence.

Central Corneal Ulcers

The corneal epithelium is a formidable barrier to potential invaders. The smooth surface of the cornea, the action of the tears and blinking, and lysozyme and beta lysin in the tears all exert an antibacterial effect. However, a number of stimuli and injuries (e.g. mechanical, thermal, chemical, ruptured bullae) can cause an epithelial defect that permits invading bacteria to gain access to the stroma once the integrity of the epithelium is broken. Infective corneal ulcers, regardless of their initial location, tend to progress in a band-like pattern toward the central cornea and away from the vascularized limbus.[77]

Description

The typical response to significant corneal inflammation is ulceration, with loss of epithelium. This area

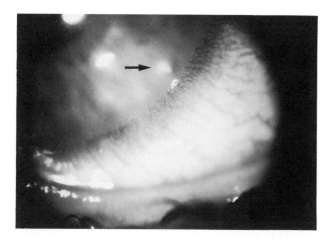

FIGURE 22.8   A marginal infiltrate (arrow) caused by hypersensitivity to exotoxins of *S. aureus*. Note the clear area between the infiltrate and the limbus. (Courtesy Jerry R. Pederson, O.D.)

stains with sodium fluorescein and represents an infection of the cornea by virus, bacteria, or fungi. Cicatrization due to corneal ulceration is a major cause of blindness throughout the world.[7] Most of this visual loss is preventable, but only if an etiologic diagnosis is made early and appropriate therapy instituted. A central corneal ulcer is an ocular emergency, since it threatens both vision and the eye itself.

Types of stimuli that can cause or worsen an ulcerative keratitis include neurotrophic, degenerative, toxic, allergic, and traumatic stimuli as well as microorganisms themselves. Exposure, lid deformities, and tear film anomalies render the host more susceptible to ulcerative keratitis. In addition, corneal degenerations, exposure to radiation, bullous keratopathy, immune disorders, diabetes, other systemic debilitations, and a phthisical eye all increase the likelihood that an ulcerative keratitis will develop. The corneal host responses to these exogenous factors include inflammation, hypersensitivity, edema, vascularization, and collagenase release. The effects of the inflammation then cause the cornea to ulcerate.

Initial Workup

MANDATORY LABORATORY TESTS

The most common cause of corneal infection in developed countries is herpes simplex.[80] If the ulcer is obviously not viral, then a bacterial or fungal etiology must be considered. Proper management requires laboratory investigation. Since etiology cannot be adequately differentiated by clinical observation alone, certain laboratory tests must be executed at once. A logical plan of antibiotic therapy should then be initiated that can be altered if necessary once the specific organism has been identified and sensitivities determined.

Stains and Cultures.   Bacteriologic or fungal cultures and smears should be obtained as part of the initial workup. Smears can be studied using staining techniques capable of yielding immediate information that can help plan effective, early treatment. However, cultures are usually more sensitive and specific in establishing a diagnosis and final therapy.

Enough slides should be prepared to allow the use of at least both Gram and Giemsa stains. The Giemsa stain is used to help rule out a fungal ulcer. It demonstrates the type of inflammatory cells, the condition of the epithelial cells, the presence or absence of cytoplasmic inclusions, and the identification of hyphae fragments.[81] A Gram stain is most important when a bacterial or yeast agent is suspected, since the impor-

tant aspect in such cases is the organism itself, and not the cytologic response.

Additional slides can be prepared should further staining procedures become necessary. If the clinical evidence indicates that the agent is a slow-growing organism such as mycobacteria, then acid-fast staining should be implemented. Eosinophilic responses may be quickly discovered using the Hansel stain. Papanicolaou's stain can reveal intranuclear inclusions.[77]

When culturing the ulcer, blood agar is an important growth medium, since it allows growth of most aerobic pathogens and some fungi. Chocolate agar is also routinely used. It will cultivate most organisms that blood agar will, in addition to various species of Neisseria, Haemophilus, and Moraxella. If a fungus is suspected, one can use Sabouraud's agar, which has a pH low enough to prevent bacterial growth. Fungi will also grow on blood agar at room temperature. Herpes simplex and adenovirus, two of the more common agents of viral infection, can usually be diagnosed by the clinical appearance alone. However, should it become necessary to culture a suspected virus, a transport medium must be inoculated, frozen, and shipped to a research virology facility or state health department laboratory.

Specimen Collection.   Before scraping the ulcerative area, a topical anesthetic should be used. Proparacaine is preferred because it has the least bacteriostatic effect of the commonly used anesthetics.[14] Since purulent exudates and necrotic surface debris are of no value for laboratory diagnosis, a sterile, dry, cotton-tipped swab should be touched to the central area of the ulcer before scraping. This applicator is then streaked onto the appropriate agar in a row of C-shaped streaks. Following this, with the aid of a slit lamp, a platinum spatula should be used to scrape the margin and base. The scraping should be deep and thorough to be certain of obtaining a sample of the organism. Multiple areas of the ulcer should be scraped.[60] The scraping action also may disrupt the cornea further, increasing the effectiveness of topical antibiotic therapy.[82] The material obtained is C-streaked directly onto the media. Organism growth is positive if the growth is on the streak area and is considered a contaminant if found on medium separated from the streak itself. Subsequent scrapings are made into smears for staining evaluations. Poor results may occur if there is insufficient specimen material, if the entire slide is not thoroughly examined, or if there has been previous antibiotic therapy.

CORNEAL SENSITIVITY TESTING

The above tests are best suited for confirming bacterial and fungal etiologies of ulcers. The diagnosis of a viral agent can, in the case of herpes infections, be aided by corneal sensitivity testing.[163] With herpes simplex, corneal anesthesia occurs early in the infection. Herpes zoster, when involving the nasociliary nerve, generally permanently impairs corneal sensation.

Corneal sensitivity can be measured qualitatively by drawing out (approximately 2 to 3 mm) a few cotton fibers from a sterile swab. The patient should look to the opposite side from the eye being tested, with the lids held open gently. The cotton wisp is then brought in from the side to touch the cornea. *A separate wisp must be used for each eye.* The examiner should carefully watch for objective signs such as increased blink rate or lacrimation.[83] The patient's subjective response to the comparison of touch between the eyes is then recorded. Should sensitivity seem diminished or absent in the involved eye, herpes infection must be suspected.

A more accurate measurement of corneal sensitivity can be made with the use of a Cochet-Bonet esthesiometer. The examiner can adjust the length of the retractable nylon thread and measure in units of length when the thread is first detected by each cornea. The readings for each eye are then compared to establish an asymmetric response.

Bacterial Corneal Ulcers

ETIOLOGY

A large number of bacteria have been identified by culture as the etiologic agents for corneal ulcers. However, the most frequently found gram-positive organisms are *S. pneumoniae, S. aureus, Staphylococcus epidermidis,* and α, γ, and β-hemolytic *Streptococcus.* The most commonly cultured gram-negative organisms are *Pseudomonas aeruginosa, Moraxella, Proteus, Escherichia coli,* and *Klebsiella.*[80]

DIAGNOSIS

Bacterial infection of the cornea can occur simultaneously with or follow bacterial infection of the conjunctiva. The intact corneal epithelium will usually present an arduous barrier even to high concentrations of the microorganisms. Besides the mechanical barrier, the cornea's smooth surface also provides protection from infection.[80] Blinking, with the flushing action of tears, helps sweep away microorganisms, while lysin and beta lysin in the tears provide an antibacterial action against gram-positive cocci[84] other than *S. aureus.*[85] Most bacteria can invade the cornea only if the epithelial layer is not intact or is in a compromised host. Organisms that can attack the cornea even though

the corneal epithelium is intact include *N. gonorrhoeae, Corynebacterium diphtheriae,* and *Listeria* species.[60,61,86]

Most bacterial ulcers are caused by opportunistic organisms normally nonpathogenic for uncompromised corneas.[80] Once the corneal epithelium has been disrupted, compromising agents or events that may precede the development of the ulcer include interference with lacrimal function, elevation of corneal temperature (as in patching), systemic immunodeficiency, or local corneal immunodeficiency (through vitamin A deficiency, existing corneal infections, corneal trophesy, or the use of anesthetic or immunosuppressive drugs).

The two main types of keratitis in which bacteria must be considered are marginal and central hypopyon. Marginal keratitis is common in bacterial conjunctivitis and blepharitis. It is not caused by the bacterial organisms themselves but is a secondary hypersensitivity response. This condition is usually not severe and will heal at about the same time as the conjunctivitis.

Central infectious keratitis is due to direct invasion by infectious organisms. The hypopyon that typically accompanies it is almost always sterile in bacterial ulcers. Central bacterial ulcers are usually characterized by stromal infiltration in the area of epithelial defect, with surrounding edema and folds in Descemet's membrane associated with endothelial fibrin plaques or anterior chamber reaction. Many types of bacterial ulcers look alike and vary only in severity. Unchecked bacterial ulcers, regardless of where they initially begin, progress toward the central cornea, away from the vascular limbus.

The severe inflammatory reaction may lead to permanent changes such as anterior polar cataracts, posterior and anterior synechiae, increased intraocular pressure, stromal scars, corneal edema, descemetocele, or corneal perforation.[87]

INITIAL MANAGEMENT

A smear and culture (as previously discussed) must be taken from the corneal ulcer. As soon as the Gram stain results become available, initial pharmacologic treatment can be chosen until the more specific culture results are known. Table 22.3 summarizes the initial antibiotic therapy based on Gram stain results. As the table suggests, the treatment of bacterial corneal ulcers is achieved with topical drops or ointments[155] and subconjunctival routes of administration. Insler and associates[88] have shown that topical administration of gentamicin achieves a level of bactericidal activity that is 3 times higher than by parenteral administration, and by using far less antibiotic.

The following sections discuss the specific therapy

TABLE 22.3
Selection of Initial Antibiotic Therapy Based on Gram Stain

Gram Stain Results		Initial Antibiotic Therapy
No organism	Topical:	Bacitracin and gentamicin
	Subconjunctival:	Methicillin and gentamicin
Gram-positive cocci or bacilli	Topical:	Bacitracin and gentamicin
	Subconjunctival:	Methicillin and gentamicin
Gram-negative cocci	Topical:	Bacitracin
	Subconjunctival:	Penicillin G
Gram-negative bacilli	Topical:	Gentamicin and carbenicillin
	Subconjunctival:	Gentamicin and carbenicillin

Modified from Jones D. Early diagnosis and therapy of bacterial corneal ulcers. In: Laibson PR, Trobe JD, eds. External ocular diseases: Diagnosis and current therapy. Int Ophthalmol Clin 1973;13:1–29.

of corneal ulcers based on the particular organism cultured.

S. AUREUS

Clinical Description. Central corneal ulcers caused by *S. aureus* are being encountered more often than in the past. This greater frequency is thought to be partially due to the increased use of topical steroids and because the ulcer occurs as a secondary infection with herpes simplex keratitis. Hence, *S. aureus* is considered to be an opportunistic organism. The aerobic, gram-positive cocci are often harbored on the conjunctiva, skin, and nares as part of the normal flora.

The gray-white, infiltrated, central ulcer due to staphylococcal infection is often round or oval and remains localized, with distinct borders, unless microabscesses occur.[87] A purulent, ropy discharge is present. The eyelids and conjunctiva are injected and chemotic. A sterile hypopyon may develop due to the increased permeability of the iris and ciliary body vessels to fibrin and polymorphonuclear leukocytes.

Management. When the *S. aureus* ulcer is less than 3 mm in diameter, is not in the axial corneal area, and is present without hypopyon, the patient can be monitored during daily office visits.

Appropriate antibiotic therapy, such as gentamicin (fortified to 9 to 13.6 mg/ml), 2 to 3 drops approximately every 2 hours should be initiated.[89] Lid hygiene procedures and warm compresses should be instituted.

If the ulcer is greater than 3 mm in diameter, presents with hypopyon, or is located in the axial cornea, the patient generally should be hospitalized in case antimicrobial sensitivities dictate a change in therapy. It also ensures compliance with around-the-clock topical medications and frequent biomicroscopic examinations.

S. PNEUMONIAE

Clinical Description. *S. pneumoniae,* often found as part of the normal flora in the upper respiratory tract, is the major bacterial pathogen that attacks disrupted corneal epithelium. The pneumococcal corneal ulcer usually occurs 24 to 48 hours after inoculation of an abraded cornea. It typically produces a gray, fairly well-circumscribed ulcer that tends to spread erratically from the original site of infection toward the center of the cornea.[7] The advancing border generally develops a shaggy undermined edge of active ulceration and infiltration as the trailing border begins to heal (Color Plate XV). The superficial corneal layers become involved first, and then the deeper parenchyma. The cornea surrounding the ulcer is often clear.

Scrapings from the leading edge of a pneumococcal corneal ulcer contain gram-positive, lancet-shaped diplococci. Sterile hypopyons tend to occur often in *S. pneumoniae* corneal ulcers.[12]

Management. Since ophthalmic bacitracin, which is very effective for this type of infection, is commercially available only as an ointment, topical drops for frequent instillation must be prepared using sterile, powdered bacitracin.[1] This is accomplished by withdrawing 9 ml of a fresh tear substitute from a 15 ml bottle with a sterile hypodermic needle and syringe through the bottle's opening. This 9 ml of artificial tear solution is then inserted, 3 ml at a time, through the rubber tops of 3 vials of bacitracin (50,000 units/vial). The reconstituted bacitracin is then drawn out and replaced into the original tear substitute bottle to rejoin the 6 ml of artificial tears that were not initially removed from the bottle. This yields a bacitracin solution of 10,000 units/ml (150,000 units/15 ml). The drops should be initially instilled every 30 minutes. As the ulcerated and infiltrated area begins to shrink, the frequency of instillation is tapered until the ulcer resolves completely. Meticulous lid hygiene and frequent warm compresses also appear to be helpful.

P. AERUGINOSA

Clinical Description.   *P. aeruginosa* is the most common gram-negative organism causing corneal ulcers.[90] It is morphologically very similar to other gram-negative enteric bacilli, making diagnosis by staining difficult. However, it is a ubiquitous organism that thrives in warm, moist environments, such as whirlpools, bath water, and swimming pools.[91] It may be found as a contaminant in ophthalmic solutions such as sodium fluorescein.[92] It may also inhabit contact lens cases[93] and eye cosmetics such as mascara.[94] In the eye, *P. aeruginosa* can cause the most destructive hypopyon keratitis.

Patients using extended wear contact lenses are at greater risk of developing bacterial corneal ulcers than are patients wearing daily wear lenses.[95] When corneal ulceration does occur, it tends to be located more centrally than peripherally and more superiorly and centrally than inferiorly. *P. aeruginosa* has become the most common organism to cause corneal infections associated with the use of extended wear contact lenses.[96,97]

Corneal ulcers due to *P. aeruginosa* may be divided into 2 groups,[3] with the less common type being the less severe. The ulcers caused by this strain of *Pseudomonas* are atypical in that they develop more slowly and remain localized off the visual axis. This strain is less virulent probably because it does not liberate a proteolytic enzyme.[3]

The more common type of ulcer is due to a corneal-virulent strain of *Pseudomonas* that produces a protease that is proteolytic against corneal collagen. The destructive process is therefore rapid and necrotic. The ocular involvement ranges from conjunctivitis and corneal abscess to endophthalmitis, orbital cellulitis, and septicemia. Soon after corneal inoculation, the eye will develop epithelial ulceration, dense stromal infiltrates, and necrosis with a greenish mucopurulent discharge. Endothelial plaques are seen, and the ulcer will spread to include most or all of the cornea. A hypopyon usually occurs. Within 24 hours, descemetocele formation, melting, and perforation may result. If the eye is to be saved, there must be immediate recognition and early treatment. To establish an early diagnosis, the characteristic signs and symptoms must be perceived and identified.[12] The patient will usually have a history of corneal injury, often by a foreign body. Also, most cases have a recent history of ocular therapy. Finally, ocular pain is almost always present 1 to 3 days after the corneal insult.

Management.   Several different antibiotics have been used with varying degrees of success. Gentamicin is generally recognized as the most effective therapeutic agent.[12] It should be administered topically in an ophthalmic solution, 13.6 mg/ml every 30 minutes. However, the clinician must recognize that some strains of *P. aeruginosa* have developed resistance to gentamicin while retaining their sensitivity to tobramycin and amikacin.[98] Topical carbenicillin (4 mg/ml) may also be used concurrently every hour. Although some practitioners advocate additional periocular antibiotics,[5,12] these medications do not seem to enhance the effectiveness of topical therapy.[99] The use of steroids does not reduce scarring and may lead to increased number of organisms.[100] Treatment should continue for several weeks after apparent clinical cure, since the infections may recur many days after therapy ceases. Since most cases occur in small sporadic epidemics, the source of contamination should be found and eliminated. Local polymyxin B therapy may be used within 3 days for individuals who have been exposed.[12]

OTHER BACTERIA

Initial treatment of corneal ulcers due to unknown or uncommon organisms may, in general, be commenced according to the results of the Gram stain. Initial antibiotic therapy should be broad and intensive. When the final culture and sensitivity reports are available, treatment may require adjustment. Should no organism be found but the clinical situation points strongly to a bacterial etiology, topical therapy should be continued. Bacitracin as 0.5% ointment or as a prepared solution of 10,000 units/ml should be used hourly on an alternate basis with gentamicin ophthalmic solution. In addition, lid hygiene and warm compresses seem to aid recovery.

Gram-positive cocci that can cause corneal ulcers are the *Staphylococcus* and *Streptococcus* species. Although some authors recommend penicillin,[7,82] these species are often penicillin-resistant,[5] so therapy should be initiated with bacitracin solution or ointment hourly and may be supplemented with gentamicin topical ophthalmic solution.

Gram-positive bacilli rarely cause corneal ulcers. Ampicillin is used against *Listeria* species. *Bacillus* and *Clostridium* species respond best to penicillin G. Erythromycin is effective against *C. diphtheriae*.

Gram-negative cocci include *Neisseria* species. Topical therapy should begin with bacitracin ointment or solution hourly. Penicillin may also be needed, keeping in mind the systemic therapy necessitated by *N. gonorrhoeae*.

Gram-negative bacilli such as *E. coli* and *Klebsiella* and *Proteus* species should be treated with gentamicin ophthalmic solution hourly or ointment every 2 hours. Until *Pseudomonas* infection is excluded by culture results, therapy of gram-negative rod infections should be approached aggressively and with close observation.

Herpes Simplex Virus Keratitis

ETIOLOGY

A dendriform, epithelial keratitis or ulceration is normally produced as an acute and chronic corneal disease by infection with herpes simplex virus type 1 (HSV-1). Despite all the advances in antiviral therapy in the past 20 years, HSV keratitis remains a leading cause of corneal blindness in the United States. This virus uses humans as its natural host and only reservoir of infection, and it is marked by its unusual ability to cause recurrent, localized lesions. Primary infection with HSV occurs most commonly between the ages of 2 and 5 years and involves about 70% to 80% of the population, yet in only 1% to 10% of infection does the disease become clinically evident.[101] Under age 6 months, an infant has neutralizing antibody against HSV from the mother.[102] The virus remains within the host for life and may be reactivated at regular or varying intervals with characteristic signs and symptoms.

Humans are so susceptible to HSV that by age 15 years, 90% of the U.S. population is infected systemically.[103] Infection usually results from contact with infected individuals, although not necessarily from those with active lesions.

Reactivation of the latent virus commonly results in herpes labialis (fever blisters) and may be precipitated by fever, shock, immunosuppressive agents (such as steroids), ultraviolet light burns, or other trigger mechanisms. The severity of the disease is indicated by the finding that 26% of the patients who develop herpetic keratitis for the first time will have a second attack. Additionally, in those who have had a history of previous disease (2 or more attacks), there is a 43% chance of its recurrence.[104]

DIAGNOSIS

A typical case of HSV keratitis often begins with a foreign body sensation. Early in the course of infection, the eye may be painful, with lacrimation and photophobia, but as the disease progresses, corneal sensitivity diminishes.[101] The cornea may also exhibit a punctate epithelial keratitis (PEK) during early onset of the disease.[103]

The HSV lesion usually begins as minute areas of opaque cells on the corneal epithelial surface. In the early stages, the vesicles rupture and appear as superficial dots. The discrete areas of epithelial involvement may then coalesce and appear in a coarse, punctate, stellate, or dendritic pattern to form the classic linear or arborescent ulcer. The dendritic ulcer of primary herpes simplex has an easily recognizable arborescent pattern (Color Plate XVI) with irregular (serrated) but sharply defined borders that are diagnostically considered to be elevated.[105] In addition, terminal end bulbs (rounded ends) may be present. Sodium fluorescein stains the ulcer crater intensely where the loss of epithelium has occurred, whereas rose bengal brightly stains the damaged epithelial cells of the ulcer border (see Color Plate XVI). A mild uveitis with keratic precipitates and ciliary injection may also occur.

The differential diagnosis is aided by several other clinical determinations. Mechanical debridement will remove the dendritic lesions only if the corneal epithelium surrounding the ulcer is removed. Additionally, associated cutaneous lesions are often of considerable diagnostic importance, since the HSV dendritic keratitis can be associated with vesicles around the lips and eyelids. Corneal sensitivity is generally considered to be reduced or absent, resulting in corneal hypoesthesia or anesthesia. This can be demonstrated by drawing wisps of cotton over each cornea and observing the diminished or absent blink response in the involved eye. Careful observation of the blink rate and lacrimation, along with the patient's subjective comparison of the "touch" in each eye, will aid in determining reduction in corneal sensitivity.

The isolation of HSV from active corneal epithelial lesions, either dendritic or dendritic-geographic ulcers, remains the most common way of confirming this viral corneal infection, aside from the clinical picture. Fortunately, HSV can generally be procured from the edges of an ulcer without much difficulty provided rose bengal, having antiviral activity, has not been instilled into the eye.[158] A cotton swab can be dipped into a test tube containing a prepoured 5 ml aliquot of Hank's modified balanced salt medium (Flow Laboratories). The wet swab is then rubbed on the ulcerated epithelium and subsequently broken into the same medium. The tube is capped and sent to a virology laboratory. The sample is injected into cell cultures of primary human embryonic kidney, diploid human lung, primary Rhesus monkey kidneys, or the continuous cell line derived from human cervical or nasopharyngeal carcinoma. The isolates of *H. hominis,* as well as the majority of all viruses, produce a morphologic alteration called a cytopathic effect (CPE) in the tissue cell cultures. *Herpesvirus* has a rapid CPE, within 24 to 48 hours, in contrast to the slow-growing varicella zoster virus, making laboratory differentiation between HSV and herpes zoster relatively simple.

Stromal herpetic keratitis that occurs in some individuals has been assumed to reflect a difference in the effects of infection on their immune systems. However, evidence is accumulating that variations in the herpetic virus genome itself may be the primary factor determining disease virulence rather than pointing to a lethargic immunologic system.[106] Some *Herpesvirus* strains produce large amounts of highly antigenic glycoproteins, which may stimulate a more severe host inflammatory reaction that involves the stroma as well as the epithelium.

In immunocompetent individuals, the disciform (stromal) keratitis is usually self-limited, lasting from several weeks to several months. However, when local or systemic immunosuppression is severe, the lesion may last for years. After repeated viral attacks, the disciform keratitis may appear as a chronic inflammation of the corneal stroma characterized by discoid edema and opacity. The stroma often becomes necrotic, and an accompanying iridocyclitis may be severe.

Hypopyon is rare. However, if present, it usually indicates a secondary bacterial or fungal infection. Focal avascular interstitial keratitis may also occur in HSV infection, but its production is usually associated with the use of steroids. Tiny areas of focal infiltration and edema are surrounded by areas of clear tissue. No vascularization is present, and any corneal level may be affected. Peripheral corneal lesions may also evolve, with a linear appearance. Epithelial loss occurs before the underlying corneal stroma becomes infiltrated. This can differentiate the herpetic marginal ulcer from the marginal ulcer of bacterial infections, in which the stroma is usually affected first. Because of the decreased corneal sensitivity, these patients are far less photophobic than patients with nonherpetic corneal infiltrates and ulcerations.

MANAGEMENT

Before the advent of chemotherapeutic methods to treat HSV keratitis, the epithelial disease was often best treated by mechanical debridement. The infected epithelial cells at the edges of the ulcer were removed mechanically by rubbing and abrading them with a cotton-tipped applicator after instillation of a suitable anesthetic, such as cocaine or tetracaine. Following debridement, the eye was pressure-patched until it healed.

Although mechanical debridement is still widely used as a management technique,[160,161] chemotherapeutic means are generally added to or have entirely replaced debridement. If mechanical debridement is used, vidarabine ointment is still liberally applied before patching. Frequent repatching (from 4 to 5 times daily) will increase the number of opportunities to instill the antiviral ointment.

Instead of initially debriding (especially in patients who must continue working or functioning visually throughout the course of treatment), it is generally preferred to begin trifluridine (Viroptic) drops every 1 to 2 hours during the day and vidarabine (Vira-A) ointment every 3 to 4 hours after bedtime. Ointment every 3 hours may be slightly more effective than hourly drops, in terms of the speed with which the epithelial lesions heal. However, some patients find use of an ointment unacceptable. If, 48 hours after the initiation of antiviral therapy, no response is noted (i.e., the defect is no smaller), the area can be debrided and repatched, with the instillation of vidarabine ointment every 2 to 3 hours. As the defect heals, the antiviral agent should be gradually tapered from 5 times a day to twice a day until day 14 of therapy, when treatment can generally be discontinued. Once the epithelium is healed, the antiviral agent must be continued at a reduced dosage for 5 to 7 days to allow latent virus to be shed. If the lesion is on the visual axis, trifluridine is the superior antiviral agent because IDU deposits can remain in the stroma underlying the previous epithelial lesion, leaving a "ghost dendrite" that may decrease visual acuity. In addition, trifluridine is the preferred antiviral agent for patients who have had multiple recurrences or in whom antiviral resistance is suspected. An alternative therapy for HSV keratitis is 400 mg of acyclovir (Zovirax) given orally 5 times daily for patients who are unable or unwilling to use topical treatment.[157]

If a superimposed bacterial blepharoconjunctivitis occurs, an antibiotic should be prescribed. Cycloplegics are sometimes beneficial in patients in whom associated anterior chamber inflammation has occurred.

Recurrent erosions may take place following healing of the epithelial ulcerative keratitis. Management should include removal of the hypertrophic and loose epithelium. The eye should then be patched with 5% sodium chloride ointment until healing occurs. Frequent use of sodium chloride drops throughout the day should be initiated for several weeks. Thereafter, instillation of sodium chloride ointment at bedtime may be sufficient.

It is generally agreed that the local administration of corticosteroids in epithelial disease causes the virus to replicate more rapidly. This produces a larger area of superficial ulceration in which there appear prolongations and knobs around the periphery characteristic of the so-called geographic or ameboid ulcer (Color Plate XVII). These "steroid-stimulated" herpetic ulcers seem harder to control, even with the new chemotherapeutic agents such as trifluridine. Thus, steroids are generally contraindicated in epithelial herpetic disease. Some evidence suggests that there are 2 different strains of *H. hominis,* with dissimilar responses to steroids. Specifically, the disease produced by either virus genome without concurrent steroid treatment is not different. However, when steroids are added, the first type does not produce an exaggerated disease, while the second genome does.[107] Since the clinician has no way of determining, at this time, which herpetic genome is responsible for the disease occurring in any particular patient, the use of steroids should be avoided.

The management of stromal herpetic disciform keratitis is very often clinically challenging. The stromal inflammatory process causes large numbers of polymorphonuclear leukocytes to accumulate, thus liberating collagenolytic enzymes that can initiate corneal destruction.[108] As the chronic inflammation continues, scarring and neovascularization may result (Fig. 22.9). Hence, steroid treatment of a stromal keratitis may reduce the inflammation and the associated sequelae. However, if initiated, the steroids may encourage existing epithelial viral disease. Since therapy often will last for many weeks or months, the possibility of complications necessitates close supervision.

Several clear indications exist for the use of topical steroids in the treatment of stromal keratitis; these include corneal destruction, neovascularization, marked intraocular inflammation, and elevated intraocular pressure.[108]

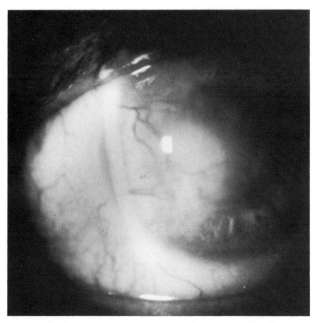

FIGURE 22.9 **Stromal HSV disease with edema, infiltration, and vascularization.**

Once it is decided to treat with steroids, the dose must be titrated according to the severity of the inflammation. A common starting point is prednisolone phosphate 0.5% drops every 6 hours.[108] After 24 hours, the dosage schedule can be adjusted. Obviously concomitant antiviral prophylactic therapy with vidarabine or trifluridine for patients with intact corneas should be prescribed approximately 2 to 3 times daily. Once the steroid dosage is significantly reduced (e.g., prednisolone phosphate 0.5% once daily), the antiviral agent can be discontinued.

Varicella Zoster Keratitis

ETIOLOGY

Herpes zoster presents as an acute vesicular eruption caused by the varicella zoster virus, which is morphologically the identical virus that causes chickenpox. The laboratory isolation of the varicella zoster virus, although possible, is rather difficult. The virus is considered to be recoverable only within the first 72 hours of the disease. Second, there is a low titer of virus in the corneal dendritic lesions.

DIAGNOSIS

Herpes zoster ophthalmicus is an infectious process of the trigeminal (gasserian) ganglion, which receives fibers from the ophthalmic nerve. A high degree of correlation exists between involvement of the eye and the tip of the nose, since the nasociliary nerve gives rise to the two long anterior ciliary nerves and the external nasal branch. The disease usually manifests itself as a severe, unilateral and dermatologically disabling neuralgia. Several days later, a peculiar vesicular eruption on an erythematous base with significant swelling and tenderness occurs on the skin (see Fig. 19.9).

Herpes zoster corneal epithelial lesions fall into 2 distinct groups: acute epithelial dendritic keratitis and delayed corneal mucous plaque keratitis. These are based on biomicroscopic appearance, time of onset, duration, behavior, and concurrent association with AIDS.[105,156]

Acute Epithelial Keratitis. This condition is characterized by small, fine, multiple dendritic or stellate lesions with slightly raised edges. These lesions appear early in the infection, within a few days of onset of the rash. They usually resolve in 4 to 6 days, and there is almost always an associated catarrhal conjunctivitis. The lesions appear in the peripheral cornea, and superficial stromal infiltrates may also be present. These acute intraepithelial lesions stain moderately well with both sodium fluorescein and rose bengal. Although corneal anesthesia is not encountered as often in acute herpes zoster as it is in HSV infection, it can occur in both diseases. This criterion may not be sufficiently specific to help in the definitive diagnosis.

Corneal Mucous Plaque Keratitis. This variation is a whitish gray plaque with sharp margins that lies on the surface of the epithelium and is linear or branching (dendriform). The plaques are usually multiple, vary in size and shape, and may appear anywhere on the cornea (Fig. 22.10). In fact, the lesions often change in shape, number, and size from day to day.

The underlying epithelium is swollen and composed of degenerated cells; thus, rose bengal stains the entire

lesion vividly. Sodium fluorescein, on the other hand, stains the lesion only minimally because no corneal epithelial ulcer exists. Stromal edema, to a certain extent, can be seen over most of the cornea. Dendriform-shaped corneal dry spots may be seen, but the Schirmer tear test is usually normal.

Corneal mucous plaques appear as early as 7 days and as late as 2 years after the first signs of cutaneous herpes zoster infection. However, the majority are seen 3 to 4 months after onset of the cutaneous lesions. These plaques are accompanied by ciliary and tarsal conjunctival injection, mild iritis, and a profuse deposition of fine keratic precipitates. Corneal sensation is almost always impaired.[105]

MANAGEMENT

Mechanical debridement of the acute corneal epithelial dendritic lesions is effective only if the involved corneal cells are removed. Mechanical debridement of the corneal mucous plaques lying on the epithelial surface can be accomplished quite easily by gently scraping with a wet cotton swab following topical anesthesia, resulting in minimal damage to the superficial epithelium.[105]

In addition to the debridement, treatment usually consists of routine administration of topical steroids or antibiotic-steroid ointment, applied to the eyelids 2 to 4 times daily. Topical steroid drops may be used from every 3 hours to once daily, depending on the severity of corneal involvement. If it is questionable whether HSV is concurrently present, vidarabine ointment or trifluridine drops, 4 times daily, may be added. Systemic steroid therapy may be useful. Since patients with acute ophthalmic herpes zoster are often very ill, aged, and infirm, hospitalization with proper therapy is often the most effective measure.

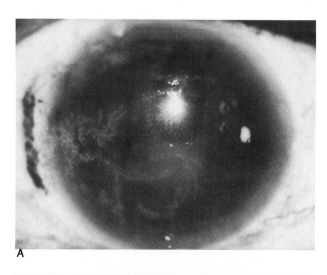

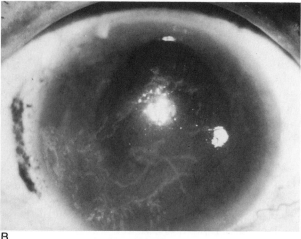

FIGURE 22.10 **Corneal mucous plaque keratitis associated with herpes zoster. *(A)* Initial presentation. *(B)* Note migratory nature of lesions 3 weeks later. (Courtesy Marc A. Michelson, M.D.)**

Fungal Corneal Ulcers

ETIOLOGY

Although fungal keratitis is extremely uncommon, it must nevertheless not be overlooked as a possible cause of corneal infection. It has a potentially devastating effect on the eye, especially if misdiagnosed or improperly treated. In the United States, the disease is more prevalent in the South and Southwest, with approximately 300 new cases occurring each year.[109] The most common causative agents are *Candida, Fusarium, Cephalosporium,* and *Aspergillus.*[110]

DIAGNOSIS

The clinical diagnosis of fungal keratitis is often very difficult by appearance alone. Positive laboratory identification of the organism by smear or culture is required before making a diagnosis and initiating antifungal therapy. One should suspect a filamentous fungal infection (e.g., *Fusarium* or *Aspergillus* species) if the cornea has been abraded or injured by any type of vegetable matter, such as a tree branch or shrub. On the other hand, the yeasts (e.g., *C. albicans*) tend to be associated with chronic corneal damage and previous long-term administration of steroids. The appearance of a fungal ulcer may mimic that of a bacterial or herpetic ulcer. The use of an antibiotic will generally serve only to enhance spread of the organism. Therefore, fungal infection must be considered in any case of persistent corneal ulcer that does not respond to antibiotic therapy or shows any signs or symptoms of HSV. A severe iritis with minimal pus is also typically seen in a fungal ulcerative keratitis. In addition, the ulcer may demonstrate hyphate margins with satellite lesions, endothelial plaques, and, occasionally, an immune ring in the presence of an elevated, ulcerative lesion. An uncontrolled fungal infection can eventually lead to corneal perforation, severe uveitis, and, in some cases, complete destruction of the eye.

MANAGEMENT

It is generally necessary to demonstrate the fungus and its hyphae on a smear or grow it on culture media before initiating antifungal therapy. Otherwise, it is most prudent to initiate therapy assuming that the ulcer is bacterial.

C. albicans infections are generally best treated with nystatin (Mycostatin) or natamycin 5% (Natacyn). The latter is available as an ophthalmic suspension and is generally administered every 2 to 4 hours.

The filamentous fungi are also generally effectively treated with natamycin 5%. Cycloplegics are used to decrease the uveal inflammation and to minimize posterior synechia formation.

Steroids should be avoided, since they enhance spread of the ulcer and can lead to loss of the eye.

Protozoan Corneal Ulcers

ETIOLOGY

Acanthamoeba is a ubiquitous protozoan found in soil, fresh and brackish water, the human throat, hot tubs, and contact lenses and their plastic cases.[111] A close causal association between *Acanthamoeba* and the use of salt tablets and distilled water is now well established.[112] Of the 22 known species of *Acanthamoeba*,[113] the 5 known to cause ocular infection have been identified as *A. castellanii, A. culbertsoni, A. hatchetti, A. polyphagia,* and *A. rhysodes*.[112] The 2 basic forms of this protozoan are a motile (trophozoite) form and a sessile (cystic) type. This latter form is double-walled, which makes it more resistant to freezing, dessication, antimicrobials, and most standard contact lens cleaning and disinfection methods. In addition, a preexisting gram-negative infection seems to enhance this protozoan's survival and infectivity.[112]

DIAGNOSIS

The 2 most common risk factors for developing an *Acanthamoeba* keratitis are contact lens wear and environmental exposure after corneal trauma resulting in an epithelial break.[111] The initial sign of infection is a patchy epithelial irregularity or pleomorphic epithelial defects assuming a stellate or dendriform pattern.[112] The infection is usually heralded by an abrupt increase in ocular pain and a decrease in vision. The pain is often disproportionate to the early clinical findings,[114] since it may be caused by radial infiltrates along the corneal nerves. The patient often has upper eyelid edema[115] and palpable preauricular adenopathy. The most common clinical signs include an annular stromal opacity that is coarsely granular with discrete lacunae occasionally appearing within the infiltrated area. The infiltrates are midstromal, normally beginning paracentrally and extending to the limbus in a radial pattern.[116] Severe iritis with hypopyon is possible. Corneal sensitivity becomes reduced later in the course of the infection. Stromal melting and corneal perforation occur in advanced infection.

Corneal scrapings of the suspected area should be accomplished thoroughly and should be as deep as possible and plated directly, in lieu of a transport medium. Giemsa and calcofluor white-stained smears; cultures on nonnutrient agar overlaid with *E. coli*, which normally become positive in three days[117]; and indirect fluorescent antibody stains for *Acanthamoeba* are all important in quickly establishing an accurate diagnosis.

The differential diagnosis may be easily confused with other corneal disorders, especially HSV epithelial and stromal keratitis. However, the ring-shaped stromal infiltrate of advanced infection is almost pathognomonic.[113]

MANAGEMENT

As a general rule, the treatment of *Acanthamoeba* keratitis is difficult. However, as in most corneal infections, early detection and treatment aid the prognosis. Medical therapy is not always satisfactory, even though propamidine isethionate 1% ointment (Brolene) has been shown to have some effect.[114] Some efficacy has been demonstrated by ketoconazole (Nizoral), miconazole (Monistat), and neomycin (Neosporin). The temporary beneficial effects seem related to reducing the bacterial growth that provides nutrition for the *Acanthamoeba*, thereby causing the protozoans to encyst. Moore and McCulley[153] have suggested the use of topical Neosporin and propamidine isethionate every 15 minutes to 1 hour around the clock for 3 days, then every hour while awake for 4 days. This is followed by use of the drugs every 2 hours for 1 week, then 4 times a day indefinitely. These authors did not recommend use of steroids, and they controlled the pain with 0.33 ml of absolute ethyl alcohol and 0.66 ml of lidocaine 2% as needed. The pain normally subsided 2 to 3 weeks after appropriate therapy.

Topical steroids have been used as supportive therapy to decrease the host immunologic response. However, the prolonged use of topical steroids in the medical management of *Acanthamoeba* keratitis may cause secondary bacterial keratitis.

Hydrophilic bandage contact lenses may be needed for persistent epithelial defects or erosions. Pain can be lessened by using ibuprofen, retrobulbar lidocaine-alcohol injections, or sulindac 200 mg twice daily.[114]

Penetrating keratoplasty is eventually needed in a large percentage of patients who develop *Acanthamoeba* keratitis.[112] Hence, it is important for the keratoplasty to be performed before the infected tissue nears the corneal periphery, since graft rejection is minimized by a smaller corneal button.[112]

Patients with contact lenses should be instructed to immediately discontinue wearing the lenses and seek primary eyecare if a red, painful eye should develop. In addition, contact lenses should never be worn in a hot tub, brackish water, or swimming pools. The lenses should not be exposed to saliva, dirty hands, tap or airplane water, soil, or nonsterile, unpreserved saline.

To best eliminate the occurrence of *Acanthamoeba* keratitis, patients should be carefully educated about proper contact lens care. This should include the recommendations to avoid distilled water (with either salt tablets or enzyme tablets), tap water, well water, saliva, or intravenous saline for either soft or hard contact lenses.[118] Commercially prepared saline solutions should be used and refrigerated when not in use. Thermal disinfection (in contrast to hydrogen peroxide) is effective against *Acanthamoeba* keratitis provided the lens is not stored in contaminated solutions or tap water after disinfection.[118]

Interstitial Keratitis

Etiology

The term interstitial keratitis (IK) refers to vascularization and nonsuppurative infiltration affecting all or part of the corneal stroma, usually associated with a systemic disease. The presence of a silvery, stromal opacification, often in a patchy or feathery configuration, is seen. Ghost vessels from previous processes of active inflammatory vascularization are common.[119]

Diagnosis

SYPHILIS

It is known that 90% of all cases of IK are secondary to syphilis.[103] Evidence indicates that the condition is an immunologic reaction to *Treponema pallidum*. The congenital form is usually bilateral (80%), with about two-thirds of the cases occurring between the ages of 5 years and the late teens. IK secondary to acquired syphilis is commonly uniocular (60%), often milder, limited to a sector of the cornea, and occasionally more amenable to treatment.[82] A positive fluorescent treponemal antibody absorption (FTA-ABS) test confirms the presence of a previous syphilitic infection.

Because of the reduction in the number of congenital syphilis cases, the practitioner seldom encounters acute IK. The acute stage begins with indistinct cellular infiltration, edema of the endothelium, keratic precipitates, miosis, and small stromal opacities. The initial symptoms include pain, lacrimation, conjunctival infection, and blurring of vision. Thereafter, gross vascularization can occur that results in the cornea's pinkish "salmon patch" appearance.

The most usual presentations of IK are congenital cases encountered during routine examination of adults when the residual effects of the active inflammation are first seen. These changes, which demonstrate a 3:1 predilection for females,[50] include diffuse stromal scarring, opacification, residual vascularization, and ghost vessels. Case histories in these adult cases reveal the recollection of severe childhood ocular inflammation that lasted several months.

TUBERCULOSIS

IK secondary to tuberculosis is believed to be due to an autoimmune reaction to the tuberculoprotein occurring in patients with systemic tuberculosis. A negative FTA-ABS and positive tuberculin skin test aid in clinical diagnosis and determination of etiology.

In tuberculosis keratitis, which is often unilateral, the cornea is typically involved in the peripheral inferior sector only, when it manifests a ring-shaped, dense, abscess-like, nodular opacity. The central cornea is relatively spared. Resolution is less rapid and less complete than that due to syphilis, leaving a dense, sector-like scar (Fig. 22.11).

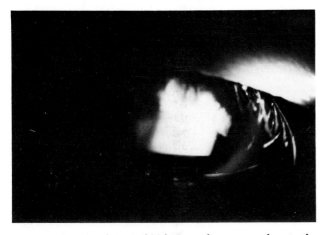

FIGURE 22.11   A dense, whitish stromal scar secondary to the interstitial keratitis of tuberculosis.

OTHER CAUSES

The most common pathologic conditions known to cause nonsuppurative, nondisciform IK are listed in Table 22.4. A nonsystemic condition that may result in IK is a chemical burn to the eye. Disciform keratitis can occur in herpes zoster, HSV, mumps, varicella, variola, and vaccinia.

Management

The more commonly encountered cases of IK generally require keratoplasty when the visual acuities are impaired enough that transplantation is necessary.

In active IK, local steroids are used to suppress the disease process and sometimes must be continued 1 or 2 years.[80] Cycloplegics are used to avoid the development of posterior synechiae and promote patient comfort. These will generally improve the final visual acuity outcome.

Treatment for the systemic problem should be initiated. This includes rifampin and isoniazid for tuberculosis and penicillin for late congenital syphilis. Penicillin does not have a pronounced effect on the

TABLE 22.4
Common Systemic Conditions Causing Interstitial Keratitis

Congenital syphilis	Mumps
Acquired syphilis	Lymphogranuloma venereum
Tuberculosis	Cogan's syndrome
Leprosy	Gold toxicity
Onchocerciasis	Herpes simplex

course of IK and may even lead to a flare-up, perhaps due to the liberation of antigen as in the systemic Herxheimer's reaction.[82] Penicillin treatment of congenital syphilis does not prevent the onset of keratitis later, nor does it prevent subsequent involvement of the fellow eye.

Degenerative Processes

Acute Ectasia Secondary to Keratoconus

ETIOLOGY

Anterior keratoconus, or ectactic corneal dystrophy, is a bilateral condition of uncertain etiology characterized by noninflammatory axial ectasia and corneal thinning. This results in a painless, progressive loss of vision due to the development of a high amount of irregular myopic astigmatism and scarring. The process generally begins at puberty and progresses for several years before stabilizing. Further progession may occur at any time. Corneal perforation can occur in advanced cases.

Keratoconus may be developmental, degenerative, or secondary to disease or nutritional disorder. It seems to have genetic influences, but no distinctive pattern of inheritance exists. A large number of environmental risk factors has been expounded. For instance, a circumstantial association does seem to exist between hard contact lens wear and the development of keratoconus. However, no cause-effect relationships can be drawn from existing data.[120] Associations have been made to many conditions, although most of them are probably invalid.[50] Although many predisposing causes may well exist, such as eye rubbing, Down's syndrome, atopic disease, connective tissue disease, and tapeto-retinal degeneration,[121] much remains to be clarified in the inheritance and etiology of keratoconus.

Histologically, there is focal disruption of Bowman's layer with patches of fibroblastic activity in that area. The epithelium is irregular with an abnormal basement membrane.[122] If Descemet's membrane tears, a condition known as acute ectasia develops. Acute hydrops may occur, with opacification and swelling of the corneal tissues due to the entrance of aqueous. There is a corresponding decrease in visual acuity. The condition resolves within 8 to 10 weeks, although some scarring may remain. If the scar is not in the pupillary area, vision can actually improve with contraction of the scar, since this may flatten the cone.[25]

DIAGNOSIS

The major symptom of keratoconus is gradual visual deterioration. The apex of the cone is usually displaced nasally and inferiorly with an oblique conical deformation of the cone. This causes vision to be distorted and blurred. Since the apex is eccentric, the patient looks through its side. Ordinary spectacle lenses cannot compensate for the parabolic curve and therefore are of little value. To overcome the distortion, the patient will tend to close the lids somewhat, converting the palpebral aperture into a stenopeic slit, thereby narrowing the circles of confusion. Using pinholes and stenopeic slits to test visual acuities may help in the diagnosis.

Other symptoms include monocular polyopia and an increase in photophobia. The patient seldom complains of pain but may report asthenopia or headaches.

Many signs are indicative of keratoconus. Munson's sign demonstrates the protrusion of the apex. This can be shown by corneal protrusion of the lower lid when the patient gazes downward. Slit-lamp examination will demonstrate thinning of the corneal apex from one-half to one-fifth its normal thickness. The thinning may be so marked as to allow the pulse beat of the intraocular pressure to be seen.[50] Vertical stress striae, known as Vogt's lines, are observed deep in the affected stroma. The increased concavity of the posterior surface may cause an endothelial "dew-drop" reflex to appear in the central portion of the cornea. There is an increased visibility of nerve fibers, and, in the advanced stages, ruptures in Descemet's membrane and Bowman's layer may be seen. Fleischer's ring, greenish yellow hemosiderin deposits at Bowman's layer, may be seen around the base of the cone. Diagnosis is also aided by noting distortion of the corneal image with the Placido's disk, keratometer, and retinoscope. Keratometric diopter readings are high, usually 48.00 D or more. Direct ophthalmoscopy is inhibited, with fundus details indistinct and unfocusable. A circular, oblong, or dumbbell-shaped shadow may appear that looks like a large indefinite cataract separating the central from the peripheral red reflex.

Posterior keratoconus has no known relationship to anterior keratoconus. The former is characterized by an absence of Descemet's membrane centrally with subsequent corneal edema. There is a slight indentation of the posterior cornea.

MANAGEMENT

Spectacles should be used as long as possible to correct the keratoconic patient's vision. When the irregular astigmatism is so advanced that visual acuity is unsatisfactory, rigid gas permeable contact lenses can be prescribed. Small, relatively thin lenses used with a 3-point touch fit (i.e., a light apical touch with peripheral touch at secondary bearing areas) are effective. Hard contact lenses do not, however, retard or halt progression of the cone.[120]

When contact lenses no longer provide adequate vision, if there is too much scarring, or if chronic edema persists after an acute attack of hydrops, keratoplasty should be considered. Penetrating keratoplasty is the most common procedure, although it is not always successful in the treatment of keratoconus, particularly in the case of extensive cones or displaced cones with limbal involvement.[123] In addition, penetrating grafts are always subject to rejection, which may be more frequent in patients receiving bilateral grafts.[124] Hence, these patients require close postoperative monitoring. Lamellar grafts are safer but have not shown the capacity to produce 20/20 (6/6) visual acuity. The epikeratophakia graft technique has produced visual acuities of 20/20 (6/6) in keratoconic patients, although this procedure is still undergoing clinical trials.[123]

Thermokeratoplasty has been used with some success.[125] This technique suffers from the problems of resteepening, scarring, and occasional epithelial defects,[126] so it should be considered a temporary measure.

As mentioned earlier, acute ectasia will usually improve spontaneously.[121] Topical steroids may be used to minimize scarring. Should perforation occur, the eye should be bandaged and the dressing changed daily until a corneal scar seals the wound. Corneal transplantation may be necessary.

Sclerokeratitis

ETIOLOGY

The etiology of sclerokeratitis is often difficult to define clearly but is part of the same mechanism that causes severe scleritis. When the anterior sclera undergoes extreme inflammation, the pathologic condition may spread to include the corneal surface. Sclerokeratitis is unilateral, and although it is rare, it is the most common corneal complication of scleral disease.

DIAGNOSIS

The patient with sclerokeratitis usually complains of pain, photophobia, and irritation. There is no discharge, but usually a severe anterior nongranulomatous uveitis is present. Sclerokeratitis is occasionally seen in conjunction with rheumatoid arthritis,[127] polyarteritis,[82] and Wegener's granulomatosis.[128]

In the area adjacent to the scleritis, corneal edema and stromal infiltration cause the cornea to thicken slightly and appear gray. The changes progress toward the axial area, but the pupillary region usually remains relatively clear. In some instances, the condition can progress to total corneal opacification. Irregular vascularization can occur at any level, and it will follow behind the advancing edge. Also trailing the leading border, spotty white opacities may develop that become crystalline. At times "precipitin rings" will appear around the white corneal opacities.[3] The cornea may appear very white, especially distal to the limbus. A yellow opacity formed by lipid deposition can occur at the outer edge of the lesion in advanced cases. The progression of sclerokeratitis may subside after months or years.

MANAGEMENT

The treatment of sclerokeratitis corresponds to that of the causative scleritis. Drugs used to treat severe scleritis include oxyphenbutazone, indomethacin, prednisolone, and immunosuppressive drugs such as azathioprine (see Chapter 23). Warm compresses and local steroid drops are used to relieve the discomfort. The pupil should be kept dilated with 1% atropine, 1 drop twice daily. Although atropine is indicated (especially in uveitis), there is a possibility of peripheral anterior synechia formation between the iris and the inflamed cornea. This may lead to iris bombé and secondary angle-closure glaucoma. Homatropine 5% can be substituted for atropine to decrease the likelihood of complications.

Bullous Keratopathy

ETIOLOGY

This noninflammatory disorder is not an independent disease but, rather, represents later stages of intense or chronic corneal edema. Consequently, bullous keratopathy is seen only in severely diseased eyes.[129] Reported causes are listed in Table 22.5. The development of bullous keratopathy depends mostly on endothelial damage, with epithelial changes remaining localized to a section of the cornea, or diffuse, depending on the extent of endothelial involvement.

TABLE 22.5
Causes of Bullous Keratopathy

- Glaucoma
- Cataract extraction/intraocular lens
- Anterior synechiae
- Vitreous touch
- Immunologic reaction after keratoplasty
- Fuchs' dystrophy
- Epithelial downgrowth
- Perforating wounds
- Birth trauma
- Anterior-posterior radial keratotomy

DIAGNOSIS

Bullous keratopathy is characterized by epithelial bullae or blebs. Filamentous tags can be observed along with epithelial bedewing, stromal edema, and endothelial changes. Ultimately, degenerative changes may appear, and blood vessels will invade the cornea from the limbus to form degenerative pannus. The condition is persistent, with the bullae enlarging, bursting, and reappearing. The recurrent cycle is associated with irritation and pain.

Pseudophakic bullous keratopathy is a relatively new clinical syndrome. In this condition, corneal endothelial dysfunction is associated with intraocular implants.[129–131]

MANAGEMENT

Most therapeutic measures are directed toward alleviating the symptoms of irritation. Soft contact lenses can protect against breakdown of the bullous lesions and thereby provide comfort for many patients, although this rarely improves visual acuity. Topical hyperosmotic agents, although they may temporarily reduce the edema, are generally unsatisfactory in reducing the corneal edema. Other methods of alleviating discomfort include chemical cauterization of the cornea, placing a conjunctival flap over the cornea, and penetrating keratoplasty. If the eye is painful and blind, retrobulbar alcohol injection or enucleation may become necessary.

Penetrating keratoplasty has been used with increasing frequency in recent years with excellent anatomic and visual results.[132] The most notable exception to this is the unsatisfactory vision achieved in some cases of aphakic bullous keratopathy.[133]

Band Keratopathy

ETIOLOGY

Band keratopathy is a condition in which a grayish white area slowly develops axially from the corneoscleral limbus in the interpalpebral aperture. This band is composed of calcium in the phosphate and carbonate salts.[134]

DIAGNOSIS

The grayish white deposits are located biomicroscopically in the epithelium, subepithelial tissue, and between the stromal lamellae.[135] These deposits are normally found in diseases causing hypercalcemia including hypervitaminosis D, in association with ocular inflammation such as acute anterior uveitis, and in dry eye syndromes. The exact mechanism by which calcium precipitates in the cornea remains unclear. However, local inflammation and hypercalcemia seem to be necessary factors. Since uveitis alters corneal metabolism, an elevation of tissue pH facilitates precipitation of the calcium salts. There has been an association between band keratopathy and the use of topical pilocarpine containing the preservative phenylmercuric nitrate, as well as the thimerosal in artificial tear solutions.[134] In addition, chronic exposure to mercury fumes has been linked with the development of band keratopathy.[134]

MANAGEMENT

Patients who have significant anterior segment inflammation, severe corneal desiccation, and a disruption of the epithelium should not use ocular medications containing a mercurial preservative, since these agents may assist in precipitating calcium.

The whitish gray opacity can be treated by carefully scraping away the calcium precipitate with a scalpel blade. In addition, partial chelation of the lesion can be achieved with ethylenediaminetetraacetic acid (EDTA). The lesion should be irrigated with 0.37% EDTA solution for 15 to 20 minutes.

Avitaminosis A

ETIOLOGY

This condition is caused by deficient levels of vitamin A.

DIAGNOSIS

The significant anterior segment findings in avitaminosis A are conjunctival xerosis and keratomalacia (corneal softening). Although many clinicians believe that xerophthalmic corneal destruction occurs clinically in "white and quiet" eyes, inflammation frequently occurs, with conjunctival injection masking the xerosis.[136] The keratomalacia leads to corneal melting and perforation. Because of systemic developments, there is a relatively high mortality rate in avitaminosis A.[137]

The initial clinical findings include a bilaterally dry, lackluster appearance of the conjunctiva and cornea that may be accompanied by abnormal night vision due to the role of vitamin A in the retinal photoreceptors. The patient usually reports a dry, sandy feeling in the eyes and has increased light sensitivity. The epithelium of the conjunctiva is keratinized, wrinkled, and often pigmented. The conjunctival changes are often associated with the presence of Bitot's spots, which appear as small, white, foamy, wedge-shaped elevations in the conjunctiva, usually on the temporal side (Fig. 22.12).

Scrapings from this area generally will show *Corynebacterium xerosis* and keratin. Although the association between Bitot's spots and vitamin A deficiency is strong, the spots are more likely to be a nonspecific manifestation of generalized malnutrition and are therefore not pathognomonic of vitamin A deficiency.

Corneal changes include infiltration, scarring, loss of sensitivity, and loss of stromal substance. Corneal involvement can be very serious, with keratomalacia occurring at a late stage of the disorder. Secondary infection and ulceration may lead to significant visual impairment and frequently to loss of the eye. Corneal ulcers associated with this condition are centrally located, bilateral, gray, and indolent. Corneal perforation is not uncommon.

MANAGEMENT

Retinoic acid 0.1% in arachis (peanut) oil applied topically 3 times daily has been shown to speed corneal

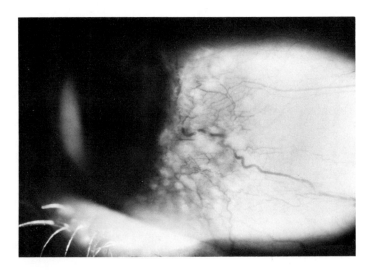

FIGURE 22.12   **Bitot's spots. (Courtesy Jimmy D. Bartlett, O.D.)**

healing significantly in a substantially larger proportion of xerophthalmia cases than systemic vitamin A alone.[138] The use of retinoic acid 3 times daily causes minimal side effects, but higher doses result in more florid vascularization and scarring.

This condition may also respond to the administration of large doses of vitamin A intramuscularly. The average daily requirement for adults is 5000 IU, and treatment dosages should be at least 20,000 IU/day.[7] Topical antibiotic drops and ointment may be used locally to prevent secondary infection. Tear substitutes or lubricating ointments should be used at frequent intervals for symptoms of irritation.

Corneal Dystrophies

A corneal dystrophy is a bilateral, symmetric, usually familial, noninflammatory condition typically involving the central portion of the cornea. Corneal dystrophies are of unknown etiology and may remain stationary or progress slowly throughout life. A large number of conditions are classified as corneal dystrophies; however, only the most common ones that are managed pharmacologically are considered in this chapter.

Epithelial Dystrophies

MEESMAN'S DYSTROPHY

Diagnosis. Meesman's corneal dystrophy (juvenile epithelial corneal dystrophy) occurs very early in life and progresses to produce bleblike epithelial vesicles that are distributed fairly uniformly throughout the epithelium. With direct slit-lamp illumination, the microcystic lesions appear as small, round, gray opacities that may stain with fluorescein if they come to the surface.[139] This condition may have associated with it symptoms of lacrimation, photophobia, and ocular irritation if the vesicles rupture. Vision is usually only minimally affected.

Management. Treatment is not usually required for this disorder. Should irritation be of consequence, soft contact lenses may be used in conjunction with artificial tear solutions and lubricating ointments. Lamellar keratoplasty is advised if visual interference becomes significant.

DYSTROPHIC RECURRENT EROSION

Diagnosis. Recurrent corneal erosions occur primarily in females and are associated with an abnormality of epithelial adhesion to the basement membrane. This causes the epithelial layers to be vulnerable to separation and erosion, the latter of which is demonstrated well by fluorescein staining (Fig. 22.13). The acute phase of the disorder may show epithelial loss, microcysts, bullae, and filament formation. Symptoms include pain (especially on awakening), photophobia, tearing, and foreign body sensation. Vision is reduced if the affected area is on the visual axis.

Recurrent episodes affect areas of the cornea previously involved. The erosions may occur at many locations on the cornea simultaneously, differentiating this from traumatic erosions, which are discussed later in this chapter. Familial bilateral erosion is rare compared with unilateral recurrent erosion associated with corneal trauma.

Management. Pressure-patching following the instillation of an antibiotic ointment should be used to aid epithelial regeneration.[140] Loose epithelium must be mechanically removed. To decrease the chance of recurrence, a hyperosmotic ointment such as 5% sodium chloride should be used at bedtime for several weeks. This will reduce lid friction and dehydrate the epithelium, allowing a tight adhesion to develop between the epithelium and the basement membrane. The use of artificial tears may help as a lubricant. Severe cases may require extended wear contact lens therapy to alleviate the pain and promote epithelial healing.

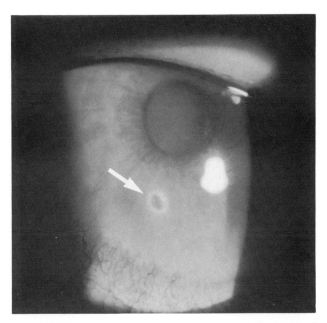

FIGURE 22.13 **Recurrent corneal erosion (arrow) characterized by well-circumscribed area of epithelial loss staining vividly with sodium fluorescein.**

COGAN'S DYSTROPHY

Diagnosis. Cogan's microcystic dystrophy is characterized by microcystic patterns in the epithelium and basement membrane and usually occurs in adult females. Dotlike opacities may be observed that appear as discrete, comma-shaped or rounded gray lesions, orderly fingerprint designs formed by concentric contoured lines, or maplike changes seen as interlacing lines. This disorder can lead to recurrent corneal erosions. Vision is virtually unaffected and symptoms are generally absent, except during acute episodes of erosion.

Management. Treatment is essentially directed toward the recurrent erosion and includes debridement of the damaged epithelium and pressure-patching as explained earlier. Therapeutic soft contact lenses may also be effective.

Endothelial Dystrophies

CORNEAL GUTTATA

Diagnosis. Corneal guttata are wartlike, mushroom-shaped hyaline excrescences of Descemet's membrane through the central endothelium. A "beaten metal" appearance of Descemet's membrane is typical when viewed with the slit lamp (Fig. 22.14). Guttata also appear as breaks in the normal hexagonal mosaic pattern of the endothelial cells when observed with spec-

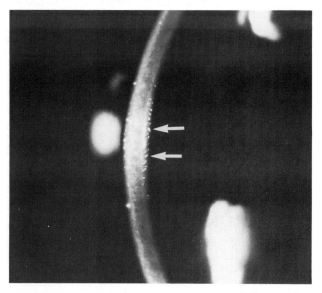

FIGURE 22.14 **Corneal guttata are seen under high magnification of the slit lamp. (Courtesy Jimmy D. Bartlett, O.D.)**

ular reflection. When located only in the periphery of the endothelium of young individuals, they are referred to as Hassall-Henle bodies. Brownish pigmentation can be seen at the level of the guttata. Because guttata represent a generalized endothelial dysfunction, they may, if numerous, lead to stromal edema and an accompanying decrease in vision. Visual acuity can also be affected if the guttata are concentrated heavily in the axial region of the cornea. Although the stromal edema can lead to epithelial edema and bullous keratopathy, most cases of corneal guttata remain stationary for years. Guttata are generally found in middle- to older-aged patients.

Management. The presence of corneal guttata does not require treatment. Should corneal edema occur, however, it can be reduced by the instillation of hyperosmotic solutions (5% sodium chloride), but treatment is rarely necessary.

FUCHS' DYSTROPHY

Diagnosis. Fuchs' dystrophy is a disorder of unknown etiology that affects primarily females in the third to fourth decades of life and continues as a slowly progressive condition. It begins with a malfunction of the endothelial pump mechanism, leading to stromal and epithelial edema (bedewing) and subsequent bullae formation. The epithelial edema is most significant in the morning on awakening, due to the reduced availability of oxygen, and during humid weather, when there is less tear evaporation, which therefore lowers tear osmolality.

The first clinical sign is a characteristic "ground glass" appearance of the endothelium, most easily seen with retroillumination. Closer inspection reveals numerous wartlike excrescences and fine pigment dusting of the endothelium. These corneal guttata begin in the central, visual axis area and progress peripherally. The edema will blur vision, and the epithelial irregularity causes light scatter, which further decreases acuity (Fig. 22.15). Once the edema has progressed to the point of epithelial bullae formation, the situation is quite problematic. If the bullae rupture, free nerve endings are exposed, resulting in a more severe foreign body sensation. Corneal infection and ulceration are possible sequelae. Eventual scarring and vascularization of the cornea occur. The end result of Fuchs' dystrophy is corneal opacification and desensitization.

Management. Treatment of this condition is generally palliative once epithelial edema occurs. The use of 5% sodium chloride ointment or drops is helpful in controlling the epithelial edema, especially in the mornings and during humid conditions when the edema

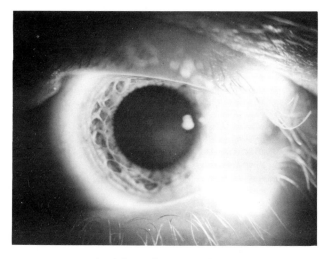

FIGURE 22.15 **The diffuse edema of Fuchs' dystrophy.**

is worse. Grayson[82] also suggests the use of a hair dryer held at arm's length and used 2 or 3 times daily to help alleviate the edema by increasing tear evaporation and thus tear osmolality. A bandage soft contact lens will relieve discomfort from the bullous keratopathy. Once progressive vision loss occurs, a penetrating kerato-plasty is the treatment of choice, and good results are usually achieved.

Injuries of the Cornea

Mechanical Trauma

ABRASIONS

Etiology.   Corneal epithelial loss is one of the more frequently encountered types of trauma in optometric practice. Corneal abrasions can result from overwear of contact lenses, foreign bodies, chemicals, fingernail scratches, and a host of other causes (Fig. 22.16). The epithelial defect can range from a mild punctate ker-atitis to total denuding of the corneal surface.

Diagnosis.   The patient usually presents with symp-toms of lacrimation, photophobia, and pain. The pain is most severe as the patient blinks, since the eyelid puts mechanical stimulation on the now free sensory nerve endings of the cornea. Slit-lamp examination of the cornea using sodium fluorescein and a cobalt blue filtered light will reveal the deepithelialized areas. In cases of severe blepharospasm, it may be necessary to use a topical anesthetic to aid in the examination.

Vertical or tracing-type linear stain is typical of the presence of a foreign body. The upper and lower forn-

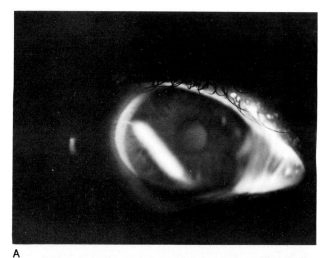

A

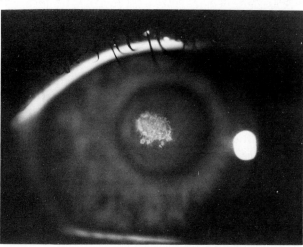

B

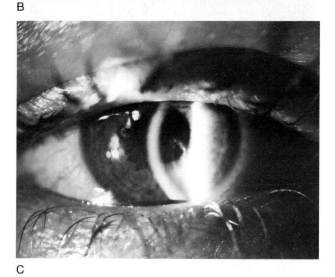

C

FIGURE 22.16 **Types of corneal abrasions. (A) Paper cut. (B) Contact lens. (C) Mascara brush.**

ices as well as the upper palpebral conjunctiva (while the lid is everted) should always be carefully examined in any corneal injury to rule out the retention of a foreign body in these areas.

Contact lens–induced abrasions may take many forms. Central punctate staining (see Figure 22.16*B*) is most often associated with overwear and is due to hypoxia. Diffuse punctate staining could indicate a reaction to the cleaning agents in the lens solutions. Small irregular abrasions may indicate epithelial damage due to poor insertion or removal techniques. Irregular linear scratches may be due to a foreign body trapped between the lens and cornea. Defective edges or cracks in the lenses can also lead to epithelial damage.[141]

Regeneration of corneal epithelium is rapid, usually beginning within 1 hour after the abrasion occurs. The defect will heal without the formation of scar tissue or an opacity if Bowman's layer remains intact. Healing is directed primarily toward reestablishing continuity of the epithelial surface and is accomplished by a cell sliding mechanism. Once the defect is covered, the cells begin to multiply and develop tight adhesions to the underlying Bowman's layer. Peripheral defects tend to heal faster, probably due to their close proximity to the limbal vascular supply.[142,143]

Some types of abrasions, particularly those due to paper, fingernail, bush, or branch scratches, are approximately 5 times more likely than other types of abrasions to spontaneously erode weeks after the initial lesion was clinically thought to be healed.[144] The size of the initial abrasion seems not to be associated with the recurrence rate. This trauma-induced recurrent erosion syndrome rarely occurs after foreign body removal or blunt trauma. Treatment is the same as that for the previously discussed dystrophic recurrent erosion.

Management.   The treatment of corneal abrasions consists of several steps. Initially, if the abrasion was caused by a foreign body, the practitioner must ensure that all the foreign material has been debrided from the wound. This is especially true of the ferrous oxide rust ring that remains after removal of a metallic foreign body. A short-acting cycloplegic, such as tropicamide 1% or cyclopentolate 1%, is generally effective in reducing the discomfort from ciliary spasm and preventing secondary iritis. Homatropine 5% is beneficial in larger, more severe abrasions. A broad-spectrum antibiotic ointment such as sodium sulfacetamide, gentamicin, or bacitracin–polymyxin B should be used to prevent potential bacterial infection. A pressure-patch should be applied (Fig. 22.17) to immobilize the eyelid and prevent it from dislodging the newly adhering cells. The patient should be instructed to remain quiet during

the initial 24 hours following the injury to lessen the chance of disturbing the newly established epithelial cells. Heat, in the form of a heating pad or hot water bottle, may be applied throughout the day in half-hour intervals to speed the temperature-dependent sliding process. All eyes patched in this manner should be examined in 24 hours, and many will be adequately repaired in this time (Fig. 22.18). If contact lenses are involved, wear should resume no sooner than 2 days after signs and symptoms have resolved. As an alternative to patching in patients who need to maintain binocularity, a bandage soft contact lens can be used.[145]

LACERATIONS

Diagnosis.   Lacerations are usually caused by sharp objects such as nails, glass slivers, knives, or scissors. The globe should be examined very carefully, since undue pressure could rupture a partial-thickness laceration or herniate intraocular contents through a full-thickness laceration. The visual acuity must be recorded for legal as well as for medical reasons. If the cut is clean and perpendicular to the corneal surface, there may be few symptoms. The patient may have little pain, lacrimation, or redness unless the wound becomes infected. A flap wound is associated with more severe symptoms, resembling those of a corneal erosion. Unless the laceration excises a large portion of the cornea, the edema will not be permanent.

Unless the examination is easy and the wound obviously not deep, it is better to defer further examination until the patient is sedated or under general anesthesia.[146] A specimen should be obtained for culture, and then a cotton pad should be gently placed over the patient's eye with a metallic shield for protection. Signs of global perforation include hypotony; anterior chamber flattening (due to aqueous leakage); alteration in pupil size, shape, or location; and prolapse of intraocular contents. A full-thickness corneal laceration will allow aqueous to leak from the wound site. After fluorescein is instilled, the dye will be diluted and washed away (Seidel's sign).

Management.   If the laceration is small and clean, it may be easily treated. Any foreign material should be eliminated, followed by prophylactic measures against infection such as the instillation of gentamicin or tobramycin. Immobilization of the lids by patching usually allows more rapid healing. Soft contact lenses or adhesives may also be used.[3] If the laceration is large and irregular, the wound must be sutured.

Surgical repair under sedation or general anesthesia may be necessary for a full-thickness laceration. If the wound is large with extensive loss of intraocular contents, enucleation may be necessary.

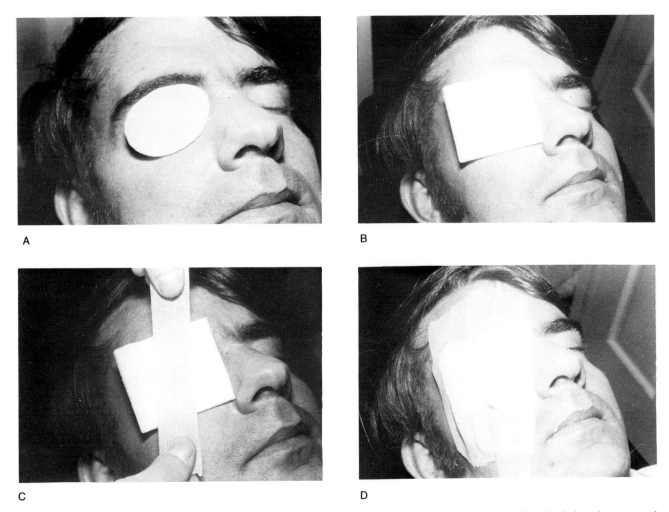

FIGURE 22.17   **Technique of pressure-patching. (A) After cleansing the skin of the forehead and cheek with an alcohol swab, an eyepad is placed over the closed eyelids. If the eye socket is deep, the pad can be folded. (B) A second eyepad is placed over the first, creating pressure against the closed eyelids and globe as tape is applied diagonally (C and D) to secure the patch.**

FOREIGN BODIES

Etiology.   Corneal foreign bodies constitute approximately 25% of all ocular injuries.[1] Metallic foreign bodies (Fig. 22.19) are very often encountered. Other materials frequently found as foreign bodies include cinders, sand, fiberglass, threads, wood particles, weeds, soil particles, briars, insect parts, and glass.

Diagnosis.   Patients with corneal foreign bodies present with the realization that there is something "in" their eyes. However, some foreign bodies cause minimal initial discomfort, especially those that are hot and traveling with moderate speed as they contact the cornea, as in the case of metal bits during drilling. In these instances, the eye becomes injected and uncom-

fortable 18 to 36 hours later. Patient history in these types of cases is extremely important; it is beneficial to know the time of injury, the probable material, and the approximate force or speed at which the object penetrated the cornea.

The patient normally reports a foreign body sensation with each blink. In addition to pain, which is usually referred to the undersurface of the upper lid, there is lacrimation and photophobia. The conjunctiva is injected to a variable degree, depending principally on composition of the material and how long it has been on the cornea. Foreign bodies frequently cause corneal track marks, abrasions, and ulcers. In the absence of infection, healing is rapid once the object is removed. If the injury has extended beneath Bowman's

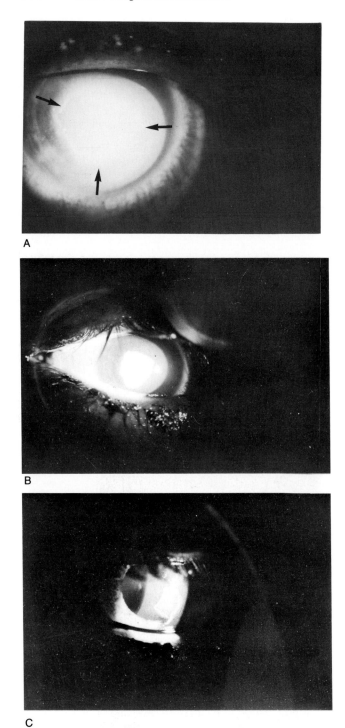

A

B

C

FIGURE 22.18 **The healing sequence of a large corneal abrasion. (A) Abrasion (arrows) occupying 30% of the cornea. (B) The abrasion occupied 20% of the cornea after 24 hours of pressure-patching. (C) After 48 hours of pressure-patching, the abrasion had well-defined edges; healing was complete after 72 hours.**

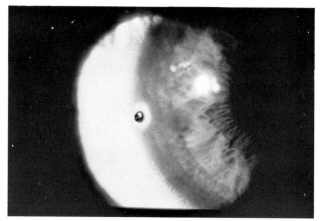

FIGURE 22.19 **A metallic foreign body embedded on the cornea.**

layer, however, some permanent opacity of the corneal stroma will occur, reducing visual acuity if it is along the visual axis.

Management. The overall goals of the treatment of corneal foreign bodies are to remove the material, instill a prophylactic antibiotic and cycloplegic, and promote comfort and healing with a well-fitting patch.[147] Visual acuities should be taken before treatment is begun.

The actual removal of the foreign body depends on its size and substance. Usually the most satisfactory method is to remove the object under slit-lamp control with a sterile spud or 26-gauge, ⅜ inch disposable, tuberculin syringe needle (Fig. 22.20). After instillation of 2 drops of 0.5% proparacaine, the needle is brought nearly tangential to the corneal surface with the bevel toward the examiner. The hand holding the needle should be positioned on the slit lamp's hand rest. As the needle point approaches the foreign body, it is positioned under the object, which is gently raised and lifted up and out. Steady fixation by the patient is absolutely crucial, and the lid must be held so that the patient cannot blink during the procedure. The foreign object generally continues to adhere to the needle. However, it is helpful to have a moistened, sterile, cotton-tipped applicator within reach so that if the foreign body becomes dislodged from the needle, it can be easily picked up with the applicator by surface tension.

In the case of a metallic foreign body, the rust ring (Fig. 22.21) that develops must be removed to allow normal healing. If the rust ring is completely and cleanly removed, healing is more rapid and the resultant irritation and scar are less than if it is left in situ. On the other hand, if excessive trauma would be needed to remove it, the rust ring is best left alone. Removal can

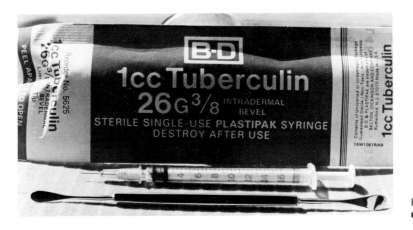

FIGURE 22.20   **A spud or 26-gauge needle can be used to remove a metallic foreign body.**

generally be accomplished with a sterile 0.5 mm spinning burr such as the Algerbrush (Fig. 22.22). The burr is placed at an angle of approximately 30° to 45° from straight on within the depression of the previously removed foreign body. The spinning burr is carefully maneuvered until the ferrous oxide rust ring is removed. Most of these types of burrs have so little power that they spontaneously stop with even minimal pressure, making it very difficult to perforate the cornea.

An anterior chamber reaction is not uncommon when the foreign body has been in place for several days or if the material is organic. Thus, it is beneficial to cycloplege the eye with 1% cyclopentolate or 5% homatropine for 1 to 3 days so that the patient does not suffer from ciliary spasm, which can be particularly bothersome at bedtime. An antibiotic ointment such as sodium sulfacetamide, gentamicin, or bacitracin–polymyxin B should be prophylactically instilled into the lower cul-de-sac to minimize the risk of bacterial infection.

The eye is then pressure-patched (see Fig. 22.17). The patient is generally most comfortable resting and using heat over the patch, which also promotes rapid

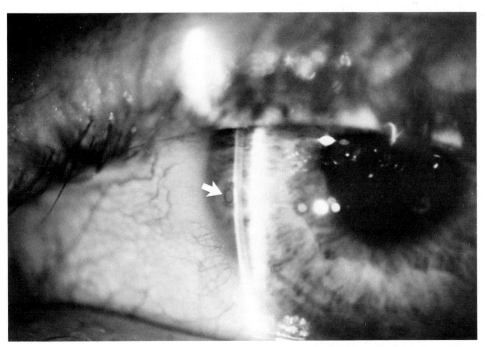

FIGURE 22.21   **Rust ring (arrow) that develops with a metallic foreign body. (Courtesy Olee J. Olsen, O.D.)**

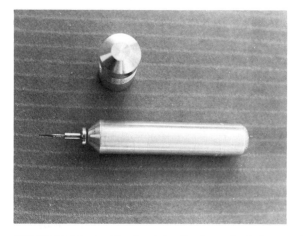

FIGURE 22.22   **An Algerbrush is effective and safe in removing corneal rust rings.**

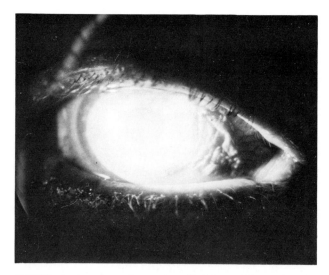

FIGURE 22.23   **Affected area of an alkali burn of the conjunctiva and cornea.**

reepithelialization. The patient should be seen the day after removal of the foreign body to ensure that healing is progressing and to search for infection.

Deep corneal foreign bodies that might penetrate the anterior chamber should be removed only in the operating theater, since complications can be anticipated.[50] Until then, the eye should be bandaged very lightly with cotton pads and covered with a protective metal shield that rests on the inferior and superior orbital bones. Manipulation of the eye and eye movement should be kept to a minimum to avoid aqueous leakage or extrusion of intraocular contents.

Burns of the Cornea

CHEMICAL BURNS

Diagnosis.   Eyes that have been contaminated with chemical agents require immediate emergency treatment. Copious flushing of the involved eye(s) using the most readily available source of water is necessary because any subsequent damage to the eye is usually directly proportional to how long the offending agent remained in contact with the ocular structures.

The insult to the eye will erode the corneal epithelium, leading to edema and possible opacification. This may also be followed by neovascularization during epithelial regeneration. The amount of injury to the perilimbal area is the most important factor in initially judging the degree of damage and prognosis for recovery.[148] Permanent visual loss depends on the degree of opacification, neovascularization, and possible proteolytic breakdown of corneal tissue. In severe burns, scarring and contraction of bulbar and adnexal tissue produce the picture of a mucous deficient dry eye.[149]

Depending on severity, there may also be ischemic necrosis of the conjunctiva (blanching) and acute iritis, along with concurrent dermal injury. In very grave cases the practitioner may also encounter cataracts, iris necrosis, secondary glaucoma, and phthisis.

Of the two main types of chemical burns (acid and alkali), alkali burns are by far the most potentially devastating to the eye. Common alkali agents that can cause serious ocular damage are lye, lime (i.e., certain plaster materials), sodium hydroxide, or ammonia. They are particularly harmful because they penetrate the cornea rapidly and continually release hydroxyl ions. Alkalis react with cell membrane lipids to form soluble compounds that disrupt the cell wall and allow rapid penetration through ocular tissues. The corneal epithelial damage (Fig. 22.23) may result in the production of collagenases, which leads to tissue necrosis, permanent scarring, and, in some cases, corneal perforation. Subsequent symblepharon and concomitant visual loss are not uncommon. Late complications can occur years after the initial injury.

Acid burns, on the other hand, cause most of their damage on initial contact and shortly thereafter and rarely penetrate the eye unless the acid contains heavy metals. Battery acid and industrial cleaning agents are common causes of acid burns. Acids cause denaturation and coagulation of all proteins with which contact is made and form insoluble acid proteinates, which limit further penetration of the cornea.

Management.   Treatment of chemical burns is initially directed toward complete removal of the noxious agent from the eye. This involves immediate irrigation with tap water or saline to dilute and wash away the chemical and may be continued for up to 1 hour if necessary.[159] Chemical antidotes should not be used, since the heat generated by the reaction may increase the degree of injury. The upper and lower fornices and the palpebral conjunctiva should then be carefully investigated for any retained solid material, which must be removed as quickly as possible to minimize progressive damage to the eye. It may be necessary to employ a topical anesthetic to perform this inspection. The eye should then be dilated with an intermediate-acting cycloplegic, such as 1% cyclopentolate or 5% homatropine, to reduce iridociliary involvement. A prophylactic antibiotic ointment should be instilled to prevent bacterial infection. Patching may be necessary. Freeing the conjunctival adhesions with a glass rod or spatula is advised to help prevent symblepharon formation. In some cases of alkali burns, either steroids or therapeutic soft contact lenses have been advocated to decrease the amount of scarring and aid in the healing process.[37] These patients must be carefully monitored daily until healing progresses, even in the less serious cases.

The final visual result depends on corneal clarity and the ability of the lids and lacrimal fluids to maintain proper protection. If the cornea is severely opacified, some authors encourage corneal transplantation,[150] while others feel that this is contraindicated.[151] Reconstructive plastic surgery may be needed for badly scarred conjunctival sacs.

THERMAL BURNS

Etiology. Thermal burns produce necrosis of the corneal tissues to any depth, depending on the heat of the offending substance and the extent and duration of contact. Mild burns can be caused by tobacco ash or hot sparks, moderate injuries from electric hair curling irons,[152,162] and severe burns from contact with molten metal or other hot liquid, especially if it contains solid bodies that retain heat while in contact with the eye. These latter cases should be treated the same as other foreign bodies, but the destruction will be greater and the healing time longer.[146]

Diagnosis. If the corneal burn is superficial, the lesion will appear as an edematous area that develops into an erosion and epithelializes in several days. Ulceration may take place, healing slowly and often with permanent scar tissue. As the burned area recovers, the necrotic tissue will be desquamated. This can lead to corneal perforation if the lesion is deep enough. Should the corneal stroma be affected, the resultant opacity will be permanent, commonly with dense, vascularized scar tissue. Usually thermal burns are asso-ciated with injury to the lids, and cicatricial ectropion and exposure keratitis may result.

Management. The immediate treatment of a thermal burn consists of gently debriding the coagulated epithelium from the lesion and removing any residual foreign material from the affected area. A cycloplegic, topical antibiotic ointment, and firm pressure-patching should be used. Topical steroids such as dexamethasone 0.1% or prednisolone acetate 1% used 4 times a day may be used to decrease symblepharon formation if the epithelium is intact.[5]

If the damage is severe, the necrotic tissue may have to be removed and grafting performed. To achieve adequate ocular protection by the lids, plastic surgery may be necessary.

RADIATION BURNS

Corneal damage will result from any form of radiation in which the surface of the eye absorbs sufficient energy. In general, the type of injury produced by irradiation of the cornea is in the form of keratoconjunctivitis. A general rule is that the shorter the wavelength, the greater the tendency for keratoconjunctivitis.[146]

ULTRAVIOLET RADIATION

Diagnosis. Ultraviolet radiation, the most common cause of light-induced ocular injury,[5] often produces a superficial keratitis even with moderate exposure. Sunlamps and electric welding arcs are common sources of this form of radiation. After exposure there is a lag time of about 6 hours before symptoms of the burn become evident. Photophobia, pain, lacrimation, and blepharospasm are the subjective findings. Objective examination reveals a keratoconjunctivitis, with fluorescein stain demonstrating punctate erosions of the corneal epithelium. There is also conjunctival hyperemia, periorbital edema, and associated burns of the face and eyelids. Damage is caused by an inhibition of mitosis, nuclear fragmentation, and loosening of the epithelial layer.[146] These changes are transient, however, and the symptoms will disappear within 1 to 2 days.

Management. Topical antibiotic ointment or drops should be used to prevent secondary infection, along with a cycloplegic such as cyclopentolate 1% to relieve ciliary spasm. Semi-pressure-patching and cold compresses may also be used to make the patient more comfortable.

INFRARED RADIATION

Diagnosis. Exposure to infrared radiation rarely results in anterior segment reaction because of the immediate discomfort the excessive heat causes. When these burns are externally evident, there are usually only transient reactions of lid edema and erythema, with perhaps a mild corneal epithelial erosion.

Management.   Therapy consists of prophylactic antibiotic ointment along with cold compresses for the discomfort.

IONIZING RADIATION

Diagnosis.   The most common causes of ionizing radiation burns are cyclotron exposure and cancer therapy involving β rays, which are selective for the cornea and conjunctiva.[146] In the mild form, this radiation keratitis consists of punctate epithelial staining, while larger dosages of radiation produce extensive epithelial loss and stromal edema. There will also be concurrent conjunctival hyperemia and circumcorneal injection.

Management.   Treatment for ionizing radiation burns is symptomatic. Cycloplegics should be used to reduce the pain of ciliary spasm and to prevent synechiae formation. Topical antibiotic ointment or drops should be used to prevent infection.

References

1. Terry JE. Ocular disease: Detection, diagnosis and treatment. Boston: Butterworths, 1985.
2. Eskridge JB, Schoessler JP, Lowther GE. A specific biomicroscopy procedure. J Am Optom Assoc 1973;44:400–409.
3. Duane TD. Clinical ophthalmology. Hagerstown, MD: Harper & Row, 1987.
4. Norn MS. Vital staining of cornea and conjunctiva. Eye Ear Nose Throat Monthly 1971;50:294.
5. Pavan-Langston D. Manual of ocular diagnosis and therapy. Boston: Little, Brown, 1980.
6. Hamilton W, Wood TO. Filamentary keratitis. Am J Ophthalmol 1982;93:466–469.
7. Vaughn D, Asbury T. General ophthalmology. Los Altos, CA: Lange, 1986.
8. Locatcher-Khorazo D, Sullivan N, Butierriey E. *Staphylococcus aureus* isolated from normal and infected eyes. Arch Ophthalmol 1967;77:370.
9. Bettman NW, Aronson SB. Host response in infectious ocular disease. Arch Ophthalmol 1969;82:30.
10. Thygeson P. Complication of staphylococcal blepharitis. Am J Ophthalmol 1969;68:446.
11. Chignell AH, Easty DL, Chestertan JR, Thomsett J. Marginal ulceration of the cornea. Br J Ophthalmol 1970;54:433.
12. Fedukowicz HB. External infections of the eye, ed. 2. New York: Appleton-Century-Crofts, 1977.
13. Valenton MJ, Okumoto M. Toxin-producing strains of *Staphylococcus epidermidis (albus)*. Arch Ophthalmol 1973; 89:186.
14. Wilson L, Julian A, Ahearn D. The survival and growth of microorganisms in mascara during use. Am J Ophthalmol 1975;79:596.
15. Ellis PP. Ocular therapeutics and pharmacology. St. Louis: C.V. Mosby Co, 1981.
16. Schacter J. Chlamydial infections. N Engl J Med 1978; 298:428–435.
17. Kordova N. Chlamydia, rickettsia and their cell wall infective variants. Can J Microbiol 1978;24:339–349.
18. Chlamydial infections of the eye (editorial). Lancet 1977;2:857–858.
19. Thygeson P. Corneal changes in TRIC agent infections. Am J Ophthalmol 1967;63:1278–1282.
20. Dawson CR, Schacter J, Ostler B, et al. Inclusion conjunctivitis and Reiter's syndrome in a married couple. Arch Ophthalmol 1970;83:300–306.
21. Dunlop E, Jane B, Khalof Al-Hussaine. Genital infections in association with TRIC virus infection of the eye. Br J Vener Dis 1964;40:33–42.
22. Markham R, Richmond S, Walshaw N, Easty D. Severe persistent inclusion conjunctivitis in a young child. Am J Ophthalmol 1977;83:414–416.
23. Schachter J. Recommended criteria for the identification of trachoma and inclusion conjunctivitis agents. J Infect Dis 1970;122:105–107.
24. Thygeson P. Historical view of oculogenital disease. Am J Ophthalmol 1971;71:975–985.
25. Johnson F, Chancerelle L, Hobson D. An improved method for demonstrating the growth of chlamydia in a tissue culture. Med Lab Sci 1978;35:67–74.
26. Darougar S, Jones B. Conjunctival swabbing for the isolation of TRIC agent (chlamydia). Br J Ophthalmol 1971; 55:585–590.
27. Drug and Therapeutics Bulletin. Consumers Assoc 1978; 16:37–39.
28. Hanna L, Jawety E, Briones D, et al. Antibodies to TRIC agents in tears and serum of naturally infected humans. J Infect Dis 1973;127:95–98.
29. Viswalingam ND, Darougar S, Yearsley P. Oral doxycycline in the treatment of adult chlamydial ophthalmia. Br J Ophthalmol 1986;70:301–304.
30. Sandstrom I. Treatment of neonatal conjunctivitis. Arch Ophthalmol 1987;105:925–928.
31. Borrie P. Rosacea with special reference to its ocular manifestations. Br J Dermatol 1953;65:458.
32. Maschella SL. Dermatology. Philadelphia: W.B. Saunders Co, 1975;1139–1142.
33. Salamon SM. Tetracyclines in ophthalmology. Surv Ophthalmol 1985;29:265–275.
34. Thygeson P. Further observations on superficial punctate keratitis. Am J Ophthalmol 1966;61:1346.
35. Abbott RL, Forster RK. Superficial punctate keratitis of Thygeson associated with scarring and Salzmann's nodular degeneration. Am J Ophthalmol 1979;87:296–298.
36. Van Bijsterveld OP, Mansour KH, Dubois FJ. Thygeson's superficial punctate keratitis. Ann Ophthalmol 1985;17:150–153.
37. Newell F, Ernest JT. Ophthalmology principles and concepts, ed. 4. St. Louis: C.V. Mosby Co, 1978.
38. Forstot SL, Binder PS. Treatment of Thygeson's superficial

punctate keratopathy with soft contact lenses. Am J Ophthalmol 1979;88:186–189.

39. Goldberg DB, Schanzlin DJ, Brown SI. Management of Thygeson's superficial punctate keratitis. Am J Ophthalmol 1980;89:22–24.

40. Expert committee on trachoma: Third report. WHO Tech Rep Ser 1964; 234.

41. Conference on trachoma and allied diseases. Am J Ophthalmol 1967;63:1027.

42. MacCallan AF. The epidemiology of trachoma. Br J Ophthalmol 1931;15:369–378.

43. Nichols RL, Bobb AA, Dahhad NA. Immunofluorescent studies of the microbiologic epidemiology of trachoma in Saudia Arabia. Am J Ophthalmol 1967;63:1372–1408.

44. Dunlop EMC. Treatment of patients suffering from chlamydial infections. J Antimicrobiol Chemother 1977;3:377–383.

45. Treatment of chlamydia trachomatis infections (editorial). Lancet 1978;1:192–193.

46. Allansmith MR, Hahn GS, Simon MA. Tissue, tear, and serum IgE concentrations in vernal conjunctivitis. Am J Ophthalmol 1976;81:506.

47. Allansmith MR, Frick OL. Antibodies to grass in vernal conjunctivitis. J Allergy 1963;34:535.

48. Neumann E, Gutman MJ, Blumenkiantz J, Michaelson IC. A review of 400 cases of vernal conjunctivitis. Am J Ophthalmol 1959;47:166.

49. Morgan G. The pathology of vernal conjunctivitis. Trans Ophthalmol Soc UK 1971;91:467.

50. Duke-Elder SS, Leigh AG. System of ophthalmology: Diseases of the outer eye. St. Louis: C.V. Mosby Co, 1965, vol. 18.

51. Foreman JC, Garland LG. Cromoglycate and other anti allergenic drugs: A possible mechanism of action. Br Med J 1976;1:820–821.

52. Tabbara KF, Arofat NT. Cromolyn effects of vernal conjunctivitis in children. Arch Ophthalmol 1977;95:2184.

53. Felius K, Van Bijsterveld OP. Effect of sodium cromoglycate on tear film break-up time. Ann Ophthalmol 1984;16:80–82.

54. Friday GA, Biglon AW, Hiles DA, et al. Treatment of ragweed allergic conjunctivitis with cromolyn sodium 4% ophthalmic solution. Am J Ophthalmol 1983;95:169–174.

55. Foster CS, Duncan J. Randomized clinical trial of topically administered cromolyn sodium for vernal keratoconjunctivitis. Am J Ophthalmol 1980;1:820–821.

56. Ostler BH. Acute chemotic reaction to cromolyn. Arch Ophthalmol 1982;100:412–513.

57. Meyer E, Kraus E, Zonis S. Efficacy of antiprostaglandin therapy in vernal conjunctivitis. Br J Ophthalmol 1987; 71:497–499.

58. Theodore F. Further observations on superior limbic keratoconjunctivitis. Trans Am Acad Ophthalmol Otolaryngol 1967;71:341.

59. Mondino BJ, Zaidman GW, Soloman SW. Use of pressure patching and soft contact lenses in superior limbic keratoconjunctivitis. Arch Ophthalmol 1982;100:1932–1939.

60. Jones DB. Early diagnosis and therapy of bacterial corneal ulcer. Int Ophthalmol Clin 1973;13:1.

61. Jones DB. A plan for antimicrobial therapy in bacterial keratitis. Trans Am Acad Ophthalmol Otolaryngol 1975; 79:95.

62. Tof FH, Wehile PF. Communicable and infectious diseases, ed. 8. St. Louis: C.V. Mosby Co, 1976;513.

63. Dawson CR. Epidemic keratoconjunctivitis. In: Fraunfelder FT, Roy FH, eds. Current ocular therapy. Philadelphia: W.B. Saunders Co, 1980;59–60.

64. Kemp MC, Hierholzer JC, Cabradilla CP, et al. The changing etiology of epidemic keratoconjunctivitis: Antigenic and restriction enzyme analyses of adenovirus types 19 and 37 isolated over a 10-year period. J Infect Dis 1983;148:24–33.

65. O'Day DM, Guyer B, Hierholzer JC, et al. Clinical and laboratory evaluation of the epidemic keratoconjunctivitis due to adenovirus types 8 and 19. Am J Ophthalmol 1976;80:475.

66. Hogan MJ, Crawford JW. Epidemic keratoconjunctivitis. Am J Ophthalmol 1942;25:1059–1078.

67. Dawson CR, Hanna L, Togni B. Adenovirus type 8 infections in the U.S. IV. Observations on the pathogenesis of lesions in severe eye disease. Arch Ophthalmol 1972;87:258–268.

68. Vass Z. Histological findings in epidemic keratoconjunctivitis. Acta Ophthalmol 1964;42:119–121.

69. Sprague JB, Hierholzer JC, Currier RW, et al. Epidemic keratoconjunctivitis (a severe industrial outbreak due to adenovirus type 8). N Engl J Med 1973;289:1341–1346.

70. Mordhorst CH, Kjer P. Studies on an epidemic of keratoconjunctivitis caused by adenovirus type 8. I. Virus isolation in human amniotic cells and serological observations. Acta Ophthalmol 1961;39:974–983.

71. Dawson CR, Hanna L, Wood TR, et al. Adenovirus type 8 keratoconjunctivitis in the U.S. III. Epidemiologic, clinical, and microbiologic features. Am J Ophthalmol 1970; 69:473–480.

72. Laibson PR, Ortolan G, Dupre-Strachan S. Community and hospital outbreak of epidemic keratoconjunctivitis. Arch Ophthalmol 1968;80:467–473.

73. Jones BR. Adenovirus infections of the eye in London. Trans Ophthalmol Soc UK 1962;82:621–640.

74. Laibson PR, Dhiri S, Oconer J, Ortolan G. Corneal infiltrates in epidemic keratoconjunctivitis. Arch Ophthalmol 1970;84:36–40.

75. Hechy S, Hanna L, Sery TW, et al. Treatment of epidemic keratoconjunctivitis with idoxuridine (IDU). Arch Ophthalmol 1965;73:49–54.

76. Goen TM, Sieboldt K, Terry JE. Cromolyn sodium in ocular allergic diseases. J Am Optom Assoc 1986;57:526–530.

77. Laibson PR, Trobe JD, eds. External ocular diseases: Diagnosis and current therapy. Int Ophthalmol Clin 1973; 13:1–242.

78. Zaidman GW, Brown SI. Orally administered tetracycline for phlyctenular keratoconjunctivitis. Am J Ophthalmol 1981;92:173–182.

79. McCulloch D, Alexander A. Phlyctenular keratoconjunctivitis. J Am Optom Assoc 1983;54:435–439.

80. Ostler H, Okumoto M, Wilkey C. The changing pattern of the etiology of central bacterial corneal (hypopyon) ulcer. Trans Pac Coast Otoophthalmol Soc 1976;57:235–246.

81. Wilson LA, Sexton RR. Laboratory diagnosis in fungal keratitis. Am J Ophthalmol 1968;66:646.

82. Grayson M. Diseases of the cornea. St. Louis: C.V. Mosby Co, 1979.

83. Terry JE. Dendriform keratitis. J Am Optom Assoc 1979;50:457–463.

84. Ford LC, DeLange R, Perry R. Identification of a nonlysosomal bactericidal factor (beta lysin) in human tears and aqueous humor. Am J Ophthalmol 1976;81:30.

85. Holt RJ. Lysozyme production by staphylococci and micrococci. J Med Microbiol 1971;4:375.

86. Chandler JW, Milam DF. Diphtheria corneal ulcers. Arch Ophthalmol 1978;96:53–56.

87. Aronson SB, Eliott JH, Moore TE, et al. Pathogenetic approach to therapy of peripheral corneal inflammatory disease. Am J Ophthalmol 1970;70:65–90.

88. Insler MS, Helm CJ, George WJ. Topical USP systemic gentamicin penetration into the human cornea and aqueous humor. Arch Ophthalmol 1987;105:922–924.

89. Glasser DB, Gardner S, Ellis JG, et al. Loading doses and extended dosing intervals in topical gentamicin therapy. Am J Ophthalmol 1985;99:329–332.

90. Bohigian GM, Escapini H. Corneal ulcer due to *Pseudomonas aeruginosa*. A comparison of the disease in California and El Salvador. Arch Ophthalmol 1971;85:405.

91. Insler MS, Gore H. *Pseudomonas* keratitis and folliculitis from whirlpool exposure. Am J Ophthalmol 1986;101:41–43.

92. Vaughan DG. Contamination of fluorescein solutions. Am J Ophthalmol 1955;39:55.

93. Golden B, Fingerman L, Allen HF. *Pseudomonas* corneal ulcers in contact lens wearers: Epidemiology and treatment. Arch Ophthalmol 1971;85:543.

94. Wilson LA, Ahearn DC. *Pseudomonas* induced corneal ulcers associated with contaminated eye mascara. Am J Ophthalmol 1977;84:112.

95. Mondino BJ, Weissman BA, Farb MD, et al. Corneal ulcers associated with daily-wear contact lenses. Am J Ophthalmol 1986;102:58–65.

96. Ormerod LD, Smith RE. Contact lens-associated microbial keratitis. Arch Ophthalmol 1986;104:79–86.

97. Alfonso E, Mandelbaum S, Fox MJ, et al. Ulcerative keratitis associated with contact lens wear. Am J Ophthalmol 1986;101:429–433.

98. Gelender H, Rettich C. Gentamicin-resistant *Pseudomonas aeruginosa* corneal ulcers. Cornea 1984;3:21–26.

99. Davis SD, Sarff LD, Hyndiuk RA. Comparison of therapeutic routes in experimental *Pseudomonas* keratitis. Am J Ophthalmol 1979;87:710–716.

100. Smolin G, Okumoto M, Leong-Sit L. Combined gentamicin-tobramycin-corticosteroid treatment. Effect on gentamicin-resistant *Pseudomonas* keratitis. Arch Ophthalmol 1980;98:473–474.

101. Howard GM, Kaufman HE. Herpes simplex keratitis. Arch Ophthalmol 1962;67:373–387.

102. Hughes WF. Treatment of herpes simplex keratitis. Am J Ophthalmol 1969;67:313–328.

103. Rubin JB, Maino JH, Carty RE. Herpes simplex virus. Rev Optom 1979;116:59–60.

104. Carroll JM, Martola EL, Laibson PR, et al. The recurrence of herpetic keratitis following idoxuridine therapy. Am J Ophthalmol 1967;63:103–107.

105. Marsh RJ, Fraunfelder FT, McGill JI. Herpetic corneal epithelial disease. Arch Ophthalmol 1976;94:1899–1902.

106. Kaufman HE. A new understanding of ocular herpetic disease. Am J Ophthalmol 1982;94:119–121.

107. Kaufman HE, Varnell ED, Centifanto YM, et al. Effect of the herpes simplex virus genome on the response of infection to corticosteroids. Am J Ophthalmol 1985;100:114–118.

108. Coster DJ, Grutzmacher RD. Herpetic eye disease. Aust J Ophthalmol 1983;11:1–14.

109. Liesegang TJ, Forster RK. Spectrum of microbial keratitis in south Florida. Am J Ophthalmol 1980;90:38–47.

110. Polack FM, Kaufman HE, Newmark E. Keratomycosis—medical and surgical treatment. Arch Ophthalmol 1971;85:410–416.

111. Davis RM, Schroeder RP, Rowsey JJ, et al. Acanthamoeba keratitis and infectious crystalline keratopathy. Arch Ophthalmol 1987;105:1524–1527.

112. Shovlin JP, DePaolis MD, Edmonds SE, et al. Acanthamoeba keratitis: Contact lenses as a risk factor, case reports and review of the literature. Int Cont Lens Clin 1987;14:349–358.

113. Jones DB. *Acanthamoeba*—The ultimate opportunist? Am J Ophthalmol 1986;102:527–530.

114. Solomon JM, Koenig SB, Hyndiuk RA. Medical and surgical treatment of *Acanthamoeba* keratitis (letter). Am J Ophthalmol 1987;104:309–311.

115. Cohen EJ, Parlato CJ, Arentsen JJ, et al. Medical and surgical treatment of *Acanthamoeba* keratitis. Am J Ophthalmol 1987;103:615–625.

116. Moore MB, McCulley JP, Kaufman HE, et al. Radial keratoneuritis as a presenting sign in *Acanthamoeba* keratitis. Ophthalmology 1986;93:1310–1315.

117. Dornic DI, Wolf T, Dillon WH, et al. Acanthamoeba keratitis in soft contact lens wearers. J Am Optom Assoc 1987;58:482–483.

118. Moore MB, McCulley JP, Newton C, et al. *Acanthamoeba* keratitis—a growing problem in soft and hard contact lens wearers. Ophthalmology 1987;94:1654–1661.

119. Smith JL. Testing for congenital syphilis in interstitial keratitis. Am J Ophthalmol 1971;72:816–820.

120. Gasset AR, Houde WL, Garcia-Bengochea M. Hard contact lens wear as an environmental risk in keratoconus. Am J Ophthalmol 1978;85:339–341.

121. Krachmer JH, Feder RS, Belin MW. Keratoconus and related noninflammatory corneal thinning disorders. Surv Ophthalmol 1984;28:293–322.

122. Teng CC. Electron microscope study of the pathology of keratoconus. I. Am J Ophthalmol 1963;55:18.

123. Kaufman HE, Werblin TP. Epikeratophakia for the treatment of keratoconus. Am J Ophthalmol 1982;93:342–347.

124. Donshik PC, Cavanagh HD, Boruchoff SA, et al. Effect of bilateral and unilateral grafts on the incidence of rejection in keratoconus. Am J Ophthalmol 1979;87:823.

125. Gasset AR, Kaufman HE. Thermokeratoplasty in the treatment of keratoconus. Am J Ophthalmol 1975;79:226.

126. Fogle JA, Kenyon KR, Stark SJ. Damage to epithelial basement membrane by thermokeratoplasty. Am J Ophthalmol 1977;83:392.

127. Jayson MI, Jones DEP. Scleritis and rheumatoid arthritis. Ann Rheum Dis 1971;30:343.

128. Goder G, Dolter J. Wegener's granulomatosis of conjunctival origin. Ophthalmologica 1971;162:321.

129. Yamaguchi T, Kanai A, Tanaka M, et al. Bullous keratopathy after anterior-posterior radial keratotomy for myopia and myopic astigmatism. Am J Ophthalmol 1982;93:600–606.

130. Waltman SR. Penetrating keratoplasty for pseudophakic bullous keratopathy. Arch Ophthalmol 1981;99:415–416.

131. Gaynes BI, Oshinskie LT. Pseudophakic bullous keratopathy. J Am Optom Assoc 1985;56:794–796.

132. Olson RJ, Waltman SR, Mattingly TP, et al. Visual results after penetrating keratoplasty for aphakic bullous keratopathy and Fuchs' dystrophy. Am J Ophthalmol 1979;88:1000–1004.

133. Farge EJ. Results of penetrating keratoplasty over a four-year period. Ophthalmology 1978;85:650–653.

134. Lemp MA, Ralph RA. Rapid development of band keratopathy in dry eyes. Am J Ophthalmol 1977;83:657–659.

135. Pouliquen Y. Ultrastructure of band keratopathy. Arch Ophthalmol 1967;27:149.

136. Sommer A. Conjunctival appearance in corneal xerophthalmia. Arch Ophthalmol 1982;100:951–952.

137. Menon K, Vijayaraghavan K. Sequelae of severe xerophthalmia—a follow-up study. Am J Clin Nutr 1980;33:218–220.

138. Sommer A. Treatment of corneal xerophthalmia with topical retinoic acid. Am J Ophthalmol 1983;95:349–352.

139. Bron AJ, Tripathi RC. Cystic disorders of the corneal epithelium. I. Clinical aspects. Br J Ophthalmol 1973;57:361.

140. Sugar A, Meyer RF, Bahn CF. A randomized trial of pressure patching for epithelial defects after keratoplasty. Am J Ophthalmol 1983;95:637–640.

141. Bergmanson JPG. Histopathological analysis of the corneal epithelium after contact lens wear. J Am Optom Assoc 1987;58:812–818.

142. Dua HS, Forrester JV. Clinical patterns of corneal epithelial wound healing. Am J Ophthalmol 1987;104:481–489.

143. Danjo S, Friend J, Thoft RA. Conjunctival epithelium in healing of corneal epithelial wounds. Invest Ophthalmol Vis Sci 1987;28:1445–1449.

144. Weene LE. Recurrent corneal erosion after trauma: A statistical study. Ann Ophthalmol 1985;17:421–524.

145. Acheson JF, Joseph J, Spalton DJ. Use of soft contact lenses in an eye casualty department for the primary treatment of traumatic corneal abrasion. Br J Ophthalmol 1987;71:285–289.

146. Sorsby A. Modern ophthalmology, ed. 2. Philadelphia: J.B. Lippincott Co, 1972.

147. Stein HA, Slatt BJ. The ophthalmic assistant, ed. 2. St. Louis: C.V. Mosby Co, 1976;296.

148. Lemp MA. Cornea and sclera. Arch Ophthalmol 1974;92:158–170.

149. Ralph RA. Conjunctival goblet cell density in normal subjects and in dry eye syndromes. Invest Ophthalmol 1975;14:299.

150. Brown SI, Tragakis MP, Pearce DB. Corneal transplantation of the alkali burned cornea. Trans Am Acad Ophthalmol Otolaryngol 1972;76:1266–1273.

151. Girard LJ, Alfor WE, Feldman GL, et al. Severe alkali burns. Trans Am Acad Ophthalmol Otolaryngol 1970;74:788–803.

152. Mannis MJ, Miller RB, Krachmer JH. Contact thermal burns of the cornea from electric curling irons. Am J Ophthalmol 1984;98:336–339.

153. Moore MB, McCulley JP. Medical and surgical treatment of *Acanthamoeba* keratitis (letter). Am J Ophthalmol 1987;104:310–311.

154. Mondino BJ. Inflammatory diseases of the peripheral cornea. Ophthalmology 1988;95:463–472.

155. Hyndiuk RA, Skorich DN, Davis SD. Fortified antibiotic ointment in bacterial keratitis. Am J Ophthalmol 1988;105:239–243.

156. Engstrom RE, Holland GN. Chronic herpes zoster virus keratitis associated with the acquired immunodeficiency syndrome. Am J Ophthalmol 1988;105:556–558.

157. Collum LMT, McGettrick P, Akhtar J, et al. Oral acyclovir (Zovirax) in herpes simplex dendritic corneal ulceration. Br J Ophthalmol 1986;70:435–438.

158. Roat MI, Romanoroski E, Araullo-Cruz T, et al. The antiviral effects of rose bengal and fluorescein. Arch Ophthalmol 1987;105:1415–1420.

159. Donzis PB, Mondino BJ. Management of noninfectious corneal ulcers. Surv Ophthalmol 1987;32:94–110.

160. Parlato CJ, Cohen EJ, Sakauye CM, et al. Role of debridement and trifluridine (trifluorothymidine) in herpes simplex dendritic keratitis. Arch Ophthalmol 1985;103:673–675.

161. Herbort CP, Matter M. Association of trifluorothymidine and debridement in herpetic dendritic keratitis. Arch Ophthalmol 1985;103:1456.

162. Bloom SM, Gittinger JW, Kazarian EL. Management of corneal contact thermal burns. Am J Ophthalmol 1986;102:536.

163. Martin XY, Safron AB. Corneal hypoesthesia. Surv Ophthalmol 1988;33:28–40.

CHAPTER 23

Diseases of the Sclera

William L. Jones

The sclera is the outer protective coat of the eye; along with the cornea, it is primarily responsible for maintaining the shape of the eye. The sclera is composed chiefly of collagen and ground substances; however, it contains a scant vascular and nervous system. Diseases of the collagen and vascular systems can manifest themselves in the sclera. This chapter will not consider all forms of scleral disease but will only discuss episcleritis, scleritis, and scleromalacia perforans.

Episcleritis

Episcleritis is usually a benign inflammation that occurs most often in young adults. It is relatively common and seems to occur spontaneously. Involvement is unilateral in approximately two-thirds of cases.[1] There may be recurrences at the same location or in a different area, and it may reappear in the fellow eye. It is found twice as often in females and has a peak incidence in the fourth decade of life.

Clinical Anatomy of the Episclera

The episclera is a thin vascular fibroelastic tissue covering the sclera. It acts as a synovial membrane for smooth movements of the globe, and, along with the check ligaments, it limits excessive eye movements.

The episclera is divided into 2 layers, the outer parietal and the inner visceral layer, both of which are loosely attached to one another by connecting fibers. Each layer is supplied with a vascular network derived from the anterior and posterior ciliary arteries. The

vessel complexes anastomose at the limbus with the conjunctival vessels. The visible vessels are usually veins derived from the superficial and deep intrascleral veins that drain the anterior region of the ciliary body and Schlemm's canal. Conjunctival, episcleral, and scleral vessels comprise the three visible vessel networks seen in the anterior segment of the eye. The topical instillation of 10% phenylephrine or 1:1000 epinephrine will blanch the superficial vessels but has little effect on the deep scleral vessels. This is an important clinical tool used in differentiating superficial from deep inflammation. Another means of distinguishing superficial from deep inflammation is by mechanically moving the conjunctival vessels when applying pressure through the lids onto the sclera. The episcleral vessels remain stationary, while the loose conjunctiva moves freely.

Etiology

In a series of patients reported by Watson,[2] 30% of the patients with episcleritis had an associated systemic condition, but the majority of cases were of unknown etiology. Of those patients with known causes, 5% were associated with collagen disease, 7% with herpes zoster, 3% with gout, 3% with syphilis, and the remainder with such conditions as Schönlein-Henoch purpura, penicillin sensitivity, erythema nodosum, and contact with industrial solvents, all of which are believed to be antigen-antibody reactions. Rheumatoid arthritis has also been associated with episodes of episcleritis.[3] Many of these patients had a strong family history of atopy, but they uniformly did not test positive themselves. Systemic diseases such as tuberculosis, gonorrhea, staphylococcal infection, and coccidioidomycosis have been implicated as sources for delayed types of bacterial allergies.[4-6] Other known causes are episcleral foreign bodies and skin diseases such as psoriasis, lichen planus, and erythema elevantum diutinum.[7] Attacks are often related to stress such as with family or with work problems.[8] It has also been found in patients with familial Mediterranean fever.[9]

Diagnosis

Episcleritis is often acute in onset (as short as half an hour), is usually unilateral, and tends to recur. The redness is often seen in a sectorial configuration within the interpalpebral fissure (Color Plate XVIII), but it can encompass the entire anterior portion of the globe. The vessels are usually tortuous, and it is not uncommon to observe saccular dilatations (Fig. 23.1). The patient may complain of a sensation of heat, prickling, photophobia, and mild discomfort. The eye is rarely tender to the touch.[2,3] Ocular pain may be absent but on occasion can be severe. The pain is usually localized to the eye, but it may radiate to the forehead. Although tearing is common, there is no ocular discharge. In rare instances, the lids may become edematous, and if photophobia is present, an associated keratitis should be suspected. Visual acuity is usually not affected, and intraocular structures are usually not involved. Pathologically, episcleritis is characterized by widespread hyperemia, edema, and lymphocytic infiltration. The lesions heal without leaving a scar.[10]

Episcleritis can be classified as either simple or nodular. Each form differs in its clinical course and appearance. Both forms, however, have areas of edema and infiltration that are localized to the episclera. Although most of the congestion is in the superficial episcleral vessels, some congestion is observed in the conjunctival and deep episcleral vessels.

The vessel injection in simple episcleritis can vary from a mild red flush to an intense fiery red. However, it does not have the bluish tinge that is so characteristic of scleritis. The congested vessels tend to retain their normal radial configuration. The edema is diffusely distributed, and there may be grayish infiltrates present that appear yellow in red-free light.

Nodular episcleritis is localized to discrete areas, each of which consists of an elevated edematous nodule associated with surrounding congestion. The nodule is mobile over the underlying sclera.[11] These nodules may be single or multiple. After many attacks of nodular episcleritis in the same location, the superficial scleral lamellae may show alterations and become slightly transparent.[2]

Management

The course of simple episcleritis is usually 10 to 21 days. It periodically reappears, but the recurrences become less frequent with time until the disease no longer recurs. Most episodes of nodular episcleritis last 5 to 10 days, but durations vary considerably. Some

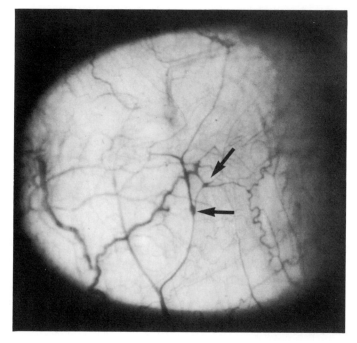

FIGURE 23.1 **Diffuse episcleritis demonstrating vessel injection, tortuosity, and saccular dilatations (arrows).**

cases may last up to 2 months. Over half the patients have intermittent attacks for 3 to 6 years, and some patients have had intermittent attacks for as long as 30 years.[12] As with simple episcleritis, recurrences of nodular episcleritis become less frequent until the disease no longer recurs.

A simple episcleritis may recur in a nodular form, or vice versa. Although episcleritis does not develop into a scleritis, scleritis will produce an overlying episcleritis. Complications of episcleritis include an occasional minor reduction in visual acuity, mild uveitis, and, in some patients with nodular episcleritis, mild changes of the pars plana.[2]

Since it is a self-limiting disease with little or no permanent damage to the eye, episcleritis generally does not require treatment.[2,12] However, many patients desire symptomatic relief from the redness and associated ocular discomfort. Treatment depends on the severity of the disease, and mild cases can be satisfactorily treated with topical decongestants or corticosteroids several times a day. With appropriate treatment, the condition generally resolves within a few days. For patients who suffer recurrent attacks, steroid treatment should be continued for several days after the condition has subsided. In severe cases of episcleritis, systemic steroids may be necessary along with the use of topical steroids. Since episcleritis is sometimes seen in association with systemic disorders, such as collagen diseases, resolution of the disease will depend on the severity of the systemic condition. An internist should assist in evaluating the patient for systemic disease.

Topical steroids may be used as frequently as 8 times a day. When administered 4 times a day, topical steroids such as dexamethasone 0.1% or prednisolone 1% frequently resolve the inflammation in 3 to 4 days.[10] As the inflammation subsides, the steroid dosage should be reduced to once or twice a day and finally discontinued as the condition completely resolves. In cases of chronic recurrence, it may be necessary to prescribe a maintenance dosage intermittently for several years.[2]

Treatment of mild episodes of episcleritis can consist of cold compresses and vasoconstrictors such as phenylephrine 0.12%. These offer symptomatic relief without greatly affecting the inflammatory process. Orally administered aspirin and other nonsteroidal anti-inflammatory agents (NSAIAs) have also been used.[13] Antihistamines and histamine desensitization have been attempted, but the response has not been nearly as effective as the response to local steroid therapy.[13] Desensitization has been known to precipitate an attack.[12] If an allergy is suspected, the definitive treatment entails elimination of the offending allergen.

Treatment of simple episcleritis usually consists of local steroids such as prednisolone 1% or dexamethasone 0.1%, which can be administered every 1 or 2 hours until the redness disappears and then 3 times a day for 4 to 5 days. Continuation of the topical steroid after the redness has dissipated prevents a rebound recurrence. However, simple episcleritis will frequently improve by 50% in the first week and completely resolve within 3 weeks without treatment. Steroid therapy serves only to hasten its resolution.[2,12]

Since nodular episcleritis tends to resolve much more slowly than does simple episcleritis, local treatment is more advantageous. Topical steroid therapy is generally used, but in more severe cases systemic therapy is sometimes necessary. All patients undergoing steroid therapy should have periodic evaluations of intraocular pressure to detect possible steroid-induced glaucoma. NSAIAs such as oxyphenbutazone and indomethacin are generally preferred over systemic steroids because of their effectiveness and less rebound phenomenon. Patients who do not respond to one of the two aforementioned drugs will often respond to the other. The recommended oral dosage of oxyphenbutazone is 100 mg 3 or 4 times daily. When used in a 10% ointment, oxyphenbutazone has been found to be of some value in the treatment of recurrent episcleritis.[13] The recommended oral dosage of indomethacin is 25 mg daily for 2 days, 50 mg daily for 2 days, then 75 mg daily until the condition is controlled.[12]

Scleritis

Unlike the more commonly encountered episcleritis, inflammation of the sclera is relatively rare. Women are more frequently affected, and scleritis is usually seen in the fourth to sixth decades of life. Scleritis is bilateral in 52% of patients. In half the bilateral cases, it occurs simultaneously in both eyes, and the remainder become bilateral in 5 or more years.[2]

Clinical Anatomy of the Sclera

The sclera is composed of collagen and elastic tissue that allow it to be resilient enough for variation in intraocular pressure, yet strong enough to prevent distortion of the globe by either the extraocular muscles or external forces. The collagen fibers are irregular in size and are spaced in a parallel and interlacing crisscross fashion, which produces a white opaque structure. The sclera is approximately 1 mm thick, except at the insertions of the recti muscles, where it is about 0.3 mm thick. It is continuous with the cornea anteriorly and with the dura sheath of the optic nerve posteriorly. A few strands of scleral tissue transgress the optic nerve, a structure known as the lamina cribrosa.

The posterior portion of the sclera is penetrated by the long and short posterior ciliary nerves and arteries; the equatorial region is penetrated by the vortex veins; and the anterior region is penetrated by the anterior ciliary arteries, veins, and nerves. Thus, the neural innervation to the sclera is through the long and short posterior ciliary nerves and the anterior ciliary nerves. Inflammation and scleral distention result in pain mediated by each of these nervous networks. Nourishment to the sclera is provided by the many branches of the long and short posterior ciliary arteries, the anterior ciliary arteries, the underlying choroid, and the overlying episclera. These vascular channels can transport various substances capable of producing inflammation within the sclera.

Etiology

A causative factor is more often found in scleritis than in episcleritis. Systemic and ocular conditions known to cause scleritis are listed in Table 23.1. In a series reported by Watson,[2] 40% of the patients with necrotizing scleritis had evidence of collagen disease, while only 20% of the patients with diffuse anterior or nodular scleritis had associated collagen disease. Of the patients with diffuse anterior and nodular scleritis, 12% had ankylosing spondylitis, and 15% occurred in patients following an attack of herpes zoster ophthalmicus. A number of other conditions such as Reiter's disease, tuberculosis, gout, and syphilis have been implicated as etiologic factors.

Experimentally, pathologic and clinical data seem to support an immunologic basis as the cause of many attacks of scleritis.[14,15] Circulating antigen-antibody complexes that involve the complement system cause inflammation at the sites where the complexes concentrate. This does not mean that the sclera is necessarily liberating the antigen, since the focus of antigen production may be at a distant tissue location. Circulating immune complexes have a predilection for the basement membranes of blood vessels, and it is there that they activate the complement system, initiate inflammation, and produce tissue damage.[16] It has been proposed that since the posterior segment of the eye has fewer blood vessels, posterior scleral inflammation is less severe than inflammation of the anterior sclera.[12,16] Examples of immune complex diseases that can have an associated scleritis include rheumatoid arthritis, systemic lupus erythematosis, and polyarteritis nodosa. Scleritis occurs in 0.7% of all patients with rheumatoid arthritis.[17] It has been found following uneventful cataract surgery.[18,19]

Diagnosis

Scleritis can be an extremely destructive disease leading to loss of vision, severe pain, perforation of the globe, and loss of the eye. Therefore, early diagnosis and treatment are crucial. Although episcleritis rarely involves the sclera, scleritis always produces a concurrent episcleritis.[2,39a]

One of the hallmark symptoms of scleritis is severe

TABLE 23.1
Systemic and Ocular Conditions Known to Cause Scleritis

Collagen Diseases	Metabolic Diseases	Granulomatous Diseases	Infectious Diseases	Ocular Conditions
Rheumatoid arthritis[a]	Thyrotoxicosis	Syphilis	Herpes zoster	Penetrating injuries
Ankylosing spondylitis	Gout	Leprosy	Herpes simplex	Thermal burns
Systemic lupus erythematosis		Tuberculosis	Onchocerciasis	Alkali and acid burns
Polyarteritis nodosa		Sarcoidosis[d]	Pseudomonas	Irradiation
Relapsing polychondritis[b]			Acanthamoeba[e]	
Wegener's granulomatosis[c]			Toxoplasmosis[f]	
Ulcerative colitis				
Crohn's disease				
Behçet's syndrome				
Dermatomyositis				
Sjögren syndrome (complete)				
Psoriatic arthritis				

[a]Barr CC, Davis H, Culbertson WW. Rheumatoid scleritis. Ophthalmology 1981;88:1269–1273.
[b]Isaak BL, Liesegang TJ, Michet CJ Jr. Ocular and systemic findings in relapsing polychondritis. Ophthalmology 1986;93:681–689.
[c]Bullen CL, Liesegang TJ, McDonald TJ, et al. Ocular complications of Wegener's granulomatosis. Ophthalmology 1983;90:279–290.
[d]Henkind P. Sarcoidosis: An expanding ophthalmic horizon. J R Soc Med 1982;75:153–159.
[e]Mannis MJ, Tamaru R, Roth AM, et al. Acanthamoeba sclerokeratitis. Determining diagnostic criteria. Arch Ophthalmol 1986;104:1313–1317.
[f]Schuman JS, Weinberg RS, Ferry AP, et al. Toxoplasmic scleritis. Ophthalmology 1988;95:1399–1403.

pain, which prompts the patient to seek eyecare. The pain may be localized to the eye, but in many instances it is much more diffuse and may be described as radiating to the jaw, sinuses, and temple. It is not uncommon for the pain to awaken the patient in the night or to prevent the patient from falling asleep during an attack. The eye can become exquisitely tender to the touch, and the slightest digital pressure through the lids can cause the patient to recoil from the examiner. The pain experienced by such patients seems much greater than can be explained by the ocular findings. This is particularly true in posterior scleritis, since the inflammation is not visible to the clinician. The pain is secondary to distension of the sensory nerve endings as they become edematous, and an even more severe pain can result from actual destruction of the nerves in necrotizing scleritis. In some cases intractable pain may be relieved only by the use of retrobulbar alcohol injections.[21]

Inflammation is a prominent feature in anterior scleritis and produces a bluish red (violaceous) color instead of the bright red injection observed in episcleritis (Color Plate XIX). Since the violaceous color is more easily seen in the daylight, the clinician may want to examine the patient next to a window or outside the office. The episcleral congestion can be differentiated from that of the sclera by instilling phenylephrine 10% or epinephrine 1:1000, which will blanch the episcleral vessels but have little effect on the deeper scleral vessels.

Another test that can be used is instillation of a topical anesthetic followed by application of a cotton swab to the inflamed site. If this elicits a pain response, then scleritis or episcleritis should be suspected. The absence of pain suggests a diagnosis of conjunctivitis or iridocyclitis.

The practitioner should be careful to exclude intraocular causes of scleral inflammation. Yeo and associates[20] have reported intraocular metastatic carcinoma that masqueraded as scleritis.

ANTERIOR SCLERITIS

Anterior scleritis can be classified into 3 types: diffuse, nodular, and necrotizing. Patients with necrotizing scleritis can be subdivided into those with and those without scleromalacia perforans.

Diffuse scleritis is more common than the other forms and involves inflammation that occurs over a small area or encompasses the entire anterior segment. The vessels of the superficial and deep layers become engorged and tortuous, losing their normal radial pattern, and they may become beaded in appearance (see Color Plate XIX).

Nodular scleritis consists of one to many immovable nodules of scleral tissue. The adjacent episclera is usually edematous and lightly affixed to the underlying sclera. The sclera may become transparent beneath the nodule. Fortunately, the sclera does not become necrotic, and the scleral inflammation does not extend beyond the nodule. About half of affected patients have a bilateral occurrence.

Necrotizing scleritis is the most serious form of scleritis and has the highest complication rate. Over 60% of patients develop complications other than scleral thinning, and 40% have loss of visual acuity.[1] The scleritis begins in a localized area with acute congestion of the vessels, which become greatly distorted or occluded. The usual presentation is that of gradual onset of a painful, injected eye. The underlying sclera becomes transparent, and the choroid may be observed when viewed in daylight. If the inflammation remains uncontrolled, it may spread to newly formed areas of scleritis in adjoining locations. Severe edema and acute congestion is known as brawny scleritis. The entire anterior segment can become involved if efforts are not made to control the inflammation. Anterior segment fluorescein angiography can be helpful in detecting early necrotizing scleritis before it advances.[21a] Serious complications generally do not occur until the necrotizing process is almost circumferential. Staphylomas are uncommon unless the intraocular pressure is above 40 mm Hg.[2,22] With successful treatment, necrotic areas may disappear or may leave a thin film of conjunctiva or episclera covering the uvea. In other cases there may be actual uveal exposure. Small defects are usually covered by new collagen, but large defects may require a scleral graft. Necrotizing scleritis may indicate a potential lethal underlying systemic vasculitis.[23]

Necrotizing anterior scleritis without accompanying inflammation is known as scleromalacia perforans. It most commonly affects women between 50 and 75 years of age who suffer from chronic polyarticular rheumatism. It is characterized by a melting of episcleral and scleral tissue with almost a total lack of symptoms. The underlying uvea may be covered by conjunctiva or be totally exposed (Fig. 23.2).

POSTERIOR SCLERITIS

Posterior scleritis is usually unilateral and is more difficult to diagnose, since it is hidden from direct view. When the patient experiences considerably more ocular pain and discomfort than can be justified by the examination, posterior scleritis should be suspected. Scleral depression can localize an area of posterior scleritis by eliciting intense pain when applied to the involved inflammatory site. Exudative retinal detachment, optic disc edema, macular edema, retinal hem-

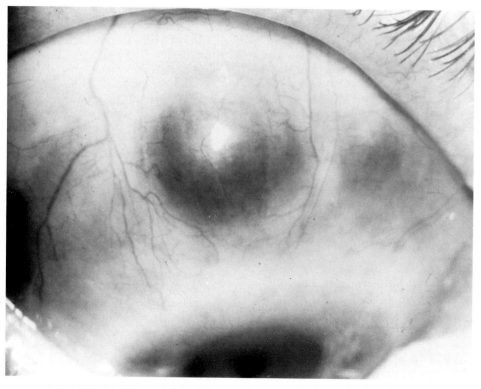

FIGURE 23.2   **Rheumatoid nodules seen in a case of scleromalacia perforans.**

orrhages, proptosis, and, rarely, angle-closure glaucoma may develop in posterior scleritis.[1,2,24–27,49] This condition can develop as a posterior extension of anterior scleritis. The diagnosis of posterior scleritis may be facilitated by ultrasonography, which shows the involvement as a clear zone immediately posterior to the globe (Fig. 23.3). This clear zone consists of transudates produced by the adjacent scleritis.[28,29] Computed tomography (CT) can also reveal the inflammation as a thickening of the sclera and a separation between the sclera and Tenon's capsule.[30] It is not uncommon for an eye to be removed because of a suspected intraocular tumor,[24,25,31] only to be discovered later by the pathologist that the lesion in question was an area of posterior scleritis.

Management

Aggressive treatment of scleritis is important to prevent complications that occur in the later stages of the disease and vary according to the degree of inflammation. They include uveitis, glaucoma, keratitis, corneal ulceration, scleral thinning, proptosis, diplopia, cataract, macular edema, optic disc edema, exudative retinal detachment, annular choroidal detachment, lid edema, chemosis, hyperemia of the conjunctiva, paresis of extraocular muscles, and myopia.[2,3,32–34] Many of these complications can result in reduced vision.

In a series reported by Watson,[2] 27% of the patients lost a significant amount of vision within a year of onset of the condition despite aggressive treatment. However, early and intensive treatment was very successful in preserving the eye; over a 6-year period in which 343 eyes were treated, only 4 were enucleated for intractable pain. All 4 patients had severe necrotizing scleritis and maintained reasonable visual acuity until the entire anterior segment became involved.

Treatment of scleritis is determined primarily by its etiology and severity of the inflammation. Associated ocular and systemic diseases are more commonly found in patients with scleritis than in those with episcleritis. A known bacterial infection or other known condition should be treated with a specific therapeutic regimen.[35–37]

Scleritis associated with brucellosis should be treated with 500 to 700 mg of tetracycline 4 times a day or 1 to 2 g of streptomycin per day for 3 to 4 weeks. Scleritis associated with syphilis should be treated with penicillin in a total dose varying from 5 to 10 million units. Scleritis associated with tuberculosis should be treated with streptomycin, 1 to 2 g daily; rifampin, 600 mg

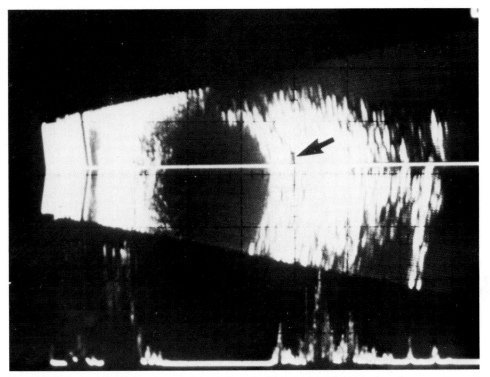

FIGURE 23.3   **B-scan ultrasonogram of posterior scleritis demonstrating the edematous zone (arrow) produced by the posterior scleritis.**

daily; or ethambutol, 15 mg/kg body weight daily. This can be administered in combination with isoniazid, 5 to 10 mg/kg body weight in 2 to 3 daily doses. Gouty scleritis can be treated with colchicine, 0.6 mg every 2 hours until the symptoms are relieved or gastrointestinal disturbances appear, but in mild cases only 0.6 mg daily may be sufficient. Phenylbutazone is used in acute cases of gout, and the initial dosage is 200 to 400 mg orally, then 200 mg every 6 hours for 4 days, followed by 100 mg 3 times a day until symptoms dissipate. Because of the risk of severe and sometimes fatal toxic reactions, therapy should not exceed 7 to 10 days. Indomethacin has been found to be effective in gout; the dosage is 50 mg 3 times daily in the acute phase and 25 mg twice daily in the quiescent phase.[13]

Scleritis secondary to leprosy should be treated with sulfone drugs, such as dapsone, in oral doses of 25 mg twice weekly and then increased by 25 mg twice weekly until a maintenance weekly dosage of 300 mg is achieved after 4 to 6 months of therapy. Sulfoxone sodium may be given for leprosy in an oral dosage of 330 mg twice weekly for the first 2 weeks and gradually increasing to 330 mg daily after 1 month of therapy. In all the systemic diseases mentioned above, the use of topical steroids can relieve pain and dramatically reduce the scleral inflammation. They may be used to treat the associated scleritis as long as the underlying systemic disease is adequately controlled.[13]

If no local or systemic disease process can be identified or if a collagen disease is discovered, then systemic anti-inflammatory or immunosuppressive agents should be administered. Scleritis is most often associated with the rheumatoid group of diseases, and the associated scleritis usually varies with the severity of the systemic condition.[38,39] The scleritis may develop while the patient is receiving salicylate or steroid therapy for the arthritis.[13]

Many parameters can be used to assess the effectiveness of treatment, including episcleral and deep scleral injection, tenderness, pain, and corneal and intraocular involvement. Pain is especially useful in determining the response of scleritis to treatment, and it is often used as an indicator to modify the treatment regimen. If the pain disappears, the steroid dosage can often be reduced with confidence.

Scleritis is usually treated with topical steroid drops or ointment. Prednisolone 1% or dexamethasone 0.1% can be used 4 times daily to once every hour depending on the severity of the inflammation. Such local steroids are used when the inflammation is mild and the pain is slight. They can be used to maintain the patient in a state of remission or may be used between severe attacks. Topical steroids can decrease symptoms and shorten the period of inflammation. However, topical steroid therapy is usually not adequate by itself to treat scleritis, and the preferred treatment plan is systemic anti-inflammatory or immunosuppressive agents. High doses of systemic anti-inflammatory drugs are necessary to achieve a therapeutic level in the poorly vascularized scleral tissue.[2]

Watson and Hayreh[22] prefer the use of NSAIAs such as oxyphenbutazone or indomethacin as the initial therapy. Oxyphenbutazone is given in divided doses of 600 mg daily for 4 days and then is tapered to 400 mg daily until all symptoms have disappeared. Indomethacin is administered in a daily 100 mg dose that is decreased to 75 mg when a therapeutic response is obtained. Patients may often respond to indomethacin if they do not respond to oxyphenbutazone, and vice versa.[12] If these two drugs fail to achieve the desired response, then oral prednisone can be administered. This is often necessary in severe attacks when an avascular area appears, as well as in recurrent attacks. Prednisone is administered in a 60 mg daily dose, but if no response is obtained, the dosage should be increased by 20 mg every 3 days until the condition is brought under control. The required dosage may be as high as 120 mg daily in severe cases of scleritis. A dosage of 300 mg daily may be effective if lower dosages have failed.[40] The dosage is gradually decreased as soon as possible to a maintenance divided dosage of 20 mg daily. Later, another anti-inflammatory drug is added, while the steroid dose is reduced by 2.5 mg steps. The steroid dosage may need to be increased if inflammation is exacerbated while the drug is being tapered.[12] An infrequently used treatment that may control more severe cases of scleritis is intravenous hydrocortisone[2] or methylprednisolone.[41]

Immunosuppressive drugs may be necessary in cases of necrotizing scleritis when high doses of steroids have failed. Azathioprine is the drug of choice and is initially administered in a dosage of 100 mg daily and increased to 150 to 200 mg daily over the following 2 weeks.[38,42,43] Since severe side effects are associated with the drug, its use should be reserved for critical situations.[12] Cyclophosphamide has produced total regression in a case of rheumatoid posterior scleritis with choroidal nodules and nonrhegmatogenous retinal detachment.[24]

Retrobulbar injections of adrenocorticotropic hormone (ACTH) have been attempted, primarily for patients who cannot tolerate systemic steroids, but the beneficial effects have usually been transient or completely nonexistent.[2,12] Subconjunctival or sub-Tenon's injections should be avoided, since the involved sclera is thin and easily perforated.[13,22] Such injections can also lead to scleral perforation due to lysis of collagen. Thus, it appears that periocular injections have little

if any beneficial effect.[44] Watson[2] has reported that the removal of a subconjunctival deposit of steroid resulted in the resolution of a progressive necrotizing scleritis.

Treatment of scleromalacia perforans consists of topical steroids such as prednisolone 0.12% 3 times daily to limit the accompanying iridocyclitis. Active cases require 40 to 80 mg of oral prednisolone daily combined with 200 mg of phenylbutazone. This approach may prevent progression of the destructive process.[12]

Surgery is rarely necessary for scleral defects because of scleral tissue's regenerative capabilities. Grafting is generally reserved for eyes in which there is an imminent danger of perforation. New collagen is readily produced in the base of small scleral defects when there is adequate medical treatment. Large defects, however, may require a scleral graft, which is usually successful when properly covered by conjunctiva. In addition to sclera, other grafting materials have included fascia lata and aortic tissue.[45–47] Unfortunately, the successful graft may also become involved in the necrotizing process if the scleral disease is out of control.[48]

Since scleritis may be the presenting sign of an underlying systemic disease, the patient must be treated in conjunction with a rheumatologist or internist. The required evaluation can be extensive, and in one series of patients, 27% died within 5 years due to underlying disease.[12]

References

1. Yannof M, Fine FS. Ocular pathology—A text and atlas. Hagerstown, MD: Harper & Row, 1982;383–388.
2. Watson P. Diseases of the sclera and episclera. In: Duane TD, Jaeger E, eds. Clinical ophthalmology. Hagerstown, MD: Harper & Row, 1987;4:1–43.
3. McGavin DDM, Williamson J, Forester JV, et al. Episcleritis and scleritis: A study of their clinical manifestations and associations with rheumatoid arthritis. Br J Ophthalmol 1976;60:192–226.
4. Scheie HG, Albert DM. Adler's textbook of ophthalmology. Philadelphia: W.B. Saunders Co, 1969;15.
5. Vaughan D, Asbury T. General ophthalmology. Los Altos, CA: Lange, 1977;102–105.
6. Hogan MJ, Zimmerman LE. Ophthalmic pathology, an atlas and textbook. Philadelphia: W.B. Saunders Co, 1962;337.
7. Roy FH. Ocular differential diagnosis. Philadelphia: Lea & Febiger, 1975;2:206–207.
8. Curtis EM. Recurrent episcleritis and emotional stress (letter). Arch Ophthalmol 1984;102:821–824.
9. Scharf J, Meyer E, Zonis S. Episcleritis associated with familial Mediterranean fever. Am J Ophthalmol 1985;100:337–339.

10. Sexton RR. Diseases of the sclera. In: Dunlap ED, ed. Gordon's medical management of ocular disease. Hagerstown, MD: Harper & Row, 1976;171–175.

11. Gold GH. Ocular manifestations of connective tissue disease. In: Duane TD, Jaeger E, eds. Clinical ophthalmology. Hagerstown, MD: Harper & Row, 1987;5:1–30.

12. Fraunfelder FT, Roy FH. Current ocular therapy. Philadelphia: W.B. Saunders Co, 1980;571–575.

13. Ellis PP. Ocular therapeutics and pharmacology. St Louis: C.V. Mosby Co, 1981;136–138.

14. Rahi AHS, Garner A. Immunopathology of the eye. Oxford: Blackwell Scientific, 1976;282.

15. Nomoto Y, Sakai H, Endoh M, et al. Scleritis and IgA nephropathy. Arch Intern Med 1980;140:783–785.

16. Bloomfield SE. Clinical allergy and immunology of the external eye. In: Duane TD, Jaeger E, eds. Clinical ophthalmology. Hagerstown, MD: Harper & Row, 1987;4:1–25.

17. Williamson J. The rheumatic eye. Practitioner 1982;226:863–874.

18. Salamon SM, Bartly JM, Zaidman GW. Peripheral corneal ulcers, conjunctival ulcers, and scleritis after cataract surgery. Am J Ophthalmol 1982;93:334–337.

19. Soong HK, Kenyon KR. Adverse reactions to virgin silk sutures in cataract surgery. Ophthalmology 1984;91:479–483.

20. Yeo JH, Jakobiec F, Iwamoto T, et al. Metastatic carcinoma masquerading as scleritis. Ophthalmology 1983;90:184–194.

21. Michels PG. Ocular manifestation in arthritis. In: Ryan SJ Jr, Smith RE, eds. Selected topics on the eye in systemic disease. New York: Grune & Stratton, 1974;365.

21a. Watson PG, Bovey FE. Anterior segment fluorescein angiography in the diagnosis of scleral inflammation. Ophthalmology 1985;92:1–11.

22. Watson PG, Hayreh SS. Scleritis and episcleritis. Br J Ophthalmol 1976;60:163–191.

23. Foster CS, Forstot SL, Wilson LA. Mortality rate in rheumatoid arthritis patients developing necrotizing scleritis or peripheral ulcerative keratitis. Effects of systemic immunosuppression. Ophthalmology 1984;91:1253–1263.

24. Hurd ER, Snyder WB, Ziff M. Choroidal nodules and retinal detachments in rheumatoid arthritis. Am J Med 1970;48:273–278.

25. Sevel D. Rheumatoid nodule of the sclera. Trans Ophthalmol Soc UK 1965;357–366.

26. Wolter JR, Bentley MD. Scleromalacia perforans and massive granuloma of the sclera. Am J Ophthalmol 1961;51:71–80.

27. Manschot WA. The eye in collagen diseases. Adv Ophthalmol 1961;11:1–16.

28. Coleman DJ, Lizzie FL, Jack RL. Ultrasonography of the eye and orbit. Philadelphia: Lea & Febiger, 1977;306.

29. Marushak D. Uveal effusion attending scleritis posterior. A case report with A-scan and B-scan echograms. Acta Ophthalmol 1982;60:773–778.

30. Trokel SL. Computed tomographic scanning of orbital inflammations. Int Ophthalmol Clin 1982;22:81–98.

31. Feldon SE, Sigelman J, Albert DM, et al. Clinical manifestations of brawny scleritis. Am J Ophthalmol 1978;85:781–787.

32. Manschot WA. Progressive scleroperikeratitis. Arch Ophthalmol 1954;52:375–384.

33. Benson WE, Shields JA, Tasman W, et al. Posterior scleritis. A cause of diagnostic confusion. Arch Ophthalmol 1979; 97:1482–1486.

34. Wilhelms KR, Grherson I, Watson PG. Histopathologic and clinical associations of scleritis and glaucoma. Am J Ophthalmol 1981;91:697–705.

35. Alfonso E, Kenyon KR, Ormerod LD, et al. *Pseudomonas* corneoscleritis. Am J Ophthalmol 1987;103:90–98.

36. Stenson S, Brookner A, Rosenthal S. Bilateral endogenous necrotizing scleritis due to *Aspergillus oryzase*. Ann Ophthalmol 1982;14:67–72.

37. Callwell DR, Kastl P, Ottman D. A fungal infection as an intrascleral abscess. Ann Ophthalmol 1981;13:841–842.

38. Jayson MI, Jones DEP. Scleritis and rheumatoid arthritis. Ann Rheum Dis 1971;30:343–347.

39. Lyne AJ, Pitkeathly DA. Episcleritis and scleritis: Association with connective tissue disease. Arch Ophthalmol 1968;80:171–176.

39a. Watson PG. The diagnosis and management of scleritis. Ophthalmology 1980;87:716–720.

40. Tessler H. Uveitis. In: Peyman GA, Sanders DR, Goldberg MF, eds. Principles and practices of ophthalmology. Philadelphia; W.B. Sanders Co, 1980;1567–1570.

41. McCluskey P, Wakefield D. Intravenous pulse methylprednisolone in scleritis. Arch Ophthalmol 1987;105:793–797.

42. Jayson MI. Rheumatoid scleritis. In: Eberl R, Rosenthal M, eds. Organic manifestations and complications in rheumatoid arthritis. Stuttgart: Schattauer, 1976;269.

43. Foster CS. Immunosuppressive therapy for external ocular inflammatory disease. Ophthalmology 1980;87:140–150.

44. Jakobic FA, Jones IS. Orbital inflammations. In: Duane TD, Jaeger E, eds. Clinical ophthalmology. Hagerstown, MD: Harper & Row, 1987;2:1–75.

45. Bick MW. Surgical treatment of scleromalacia perforans. Arch Ophthalmol 1959;61:907–917.

46. Torchia RT, Dunn RE, Pease PJ. Fascia lata grafting in scleromalacia perforans. Am J Ophthalmol 1968;66:705–709.

47. Merz EH. Scleral reinforcement with aortic tissue. Am J Ophthalmol 1964;57:766–790.

48. Jayson MI, Easty DL. Ulceration of the cornea in rheumatoid arthritis. Ann Rheum Dis 1977;36:428–432.

49. Benson WE. Posterior scleritis. Surv Ophthalmol 1988;32:297–316.

CHAPTER 24

Uveitis

Murray Fingeret
John W. Potter

The iris, ciliary body, and choroid comprise the uvea, a highly vascularized structure that can be affected by numerous disease processes. Pharmacologically, a variety of drugs may be used in the treatment of uveal inflammation, and this chapter considers how these drugs can be used to modify the natural course of uveitis to prevent serious complications from the disease.

Definition and Classification

Uveitis is an inflammation of the iris, ciliary body, or choroid of the eye. The inflammation can be limited to the anterior or to the posterior structures, or it can affect both, and clinical features will depend on the site of involvement. The etiology of many cases of uveitis is often unknown or presumed,[1] and treatment is often nonspecific, aimed at reducing inflammation and preventing ocular complications.

A variety of methods are used to classify uveitis.[2,3] One method is based on the anatomic site of inflammation. For example, uveitis that involves the iris only is termed iritis. Another method is to classify the uveal inflammation based on whether it affects the anterior, intermediate, or posterior structures of the eye. A third method is to classify the inflammation as either granulomatous or nongranulomatous. A granulomatous uveal inflammation may present acutely, or, more likely, be chronic. It may involve either the anterior or the posterior uvea, have an insidious onset, and often presents with a white eye.[4] Such inflammation can involve the choroid or the retina and may produce large, greasy keratic precipitates that can be observed along with epithelioid cells and macrophages in the anterior chamber. In contrast, a nongranulomatous uveal inflammation usually involves the anterior segment of the eye and has an acute onset accompanied by a cellular reaction in the anterior chamber that represents smaller cell types (lymphocytes) than those in granulomatous inflammation. There is considerable overlap in any clinical classification system, but these classifications provide some opportunity to differentiate various presentations and predict the natural course of the inflammation.

On the forefront of a better understanding of the etiology and course of uveitis is the role of immunology.[2] In almost all cases of uveitis, there is limited response to antimicrobial therapy, and the cause of the inflammation is rarely discovered.[5] Concepts in immunology, including human leukocyte antigen (HLA) typing, may add much to our knowledge of uveal inflammation. Many cases show that specific HLAs and certain types of uveitis are associated, indicating that a specific subset of the population might be at greater risk for certain types of uveal inflammation.[6]

Epidemiology

Anterior uveitis is more common than posterior uveitis. Anterior uveal inflammation accounts for about 12 cases per 100,000 population, whereas posterior uveitis accounts for only about 3 cases per 100,000 population.

Thus, anterior uveitis is about 4 times as common as posterior uveitis.[7]

The peak prevalence for cases of uveitis is in persons age 20 to 50 years.[8] This age group also parallels the peak activity of T-lymphocytes.

Uveitis may have a sexual predilection depending on the specific condition.[9,10] Reiter's syndrome and ankylosing spondylitis, for example, are more common in males, whereas sarcoid and juvenile rheumatoid arthritis are more common in females. Race can also be a factor. Ocular toxoplasmosis and histoplasmosis are more frequently observed in whites, while ocular sarcoidosis occurs more often in blacks. In addition, there may be a geographic predisposition for certain uveal inflammations.[9,10] Ocular histoplasmosis is observed in persons from the midwestern United States, Behçet's disease is more typically observed in persons from Mediterranean countries and Japan, and sarcoid is seen in whites from Scandinavia.

Etiology

At one time an infectious agent was thought to cause most uveitis. Currently, however, uveitis is thought to be an immune-complex disorder with some type of T-cell antigen dysfunction playing a major role. A previous infection may alter the patient's immunologic condition, or a primary immunologic condition can underly the presenting uveitis.[11] HLA studies are being undertaken to identify persons who might be predisposed to recurrent episodes of uveitis or whose uveitis might be associated with immunologic conditions. HLA systems are the antigenic complexes involved with histocompatibility, including graft rejection. There are four groups of HLA antigens, A, B, C, and D, but types A and B are observed most frequently.[11] They are present on the surface membranes of leukocytes and are regulated by the gene loci on chromosome 6. The HLA system is a genetic marker for cell surface antigens and can be used to identify the subgroup that may be at risk for a certain condition. Certain HLA phenotypes are at a greater risk for specific inflammatory conditions.

About 35% of patients with ankylosing spondylitis will have uveitis at some point in the natural course of the disease.[2] Of patients with ankylosing spondylitis, about 90% will have HLA-B27,[12,13] and HLA-B27 has also been found in Reiter's syndrome, juvenile rheumatoid arthritis, and persons with acute iridocyclitis of unknown etiology.[5] In addition, HLA-B27 has been observed in 50% to 70% of patients with acute iridocyclitis compared with a control group manifesting 4% to 8% HLA-B27.[12] However, an individual with HLA-B27 has only a 1% chance of developing uveitis, which suggests that other factors exist in the etiology of uveal inflammation.[5] Such risk factors remain unknown. An individual may have no HLA-B27 and incur ankylosing spondylitis, but the chance of acquiring uveitis is only 7%, compared with 35% if the gene is present.[5]

Diagnosis

The symptoms and signs of uveitis depend on the anatomic site of inflammation. An acute anterior uveitis is usually characterized by a painful, often photophobic, red eye. The redness, known as ciliary flush, occurs in a circumcorneal fashion (Color Plate XX). The pupil may be miotic, the intraocular pressure may be reduced, and there can be slit-lamp findings of posterior synechiae (Fig. 24.1) or of keratic precipitates on the corneal endothelium (Fig. 24.2). Such keratic precipitates can vary in size and appearance from small and pinpoint to large and waxy.

The hallmark anterior segment reaction that is virtually pathognomonic of anterior uveitis is the appearance of cells and flare in the anterior chamber (Fig. 24.3). Cells appear as small individual white particles floating in the anterior chamber. They represent the passage of lymphocytes through the dilated spaces of the iris blood vessels into the anterior chamber. Flare represents transudation of protein into the aqueous and appears as a haziness or milkiness in the anterior chamber. Cells and flare are best detected by using the biomicroscope and carefully observing the aqueous in the anterior chamber using the dilated pupil as the

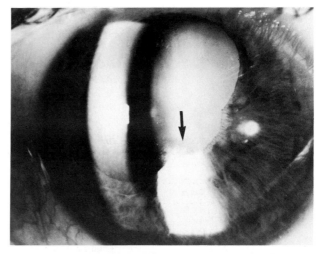

FIGURE 24.1   **Posterior synechia (arrow) associated with anterior uveitis. (Courtesy Scott Richter, O.D.)**

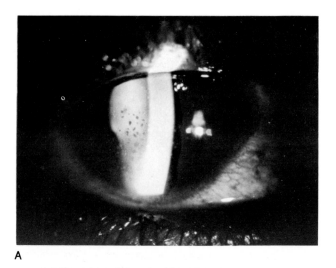

A

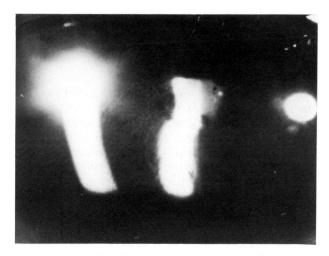

FIGURE 24.3 **Cells and flare in anterior chamber associated with anterior uveitis.**

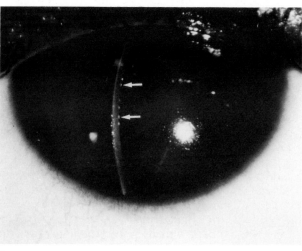

B

FIGURE 24.2 **Large keratic precipitates associated with anterior uveitis. (A) As seen with wide slit-lamp beam. (B) Viewed with thin optic section. (Courtesy Scott Richter, O.D.)**

background. It is best done in a dark room, allowing time for the examiner to dark-adapt. A bright conical or short parallelpiped beam under moderate to high magnification (10 to 20X) is oscillated back and forth and up and down in the anterior chamber while searching for the cells and flare to come into focus. A typical grading system for cells and flare is shown in Table 24.1.

Patients with anterior uveitis often present with symptoms of ocular pain, photophobia, and blurred vision. Pain is usually acute in onset, isolated deep in the eye, and dull or pulsating. Photophobia is a constant symptom in many cases and may present as the first sign of the condition. Photophobia can be reduced with cycloplegia, which places the iris and ciliary body muscles at rest. Blurred vision results from lacrimation or the accumulation of cells and flare in the anterior chamber.

TABLE 24.1
Grading Scale for Anterior Chamber Cells and Flare

Anterior Chamber Sign	Grade				
	Trace	*+*	*+ +*	*+ + +*	*+ + + +*
Cells	1–3 cells noted in beam	4–8 cells	9–15 cells	Too many cells to count	Appearance of snowstorm
Flare	None to questionable	Faint haze just detectable	Moderate haze; iris detail clear	Marked haze; iris detail fuzzy	Plastic iritis; fibrin clot

Cases of anterior uveitis that are bilateral, recurrent, or refractory to treatment necessitate a more extensive diagnostic evaluation. Such anterior uveitis often results from an endogenous condition, and the more common etiologies include tuberculosis, syphilis, arthritic and rheumatologic conditions, herpetic disease, and sarcoidosis.

Posterior uveitis is characterized by a white eye with little or no pain. Although there may be some cell and flare reaction in the anterior chamber, if present it is most remarkable in the vitreous. Histoplasmosis is an example of a posterior uveitis without cells or flare. Blurred vision is present if the macula is involved or if the vitreous is sufficiently hazy to diminish vision. Once the uveitis has diminished, there may be observable cells attached to relatively immobile vitreous fibrils. In addition, there may be flare in the posterior chamber, which can be noted with a conical beam from the slit lamp. When viewed with the binocular indirect ophthalmoscope, flare in the posterior chamber can appear as a green-tinted haze.

The most frequently encountered cases of posterior uveitis are from endogenous causes that include toxoplasmosis, histoplasmosis, and toxocariasis. The immune system may be altered by the suspected endogenous cause, or it may respond to an underlying systemic disease that predisposes the person to other immunologic disease.[14] It is only rarely that an infectious agent is identified in the ocular tissues. Instead, the uveitis may represent the immunologic focus of an endogenous condition.

Many of the endogenous causes can be identified or suspected based on laboratory tests. Some of the most common tests employed are skin and blood tests and x-ray films of the chest and joints (Table 24.2). Procedures such as the enzyme-linked immunosorbent assay (ELISA) have been introduced to detect antibodies that are present in extremely small quantities.[9] In addition to these tests, HLA typing has added to the diagnostic armamentarium by identifying persons who are at greater risk for certain inflammations.

Management

Anterior Uveitis

The objectives in the treatment of anterior uveitis are to (1) reduce the severity of the attack(s) or exacerbations, (2) prevent posterior synechiae, (3) prevent damage to the iris blood vessels and blood-aqueous barrier, (4) reduce the frequency of attacks, (5) prevent the development of secondary cataracts, and (6) prevent phthisis bulbi.

TABLE 24.2
Laboratory Tests in the Etiologic Diagnosis of Uveitis

Suspected Etiology	Laboratory Test
Ankylosing spondylitis	Sacroiliac joint x-ray film
	Sedimentation rate
Histoplasmosis	Chest x-ray film
	HLA-B7 test
Tuberculosis	Purified protein derivative (PPD) skin test
	Chest x-ray film
	Sedimentation rate
Sarcoidosis	Serum angiotensin converting enzyme (ACE)
	Kveim test
	Serum lysozyme
	Limited gallium scan
	Biopsy of suspected lesion (skin, conjunctiva, lacrimal gland)
	Chest x-ray film
Syphilis	Fluorescent treponemal antibody absorption (FTA-ABS) test
	Venereal Disease Research Laboratory (VDRL) test
Rheumatoid conditions	Rheumatoid factor
	Sedimentation rate
	HLA-B27 test
Toxocara	Enzyme-linked immunosorbent assay (ELISA)
Toxoplasmosis	*Toxoplasma* dye test
	Fluorescent antibody test
	ELISA test
Juvenile rheumatoid arthritis	Antinuclear antibody (ANA)
	Sedimentation rate
Reiter's syndrome	HLA-B27 test
	Sedimentation rate
	Sacroiliac joint x-ray film
Behçet's disease	HLA-B5 test

Posterior synechiae can often be prevented with use of cycloplegics. Cycloplegia places the ciliary body and iris at rest and reduces many of the associated symptoms. Table 24.3 lists the spectrum of drugs that can be used for therapeutic cycloplegia. At one end of the spectrum is tropicamide 1%, cycloplegia from which can last up to 6 hours. This drug, as well as homatropine 2%, may be useful in very mild forms of anterior uveitis. Cyclopentolate 1% is a more effective cycloplegic and is useful when administered 2 or 3 times daily in mild to moderate cases of anterior uveitis. Homatropine 5% is an intermediate-strength cycloplegic usually employed 3 to 4 times daily or, in more severe cases, up to every 2 hours. Atropine 1% is the strongest cycloplegic. Although atropine cycloplegia can last up to 2 weeks in a healthy eye, the drug must be instilled twice daily to induce cycloplegia in the inflamed eye. If atropine is contraindicated because of hypersensitivity, scopolamine 0.25%, another strong

TABLE 24.3
Drugs for Therapeutic Cycloplegia

Drug	Indication
Tropicamide 1%	Mild anterior uveitis
Homatropine 2%	
Cyclopentolate 1%	Mild to moderate anterior uveitis
Homatropine 5%	Moderate anterior uveitis
Atropine 1%	Severe anterior uveitis
Scopolamine 0.25%	

cycloplegic, can be used. Patients with uveitis with an excessive protein (flare) component are at greater risk for posterior synechiae and must therefore be more aggressively managed with cycloplegics. The cycloplegia should be reduced as the inflammation begins to subside.

It is helpful to use a cycloplegic that will provide some iris movement, keeping the pupil somewhat mobile.[15] This will prevent posterior synechiae. A drug that will keep the pupil dilated and fixed in an 8 mm state may promote synechia formation just as a fixed 3 mm pupil would. Because of this, atropine is often avoided in favor of homatropine 5%, which will permit some movement of the pupil. In cases of suspected noncompliance, it is better to use a longer-acting cycloplegic such as atropine. When in doubt, it is better to use a stronger rather than weaker cycloplegic.

It is necessary to measure the intraocular pressure in uveitis. Inflammation of the ciliary body will often reduce aqueous production, and intraocular pressure will be low. On the other hand, an increased intraocular pressure may be measured if the trabeculum becomes inflamed and does not allow the aqueous to filter properly, or if cells block the meshwork. In addition, a high intraocular pressure may occur if there is formation of posterior synechiae with iris bombé, or if anterior synechiae form and block aqueous outflow. The treatment of uveitic glaucoma is discussed in Chapter 29.

Steroid therapy can be delivered to the eye by several routes. Topical steroid administration is the most common method for treatment of anterior uveitis. In more severe cases, however, periocular injections or oral steroids may be indicated. For posterior uveitis, topical steroids have little effect, and periocular and oral steroids are the methods of choice.

The most effective steroid topically administered is 1% prednisolone acetate because it can most effectively penetrate the intact epithelium of the cornea to gain access to the anterior chamber (Table 24.4).[16] Since they are suspensions, prednisolone acetate preparations should be shaken vigorously to resuspend the steroid particles before the medication is instilled. Dosage frequency may be as often as every hour for severe inflammations but is usually 4 times daily for mild to moderate involvements. Weaker preparations and less frequent instillation will depend on the severity of the inflammation. Frequently administered, high-concentration steroids should be tapered to prevent a rebound phenomenon. The tapering is done over 1 to 2 weeks to try to preserve the remission. Patients should be monitored at 1- to 2-week intervals during the active phase of the uveitis until all signs of inflammation have disappeared.

Any uveal inflammation must be aggressively managed to minimize damage to the iris blood vessels and the blood-aqueous barrier, which, if affected, can allow an acute presentation to become chronic and difficult to manage. Once the active inflammation has subsided, the steroid dosage should be tapered to preserve the remission. If the patient has been receiving the steroid more than 4 times daily, the medication should be reduced to 4 times daily for 4 days, 3 times daily for 3 days, 2 times daily for 2 days, once for 1 day, and then discontinued. Further modification may be needed depending on circumstances, since too sudden withdrawal can reactivate the uveitis.

Occasionally, a case of chronic anterior uveitis requires continual low-dose topical steroids to maintain the quiet eye. The risks of once to twice daily topical steroid used indefinitely must be weighed against the potential damage due to further exacerbations or attacks of uveitis.

Many side effects of systemic steroid use can be avoided by using periocular injections. In particular, periocular steroids are useful in the treatment of pos-

TABLE 24.4
Anti-Inflammatory Effectiveness of Topical Steroids with Intact Corneal Epithelium

Minimal Effectiveness	Moderate Effectiveness	Maximal Effectiveness
Dexamethasone sodium phosphate 0.05% (ointment)	Prednisolone sodium phosphate 1.0%	Dexamethasone alcohol 0.1%
Dexamethasone sodium phosphate 0.1%	Fluorometholone alcohol 0.1%	Prednisolone acetate 1.0%

Modified from Leibowitz HM, Kupferman A. Int Ophthalmol Clin 1980; 20:117–134.

terior uveitis. They can be administered by injection in the anterior subconjunctiva, posterior sub-Tenon's capsule, or in a retrobulbar fashion. Periocular steroids can be injected so that they are placed close to the site of inflammation.

Oral steroids may reach all parts of the eye in high concentration. They are easily administered but can lead to significant systemic side effects. An alternate-day dosage can be used when the condition is stabilized because the anti-inflammatory effect is comparable to daily dosage, and the depressive effects on immunity and the adrenal glands are much less intense.[15]

Pulse dosages of intravenous methylprednisolone have been shown to be effective for severe or recalcitrant forms of uveitis while minimizing the side effects associated with more conventional routes of steroid administration.[17,18]

Oral nonsteroidal anti-inflammatory agents (NSAIAs) (e.g., indomethacin, aspirin, ibuprofen) have held great promise but up to now have been a clinical disappointment. They do not appear to be potent enough for use during an attack of uveitis. Flurbiprofen (Ocufen), a topical NSAIA, is now available to prevent miosis during cataract surgery. Miosis during cataract surgery is due to the release of prostaglandins during surgery, and flurbiprofen inhibits the synthesis of prostaglandins, decreasing miosis and presumably the inflammatory component mediated by prostaglandins. This agent may be available in the near future for use as a topical anti-inflammatory agent. If flurbiprofen can be shown to decrease inflammation, its potential is great, since it does not elevate intraocular pressure or cause cataracts, side effects associated with steroid use.

Immunosuppressive therapy can be used in severe cases where steroids may not be effective and the eye is worsening. Chlorambucil has been effective in Behçet's disease and other types of uveitis, including juvenile rheumatoid arthritis and sympathetic ophthalmia.[15] However, these immunosuppressive agents have many serious side effects and require immunologic consultation.

Cyclosporine is a second-generation immunosuppressive drug that attempts to modify the immune response without destroying cells from the immune system. An 11-amino acid cyclic peptide, it has been extensively used in the field of organ transplantation with dramatic results.[19] Unfortunately, at the dosage levels used to prevent organ rejection, nephrotoxicity almost always occurs. This is acceptable for the liver or heart patient near death but is unacceptable for patients with uveitis. The dosage levels of cyclosporine have been reduced by using it with other medications such as systemic steroids or bromocriptine.[19]

Patients receiving cyclosporine have chronic autoimmune conditions and will require treatment for a long time, further increasing the risk of side effects. Thus, cyclosporine is now viewed as a second-line medication for Behçet's disease and other sight-threatening uveitic conditions not responding to topical, periocular, or systemic steroids.

Posterior Uveitis

Management of the patient with posterior uveitis is quite different from management of one with anterior uveitis. The objectives of treating and managing posterior uveitis include (1) protecting the macula, (2) protecting the optic nerve, (3) protecting the vitreous, (4) preventing loss of ciliary body or retinal function, and (5) preventing cataract formation.

Uveitis posterior to the iris and lens has little chance of creating posterior synechiae, so cycloplegia is not necessary. Because of the posterior inflammatory site, topical steroids are not effective in therapeutic doses, and systemic or periocular administration is necessary. Systemic and periocular steroids have greater risks and must be used carefully. It is important that the uveitis not be of an infectious origin that can be worsened by steroids if not covered concurrently with the appropriate antimicrobial agent(s). Periocular steroids should not be used in an infectious condition because of the risks of reactivation to an uncontrollable level. If periocular steroids are used, a sub-Tenon's injection of a repository form may be given up to every 2 weeks. Systemic steroids are usually started with a full dose divided into 4 parts per 24 hours. When the condition stabilizes, the medication can be given every other morning to reduce the amount of immune system suppression. If used for less than 2 weeks, the dose of systemic steroid may be quickly reduced, but in most cases a slower withdrawal of steroid will preserve the remission.

Each encounter with uveitis, either anterior or posterior, must be considered individually. The decision to treat with cycloplegics, steroids, or immunosuppressive agents should be made carefully. Patients with uveitis that is bilateral, recurrent, or refractory to treatment should undergo more extensive evaluation for underlying systemic disease.

Specific Uveitides

Trauma

Trauma to the eye can result in anterior uveitis. Contusion injury can create a mild to severe iridocyclitis with moderate cases requiring only cycloplegia for a short time. Severe inflammation will require more aggressive therapy, including the use of topical steroids. In addition to uveitis, trauma may cause other ocular problems, including perforating injury, angle recession glaucoma, and retinal breaks with or without retinal detachment.

A traumatic corneal abrasion can cause anterior uveitis from vasodilation and increased permeability of the iris blood vessels in response to the primary insult. As the corneal abrasion resolves with treatment that might include antibiotics and patching, the uveitis also will resolve. Some patients may require cycloplegia to reduce ocular pain associated with the anterior segment inflammation (see Chapter 22).

Trauma can lead to bleeding in the anterior chamber, be it only a few red blood cells or frank hemorrhage. Such hemorrhage, or hyphema, will usually fill less than one-third of the anterior chamber[20] (Fig. 24.4). So-called microscopic hyphemas may be observable only with the slit lamp and consist of a few red blood cells in the anterior chamber. This may be difficult to differentiate from the cells seen in anterior uveitis, but use of the green filter may enable differentiation—red cells will not be apparent with the green filter, but the white cells of uveitis can be observed.

The clinician should also investigate for associated conditions, including blow-out fractures of the orbit, corneal edema, subluxated lens, retinal breaks, or retinal detachment. Gonioscopy, to rule out the possibility of angle recession, and binocular indirect ophthalmoscopic examination should be delayed until the hyphema has cleared enough to permit adequate visualization of ocular structures without reinjury to any tissue.

The majority of hyphemas last about 5 days, and from 2% to 38% rebleed.[52] This 5-day period represents the period of greatest risk for a rebleed.[20] If after 5 days no rebleed has occurred, the chances of rebleed decrease significantly. Conversely, with each episode of rebleed, the chances of good visual recovery diminish.

The initial height of the hyphema tends to correlate with the chance for rebleeding, with a significantly higher rate of secondary hemorrhage among patients with larger initial hyphemas,[52] but the severity of the injury cannot be determined from the height of the hyphema at initial presentation.

Treatment of hyphema is controversial. Miotics have been used to increase the area of absorption on the iris.[21] However, because most of the resorption of hyphema probably takes place in the angle rather than in the iris, cycloplegics and mydriatics are now advocated.[22] Cycloplegics may aid in resolving associated iritis, and mydriatics may reduce the likelihood of secondary synechiae. However, some authors contend that any manipulation of the iris, even with medication, increases the potential for rebleed.[20] Topical steroid therapy may be implemented in protracted cases,[20] and topical β blockers or systemic carbonic anhydrase inhibitors can be used in cases where the intraocular pressure is elevated.

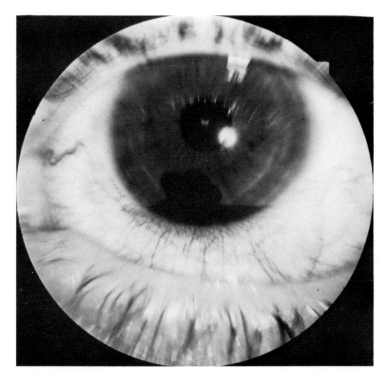

FIGURE 24.4 **Traumatic hyphema filling less than one-third of anterior chamber.**

Oral antifibrinolytic agents have been advocated for use in the medical management of hyphemas.[22–24] Aminocaproic acid (Amicar) has lowered the rate of rebleeding from about 30% to 3%.[25] The full dose is 100 mg/kg body weight every 4 hours up to a maximal dose of 30 g daily. The drug is expensive and causes numerous side effects, including dizziness, hypotension, syncope, nausea, and vomiting. In one study[25] the dose was reduced by half while maintaining the impressive low rate of rebleeding and causing fewer side effects, except for nausea and vomiting.

Aminocaproic acid has been shown to be ineffective for traumatic hyphemas in children,[26] but another antifibrinolytic agent, tranexamic acid (Cyklokapron), has been shown to reduce the incidence of secondary hemorrhage significantly in the pediatric population.[53] Because of the cost of therapy and its side effects, some investigators have questioned the value of systemic treatment with aminocaproic acid.[52] When topically applied,[54] however, the drug may reduce the incidence of secondary hemorrhage with fewer systemic side effects.

There is general agreement that patients with hyphema should be at rest, but there is controversy over the methods to be implemented. Some practitioners place patients in the hospital with complete bedrest, bilateral patches, and sedation. Evidence, however, suggests that there is no difference in prognosis if the patient is not hospitalized.[27] If the patient is not hospitalized, the eye should be protected with a shield at bedtime, and the patient should have periodic bedrest with the head elevated at a 30° to 45° angle.[20] The angle of the head helps settle the hyphema in the inferior anterior chamber angle.

Cataract Surgery

Immediately following cataract extraction, with or without the implantation of an intraocular lens, prophylactic antibiotic and steroid eyedrops are used. Antibiotics are generally discontinued within the first 3 weeks, and steroids are used for 3 to 6 weeks. Antibiotics are usually discontinued abruptly, whereas topical steroids must be gradually tapered (Table 24.5). In general, 1 less daily drop is used each week once tapering of topical steroids has begun. As an example, during weeks 1 through 3 the steroid dosage frequency might be 4 times daily, and during week 4 it would be 3 times daily. Then, during week 5 the frequency would be twice daily, and for week 6 it would be only 1 drop daily. During the first 3 weeks the cells and flare should diminish from grade 3+ to 1+ (or only trace). By the sixth week no anterior chamber reaction should be observed.

Retinal Tears

A patient presenting with anterior uveitis, especially one resistant to treatment, requires a careful dilated fundus examination with the binocular indirect ophthalmoscope. Small, peripheral, hitherto asymptomatic retinal tears, with or without accompanying retinal detachment, may be the causative agent. Repair of the retinal disorder will usually cause the anterior uveitis to resolve.

Arthritis

Although the relationship is not fully understood, uveitis and arthritis are related. Uveitis occurs more frequently in patients with arthritis than in the general population.[28] An immunologic basis has been implicated, and data from HLA testing have substantiated such a relationship.[28]

In children, especially girls, a higher prevalence of iritis is associated with juvenile rheumatoid arthritis.[29] Children affected with uveitis have limited debilitation from the systemic condition. In juvenile rheumatoid arthritis, the onset of uveitis is insidious, and affected children may have cells, flare, and synechiae without ocular symptoms. Because the eye is not injected and there may be no symptoms, the uveitis, which is generally bilateral, may be an elusive diagnosis. Such uveitis is typically chronic, with the child developing a secondary cataract or band keratopathy before the diagnosis is established.[30] In fact, loss of vision from either band keratopathy or secondary cataract may be the reason for the child's eye examination. The treatment for uveitis in children with rheumatoid arthritis is cycloplegia and careful use of topical or systemic steroids. Because steroids do not always control the inflammation adequately, immunosuppressive drugs may be required in some cases.[31]

Ankylosing spondylitis (Marie-Strumpell disease) is a chronic form of arthritis involving the sacroiliac joint, spine, and soft surrounding tissue (Fig. 24.5). The condition is found most frequently in young men, and the characteristic uveitis is an iridocyclitis presenting as an acute anterior, nongranulomatous inflammation. It is uncommon for this nongranulomatous anterior segment inflammation to become chronic, but the patient may have the uveitis many years before having back pain. About one-third of all patients will have iridocyclitis at some point in the course of this systemic disease.[11]

Adult males who have recurrent episodes of bilateral, acute nongranulomatous anterior uveitis should have x-ray studies of the sacroiliac joints. HLA-B27 has been observed in 80% to 90% of patients with

TABLE 24.5
Postoperative Management of the Aphakic/Pseudophakic Patient

Examination Schedule	Medications	Examination	Patient Instructions
Immediately postoperative	• Topical antibiotic ointment or • Topical antibiotic-steroid ointment		• Eye shield—to be removed by practitioner • Return in 1 day • Acetaminophen or ibuprofen p.r.n.
Day 1	• Topical antibiotic and steroid drops q.i.d. • If IOP elevated, topical antiglaucoma therapy	• History • Visual acuity (pinhole) • Slit-lamp examination • Tonometry	• Gently clean lids daily • Use medications as prescribed • Acetaminophen or ibuprofen p.r.n. • Eye shield at bedtime • Wear glasses during the day • No lifting or straining • Bathe and wash hair with assistance • Return in 2 weeks
2 weeks	• Taper antibiotic and steroid drops to b.i.d.	• History • Visual acuity (pinhole) • Slit-lamp examination • Tonometry • Keratometry • Refraction • Fundus examination if vision less than 20/50	• Same as day 1 instructions • Return in 1 month
6 weeks	• Discontinue medications	• History • Visual acuity (pinhole) • Slit-lamp examination • Tonometry • Keratometry • Refraction • Fundus examination • If high astigmatism, cut suture • Check clarity of posterior capsule	• Discontinue eye shield • Prescribe spectacles or contact lens if refraction stable • Assume normal activity • Return in 6 weeks
12 weeks		• Check clarity of posterior capsule	• Return in 6 months

IOP, intraocular pressure.

iridocyclitis in ankylosing spondylitis.[6] Treatment, as in other forms of nongranulomatous anterior uveitis, is aimed at decreasing inflammation and preventing complications. Topical steroids and cycloplegics can be used to accomplish these therapeutic goals.

Inflammatory Bowel Disease (Crohn's Disease and Ulcerative Colitis)

Patients with manifest ulcerative colitis have an increased frequency of acute, bilateral, nongranulomatous iridocyclitis—0.5% to 12% level.[11] This iridocyclitis occurs between the second and fourth decades of life. In patients with both ulcerative colitis and sacroilitis, the frequency of iridocyclitis is about 50%.[11]

Reiter's Syndrome

Reiter's syndrome is a triad of nongonococcal urethritis, polyarthritis, and acute conjunctivitis. It has been observed most often in young men, with 8% to 40% having an acute anterior uveitis. The arthritis is usually oligoarticular and asymmetric, affecting the large, weight-bearing joints of the lower extremities. Inflammation of the axial skeleton presenting as a sacroilitis may be seen. The etiology of Reiter's syndrome is obscure, but an infectious cause has been suggested. A history of dysenteric or venereal disease can often be elicited.[9] The conjunctivitis is often bilateral and mucopurulent and may be accompanied by keratodermia blenorrhagica (see Fig. 21.24) and a circinate balanitis. In addition, HLA-B27 is seen in 63%

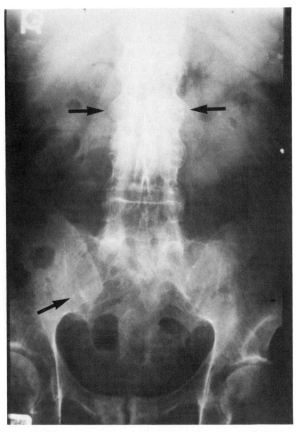

FIGURE 24.5 **X-ray film of spine of patient with ankylosing spondylitis. The sacroiliac joint margin (lower arrow) is blurred and poorly defined. This anteroposterior view also reveals the appearance of a bamboo spine (upper arrows), diagnostic of ankylosing spondylitis.**

to 96% of patients with Reiter's syndrome compared with 4% to 8% in a control population.[6] The correct diagnosis is important because the condition is self-limiting. Systemic tetracycline can be used for patients with Reiter's syndrome, since this drug is effective against *Chlamydia*. For the anterior uveitis, topical steroids and cycloplegics are indicated to limit the inflammation.

Behçet's Disease

Behçet's disease is a condition consisting of major findings that include nongranulomatous, bilateral, hypopyon uveitis; aphthous ulcers of the tongue and mouth; genital ulcers; and nonulcerative skin lesions. Minor findings include arthritis, thrombophlebitis, cardiovascular disease, gastrointestinal disease, and central nervous system (CNS) disorders. The ocular

components account for a great deal of the morbidity, but the so-called minor findings can be extremely serious. A vasculitis appears to be the underlying pathology.

Behçet's disease occurs in persons of Mediterranean and Japanese ancestry.[9,32,33] The etiology is unknown, but some evidence suggests a viral, immunologic, and hereditary condition. HLA-B5 has been demonstrated in Japanese patients with the disease.[34] Ocular lesions occur in 75% of cases.[35] Complications include occlusive retinal vasculitis, cataract formation, and glaucoma. Almost half the cases with retinal involvement will lead to blindness in 4 to 8 years if untreated.[35] Steroids have not proved effective, but the use of immunosuppressive agents such as chlorambucil or cyclosporine, for at least 1 year after the inflammation has subsided, may reduce the morbidity in most cases.[9]

Cyclosporine, because of reduced toxicity, has become the immunosuppressive agent of choice for patients with Behçet's disease with ocular or CNS involvement.[19] Topical and systemic steroids are often used concurrently.

Sarcoidosis

Sarcoid disease is a granulomatous condition of unknown etiology. It can affect any organ, and 25% to 50% of patients with the condition will have ocular problems, usually uveitis.[11] Sarcoid disease occurs more often in females[11] and is more common among black Americans than in black Africans, but it also occurs in white Scandinavians.

The most frequent ocular presentation of sarcoid disease is an acute, granulomatous iridocyclitis. With chronicity, mutton-fat keratic precipitates, synechiae, and cataracts may form. A retinochoroiditis may develop with retinal lesions characterized by "candle-wax drippings" beginning in the peripheral retina around the equator. In addition, a vitritis may be present, and retinal periphlebitis can occur, leading to macular edema.

The primary method by which to establish the diagnosis of sarcoid disease is the chest x-ray film. The classic picture is one of bilateral hilar adenopathy (Fig. 24.6). When findings are questionable, a conjunctival biopsy may prove useful. Even if there is no ocular disease, a conjunctival biopsy will be positive in about one-third of patients with sarcoid disease.[11] If the x-ray studies and conjunctival biopsy are equivocal, a biopsy of the liver or mediastinum can be performed, and noninvasive tests useful in determining the diagnosis include angiotensin-I-converting enzyme (ACE), gallium scan, and serum lysozyme levels.[9,36,37]

Topical and periocular steroids along with cyclo-

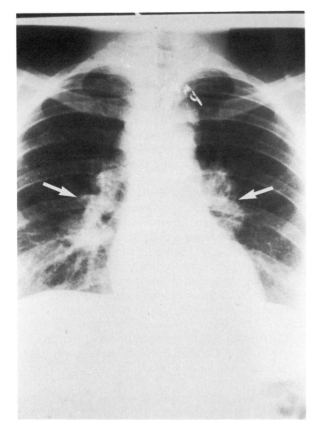

FIGURE 24.6   Chest x-ray film showing bilateral hilar adenopathy (arrows) in patient with sarcoidosis.

plegics remain the therapy of choice for the anterior uveitis, but many patients require the long-term use of systemic steroids to control the inflammation. Because uveitis in sarcoid disease is chronic, drug therapy for each patient must be individualized.

Fuchs' Heterochromic Iridocyclitis

Fuchs' heterochromic iridocyclitis is a mild, unilateral anterior uveitis with onset in early adulthood. The involved iris is heterochromic, usually lighter, and appears moth-eaten. The heterochromia occurs because the iris stroma is atrophic. In fact, the heterochromia is often the first sign of the disease, since the eye is usually white with some cells and little flare. Clear or white clumps of lymphocytes, which do not accumulate pigment, are seen on the corneal endothelium. Synechia formation is uncommon in Fuchs' heterochromic iridocyclitis, but complications can include posterior subcapsular cataract formation and glaucoma.

The associated cataract can be removed surgically because synechiae rarely form. The secondary glaucoma can occur from two causes. First, a trabeculitis may lead to decreased aqueous outflow and glaucoma. The trabeculitis can be controlled with topical or periocular steroids. Second, iris neovascularization may lead to neovascular glaucoma. In these cases vessels grow from the iris root to the trabecular meshwork and close the angle. Iris laser photocoagulation can be used to control the glaucoma.

Since Fuchs' heterochromic iridocyclitis occurs in young persons, patients will require a lifetime of follow-up including periodic angle evaluation to rule out neovascular growth. Many cases of Fuchs' heterochromic iridocyclitis are difficult to diagnose in the early stages because the eye is white, and the condition is rare enough to escape initial recognition. However, because the iridocyclitis does not respond well to steroids, and because steroids can cause cataract formation, an early and timely diagnosis is important. Steroids are indicated only if the inflammation becomes symptomatic or if trabeculitis occurs. Finally, cycloplegia is not usually required because there is little risk of synechia formation.

Herpes Simplex

Anterior uveitis associated with herpes simplex virus (HSV) is generally of two types. First, anterior uveitis can result from corneal epithelial dendritic formation, which causes an axonal reflex with vasodilation of the blood vessels of the iris and ciliary body. This produces the characteristic cells and flare. Second, and more severe, is anterior uveitis resulting from corneal stromal involvement from HSV. Although the virus is not the direct cause, it may alter the immune system and lead to inflammation. This more severe uveitis is unilateral and quite painful. In addition to the uveitis, there may be hemorrhage or red blood cells in the anterior chamber. This second form of anterior uveitis may last for months, whereas the epithelial herpetic uveitis is limited to the duration of the epitheliopathy. Synechiae, keratic precipitates, and occasionally trabeculitis with resulting glaucoma can result from anterior uveitis associated with stromal HSV.

The most appropriate therapy for anterior uveitis associated with epithelial HSV is topical antiviral agents and cycloplegia. As the epithelium heals, the anterior uveitis resolves. In contrast, stromal herpetic keratitis can cause an anterior uveitis that may be quite difficult to manage. Because such uveitis can readily cause synechia formation, cycloplegia is imperative. In addition, high dosages of topical steroids may be required to control the anterior segment inflammation, with topical antiviral agents administered concomitantly to combat the steroid-induced viral replication. Trabeculitis may precipitate a secondary glaucoma that should be managed with oral carbonic anhydrase inhibitors such as acetazolamide, or topical β blockers. Miotics should be avoided, since they can exacerbate the uveitis.

Herpes Zoster

Like HSV, herpes zoster can present with two different forms of anterior uveitis. First, anterior uveitis can occur from a corneal axonal reflex as in HSV uveitis. The second form is seen in older persons with herpes zoster and consists of an immunologic uveitis characterized by intense iridocyclitis. This second form of uveitis eventually leads to patchy necrosis of the iris and secondary segmental iris atrophy that will easily transilluminate. This characteristic wedge defect in the iris can be helpful in confirming the clinical diagnosis of herpes zoster uveitis. The chronic form of herpes zoster uveitis is felt to be an immune reaction[9] and is therefore quite difficult to control with steroids.

Treatment is aimed at reducing the local hypersensitivity to the zoster virus and includes the use of oral acyclovir, topical cycloplegics, topical antivirals, and topical or oral steroids.

Intermediate Uveitis

Intermediate uveitis is a recent term[3] describing a collection of conditions having inflammatory cells in the vitreous (Fig. 24.7), little, if any, anterior segment reaction, no synechia, and mild periphlebitis.[38] Fundus lesions are not present, but macular and optic disc edema are part of the presentation. Symptoms may be absent but can include blurred vision or floaters. Pain or redness of the eye is rarely seen.

Subclassifications of intermediate uveitis include pars planitis, chronic cyclitis, and senile vitritis. Several systemic conditions may present with intermediate uveitis. These include multiple sclerosis, reticulum cell sarcoma, sarcoidosis, or Whipple's disease. A retinal detachment may appear with cells or pigment in the anterior vitreous and mimic the appearance of intermediate uveitis.

Pars planitis is a condition of unknown etiology usually occurring in teenagers or young adults. The signs and symptoms are typical of those of intermediate uveitis but also include a cellular exudation or cyclitic membrane forming over the inferior pars plana.[39] The binocular indirect ophthalmoscope with scleral depression is required to see these "snowbanks" in the far periphery (Fig. 24.8). Cystoid macular edema is often the cause of decreased vision in patients with pars planitis. Pars plana snowbanks are not necessary for the diagnosis of intermediate uveitis, but the presence of snowbanks is associated with a more severe vitreal disease and an increased incidence of cystoid macular edema.[40]

Many cases of intermediate uveitis do not require therapy. If cystoid macular edema is present but mild (visual acuity better than 20/40), the condition may be periodically monitored with visual acuity measurements and fluorescein angiography.[39] However, if the vision drops below 20/40 or the patient is extremely symptomatic, then treatment should be instituted using oral or periocular steroids. Since intermediate uveitis will often persist for 10 to 20 years with periods of

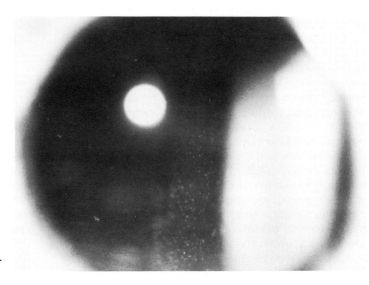

FIGURE 24.7 **Cells in vitreous associated with pars planitis. (Courtesy Scott Richter, O.D.)**

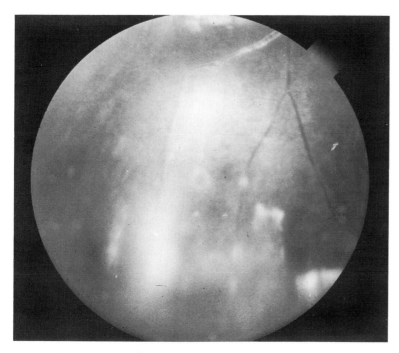

FIGURE 24.8 **Inferior peripheral exudates (snow-banks) associated with pars planitis. (Courtesy Scott Richter, O.D.)**

exacerbations and remissions, the risks of long-term systemic steroid use must be weighed against the potential benefits.

Tuberculosis

Both anterior and posterior uveitis have been associated with tuberculosis, and uveitis from tuberculosis has been observed in 3% of the population of a clinic specializing in uveitis.[9] Two types of uveitis are related to tuberculosis. The first is due to perforated tuberculosis lesions with direct infection of the uveal tissues. Second, tuberculosis may alter the immune status in an individual who has been previously infected with the disease. Such alteration of the immune system in persons with tuberculosis creates a nongranulomatous uveitis. The diagnosis of tuberculosis is often presumptive and is based on a positive purified protein derivative (PPD) skin test and positive chest x-ray films[41] but without obtaining cultures of the organism. Anterior uveitis can vary from an acute onset of a painful red eye to a smoldering, chronic, low-grade inflammation. The latter manifestation leads to formation of cataract, glaucoma, and phthisis and responds very poorly to therapy. Finally, a fulminating reaction may occur leading to corneal perforations. In addition to the anterior uveitis with its attendant synechiae and mutton-fat keratic precipitates, a posterior uveitis may occur that is characterized by diffuse chorioretinitis.

Because it penetrates the eye so well, isoniazid (INH) is the drug of choice for therapy of uveitis in tuberculosis. However, INH can cause hepatitis or peripheral neuropathy, and many patients may develop tolerance to the medication. For some patients, ethambutol can be used in combination with INH, and in those patients who develop tolerance to INH, rifampin can be used. INH is used for 1 year, and ethambutol is used for at least 2 months while the patient is monitored monthly for liver toxicity. If peripheral neuropathy occurs during therapy, pyridoxine (vitamin B_6) can be used for prevention. Steroids have been used on occasion, but only with extreme caution, since they can aggravate or precipitate a local or systemic tuberculosis reaction.

Syphilis

Either congenital or acquired syphilis can cause uveitis. Because of transplacental transfer in the congenital form, an acute anterior uveitis can be seen in the newborn with congenital syphilis. However, the acute anterior uveitis is usually observed at about 6 months. The uveitis is generally bilateral, and the diagnosis is established by obtaining a positive fluorescent treponemal antibody absorption (FTA-ABS) test from both child and mother. The therapy for syphilis is penicillin, but despite therapy the patient may develop interstitial keratitis, a bilateral immunologic corneal reaction usually seen between 6 and 12 years. A secondary anterior uveitis may occur in patients with interstitial keratitis.

The most common ocular finding in congenital syphilis is chorioretinitis, which occurs in about half the cases.[42] The chorioretinitis represents an inflammation of the retinal pigment epithelium, with the pigment migrating in a perivascular pattern, revealing a bone spicule or "salt and pepper" appearance similar to that seen in retinitis pigmentosa. This fundus picture and the occurrence of associated deafness in congenital syphilis can lead the clinician to suspect a diagnosis of Usher's syndrome. However, normal acuities, laboratory testing, and full visual fields help provide the diagnosis.

In the secondary stages of acquired syphilis there may be a chorioretinitis and an iridocyclitis. The condition may be unilateral and be associated with excellent visual acuities and full visual fields.

In any recurrent or bilateral anterior uveitis not responding to therapy, Venereal Disease Research Laboratory (VDRL) and FTA-ABS tests should be considered. If the tests are positive for syphilis, penicillin therapy should be instituted to eradicate potential treponemes and prevent the onset of tertiary syphilis and its associated neurosyphilis. Since penicillin will not diminish the inflammation, steroids and cycloplegics are necessary to treat the anterior uveitis.

Phakoantigenic Uveitis

Phakoantigenic uveitis can be seen in traumatic conditions where the capsule of the lens has been ruptured, or in mature cataract that leaks protein into the anterior chamber. The severe anterior uveitis that results is due to the antigenic nature of the lens proteins, which stimulate an inflammatory reaction. Although such a uveitis is quite severe, it is rare. Generally, the history is most useful in the diagnosis. The patient usually reports a traumatic incident or is elderly and has a history of poor vision with one eye for years. The anterior chamber is filled with flare so pronounced that it is often difficult to visualize the lens. Until the lens is surgically removed, the patient can receive topical cycloplegics and steroids to reduce the inflammation, but the best treatment is removal of the lens. If there is severe inflammation, macrophages laden with lens material may clog the trabeculum and lead to phakolytic glaucoma. Although there is no clear understanding of the etiology, immunology may play an important role in the pathogenesis of phakoantigenic uveitis.

Sympathetic Ophthalmia

Sympathetic ophthalmia is a bilateral, granulomatous uveitis that may occur after ocular trauma or surgery,

with the inflammation usually occurring from 2 to 8 weeks after the antecedent event. It has been reported to occur as early as 9 days to as late as 50 years after the initial insult.[2] Because of the autoimmune processes involved in sympathetic ophthalmia, the pathogenesis has been studied extensively. The inflammation of sympathetic ophthalmia is a delayed hypersensitivity reaction that causes a panuveitis of insidious onset in the uninvolved eye. There is evidence to suggest that retinal S antigens from the retinal photoreceptors may be the cause of the delayed hypersensitivity reaction.[43,44] Affected patients become sensitized to their retinal rod outer segments, a type of cell-mediated hypersensitivity occurs, and uveitis that affects the entire uvea ensues.[44]

Treatment of sympathetic ophthalmia involves reducing the body's immune response.[45] Early, high dosages of steroids should be employed, but in cases where steroid therapy is unsuccessful or contraindicated, immunosuppressive therapy may be used with some success.[9,46] Methotrexate, chlorambucil, cyclophosphamide, and cyclosporine have been used,[46] but they are extremely toxic. Cycloplegia is needed to prevent synechiae, and steroids may be required topically, subconjunctivally, or orally. Because sympathetic ophthalmia occurs only rarely, and because it may not occur until many years after the initial insult, prophylactic steroid therapy is controversial.[9] The uveal inflammation of sympathetic ophthalmia occurs in only 0.1% of patients with significant ocular trauma,[47] but because it affects the uninvolved eye, it causes great concern. Often the fellow eye may be so damaged from the panuveitis that the first, traumatized eye may have better resulting vision. Occasionally a perforated, painful eye must be enucleated because of the threat of sympathetic ophthalmia, but each case should be considered on its own merits, since sympathetic ophthalmia is rare. If enucleation is indicated, it must be done within 2 weeks of the injury. If panuveitis has begun in the sympathizing eye, removal of the injured eye will not alter the course.

Histoplasmosis

Histoplasmosis is an infection that occurs both systemically and ocularly, and is caused by the fungus *Histoplasma capsulatum*. Both the systemic and the ocular diseases are most frequently encountered in the Ohio and Mississippi river valleys in the United States. The systemic disease occurs in all races and age groups, with an acute pulmonary reaction being the most frequently observed manifestation of the disease.

Ocular histoplasmosis consists of a triad of peripapillary chorioretinal atrophy, peripheral atrophic scars, and macular scarring noted in young adults (Fig. 24.9).

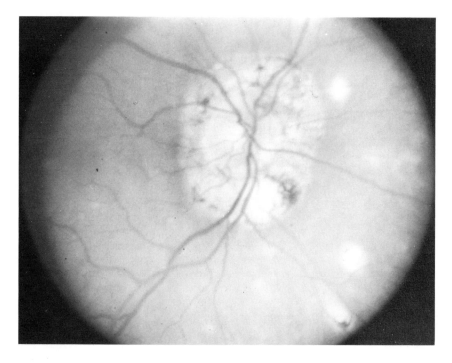

FIGURE 24.9 **Peripapillary chorioretinal atrophy and peripheral atrophic scars in presumed ocular histoplasmosis syndrome.**

The fundus scars predispose the patient to active macular disease, best noted by the fluid and hemorrhage surrounding the old scars. Interestingly, ocular histoplasmosis is uncommon in blacks.[48] The choroiditis occurs in both eyes, and there is no anterior uveitis or vitritis. Most cases are called presumed ocular histoplasmosis syndrome (POHS) because it is rare for the fungus to be isolated from affected choroidal tissue. The diagnosis is based on the ophthalmoscopic findings. Although characteristic lung lesions are usually noted on the chest x-ray film, it is rarely needed for diagnostic purposes. Skin tests are not recommended because they may reactivate the ocular lesions and lead to vision loss.

The systemic condition is treated with amphotericin B, which is extremely toxic and has no effect on the eye.[49] For ocular histoplasmosis, the major concern is the potential for loss of vision from both atrophic and hemorrhagic lesions at the maculae. Because the atrophic lesions can provide an environment where subretinal neovascularization can occur, resulting in hemorrhagic maculopathy, therapy for the ocular manifestations of histoplasmosis is aimed at preserving macular function. High dosages of systemic steroids are used, and argon laser photocoagulation is implemented to control the subretinal neovascularization. No therapy is indicated for inactive scars.

There may be an altered immune mechanism in histoplasmosis, and HLA-DRW-2 and HLA-B7 have been observed in cases of ocular histoplasmosis.[48,50] In addition, there may be a trigger mechanism in some cases, since both emotional and physical stress have been known to reactivate ocular histoplasmosis.[51]

References

1. Hendly DE, Genetler AJ, Smith RE, Rao NA. Changing patterns of uveitis. Am J Ophthalmol 1987;103:131–136.
2. Schlaegel TF. Essentials of uveitis. Boston: Little, Brown, 1969.
3. Bloch-Michel E, Nussenblatt RB: International uveitis study group recommendations for evaluations of intraocular inflammatory disease. Am J Ophthalmol 1987;103:234–235.
4. Tessler HH. Classification and symptoms and signs of uveitis. In: Duane TD, Jaeger EA, eds. Clinical ophthalmology. Hagerstown, MD: Harper & Row, 1987;4: Chap. 32, pp. 1–10.
5. Schlaegel TF. Etiologic diagnosis of uveitis. In: Duane TD, Jaeger EA, eds. Clinical ophthalmology, Hagerstown, MD: Harper & Row, 1987;4: Chap. 41, pp. 1–5.
6. Scharf Y, Zonis S. Histocompatibility antigens (HLA) and uveitis. Surv Ophthalmol 1980;24:220–228.
7. Darrell RW, Kurland L, Wagenerti P. Epidemiology of uveitis. Incidence and prevalence in a small community. Arch Ophthalmol 1962;68:4.
8. Schlaegel TF. General factors in uveitis. In: Duane TD, Jaeger EA, eds. Clinical ophthalmology. Hagerstown, MD: Harper & Row 1987;4: Chap. 39, pp. 1–6.
9. Schlaegel TF. Perspectives in uveitis. Ann Ophthalmol 1981;13:799–806.
10. Rothova MD, vanVeenendall WG, Linssen A, et al. Clinical features of anterior uveitis. Am J Ophthalmol 1987;103:137–145.

11. Friedlander MH. Allergy and immunology of the eye. Hagerstown, MD: Harper & Row, 1979.

12. Brewerton DA, Caffrey M, Nicholls A, et al. Acute anterior uveitis and HLA-27. Lancet 1973;2:994–996.

13. Khan MA, Kushner I, Braun WE. Association of HLA-A2 with uveitis in HLA-B27 patients with ankylosing spondylitis. J Rheumatol 1981;8:295–298.

14. Golden B, Givoiset MM. Uveitis, immunologic, and allergic phenomena. Springfield, IL: Charles C Thomas, 1973.

15. Schlaegel TF. Nonspecific treatment of uveitis. In: Duane TD, Jaeger EA, eds. Clinical ophthalmology. Hagerstown, MD: Harper & Row, 1987;4: Chap. 43, p 1–13.

16. Leibowitz HM, Kupferman A. Anti-inflammatory medications. Int Ophthalmol Clin 1980;20:117–134.

17. Wakefield D. Methylprednisolone pulse therapy in severe anterior uveitis. Aust NZ J Ophthalmol 1985;13:411–415.

18. Wakefield D, McCluskey P, Penny R. Intravenous pulse methylprednisolone therapy in severe inflammatory eye disease. Arch Ophthalmol 1986;104:847–851.

19. Nussenblatt RB, Palestine AG. Cyclosporine: Immunology, pharmacology and therapeutic uses. Surv Ophthalmol 1986;31:159–169.

20. Read JE, Crouch ER. Trauma: Ruptures and bleeding. In: Duane TD, Jaeger EA, eds. Clinical ophthalmology. Hagerstown, MD: Harper & Row, 1987;4: Chap. 61, pp 6–18.

21. O'Neal JC. Treatment of traumatic hyphema. Eye Ear Nose Throat Monthly 1952;31:481.

22. Kutner B, Fourman S, Brein K, et al. Aminocaproic acid reduces the risk of secondary hemorrhage in patients with traumatic hyphema. Arch Ophthalmol 1987;105:206–208.

23. Crouch ER Jr, Frenkel M. Aminocaproic acid in the treatment of traumatic hyphema. Am J Ophthalmol 1976;81:355–360.

24. McGetrick JJ, Jampol LM, Goldberg MF, et al. Aminocaproic acid decreases secondary hemorrhage after traumatic hyphema. Arch Ophthalmol 1983;101:1031–1033.

25. Palmer DJ, Goldberg MF, Frenkel M, et al. A comparison of two dose regimens of epsilon aminocaproic acid in the prevention and management of secondary traumatic hyphemas. Ophthalmology 1986;93:102–108.

26. Kraft SP, Christianson MD, Crawford JS, et al. Traumatic hyphema in children. Treatment with epsilon-aminocaproic acid. Ophthalmology 1987;94:1232–1237.

27. Read JE, Goldberg MF. Traumatic hyphema: Comparison of medical treatment. Trans Am Acad Ophthalmol Otolaryngol 1974;78:799.

28. Schlaegel TF, Coles RS. Uveitis and miscellaneous general diseases. In: Duane TD, Jaeger EA, eds. Clinical ophthalmology. Hagerstown, MD: Harper & Row, 1987;4: Chap. 53, pp. 1–13.

29. Lenoch F, Kralik V, Bartos J. Rheumatic iritis and iridocyclitis. Ann Rheum Dis 1959;18:45.

30. Wolf MD, Lichter PR, Ragsdale CR. Prognostic factors in the uveitis of juvenile rheumatoid arthritis. Ophthalmology 1987;94:1242–1248.

31. Mehra R, Moore T, Catalano JD, et al. Chlorambucil in the treatment of iridocyclitis in juvenile rheumatoid arthritis. J Rheumatol 1981;8:141–144.

32. Abdulla MI, Bahgat NE. Long-lasting remission of Behçet's disease after chlorambucil therapy. Br J Ophthalmol 1973;57:706.

33. Mamo JG, Azzam SA. Treatment of Behçet's disease with chlorambucil. Arch Ophthalmol 1970;84:446.

34. Ohno S, Nakayama E, Sugira S, et al. Specific histocompatibility antigens associated with Behçet's disease. Am J Ophthalmol 1975;80:636–641.

35. Chajek T, Fainru M. Behçet's disease. Report of 41 cases and a review of the literature. Medicine 1975;54:179–196.

36. Baarsma GS, Lahey E, Glasuis E, et al. The predictive value of serum converting enzyme and lysozyme levels in the diagnosis of ocular sarcoidosis. Am J Ophthalmol 1987;104:211–217.

37. Weinreb RN, Tessler H. Laboratory diagnosis of ophthalmic sarcoidosis. Surv Ophthalmol 1984;26:653–664.

38. Tessler H. The uvea—what is intermediate uveitis. In: Ernest JT, ed. The yearbook of ophthalmology 1985. Chicago: Year Book Publishers, 1985;155–156.

39. Henderly DE, Genstler AJ, Smith RE, Rao NA. Pars planitis. Trans Ophthalmol Soc UK 1986;105:227.

40. Smith RE, Nozik RA. Uveitis: A clinical approach to diagnosis and management. Baltimore: Williams & Wilkins, 1983;147–150.

41. Abrams J, Schlaegel TF. The tuberculin skin test in the diagnosis of tuberculosis uveitis. Am J Ophthalmol 1983;96:295–298.

42. Schlaegel TF. Bacterial uveitis (tuberculosis and syphilitic). In: Duane TD, Jaeger EA, eds. Clinical ophthalmology. Hagerstown, MD: Harper & Row, 1987;4: Chap. 44, pp. 1–10.

43. Wacker WB, Rao NB, Marak GE. Experimental sympathetic ophthalmia. In: Silverstein AM, O'Connor GR, eds. Immunology and immunopathology of the eye. New York: Masson; 1979;121–126.

44. Wacker WB. Experimental allergic uveitis. J Immunol 1977;199:1949–1950.

45. Perry HD, Yanoff M, Scheie HG. Rubeosis in Fuchs' heterochromic iridocyclitis. Arch Ophthalmol 1975;93:337.

46. Corwin JM, Weiter JJ. Immunology of chorioretinal disease. Surv Ophthalmol 1981;25:287–305.

47. Aronson SB, Elliot JH. Ocular inflammation. St. Louis: C.V. Mosby Co, 1972.

48. Meridith TA, Smith RE, Duguesnoy RJ. Association of HLA-DRW2 antigen with presumed ocular histoplasmosis. Am J Ophthalmol 1980;89:70–76.

49. Schlaegel TF. Ocular histoplasmosis. New York: Grune & Stratton, 1977.

50. Meridith TA, Smith RE, Braley RE, et al. The prevalence of HLA-B7 in presumed ocular histoplasmosis in patients with peripheral atrophic scars. Am J Ophthalmol 1978;86:325–328.

51. Schaegel TF. Presumed ocular histoplasmosis. In: Duane TD, Jaeger EA, eds. Clinical ophthalmology. Hagerstown, MD: Harper & Row, 1987;4: Chap. 48, pp. 1–19.

52. Kennedy RH, Brubaker RF. Traumatic hyphema in a defined population. Am J Ophthalmol 1988;106:123–130.

53. Uusitalo RJ, Ranta-Kemppainen L, Tarkkanen A. Management of traumatic hyphema in children. An analysis of 340 cases. Arch Ophthalmol 1988;106:1207–1209.

54. Allingham RR, Crouch ER, Williams PB, et al. Topical aminocaproic acid significantly reduces the incidence of secondary hemorrhage in traumatic hyphema in a rabbit model. Arch Ophthalmol 1988;106:1436–1438.

CHAPTER 25

Diseases of the Retina

Larry J. Alexander

Although diseases of the retina, specifically of the macular area, represent a serious threat to vision, successful pharmacologic management of these conditions has been disappointing. Since a discussion of all diseases of the retina is beyond the scope of this text, this chapter will consider only retinal conditions that are either amenable to pharmacologic intervention or that show some potential for new therapeutic procedures.

Specialized Clinical Testing Techniques for Retinal Disease

Fluorescein Angiography

Fluorescein angiography and oral fluorography are gaining importance as diagnostic tools now that new developments are being made in laser treatment of retinal vascular disease. Laser modifications and a better understanding of ocular vasculopathy are allowing for earlier therapeutic intervention, treatment closer to the foveal avascular zone (FAZ), and better visual results.

Fluorescein has been used in vision care for over 100 years.[1] The use of fluorescein to study the retinal vasculature was attempted in 1910. The oral route of administration was chosen.[2] The first use of intravenous fluorescein was reported in 1930,[3] and several other reports followed over the next 30 years. The most significant work, however, came in 1961 with the photodocumentation of fluorescein studies. The photographs allowed a more detailed and logical approach to understanding fluorescein angiography.[4] The first

comprehensive text on fluorescein studies was published in 1977[5] and was soon followed by other works.[6]

The concept of oral fluorography was reintroduced in 1979 to allow fluorescein studies without potential systemic side effects.[7] Further studies in oral fluorography established the technique as a viable alternative in diagnosis of retinal vascular diseases.[8,9] The Oral Fluorescein Study Group was formed in 1984 to further evaluate the orally administered fluorescein technique. The report in 1985 concluded that oral fluorography was not a substitute for the diagnostic capabilities of intravenous fluorescein angiography but was a significant diagnostic tool, especially for fundus disorders that demonstrated fluorescein leakage. That report also established the fact that minimal side effects occur with oral fluorescein administration.[10]

Fluorescein angiography is especially useful in detecting subclinical retinal changes in diabetic patients. Yamana and associates[11] reported that of 272 eyes of 166 patients with no ophthalmoscopically visible vascular changes, fluorescein angiography demonstrated diabetic vascular changes in 66.5%. Other studies have found angiographic changes in diabetic children that were not observed by ophthalmoscopy alone.[12,13] Fluorescein studies have also demonstrated significant vascular changes in the mid-periphery that were previously overlooked.[14] Prudent clinical judgment dictates that fluorescein studies be performed in diabetic patients with any unexplained reduction in macular function, with encroachment of diabetic retinopathy into the macular area, with any sign of proliferative retinopathy, with the appearance of intraretinal microvascular abnormalities (IRMA), and with the appearance of 3 or more signs of preproliferative diabetic retinopathy.

Table 25.1 lists some ocular disease processes that indicate the need for fluorescein angiography to assist in the differential diagnosis and management.

TECHNIQUE

Fluorescein studies may be performed with or without an appropriate fundus camera. If performed with a binocular indirect ophthalmoscope, the technique is known as fluorescein angioscopy. To perform fluorescein angioscopy successfully, the binocular indirect ophthalmoscope must be equipped with a high-intensity light source and appropriate filters.

If fluorescein photographic studies are desired, it is necessary to use a fundus camera equipped with a high-intensity flash system with a rapid recycle time as well as with appropriate blue excitation and yellow-green barrier filters. The excitation filter should be either the Baird Atomic B4 470 or Kodak Wratten 47 to create wavelengths to stimulate fluorescence. The barrier filter should be either an Ilford 109 Delta Chromatic 3 or Kodak Wratten G15 to block the exciting light from the film plane, allowing only visualization of the fluorescing blood.[15] Note that both barrier and excitation filters lose specificity (fade) with age and should be

TABLE 25.1
Ocular Diseases Indicating the Need for Fluorescein Angiography

Acute posterior multifocal placoid pigment epitheliopathy (APMPPE)
Angiomatosis retinae
Anterior ischemic optic neuropathy
Behçet's disease
Branch retinal vein occlusion
Cavernous hemangioma of the retina
Choroidal rupture (when developing choroidal neovascularization)
Coat's disease (Retinal Telangiectasia)
Cystoid maculopathy (Irvine-Gass syndrome)
Diabetic retinopathy
Eale's disease
Fuch's spot (degenerative myopia)
Hemicentral retinal vein occlusion
Idiopathic central serous choroidopathy
Iris neovascularization
Maculopathy of angioid streaks
Malignant choroidal melanoma
Preretinal macular fibrosis
Presumed ocular histoplasmosis (macular changes)
Proliferative peripheral retinal disease
Retinal capillary hemangioma
Retinal macroaneurysm
Retinal pigment epithelial dystrophies (central)
Retinal pigment epithelial detachment
Retinal tumors
Sensory retinal detachments
Tumors of the iris and ciliary body

replaced according to manufacturer's guidelines. It is also advisable to fit the camera back with a power winder, since the early phases of fluorescein studies necessitate rapid-fire photography.

Several films and developing processes are available to enhance study results. Although any high-speed 200 to 400 ASA black-and-white film can be used, it is difficult to advise on processing. It is best to simply contact a local film processing laboratory or an experienced angiographer regarding optimal processing and film use. Some practitioners advocate color film because then the studies can eliminate autofluorescence,[16] but adoption of this technique has met with resistance.

Although other dyes have been used,[17] sodium fluorescein is still the accepted standard. Sodium fluorescein for intravenous injection is available in 10% and 25% concentrations. Generic brands are available at considerably reduced cost and may be used without fear. One study does, however, report the presence of a toxic substance, dimethyl formamide, an industrial solvent, in commercially prepared sodium fluorescein for injection.[18] Moreover, outdated fluorescein carries the potential for side effects, such as an increase in the incidence of nausea.

Sodium fluorescein is considered pharmacologically inert and fluoresces when stimulated by an excited light source. Fluorescein is injected into a suitable vein in the antecubital space or on the hand. It reaches ocular circulation bound to serum albumin and in a free, unbound state. This then fluoresces, allowing for easy visualization of vascular alterations and leakage from altered vessels. Factors affecting the quality of the results include clarity of the ocular media, maximal dilation of the pupil, and especially the concentration of fluorescein reaching the retinal-choroidal vascular system.[19] Improper injection is the most significant factor contributing to decreased retinal-choroidal concentration. The injection must be into the vein and performed within 10 to 15 seconds.

A crash cart (cardiopulmonary resuscitation unit) must be available on site to accommodate any potential side effects. Before the procedure it must be ensured that (1) an informed consent form has been read and signed by the patient (see Chapter 33), (2) the patient is aware of what is about to happen, (3) the patient's pupils are maximally dilated, (4) color photographs of the fundus have been taken, (5) red-free photographs of the fundus have been taken on the black-and-white angiographic film, (6) the fundus camera and patient are adjusted to a comfortable height, (7) the filters are placed in the camera, (8) the proper flash settings are made, and (9) an appropriate intravenous line has been established and maintained with heparinized saline. Next, 5 ml of 10% sodium fluorescein should be ready in a syringe to replace the heparinized saline. The patient should be situated in the camera and the syringe of fluorescein should be attached. When the appropriate area of the fundus is in focus and the filters are moved into place, the bolus of fluorescein should be injected rapidly. The photography usually begins within about 15 seconds, which is the choroidal flush phase. Rapid sequence photographs are taken within the first few minutes, then intermittently for the next 10 to 20 minutes. Late phase photographs will detect leakage problems such as sensory retinal detachments associated with choroidal neovascular nets. Particular timing sequences depend on the suspected disease being investigated.

COMPLICATIONS

Complications are inherent in any procedure such as fluorescein angiography. Fortunately, the more common complications can easily be managed without aborting the diagnostic procedure. One study[20] reported adverse reactions in 4.82% of 5000 procedures. Of these, nausea was most frequent (2.24%), followed by vomiting (1.78%) and urticaria and pruritus (0.34%). No higher rate of side effects was found when 25% sodium fluorescein was used than when 10% sodium fluorescein was employed.[20] The itching and hives are thought to be associated with a change in the plasma complement associated with a rise in the histamine level.[21] In another study[22] of 2631 procedures it was found that males and young patients experienced side effects at a higher rate. In this study, only one life-threatening event, acute pulmonary edema, was reported.[22] Although some clinicians[23] discount the beneficial effect of prophylaxis against the side effects of fluorescein, a recent double-blind study reported that 20 mg of intravenous metoclopramide hydrochloride significantly decreased the incidence of nausea and vomiting.[24] The primary side effect of nausea or warm flush usually occurs within the first 30 seconds after injection and is transient. If the patient is advised of this potential side effect in advance, the procedure can usually be completed without difficulty. It is also wise to advise the patient that the skin and urine will be discolored for several days following the procedure.

ORAL FLUOROGRAPHY

Oral fluorography can offer results similar to those obtained with intravenous fluorescein angiography but without the potential side effects. Oral fluorography is especially useful in cases where late dye leakage is expected. Oral fluorography can be performed using either USP bulk powder sodium fluorescein or commercially available 5 ml vials of 10% injectable sodium fluorescein. The powdered form is difficult to obtain, but using 2 to 3 of the 5 ml vials of 10% fluorescein is usually sufficient to obtain good results. The fluorescein is mixed with a citrus drink and allowed to cool in crushed ice. The patient is asked to fast for about 8 hours before the test. The patient then is instructed to remove any dentures, since the solution will discolor these prosthetic devices. Before the procedure it must be ensured that (1) an informed consent form has been read and signed by the patient (see Chapter 33), (2) the patient is aware of what is about to happen, (3) the patient's pupils are maximally dilated, (4) color photographs of the fundus have been taken, (5) red-free photographs have been taken, (6) the fundus camera has been adjusted, and (7) the proper film has been loaded, filters put in place, and flash settings set. The patient is then instructed to drink the solution rapidly through a straw to prevent staining the lips.

Photography begins at the first sign of retinal circulation (15 to 30 minutes), with the late phase showing in about 1 hour. As with intravenous studies, the skin and urine will be slightly discolored for several days.

Reported complications of oral fluorography are few and minor.[25–28] It has been suggested that it would require ingestion of 90 g of fluorescein by a 100-pound person to produce a toxic effect.[26]

The technique of oral fluorescein studies can be beneficial in aphakic children,[29] in patients with vaso-occlusive diseases of the retina,[30] and in patients with many other retinal diseases that manifest late-stage leakage such as idiopathic central serous choroidopathy (ICSC) and cystoid macular edema (CME) (Fig. 25.1).[31]

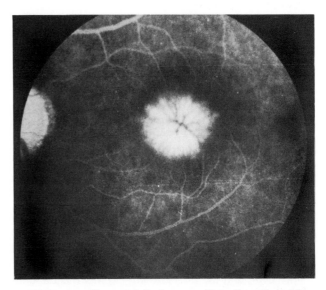

FIGURE 25.1 **Characteristic "rose petal" configuration of fluorescein staining in cystoid macular edema (CME) following administration of oral fluorescein sodium. (Courtesy James Hunter, O.D.)**

INTERPRETATION

A fundamental understanding of retinal-choroidal anatomy and vasculature is crucial in interpreting fluorescein angiography. Some basic features of the retinal and choroidal system create the diagnostic capabilities of fluorescein angiography. These features are as follows: (1) healthy retinal vessels do not leak fluorescein because the vessel walls are not fenestrated, (2) healthy choriocapillaris vessels are fenestrated and freely leak, creating a sponge-like tissue; (3) in a healthy retina the fluid in the choriocapillaris is kept away from the sensory retina by an intact retinal pigment epithelium (RPE)/Bruch's membrane barrier. The RPE also serves as a filter to allow only part of the choroidal glow to show through. If the RPE is absent, more glow (hyperfluorescence) will be visible, and if there is an excess of RPE, less glow (hypofluorescence) will be visible. Dense RPE and xanthophyl mask the choroidal flush in a healthy macula.

In addition to the basic anatomic characteristics, the time-related stages of the angiogram are also important. The stages are classically described as the choroidal flush (prearterial phase), the arterial-venous phase, and the late phase. The choroidal flush occurs within seconds after injection. The posterior ciliary arteries supply the choroidal system in a patchy pattern, which is quickly masked by the fluorescein leaking into the choroidal swamp through fenestrated vasculature. This fluorescein will stay within the swamp if the RPE/Bruch's membrane barrier is healthy. Observation of the choroidal flush stage is especially useful in detecting diseases of the choroidal vasculature or the RPE/Bruch's membrane barrier, such as choroidal neovascularization in age-related maculopathy.

Within a few more seconds the retinal arteries start to fill in a laminar flow pattern. The central core of the artery glows first, followed by filling to the limits of the walls. The capillaries then fill, followed by the laminar filling of the veins. With the veins, the area of the blood column near the walls glows first, followed by filling to the center. The walls of the arteries, capillaries, and veins in the healthy retina are not fenestrated and therefore should demonstrate no leakage. Any condition that creates breakdown of vessel walls with subsequent leakage or neovascularization would be most apparent in this stage. An example is leaking microaneurysms in diabetic retinopathy.

The late stages of fluorescein angiography usually occur about 10 minutes after injection. During this stage the arteries and veins have almost emptied of fluorescein, and the underlying choroidal flush is minimized. The optic nerve remains hyperfluorescent because the dye adheres to the nerve tissue. During this stage leakage of choroidal and retinal vessels becomes more apparent by the diffusely spreading staining pattern overlying the vascular lesion. Late staining also occurs in sensory retinal detachments and RPE detachments due to choriocapillaris leakage.

Application of the time-stages of fluorescein angiography and the basic retinal-choroidal anatomy will allow for effective interpretation of fluorescein angiograms. The practitioner must realize that 2 basic situations occur in diseased conditions: (1) hypofluorescence, or a blockage of the glow, where one would normally expect it; and (2) hyperfluorescence, or an excessive glow, where one would not normally expect it. Table 25.2 outlines conditions that create hypofluorescence and hyperfluorescence, and Figure 25.2 illustrates some of the conditions best interpreted with fluorescein angiography.

Vitreous Fluorophotometry

Vitreous fluorophotometry is a technique used to detect the breakdown of the blood-retinal barrier at its earliest stages. This procedure allows the practitioner to detect minimal amounts of fluorescein that have escaped from the retinal vasculature into the vitreous.[32] This can be detected as early as 1 year after the onset of diabetes, whereas maculopathy does not appear until more than 10 years later.[33] At present, fluorophotometry merely confirms what the clinician would expect and adds little to the clinical management of diabetic retinal vascular disease.

Electrodiagnostic Testing

Electrodiagnostic evaluation has been used as a possible means of assessing retinal vasculopathy as well as of predicting the outcome of patients with diabetic retinopathy. Classic methods of testing retinal function have shown changes in the electroretinogram (ERG) and electro-oculogram (EOG) only after vasculopathy has advanced.[34] The oscillatory potentials of the ERG, which originate in the inner nuclear layers of the retina, are assumed to be very sensitive to impaired retinal circulation and are possibly insulin-sensitive.[35-39] Further studies indicate that the latency of the oscillatory potential is delayed in diabetics. The oscillatory potentials may have some prognostic value in predicting progression to proliferative diabetic retinopathy in juvenile onset diabetics.[40] Other studies have proved the effectiveness of electrodiagnostic studies in the early detection of diabetic retinopathy before clinically observable changes.[41-46]

One other area of interest is the recent development of methods to generate objective contrast sensitivity

TABLE 25.2
Common Ocular Conditions Creating Hypofluorescence or Hyperfluorescence during Fluorescein Angiography

	Hypofluorescence	*Hyperfluorescence*
RPE/Bruch's membrane	APMPPE (early) Congenital hypertrophy of RPE RPE hyperplasia	Age-related maculopathy (dry) Angioid streaks APMPPE (late) Choroidal folds Chorioretinal scars Drusen ICSC (cystoid maculopathy) Retinal hole RPE detachment RPE window defects Serous sensory retinal detachment
Choroid	Benign choroidal melanoma with no overlying serous detachment	Choroidal neovascularization Malignant choroidal melanoma
Retina	BAO CAO Cotton wool spots Preretinal hemorrhages Retinal exudates Subretinal hemorrhages	Angiomatosis retinae Capillary hemangioma Cavernous hemangioma (stasis) Leaking compromised veins Macroaneurysms Microaneurysms Neovascularization (retinal) Periphlebitis Telangiectasia
Optic nerve		Anterior ischemic optic neuropathy Neovascularization (disc) Papilledema

RPE, retinal pigment epithelium; APMPPE, acute posterior multifocal placoid pigment epitheliopathy; ICSE, idiopathic central serous choroidopathy; BAO, branch artery occlusion; CAO, central artery occlusion.

readings and objective visual field plottings through visually evoked cortical potentials (VECP).[47-55] Although these projects are in their infancy, VECP would have tremendous impact in establishing an objective predictive factor and may have potential in evaluating noncommunicative patients.

Retinal Vascular Occlusive Disease

Retinal vascular occlusive disease is important from the standpoint of both vision loss and associated systemic disease. The retinal process invariably compromises some vision and reflects an underlying systemic disease condition. Although there is an intimate relationship among all retinal vaso-occlusive diseases, they are often divided into 5 categories: (1) branch vein occlusion (BVO), (2) central vein occlusion (CVO), (3) hemicentral vein occlusion (HCVO), (4) branch artery occlusion (BAO), and (5) central artery occlu-

sion (CAO). The vein occlusion categories are then subdivided into ischemic and nonischemic categories depending on the degree of retinal hypoxia present.

Branch Vein Occlusion

BVO is the most common of the retinal vascular occlusive diseases. It has a peak incidence in the fifth to sixth decade with no racial or sexual predilection.[56-57] This is contrasted with CVO, which has a strong male predominance. There is a 4% to 5% incidence of bilaterality.[58]

ETIOLOGY

Although the specific microscopic events surrounding BVO are somewhat obscure, a few general statements can be made. Although arterial disease plays a part in the process, it may not initiate the condition.[54-60] BVO does, however, have a strong association with systemic

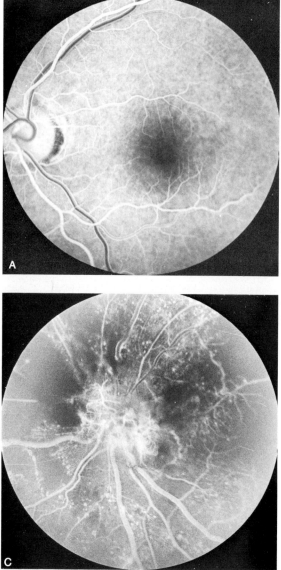

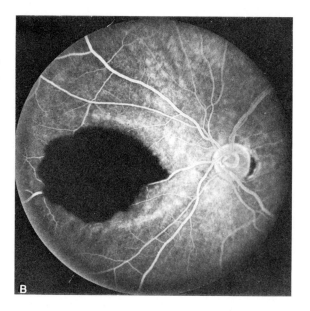

FIGURE 25.2   **Examples of fluorescein angiography. (A) Choroidal-arterial phase showing laminar flow in the veins. (B) Blockage of background choroidal fluorescence as well as arteries and veins by a preretinal hemorrhage. (C) Early-phase angiogram of disc neovascularization. (D) Later-phase angiogram of disc neovascularization demonstrating leakage into the vitreous. (E) Microaneurysms surrounding the macula. (F) Demonstration of the intraretinal edema caused by leaking microaneurysms. (G) Subretinal pigment epithelial neovascularization, early phase. (H) Subretinal pigment epithelial neovascularization, early phase. (I) Subretinal pigment epithelial neovascularization, late phase, demonstrating fluid accumulation in overlying sensory retinal detachment.**

diseases (57% of patients).[56] Hypertension, glucose intolerance, hyperlipidemia, and hypercholesterolemia all have been implicated in BVO.[61,62] Recent work implicates platelet coagulation activities in early thrombosis formation in retinal vein occlusion.[63] Table 25.3 summarizes the common systemic factors in BVO. The association with systemic disease emphasizes the importance of diagnosis and appropriate management of the underlying systemic vascular condition.

DIAGNOSIS

BVO can present as 2 distinct clinical entities—nonischemic retinopathy and ischemic retinopathy. The distinction is a clinical impression depending on the degree of superficial hemorrhage, cotton wool spots, and associated arterial changes. The superior temporal veins are affected most often, this being attributed to the fact that there are more artery/vein (A/V) crossings in the superior temporal retinal than elsewhere.[60]

The clinical picture will vary considerably depending on the site of occlusion, the degree of ischemia created, and the time elapsed since the occlusion. Often a prodromal sign (Bonnet's sign) will present as small splinter hemorrhages around an area of A/V nicking.[64] Should an occlusion occur either at an A/V crossing or elsewhere, the classic BVO develops. The clinical picture is that of dilated, tortuous veins and dot/blot

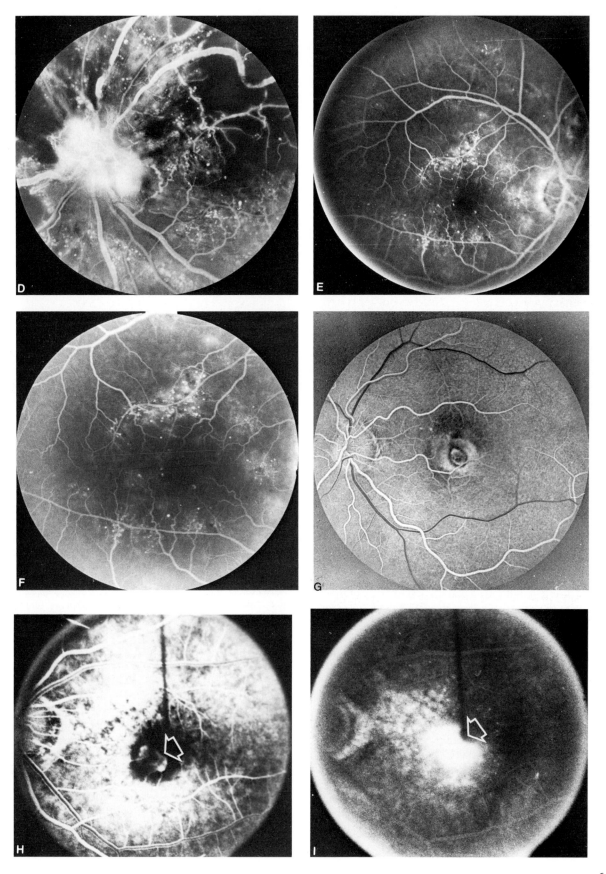

TABLE 25.3
Common Systemic Factors in Branch Vein Occlusion

- Hypertension
- Diabetes
- Hyperlipidemia and hypercholesterolemia
- Hyperviscosity syndromes and altered platelet function
- Estrogens
- Chronic lung disease
- Trauma
- Elevated serum immunoglobulins
- Elevated intraocular pressure

hemorrhages from the site of the obstruction to the retinal periphery in the sector of retina normally drained by the affected vein. Microaneurysms also occur in the affected area, leaking and creating retinal edema. As more retinal hypoxia is created, cotton wool spots and flame-shaped hemorrhages are added to the picture (Fig. 25.3). Lipid infiltrates often occur near the site of the occlusion about 2 months after onset. If the macular area is not adequately drained, partial or complete macular edema (48% to 56% of cases) may develop, compromising vision.[65] As the BVO progresses, collateral channels open to shunt blood around the occluded zone. The development of effective collaterals is important in the prognosis. Collaterals observed temporal to the macula crossing the horizontal raphe are pathognomonic of an old BVO. Pupillary margin neovascular tufts may occur in BVO,[66] and other sequelae include preretinal neovascularization (24% to 80%), disc neovascularization, and vitreous hemorrhage (10% to 40%).[67,68]

Trempe and associates[69] have identified additional findings associated with BVO and its effect on the vitreous. When retinal occlusive disease occurs, the vitreous overlying the process appears to change. When the vitreous is totally attached to the retina in eyes with BVO, the vitreous adjacent to and overlying the area becomes liquified. In the early stages the gel exhibits white degenerative opacities that become larger as the retinal hemorrhage is reabsorbed. Vitreous detachment also affects the development of complications.[69]

An additional finding that may assist in the diagnosis of BVO is the effect of venous occlusive disease on intraocular pressure. It has been found that 80% of patients have reduced intraocular pressure in the eye with venous occlusive disease.[70] There is a greater decrease in CVO than in BVO, a greater decrease in ischemic CVO than in nonischemic CVO, and a greater decrease in patients with relatively high pressure in the fellow eye. The duration of the hypotensive effect is about 3 months in ischemic CVO, 18 months in nonischemic CVO, and 24 months in BVO.[70]

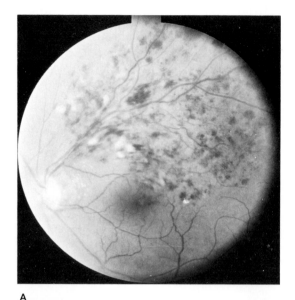

A

B

FIGURE 25.3 **(A) Superior temporal branch vein occlusion (BVO). Deep retinal hemorrhages emanate to the periphery, and isolated cotton wool spots are present. (B) An inferior temporal BVO of the ischemic variety. Superficial dense hemorrhages dominate the clinical picture.**

MANAGEMENT

Much of the controversy surrounding the treatment of BVO results from the controversy surrounding the natural course of the disease. Untreated patients often have similar outcomes to patients treated medically or surgically.

In general, visual acuities of 20/40 (6/12) or better are obtained in 53% to 60% of untreated BVO patients who have been monitored for at least 1 year.[58,71] If initial visual acuity is 20/40 or better, the prognosis is excellent, but with poor initial acuity (20/200 or worse), the visual outcome is uncertain.[71]

Various complications can develop. Neovascularization develops in 22% to 80% of cases, and vitreous hemorrhage occurs in 10% to 40% of patients developing neovascularization.[67,68] Macroaneurysms can develop in areas of ischemic retina and may leak, causing retinal edema.[57] Primary open-angle glaucoma is thought to develop in about 14% of patients with BVO.[67] Retinal breaks have been reported in the area affected by retinal occlusive disease. These present as round or oval, 0.5 to 1 DD holes with smooth edges in the postequatorial retina.[72] Rhegmatogenous retinal detachments have also been linked to BVO of long duration.[73] Iris neovascularization is uncommon, as contrasted to this complication in patients with ischemic CVO.

Management of BVO is quite controversial. This is because the natural course of the disease has a relatively good prognosis. One noncontroversial aspect is the need to investigate each patient for the presence of associated systemic diseases. Every patient should have a complete physical examination including blood pressure, blood glucose, lipid profile, coagulation profile, complete blood count (CBC) with differential and smear, and electrocardiogram with blood chemistry if systemic hypertension is present.

Several medical management approaches have been advocated for BVO. Low molecular weight dextran in combination with papaverine hydrochloride,[74] anticoagulants, fibrinolytic agents, antithrombotic agents, steroids, and vasodilators have been tried, but no proof exists as to their efficacy.[60]

Ticlopidine has been evaluated for its action as a platelet aggregation inhibitor in the treatment of BVO and has been shown to be effective if the occlusion is fresh. It has also shown similar results in the treatment of CVO.[75]

Laser photocoagulation has a role in the management of BVO. The rationale for photocoagulation of nonproliferative BVO is threefold: (1) the scar tissue formed in photocoagulation acts as a barrier to prevent retinal edema from spreading to the fovea; (2) areas of leakage (aneurysms) are sealed to prevent further leakage; and (3) destruction of the capillary bed reduces the input of arterial blood to obstructed areas, which reduces edema and allows the intact bed to drain more effectively.[76]

The rationale for photocoagulation of proliferative BVO is to destroy retina/choroid, which minimizes hypoxia. This facilitates regression of neovascularization. The accepted method of photocoagulation is a combination of scatter burns from the affected area to the equator, and focal photocoagulation of identifiable neovascularization elsewhere. If the neovascularization is confined to the disc, the scatter quadrantic method is recommended. In all cases the burns should be confined to the area outside a 1 DD zone around the fovea.[60]

Before photocoagulative intervention, fluorescein angiography should be performed to assess the damage and provide a blueprint or map for the procedure. Although controversy still exists regarding the benefit of photocoagulation,[77,78] the majority of clinical studies support photocoagulative intervention to retain or to improve visual results in many cases of BVO.[79–83] This intervention is especially important in cases of macular edema or neovascularization.

Central Vein Occlusion

CVO is a visually debilitating condition with a strong association with systemic cardiovascular disease. CVO has a strong male predominance, with peak occurrences in the fifth to sixth decades. As with BVO, there is an ischemic and nonischemic presentation, with degree of retinal hypoxia being the determining factor.

ETIOLOGY

CVO presents as a sudden, variable loss of vision. The etiology is complex and is age-dependent. Table 25.4 categorizes systemic factors as related to age. Several causes for CVO have been reported[84]: antithrombin deficiency,[85] associated with spontaneous carotid-cavernous fistula,[86] secondary to hemodialysis,[87] increase in platelet aggregability,[88,89] elevation of throm-

TABLE 25.4
Systemic Factors in Central Vein Occlusion as Related to Age

Age (yr)	Causes
Under 50	Head injuries
	Hyperlipidemia
	Estrogen-containing preparations
	Hyperviscosity syndromes
	Cryofibrinogenemia
Over 50	Hypertension
	Abnormal GTT
	Hyperlipidemia
	Chronic lung disease
	Elevated serum IgA
	Hyperviscosity syndromes
	Cryofibrinogenemia

GTT, glucose tolerance test.
Adapted from McGrath MA, Wechsler F, Hunyor AB, et al. Systemic factors contributory to retinal vein occlusion. Arch Intern Med 1978;138:216–220.

bocyte aggregation,[90] hypercholesterolemia, hypertriglyceridemia, and hyperlipidemia.[91]

Predisposing factors for CVO include glaucoma, papilledema, subdural hematoma, hemorrhage within the optic nerve, drusen of the optic nerve, hypertension, cardiovascular and cerebrovascular disease, diabetes, leukemia, thrombocytopenia, mitral valve prolapse, sclerodermatous vascular disease, Reye's syndrome, systemic lupus erythematosus, and trauma.[92–100]

DIAGNOSIS

From an ophthalmoscopic standpoint, CVO can present as 2 distinct clinical entities. These are not always easily differentiated, however, since the conditions exist as part of a continuum. The recognized types are nonischemic retinopathy and ischemic retinopathy. The primary difference is determined by the presence of significant retinal ischemia.[101] The CVO in either case can present with the prodromal symptom of transient obscurations (brief blurring of vision associated with postural changes) and the prodromal sign of a yellowish hue in the posterior pole when comparing one eye with the other. The prodromata may last months, with the active phase being heralded by dot and blot hemorrhages and intraretinal edema. The hemorrhages extend from the posterior pole to the retinal periphery. Evidence of capillary dilation may occur near the optic disc or temporal vascular arcade as seen by fluorescein angiography. Vision loss is relatively sudden, since the macular area is very susceptible to intraretinal edema.

The two major types of CVO have specific characteristics, prognosis, and management procedures. Non-ischemic CVO is characterized by dot and blot hemorrhages, intraretinal edema, and various degrees of macular edema (Fig. 25.4). The ischemic CVO presents as dot and blot hemorrhages, superficial flame-shaped hemorrhages, cotton wool spots, silver wire or sheathed arteries, and very dense intraretinal and macular edema (Fig. 25.5). Another clinical finding that accompanies the acute stage of the occlusion is lowered intraocular pressure. There is a greater initial reduction of pressure in ischemic CVO than in nonischemic CVO, and both have a greater reduction than do BVO.[102,103] Two cases of transient angle-closure glaucoma have been reported in patients with CVO.[104] It has also been reported that there is a difference in relative afferent pupillary defects between ischemic and nonischemic CVO.[105]

Fluorescein angiographic findings in CVO will vary considerably depending on the type of occlusion as well as the elapsed time after onset. Initially there will be blockage of background choroidal fluorescence by the intraretinal and flame-shaped hemorrhage. The retina will be stained with fluorescein because of intraretinal leakage, and the macula will demonstrate varying degrees of edema. Neovascularization may develop along with its classic fluorescein angiographic picture.

MANAGEMENT

The visual prognosis of CVO is guarded, but one can expect a more favorable outcome in nonischemic CVO than in ischemic CVO.[106–108] Although recovery of visual acuity is variable, neovascular glaucoma is an identified complication in 14% to 20% of all CVO

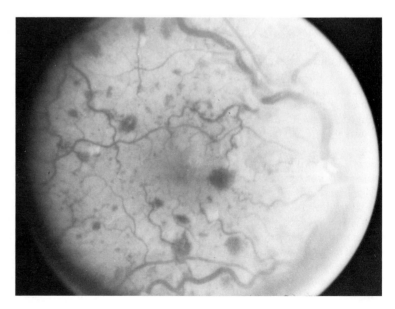

FIGURE 25.4 **Nonischemic central vein occlusion (CVO). Note tortuosity and dilation of veins and deep retinal hemorrhages.**

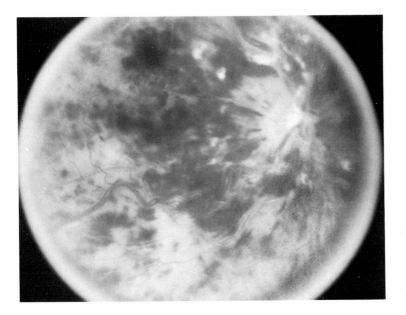

FIGURE 25.5   **Ischemic CVO. Note cotton wool spots and nerve fiber layer hemorrhages.**

cases.[109] The risk of neovascular glaucoma is even higher (60%) in ischemic CVO.[110,111] The incidence of primary open-angle glaucoma in patients with CVO is 5.7% to 66%, and CVO occurs in 3.5% to 5% of patients with primary open-angle glaucoma and in 3% of patients with ocular hypertension.[112] Disc and retinal neovascularization do not represent as significant a threat in CVO as in BVO because of the retinal capillary endothelial death that occurs in the former.

Although management of the ocular disorder is somewhat controversial, diagnosis and management of the underlying systemic condition is imperative.

Anticoagulants do not actively dissolve a thrombus once it has formed, but they may prevent its propagation. Monitoring of anticoagulant levels is essential once therapy has been instituted. Heparin is often the drug of choice, but hospitalization is required because of the intravenous or intramuscular route of administration. The usual dosage of heparin is 100 mg followed by 50 mg every 4 to 6 hours to stabilize the anticoagulant level.

Coumarin drugs are then instituted because they may be given orally on an outpatient basis. Since this drug group specifically depresses prothrombin levels, these levels should be monitored. There should be a 24- to 48-hour overlap of heparin therapy to ensure establishment of coumarin activity.

Warfarin may be administered in an initial dosage of 20 to 25 mg followed by 2 to 10 mg daily as a maintenance dosage. Oral prednisone therapy can be used to treat the inflammatory component.[113]

Anticoagulation therapy, although controversial, does seem to give slightly more favorable results than no therapy at all. Anticoagulation therapy may minimize the progression from nonischemic to ischemic CVO, actually reducing the incidence of development of neovascular glaucoma.[114,115] Monitoring of blood prothrombin times is a crucial aspect of any anticoagulation therapy.

Despite good results with retrobulbar injections of lidocaine and acetylcholine, coupled with systemic administration of low molecular weight dextran and papaverine hydrochloride, investigators suggest that this therapy is only moderately beneficial.[116]

Recent work has indicated that isovolemic hemodilution improves the visual outcome of patients with CVO and does offer some hope.[117]

One indisputable mode of therapy is the use of panretinal photocoagulation to prevent the development of neovascular glaucoma. Visual outcome is not necessarily improved by photocoagulation,[118] but the chance of development of neovascular glaucoma is minimized.[119–122] Panretinal photocoagulation has little effect in nonischemic CVO unless it is secondary to ipsilateral carotid artery occlusion,[123] but it is of significant benefit in ischemic CVO. Photocoagulation minimizes the vasoproliferative stimulus created by the hypoxic retina, which minimizes iris neovascularization.[124] The practitioner should recognize, however, that retinal neovascularization can recur even after panretinal photocoagulation.[125]

If nonischemic retinopathy appears to be worsening and there is associated orbital pain, bypass surgery of the carotid system may produce beneficial results.[126,127] It is important to note that patients with neovascular glaucoma but without an obvious precipitating fundus condition should be suspected of having ipsilateral ca-rotid artery disease until proven otherwise.[128,129]

Hemicentral Vein Occlusion

The basis of an HCVO lies in the fact that a 2-trunked central retinal vein exists in some patients.[130] This oc-curs when the vein bifurcates in the anterior portion of the optic nerve before piercing the lamina cribrosa. One of the 2 trunks may become occluded to produce the picture of an HCVO. Although the clinical findings may resemble a BVO, from a pathogenesis standpoint the condition is more related to CVO. This analysis, however, is controversial, since some clinicians believe that HCVO is actually simultaneous BVOs of different branches.[131] The HCVO may present in either a non-ischemic or ischemic form and usually involves half the retina (Fig. 25.6).

Prognosis depends on macular involvement and the development of neovascularization. Neovasculariza-tion is not expected in the nonischemic form but can develop in the ischemic variety within 6 months.[132]

Retinal Arterial Occlusion

Retinal arterial occlusions occur in 2 forms—CAO and BAO. Both conditions have similar origins and similar treatment modalities, although prognosis differs in the 2 conditions.

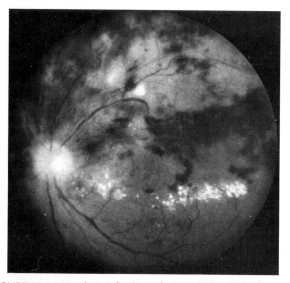

FIGURE 25.6   **Hemicentral vein occlusion (HCVO). The superior half of the retina is involved with hard exudates demarcating the retinal edema.**

CENTRAL ARTERY OCCLUSION

Etiology.   Patients with increased vascular resistance, such as internal carotid artery obstruction, are highly susceptible to CAO.[133,134] Any condition contributing to this increased resistance may act as a causative factor. These include emboli from cardiac lesions,[135,136] mitral valve prolapse,[137] emboli from artificial cardiac valves,[138] emboli from bacterial endocarditis,[139] thrombi secondary to giant cell arteritis, syphilis, and fungal infections of the ethmoid or sphenoid sinuses,[140] occlu-sion secondary to oral contraceptives,[141] and occlusion secondary to polyarteritis nodosa.[142] Both CAO and BAO may occur secondary to methylprednisolone ace-tate injections of the head and neck soft tissue.[143,144] Additional reports implicate cardiac catherization,[145] Sneddon's disease associated with antiphospholipid an-tibodies,[146] complications of rhinoplasty,[147] endarter-ectomy,[148] pregnancy,[149] and osteogenesis imperfecta.[150]

Diagnosis.   The typical clinical presentation of a CAO is a sudden, painless loss of vision in a nondiseased eye. The visual acuity loss is severe, and there is loss of the direct pupillary response. If there remains a patent cilioretinal artery (origin from the choroidal vascular supply), a variable central island of vision may be maintained.

The ophthalmoscopic appearance of the retina de-pends on time elapsed since the occlusion. Initially the retinal arteries appear narrowed in contrast to the veins, and there is a subtle haziness of the retinal tissue. The veins may become distended and may exhibit a box car segmentation. Within hours the inner retinal tissue becomes milky white (Fig. 25.7) and contrasts markedly with the red-appearing macula, which re-ceives its nutrition from the choroid.

After weeks, the retina is replaced by glial tissue, the arterial tree assumes a more normal appearance except for irregular narrowing, and optic atrophy may ensue. Neovascular glaucoma is rare in CAO. The presence of neovascular glaucoma associated with ar-terial obstructive disease usually indicates the ocular ischemic syndrome, which includes aqueous flare, ru-beosis iridis, mid-peripheral intraretinal hemorrhages, narrowed retinal arteries, cherry red spot, neovascu-larization of the disc or retina, and ipsilateral or bilat-eral common carotid artery obstruction.[151]

Management.   From a visual standpoint prognosis is grim unless therapy is begun within 1 to 2 hours after the occlusion. Management of the underlying systemic condition is also of immediate concern.

Management of CAO depends on the precipitating factor. If CAO is secondary to facial trauma resulting in retrobulbar hemorrhage, the treatment is surgical

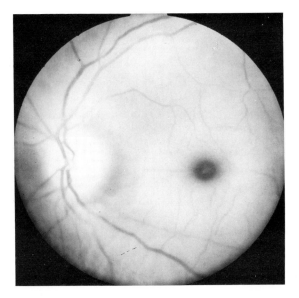

FIGURE 25.7 **Central artery occlusion (CAO). (Courtesy Hernan Benavides, O.D.)**

drainage of the hematoma.[152] If the CAO is due to sickle cell occlusion, exchange transfusions have offered some success.[153]

Some general statements regarding therapy can be made. The occlusions caused by emboli may exhibit some recovery if therapy is instituted within 1 to 2 hours. Digital massage of the globe through the eyelid may dislodge the embolus. Massage coupled with inhalation of a mixture of 5% CO_2 (vasodilator) combined with 95% O_2 for 15 minutes followed by breathing room air for 15 minutes over 6 to 12 hours may be of value. However, when considering the fact that CAO occurs at the lamina and that vasodilators will not affect this collagen-like structure, the use of vasodilators is illogical. Deutsch and associates[154] have concluded that attempts at vasodilation are of little benefit.[154] Paracentesis of the anterior chamber will quickly lower the intraocular pressure and facilitate dislodgement of the embolus. The intraocular pressure should be maintained low for several days by oral administration of acetazolamide, 250 mg every 6 hours.[140] Retrobulbar injections of acetylcholine, atropine, or tolazoline may be beneficial. Papaverine plus heparin through the infraorbital artery has been attempted.[155]

Any attempt to restore circulation is worthwhile, since the prognosis is otherwise grim. Particular attention must be given to the patient's general health status, since CAO implies generalized cardiovascular compromise. A recent report[156] concluded that over 50% of patients with CAO who undergo carotid angiography have an ipsilateral carotid lesion. This sug-

gests that CAO is a significant marker for extracranial carotid disease.[156]

BRANCH ARTERY OCCLUSION

Etiology. Etiology of BAO is similar to that of CAO, with the additional precipitating factors of self-injected emboli or emboli secondary to diagnostic procedures.[157,158] In general, individuals with BAO secondary to generalized cardiovascular disease have lesions that are more amenable to surgical intervention than do individuals with CAO.[134] It has also been suggested that there is an idiopathic form of BAO, and it is thought that this may be a variety of focal arteritis.[159]

Diagnosis. The most frequently affected region of the retina is the superior temporal area. Vision and visual fields are variable, but the ophthalmoscopic appearance is similar to that of CAO. The major difference in the evolution is the tendency toward development of arterial shunts in CAO. The vision remains compromised in the affected area, and segmental optic atrophy may be a complication.

Management. The likelihood for return of vision or visual field is minimal unless therapy is instituted within 1 to 2 hours. The visual field that remains is sharp-edged along the horizontals, representing termination of the inner retinal arterial supply at the horizontal raphé.

Management of BAO depends on the extent of visual loss. If vision is severely compromised, aggressive therapy should be used as in CAO.[160] If loss of visual field occurs without severe loss of vision, the procedure of greatest importance is an aggressive search for the cause of the BAO.

Some clinicians advocate pentoxifylline, 300 to 600 mg daily over a 3-month period, to prevent retinal or intravitreal neovascularization caused by retinal ischemia.[161] This method of management of retinal occlusive disease is still under investigation and has yet to be proved as a beneficial therapeutic procedure.

Diabetes and Diabetic Retinopathy

Approximately 5.5 million persons in the United States are known to have diabetes.[162–164] The numbers of patients with diabetes will increase because of the increase in the number of elderly people. It is estimated that beyond age 60, the prevalence of diabetes is 10% and rises to 16% to 20% over age 80.[165,166]

The complication of diabetic retinopathy accounts for about 50,000 cases of legal blindness in the United

States, with approximately 5800 new cases per year.[163] Diabetic retinopathy is responsible for 10% of new cases of legal blindness in all age groups and 20% of new cases of blindness in the age group 45 to 74 years. Diabetic retinopathy is present in about 50% of patients with diabetes of 10 years' duration and in 100% of patients with diabetes of 17 years' duration.[167] The prevalence of diabetic retinopathy is related to age, duration, pregnancy, and type. The most common loss of vision is related to maculopathy in type-2 diabetes.[169–175]

Etiology

Diabetes mellitus is a systemic disease of altered carbohydrate metabolism resulting in alterations of the vasculature throughout the body. Although the exact trigger mechanism is unknown, it is accepted that alterations in vascular structure coupled with alterations in blood composition lead to the development of diabetic retinopathy.[176–185]

In addition to changes in the blood, there are accompanying alterations in vascular structure. Basement membrane thickening of the capillaries has long been implicated in the development of diabetic retinopathy.[186] There is a reduction in mural cells, resulting in microaneurysms.[187] Both of these alterations are thought to be secondary to increased lactate concentration.[188,189] The genesis of all visually debilitating retinopathy is thought to be sluggishness of the blood and occlusion of the microcirculatory system.[190]

Increasing evidence is accumulating to implicate sorbitol as a contributing factor in the pathogenesis of diabetic retinopathy. When excess glucose accumulates in the tissues of the patient with diabetes, it is converted by aldose reductase to the sugar alcohol, sorbitol. Sorbitol then irreversibly accumulates in tissues such as the mural cells along the retinal capillaries and subsequently alters the mural cells, resulting in death, degeneration, and eventual compromise of the retinal capillaries. This alteration of structure also occurs within other ocular and systemic tissues.[191–194]

The microcirculatory changes either result in leakage, causing edema, or create a hypoxic situation that stimulates release of the vasoproliferative biochemical stimulus that initiates the neovascular response.[195]

Diagnosis

Three basic stages of diabetic retinopathy are now defined, but many variations exist within these classifications. For purposes of this discussion the 3 stages of diabetic retinopathy will be considered to be back-

ground diabetic retinopathy, preproliferative diabetic retinopathy, and proliferative diabetic retinopathy. Background diabetic retinopathy includes microaneurysms, intraretinal (dot-blot) hemorrhages, intraretinal (macular) edema, and hard exudates (Fig. 25.8A). Pre-

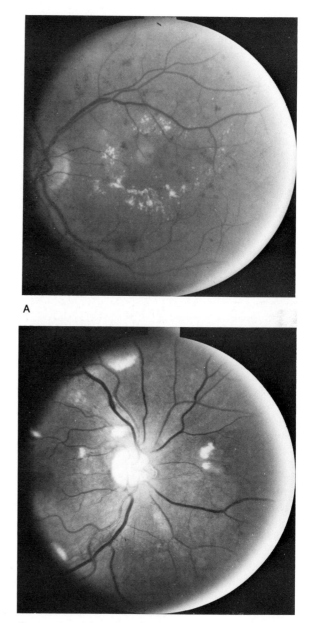

A

B

FIGURE 25.8   *(A)* **Background diabetic retinopathy with dot-blot deep retinal hemorrhages and hard exudates surrounding the macula.** *(B)* **Preproliferative diabetic retinopathy: cotton wool spots.** *(C)* **Preproliferative diabetic retinopathy. Increased venous tortuosity indicates relative hypoxia.** *(D)* **Fluorescein angiography of preproliferative diabetic retinopathy shows areas of capillary dropout.** *(E)* **Fibrotic proliferation emanating from the disc. Note areas of photocoagulation scars.**

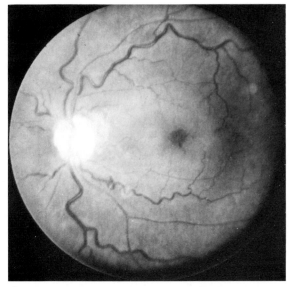

C

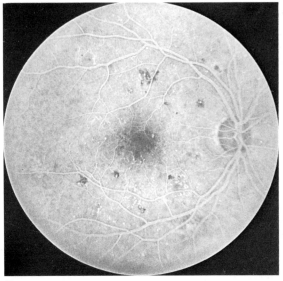

D

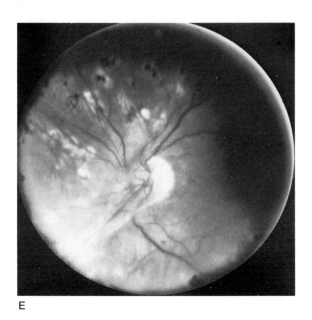

E

proliferative diabetic retinopathy is defined by cotton wool spots, increased venous tortuosity, venous looping, IRMA, flame-shaped hemorrhages, and areas of capillary shutdown (visible only on fluorescein angiography) (Fig. 25.8B to D). Proliferative diabetic retinopathy includes neovascularization of the disc, neovascularization elsewhere in the retina, vitreous hemorrhage, fibrotic proliferation, and subsequent retinal detachment (Fig. 25.8E).

Since the diabetic patient also has other systemic problems, the clinician should be alert to the increased incidence of all systemic vascular anomalies.

Management

Although the benefits of careful blood glucose control are controversial, it is strongly suggested that early detection and effective treatment positively affects overall prognosis.[196-199] It has been well established that strict control of diabetes during the first 5 years after diagnosis may reduce the frequency and delay the onset of diabetic retinopathy.[200] It has also been shown that there is a high correlation between degree of metabolic control, as measured by glycosylated hemoglobin level (A_1C), and the presence of early retinopathy as defined by angiography.[201,202] Other clinical studies, although not totally conclusive, seem to indicate that strict metabolic control may favorably affect the development of retinopathy.[203,204]

Strict control using multiple daily injections of insulin or the portable insulin pump may have a positive effect on retinopathy.[205,206] If, however, retinopathy advances too far too fast, conventional means of controlling blood glucose have a minimal effect.

Although metabolic control and diet undeniably have some effect on the development of diabetic retinopathy, work has been conducted to alter some of the precursors to microcirculatory changes. Salicylates such as acetylsalicylic acid (aspirin), salicylic acid, methyl salicylate, and sodium salicylate act to interfere with the second stage of platelet aggregation,[178,207] suppress increased capillary permeability as an anti-inflammatory agent,[208] and in nontoxic doses enhance glucose uptake into muscle, which reduces glycosuria and hyperglycemia.[209,210] Para-amino salicylate has been shown to effectively reduce blood lipids and thus the hard exudates of diabetic retinopathy.[176,211,212] Because the typical dosage required for favorable results in most studies is low (300 to 600 mg daily), the side effects are minimal, assuming the patient has no inherent condition in which aspirin is contraindicated. Clofibrate (Atromid-S) has been used to reduce hard exudates. However, no controlled studies have verified its efficacy. Calcium dobesilate (Doxium) has been reported to be beneficial for the treatment of diabetic retinopathy, but a well-controlled study did not validate this claim.[195] Vitamin C, flavinoids, and etamsylate did not have a positive proved effect on diabetic retinopathy.[213] Cinnarizine and flurarizine exert an antiedematous action and may improve visual function in diabetic retinopathy.[214] These calcium entry blockers may have potential for preventive treatment in diabetic retinopathy.

Further work is being conducted regarding medical management with specific emphasis on antiplatelet aggregator drugs and aldose reductase inhibitors. There is increasing evidence that supports therapeutic intervention using aldose reductase inhibitors or supplementations of dietary myoinositol.[215–219] Other experimental systemic modalities offering promise include pentoxifylline,[220] thromboxane synthetase inhibitors,[221,222] oral buflomedil,[223] vitamin E,[224] and sulindac.[225]

Currently the primary method of management for diabetic retinopathy involves the use of laser photocoagulation and vitrectomy. Specific methods of management for each of the three clinical phases of diabetic retinopathy will now be considered. Although simplification of diabetic retinopathy into categories can be misleading, certain guidelines do exist.

BACKGROUND DIABETIC RETINOPATHY

Background diabetic retinopathy may be managed by photocoagulation when areas of leaking microaneurysms, in the form of diabetic maculopathy, alter vision. Laser photocoagulation is indicated when there is (1) progressive vision loss secondary to intraretinal edema, (2) a photodocumented increase in hard exudates, and (3) identifiable areas of leakage as demonstrated by fluorescein angiography. Most studies point to the benefits of photocoagulative intervention when guidelines are followed carefully.[226–233] If there is no macular edema, background diabetic retinopathy can be monitored at 6- to 12-month intervals depending on the patients' general health status.

PREPROLIFERATIVE DIABETIC RETINOPATHY

The signs of preproliferative disease have no specific treatment but have taken on special importance in current management of diabetic retinopathy. Preproliferative diabetic retinopathy (PPDR) is also known as nonproliferative diabetic retinopathy (NPDR) and consists of (1) extensive intraretinal hemorrhages or microaneurysms, (2) cotton wool spots, (3) IRMA appearing as tortuous small vessels, (4) venous caliber abnormalities (beading) and increased tortuosity, (5) arteriolar abnormalities including caliber irregularities or vessel wall changes, and (6) capillary dropout, or the featureless retina.[234] The IRMA may even be seen clinically as a germination bed for neovascularization elsewhere. All the ophthalmoscopic signs indicate relative retinal hypoxia and the imminent possibility of progression toward proliferative diabetic retinopathy.

If IRMA or 3 or more signs of PPDR occur, fluorescein angiography is indicated. If, however, only isolated signs of PPDR are present, the patient should be followed at 3-month intervals and his or her general health status evaluated.

PROLIFERATIVE DIABETIC RETINOPATHY

Proliferative diabetic retinopathy (PDR) is the result of retinal hypoxia and includes all ocular neovascularization, the accompanying scaffolding, and the subsequent hemorrhaging of the new vessel growth. When signs of PDR are present, it has been proved that photocoagulative intervention is the indisputable treatment of choice to prevent severe vision loss.[234–241] Intervention is considered appropriate regardless of the presence of high-risk characteristics. Fluorescein angiography must be performed before initiation of treatment.[234–241]

Vitrectomy has enjoyed limited success and carries a relatively high complication rate. Vitrectomy is, however, one of two viable treatment modalities in cases of long-standing vitreous hemorrhage and traction retinal detachment. If vitreous hemorrhage lasts for 3 to 6 months, vitrectomy may be used. Vitrectomy for traction retinal detachment should be reserved for traction involving the macula.[195] Vitrectomy combined with argon laser endophotocoagulation offers some promise in improving postoperative vision.[242–245]

Another option for the treatment of vitreous hemorrhage involves intravitreal injection of 25,000 Ploug units of urokinase dissolved in 0.3 ml of distilled water. Preoperative medication of 500 mg of oral acetazolamide, pupillary dilation, and anterior chamber paracentesis are performed before the injection. Should the hemorrhage not resolve within 6 to 8 weeks, another injection is recommended. Note that intravitreal urokinase produces a hypopyon for 3 to 6 days, creating a transient rise in intraocular pressure. Acetazolamide, 250 mg every 6 hours during the first to second week postoperatively, will control the pressure.[247]

Hereditary Diseases

Hereditary Gyrate Atrophy of the Choroid and Retina with Hyperornithinemia

ETIOLOGY

This autosomal recessive and progressive dystrophy is associated with hyperornithinemia (plasma ornithine levels are typically 800 to 1300 μM) and deficient ornithine ketoacid aminotransferase activity. Serum lysine levels are typically lower than normal. A deficiency of creatinine or phosphocreatinine may also be involved in the pathogenesis.[248]

However, there are cases of gyrate atrophy with normal plasma ornithine levels and cases of hyperornithinemia without gyrate atrophy.[249]

DIAGNOSIS

The classic clinical presentation is myopia in the first decade, night blindness in the second decade, cataracts of such severity that extraction is needed in the third decade, and progressive visual impairment caused by macular changes in the fourth to fifth decades. However, there appear to be variations depending on serum ornithine levels.[250]

The fundus has a characteristic appearance with irregular, sharply defined areas of chorioretinal atrophy beginning in the periphery and progressing toward the posterior pole. The areas of atrophy tend to merge and take on scalloped borders. The fundus takes on a yellowish appearance, as does the disc, as pigment migrates and retinal vessels attenuate. The cataract that occurs in 40% of patients begins as a posterior subcapsular complicated variety. Abnormal electrodiagnostic signs are present. Seizure disorders may become a problem.[249,251]

MANAGEMENT

Visual acuity remains intact until macular encroachment occurs, but visual fields exhibit a concentric constriction with accompanying night vision problems. Color vision loss eventually ensues.

Since this is a hereditary disorder, genetic counseling and examination of siblings is crucial. Otherwise, management is directed at reducing serum ornithine levels. This can be achieved by restricting protein.[252,253] Arginine-deficient diets may reduce serum ornithine levels, especially in patients who do not respond to oral pyridoxine therapy. Oral pyridoxine (vitamin B_6), 15 to 18 mg daily, may reduce serum ornithine, while massive doses (600 to 750 mg) may improve retinal function.[254–255] Orally administered α-aminoisobutyric acid aids the reduction in serum ornithine.[252]

If serum ornithine is maintained between 55 and 355 μM by any means, it appears that chorioretinal degeneration does not progress.[252] No direct evidence exists to firmly support any particular therapy, but any method that reduces serum ornithine levels will improve the prognosis of hereditary gyrate atrophy. Dietary restrictions are safe as long as amino acid requirements are met by supplements. High doses of vitamin B_6 have no known adverse effects.

Acquired or Degenerative Diseases

Cystoid Macular Edema

ETIOLOGY

Cystoid macular edema (CME) occurs secondary to many ocular conditions. The most familiar form is associated with cataract surgery and is referred to as the Irvine-Gass syndrome. Other causes include BVO,[256] retinitis pigmentosa,[257] progressive pigmentary degeneration,[258] YAG laser capsulotomy,[259] pars planitis,[260] severe carotid artery obstruction,[261] corneal relaxing incision,[262,263] long-standing venous stasis retinopathy,[264] retinal surgery, ocular inflammation,[265] and ocular tumors. In general, any condition that can produce intraretinal fluid accumulation, including drug toxicities such as with epinephrine, can cause CME.

Cystoid maculopathy occurs when fluid seeps into Henle's fiber layer of the fovea. It is obvious that the leakage occurs as the result of venous stasis in vascular disease and inflammatory conditions, but the etiology in dystrophic conditions and toxic reactions is not as easily identified. Following cataract surgery with vitreous face complications, cystoid maculopathy may develop (Irvine-Gass syndrome). There is usually a delay in the onset of this condition postsurgically, with the peak incidence occurring at about the sixth postoperative week. By fluorescein studies, it has been shown that about 40% to 50% of phakic eyes develop cystoid maculopathy, but only 2% to 3% present a significant problem.[266,267] The prognosis is reasonably good because about 50% of affected patients recover normal vision within about 6 months. Twenty percent have the condition for 1 to 3 years.[268]

DIAGNOSIS

As mentioned previously, it is well known that cystoid maculopathy may result from any number of ocular conditions. The majority of these conditions are related to systemic disease processes such as hypertension, atherosclerosis, hyperlipidemia, and hypercholesterolemia and their ocular manifestations. The clinical picture will be characteristic in these conditions. In the Irvine-Gass syndrome, the fundus may reveal only a loss of foveal reflex or, in more severe cases, a retinal elevation. Visual acuity will be reduced, there will be a prolonged macular photostress recovery time, and metamorphopsia will be revealed by the Amsler grid. The definitive clinical diagnosis can be made by fluorescein studies.

Differential diagnosis is best accomplished by fluorescein angiography, which assists in differentiating cystoid maculopathy from dystrophic or degenerative conditions as well as from subretinal pigment epithelial neovascularization.

MANAGEMENT

Management of CME is controversial because the disease is difficult to study. The condition appears to be quite prevalent by angiographic studies, but true clinical manifestations appear to be rare.[266–268] However, management of any condition that can precipitate CME is mandatory.

The controversy arises when CME occurs as the primary condition. Oral inhibitors of prostaglandin synthesis, such as indomethacin, have been advocated, but their efficacy is not proved. Topical steroids are inadequate, and oral steroids have numerous and sometimes serious side effects. Periocular steroid injections may be attempted in cases where there is an immediate, severe threat to vision. A sub-Tenon's injection of methylprednisolone, 40 to 80 mg, is placed in the superior temporal quadrant posterior to the equator after topical anesthesia is achieved with 4% lidocaine. One or two treatments may result in remission, but edema often returns after the therapeutic effect has resolved.[267]

Many studies have reported the benefits to aphakic CME of prostaglandin inhibitors such as 1% topical indomethacin drops 4 times daily for 1 to 4 months. Actual prophylaxis against angiographically proved aphakic CME has also been achieved by topical indomethacin.[269–271] Some authors have advocated combining topical 1% indomethacin with 1% prednisolone.[272–274] The question remains whether management of angiographically proved CME is necessary, since there is usually no statistically significant difference in visual outcome with or without pharmacologic intervention.[275] Other prostaglandin inhibitors such as fenoprofen sodium have produced similar, equivocal results.[276] Flach and associates[277] recently used 0.5% topical ketorolac tromethamine solution and demonstrated that this nonsteroidal anti-inflammatory agent (NSAIA) may reverse vision loss in some patients with long-standing aphakic and pseudophakic CME.

Pars plana vitrectomy may be considered if vitreous strands are apparent. Laser photocoagulation has been used in an attempt to drain the macular area, with some positive results attained with grid photocoagulation.[278–280]

Inflammatory Diseases

Ocular Toxoplasmosis

ETIOLOGY

Toxoplasma gondii is an obligate intracellular protozoan parasite that is one of the most likely causes of posterior uveitis in the United States. *T. gondii* uveitis is rarely acquired but, rather, is thought to be congenital with a delayed ocular onset.[281] The factors that lead to reactivation as well as the occasional acquired infection involve a compromise of the patient's immune status.

The prevalence of toxoplasmosis varies considerably in different studies. In general, it is accepted that 70% to 80% of females are at risk during child-bearing years.[282] Congenital infection occurs as a consequence of primary maternal infection during pregnancy.[283] The rate of fetal infection increases throughout the pregnancy,[284,285] and the incidence of congenital infection is 0.01% of live births.[286] Toxoplasmosis can, however, be transmitted to the fetus only during maternal parasitemia.[287] When the parasite reaches the ocular circulatory system, it lodges in retinal vessels, often in the nerve fiber layer. When active parasites are present, a necrotizing retinitis ensues. It is thought that the live organism rather than the toxins is the cause of the retinochoroiditis.[287,288] Humoral and cell-mediated immunity inhibit the active process that results in encystation of still viable *T. gondii*. It has been suggested that the body produces an antibody that protects the parasite.[289] The encysted *T. gondii* then await a future compromise of the immune system, which leads to successful reactivation.[290] This results in the typical toxoplasmosis scar with satellites of reactivated lesions. The compromised immune system in the patient with acquired immunodeficiency syndrome (AIDS) significantly increases the risk of reactivation of toxoplasmic encystations. Toxoplasmosis in patients with AIDS is discussed later in this chapter.

The anterior uveitis that accompanies the retinal lesion is believed to be a manifestation of hypersensitivity, since *T. gondii* have never been recovered from the anterior chamber.[289]

In the past, acquired *T. gondii* retinochoroiditis was considered to be rare. Fewer than 1% of patients with acquired systemic toxoplasmosis manifest retinal lesions.[286] However, more reports are surfacing that suggest an increase in the acquired form. There are even reports of miniepidemics of acquired toxoplasmosis that involve retinal lesions.[291–295] It has been suggested that the incidence of acquired toxoplasmic retinochoroiditis will increase because of the increased use of immunosuppressive therapy.[292,296]

DIAGNOSIS

Reactivated congenital toxoplasmic retinochoroiditis typically occurs as an indistinct yellow-white lesion with an overlying vitritis (Fig. 25.9). The active lesion usually occurs at the margin of an old toxoplasmic scar, which suggests a rupture of an encysted toxoplasmic colony. There may be an associated posterior vitreous detachment with keratic precipitates on the vitreous face. The frequent association of retinal arteritis,[297,298] occlusive vasculitis,[299,300] iridocyclitis, optic neuritis (papillitis), and macular edema[301] reflects the inflammatory aspect of the disease. The inflammatory response indicates the need to incorporate steroids into the treatment regimen. One additional consideration is the possibility of subretinal pigment epithelial neovascularization in active toxoplasmic retinochoroidopathy.[295]

It has been suggested that reactivation of congenital toxoplasmosis can manifest itself neurologically. Robinson and Bauman[302] have described a girl with focal encephalitis associated with a reactivation of ocular toxoplasmic retinochoroidopathy. The brain and eye share a similar vascular system, resulting in the following characteristics of congenital toxoplasmosis: (1) convulsions, (2) intracranial calcification, and (3) retinochoroiditis.

Active toxoplasmosis is common in the teen years but is rare over age 40 years. An active attack lasts 1 week to 2 years, with an average of 4.2 months.[286] Several laboratory tests are available to assist in the diagnosis of toxoplasmic retinochoroidopathy. The Sabin-Feldman methylene blue dye test (SFDT) is the diagnostic test used most often in toxoplasmosis.

The SFDT is of limited usefulness in congenital toxoplasmosis, since the mother's antibodies cross the placenta whether or not the infection is transmitted. The SFDT does, however, measure antibodies that are detectable for decades.[303] The complement fixation test (CFT) measures antibodies of comparatively short duration after infection and therefore has value in indicating which children have been infected during the first 6 years of life.[304] The indirect fluorescent antibody test is a useful adjunct to the SFDT but has some limitations due to availability. The presence of an IgM antibody is significant because this antibody will not pass the placental barrier; therefore, its presence indicates infection.[305–308] The lymphocyte transformation test may also be of some benefit for detecting infection in the first year of life.[286]

Since many diseases may mimic toxoplasmic retin-

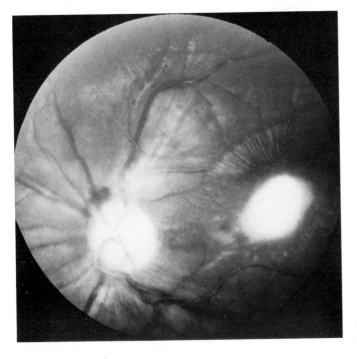

FIGURE 25.9 **Active ocular toxoplasmosis involving the macula. (Courtesy John F. Amos, O.D.)**

ochoroidopathy, other laboratory tests should be routinely performed, including routine screening for AIDS. A PPD coupled with a chest x-ray film will rule out tuberculosis. FTA-ABS will assist in the differential diagnosis of syphilitic retinitis. Other conditions necessitate more sophisticated laboratory analyses.

MANAGEMENT

Visual prognosis in cases of ocular toxoplasmosis depends on the time elapsed between activation or reactivation of the retinitis and initiation of therapy. If the lesion progresses to necrosis (even 5 or 6 days), therapy will act only to limit the extent of damage. Indications for treatment of ocular toxoplasmosis are[309] (1) active lesions near the macula or papillomacular bundle, (2) lesions threatening or involving the optic nerve, (3) lesions severe enough to cause significant vitreous traction or retinal detachment, and (4) peripapillary lesions, especially those closer to the disc because of the associated sectorial visual field loss.

Accepted systemic therapy is the use of antitoxoplasmic agents with the addition of oral steroids when an inflammatory reaction exists. The synergistic use of triple sulfonamides with pyrimethamine has been shown to be an effective antitoxoplasmic regimen because each works at a different point in the toxoplasmosis cycle.[310]

Pyrimethamine (Daraprim) is typically prescribed in an initial loading dose of 100 to 150 mg orally followed by 25 to 50 mg daily for 4 to 6 weeks.[311,312] Pyrimethamine is a folate antagonist and therefore can cause white blood cell and platelet depression as well as megaloblastic anemia. Should the platelet count drop below 100,000/mm³, 10 mg of folinic acid (leucovorin) can be administered intramuscularly or orally in orange or tomato juice to reverse the effect without affecting the action of the pyrimethamine. Some authors advocate using 2 to 3 mg of leucovorin 3 times per week as a preventive measure.[313,314] One may also use 1 tablet of brewer's yeast 3 times daily as a substitute for folinic acid.[315]

Chlortetracycline can be used as a substitute for pyrimethamine at a loading dose of 2 g followed by 250 mg 4 times daily for 1 month. Spiramycin at 2 g daily can be used as a substitute in pregnant women because it does not cross the placental barrier.[283]

Triple sulfonamides (sulfadiazine-sulfamerazine-sulfamethazine) lessen the chance of renal calculus formation while being effective antitoxoplasmic agents. The loading dose is 2 to 4 g followed by 1 g 4 times daily. Therapy should be continued for 4 to 6 weeks.[316]

Clindamycin (Cleocin) is an antitoxoplasmic drug with a high rate of ocular penetration but that is not yet approved for routine use in the treatment of ocular

toxoplasmosis.[288,312] If oral clindamycin is given, the dosage is 300 mg 4 times daily for 4 weeks. The alternative to this dosage is 50 mg administered subconjunctivally on alternate days for 4 weeks.[317] The major concern with clindamycin is the side effect of severe colitis, which can prove fatal. Should bowel movement exceed 4 times daily beyond normal, the drug should be discontinued and the patient should notify the physician. Vancomycin, 500 mg every 6 hours for 10 days, has been reported to be effective in controlling the colitis.[318]

Steroids have some value in the management of ocular toxoplasmosis. However, it is likely that all toxoplasmic retinochoroiditis is infectious and that the steroid's immunosuppressive action is potentially dangerous.[319] When used alone in either injectable or oral form, steroids will cause a brief improvement in the inflammatory process followed by a worsening.[311] However, when used in conjunction with antitoxoplasmic agents, steroids will improve some of the inflammatory responses and allow for less overall damage. The standard therapeutic dosage is 100 mg of oral prednisone daily for 7 to 10 days followed by a tapering of dosage on alternate days.[316]

Tessler[316] has proposed a variation on antitoxoplasmosis therapy that he contends minimizes the hematologic problems associated with pyrimethamine therapy. He calls this approach quadruple therapy:

Pyrimethamine	75 mg loading dose followed by 25 mg daily, discontinued in 1 to 2 weeks
Triple sulfonamides	2 g loading dose followed by 1 g 4 times daily, discontinued in 3 weeks
Clindamycin	300 mg 4 times daily, discontinued in 3 weeks
Oral prednisone	60 to 80 mg every other day at breakfast, tapering off in 3 to 4 weeks

One other aspect of ocular toxoplasmosis that must be managed is that of associated iridocyclitis. The degree of cells, flare, and keratic precipitates dictates the mode of therapy. Mydriatic-cycloplegic agents such as cyclopentolate 1% or homatropine 5% should be instilled 2 to 4 times daily in less severe cases and atropine 1% instilled twice daily in severe cases. Topical steroids assist in alleviating the inflammatory process. Prednisolone acetate 0.5% to 1% has the best ocular penetration and may be used at intervals that correspond to the degree of inflammation.

Nonmedical therapeutic modalities have been attempted without overwhelming success. Photocoagulation has been performed in healed lesions to prevent recurrences.[320] Photocoagulation and cryopexy should, however, not be applied in active cases unless all other therapeutic modalities have been exhausted.[321] There are instances when either vitrectomy—in the case of traction—or lensectomy in the case of complicated cataract—may be needed.[322]

Ocular Toxocara canis

ETIOLOGY

Toxocara is a parasite that infects dogs, wolves, foxes, and other canids and is transferrable to humans through feces. The human infestation is manifest in 2 forms, ocular larva migrans and visceral larva migrans. Affected patients are usually between 2 and 40 years, with an average age of 7.5 years.[323] The syndrome of visceral larva migrans is diagnosed most frequently in the southcentral and southeastern region of the United States.[324]

It has been shown that the major risk factor is exposure to dogs in the household or contact with puppies. Pica has been implicated, and this is conceivable, since 10% to 30% of soil samples in public playgrounds and parks has been found contaminated with *Toxocara* eggs.[325] It is not known if larval invasion of the eye occurs immediately after ingestion of the eggs or after months or years.[326] It is believed, however, that the number of eggs ingested may determine whether the ocular, visceral, or oculovisceral form of *Toxocara* infection develops.[327]

DIAGNOSIS

Visceral larva migrans is rarely acute. The patient usually complains of a wheezy cough, chest pain, intermittent fever, loss of appetite, and sometimes right upper abdominal pain. In children pruritic eruptions occasionally occur over the trunk and lower extremities, accompanied by transient tender nodules. There also may be some focal or generalized seizures. In the systemic condition eosinophils and neutrophils are predominant in the peripheral blood smear.[328]

Ocular larva migrans can occur up to 3 years after the time of presumed infection. Ocular toxocariasis may vary from a low-grade iritis with peripheral anterior synechiae to posterior pole or peripheral retinal granulomas. There have also been cases reported of a BAO secondary to a neuroretinitis,[329] and hypopyon with an iris nodule.[330]

The posterior pole lesion may be characterized by decreased vision or strabismus, depending on the location of the lesion. The lesion is typically round, raised, and white and is about 1 disc diameter in size (Fig. 25.10). There can be surrounding pigmentary

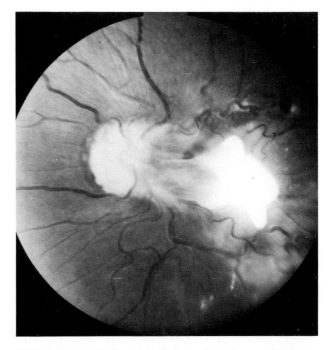

FIGURE 25.10   **Ocular toxocariasis involving the macular region. (Courtesy Randall Coshatt, O.D.)**

migration. Fibrous bands may radiate from the lesion, and a crescentic dark area in the lesion is thought to be the larval position within the granuloma.[331]

Tables 25.5 and 25.6 summarize the differences between the ocular and the visceral larva migrans syndromes. It should be noted that it is rare to have concurrent ocular and visceral syndromes.

The clinical diagnosis is based on the enzyme-linked immunosorbent assay (ELISA). The ELISA gives a diagnostic sensitivity of 78% with a 92% specificity.[324] This test is performed in a communicable disease center on 10 ml of clotted blood.[332,333] In an instance where the differential diagnosis of a posterior pole lesion is uncertain and a nondiagnostic ELISA is performed on blood, it is suggested that an anterior chamber tap be performed, since the antibody level is higher in the aqueous than in the blood. This can often prevent an unnecessary enucleation.[334] It is also suggested that ultrasonography may be of some assistance in differential diagnosis.[335] When *Toxocara* is found in 1 family member, all other family members should be examined.[336]

MANAGEMENT

Management of ocular toxocariasis is controversial. The best management is elimination of the nematodes.

TABLE 25.5
Differences between Ocular and Visceral Toxocariasis

Characteristic	Ocular Larva Migrans	Visceral Larva Migrans
Average age of patient	7.5 years	2 years
White blood cell count	Normal	Elevated
Eosinophilia	Normal	Elevated (>30%)
Hepatomegaly	None	Usually present
Splenomegaly	None	Usually present
Ocular findings	Posterior pole granuloma Endophthalmitis Peripheral granulomas	Very rare

From Schlaegel TF. Uveitis and miscellaneous parasites. Int Ophthalmol Clin 1977;17:177–194.

Diethylcarbamazine is the drug used most often in treatment of visceral larva migrans. The initial dosage is 0.5 mg/kg body weight according to tolerance. The dosage is then increased over 3 or 4 days to achieve a final dosage of 3 mg/kg administered 3 times daily. This dosage level is maintained for 21 days.[337,338]

Steroid therapy, such as oral prednisone 40 mg daily for several weeks, may be of some value in managing the accompanying inflammatory response in the visceral form. The steroid must then be tapered. Although subconjunctival injections of steroids have been reported to aid improvement,[332,338] no proof exists.

Thiabendazole has been tried in systemic *Toxocara* infection with variable success. The usual dosage is 1.5 g twice daily for patients over 70 kg. The dosage is decreased proportionally for patients under 70 kg. This agent is thought to have more of an anti-inflammatory and analgesic effect than an anthelmintic effect.

Photocoagulation and cryopexy may be of some value in isolating the organism if the granuloma is out of the capillary-free zone of the macula. When the granuloma occurs in the macular area and these methods are employed, resultant visual acuity is usually less than 20/200 (6/60).[339]

Should a traction retinal detachment occur secondary to the inflammatory reaction to ocular larva migrans, vitreoretinal surgical intervention may be successful.[340]

Sarcoid Ophthalmopathy

ETIOLOGY

Sarcoidosis is a systemic disease of unknown etiology. It is probably an antigenic reaction of the reticuloendothelial system, but recent work also implicates genetically linked cofactors in the etiology of sarcoidosis.[341] Sarcoidosis is a granulomatous disease that affects many bodily functions. The process may be acute, which indicates a more favorable prognosis than does the chronic presentation. Onset usually occurs between the second and fifth decades, and approximately 27% to

TABLE 25.6
The Relationship between Ocular and Visceral Larva Migrans Syndromes: A Hypothetical Model Based on Observations in Human and Experimentally Infected Animals

Toxocariasis	Infectious Dose	Incubation Period	ELISA Antibody Titer
Visceral	Moderate to high	Short (days to months)	High (>1:16)
Ocular	Low	Long (months to years)	Low (<1:512)
Visceral and ocular	Very high	Very short (days)	Very high (>1:1024)

ELISA, enzyme-linked immunosorbent assay.
From Glickman LT, Shantz PM. Epidemiology and pathogenesis of zoonotic toxocariasis. Epidemiol Rev 1981; 3:230–250.

50% of patients have ocular involvement.[342,343] The most common ocular manifestation is chronic granulomatous anterior uveitis, but the vitreous and retina may also be involved. Blacks are affected more often than are whites.[344]

DIAGNOSIS

Granulomatous anterior uveitis is often the first manifestation. Posterior ocular involvement occurs in about 25% to 37% of patients with ocular sarcoid. The vitreous may be involved, showing fluffy snowball infiltrates near whitish chorioretinal nodules in the inferior retinal periphery. These nodules can vary in size from a disc diameter to large masses.[345,346]

Periphlebitis is the most common fundus feature, and the equatorial retinal veins are most often involved. These changes range from marked, creamy-white perivascular exudation to changes present only in a fluorescein angiogram.[347] Focal subretinal lesions that could be choroidal granulomas may be seen most commonly in the equatorial retina. It is known that patients with extensive subretinal lesions have less severe periphlebitis. Optic disc edema, neovascularization, or angiomas may occur as components of sarcoid retinopathy.[348,349] Subretinal neovascularization has also been reported as a complication.[350]

The diagnosis of sarcoidosis can be elusive. The Kveim biopsy test is not 100% diagnostic,[345] but it is still the most efficient test available. Chest x-ray studies also assist in the diagnosis. The elevation of ACE in some patients with granulomatous uveitis is strongly suggestive of sarcoidosis.[351,352]

The systemic implications of sarcoidosis are crucial because the disease can affect numerous systems. Neurologic[353,354] and cardiovascular[355,356] complications can be severe. When managing the patient with ocular manifestations of sarcoidosis, the practitioner must not ignore the potential systemic morbidity of the disease.

In addition to evaluating serum ACE, it has been recommended that limited gallium scans of the head, neck, and chest be used for patients with granulomatous uveitis.[357] Conjunctival lesions occur in 50% of patients with ocular sarcoid, and biopsy of these lesions may aid in diagnosis.[358,359]

MANAGEMENT

The course of the disease is variable, characterized by frequent remissions in the first 3 years, but may become chronic and progressive.[360] As previously mentioned, an acute onset has a more favorable prognosis than does the chronic disease. Visual prognosis is reasonably good if neovascularization does not develop. A final visual acuity of 20/30 (6/9) can be expected if the intraocular inflammation can be controlled.[345]

It must be remembered that sarcoidosis is a disease of remissions and exacerbations. This also applies to the ocular involvement. If active fundus involvement becomes a part of the disease complex, oral steroid therapy should be initiated. Prednisone is started at 60 mg daily and tapered as the inflammatory response diminishes. If the disease is unresponsive to steroids, chlorambucil may be used. This is started at a single daily dose of 4 to 6 mg, increasing weekly by 2 mg if necessary to a maximal dose of 12 mg daily. White blood cell count and platelet activity must be monitored while the patient is taking chlorambucil.[360]

Other options include phenylbutazone or oxyphenbutazone, 600 mg daily in divided doses during the first few days followed by a reduction to 300 mg daily. Other drugs include immunosuppressive agents, chloroquine, and potassium paraaminobenzoate.[361] It has recently been suggested that with proper surveillance for ocular side effects, chloroquine may be used to control the calcium abnormalities of sarcoidosis.[362]

The most severe ocular complication of sarcoidosis is neovascularization. Whether this appears in the subretinal or supraretinal form, laser photocoagulation may avert potential loss of vision.

Management of the accompanying granulomatous anterior uveitis is achieved through use of topical steroids and mydriatic-cycloplegic agents. The cycloplegic of choice will vary according to severity of the inflammation, with 1% atropine reserved for the stubborn cases. If better mydriasis is needed, 2.5% phenylephrine may be used in conjunction with the cycloplegic. Prednisolone acetate 1% every 2 hours during the day is used initially and should be tapered slowly as the inflammation subsides. If improvement is not noted after a few days, subconjunctival or oral steroids should be used.

Retinal Periphlebitis (Eales' Disease)

ETIOLOGY

Retinal periphlebitis refers to a primary inflammation of the walls of peripheral retinal veins that may result in intraretinal or intravitreal hemorrhages. Retinal periphlebitis is considered to be a nonspecific inflammatory reaction to antigens, most likely tubercular in origin. However, other causes have been reported, which focuses on the necessity to carefully investigate the patient's general medical status.[363,364]

Retinal periphlebitis most often occurs in young men in the third decade. It is most often bilateral, but when unilateral it has been described as affecting the left eye more frequently.

DIAGNOSIS

Early in the course of the disease visual acuity is often unaffected, but the patient complains of floaters. Usually hemorrhages occur near veins in the periphery, and there is marked perivascular sheathing. At times, hemorrhages may emanate into the vitreous. Vitreous haze may occur above the lesions. Vision is eventually compromised by vitreous hemorrhage, retinal traction, or macular edema due to eventual engorgement and leakage of vessels of the posterior pole. Hemorrhages may occur in the posterior pole in combination with optic disc edema.

MANAGEMENT

With the advent of fluorescein angiography and photocoagulation, the prognosis for this disease has significantly improved. Before this, vitreous hemorrhage and retinal traction often caused some degree of permanent visual impairment. Although floaters and recurrent hemorrhage still present a threat to the patient with retinal periphlebitis, intervention is of substantial benefit if the disease is diagnosed early.

As previously mentioned, a complete medical workup, including PPD, chest x-ray study, and complete blood studies, is indicated. Vitreous hemorrhages often clear spontaneously with bed rest. Should vitreous hemorrhages persist, vitrectomy has proved to be an acceptable mode of therapy.[365]

There are some advocates of massive doses of systemic steroids to be given in the active vasculitis stage, but no proof exists of their efficacy.[366]

Fluorescein angiography is indicated in retinal periphlebitis to establish areas of leakage or neovascularization. These areas are amenable to laser photocoagulation to limit intravitreal hemorrhage.[367] Since retinal periphlebitis can progress very rapidly, treatment should begin as soon as possible.[368]

Acute Posterior Multifocal Placoid Pigment Epitheliopathy

ETIOLOGY

Acute posterior multifocal placoid pigment epitheliopathy (APMPPE) is a relatively benign, bilateral condition affecting young adults. The sudden appearance of multifocal, yellow-white, placoid lesions in the posterior pole of 1 eye, followed by similar development in the fellow eye, is characteristic.[369,370] Scotomas occur in the visual field corresponding to the affected areas, and vision decreases if the fovea is involved. APMPPE has a rapid onset and resolves over a period of weeks,

the scotomas and visual acuity resolving more slowly than does the ophthalmoscopic appearance.

The specific etiology of APMPPE is obscure. It seems that the condition has vaso-occlusive disease overtones because of its association with many systemic disease processes. Toxoplasmosis, viruses, tuberculosis, and erythema nodosum have been suggested as possible etiologic agents.[371] The associated ocular and systemic conditions are listed below:

- Headache
- Cerebral vasculitis
- Cerebrospinal fluid pleiocytosis
- Erythema multiforme[372]
- Thyroiditis[373]
- Papillitis
- Posterior uveitis
- Retinal vasculitis with serous retinal detachment[374]
- Serous retinal detachments
- Iridocyclitis
- Marginal corneal thinning
- Episcleritis
- Adenovirus type 5
- Harada's disease[375]
- Tuberculosis[376]
- Meningoencephalitis[377]

Controversy surrounds the specific pathogenic process as well as the specific etiologic agent. Originally APMPPE was attributed to a primary inflammatory process of the retinal pigment epithelium.[378–380] There has been some support for this theory, but evidence now favors primary pathology of the choriocapillaris. Fluorescein angiographic findings coupled with the $\frac{1}{8}$ to $\frac{1}{4}$ disc diameter size of the lesions (the typical size of the compartments of the choriocapillaris) would seem to implicate the choriocapillaris.[381,382]

DIAGNOSIS

Assessing the depth of the lesions by fluorescein angiography is crucial in the differential diagnosis of APMPPE. The yellow-white, placoid lesions lie deep within the retina, and there is retinal pigment epithelial involvement (Fig. 25.11A). The retinal-vitreous interface is usually unaffected, but papillitis, episcleritis, and marginal corneal thinning have been reported in association with APMPPE.[369] Holt and associates[383] have suggested that some degree of uveitis is present in most cases of APMPPE.

Fluorescein angiography exhibits a pattern that is diagnostic of APMPPE. In the early phases of angiography there is blockage of background choroidal fluorescence in the affected areas (Fig. 25.11B). This is

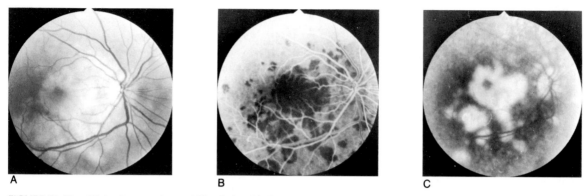

FIGURE 25.11   *(A)* Acute posterior multifocal placoid pigment epitheliopathy (APMPPE), showing retinal pigment epithelial involvement surrounding the macular area. *(B)* APMPPE in the early phase of fluorescein angiography demonstrating blockage of background choroidal fluorescence. *(C)* APMPPE in the late phase of fluorescein angiography demonstrating staining of the lesions. (Courtesy Paul Ajamian, O.D., and Jeffrey Coughran, O.D.)

followed by a late-stage staining of the lesions (Fig. 25.11*C*).

Although differential diagnosis is best attained through careful case history, fundus appearance, and fluorescein angiography, some practitioners use systematic laboratory studies directed toward special viral culturing techniques and serologic screening for antibodies.[383] This approach, however, has not met with widespread support.

The following conditions should be considered in the differential diagnosis: Dawson's subacute sclerosing panencephalitis, detachment of the retinal pigment epithelium, presumed ocular histoplasmosis, retinal pigment epithelitis, Best's vitelliruptive degeneration, and acute herpes simplex retinitis.[369]

MANAGEMENT

APMPPE is a condition that resolves spontaneously in 2 to 12 weeks, with a dramatic improvement in acuity and scotomatous areas in the first 2 weeks. Further improvement continues during the following weeks, with the vision resolving more slowly than does the ophthalmoscopic picture. The visual recovery is usually good but may not be totally complete. The resultant ophthalmoscopic picture consists of areas of depigmentation with some pigment clumping. Systemic steroids seem to have no effect on rate of recovery, although there are no controlled studies to confirm this.[384]

Although APMPPE is recognized as a relatively benign, self-limited condition, 1 author[385] has suggested that the condition may be part of a continuum that results in extensive chorioretinal atrophy and reduced acuity. The clinician must also be alert to the possibility of subretinal pigment epithelial neovascularization, since the retinal pigment epithelial–Bruch's membrane barrier is altered.

Acquired Immunodeficiency Syndrome

Etiology

Of the cumulative total of AIDS cases reported as of early 1988, 70% had occurred in homosexual or bisexual males and 14% had occurred in intravenous drug abusers.[386] The probable cause of AIDS is a retrovirus of the human T-cell lymphotrophic family (HTLV-III). The virus was formerly known as lymphadenopathy-associated virus (LAV) and is now referred to as the human immunodeficiency virus (HIV). The Centers for Disease Control (CDC) define a case of AIDS as an illness characterized by (1) one or more opportunistic diseases (Table 25.7) that at least moderately indicate underlying cellular immunodeficiency and (2) absence of all known underlying causes of cellular immunodeficiency, and absence of all other causes of reduced resistance reported to be associated with at least one of those opportunistic diseases.[387]

Only a minority of individuals currently infected with HIV has AIDS. Up to 25% of individuals infected have lymphadenopathy syndrome: chronic generalized lymphadenopathy, fever, fatigue, malaise, night sweats, weight loss, thrush, or diarrhea. About 10% to 30% of these individuals progress to AIDS within 2 to 3 years.[387] Patients with AIDS rarely survive longer than 3 years.

HIV has been isolated from blood, semen, saliva, bone marrow, lymph nodes, brain, peripheral nerves, cerebrospinal fluid, and conjunctival and corneal epithelium.[388] Fortunately, although the virus is omnipresent, it is also eliminated by several conventional sterilization methods. Transmission is by (1) sexual contact with exchange of body secretions, (2) infusion of blood or blood products, or (3) infected mother to child.

TABLE 25.7
**Diseases Indicating Underlying
Cellular Immunodeficiency**

Protozoal and helminthic infections
   Cryptosporidiosis
   Pneumocystis carinii
   Strongyloidosis
   Toxoplasmosis
Fungal infections
   Candidiasis
   Cryptococcosis
Bacterial infections
   Mycobacterium avium
   Mycobacterium tuberculosis
Viral infections
   Herpes zoster
   Cytomegalovirus
   Herpes simplex
Cancer
   Kaposi's sarcoma
   Diffuse lymphoma (undifferentiated)
   Lymphoma
   Hodgkin's disease
Other opportunistic infections
   Histoplasmosis
   Isosporiasis

Diagnosis

It is estimated that patients with AIDS will have at least one ophthalmic or neuro-ophthalmic manifestation at some point in their illness.[389] Cotton wool spots are the most common retinal manifestation of AIDS, occurring in at least two-thirds of patients. These lesions occur as the result of capillary damage, creating localized ischemia. The cotton wool spots are transient, lasting 4 to 6 weeks. Cotton wool spots have no particular prognostic significance.

Flame, white-centered, or dot-blot hemorrhages may also occur as a manifestation of the retinal microvasculopathy. These are seen in 15% to 40% of patients. Ischemic maculopathy may be present in about 6% of patients and is characterized by macular edema and macular star formation.[390]

Ocular opportunistic infections are usually associated with disseminated systemic disease and are often severe. Cytomegalovirus (CMV) retinopathy is the most common severe ocular manifestation of AIDS, affecting 25% to 45% of patients.[389] CMV retinopathy has also been reported as the initial manifestation of AIDS.[391] Although most adults have been exposed to CMV, the intact immunosuppressive system keeps the infection at bay. CMV retinopathy is a necrotizing infection that leads to full-thickness retinal destruction. It may be multifocal and bilateral in 50% of patients. Early CMV lesions are white and granular, appearing near major vascular arcades and usually near the disc. The virus spreads in a "brushfire" fashion accompanied by hemorrhage (Fig. 25.12). In contrast to toxoplasmosis, the overlying vitreous in CMV retinopathy is clear. Once established, the CMV spreads and within 6 months destroys the entire retina. Not only is CMV visually devastating, but it is also associated with the end stage of AIDS.[390]

Although toxoplasmosis is the most common cause of posterior uveitis among healthy individuals, it is rare in patients with AIDS. Nevertheless, should a patient present with reactivated toxoplasmosis, all immunosuppressive conditions should be considered, including AIDS. Toxoplasmosis is, however, the most common cause of neurologic complication in AIDS.[392–395] It has also been reported that testicular toxoplasmosis may occur in patients with AIDS.[396]

All opportunistic infections can involve the eye in patients with AIDS. These include herpes zoster ophthalmicus, herpes simplex, *Cryptococcus neoformans*, *Histoplasma capsulatum*, *Mycobacterium avium*, and *Candida*. All these infections must be recognized as potential components of the AIDS complex.

Kaposi's sarcoma may also occur in the ocular adnexal area. These reddish purple, nodular tumors tend to appear near the medial canthus or inferior cul-de-sac. These tumors may be the first sign of AIDS. Kaposi's sarcomas occur in about 25% of patients with AIDS, and about 18% of patients with the sarcomas have conjunctival lesions.[390]

Neuro-ophthalmic abnormalities may occur in AIDS. Cranial nerve palsies are the most common sequelae of neurologic lesions and may be the first or a later sign of neurologic involvement. Visual field loss and vision loss may also be a manifestation of either intracranial infection or neoplasia. Papilledema is a frequent sign of intracranial involvement, but ischemic optic neuropathy is a more rare manifestation. Pupillary abnormalities may be associated with all neurologic manifestations of AIDS.[388,390]

The laboratory diagnosis of AIDS is made by ELISA for HIV. ELISA is a highly specific screening test for the presence of antibodies to the HIV virus. Positive results on the ELISA must then be confirmed by a Western blot test or immunofluorescent assay (IFA). A positive ELISA means only that antibodies to the HIV virus are present and does not imply that the patient will necessarily progress to the full-blown AIDS complex.

Management

Although much research is ongoing regarding therapeutic management of AIDS, no well-defined regimen

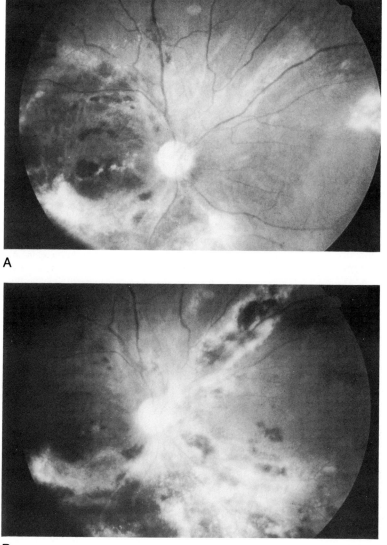

A

B

FIGURE 25.12 *(A)* CMV retinitis in a 27-year-old male with AIDS. *(B)* One month later, showing marked progression of retinitis. (Courtesy Brian P. Den Beste, O.D.)

has been developed. Drugs currently under investigation include hydroxyacyclovir, HPA-23, interferon, suramin, zidovudine, PFA, dapsone, fansidar, and ansamycin. The opportunistic infections must be managed separately, and often the infection reappears when treatment ceases. For toxoplasmic retinitis and encephalitis, pyrimethamine and sulfadiazine are effective against the active organism, but there is a high recurrence rate when treatment is discontinued.[397,398]

There are many reports regarding the treatment of CMV retinitis. Intravenous ganciclovir in dosages ranging from 5 to 14 mg/kg body weight daily for 10 to 20 days appears to effectively halt the progression of CMV retinitis. The only serious side effect is reversible neu-

tropenia. However, since reactivation is inevitable at cessation of treatment, therapy must be continued indefinitely.[399–405] Several authors[406,409] have recommended intravitreal injections of ganciclovir.

Clearly the best possible management for AIDS is prevention through appropriate education and prophylaxis. The following is a summary of current recommendations to prevent transfer of HIV.[407,408]

1. Special care must be exercised regarding all sexual contacts.
2. Gloves should be worn when there is potential contact with body secretions or blood. Otherwise, rou-

tine examination followed by careful handwashing are sufficient.

3. Masks may be worn in the examination of patients suspected of having airborne opportunistic organisms.

4. Goggles or eye shields should be worn when infected fluids might be splashed into the eyes.

5. All needles and syringes should be disposed of properly in "contaminant" containers.

6. Tonometer tips and all other instruments making contact with the eye should be disinfected after use. HIV is inactivated by 5 to 10 minute exposure to 3% hydrogen peroxide, a 1:10 dilution of household bleach, or 70% ethanol or isopropyl alcohol. Environmental surfaces may be disinfected in the same manner.

7. Rigid polymethylmethacrylate (PMMA) contact lenses and rigid gas-permeable lenses should be disinfected with commercially available hydrogen peroxide systems. Soft contact lenses may be heat-disinfected or disinfected with commercially available hydrogen peroxide systems.

References

1. Von Bayer A. Ber Deutsch Chemistrie. Ges 1871;4:555.
2. Burk A. Die Klinische, physiologische und pathologische bedeutung der fluoreazenz in augenach darreichung von uranin. Klin Monatsbl Augenheilkd 1910;48:454–455.
3. Kikai K. Ueber die vitalfarbung des hinteren bulbussabschnittes. Arch Augenheilkd 1930;103:541.
4. Novotny HR, Alvis DL. A method of photographing fluorescein in circulating blood in the human retina. Circulation 1961;24:82–86.
5. Patz A, Fine SL. Interpretation of the fluorescein angiogram. Boston: Little, Brown, 1977.
6. Schatz H. Interpretation of fundus fluorescein angiography. St. Louis: C.V. Mosby Co, 1978.
7. Kelley JS, Kincaid M. Retinal fluorography using oral fluorescein. Arch Ophthalmol 1979;97:2331–2332.
8. Hunter JE. Oral fluorography in retinal pigment epithelial detachment. Am J Optom Physiol Opt 1982;59:926–928.
9. Hunter JE. Oral fluorography in papilledema. Am J Optom Physiol Opt 1983;60:908–910.
10. The Oral Fluorescein Study Group. Oral fluorography. J Am Optom Assoc 1985;10:784–792.
11. Yamana Y, Ohnishi Y, Taniguchi Y, Ikeda M. Early signs of diabetic retinopathy by fluorescein angiography. Jpn J Ophthalmol 1983;27:218–227.
12. Starup K, Larsen HW, Enk B, Vestermark S. Fluorescein angiography in diabetic children. Acta Ophthalmol 1980;58:347–354.
13. Klemen UM, Freyler H, Schober E, Frisch H. Diagnosis of retinal vascular changes in diabetic children by means of fluorescein angiography. Monatsschr Kinderheilkd 1980;128:502–505.
14. Schimizu K, Kobayashi Y, Muraoka K. Midperipheral fundus involvement in diabetic retinopathy. Ophthalmology 1981;88:601–612.
15. Terry J. Ophthalmic photography and fluorescein angiography. In: Terry J, ed. Ocular disease. Boston: Butterworths, 1984.
16. Bianchi C. Fluorescein angiography. Why not in color? J Fr Ophthalmol 1980;3:715–718.
17. Hyvarinen L, Flower RW. Indocyanine green fluorescein angiography. Acta Ophthalmol 1980;58:528–538.
18. Jacob JS, Rosen ES, Young E. Report of the substance, dimethyl formamide, in sodium fluorescein used for fluorescein angiography. Br J Ophthalmol 1982;66:567–568.
19. Romanchuk KG. Fluorescein. Physiochemical factors affecting its fluorescence. Surv Ophthalmol 1982;26:269–283.
20. Butner RW, McPherson AR. Adverse reactions in intravenous fluorescein angiography. Ann Ophthalmol 1983;15:1084–1086.
21. Arroyave CM. Plasma complement and histamine changes after intravenous administration of sodium fluorescein. Am J Opthahlmol 1969;87:474–479.
22. Pacurariu RI. Low incidence of side effects following fluorescein angiography. Ann Ophthalmol 1982;14:32–36.
23. Ellis PP, Schoenberger M, Rendi MA. Antihistamines as prophylaxis against side reactions to intravenous fluorescein. Trans Am Ophthalmol Soc 1980;78:190–205.
24. Brown RE, Sabates R, Drew SJ. Metoclopramide as prophylaxis for nausea and vomiting induced by fluorescein. Arch Ophthalmol 1987;105:658–659.
25. Irwin R. Practical aspects of oral fluorography. J Ophthal Photog 1981;4:16–18.
26. Noble MJ, Cheng H, Jacobs PM. Oral fluorescein and cystoid macular edema: Detection in aphakic and pseudophakic eyes. Br J Ophthalmol 1984;68:221–224.
27. Emerson GA, Anderson HH. Toxicity of certain proposed antileprosy dyes: Fluorescein, eosin, erythrosin and others. Int J Leprosy 1934;2:257–263.
28. Kelley JS, Kincaid M, Hoover RE, McBeth C. Retinal fluorograms using oral fluorescein. Ophthalmology 1980;87:805–811.
29. Morgan KS, Franklin RM. Oral fluorescein angioscopy in aphakic children. J Pediatr Ophthalmol Strabismus 1984;21:33–36.
30. El-Mofty A, Barada A, Yaqoub M. Fundus fluorescein angioscopy in vaso-occlusive diseases of the retina. Bull Ophthalmol Soc Egypt 1982;75:237–241.
31. Balogh VJ. The use of oral fluorescein angiography in idiopathic central serous chorioretinopathy. J Am Optom Assoc 1986;57:909–913.
32. Cunha-Vaz JG, Fonseca JR, Hagenouw JRB. Treatment of early diabetic retinopathy with cyclandelate. Br J Ophthalmol 1976;61:399–404.
33. Davis MD, Meyers FL, Bresnick GH, DeVenecia G. Natural evolution. In: L'Esperance FA, ed. Current diagnosis and management of chorioretinal disease. St. Louis: C.V. Mosby Co, 1977;179–184.
34. Henkes HE. Advances in electro-ophthalmology. Its use in retinal vascular diseases. In: Deutman AF, ed. Doc Ophthalmol Proc Series 1976;7:181–186.
35. Yonemura D, Aoki T, Tsuzuki K. Electroretinogram in diabetic retinopathy. Arch Ophthalmol 1962;68:19–24.

36. Yonemura D, Kawasabo K. The early receptor potential in the human electroretinogram. Jpn J Physiol 1967;17:235–244.

37. Yonemura D, Tsusuki K, Aoki T. Clinical importance of the oscillatory potential in the human ERG. Acta Ophthalmol (Suppl) 1963;70:115–123.

38. Simonsen SE. ERG in diabetics. In: Francois J, ed. The clinical value of electroretinography. ISCERG Symposium, Ghent 1966; New York: Karger, 1968;403–412.

39. Schmoeger E. ERG and EOG in systemic diseases (main report). In: Schmoeger E, Kelsey JH, eds. Doc Ophthal Proc Series 1980;23:3–7.

40. Biersdorf WR, Grizzard WS, Malone JI. Early detection of diabetic retinopathy in children. In: Niemeyer G, Huber CH, eds. Doc Ophthal Proc Series 1982;31:185.

41. Simonsen SE. ERG in juvenile diabetics. In: Goldberg MF, Fine SL, eds. Symposium on the treatment of diabetic retinopathy 1969. U.S. Public Health Service pub. no. 1980. Washington, DC: U.S. Government Printing Office, 1969;681–689.

42. Nemtseev HJ, Mikhaliloua NA, Makarskaya NV, et al. Electroretinography and chronoperimetry in the treatment of diabetic retinopathy by drugs and light coagulation. In: Schmoeger E, Kelsey JH, eds. Doc Ophthal Proc Series 1980;23:63–66.

43. Marquez MC, Santiesteban R, Castro A, et al. The significance of some electrophysiological methods in the diagnosis of the diabetic retinopathy. In: Schmoeger E, Kelsey JH, eds. Doc Ophthal Proc Series 1980;23:77–78.

44. Bresnick GH, Jones RM, Mattson D, et al. The relationship between ERG abnormalities and fundus lesions in diabetic retinopathy. In: Niemeyer G, Huber CH, eds. Doc Ophthal Proc Series 1982;31:186.

45. Speros P, Price J. Oscillatory potentials: History, techniques and potential use in the evaluation of disturbances of retinal circulation. Surv Ophthalmol 1981;25:237–252.

46. Frost-Larsen K, Larsen H, Simonsen SE. Oscillatory potential and nyctometry in insulin-dependent diabetics. Acta Ophthalmol 1980;58:879–888.

47. Steno Study Group. Effect of 6 months of strict metabolic control on eye and kidney function in insulin-dependent diabetics with background retinopathy. Lancet 1982;121–124.

48. Coupland SG, Kirkham TH, Evans G. Electrophysiological determination of contrast sensitivity function in the clinical setting. In: Niemeyer G, Huber CH, eds. Doc Ophthal Proc Series 1982;31:361–369.

49. Kakisu Y, Adachi-Usami E, Chiba J, Kuroda N. Central visual field tests by means of checker board pattern VECPs. In: Niemeyer G, Huber CH, eds. Doc Ophthal Proc Series 1982;31:407–413.

50. Yamazaki H, Adachi-Usami E, Chiba Y. Contrast thresholds of diabetic patients determined by means of the VECP and psychophysical measurements. In: Niemeyer G, Huber CH, eds. Doc Ophthal Proc Series 1982;31:446.

51. Roever J, Schaubele G, Huettel M. Computer assisted evaluation of clinical applied VEP in some ophthalmological and neurological diseases. In: Schmoeger E, Kelsey JH, eds. Doc Ophthal Proc Series 1980;23:127–132.

52. Mueller W, Haase E, Gauss J, Henning G. Experience and results of perimetric investigation by means of VECP. In: Schmoeger E, Kelsey JH, eds. Doc Ophthal Proc Series 1980;23:263–268.

53. Walther A. A new perimeter for electroperimetry. In: Schmoeger E, Kelsey JH, eds. Doc Ophthal Proc Series 1980;23:269–271.

54. Weber P, Henning G. First experience gathered in computer-aided detection of electroperimetric VECP. In: Schmoeger E, Kelsey JH, eds. Doc Ophthal Proc Series 1980;23:273–276.

55. Henning G, Spittel U, Mueller W, Weber P. An attempt to computer-aided detection of VECP for electroperimetry. In: Schmoeger E, Kelsey JH, eds. Doc Ophthal Proc Series 1980;23:279–282.

56. Gutman FA. Discussion of macular branch vein occlusion. Ophthalmology 1980;87:98–104.

57. Shulman J, Jampol LM, Goldberg MF. Large capillary aneurysms secondary to venous obstruction. Br J Ophthalmol 1981;65:36–41.

58. Joffe L, Goldberg RE, Magaragal LE, Annesley WH. Macular branch vein occlusion. Ophthalmology 1980;87:91–97.

59. Editorial. Retinal vein occlusion. Br J Ophthalmol 1979;63:375–376.

60. Orth DH, Patz A. Retinal branch vein occlusion. Surv Ophthalmol 1978;22:357–376.

61. Dodson PM, Galton DJ, Hamilton JM, Blach RK. Retinal vein occlusion and the prevalence of lipoprotein abnormalities. Br J Ophthalmol 1982;66:161–164.

62. McGrath MA, Wechsler F, Hunyor ABL, Penney R. Systemic factors contributory to retinal vein occlusion. Arch Intern Med 1978;138:216–220.

63. Walsh PN, Goldberg RE, Tax RL, Magargal LE. Platelet coagulant activities and retinal vein thrombosis. Thromb Haemostas 1977;38:399–406.

64. Bonnet P. Le "signe de prethrombose" observe sur les vaisseaux de la retine dans l'hypertension arterielle. Arch Ophthalmol 1951;11:12–34.

65. Gutman FA, Zegarra H. The natural course of temporal retinal branch vein occlusion. Trans Am Acad Ophthalmol Otolaryngol 1974;78:178–192.

66. Mason G. Iris neovascular tufts. Ann Ophthalmol 1980;12:420–422.

67. Blankenship GW, Okun E. Retinal tributary vein occlusion. History and management by photocoagulation. Arch Ophthalmol 1973;89:363–368.

68. Michels RG, Gass JDM. The natural course of retinal branch vein obstruction. Trans Am Acad Ophthalmol Otolaryngol 1974;78:166–177.

69. Trempe CL, Takahashi M, Topilow HW. Vitreous changes in retinal branch vein occlusion. Ophthalmology 1981;88:681–687.

70. Hayreh SS, March W, Phelps CD. Ocular hypotony following retinal vein occlusion. Arch Ophthalmol 1978;96:827–833.

71. Orth DH. Vascular occlusions. In: Patz A, Fine SL, eds. Intrepretation of the fundus fluorescein angiogram. Int Ophthalmol Clin 1977;17:97–112.

72. Regenbogen L, Godel V, Feiler-Ofry V, et al. Retinal breaks secondary to vascular accidents. Am J Ophthalmol 1977;84:187–196.

73. Ramos-Umpierre A, Berrocal JA. Retinal detachment fol-

lowing branch vein occlusion. Ann Ophthalmol 1977;9:339–340.

74. Gombos GM. Retinal vascular occlusions and their treatment with low molecular weight dextran and vasodilators: Report of six years' experiences. Ann Ophthalmol 1978;10:579–583.

75. Houtsmuller AJ, Vermeulen JA, Klompe M, et al. The influence of ticlopidine on the natural course of retinal vein occlusion. Agents Actions (Suppl) 1984;15:219–229.

76. Wetzig PC. The treatment of acute branch vein occlusion by photocoagulation. Am J Ophthalmol 1979;87:66–73.

77. Laatikainen L. Photocoagulation in retinal venous occlusion. Acta Ophthalmologica 1977;55:478–488.

78. Shilling JS, Jones CA. Retinal branch vein occlusion: A study of argon laser photocoagulation in the treatment of macular edema. Br J Ophthalmol 1984;68:196–198.

79. Gutman FA, Zegerra H, Rauer A, Zakov N. Photocoagulation in retinal branch vein occlusion. Ann Ophthalmol 1981;13:1359–1363.

80. Gutman FA, Zegarra H. Macular edema secondary to occlusion of the retinal veins. Surv Ophthalmol 1984;28 Suppl:462–470.

81. Jalkh AE, Avila MP, Zakka KA, et al. Chronic macular edema in retinal branch vein occlusion; role of laser photocoagulation. Ann Ophthalmol 1984;16:526–529, 532–533.

82. The Branch Vein Occlusion Study Group. Argon laser photocoagulation for macular edema in branch vein occlusion. Am J Ophthalmol 1984;98:271–282.

83. Branch Vein Occlusion Study Group. Argon laser scatter photocoagulation for prevention of neovascularization and vitreous hemorrhage in branch vein occlusion. Arch Ophthalmol 1986;104:34–41.

84. McGarth MA, Wechsler F, Hunyor AB, Penney R. Systemic factors contributory to retinal vein occlusion. Arch Intern Med 1978;2:216–220.

85. Ririe DG, Cosgriff TM, Martin B. Central retinal vein occlusion in a patient with familial antithrombin III deficiency: Case report. Ann Ophthalmol 1979;11:1841–1845.

86. Brunette I, Boghen D. Central retinal vein occlusion complicating spontaneous carotid cavernous fistula. Case report. Arch Ophthalmol 1987;105:464–465.

87. Barton CH, Viziri ND. Central retinal vein occlusion associated with hemodialysis. Am J Med Sci 1979;277:39–47.

88. Priluck IA. Impending central retinal vein occlusion associated with increased platelet aggregability. Ann Ophthalmol 1979;11:79–84.

89. Walsh PN, Goldberg RE, Tax RL, Magargal LE. Platelet coagulant activities and retinal vein thrombosis. Thromb Haemostas 1977;38:399–406.

90. Heidrich H, Hofner J, Wollensak J, Schneider D. Retinal vascular occlusion and thrombocyte aggregation. J Med 1980;11:127–131.

91. Dodson PM, Galton DJ, Hamilton AM, Black PK. Retinal vein occlusion and the prevalence of lipoprotein abnormalities. Br J Ophthalmol 1982;66:161–164.

92. Hedges TR Jr, Giliberti OL, Magargal LE. Intravenous digital subtraction angiography and its role in ocular vascular disease. Arch Ophthalmol 1985;103:666–669.

93. Brown GC, Shah HG, Magargal LE, Savino PJ. Central retinal vein obstruction and carotid artery disease. Ophthalmology 1984;91:1627–1633.

94. Gonder JR, Magargal LE, Walsh PN, et al. Central retinal vein obstruction associated with mitral valve prolapse. Can J Ophthalmol 1983;18:220–222.

95. Green WR, Chan CC, Hutchins GM, Terry JM. Central retinal vein occlusion: A prospective histopathologic study of 29 eyes in 28 cases. Trans Am Ophthalmol Soc 1981;79:371–422.

96. Priluck IA, Robertson DM, Holenhorst RW. Long-term follow-up occlusion of the central retinal vein in young adults. Am J Ophthalmol 1980;2:190–202.

97. Littlejohn GO, Urowitz MB, Paulin CJ. Central retinal vein occlusion and scleroderma: Implications for sclerodermatous vascular disease. Ann Rheum Dis 1981;40:96–99.

98. Smith P, Green WR, Miller NR, Terry JM. Central retinal vein occlusion in Reye's syndrome. Arch Ophthalmol 1980;98:1256–1260.

99. Silverman M, Lubeck MJ, Briney WG. Central retinal vein occlusion complicating systemic lupus erythematosus. Arthritis Rheum 1978;21:839–843.

100. Kline LB, Kirkham TH, Belanger G, Remillard G. Traumatic central retinal vein occlusion. Ann Ophthalmol 1978;10:587–591.

101. Hayreh SS, van Heuven WA, Hyareh MS. Experimental retinal vascular occlusion. Pathogenesis of central retinal vein occlusion. Arch Ophthalmol 1978;96:311–323.

102. Frucht J, Shapiro A, Merin S. Intraocular pressure in retinal vein occlusion. Br J Ophthalmol 1984;68:26–28.

103. Hayreh SS, March W, Phelps CD. Ocular hypotony following retinal vein occlusion. Arch Ophthalmol 1978;96:827–833.

104. Bloome MA. Transient angle-closure glaucoma in central retinal vein occlusion. Ann Ophthalmol 1977;9:44–48.

105. Servais GE, Thompson HS, Hayreh SS. Relative afferent pupillary defect in central retinal vein occlusion. Ophthalmology 1986;93:301–303.

106. Zegarra H, Gutman FA, Conforto J. The natural course of central retinal vein occlusion. Ophthalmology 1979;86:1931–1942.

107. Frucht J, Hanko L, Norin S. Central retinal vein occlusions in young adults. Acta Ophthalmol 1984;62:780–786.

108. Zegarra H, Gutman FA, Zakov N, Carim M. Partial occlusion of the central retinal vein. Am J Ophthalmol 1983;96:330–357.

109. Little HL, Chan CC. Infrequency of retinal neovascularization following central retinal vein occlusion attributed to endothelial death. Mod Probl Ophthalmol 1979;20:121–126.

110. Magargal LE, Brown GC, Augsburger JJ, Parrish RK. Neovascular glaucoma following central retinal vein obstruction. Ophthalmology 1981;88:1095–1101.

111. Tasman W, Magargal LE, Augsburger JJ. Effects of argon laser photocoagulation on rubeosis iridis and angle neovascularization. Ophthalmology 1980;87:400–402.

112. Lunta MH, Schenker HI. Retinal vascular accidents in glaucoma and ocular hypertension. Surv Ophthalmol 1980;25:163–167.

113. Ellis PP. Retinal vein occlusion. In: Fraunfelder FT, Roy FH, eds. Current ocular therapy. Philadelphia: W.B. Saunders Co, 1980;561–562.

114. Minturn J, Brown GC. Progression of nonischemic central retinal vein obstruction to the ischemic variant. Ophthalmology 1986;93:1158–1162.

115. Jaeger EA. Venous obstructive disease of the retina. In: Duane TD, ed. Clinical ophthalmology. Philadelphia: Harper & Row, 1981;3:Chap. 15, pp. 12–13.

116. Gombos GM. Retinal vascular occlusions and their treatment with low molecular weight dextran and vasodilators: Report of six years' experience. Ann Ophthalmol 1978; 10:579–583.

117. Hansen LL, Daniseyski P, Arntz HR, et al. A randomized prospective study on treatment of central retinal vein occlusion by isovolemic hemodilution and photocoagulation. Br J Ophthalmol 1985;69:108–116.

118. Laatikainen L. Photocoagulation in retinal venous occlusion. Acta Ophthalmol 1977;55:478–488.

119. Laatikainen L. Preliminary report on effect of panphotocoagulation on rubeosis iridis and neovascular glaucoma. Br J Ophthalmol 1977;61:278–284.

120. Smith RJ. Rubeotic glaucoma. Br J Ophthalmol 1981;65:606–609.

121. Demeler U. Management of retinal venous occlusion. Ophthalmologica 1980;180:61–67.

122. May DR, Klein ML, Peyman GA, Raichand M. Xenon arc panretinal photocoagulation for central retinal vein occlusion: A randomized prospective study. Br J Ophthalmol 1979;63:725–734.

123. Carter JE. Panretinal photocoagulation for progressive ocular neovascularization secondary to occlusion of the common carotid artery. Ann Ophthalmol 1984;16:572–576.

124. Laatikainen L, Kohner EM, Khoury D, Black RK. Panretinal photocoagulation in central retinal vein occlusion: A randomized controlled clinical study. Br J Ophthalmol 1977;61:741–753.

125. Manschot WA. Retinal neovascularization after retinal vaso-obliteration. Frequency-origin-morphology. Doc Ophthalmol 1983;55:117–120.

126. Kerns TP, Siekert RG, Sandt TM. The ocular aspects of bypass surgery of the carotid artery. Mayo Clin Proc 1979;54:3–11.

127. Kerns TP, Younge BR, Piepgras DG. Resolution of venous stasis retinopathy after carotid bypass surgery. Mayo Clin Proc 1980;55:342–346.

128. Cowan CL Jr, Butler G. Ischemic oculopathy. Ann Ophthalmol 1983;15:1052–1057.

129. Brown GC, Magargal LE, Schachat A, Shah H. Neovascular glaucoma. Etiologic considerations. Ophthalmology 1984;91:315–320.

130. Chopdar A. Dual trunk central retinal vein incidence in clinical practice. Arch Ophthalmol 1984;102:85–87.

131. Sanborn GE, Magargal LE. Characteristics of the hemispheric retinal vein occlusion. Ophthalmology 1984;91:1616–1626.

132. Hayreh SS, Hayreh MS. Hemi-central retinal vein occlusion. Pathogeneses, clinical features, and natural history. Arch Ophthalmol 1980;98:1600–1609.

133. Sayegh F. Obstruction of the central retinal artery. Comparison of the ophthalmodynamometry measurements in relation to the time. Ophthalmologica 1979;179:322–329.

134. Wilson LA, Warlow CP, Russell RW. Cardiovascular disease in patients with retinal arterial occlusion. Lancet 1979;1:292–294.

135. Cullen JG, Korcusba K, Masser G, et al. Calcified left ventricular thrombus causing repeated retinal arterial emboli: Clinical, echocardiographic, and pathologic features. Chest 1981;79:708–710.

136. Brockmeier LB, Adolph RJ, Gustin BW, et al. Calcium emboli to the retinal artery in calcific aortic stenosis. Am Heart J 1981;101:32–37.

137. Baker RS, Tibbs PA, Millett AJ. Carotid-retinal embolism with coexistant mitral valve prolapse. Neurology 1981; 31:1192–1193.

138. Rush JA, Kearns TP, Danielson GK. Cloth-particle retinal emboli from artificial cardiac valves. Am J Ophthalmol 1980;89:845–850.

139. Reese LT, Shafer D. Retinal embolization from endocarditis. Ann Ophthalmol 1978;10:1655–1657.

140. Appen RE. Central retinal artery occlusion. In: Fraunfelder FT, Roy FH, eds. Current ocular therapy. Philadelphia: W.B. Saunders Co, 1980;549–550.

141. Stowe GC III, Zakov ZN, Albert DM. Central retinal vascular occlusion associated with oral contraceptives. Am J Ophthalmol 1978;86:798–801.

142. Solomon SM, Solomon JH. Bilateral central retinal artery occlusions in polyarteritis nodosa. Ann Ophthalmol 1978;10:567–569.

143. Wilson RS, Havener WH, McGrew RN. Bilateral retinal artery and choriocapillaris occlusion following the injection of long-acting corticosteroid suspension in combination with other drugs. I. Clinical studies. Ophthalmology 1978;85:967–973.

144. Whiteman DW, Rosen DA, Pinkerton RM. Retinal and choroidal microvascular embolism after intranasal corticosteroid injection. Am J Ophthalmol 1980;89:851–853.

145. Hallerman D, Singh B. Iatrogenic central retinal artery embolization: A complication of cardiac catherization. Ann Ophthalmol 1984;16:1025–1027.

146. Jonas J, Kolbe K, Volcker HE, et al. Central retinal artery occlusion in Sneddon's disease associated with antiphospholipid antibodies. Am J Ophthalmol 1986;102:37–40.

147. Cheney ML, Blair PA. Blindness as a complication of rhinoplasty. Arch Otolaryngol Head Neck Surg 1987;113:768–769.

148. Etre JM, Magnus DE, Jones WL. Central retinal artery occlusion with an irido-embolus following carotid endarterectomy. J Am Optom Assoc 1987;58:419–422.

149. LaMonica CB, Foye GJ, Silberman L. A case of sudden retinal artery occlusion and blindness in pregnancy. Obstet Gynecol 1987;69:433–435.

150. Bradish CF, Flowers M. Central retinal artery occlusion in association with osteogenesis imperfecta. Spine 1987;12:193–194.

151. Brown GC, Magargal LE, Simeone FA, et al. Arterial obstruction and ocular neovascularization. Ophthalmology 1982;89:139–146.

152. Hodes BL, Edelman D. Central retinal artery occlusion after facial trauma. Ophthalmic Surg 1979;10:21–23.

153. Weissman H, Nadel AJ, Dunn M. Simultaneous bilateral retinal arterial occlusions treated by exchange transfusions. Arch Ophthalmol 1979;97:2151–2153.

154. Deutsch TA, Read JS, Ernest JT, et al. Effects of oxygen and carbon dioxide on the retinal vasculature in humans. Arch Ophthalmol 1983;101:1278–1280.

155. Henbink P, Chambers JK. Arterial occlusive disease of the

retina. In: Duane TD, ed. Clinical ophthalmology. Philadelphia: Harper & Row, 1981;3; Chap. 14, p. 14.

156. Sheng FC, Quinones-Baldrich W, Machleder HI, et al. Relationship of extracranial carotid occlusive disease and central retinal artery occlusion. Am J Surg 1986;152:175–178.

157. Schatz H, Drake M. Self-injected retinal emboli. Ophthalmology 1979;86:468–483.

158. Nehen AM, Damgaard-Jensen L, Hansen PE. Foreign body embolism of retinal arteries as a complication of carotid angiography. Neuroradiology 1978;15:85–88.

159. Gass JD, Tiedeman J, Thomas MA. Idiopathic recurrent branch retinal arterial occlusion. Ophthalmology 1986; 93:1148–1157.

160. Nielsen NV. Treatment of acute occlusion of the retinal arteries. Acta Ophthalmologica 1979;57:1078–1081.

161. Iwafune Y, Yoshimoto H. Clinical use of pentoxifylline in haemorrhagic disorders of the retina. Pharmatherapeutica 1980;2:429–438.

162. Herman WH, Sinnock P, Brenner E, et al. An epidemiologic model for diabetes mellitus: Incidence, prevalence and mortality. Diabetes Care 1984;7:367–371.

163. Mazze RS, Sinnock P, Deeb L, et al. An epidemiological model for diabetes mellitus in the United States: Five major complications. Diabetes Res Clin Pract 1985;1:185–191.

164. Drury TF, Powell AL. Prevalence, impact, and demography of known diabetes in the United States. NCHS Advance Data 1986;14:1–14.

165. Wilson PM, Anderson KM, Kannel WB. Epidemiology of diabetes mellitus in the elderly. The Framingham Study. Am J Med 1986;80:3–9.

166. Lipson LG. Diabetes in the elderly: Diagnosis, pathogenesis, and therapy. Am J Med 1986;80:10–21.

167. Kahn HA, Moorehead HB. Statistics on blindness in the model reporting area 1969 to 1970. U.S. Department of Health, Education and Welfare pub. no. 73–427. Washington, DC: U.S. Government Printing Office, 1971.

168. Vision Research Center. A national plan: 1978–1982. National Advisory Eye Council 1977. U.S. Department of Health, Education and Welfare pub. no. 78-1258. Washington, DC: U.S. Government Printing Office, 1977.

169. Dwyer MS, Melton LJ, Ballard DJ, et al. Incidence of diabetic retinopathy and blindness: A population-based study in Rochester, Minnesota. Diabetes Care 1985;8:316–322.

170. Klein R, Klein BE, Moss SE, et al. Retinopathy in young-onset diabetic patients. Diabetes Care 1985;8:311–315.

171. Mitchell P. Development and progression of diabetic eye disease in Newcastle (1977–1984): Rates and risk factors. Aust NZ J Ophthalmol 1985;13:39–44.

172. Grey RH, Malcolm N, O'Reilly D, Morris A. Ophthalmic survey of a diabetic clinic. I. Ocular findings. Br J Ophthalmol 1986;70:797–803.

173. Klein R, Davis MD, Moss SE, et al. The Wisconsin epidemiological study of diabetic retinopathy. Adv Exp Med Biol 1985;189:321–335.

174. Jerneld B, Algvere P. The prevalence of retinopathy in insulin-dependent juvenile-onset diabetes mellitus—a fluorescein angiographic study. Acta Ophthalmol 1984;62:617–630.

175. Phelps RL, Sakol P, Metzger BE, et al. Changes in diabetic retinopathy during pregnancy. Correlations with regulation of hyperglycemia. Arch Ophthalmol 1986;104:1806–1810.

176. Esmann U, Jensen HJ, Lundbaek K. Disappearance of waxy exudates in diabetic retinopathy during administration of p-amino salicylate (PAS). Acta Med Scand 1963;174:99–104.

177. Dobbie JG. Increased platelet aggregation in diabetes mellitus. J Lab Clin Med 1972;80:236–246.

178. Dobbie JC, Kwaan HC, Colwell J, Suwanwela N. Role of platelets in pathogenesis of diabetic retinopathy. Arch Ophthalmol 1974;91:107–109.

179. Bridges JM, Dolby AM, Millar JHD, Weaver JA. An effect of D-glucose on platelet stickiness. Lancet 1965;1:75–77.

180. Fields WS, Hass WK. Aspirin, platelets, and stroke. St. Louis: Green, 1971;51–52.

181. Fahraeus R. Suspension stability of the blood. Acta Med Scand 1921;55:1.

182. Ditzel J, Moinat P. Changes in serum proteins, lipoproteins, and protein-bound carbohydrates in relation to pathologic alterations in microcirculation of diabetic subjects. J Lab Clin Med 1959;54:843.

183. Van Haeringer NJ, Oosterhuis JA, Terpstra J, Glasius E. Erythrocyte aggregation in relation to diabetic retinopathy. Diabetologia 1973;9–20.

184. Skovborg F, Nielson AV, Schlichtkrull J, Dizel J. Blood viscosity in diabetic patients. Lancet 1966;1:129.

185. Little HL. Pathogenesis. In: L'Esperance FA, James WA, eds. Diabetic retinopathy: Clinical evaluation and management. St. Louis: C.V. Mosby Co, 1981:58–88.

186. Bloodworth JM. Diabetic microangiopathy. Diabetes 1963; 12:99–114.

187. Cogan G, Merola L, Laibson PR. Blood viscosity, serum hexosamine, and diabetic retinopathy. Diabetes 1961;10:393.

188. Keen H, Chlouverakis C. Metabolic factors in diabetic retinopathy. In: Graymore CN, ed. First international symposium on the biochemistry of the retina. New York: Academic Press, 1964:121–136.

189. Carol WW, Geeraets WJ. Diabetic retinopathy and salicylates. Ann Ophthalmol 1972;4:1019–1046.

190. Kornzweig AL. Capillary microaneurysms and shunt vessels in diabetic retinopathy. Ann Ophthalmol 1972;4:589.

191. Cogan DG (moderator). Aldose reductase and complications of diabetes. Ann Intern Med 1984;101:82–91.

192. Buzney SM, Frank RN, Varma SD, et al. Aldose reductase in retinal mural cells. Invest Ophthalmol Vis Sci 1977;16:392–396.

193. Kinoshita JH. Aldose reductase in the diabetic eye. Am J Ophthalmol 1986;102:685–692.

194. Dvornik D. Aldose reductase inhibition. An approach to the prevention of diabetic complications. New York: Biomedical Information Corporation, 1987.

195. Benson WE, Tasman W, Duane TD. Diabetic retinopathy. In: Duane TD, ed. Clinical ophthalmology. Philadelphia: Harper & Row; 1981; 3:Chap. 30, pp. 1–24.

196. Engerman R, Bloodworth JMB, Nelson BS. Relationship of microvascular disease in diabetes to metabolic control. Diabetes 1977;26:760–769.

197. Cahil GF, Etzwiler DD, Freinke N. Blood glucose control in diabetes. Diabetes 1976;25:237–239.

198. Blankenship GW. Diabetic retinopathy, present and future.

Conclusion of diabetic retinopathy symposium. Ophthalmology 1981;88:658.

199. Friberg TR, Rosenstock J, Sanborn G, et al. The effect of long-term near normal glycemic control on mild diabetic retinopathy. Ophthalmology 1985;92:1051–1058.

200. Caird FT. Control of diabetes and diabetic retinopathy. In: Goldberg MF, Fine SL, eds. Symposium on the treatment of diabetic retinopathy. U.S. Public Health Service pub. no. 1890. Washington, DC: U.S. Government Printing Office, 1969;115–118.

201. Doft BH, Kingsley LA, Orchard TJ, et al. The association between long-term diabetic control and early retinopathy. Ophthalmology 1984;91:763–769.

202. Rosenstock J, Friberg T, Raskin P. Effect of glycemic control on microvascular complications in patients with type I diabetes mellitus. Am J Med 1986;81:1012–1018.

203. Colwell JA. Effect of diabetic control on retinopathy. Diabetes 1966;15:497–499.

204. Eschwege E, Gugot-Argenton C, Aubry JP, Tchobroutsky G. Effect of multiple daily injections on the course of diabetic retinopathy. Diabetes 1976;25:463–469.

205. Waltman SR, Santiago J, Krupin T, et al. Vitreous fluorophotometry and blood-sugar control in diabetics. Lancet 1979;2:1068.

206. Irsigler K, Kritz H, Najemnik C, Freyler H. Reversal of florid diabetic retinopathy (letter). Lancet 1979;2:1068.

207. Seeman P, Sellers EM, Roschlau WHE. Principles of medical pharmacology. Toronto: University of Toronto Press, 1980;3:527.

208. Smith MJH, Smith PK. The salicylates. New York: John Wiley & Sons, 1966;70.

209. Smith PK. The pharmacology of salicylates and related compounds. Ann NY Acad Sci 1960;86:38–63.

210. Nillson S. Treatment of diabetes mellitus with a preparation containing salicylic acid, para-amino benzoic acid, and ascorbic acid (PASCON). Acta Med Scand 1959;165:273–278.

211. Riska N. The effect of PAS on the cholesterol level in the blood. Acta Tuberc Scand 1955;30:134.

212. Mooney AJ. Diabetic retinopathy—a challenge. Br J Ophthalmol 1963;47:513–520.

213. Goldberg MF, Liang JC. Treatment of diabetic retinopathy. Review. Diabetes 1980;29:841–851.

214. Nihard P. Effect of calcium entry blockers on arterioles, capillaries and venules of the retina. Angiology 1982;33:37–45.

215. Clements RS Jr. New therapies for the chronic complications of older diabetic patients. Am J Med 1986;80:54–60.

216. Cunha-Vaz JG, Mota CC, Leite EC, et al. Effect of sorbinil on blood-retinal barrier in early diabetic retinopathy. Diabetes 1986;35:574–578.

217. Pitts NE, Vreeland F, Shaw GL, et al. Clinical experience with sorbinil—an aldose reductase inhibitor. Metabolism 1986;35(4 Suppl 1):96–100.

218. Pfiefer MA. Clinical trials of sorbinil on nerve function. Metabolism 1986;35(4 Suppl 1):78–82.

219. Christensen JE, Varnek L, Gregersen G. The effect of an aldose reductase inhibitor (sorbinil) on diabetic neuropathy and neural function of the retina: A double blind study. Acta Neurol Scand 1985;71:164–167.

220. Solerte SB, Ferrari E. Diabetic retinal vascular complications and erythrocyte filtrability; results of a 2-year follow-up study with pentoxifylline. Pharmatherapeutica 1985;4:341–350.

221. Barnett AH, Armstrong S, Wakelin K, et al. Specific thromboxane synthetase inhibition and retinopathy in insulin-dependent diabetics. Diabetes Res 1986;3:131–134.

222. Takahashi R, Shiraki M, Morita I, et al. Platelet thromboxane synthesizing activity in non-insulin-dependent diabetes: Correlation with diabetic retinopathy and diabetic treatment. Prostaglandins Leukotrienes Med 1985;17:149–158.

223. Ducrey N, Curchod B. Oral buflomedil in diabetic background retinopathy: Results of a preliminary controlled study. J Int Med Res 1984;12:184–187.

224. Watanabe J, Umeda F, Wakasugi H, Ibayashi H. Effect of vitamin E on platelet aggregation in diabetes mellitus. Thromb Haemost 1984;59:313–316.

225. Cunha-Vas JG, Mota CC, Leite EC, et al. Effect of sulindac on the permeability of the blood-retinal barrier in early diabetic retinopathy. Arch Ophthalmol 1985;103:1307–1311.

226. Patz A, Schatz H, Berkow JW, et al. Macular edema: An overlooked complication of diabetic retinopathy. Trans Am Acad Ophthalmol Otolaryngol 1973;77:34–42.

227. Cheng H. Photocoagulation and diabetic retinopathy. Br Med J 1979;365–366.

228. Rubenstein K, Myska V. Pathogenesis and treatment of diabetic maculopathy. Br J Ophthalmol 1974;58:76–84.

229. Blankenship GW. Diabetic macular edema and argon laser photocoagulation: A prospective randomized study. Ophthalmology 1979;86:69–75.

230. Ferris FL, Podgor MJ, Davis MD. Macular edema in diabetic retinopathy study patients. Diabetic retinopathy study report number 12. Ophthalmology 1987;94:754–760.

231. Early Treatment Diabetic Retinopathy Study Research Group. Photocoagulation for diabetic macular edema. Report number 1. Arch Ophthalmol 1985;103:1796–1806.

232. Early Treatment Diabetic Retinopathy Study Research Group. Treatment techniques and guidelines for photocoagulation of diabetic macular edema. Report number 2. Ophthalmology 1987;94:761–774.

233. Olk RJ. Modified grid argon (blue-green) laser photocoagulation for diffuse diabetic macular edema. Ophthalmology 1986;93:938–950.

234. The Diabetic Retinopathy Study Research Group. Indications for photocoagulation treatment of diabetic retinopathy. Report number 14. Int Ophthalmol Cl 1987;27:239–253.

235. The Diabetic Retinopathy Study Research Group. Photocoagulation treatment of proliferative diabetic retinopathy: The second report of diabetic retinopathy study findings. Ophthalmology 1978;85:82–106.

236. The Diabetic Retinopathy Study Research Group. Design, methods and baseline results. Report number 6. Invest Ophthalmol Vis Sci 1981;21:149–209.

237. The Diabetic Retinopathy Study Research Group. A modification of the Airlie House classification of diabetic retinopathy. Report number 7. Invest Ophthalmol Vis Sci 1981;21:210–226.

238. The Diabetic Retinopathy Study Research Group. Four risk factors for severe visual loss in diabetic retinopathy. The

third report from the diabetic retinopathy study. Arch Ophthalmol 1979;97:654–655.

239. The Diabetic Retinopathy Study Research Group. Preliminary report on effects of photocoagulation therapy. Am J Ophthalmol 1976;81:383–396.

240. The Diabetic Retinopathy Study Research Group. Photocoagulation therapy of proliferative diabetic retinopathy: The second report of diabetic retinopathy study findings. Ophthalmology 1978;85:82–106.

241. Wolbarsht ML, Landers MB. The rationale of photocoagulation therapy for proliferative diabetic retinopathy: A review and a model. Ophthalmic Surg 1980;11:235–245.

242. Liggett PE, Lean JS, Barlow WE, Ryan SJ. Intraoperative argon endophotocoagulation for recurrent vitreous hemorrhage after vitrectomy for diabetic retinopathy. Am J Ophthalmol 1987;103:146–149.

243. Thompson JT, de Bustros S, Michels RG, Rice TA. Results and prognostic factors in vitrectomy for diabetic traction detachment of the macula. Arch Ophthalmol 1987;105:497–502.

244. Thompson JT, de Bustros S, Michels RG, et al. Results of vitrectomy for proliferative diabetic retinopathy. Ophthalmology 1986;93:1571–1574.

245. Ramsay RC, Knobloch WH, Cantrill HL. Timing of vitrectomy for active proliferative diabetic retinopathy. Ophthalmology 1986;93:283–289.

246. The DRVS Research Group. Two-year course of visual acuity in severe proliferative diabetic retinopathy with conventional management. Ophthalmology 1985;92:492–501.

247. Crock GW. Vitreous hemorrhage. In: Fraunfelder FT, Roy FH, eds. Current ocular therapy. Philadelphia: W.B. Saunders Co, 1980;579–580.

248. Sipila I. Inhibition of arginino-glycine aminotransferase by ornithine. A possible mechanism for the muscular and chorioretinal atrophies in gyrate atrophy of the choroid and retina with hyperornithinemia. Biochem Biophys Acta 1980;613:79–84.

249. Francois J. Gyrate atrophy of the choroid and retina. Ophthalmologica 1979;178:311–320.

250. Kaiser-Kupfer MI, Valle D, Bron AJ. Clinical and biochemical heterogeneity in gyrate atrophy. Am J Ophthalmol 1980;89:219–222.

251. McCulloch C. Choroideremia and gyrate atrophy. In: Duane TD, ed. Clinical ophthalmology. Philadelphia: Harper & Row; 1981;3:Chap. 25, pp. 6–9.

252. Valle D, Walser M, Brusilow SW, Kaiser-Kupfer M. Gyrate atrophy of the choroid and retina. Amino acid metabolism and correction of hyperornithinemia with an arginine-deficient diet. J Clin Invest 1980;63:371–378.

253. Kaiser-Kupfer M, deMonasterio FM, Valle D, et al. Gyrate atrophy of the choroid and retina: Improved visual function following reduction of plasma ornithine by diet. Science 1980;210:1128–1131.

254. Vannus-Sulonen K, Sipilä I, Vannus A, et al. Gyrate atrophy of the choroid and retina: A five-year follow-up of creatine supplementation. Ophthalmology 1985;92:1719–1727.

255. Kennaway NG, Weleber RG, Buist NRM. Gyrate atrophy of the choroid and retina with hyperornithinemia: Biochemical and histologic studies in response to vitamin B_6. Am J Hum Genet 1980;32:529–541.

256. Ogura Y, Takahashi M, Ueno S, Honda Y. Hyperboric oxygen treatment for chronic cystoid macular edema after branch retinal vein occlusion. Am J Ophthalmol 1987; 104:301–302.

257. Heckenlively JR. Grid photocoagulation for macular edema in patients with retinitis pigmentosa (letter). Am J Ophthalmol 1987;104:94–95.

258. MacKay CJ, Shek MS, Carr RE, et al. Retinal degeneration with nanophthalmos, cystic macular degeneration, and angle closure glaucoma. A new recessive syndrome. Arch Ophthalmol 1987;105:366–371.

259. Lewis H, Singer TR, Hanscom TA, Straatsma BR. A prospective study of cystoid macular edema after neodymium: YAG laser posterior capsulotomy. Ophthalmology 1987; 94:478–482.

260. Henderly DE, Hammond RS, Rao NA, Smith RE. The significance of the pars plana exudate in pars planitis. Am J Ophthalmol 1987;103:669–671.

261. Brown GC. Macular edema in association with severe carotid artery obstruction. Am J Ophthalmol 1986;102:442–448.

262. Dulaney DD. Cystoid macular edema and corneal-relaxing incisions (letter). Arch Ophthalmol 1987;105:742–743.

263. Carter J, Barron BA, McDonald MB. Cystoid macular edema following corneal-relaxing incisions. Arch Ophthalmol 1987;105:70–72.

264. Brough GH, Jones WL. Long-standing venous stasis retinopathy with resultant cystoid macular edema. J Am Optom Assoc 1987;58:423–425.

265. Nussenblatt RB. Macular alterations secondary to intraocular inflammatory disease. Ophthalmology 1986;93:984–988.

266. Irvine AR. Cystoid maculopathy. Surv Ophthalmol 1976;21:1–17.

267. Irvine AR. Cystoid maculopathy (cystoid macular edema, Irvine-Gass syndrome). In: Fraunfelder FT, Roy FH, eds. Current ocular therapy. Philadelphia: W.B. Saunders Co, 1980;517–519.

268. Watzke RC. Acquired macular disease. In: Duane TD, ed. Clinical ophthalmology. Philadelphia: Harper & Row, 1981;3:Chap. 23, pp. 22–24.

269. Yamaaki H, Hendrikse F, Deutman AF. Iris angiography after cataract extraction and the effect of indomethacin eyedrops. Ophthalmologica 1984;188:82–86.

270. Urner-Bloch U. Prävention des zystoiden Makulaödems nach Kataraktextraktion durch lokale Indomethacin Applikation. Klin Monatsbl Augenheikd 1983;183:479–484.

271. Miyake K. Indomethacin in the treatment of postoperative cystoid macular edema. Surv Ophthalmol 1984;28:554–568.

272. Yannuzzi LA. A perspective on the treatment of aphakic cystoid macular edema. Surv Ophthalmol 1984;28:540–553.

273. Sanders DR, Kraff M. Steroidal and nonsteroidal anti-inflammatory agents; effect on postsurgical inflammation and blood-aqueous humor barrier breakdown. Arch Ophthalmol 1984;102:1453–1456.

274. Jampol LM. Pharmologic therapy of aphakic and pseudophakic cystoid macular edema. Ophthalmology 1985;92:807–810.

275. Kraff MC, Sanders DR, Jampol LM, et al. Prophylaxis of pseudophakic cystoid macular edema with indomethacin. Ophthalmology 1982;89:886–889.

276. Burnett J, Tessler H, Isenberg S, Tso MOM. Double-masked

trial of fenoproxen sodium: Treatment of chronic aphakic cystoid macular edema. Ophthalmic Surg 1983;14:150–152.

277. Flach AJ, Dolan BJ, Irvine AR. Effectiveness of ketorolac tromethamine 0.5% ophthalmic solution for chronic aphakic and pseudophakic cystoid macular edema. Am J Ophthalmol 1987;103:479–486.

278. Watzke RC, Burton TC, Woolson RF. Direct and indirect laser photocoagulation of central serous choroidopathy. Am J Ophthalmol 1979;88:914–918.

279. Braustein RA, Gass JDM. Serous detachments of the retinal pigment epithelium in patients with senile macular disease. Am J Ophthalmol 1979;88:652–660.

280. Newsome DA, Blackarski PA. Grid photocoagulation for macular edema in patients with retinitis pigmentosa. Am J Ophthalmol 1987;103:161–166.

281. Perkins ES. Ocular toxoplasmosis. Br J Ophthalmol 1973;57:1–17.

282. Feldman HA. Toxoplasmosis. N Engl J Med 1968;279:1431–1437.

283. Desmonts F, Couvreur J. Congenital toxoplasmosis. A prospective study of 378 pregnancies. N Engl J Med 1974;290:1110–1116.

284. Kimball AC, Kean BH, Fuchs F. Congenital toxoplasmosis. A prospective study of 4,048 obstetric patients. Am J Obstet Gynecol 1971;111:211–218.

285. Amos CS. Posterior segment involvement in selected pediatric infectious diseases. J Am Optom Assoc 1979;50:1211–1220.

286. Schlaegel TF. Toxoplasmosis. In: Duane TD, ed. Clinical ophthalmology. Philadelphia: Harper & Row, 1981;4 Chap. 51, pp. 1–17.

287. Carter AD, Frank JW. Congenital toxoplasmosis: Epidemiologic features and control. Can Med Assoc J 1986;135:618–623.

288. Corwin JM, Weiter JJ. Immunology of chorioretinal disorders. Surv Ophthalmol 1981;25:287–305.

289. O'Conner GR. Protozoan diseases of the uvea. Int Ophthalmol Clin 1977;17:163–176.

290. Streilein JW, Kaplan HJ. Immunologic privilege in the anterior chamber. In: Silverman AM, O'Connor GR, eds. Immunology and immunopathology of the eye. New York: Masson, 1979;174–179.

291. O'Connor GR. Manifestations and management of ocular toxoplasmosis. Bull NY Acad Med 1974;50:192–210.

292. Reese LT, Shafer DM, Zweifach P. Acute acquired toxoplasmosis. Ann Ophthalmol 1981;13:467–470.

293. Masur H, Lempert JA, Cherubini TD. Outbreak of toxoplasmosis in a family and documentation of acquired retinochoroiditis. Am J Med 1978;64:396–402.

294. Gump DW, Holden RA. Acquired chorioretinitis due to toxoplasmosis. Ann Intern Med 1979;90:58–60.

295. Willerson D, Aaberg TM, Reeser F, Meredith TA. Unusual ocular presentation of acute toxoplasmosis. Br J Ophthalmol 1971;61:693–698.

296. Hoerni B, Vallat M, Durand M, Pesme D. Ocular toxoplasmosis and Hodgkin's disease. Arch Ophthalmol 1978;96:62–63.

297. Orzalesi N, Ricciardi L. Segmental retinal periarteritis. Am J Ophthalmol 1971;72:55–59.

298. Schwartz PL. Segmental retinal periarteritis as a complication of toxoplasmosis. Ann Ophthalmol 1977;9:157–162.

299. Nicholson D. Ocular toxoplasmosis in an adult receiving long-term corticosteroid therapy. Arch Ophthalmol 1976;94:248–254.

300. Braunstein RA, Gass JDM. Branch artery obstruction caused by acute toxoplasmosis. Arch Ophthalmol 1980;98:512–513.

301. Saari M. Toxoplasmic chorioretinitis affecting the macula. Acta Ophthalmologica 1977;55:539–547.

302. Robinson RO, Bauman RJ. Late cerebral relapse of congenital toxoplasmosis. Arch Dis Child 1980;55:231–232.

303. Kean BH, Kimball AC. The complement-fixation test in the diagnosis of congenital toxoplasmosis. Am J Dis Child 1977;131:21–28.

304. Sabin A. Complement fixation test in toxoplasmosis and persistence of the antibody in human beings. Pediatrics 1949;4:443–452.

305. Potasman I, Araujo FG, Remington JS. Toxoplasma antigens recognized by naturally occurring human antibodies. J Clin Microbiol 1986;24:1050–1054.

306. Lindenschmidt EG. Demonstration of immunoglobulin M class antibodies to toxoplasma gondii antigenic component p 35000 by enzyme-linked antigen immunoabsorbent assay. J Clin Microbiol 1986;24:1045–1049.

307. Tomasi JP, Schlit AF, Stadtsbaeder S. Rapid double-sandwich enzyme-linked immunoabsorbent assay for detection of human immunoglobulin M anti-*Toxoplasma gondii* antibodies. J Clin Microbiol 1986;24:849–850.

308. Lin TM, Chin-See MW, Halbert SP, Joseph JM. An enzyme immunoassay for immunoglobulin M antibodies to *Toxoplasma gondii* which is not affected by rheumatoid factor or immunoglobulin G antibodies. J Clin Microbiol 1986;23:77–82.

309. Martin WG, Grown GC, Parris RK, et al. Ocular toxoplasmosis and visual field defects. Am J Ophthalmol 1980;90:25–29.

310. Schlaegel TF. Perspectives in uveitis. Ann Ophthalmol 1981;13:799–806.

311. Sabates R, Pruett RC, Brockhurst RJ. Fulminant ocular toxoplasmosis. Am J Ophthalmol 1981;92:497–503.

312. O'Connor GR. Toxoplasmosis (ocular toxoplasmosis, toxoplasmic retinochoroiditis). In: Fraunfelder FT, Roy FH, eds. Current ocular therapy. Philadelphia: W.B. Saunders Co, 1980;99–101.

313. Schlaegel TF. Essentials of uveitis. Boston: Little, Brown, 1969;181–207.

314. Fenkel JK, Jacobs L. Ocular toxoplasmosis. Arch Ophthalmol 1958;59:260–279.

315. Sabates R, Pruett RC, Brockhurst RJ. Ocular toxoplasmosis treated with pyrimethamine (letter). Am J Ophthalmol 1982;93:371–372.

316. Tessler HH. Ocular toxoplasmosis. Int Ophthalmol Clin 1981;21:185–189.

317. Ferguson JG. Clindamycin therapy for toxoplasmosis. Ann Ophthalmol 1981;13:95–100.

318. Antibiotic colitis—new cause, new treatment. Med Lett Drugs Ther 1979;21:97.

319. Nozik RA. Results of treatment of ocular toxoplasmosis with injectable corticosteroids. Trans Am Acad Ophthalmol Otolaryngol 1977;83:811–818.

320. Spalter HF, Campbell CJ, Noyori KS, et al. Prophylactic photocoagulation of recurrent toxoplasmic retinochoroiditis. A preliminary report. Arch Ophthalmol 1966;75:21–31.

321. Ghartey KN, Brockhurst RJ. Photocoagulation of active toxoplasmic retinochoroiditis. Am J Ophthalmol 1980;89:858–864.

322. Fitzgerald CR. Pars plana vitrectomy for vitreous opacity secondary to presumed toxoplasmosis. Arch Ophthalmol 1980;98:321–323.

323. Brown DH. Ocular *Toxocara canis*. J Pediatr Ophthalmol 1970;7:182–191.

324. Schantz PM, Glickman LT. Current concepts in parasitology. Toxocaral visceral larva migrans. N Engl J Med 1978;298:436–439.

325. Berrocal J. Prevalence of *Toxocara canis* in babies and in adults as determined by the ELISA test. Trans Am Ophthalmol Soc 1980;78:376–413.

326. Shantz PM, Weis PE, Pollard ZF, White MC. Risk factors for toxocaral ocular larval migrans. A case-control study. Am J Public Health 1980;70:1269–1272.

327. Glickman LT, Shantz PM. Epidemiology and pathogenesis of zoonotic toxocariasis. Epidemiol Rev 1981;3:230–250.

328. Morris PD, Katerndahl DA. Human toxocariasis. Review with report of a probable cause. Postgrad Med 1987;81:263–267.

329. Brown GC, Tasman WS. Retinal arterial obstruction in association with presumed *Toxocara canis* neuroretinitis. Ann Ophthalmol 1981;1385–1387.

330. Liesegang TJ. Atypical ocular toxocariasis. J Pediatr Ophthalmol 1977;14:349–353.

331. Dugid IM. Features of ocular infestation by *Toxocara*. Br J Ophthalmol 1961;45:789–796.

332. Schlaegel TF. Uveitis and miscellaneous parasites. Int Ophthalmol Clin 1977;17:177–194.

333. Pollard ZF, Jarrett WH, Hagler WS, et al. ELISA for diagnosis of ocular toxocariasis. Ophthalmology 1979;86:743–752.

334. Felberg NT, Shields JA, Federman JF. Antibody to *Toxocara canis* in the aqueous humor. Arch Ophthalmol 1981;99:1563–1564.

334. Kennedy JJ, Defeo E. Ocular toxocariasis demonstrated by ultrasound. Ann Ophthalmol 1981;13:1357–1358.

336. Pollard ZF. Ocular *Toxocara* in siblings of two families. Diagnosis confirmed by ELISA test. Arch Ophthalmol 1979;97:2319–2320.

337. Woodruff AW. Toxocariasis (visceral larva migrans). In: Fraunfelder FT, Roy FH, eds. Current ocular therapy. Philadelphia: W.B. Saunders Co, 1980;98–99.

338. Nolan J. Chronic toxocaral endophthalmitis: Successful treatment of a case with subconjunctival depot corticosteroids. Br J Ophthalmol 1976;60:365–370.

339. Crane TB, Christensen GR. Presumed subretinal nematode infestation with visual recovery. Ann Ophthalmol 1981;13:345–348.

340. Hagler WS, Pollard ZF, Jarrett WH, Donnelly EH. Results of surgery for ocular *Toxocara canis*. Ophthalmology 1981;88:1081–1086.

341. Nowack D, Goebel KM. Genetic aspects of sarcoidosis. Class II histocompatability antigens and a family study. Arch Intern Med 1987;147:481–483.

342. Bernardino VB, Naidoff MA. Retinal inflammatory disease. In: Duane TD, ed. Clinical ophthalmology. Philadelphia: Harper & Row, 1981;3:Chap. 10, p. 7.

343. Jabs DA, Johns CJ. Ocular involvement in chronic sarcoidosis. Am J Ophthalmol 1986;102:297–301.

344. Obenauf CD, Shaw HE, Sydnor CF. Klintworth GK. Sarcoidosis and its ophthalmic manifestations. Am J Ophthalmol 1978;86:648–655.

345. Spalton DJ, Sanders MD. Fundus changes in histologically confirmed sarcoidosis. Br J Ophthalmol 1981;65:348–358.

346. Mizuno K, Takahashi J. Sarcoid cyclitis. Ophthalmology 1986;93:511–517.

347. O'Day J, Schilling JS, Ffytche TJ. Retinal vasculitis. Trans Ophthalmol Soc UK 1979;99:163–166.

348. Noble KG. Ocular sarcoidosis occuring as a unilateral optic disk vascular lesion. Am J Ophthalmol 1979;87:490–493.

349. Doxanas MT, Kelley JS, Prout TE. Sarcoidosis with neovascularization of the optic nerve head. Am J Ophthalmol 1980;90:347–351.

350. Gragoudas ES, Regan CDJ. Peripapillary subretinal neovascularization in presumed sarcoidosis. Arch Ophthalmol 1981;99:1194–1197.

351. Weinreb RN, Kimura SJ. Uveitis associated with sarcoidosis and angiotensin converting enzyme. Trans Am Ophthalmol Soc 1979;77:280–293.

352. Lieberman J, Sastree A. An angiotensin-converting enzyme (ACE) inhibitor in human serum. Increased sensitivity of the serum ACE assay for detecting active sarcoidosis. Chest 1986;90:869–875.

353. Stern BJ, Griffin DE, Luke RA, et al. Neurosarcoidosis: Cerebrospinal fluid lymphocyte subpopulations. Neurology 1987;37:878–881.

354. Sethi KD, el Gammal T, Patel BR, Swift TR. Dural sarcoidosis presenting with transient neurologic symptoms. Arch Neurol 1986;43:595–597.

355. Valantine H, McKenna WJ, Nihoyannopoulas P, et al. Sarcoidosis: A pattern of clinical and morphological presentation. Br Heart J 1987;57:256–263.

356. Ohtahara A, Kotake H, Hisatome I, et al. Mashiba H. Complete atrioventricular block with a 22 month history of ocular sarcoidosis: A case report. Heart Lung 1987;16:66–68.

357. Weinreb RN, Barth R, Kimura SJ. Limited gallium scans and angiotensin coverting enzyme in granulomatous uveitis. Ophthalmology 1980;87:202–209.

358. Merritt JC, Lipper SL, Peiffer RL, Hale LM. Conjunctival biopsy in sarcoidosis. J Natl Med Assoc 1980;72:347–349.

359. Nicols CW, Eagle RC, Yanoff M, Menocal NG. Conjunctival biopsy as an aid in the evaluation of the patient with suspected sarcoidosis. Ophthalmology 1980;87:287–289.

360. Kataria YP. Chlorambucil in sarcoidosis. Chest 1980;78:36–43.

361. Letocha CE, Sarcoidosis. In: Fraunfelder FT, Roy FH, eds. Current ocular therapy. Philadelphia: W.B. Saunders Co, 1980;320–321.

362. O'Leary TJ, Jones G, Yip A, et al. The effects of chloroquine on serum 1, 25-dihydroxyvitamin D and calcium metabolism in sarcoidosis. N Engl J Med 1986;315:727–730.

363. Lobes LA, Folk JC. Syphilitic phlebitis simulating branch vein occlusion. Ann Ophthalmol 1981;13:825–827.

364. Martin NF, Green WR, Martin LW. Retinal periphlebitis in the Irvine-Gass syndrome. Am J Ophthalmol 1977;83:377–386.

365. Algvere P, Alanko H, Kickhoff K, et al. Pars plana vitrectomy in the management of intraocular inflammation. Acta Ophthalmol 1981;59:727–736.

366. Klein ML. Eales' disease. In: Fraunfelder FT, Roy FH, eds. Current ocular therapy. Philadelphia: W.B. Saunders Co, 1980;552–553.

367. Elliot AJ. Periphlebitis retinae. In: Duane TD, ed. Clinical ophthalmology. Philadelphia: Harper & Row, 1981;3:Chap. 16, pp. 1–6.

368. Katzman B, Tiwari RD. Eales' disease: A case of rapid progression. Ann Ophthalmol 1979;11:1323–1326.

369. Sigelman J, Behrens M, Hilal S. Acute posterior multifocal placoid pigment epitheliopathy associated with cerebral vasculitis and homonymous hemianopsia. Am J Ophthalmol 1979;88:919–924.

370. Goen TM, Terry JE. Acute posterior multifocal placoid pigment epitheliopathy. J Am Optom Assoc 1987;58:112–117.

371. Azar P, Gohd RS, Waltman D, Gitter KA. Acute posterior multifocal placoid pigment epitheliopathy associated with adenovirus type 5 infection. Am J Ophthalmol 1975;80:1003–1005.

372. Van Buskirk M, Lessell S, Friedman E. Pigment epitheliopathy and erythema nodosum. Arch Ophthalmol 1971;85:369–372.

373. Jacklin HN. Acute posterior multifocal placoid pigment epitheliopathy and thyroiditis. Arch Ophthalmol 1977;95:995–997.

374. Kirkham TH, Ffytche TJ, Sanders MD. Placoid pigment epitheliopathy with retinal vasculitis and papillitis. Br J Ophthalmol 1972,56:875–886.

375. Wright BE, Bird AC, Hamilton AM. Placoid pigment epitheliopathy and Harada's disease. Br J Ophthalmol 1978;62:609–621.

376. Deutman AF, Lion F. Choriocapillaris nonperfusion in acute multifocal placoid pigment epitheliopathy. Am J Ophthalmol 1977;84:652–657.

377. Kersten DH, Lessell S, Carlow TJ. Acute posterior multifocal placoid pigment epitheliopathy and late onset meningo-encephalitis. Ophthalmology 1987;94:393–396.

378. Gass JDM. Acute posterior multifocal placoid pigment epitheliopathy. Arch Ophthalmol 1968;80:177–185.

379. Ryan SJ, Maumenee AE. Acute posterior multifocal placoid pigment epitheliopathy. Am J Ophthalmol 1972;74:1066–1074.

380. Bird AC, Hamilton AM. Placoid pigment epitheliopathy. Presenting with bilateral serous retinal detachment. Br J Ophthalmol 1972;56:881–886.

381. Hedges TR, Sinclair SH, Gragoudas ES. Evidence for vasculitis in acute posterior multifocal placoid pigment epitheliopathy. Ann Ophthalmol 1979;11:539–542.

382. Young NJA, Bird AC, Sehmi K. Pigment epithelial diseases with abnormal choroidal perfusion. Am J Ophthalmol 1980;90:607–618.

383. Holt WS, Regan CDJ, Trempe C. Acute posterior multifocal placoid pigment epitheliopathy. Am J Ophthalmol 1976;81:404–412.

384. Annesley WH, Tomer TL, Shields JA. Multifocal placoid pigment epitheliopathy. Am J Ophthalmol 1973;76:511–518.

385. Murray SB. Acute posterior multifocal placoid pigment epitheliopathy. Not so benign? Trans Ophthalmol Soc UK 1979;99:497–500.

386. Report. AOA News. Jan. 15, 1988; 3.

387. Spira TJ. The acquired immunodeficiency syndrome. In: Inslor MS, ed. AIDS and other sexually transmitted diseases and the eye. Orlando, FL: Grune & Stratton, 1987;119–144.

388. Den Beste BP, Hummer J. AIDS: A review and guide for infection control. J Am Optom Assoc 1986;57:675–682.

389. Springer M. Ophthalmologists on the front line treating AIDS patients. Arch Ophthalmol 1987;105:325.

390. Holland GN. Ophthalmic disorders associated with the acquired immunodeficiency snydrome. In: Inslor MS, ed. AIDS and other sexually transmitted diseases and the eye. Orlando, FL: Grune & Stratton, 1987;145–172.

391. Henderly DE, Freeman WR, Smith RE, et al. Cytomegalovirus retinitis as the initial manifestation of the acquired immunodeficiency syndrome. Ann Ophthalmol 1987;103:316–320.

392. Rotterdam H. Tissue diagnosis of selected AIDS-related opportunistic infections. Am J Surg Pathol 1987;11 Suppl:3–15.

393. Levy RM, Rosenbloom S, Perrett LV. Neuroradiologic findings in AIDS: A review of 200 cases. Am J Radiol 1986;147:977–983.

394. Berger JR, Maskowitz L, Fisch IM, Kelley RE. Neurologic disease as the presenting manifestation of acquired immunodeficiency syndrome. South Med J 1987;80:683–686.

395. Mills J. Pneumocystis carinii and Toxoplasma gondii infections in patients with AIDS. Rev Infect Dis 1986;8:1001–1011.

396. Nistal M, Santana A, Paniaqua R, Palacios J. Testicular toxoplasmosis in two men with the acquired immunodeficiency syndrome (AIDS). Arch Pathol Lab Med 1986;110:744–746.

397. Meredith JT. Toxoplasmosis of the central nervous system. Am Fam Physician 1987;35:113–116.

398. Haverkos HW. Assessment of therapy for Toxoplasma encephalitis. The TE Study Group. Am J Med 1987;82:907–914.

399. Pepose JS, Newman C, Bach MC, et al. Pathologic features of cytomegalovirus retinopathy after treatment with the antiviral agent ganciclovir. Ophthalmology 1987;94:414–424.

400. Henderley DE, Freeman WR, Causey DM, Rao NA. Cytomegalovirus retinitis and response to therapy with ganciclovir. Ophthalmology 1987;94:425–434.

401. Rosecan LR, Laskin OL, Kalman CM, et al. Antiviral therapy with ganciclovir for cytomegalovirus retinitis and bilateral exudative retinal detachments in an immunocompromised child. Ophthalmology 1986;93:1401–1407.

402. Holland GN, Sidikaro Y, Kreiger AE, et al. Treatment of cytomegalovirus retinopathy with ganciclovir. Ophthalmology 1987;94:815–823.

403. Jabs DA, Newman C, De Bustros S, Polk BF. Treatment of cytomegalovirus retinitis with ganciclovir. Ophthalmology 1987;94:824–830.

404. Orellana J, Teich SA, Friedman AH, et al. Combined short- and long-term therapy for the treatment of cytomegalovirus

retinitis using ganciclovir (BWB759U). Ophthalmology 1987;94:831–838.

405. Laskin OL, Stahl-Bayliss CM, Kalman CM, Rosecan LR. Use of ganciclovir to treat serious cytomegalovirus infections in patients with AIDS. J Infect Dis 1987;155:323–327.

406. Henry K, Cantrill H, Fletcher C, et al. Use of intravitreal ganciclovir (dihydroxy propoxymethylquanine) for cytomegalovirus retinitis in a patient with AIDS. Am J Ophthalmol 1987;103:17–23.

407. Centers for Disease Control. Recommendations for preven-

tion of HIV transmission in health-care settings. MMWR 1987;36(Suppl no. 25):3–18.

408. Centers for Disease Control. Recommendations for preventing possible transmission of human T-lymphotropic virus type III/lymphadenopathy-associated virus from tears, MMWR 1985;34:533–534.

409. Ussery FM, Gibson SR, Conklin RH, et al. Intravitreal ganciclovir in the treatment of AIDS-associated cytomegalovirus retinitis. Ophthalmology 1988;95:640–648.

CHAPTER 26

Diseases of the Optic Nerve

Larry J. Alexander

Recognition of diseases of the optic nerve is crucial because of the neurologic implications. Differential diagnosis of clinical signs and symptoms is extremely important because secondary neurologic testing can be expensive, and treatment of most optic neuropathies involves the use of steroids that have inherent risks. This chapter considers methods of differential diagnosis of optic nerve anomalies as well as the therapeutic management of these disorders.

Clinical Anatomy of the Optic Nerve

Gross Anatomy

To understand the various aspects of optic nerve compromise, one must have a working knowledge of relevant optic nerve anatomy. The optic nerve is actually a white-matter tract of the brain rather than a true cranial nerve. The nerve can be divided into 4 portions: (1) intraocular—1 mm length and 1.5 mm diameter; (2) intraorbital—25 to 30 mm length and about 3 to 4 mm diameter; (3) intraosseus—4 to 10 mm length; (4) intracranial—14 to 20 mm length. One important fact to recognize is that the intraorbital portion is 25 to 30 mm long while the distance from the posterior aspect of the globe to the optic foramen is only 20 mm. The nerve must therefore have a somewhat tortuous course. This becomes important clinically when one attempts to elicit pain on gross ocular excursions associated with optic neuritis. The nerve must straighten before it can tug on the pain receptors of the basal meninges attachment of the nerve to the orbital wall. To accom-

plish this the nerve must be straightened by full excursions to one side or the other.

Microscopic Anatomy

The optic nerve head is separated into several regions. The surface nerve fiber layer is the most superficial layer. The prelaminar or glial region is a supportive and nutritive region for the nerve fibers. This area occupies over half the optic nerve head volume. The lamina is connective and glial tissue that bridges the scleral canal. The retrolaminar optic nerve is about twice the diameter of the intraocular portion due to the presence of myelin. This part of the optic nerve is enclosed in a sheath of dura, arachnoid, and pia—a direct continuation of the brain.

Vascular Supply

The vascular supply of the optic nerve originates from the ophthalmic artery, a branch of the internal carotid system. The central retinal artery enters the nerve posterior to the globe and courses forward to the papillary branches to serve the inner retinal layers. The majority of the arterial blood supply to the nerve emanates from an incomplete circle of Zinn, which consists of short posterior ciliary arteries, the posterior ciliary arteries, the pial arterial network, and small branches of the central retinal artery. The compartmentalized concept of blood supply to the nerve head is important in understanding such entities as anterior ischemic optic neuropathy, in which isolated areas of the nerve head are destroyed.

Diagnosis of Optic Nerve Disease

Case History

An informative case history is extremely important for the differential diagnosis and subsequent management of diseases of the optic nerve. Rarely will a patient present with an acquired problem of the optic nerve without some degree of subjective symptomatology. The most informative means of assessing the signs and symptoms is to establish a temporal profile. The temporal profile of the problem establishes when, where, and how (under what circumstances) the signs and symptoms first occurred. How long did the problem last? What followed the problem? Did it recur? Were there associated signs and symptoms? All these factors contribute to the establishment of this profile.

Figure 26.1 illustrates the thought process involved in establishing a temporal profile. Each answer to questions posed should provoke either another question or initiate further testing procedures.

In addition to the temporal profile, the clinician must ascertain family and personal medical and ocular history. Table 26.1 illustrates some examples of temporal profile symptomatology.

Visual Acuity

Visual performance analysis is vital in the assessment of optic nerve disease. All tests of visual performance must be carried out through the best refractive correction. A significant aspect of any visual acuity assessment is the refraction to best visual acuity or a pinhole test over the current prescription.

Visual acuity can be tested in a variety of ways (Snellen, illiterate E, etc.) depending on the situation. In testing for optic nerve disease one must also consider assessment of functional visual acuities. Functional acuity can be defined as the ability to perform a visual task such as reading. A patient with a right homonymous hemianopsia, for example, might very well be able to recognize isolated letters but would have noticeable difficulty reading a line of print. Such monocular functional acuities act as an effective means of detecting subtle optic nerve abnormalities.

Another method of evaluating visual function is contrast sensitivity. Arden and Gucukoglu[1] have reported greater sensitivity using printed sinusoidal gratings as an indicator of reduced acuity in retrobulbar neuritis than by using visually evoked responses (VER). Their findings support the suggestion by Regan and associates[2] that grating (contrast sensitivity) tests permit earlier diagnosis of multiple sclerosis.

Color Vision

When retinal disease affects the photoreceptors, there is a reduction or loss of function. When the cones are involved, this is manifest clinically as some degree of color vision loss or desaturation. Retinal lesions that

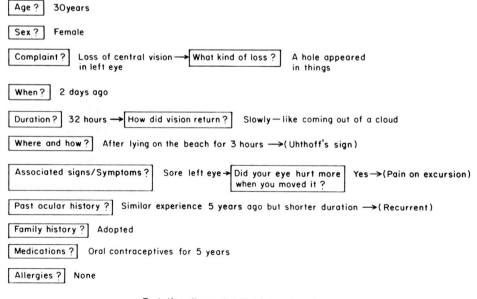

Tentative diagnosis : Multiple sclerosis

FIGURE 26.1   **Example of questioning needed to generate a temporal profile.**

TABLE 26.1
Examples of Temporal Profile Symptomatology

Symptom	Probable Cause
Loss of vision over night	Common in thrombosis
5- to 15-second losses or blurring of vision	Transient obscurations of papilledema or impending central retinal vein occlusion
Abrupt loss of vision progressively worsening	Hemorrhage
Loss of vision for a few days, followed by partial return of vision	Demyelinizing disease
5 to 15 (up to 60)-minute losses of vision returning to normal	Transient monocular blindness of internal carotid stenosis (Retinal stroke)
Slowly progressive loss of vision	Neoplasm
Sudden bilateral contraction of fields (tubular)	Vertebrobasilar stroke sparing macular fibers
Sudden hemianopic field loss	Contralateral postchiasmal interruption of blood flow
Sudden fading of vision with postural change	Hypotensive attack—may also occur with mitral valve prolapse

reduce visual acuity do not necessarily cause a proportionate reduction in color perception. Often in-depth testing will demonstrate only mild defects.[3] However, defects in the optic nerve will create faulty conduction of the nerve impulse, leading to reduced color perception. Glaser[4] has described the concept of optic nerve defects "as a barrier to conduction in the optic nerve and to which the nerve fibers associated with cone function are preferentially sensitive." He points out that a "focal fundus lesion corresponds only to an isolated hole in the color sensitive retina." This barrier concept can also be used to explain the results of evaluation procedures such as light comparison testing, contrast sensitivity, Pulfrich stereo phenomenon, neutral density filter testing, and VER. In all cases the optic nerve exhibits a delayed or diminished response to stimulation. Figure 26.2 illustrates a schematic representation of the barrier concept of optic nerve conduction defects.

Of all manifestations of optic nerve conduction defects in idiopathic retrobulbar neuritis, Linksz[5] reports that color vision is the first visual function to be involved and the last to be restored. Wildberger and Van Lith[6] found that the Farnsworth-Munsell 100-hue test and the VER were more reliable tests of damage to the optic nerve than were standard visual acuity testing techniques. Griffin and Wray[7] confirmed the validity of the 100-hue test and added that performance on the test can quantify the degree of involvement. Although such standardized color vision tests have value in assessing diseases of the optic nerve, a test of color comparison provides a rapid appraisal of the general status of color vision. After the patient's eyes have been equally light-adapted, the clinician can alternately present to each eye a red-colored target, such as a red cycloplegic bottle cap. The patient is then asked to compare the intensity or quality of the color. The patient with a lesion of the optic nerve will report that the color is desaturated or grayish with the involved

eye. This test can also be used to investigate quadrantic visual field defects associated with optic nerve disease by placing the test object in the appropriate part of the visual field.

Light Comparison Test

This test is a subjective evaluation of optic nerve conduction quality. It is similar to color comparison in

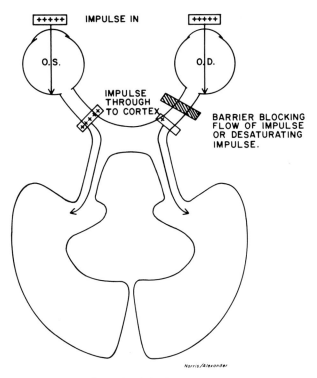

FIGURE 26.2 **Schematic of the barrier concept of optic nerve conduction defects.**

that a bright light is alternately presented to each eye, and the patient is asked to compare his or her perception of the intensity or quality of the light. A patient with an optic nerve conduction defect will report a reduction of light intensity with the involved eye.

The clinician typically presents the light first to the "good eye" and states, "This light is worth a dollar." The light is then moved to the involved eye and the patient is asked, "How much is the light worth now?"

Neutral Density Filter Test

The clinician may employ a 2 log unit neutral density (ND) filter to distinguish a normal eye, an eye with functional amblyopia, and an eye with an optic nerve conduction defect (Table 26.2).[8]

Macular Photostress Test

Macular photostress testing is a noninvasive method of evaluating macular physiologic function. It is a dynamic test of macular performance that is based on measuring the time required for an eye to recover sufficient visual function to perform a defined visual task after it has been dazzled with an intense light.[9] A prolonged photostress recovery time is thought to be associated with altered retinal adaptation. Several studies have proved that the efficiency of retinal adaptability to stress depends not only on the photochemical mechanism of vision but also on the anatomic relationship of the photoreceptors to the retinal pigment epithelium.[10–13] The photostress test serves as a sensitive discriminator between subtle maculopathy and optic neuropathy.[14]

A suggested procedure for performing the macular photostress test is as follows:

1. Determine the best refractive correction and place it in a trial frame.
2. Ensure equal light adaptation in a darkened room.
3. Occlude 1 eye and project the line of best visual acuity.
4. Bleach the patient's eye by projecting the fixation

target of a direct ophthalmoscope on the patient's macula for 10 seconds.
5. After removing the light, time the recovery to the line above the best acuity line.
6. Repeat with the other eye after readaptation to the dark.

The average normal recovery time using this technique is about 50 seconds. A patient with macular dysfunction will have a significantly prolonged photostress recovery time. A recovery time significantly longer with 1 eye compared with its fellow is probably more important than are bilaterally delayed recoveries. A commercially available brightness acuity tester will also provide acceptable results, with some latitude in testing techniques.

Elicitation of Pain on Gross Excursion

Pain on rotation of the eyes is often associated with optic neuritis. From 20% to 50% of patients with optic neuritis have pain on rotation of the globe.[15] It must be emphasized, however, that this is not an absolute sign of optic neuritis. The clinician must elicit large movements of the eyes to put enough stretch on the nerve to stimulate the pain receptors.

Uhthoff's Symptom

Uhthoff's symptom is the reduction of vision function associated with an increase in body temperature. This symptom is most often associated with chronic demyelinizing disease (multiple sclerosis).[16] Goldstein and Cogan[17] even reported enlargement of a preexisting scotoma associated with overheating.

L'Hermitte's Symptom

L'Hermitte's symptom is the sensation of electriclike shocks in the limbs and trunk when the head is flexed forward placing the chin on the chest. This symptom is strongly suggestive of demyelinizing disease.[18]

TABLE 26.2
Expected Results of 2 Neutral Density (ND) Filter Test

Normal	Functional Amblyopia	Optic Nerve Conduction Defect
2- to 3-line reduction in visual acuity	Minimal, if any, reduction in visual acuity	Severe reduction in visual acuity

The Pulfrich Stereo Phenomenon

The Pulfrich stereo phenomenon is the binocular perception of a pendulum swinging in an elliptical path when, in fact, the pendulum is swinging in a straight path. This illusion is created by a difference between the eyes in latency of the visual signal to the cortex. It can be produced artificially by placing a neutral density filter in front of 1 eye, but it can also be created by an optic nerve conduction defect such as optic neuritis.[19]

Pupillary Testing

Pupillary testing is absolutely essential in the differential diagnosis of optic nerve disease. Rather than discuss all possibilities of pupillary abnormalities, this section will address the Marcus Gunn pupil, which reflects an afferent defect of the optic nerve. The best method for demonstrating the Marcus Gunn pupil is the swinging flashlight test.

The swinging flashlight test is performed as follows (assume the left eye has optic neuritis).

1. Penlight to O.D. → O.D. constricts; O.S. constricts
2. Swing penlight to O.S. → O.D. dilates, O.S. dilates
3. Swing penlight to O.D. → O.D. constricts, O.S. constricts

Conclusion → O.S. optic nerve conduction defect (positive Marcus Gunn pupil)

Visual Fields

In differentiating any disease process of the visual pathway, visual field testing is crucial. The subject of visual field testing is beyond the scope of this text. However, the clinician should note that (1) optic nerve disease creates a "hole" in the visual field, while macular disease creates a "mask" over the visual field; (2) the Amsler grid is an excellent central field test where metamorphopsia indicates macular disease; and (3) the vertical meridians are crucial in neurologic testing— field defects associated with retinal disease can cross the vertical meridians, but field defects associated with neurologic disease usually do not do so.

With the advent of automated threshold testing devices, new techniques are now available to assist in the differential diagnosis of optic nerve disease. Automated threshold perimetry is a more sensitive procedure and has led some investigators to conclude that visual field defects in optic nerve disease may be more common than previously thought.[20]

Other Clinical Testing Procedures

Many procedures are available for the clinical differential diagnosis of diseases of the optic nerve. Among these are stereoscopic fundus examination techniques, ultrasonography, fluorescein angiography, and electrodiagnostic procedures. Beyond clinical testing is laboratory assessment, radiologic studies, and neuroradiologic evaluations.

Relatively new testing techniques or modifications of existing techniques show great promise in assisting in differential diagnosis of optic neuropathies. The most effective new procedures include magnetic resonance imaging (MRI), brain stem auditory evoked potentials (BAEP), evaluation of oligoclonal bands in cerebrospinal fluid, and contrast sensitivity testing.[21–31]

Figure 26.3A illustrates a B-scan ultrasonography of an eye with a flat optic nerve head, while Fig. 26.3B illustrates optic nerve head elevation secondary to papilledema. Figure 26.4 shows fluorescein angiographic findings in active ischemic optic neuropathy.

Table 26.3 summarizes the clinical tests available for differentiating between diseases of the macula and diseases of the optic nerve.

The Optic Neuropathies

Acquired optic nerve disease can be the result of numerous afflictions. In the past, terms such as optic neuritis and papilledema have erroneously been applied to optic neuropathy. This discussion will consider all acquired diseases of the optic nerve under the heading of optic neuropathy. Terminology will then be applied that specifically defines the pathologic process. The suffix "-itis" will refer only to proven inflammatory processes, and the term optic disc edema will refer to any swelling of the nerve fibers of the optic nerve. Table 26.4 summarizes the general etiologies of optic neuropathy, while Table 26.5 lists the causes of optic disc edema. Table 26.6 is a simplified summary of typical causes of optic neuropathy by age.

Demyelinizing Optic Neuropathy

ETIOLOGY

Demyelinizing optic neuropathy is classically referred to as retrobulbar neuritis. Demyelinizing optic neuropathy is an inflammatory process of the optic nerve posterior to the globe. The etiology of this condition remains obscure. The association of retrobulbar neuritis with demyelinizing disease is irrefutable,[32,33] but

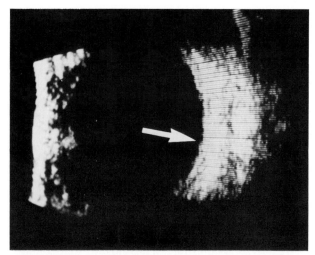

A

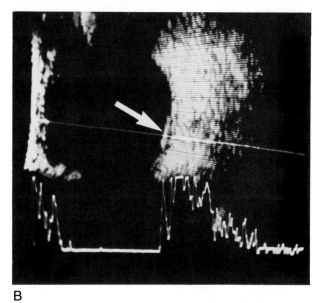

B

FIGURE 26.3 *(A)* B-scan ultrasonography demonstrating a flat optic nerve head (arrow). *(B)* B-scan ultrasonography demonstrating an elevated optic nerve head (arrow) secondary to papilledema.

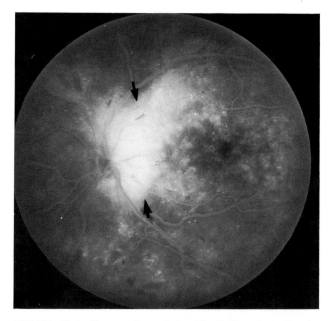

FIGURE 26.4 **Fluorescein angiographic findings in active ischemic optic neuropathy. The inflammed nerve head readily leaks fluorescein.**

other conditions have also been implicated, especially those of viral origin such as herpes zoster[34] and the Guillain-Barré syndrome.[35] In addition, environmental factors such as carbon monoxide poisoning have been reported in a delayed-reaction case of retrobulbar neuritis.[36] Metabolic causes such as diabetes, thyroid disease, and vitamin deficiencies are potential causes of retrobulbar neuritis.[18]

From an epidemiologic standpoint, retrobulbar neuritis is usually a disease of the young. Viral conditions in the active or postinfectious stage can incite the inflammation in children or young adults. Optic neuritis in an individual under 40 years of age should create some concern about the possibility of a demyelinizing disease.

DIAGNOSIS

Diagnosis in the classic sense—"patient sees nothing, doctor sees nothing"—reflects the absence of ophthalmoscopic changes of the optic nerve head. Retrobulbar neuritis is most often unilateral, presenting as an impairment of vision and progressing to maximum loss after 1 week. Tenderness of the globe, especially above the superior rectus muscle, and pain on gross extraocular muscle excursions may also precede or run concurrently with the vision loss. A Marcus Gunn pupil is always present as well, as are variable central or centrocecal scotomas. Diagnostic tests such as color vision, light comparison, Pulfrich stereo phenomenon, and VER are often positive. Uhthoff's and L'Hermitte's symptoms may also be reported. Further neurologic assessment such as Romberg's sign may aid in the differential diagnosis. In addition, double-flash resolution tests may be of benefit in detecting subclinical demyelinization of the visual pathway.[37] As previously mentioned, ophthalmoscopic observation of the nerve head typically reveals normal findings in the active stage. However, if the inflammatory process is near the nerve head, it may be possible to observe some optic disc edema secondary to axoplasmic stasis.

TABLE 26.3
Tests for Differential Diagnosis between Optic Nerve and Retinal (Macular) Disease

Test	Optic Nerve Disease	Macular Disease
Visual acuity	Reduced	Reduced
Contrast sensitivity	Reduced	Reduced
Color vision	Desaturated	May be altered depending on severity
Light comparison test	Positive	Negative
Neutral density filter test	Positive	Negative
Macular photostress test	Negative	Positive
Pain on gross excursions	Positive	Negative
Uhthoff's symptom	Positive	Negative
L'Hermitte's symptom	Positive	Negative
Marcus Gunn pupil	Positive	Negative
Pulfrich stereo phenomenon	Positive	Negative
Visual fields	Hole in field	Shadow over field
Fluorescein angiography	Often negative	Positive

MANAGEMENT

Prognosis for return of vision function is good. Vision characteristically begins to improve within 2 to 3 weeks, with stabilization at near normal by the fourth to fifth week. Some patients improve rapidly to a moderate acuity level, stabilize, then experience a return of vision to near normal over a prolonged period. Recurrences characterize the disease, and with each recurrence there is further compromise of acuity or visual field. Each attack of retrobulbar neuritis can produce optic atrophy, although the incidence of such optic atrophy is as low as 36%.[38]

One additional consideration in prognosis is neuromyelitis optica (Devic's disease), which is considered a variant of multiple sclerosis in children and young adults. This disease is characterized by a rapid, bilateral loss of vision and has a poorer prognosis for visual recovery.

Differential diagnosis is vital. Although most optic neuropathy in the 20- to 40-year age group can be attributed to a demyelinizing disease, the clinician must rule out other potential causes.

TABLE 26.4
Etiology of Optic Neuropathy

- Hereditary or familial
- Inflammatory
- Demyelinizing
- Toxic
- Ischemic
- Compressive

TABLE 26.5
Known Causes of Unilateral Optic Disc Edema

Anterior ischemic optic neuropathy
Carotid cavernous fistula
Cavernous sinus thrombosis
Central retinal vein occlusion
Diabetic papillopathy
Drusen of the nerve head
Foster-Kennedy syndrome
Hemicentral retinal vein occlusion
Leukemic infiltrates of the optic nerve
Orbital cellulitis
Papilledema secondary to intracranial mass or hemorrhage
Papilledema secondary to benign intracranial hypertension
Papillitis
Papillophlebitis
Primary optic nerve tumors
Primary orbital tumors
Thyroid eye disease

TABLE 26.6
Typical Causes of Optic Neuropathy, by Age of Onset

Age (yr)	Typical Cause
1–10	Inflammatory
10–20	Postinfectious
20–40	Demyelinization
50–70	Atherosclerotic anterior ischemic optic neuropathy or toxic optic neuropathy
60–80	Temporal arteritic optic neuropathy

Multiple sclerosis does not always present systemically after demyelinizing optic neuropathy. Reports in the literature vary from 0% to 85% of cases of multiple sclerosis developing after a case of retrobulbar neuritis. Some of the discrepancy involves inappropriate diagnoses of either demyelinizing optic atrophy or multiple sclerosis.

The criteria for the diagnosis of multiple sclerosis are very controversial. The Medical Research Council Committee has developed a set of criteria for classification of the disease (Table 26.7).

Pharmacologic management of all the optic neuropathies is extremely controversial because such neuropathies often spontaneously resolve, and there are no definitive, controlled studies to support therapeutic intervention. Certainly every attempt should be made to ascertain the underlying cause of the neuropathy. If the cause is systemic or neurologic, treatment for that specific condition must be instituted.

The proponents of therapeutic intervention in the optic neuritides cite the fact that significantly more damage can be expected if edema associated with the inflammation is allowed to progress. Photographs after treatment of disc edema in acute papillitis have demonstrated the efficacy of steroid therapy. Reduced edema is thought to lessen the extent of scarring.[39] The "treaters" consider the euphoria-inducing effect of steroids to be beneficial and believe that patients perceive that drugs are necessary in managing a disease that is causing them to "go blind."[40] The medicolegal standards often force the issue toward treatment, since it is often difficult to prove that withholding treatment may be more beneficial than providing it.

The opponents of therapeutic intervention in optic neuritis cite the fact that there is no clinical model to support the theory that edema or inflammation are implicated in the evolution of optic neuritis. It is felt that if edema were involved, more dramatic resolution would be expected after institution of steroid therapy. Even proponents admit no statistical significance in ultimate visual acuities achieved with treatment compared with no treatment, although they report that short-term recovery is enhanced.[41,42] All arguments advocating therapy must be tempered by the inherent risks of adrenocorticotropic hormone (ACTH) or steroid therapy.[43]

If one chooses to institute ACTH or steroid therapy, several precautionary measures must be observed. Before therapy the practitioner must consider the systemic ramifications of such therapy. Several methods of therapy have been used, all intended to produce improvement without creating side effects.

ACTH therapy may be employed through the parenteral route and is advantageous in that it does not suppress adrenal function. Its disadvantage lies in the necessity of hospitalization. Wray[40] uses the following treatment regimen:

> ACTH 20 units/ml, 80 units IV every 6–8 hours in 500 ml of 5% dextrose in water for 3 days. Then ACTH gel (40 units/ml), 40 units IM every 12 hours for 7 days, then the dose is reduced by 10 units every 3 days as follows:

- 35 units b.i.d. × 3 days
- 30 units b.i.d. × 3 days
- 50 units q.d. × 3 days
- 40 units q.d. × 3 days
- 30 units q.d. × 3 days
- 20 units q.d. × 3 days
- 20 units q.o.d. × 3 days

Oral therapy can be provided in the form of prednisone. This approach has economic as well as convenience benefits. Oral prednisone therapy may be instituted as follows: 100 mg the first day, decreasing to 80 mg the second day, 60 mg the following 3 days, and finally 30 mg for the sixth and seventh days. The therapeutic benefit can be assessed after 7 days. If positive, the steroid may be tapered. If the response is negligible, the therapy is discontinued. Other regimens that have been recommended include massive dosages of prednisone (200 mg daily) for 36 to 72 hours to abort the attack, without follow-up treatment, or 60 to 80 mg of prednisone equivalent as alternative-day therapy. All proponents of therapy emphasize the importance of early treatment.

Sub-Tenon's injections of steroids offer another therapeutic approach.[44–46] A sterile, disposable 1 ml tuberculin syringe with a 27-gauge, $\frac{1}{2}$ inch needle is used to inject 1 ml of triamcinolone (Kenalog). The effect of the injection usually lasts for 1 to 2 weeks. Complications include perforation of the globe, pain, hemorrhage, and steroid-induced glaucoma.

TABLE 26.7
Diagnostic Classification Criteria for Multiple Sclerosis

Classification	Clinical Signs or Symptoms
Proven	Pathologic proof
Clinically definite	Some physical disability, remissions and relapses greater than 2 episodes
Early or probable	Signs of lesions at two or more sites
	Age of onset 10–50 years
	No better explanation
	Lesions predominantly in white matter
	Remissions and relapses
	Early single episode suggesting multiple sclerosis with signs of multiple lesions
	Slight or no disability

Fraunfelder and Roy[47] restate the above modes of therapy, pointing out that half the practitioners employ a wait-and-see attitude while the other half use 1 of the 3 suggested methods of treatment. The answer probably lies somewhere between these extremes. If the optic neuritis is severe or if it occurs in the only eye with usable vision, some intervention must be attempted despite the lack of definitive supportive studies.[48]

More recently, attempts have been directed toward the treatment of the demyelinizing disease at a systemic level. These modalities have often demonstrated transient therapeutic benefit to the patients. Forms of interferon therapy have given equivocal results.[49–52] Plasmapheresis still remains controversial.[53] Use of 4-aminopyridine (4-AP) intravenously appears to have transient benefits.[54] Hyperbaric oxygen therapy has not proved to be of benefit.[55]

Inflammatory Optic Neuropathy

ETIOLOGY

Inflammatory optic neuropathy, classically referred to as papillitis, occurs when the optic nerve is affected by a localized inflammatory process that may also secondarily affect the retina (neuroretinitis).

Inflammatory optic neuropathy is the most common form of optic neuropathy in children, and bilateral presentation is more common in children than in adults.[56] From an etiologic standpoint papillitis has been associated with a variety of conditions. Intraocular inflammatory conditions such as juxtapapillary choroiditis, sympathetic ophthalmia, syphilis, toxoplasmosis,[18] and toxocariasis have been implicated. Meningitis, both acute and chronic, has been cited as a cause.[57,58] Viral syndromes such as mumps have been associated with papillitis.[4] There have also been reports of drug-induced papillitis secondary to Cafergot therapy[59,60] (Table 26.8).

DIAGNOSIS

The clinical characteristics of papillitis make the entity easily distinguishable from other conditions of optic disc edema. Symptoms include a rapid loss of vision (central scotoma) and, at times, ocular or orbital pain. The vision loss in papillitis is similar to the pattern experienced in retrobulbar neuritis. There is a rapid decrease in acuity during the first 2 or 3 days, followed by stabilization over 7 to 10 days, leading to a gradual improvement of vision.[61] Some degree of secondary optic atrophy is always possible 4 to 8 weeks after the inflammation.[47] Signs include:

- Optic disc edema varying from subtle to severe
- Marcus Gunn pupil
- Cells in the vitreous
- Obscuration of the central cup
- Vascular alterations depending on elapsed time

There exist 2 distinctive types of papillitis with surrounding retinal changes. The type of papillitis associated with viral infections in children (e.g., mononucleosis) exhibits dirty-yellow, globular exudates scattered throughout the papillomacular bundle. These exudates are usually about the size of a retinal vessel and may coalesce to form a macular wing or star. There is associated superficial retinal edema. This condition carries a good visual prognosis, resolving spontaneously without treatment over weeks to months. The other type of papillitis is nonspecific in origin and is characterized by a yellowish swollen disc. There is considerable spread of retinal edema, vessels may be obscured, and there may be small linear hemorrhages adjacent to the disc (Fig. 26.5). This form often resolves with residual perivascular sheathing, gliosis, and disc pallor, but visual acuity is often severely reduced.[18]

MANAGEMENT

Prognosis for inflammatory optic neuropathy varies considerably. Reducing the inflammation by use of ACTH or steroids has both proponents and opponents.

TABLE 26.8
Common Etiologic Factors Associated with Inflammatory Optic Neuropathy

Toxoplasmosis	Presumed ocular histoplasmosis	Crohn's disease
Toxocariasis	Chickenpox	Ulcerative colitis
Meningitis	Herpes zoster	Polio
Measles	Cat-scratch fever	Mononucleosis
Mumps	Behçet's disease	Reiter's disease
Syphilis	Postvaccination reaction	Bacterial infections
Tuberculosis	Pharmacologic idiosyncrasies	Fungal infections
Collagen vascular disease		

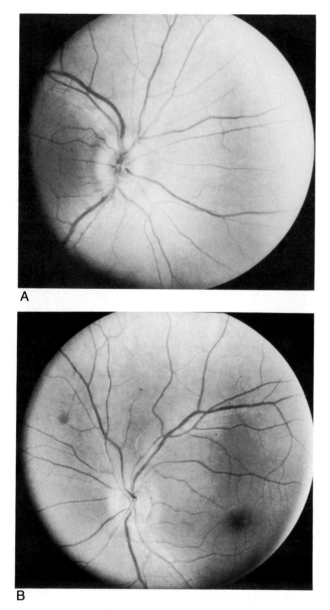

FIGURE 26.5 **Unilateral inflammatory optic neuropathy demonstrating significant optic disc edema in the right eye (A) compared with the left (B).**

Diagnosis of the underlying causative agent or condition is crucial to specify the proper therapeutic intervention. The sooner the resolution, the better the prognosis for improved vision.

The most important aspect of management of inflammatory optic neuropathy is rapid diagnosis with emphasis placed on attempting to ascertain the etiology. Adjunctive diagnostic tests should be ordered and other tests added when a specific etiologic agent is suspected. Basic tests should include erythrocyte sedi-

mentation rate (ESR) (to rule out temporal arteritis), complete blood count (CBC), fluorescent treponemal antibody absorption test (FTA-ABS) (to rule out syphilis), collagen vascular screen, computed tomography (CT) or MRI. Supplementary tests may include specific antibody titer tests for infection.

Therapeutic intervention must occur as soon as the etiologic factor is determined. If therapy is insufficient to reduce the inflammation, steroids may be incorporated into the treatment regimen. The decision to initiate steroid or ACTH therapy must be tempered by the associated risks.

Ischemic Optic Neuropathy

Ischemic optic neuropathy (ION) is a clinical diagnosis that describes compromise of the optic nerve with ensuing vision or visual field loss in the absence of identifiable inflammation, demyelinization, or cranial-orbital compression by a mass lesion. The condition is usually acute and involves the prelaminar region of the optic nerve, although it may also occur chronically in the retrolaminar position. Although many classifications have been assigned to this condition, 3 categories are distinct with regard to etiology: (1) arteriosclerotic-hypertensive ION, (2) temporal or cranial arteritic ION, and (3) diabetic ION or diabetic papillopathy. Each of these conditions will be discussed separately, since management of each differs distinctly.

ARTERIOSCLEROTIC-HYPERTENSIVE ION

Etiology. Arteriosclerotic-hypertensive ION is considered to be a small vessel disease causing impaired perfusion in the optic nerve head.[61-63] Hayreh[64] contends that the lesion occurs in the short posterior ciliary arteries that supply the choroid and distal optic nerve. Regardless of the pathogenesis, however, it is known that sudden systemic hypotension[65] and a high prevalence of associated systemic hypertension[66,67] lend credence to the claim that this condition is simply an acute alteration of the pressure-perfusion ratio at the nerve head.[68] The underlying causes of the altered pressure perfusion include Lyme disease, complications of general surgery, radiation therapy, relapsing polychondritis, and tamoxifen therapy.[69-73] Intraocular pressure, blood pressure, and cerebrospinal fluid pressure must be precisely balanced to maintain nerve head tissue. Should this balance be altered, optic nerve tissue is compromised. The corollary for chronically altered pressure-perfusion ratio is low-tension glaucoma.

Diagnosis. There is a broad range of ages of patients presenting with arteriosclerotic-hypertensive ION. In general, age may range from 40 to 80 years, but only

TABLE 26.9
Systemic Diseases Associated with AHION

Generalized atherosclerosis and arteriosclerosis	Polyarteritis nodosa
Carotid artery disease	Systemic lupus erythematosus
Systemic hypertension	Blood loss
Systemic hypotension	Vasomotor problems (migraine)
Myocardial infarction	Syphilis
Cardiac emboli	Allergic disorders
Mitral valve prolapse	Hematologic disorders (polycythemia, sickle cell)
Diabetes	
Lyme disease	Glaucoma
General surgery	Radiation therapy
Tamoxifen therapy	Relapsing polychondritis

about 5% of patients are older than age 70 years. The majority of patients are between 55 and 77 years of age.[66]

The clinical presentation includes:

- Acute visual acuity or visual field loss.
- Marcus Gunn pupil.
- Inferonasal visual field defect, a variety of altitudinal defects, or a central scotoma.
- Family history of diabetes or hypertension, but no associated transient ischemic attacks, ischemic cerebral infarction, or complications of large-vessel arteriosclerosis or cardiac disease with embolism.[67]
- Optic disc edema that is usually sectorial but rarely extending beyond the edge of the disc when in the early phase.
- Hyperemic disc with small, linear, flame-shaped hemorrhages on the disc margin that disappear in 3 to 5 weeks or that may present as pale optic disc edema.
- As the condition progresses, optic atrophy with subsequent cupping in some instances.

The condition progresses to a decrease of vision over 24 hours to 4 weeks, but in most cases this occurs in less than 9 days without remission. There are usually no systemic complaints associated with the episode.[8] Stabilization of vision then occurs, but optic atrophy ensues within about 3 months. Visual acuity stabilizes at 20/60 (6/18) or better in 45% to 50% of cases and is worse than 20/200 (6/60) in about 40% of cases.[57,66] The primary concern is subsequent involvement in the fellow eye, which can occur months to years later.[67] The incidence of involvement of the fellow eye is between 16% and 40%.[57,62] The coincident occurrence of central retinal artery occlusion is a possible complication.[74]

Management. The management of ION is multifactorial. Recognition and management of the underlying systemic condition is imperative. Table 26.9 summarizes some of the more common systemic diseases associated with ischemic optic neuropathy. One other rare but important concern is differentiation of the Foster-Kennedy syndrome from ischemic optic neuropathy. Table 26.10 summarizes the primary differences between the 2 entities. The success of therapy for the optic nerve lesion depends on the rapidity of diagnosis. Proponents of steroid therapy contend that treatment must be instituted at the earliest possible moment to reduce optic disc edema. The reduction of edema is thought to help by reducing capillary permeability and thus improving circulation. This, coupled with reduction of intraocular pressure, is thought to improve the pressure-perfusion ratio, which will minimize optic atrophy. Once atrophy has occurred, nothing can be done to improve the outcome.

Patients with ION associated with collagen vascular disease should be promptly treated with high dosages of systemic steroids. A typical therapeutic regimen consists of oral prednisone, 80 mg daily for 10 to 14 days, tapering to 40 mg daily for 4 to 8 weeks until the optic disc edema subsides.

The diabetic patient with ION may also be treated with high dosages of steroids in the early phase of disc edema, provided that the patient's diabetic status is carefully monitored.

TABLE 26.10
Differential Diagnosis between Foster-Kennedy Syndrome and Ischemic Optic Neuropathy

	Ischemic Optic Neuropathy	*Foster-Kennedy Syndrome*
Onset	Sudden vision loss or field defect in 1 eye followed by stabilization	Insidious progression of reduced vision with papilledema in fellow eye
Visual fields	Altitudinal hemianopsia, arcuate scotoma, central scotoma	Central scotoma in eye with optic atrophy and enlarged blind spot in fellow eye
Fundus	Sector optic disc edema followed by sector atrophy	Uniform optic atrophy with optic disc edema in fellow eye
Associated systemic signs and symptoms	May be a family or personal history of hypertension, diabetes, or stroke	Hemiplegia, loss of smell, personality change

If the ION is not secondary to a frank vasculitis, steroid (even anticoagulant) therapy is often instituted. However, there is no proved benefit to this approach[66,75,76] although some authors argue that if optic disc edema is present, therapeutic intervention is invaluable.[76] In addition, it has been suggested that aspirin may be useful in the treatment of ION.[75,76]

TEMPORAL ARTERITIC ION

Etiology. Temporal arteritic ION is a true ocular emergency. Immediate recognition of this condition is crucial to prevent involvement of the fellow eye, with the possible consequence of bilateral blindness. Temporal arteritic ION is associated with giant cell arteritis, a systemic disease with special predilection for arteries of the head and neck. The condition most often occurs in patients over 70 years of age.

Diagnosis. One to 2 weeks before actual onset of the condition, the patient may experience prodromal symptoms. These can consist of hazy vision, visual field defects, flashing lights, color vision disturbances, temporal headaches, an unexplained weight loss, suboccipital neck pains, scalp tenderness, and jaw aches associated with chewing and talking. Polymyalgia rheumatica also may be a prodromal symptom complex.[77] The attack is heralded by an acute vision loss to the 20/60 (6/18) to NLP level.[66] Ophthalmoscopically, the disc shows pallid edema. In about 50% of cases there is a chalky-white swelling of the disc with an occasional hemorrhage.[47] Clinically leukocytosis, elevated ESR, serum globulins on serum electrophoresis, and a hard nonpulsating temporal artery are reliable indicators of a positive diagnosis. An ESR over 40 (Westergren) should indicate the need for temporal artery biopsy. A positive temporal artery biopsy provides the definitive diagnosis. However, *the delay for a biopsy should not delay initiation of therapy.*

Prognosis is grim with regard to ocular involvement. The process will usually involve the fellow eye within 1 year unless there is therapeutic intervention. Even with therapy some patients proceed to total blindness. The ultimate outcome of an active case is optic atrophy.

Management. Management of temporal arteritic ION involves massive doses of systemic steroids to prevent vision loss in the fellow eye. Vision function in the affected eye may deteriorate,[66] improve, or remain stable after systemic steroid therapy is initiated.[78–81] Steroid intervention is necessary because of the true inflammatory nature of this condition. Steroids decrease capillary permeability so that the anoxic and toxic destruction by edema of the nerve fiber layer is

reduced to a minimum. The typical recommended treatment regimen varies considerably among clinicians. The treatment recognized by most clinicians consists of high initial dosages of prednisone (80 to 120 mg daily).[82] The precise amount should be determined by relief of symptomatology and reduction of the ESR. Once the appropriate dosage level has been established, therapy must be maintained and regulated according to the ESR. Therapy may continue for years unless there are strong contradictions to steroid therapy.

Anticoagulants (heparin, streptokinase) should be given only in cases of confirmed hyperviscosity syndromes and then only in consultation with an internist. The use of anticoagulants in the elderly carries the risk of cerebral hemorrhage. Vasodilators, such as theophylline and nicotinic acid derivatives, apparently are of no benefit in ischemic conditions.[77]

DIABETIC PAPILLOPATHY

Etiology. Diabetic papillopathy is an enigmatic form of optic neuropathy in a juvenile-onset diabetic of several years' duration. It can be characterized as neither anterior ischemic optic neuropathy nor papilledema because it lacks several characteristics of both. The etiology of the process is somewhat obscure except for the fact that diabetes is itself a small-vessel disease, and diabetic papillopathy may be a manifestation of diffuse microangiopathy.

Diagnosis. The clinical presentation includes optic disc edema that may be sectorial or total (Fig. 26.6). The pupils are usually fully reactive, and there is typically a lack of visual symptoms because vision loss is only mild to moderate. Visual field loss varies from enlarged blind spots to isolated scotomas. There is typically only background diabetic retinopathy as an associated finding, although there have been 2 cases reported with coincident disc neovascularization.[83] Any vision loss or visual field compromise characteristically resolves in months without specific therapy. There are reports, however, of patients who have retained arcuate nerve fiber bundle defects and optic atrophy.[83]

Management. Management consists of a combination of accurate recognition and diagnosis, the exclusion of increased intracranial pressure causing papilledema, and the exclusion of disc neovascularization. Disc neovascularization and diabetic papillopathy appear very similar on fluorescein angiography, since both demonstrate freely leaking vessels. The clinician must also ascertain how well controlled is the patient's diabetes.

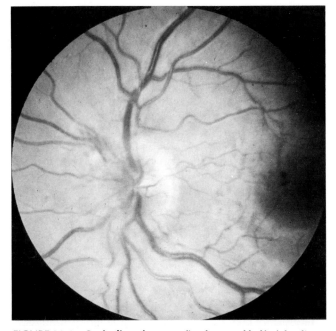

FIGURE 26.6   **Optic disc edema confined to nasal half of the disc in a case of diabetic papillopathy.**

Leber's Optic Neuropathy

ETIOLOGY

Like diabetic papillopathy, Leber's optic neuropathy is an enigma and is considered to be a distinct clinical entity. It is classically defined as a visually debilitating optic atrophy that occurs as a sequel to acute or subacute optic neuritis. The etiology is somewhat obscure, but some authors have proposed that it may be an inherited inability to detoxify cyanide.[84] Further studies have implicated a deficiency of thiosulfate sulfurtransferase (Rhodanese) as a cause for this defect in the detoxification of cyanide.[85] Others have suggested that Leber's optic neuropathy is a mitochondrial disease.[86]

The hereditary aspect of this disease is equally obscure. In the United States men are more often affected than women (6.7:1), with age of onset for men at 18 to 30 years and women at 10 to 40 years.[87] The following characteristics summarize the inheritance patterns that do not conform to Mendelian principles.[88–91]

- Males are predominantly affected.
- Affected males cannot transmit the disease.
- The sister of an affected male is a carrier.
- Affected females all have normal fathers.
- All women born into families with only females affected are carriers.

- The heterozygous female can transmit the trait to her sons and the carrier state to her daughters.

DIAGNOSIS

The disease is characterized by acute or subacute vision loss. Usually both eyes are affected simultaneously, but there may be an interval of 1 to 6 months between involvement of the 2 eyes. Preacute signs and symptoms do occur. In some patients there is atrophy of retinal nerve fibers before the actual attack, as well as an altered Farnsworth-Munsell 100-hue test and VER.[92–94] When the actual attack occurs, there is mild optic disc edema with early circumpapillary telangiectatic microangiopathy.[95] There is a predilection for the nerve fibers of the macula, thereby causing an early vision loss and a central scotoma that can break out to the periphery. This vision loss is to the 20/200 (6/60) to 20/400 (6/120) level, and the condition eventually settles into a permanent optic atrophy that most often affects the temporal sector of the disc. When the condition is active, there may be headaches associated with meningitis, cerebral edema, swelling of the optic nerves, and opticochiasmatic arachnoiditis.

MANAGEMENT

The prognosis for Leber's optic neuropathy is grim. The condition usually becomes stationary, although there have been reports of spontaneous improvement of vision in 16% to 75% of affected patients. There also may be further progression of the vision loss even after years of stability.[87] No treatment has been shown to be effective in symptomatic cases. However, in view of the suspected defect in cyanide metabolism, it has been suggested that hydroxocobalamin (vitamin B_{12A}) and cyanocobalamin (vitamin B_{12}), 1 mg parenterally daily for 7 days, may be an effective therapeutic approach. This vitamin therapy has no side effects, but no proof of its efficacy exists. Advocates of such vitamin therapy cite the similarity of Leber's disease to toxic optic neuropathies that respond favorably to vitamin therapy. Such therapy is used because of the belief that a thiamine-dependent transferase catalyzes a step in the pentose shunt. When this is compromised, nerve fiber loss ensues.[96]

Papillophlebitis

ETIOLOGY

Papillophlebitis is a relatively benign condition presenting as optic disc edema presumably secondary to occlusion of the central retinal vein. This occlusion is thought to be initiated by phlebitis.[97] Papillophlebitis occurs in otherwise healthy young adults (20 to 40 years) with no predilection for either sex.

DIAGNOSIS

Clinically, the patient may report vague symptoms of reduced visual acuity that is usually no worse than 20/30 (6/9). Hayreh[98] has classified 2 distinct ophthalmoscopic presentations: (1) type 1, optic disc vasculitis characterized by gross unilateral disc edema without retinal vascular abnormalities; and (2) type 2, optic disc vasculitis characterized by disc edema with hemorrhages on and surrounding the disc in the early stages and with grossly dilated and tortuous retinal veins (Fig. 26.7), more pronounced than one would anticipate in the equivalent stage in the development of papilledema. Other clinical findings include enlarged blind spots with some variability in the central scotoma.[99] Laboratory tests and neuroradiologic findings are unrevealing, but they should be ordered to exclude other causes of optic disc edema (see Table 26.5).

MANAGEMENT

Papillophlebitis is a self-limiting condition, resolving over 6 to 18 months, with no vision-threatening sequelae. Perivenous sheathing of the large veins may occur many months after the onset of optic disc edema. Dilated venules on the disc surface as well as optociliary shunts can develop to drain the congested disc, and these may remain after the process has subsided.[100] Macular pigmentary changes may also persist due to macular involvement.

Active management is controversial, since there are avid proponents of the conservative, "no-treatment" approach as well as those who advocate aggressive

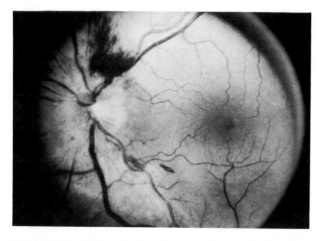

FIGURE 26.7   **Mild optic disc edema associated with dilated tortuous veins and hemorrhage in papillophlebitis.**

steroid therapy. Because papillophlebitis is viewed as a vasculitis, steroid therapy should theoretically be of benefit, especially when one considers the associated optic disc edema. There has been an occasional report of dramatic response with steroid therapy similar to that used in cases of optic disc edema secondary to optic neuritis, but no controlled studies exist to substantiate the effectiveness of this therapy.[99] Indeed, case reports often acknowledge that optic disc edema is unaffected by steroid or anticoagulant therapy. Controversy even exists on the value of ordering routine laboratory studies including CBC, urinalysis, LE prep, ANA, ESR, RPR, FTA-ABS, Venereal Disease Research Laboratory (VDRL), skull films, LP, and chest x-ray.[100]

In summary, steroid therapy appears to be ineffective in papillophlebitis. Moreover, such therapy can mask a much more serious condition that may be producing the optic disc edema. Patients suspected of having papillophlebitis should be monitored carefully, since unilateral optic disc edema can be secondary to many other conditions. Routine follow-up examination will confirm the stability and subsequent remission of papillophlebitis.

Papilledema

Papilledema is best defined as optic disc edema occurring secondary to increased intracranial pressure. Although the exact etiopathogenesis is somewhat obscure and may involve both mechanical as well as vascular factors, the mechanical theory proposed by Hayreh[101] seems most plausible.[102] Visual symptoms are rare in the early phases of papilledema, since the axoplasmic stasis has little to do with transfer of the nerve impulse along the outer membrane of the nerve fibers.[103] The reduction in vision does not occur until there is frank ischemia of nerve fibers associated with the vascular phase of the optic disc edema.[102,104]

Etiology

The causes of increased intracranial pressure are many. Any intracranial space-occupying lesion may produce papilledema. Other causes include intracerebral or subarachnoid hemorrhage,[105] tumors of the spinal cord,[106] inflammatory polyneuritis,[107] infectious disease, toxic metabolic diseases, trauma, congenital malformations of the brain, therapeutic doses of lithium carbonate,[9,108] amiodarone,[109] transient erythroblastopenia of childhood,[110] or radical neck dissection.[111] Benign intracranial hypertension (pseudotumor cerebri) is another important cause of papilledema. This condition is characterized by bilateral papilledema associated with headache, some compromise of visual acuity or fields, occasional sixth-nerve palsy with absence of frank focal neurologic signs, and depressed plasma steroid levels.[112] Although not life threatening, there is a definite potential for blindness.[113,114] Benign intracranial hypertension may occur secondary to middle ear disease, minor head injury, childhood systemic lupus erythematosus,[115] or toxic conditions such as hypervitaminosis A or tetracycline and nalidixic acid toxicity, although the condition appears to be due to poor resorption of the cerebrospinal fluid.[116] In over 50% of cases, the underlying etiology is unknown. The cases with no apparent etiology are dominated by females aged 10 to 50 years.[117]

Diagnosis

The diagnosis of papilledema in the early stages is often a significant clinical challenge. It is made by a combination of stereoscopic observation of the optic disc (see Chapter 16), visual field analysis, evaluation of focal neurologic signs, and the patient's history of transient obscurations (5 to 30 *seconds* of blurring or loss of vision usually associated with postural changes). The optic disc edema itself has been shown experimentally to occur about 1 to 7 days after increased intracranial pressure,[118] but papilledema can occur much sooner (within 2 to 48 hours) because of intracranial hemorrhage.[119,120] The absence of a venous pulsation is thought to be a sign of increased intracranial pressure[121] although this concept has been questioned.[122]

The differential diagnosis between papilledema and pseudopapilledema is crucial for proper patient management (Table 26.11, Fig. 26.8). Pseudopapilledema is a congenital anomalous elevation of the optic nerve head that may be associated with high hyperopia, hyaloid remnants, myelinated nerve fibers, hyaline bodies (drusen), or other, unexplainable, congenital elevations. This condition is often misdiagnosed, resulting in unnecessary invasive and expensive neurologic evaluations. Fluorescein angiography is of some value in differentiating true papilledema from pseudopapilledema, but a normal fluorescein angiogram does not rule out papilledema. Stereoscopic fundus photography and observation of the peripapillary reflex with a red-free filter are also of value in the differential diagnosis.[123]

Optic disc edema is the first observable sign of papilledema. The swelling of the nerve fibers and subsequent transudation of the debris first appear in the inferior aspect of the disc, followed by the superior, then the nasal aspects, with the temporal aspect least susceptible to swelling. This swelling eventually spreads into the surrounding retina. The disc margins then blur with later involvement of the small vessels of the disc.[118,124,125] As the process progresses there may be hemorrhage on or near the disc at any retinal level, but rarely beyond the radius of the macula. There have been some reports of diffuse hemorrhagic retinopathy similar to venous stasis disease. As the papilledema progresses, vision is maintained. Later, visual field defects occur that progress to involve fixation. The enlarged blind spot may eventually expand to involve fixation.

Other complications that may lead to reduced visual acuity are subretinal pigment epithelial neovascularization,[126] choroidal folds,[127] preretinal macular hemorrhage, choroidal and subretinal hemorrhages, macular star formation, and retinal pigment epithelial disease.[128] Another fundus sign of long-standing papillede-

TABLE 26.11
Differential Diagnosis between Papilledema and Pseudopapilledema

Characteristic	Papilledema	Pseudopapilledema
Abnormal vasculature	No	Yes
Familial patterns	No	Yes
Hemorrhages	Yes	Only when drusen shear vessels
Nerve fiber layer swelling	Yes, into retina	No
Exudates and cotton wool spots	Yes	No
Enlarged blind spot	Yes	No
Transient obscurations of vision	Yes	No
Spontaneous venous pulsation	Usually no	Usually yes
Maintenance of central cup	Yes, until late	No
Buried drusen	No	Yes at times
Headache	Postural and severe	Possibly migraine
Other neurologic signs or symptoms	Yes	No
Fluorescein leakage	Yes	No

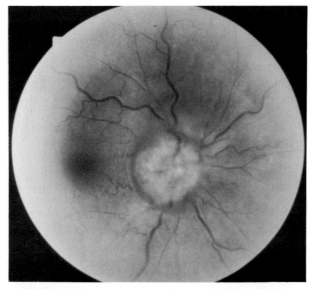

A

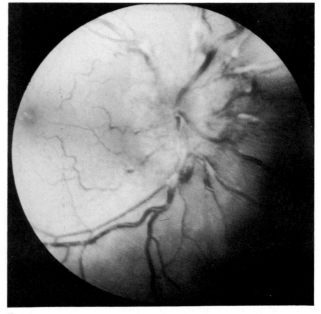

B

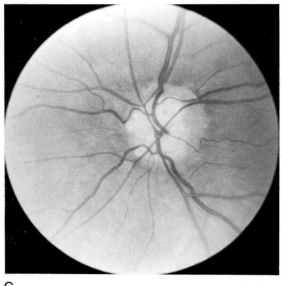

C

FIGURE 26.8   *(A)* Compensated papilledema in a case of benign intracranial hypertension. *(B)* Noncompensated papilledema in a case of acute aqueductal stenosis. *(C)* Pseudopapilledema secondary to buried drusen of the optic nerve head.

ma is the development of optociliary shunt vessels that are most often associated with sphenoid ridge meningiomas.[129]

Management

If left untreated, papilledema can progress to intractable optic atrophy. Clearly the most important aspect of treatment is management of the underlying cause of increased intracranial pressure. A diagnosis of true papilledema should always imply emergency hospital admission. If the underlying cause cannot be readily determined, medical or surgical intervention must be undertaken.

Medical treatment must be used with caution, since the papilledema may resolve while the underlying condition continues untreated. Should cerebral edema exist, causing severe neurologic signs and optic disc edema, treatment may be instituted until the underlying cause can be managed. The edema can be controlled by using 2 to 4 g of acetazolamide daily in addition to 40 to 100 mg (usually 60 mg) of oral prednisone daily. Lumbar punctures may also be employed in skilled hands.

Should this regimen not alleviate the problem, neurosurgical shunting procedures or optic nerve decompression must be undertaken. Neurosurgical shunting procedures (lumboperitoneal shunt) alleviate the problem of elevated intracranial pressure but may be compromised by infection, plugs, or resultant low intracranial pressure with headache and dizziness. Optic nerve decompression involves invasion of the subarachnoid space of the optic nerve with direct relief of intracranial pressure.[47,130,131] Hupp and associates[132] reported that 7 of 19 eyes showed improvement in vision function after optic nerve sheath decompression.

Treatment of benign intracranial hypertension is related to cause, initial severity, and success of long-term controllability. If the cause is amenable to treatment, such as otitis or hypervitaminosis A, that must take precedence. Because benign intracranial hypertension is self-limited, usually resolving in 3 to 9 months, there are generally only 2 reasons to employ treatment—severe headaches or evidence of optic neuropathy.[112] If there exists a depressed plasma steroid level, daily dosages of oral prednisone, 80 to 100 mg, in conjunction with acetazolamide, 250 mg 4 times daily, may be necessary.[47] Jefferson and Clark[133] advocate abstention from steroid therapy and surgical intervention. These authors favor dehydration therapy and monitor resolution by measuring the blind spot. The patient is required to limit fluid intake to 900 ml daily. The dehydrating agents employed may be 1 or a combination of the following: oral urea (1 g/kg body weight daily until resolution), oral glycerol (1 to 1.5 g/kg daily until resolution), hydroflumethiazide (100 mg on alternate days until resolution), and chlorthalidone (200 mg on alternate days until resolution). The authors prefer chlorthalidone because of rapid resolution with a mean time-to-cure of 12 weeks. If medical therapy is unsuccessful in controlling the condition, a theroperitoneal shunt may be needed.[134] Techniques of medical therapy are constantly improving. With the introduction of in-dwelling intracranial pressure monitoring devices, therapy may be modified to maximize results.[135]

Nutritional and Toxic Optic Neuropathy

Etiology

Nutritional and toxic optic neuropathy refers to vision loss secondary to degenerative changes of the optic nerve fibers in response to exogenous metabolic stimuli. This may occur in deficiency states (thiamine or vitamin B$_{12}$) as a toxic response to certain drugs or substances (Table 26.12). In most cases one can establish that the patient has been exposed to toxins or has

TABLE 26.12
Drugs or Substances Responsible for Toxic Optic Neuropathy

Alcohol	Isoniazid
Barbiturates	Lead
Carbon monoxide	Placidyl
Chloramphenicol	Phenothiazines
Chloroquine	Steroids
Cyanide	Streptomycin
Digitalis	Tobacco
Diiodohydroxyquin	Tryparsamide
Disulfiram	Vitamin D
Ethambutol	Disulfiram
Heavy metals	Ethchlorvynol
Hydroxychloroquine	Hexamethonium
Iodochlorhydroxyquin	Iodide compounds

had some dietary deficiency. The precise pathogenesis of the atrophic process is somewhat obscure, although there appears to be an alteration in adenosine triphosphate (ATP) formation. This leads to a stasis of axoplasmic flow with subsequent optic disc edema, eventually resulting in axonal death.[136–138]

Diagnosis

The atrophies are characterized clinically by a gradual, bilateral painless reduction of visual acuity with eventual centrocecal scotomas. The scotomas have variable margins that are better defined and much larger with red targets. There are no specific nerve fiber bundle defects, but often a dense scotoma occurs in the area corresponding to the papillomacular bundle. The defects characteristically do not cross the vertical meridian, although ethambutol toxicity may demonstrate a bitemporal hemianopsia, since the chiasm may be implicated in the process. The visual field changes are usually progressive, although they are somewhat reversible. There is also an associated dyschromatopsia, but the patient may be unaware of the color vision loss. Even though this condition can cause reduced vision, it is unusual for vision to be reduced below hand motion. Ophthalmoscopically the optic disc may be edematous with isolated splinter hemorrhages in the early stages, but the nerve head eventually becomes atrophic.

Management

The condition is reversible and has a favorable prognosis if the toxic agent or nutritional deficiency is detected and removed. It is especially important to recognize that patients treated with ethambutol can develop atrophy because of the chelation of zinc and other metals necessary for optic nerve function. Serum zinc levels should be evaluated in these patients. It has even been shown that children with hereditary optic atrophy may have reduced serum zinc levels.[139] Zinc sulfate, 100 to 250 mg 3 times daily, may promote reversal of the neuropathy. The dosage of oral zinc sulfate depends on the individual's ability to absorb the drug as well as the possible side effects such as nausea, vomiting, diarrhea, and bleeding secondary to gastric erosion. It should be emphasized that such zinc therapy is not yet approved by the Food and Drug Administration.[140,141]

It has been suggested that if isoniazid is implicated in optic neuropathy or other neurologic signs, pyridoxine (vitamin B_6), 25 to 100 mg daily, may be used. Prophylactic administration of this agent in combination with isoniazid and monoamine oxidase inhibitor therapy has been suggested.[4,47]

The patient with tobacco or alcohol amblyopia usually has either low serum levels of vitamin B_{12} or is unable to absorb this vitamin in sufficient amounts. Thus, the treatment for this condition involves supplemental vitamin therapy. After the serum vitamin B_{12} deficiency has been documented, the patient should be given 300 mg of oral thiamine each week and 1000 µg of intramuscular hydroxocobalamin each week for 10 weeks. The sooner this therapy is instituted, the better the prognosis. The hydroxocobalamin form of vitamin B_{12} appears to be more effective than cyanocobalamin.[142] In terms of recovery from the amblyopia, cessation of smoking or drinking does not appear to produce remission unless the patient concurrently improves his or her diet. Thus, it is unnecessary, and in practice difficult, to persuade patients who are habitual abusers of these agents to stop. Improvement of dietary status seems to be the most important factor.[143]

Vitamin B_{12} deficiency can also cause megaloblastic anemia. White-centered hemorrhages can occur in the posterior pole, and there may be disc pallor. If the ischemia is severe enough, cotton wool spots may occur. A CBC will confirm the diagnosis, but the clinician should realize that visual-neurologic symptoms can occur before the clinical laboratory changes. Serum folate and vitamin B_{12} levels should be determined and appropriate therapy (IM injections of hydroxocobalamin) instituted at the earliest sign of megaloblastic anemia.

The crucial feature of all optic neuropathies that must never be ignored is the possibility of an underlying neoplasm. Visual field analysis at regular intervals will aid in excluding the possibility of an optic nerve or chiasmal neoplasm.

References

1. Arden GB, Gucukoglu AG. Grating test of contrast sensitivity in patients with retrobulbar neuritis. Arch Ophthalmol 1978;96:1626–1629.
2. Regan D, Silver R, Murray TJ. Visual acuity and contrast sensitivity in multiple sclerosis—hidden visual loss: An auxiliary diagnostic test. Brain 1977;100:563–579.
3. Krill AE, Fishman GA. Acquired color vision defects. Trans Am Acad Ophthalmol Otolaryngol 1971;75:1095–1111.
4. Glaser JS. Neuro-ophthalmologic examination: General considerations and special techniques. In: Duane TD, Jaeger EA, eds. Clinical ophthalmology. Philadelphia: Harper & Row, 1987;2:Chap. 2, pp. 1–38.
5. Linksz A. The clinical characteristics of acquired color-vision defects. In: Straatsma BR, Hall MO, Allen RA, Crescitelli F, eds. The retina, morphology, function and clinical characteristics. Berkeley: University of California Press; 1969;583–592.
6. Wildberger HGH, Van Lith GHM. Color vision and visually evoked response (VECP) in the recovery period of optic neuritis. Mod Probl Ophthalmol 1976;17:320–324.
7. Griffin JF, Wray SH. Acquired color vision defects in retrobulbar neuritis. Am J Ophthalmol 1978;86:193–201.
8. Von Noorden GK, Burian HM. Visual acuity in normal and amblyopic patients under reduced illumination. I. Behavior of visual acuity with and without neutral density filter. Arch Ophthalmol 1959;61:533–535.
9. Severin SL, Harper JY Jr, Culver JF. Photostress test for the evaluation of macular function. Arch Ophthalmol 1963;70:593–597.
10. Wald G. The photoreceptor process in vision. Am J Ophthalmol 1955;40(5, pt. 2):18–41.
11. Futterman S. Metabolism of the retina. III. The role of reduced triphosphopyridine nucleotide in the visual cycle. J Biol Chem 1963;238:1145–1150.
12. Dowling JE. Chemistry of visual adaptation in the rat. Nature 1960;188:114–118.
13. Brindley GS. The discrimination of afterimages. J Physiol 1959;147:194–203.
14. Glaser JS, Savino PJ, Sumers KD, et al. The photostress recovery test in the clinical assessment of visual function. Am J Ophthalmol 1977;255–260.
15. Smith JL. The optic nerve. Miami: Neuro-Ophthalmology Tapes, 1977;8.
16. Perkin GD, Rose FC. Uhthoff's syndrome. Br J Ophthalmol 1976;60:60–63.
17. Goldstein JE, Cogan DG. Exercise and the optic neuropathy of multiple sclerosis. Arch Ophthalmol 1964;72:168–170.
18. Walsh FB, Hoyt WF. Clinical neuro-ophthalmology, ed. 3. Baltimore: Williams & Wilkins 1969;1:991.
19. Sokol S. The Pulfrich stereo-illusion as an index of optic nerve dysfunction. Surv Ophthalmol 1976;20:432–434.
20. Smith TJ, Baker RS. Perimetric findings in pseudotumor cerebri using automated techniques. Ophthalmology 1986;93:887–894.
21. Johns K, Lavin P, Elliot JH, et al. Magnetic resonance imaging of the brain in isolated optic neuritis. Arch Ophthalmol 1986;104:1486–1488.

22. Lorance RW, Kaufman D, Wray SH, et al. Contrast sensitivity testing in neurovisual diagnosis. Neurology 1987;37:923–929.

23. Iragui VJ, Wiederholt WC, Romine JS. Evoked potentials in trigeminal neuralgia associated with multiple sclerosis. Arch Neurol 1986;43:444–446.

24. Edwards MK, Farlow MR, Stevens JC. Multiple sclerosis: MRI and clinical correlation. AJR 1986;147:571–574.

25. Cutler JR, Aminoff MJ, Brant-Zawadski M. Evaluation of patients with multiple sclerosis by evoked potentials and magnetic resonance imaging: A comparative study. Ann Neurol 1986;20:645–648.

26. Stevens JC, Farlow MR, Edwards MK, et al. Magnetic resonance imaging: Clinical correlation in 64 patients with multiple sclerosis. Arch Neurol 1986;43:1145–1148.

27. Reese L, Carr TJ, Nicholson RL, et al. Magnetic resonance imaging for detecting lesions of multiple sclerosis: Comparison with computed tomography and clinical assessment. Can Med Assoc J 1986;135:639–645.

28. Rollins DW. Multiple sclerosis and vision. J Am Optom Assoc 1986;57:904–908.

29. Kempster PA, Iansek R, Balla JI, et al. Value of visual evoked response and oligoclonal bands in cerebrospinal fluid in diagnosis of spinal multiple sclerosis. Lancet 1987;1:769–771.

30. Stewart JM, Houser OW, Baker HL Jr, et al. Magnetic resonance imaging and clinical relationships in multiple sclerosis. Mayo Clin Proc 1987;62:174–184.

31. Golden GS, Woody RC. The role of nuclear magnetic resonance imaging in the diagnosis of MS in childhood. Neurology 1987;37:689–693.

32. Burde RM, Keltner JL, Gittinger JW, Miller NR. Optic neuritis—etiology? Surv Ophthalmol 1980;24:307–314.

33. Lessell S. Current concepts in ophthalmology. Optic neuropathies. N Engl J Med 1978;299:533–537.

34. Godel V, Blumenthal M, Regenbogen L. Retrobulbar neuritis and central serous chorioretinopathy. J Pediatr Ophthalmol 1977;14:296–298.

35. Nikoskelainen E. Symptoms, signs and early course of optic neuritis. Acta Ophthalmol 1975;53:254–271.

36. Reynolds NC Jr, Shapiro I. Retrobulbar neuritis with neuroretinal edema as a delayed manifestation of carbon monoxide poisoning: Case report. Milit Med 1979;144:472–473.

37. Galvin RJ, Heron JR, Regan D. Subclinical optic neuropathy in multiple sclerosis. Arch Neurol 1977;34:666–670.

38. Marshall D. Ocular manifestations of multiple sclerosis and relationship to retrobulbar neuritis. Trans Am Ophthalmol Soc 1950;48:487–575.

39. Lubow M, Adams L. The changing management of acute optic neuritis. In: Smith JL, ed. Neuro-ophthalmology. Symposium of the University of Miami and the Bascom Palmer Eye Institute. St Louis: C.V. Mosby Co, 1972;6:44–50.

40. Wray SH. The treatment of optic neuritis. Sight Sav Rev 1972;42:5–13.

41. Rawson MD, Liversedge LA, Goldfarb G. Treatment of acute retrobulbar neuritis with corticotrophin. Lancet 1966;2:1044–1046.

42. Rose AS, Kuzma JW, Kurtzke JF, et al. Cooperative study in the evaluation of therapy in multiple sclerosis: ACTH versus placebo. Final report. Neurology 1970;20 (5, pt. 2):1–59.

43. Rawson MD, Liversedge LA. Treatment of retrobulbar neuritis with corticotrophin (letter). Lancet 1969;2:222.

44. Gould ES, Bird AC, Leaver PK, McDonald WI. Treatment of optic neuritis by retrobulbar injection of triamcinolone. Br Med J 1977;1:1495–1497.

45. Bird AC, Leaver PK, Gould E, McDonald I. Assessment of intraconal steroids in the treatment of retrobulbar neuritis. In: Glaser JS, ed. Neuro-opthalmology. Symposium of the University of Miami and the Bascom Palmer Eye Institute. St Louis: C.V. Mosby Co, 1977;9:154–159.

46. Bowden AN, Bowden PMA, Friedmann AI, et al. A trial of corticotropin gelatin injection in acute optic neuritis. J Neurol Neurosurg Psychiatry 1974;37:869–873.

47. Fraunfelder FT, Roy FH. Current ocular therapy. Philadelphia: W.B. Saunders Co, 1980;528–529.

48. Hepler RS. Management of optic neuritis. Surv Ophthalmol 1976;20:350–357.

49. Panitch HS. Systemic alpha-interferon in multiple sclerosis. Long-term patient follow-up. Arch Neurol 1987;44:61–63.

50. Camenga DL, Johnson KP, Alter M, et al. Systemic recombinant alpha-2 interferon therapy in relapsing multiple sclerosis. Arch Neurol 1986;43:1239–1246.

51. Panitch HS, Hirsch RL, Haley AS, et al. Exacerbations of multiple sclerosis in patients treated with gamma interferon. Lancet 1987;1:893–895.

52. Jacobs L, Salazar AM, Herndon R, et al. Multicentre double-blind study of effect of intrathecally administered natural human fibroblast interferon on exacerbations of multiple sclerosis. Lancet 1986;2:1411–1413.

53. Tindal RS, Rollins JA. Assessment of therapeutic plasmapheresis in demyelinating neurologic disorders. South Med J 1986;79:991–997.

54. Stefoski D, Davis FA, Faut M, et al. 4-Aminopyridine improves clinical signs in multiple sclerosis. Ann Neurol 1987;21:71–77.

55. Harpur GD, Suke R, Bass BH, et al. Hyperbaric oxygen therapy in chronic stable multiple sclerosis: Double blind study. Neurology 1986;36:988–991.

56. Kennedy C, Carroll FD. Optic neuritis in children. Trans Am Acad Ophthalmol Otolaryngol 1960;64:700–712.

57. Miettinen P, Wasz-Hockert O. Ophthalmological aspects of tuberculous meningitis. Acta Ophthalmol Suppl 1960;61:1–54.

58. Okun E, Butler WT. Ophthalmological complications of cryptococcal meningitis. Arch Ophthalmol 1964;71:52–57.

59. Gupta DR, Strobas RJ. Bilateral papillitis associated with Cafergot® therapy. Neurology 1972;22:793–797.

60. Wollensak J, Grajewski O. Bilateral vascular papillitis following ergotamine medication. Klin Monatsbl Augenheikd 1978;173:731–737.

61. Bajandas FJ. Neuro-ophthalmology board review manual. Thorofore, NJ: Charles B. Slack, 1980.

62. Lieberman MF, Shahi A, Green WR. Embolic ischemic optic neuropathy. Am J Ophthalmol 1978;86:206–210.

63. Anderson DR, Davis EB. Retina and optic nerve afer posterior ciliary artery occlusion. Arch Ophthalmol 1974;92:422–426.

64. Hayreh SS. Anterior ischemic optic neuropathy. New York: Springer-Verlag, 1975;126.

65. Drance SM, Morgan RW, Sweeney VP. Shock-induced optic neuropathy: A cause of non-progressive glaucoma. N Engl J Med 1973;288:392–395.

66. Boghen DR, Glaser JS. Ischaemic optic neuropathy. Brain 1975;98:689–708.

67. Ellenberger C Jr. Ischemic optic neuropathy as a possible early complication to vascular hypertension. Am J Ophthalmol 1979;88:1045–1051.

68. Burde RM. Ischemic optic neuropathy. In: Smith JL, Glaser JS, eds. Neuro-opthalmology. Symposium of the University of Miami and the Bascom Palmer Eye Institute. St Louis: C.V. Mosby Co, 1973;7:38–62.

69. Schechter SL. Lyme disease associated with optic neuropathy. Am J Med 1986;81:143–145.

70. Rizzzo JF, Lessell S. Posterior ischemic optic neuropathy during general surgery. Am J Ophthalmol 1987;103:808–811.

71. Guy J, Schatz NJ. Hyperbaric oxygen in the treatment of radiation-induced optic neuropathy. Ophthalmology 1986;93:1083–1088.

72. Isaak BL, Liesegang TJ, Michet CJ Jr. Ocular and systemic findings in relapsing polychondritis. Ophthalmology 1986;93:681–689.

73. Pugesgaard T, Von Eyben FE. Bilateral optic neuritis evolved during tamoxifen treatment. Cancer 1986;58:383–386.

74. Quigley H, Anderson DR. Cupping of the optic disc in ischemic optic neuropathy. Trans Am Acad Ophthalmol Otolaryngol 1977;83:755–762.

75. Miller NR. Anterior ischemic optic neuropathy: Diagnosis and management. Bull NY Acad Med 1980;56:643–654.

76. Hayreh SS. Anterior ischemic optic neuropathy. III. Treatment, prophylaxis, and differential diagnosis. Br J Ophthalmol 1974;58:981–989.

77. Boke W, Voigt GJ. Circulatory disturbances of the optic nerve. Ophthalmologica 1980;180:88–100.

78. Cohen DN. Temporal arteritis: Improvement in visual prognosis and management with repeat biopsies. Trans Am Acad Ophthalmol Otolaryngol 1973;77:Op. 74–85.

79. Mosher HA. The prognosis in temporal arteritis. Arch Ophthalmol 1959;62:641–644.

80. Schneider HA, Weber AA, Ballen PH. The visual prognosis in temporal arteritis. Ann Ophthalmol 1971;3:1215–1230.

81. Whitfield AGW, Bateman M, Cooke WT. Temporal arteritis. Br J Ophthalmol 1963;47:555–566.

82. Eshaghian J. Controversies regarding giant cell (temporal, cranial) arteritis. Doc Ophthalmol 1979;47:43–67.

83. Appen RE, Chandra SR, Klein R, Myers FL. Diabetic papillopathy. Am J Ophthalmol 1980;90:203–209.

84. Wilson J, Linnell JC, Matthews DM. Plasma-cobalamins in neuro-ophthalmological diseases. Lancet 1971;1:259–261.

85. Poole CJ, Kind PR. Deficiency of thiosulphate sulphurtransferase (Rhodanese) in Leber's heredity optic neuropathy. Br Med J 1986;292:1229–1230.

86. Novotny EJ Jr, Singh G, Wallace DC, et al. Leber's disease and dystonia: A mitochondrial disease. Neurology 1986;94:213–218.

87. Francois J. Hereditary optic atrophy. Int Ophthalmol Clin 1968;8:1016–1054.

88. Waardenburg PJ. Some remarks on the clinical and genetic puzzle of Leber's optic neuritis. J Hum Genet 1969;17:47996.

89. Went LN. Leber disease and variants. In: Vinken PJ, Brugn GW, eds. Handbook of clinical neurology. New York: American Elsevier, 1972.

90. Seedorff T. Leber's disease IV. Acta Ophthalmol 1969;47:813–821.

91. Seedorff T. Leber's disease V. Acta Ophthalmol 1970;48:186–213.

92. Nikoskelainen E, Sogg RL, Rosenthal AR, et al. The early phase in Leber hereditary optic atrophy. Arch Ophthalmol 1977;95:969–978.

93. Crutz-Coke R. Diagnosis in color blindness: An evolutionary approach. Springfield, IL: Charles C Thomas, 1970.

94. Livingstone IR, Mastaglia FL, Howe JW, Aherne GES. Leber's optic neuropathy: Clinical and visual evoked response studies in asymptomatic and symptomatic members of a 4-generation family. Br J Ophthalmol 1980;64:751–757.

95. Smith JL, Hoyt WF, Susac JO. Ocular fundus in acute Leber optic neuropathy. Arch Ophthalmol 1973;90:349–354.

96. Lessell S. Toxic and deficiency optic neuropathies. In: Smith JL, Glaser JS, eds. Neuro-ophthalmology. Symposium of the University of Miami and the Bascom Palmer Eye Institute. St Louis: C.V. Mosby Co, 1973;7:21–37.

97. Lyle TK, Wybar K. Retinal vasculitis. Br J Ophthalmol 1961;45:778–788.

98. Hayreh SS. Optic disc vasculitis. Br J Ophthalmol 1972;56:652–670.

99. Laibovitz RA. Presumed phlebitis of the optic disc. Ophthalmology 1979;86:313–319.

100. Lonn LI, Hoyt WF. Papillophlebitis: A cause of protracted yet benign optic disc edema. Eye Ear Nose Throat Monthly 1966;45:62–68.

101. Hayreh SS. Optic disc edema in raised intracranial pressure. VI. Associated visual disturbances and their pathogenesis. Arch Ophthalmol 1977;95:1566–1579.

102. Wirtschafter JD, Rizzo FJ, Smiley BC. Optic nerve axoplasm and papilledema. Surv Ophthalmol 1975;20:157–189.

103. Hayreh SS. Optic disc edema in raised intracranial pressure. Arch Ophthalmol 1977;95:1553–1565.

104. Green GJ, Lessell S, Loewenstein JI. Ischemic optic neuropathy in chronic papilledema. Arch Ophthalmol 1980;98:502–505.

105. Pagani LF. The rapid appearance of papilledema. J Neurosurg 1969;30:247–249.

106. Raynor RB. Papilledema associated with tumors of the spinal cord. Neurology 1969;19:700–704.

107. Morley JB, Reynolds EH. Papilloedema and the Landry-Guillain-Barre syndrome. Brain 1966;89:205–222.

108. Lobo A, Pilek E, Stokes PE. Papilledema following therapeutic dosages of lithium carbonate. J Nerv Ment Dis 1978;166:526–529.

109. Gittinger JW Jr, Asdourian GK. Papillopathy caused by amiodarone. Arch Ophthalmol 1987;105:349–351.

110. Green NS, Garvin JH Jr, Chutorian A. Transient erythoblastopenia of childhood presenting with papilledema. Clin Pediatr 1986;25:278–279.

111. de Vries WA, Balm AJ, Tiwari RM. Intracranial hypertension following neck dissection. J Laryngol Otol 1986;100:1427–1431.

112. Boddie HG, Banna M, Bradley WG. "Benign" intracranial hypertension: A survey of the clinical and radiological features, and long-term prognosis. Brain 1974;97:313–326.

113. Bowman MA. Pseudotumor cerebri. Am Fam Physician 1987;35:177–182.

114. Bence BG, Grala PE. Pseudotumor cerebri. J Am Optom Assoc 1986;57:751–754.

115. DelGiudice GC, Scher CA, Athreya BH, Diamond GR. Pseudotumor cerebri and childhood systemic lupus erythematosus. J Rheumatol 1986;13:748–752.

116. Johnson I, Paterson A. Benign intracranial hypertension. II. CSF pressure and circulation. Brain 1974;97:301–312.

117. Johnson I, Paterson A. Benign intracranial hypertension. I. Diagnosis and prognosis. Brain 1974;97:289–300.

118. Hayreh MS, Hayreh SS. Optic disc edema in raised intracranial pressure. I. Evolution and resolution. Arch Ophthalmol 1977;95:1237–1244.

119. Cogan DC. Neurology of the visual system. Springfield, IL: Charles C Thomas, 1966;142–143.

120. Walsh TJ, Garden JW, Gallagher B. Obliteration of retinal venous pulsations during elevation of cerebrospinal-fluid pressure. Am J Opthalmol 1969;67:954–956.

121. Hayreh SS, Hayreh MS. Optic disc edema in raised intracranial pressure. II. Early detection with fluorescein fundus angiography and stereoscopic color photography. Arch Ophthalmol 1977;95:1245–1254.

122. Savino PJ, Glaser JS. Pseudopapilledema versus papilledema. Int Ophthalmol Clin 1977;17:115–137.

123. Tso MOM, Hayreh SS. Optic disc edema in raised intracranial pressure. III. A pathologic study of experimental papilledema. Arch Ophthalmol 1977;95:1448–1457.

124. Tso MOM, Hayreh SS. Optic disc edema in raised intracranial pressure. IV. Axoplasmic transport in experimental papilledema. Arch Ophthalmol 1977;95:1458–1462.

125. Galvin R, Sanders MD. Peripheral retinal haemorrhages with papilloedema. Br J Ophthalmol 1980;64:262–266.

126. Jamison RR. Subretinal neovascularization and papilledema associated with pseudotumor cerebri. Am J Ophthalmol 1978;85:78–81.

127. Bird AC, Sanders MD. Choroidal folds in association with papilloedema. Br J Ophthalmol 1973;57:89–97.

128. Morris AT, Sanders MD. Macular changes resulting from papilloedema. Br J Ophthalmol 1980;64:211–216.

129. Eggers HM, Sanders MD. Acquired optociliary shunt vessels in papilloedema. Br J Ophthalmol 1980;64:267–271.

130. Smith JL, Hoyt WF, Newton TH. Optic nerve sheath decompression for relief of chronic monocular choked disc. Am J Ophthalmol 1969;68:633–639.

131. Galbraith JEK, Sullivan JH. Decompression of the perioptic meninges for relief of papilledema. Am J Ophthalmol 1973;76:687–692.

132. Hupp SL, Glaser JS, Frazier-Byrne S. Optic nerve sheath decompression. Review of 17 cases. Arch Ophthalmol 1987;105:386–389.

133. Jefferson A, Clark J. Treatment of benign intracranial hypertension by dehydrating agents with particular reference to the measurement of the blind spot area as a means of recording improvement. J Neurol Neurosurg Psychiatry 1976;39:627–639.

134. Keltner JL, Miller NR, Gittinger JW, Burde RM. Pseudotumor cerebri. Surv Ophthalmol 1979;23:315–322.

135. Gucer G, Viernstein L. Long-term intracranial pressure recording in the management of pseudotumor cerebri. J Neurosurg 1978;49:256–263.

136. Martin-Amat G, Tephly TR, McMartin KE, et al. Methyl alcohol poisoning. II. Development of a model for ocular toxicity in methyl alcohol poisoning using the rhesus monkey. Arch Ophthalmol 1977;95:1847–1850.

137. Hayreh MS, Hayreh SS, Baumbach GL, et al. Methyl alcohol poisoning. III. Ocular toxicity. Arch Ophthalmol 1977;95:1851–1858.

138. Baumbach GL, Cancilla PA, Martin-Amat G, et al. Methyl alcohol poisoning. IV. Alterations of the morphological findings of the retina and optic nerve. Arch Ophthalmol 1977;95:1859–1865.

139. Leopold IH. Zinc deficiency and visual impairment? (editorial.) Am J Ophthalmol 1978;85:871–875.

140. Moynahan EJ. Zinc deficiency and disturbances of mood and visual behaviour (letter). Lancet 1976;1:91.

141. Moore R. Bleeding gastric erosion after oral zinc sulphate. Br Med J 1978;1:754.

142. Faigenbaum SJ, Leopold IH. Ophthalmology in nutritional support of medical practice. Hagerstown, NJ: Harper & Row, 1977:422–431.

143. Lessell S, Coppeto JM. The management of optic neuritis and nutritional amblyopia. In: Srinivasan BD, ed. Ocular therapeutics. New York: Masson, 1980;201–208.

CHAPTER 27

Thyroid-Related Eye Disease

Jimmy D. Bartlett
Eduardo Gaitan

Robert Graves,[1] an Irish physician, is usually credited with the first publication describing the suspected association between thyroid disease and the eye. The eponym "Graves' ophthalmopathy" has accordingly been proposed as the standard term describing the orbital disease that may result from or relate to abnormalities of the thyroid gland. Although approximately 75% of patients with Graves' disease have some degree of ocular involvement, only 15% of those patients ever develop serious functional impairment of vision.[2] Nevertheless, the diagnosis and management of thyroid-related eye disease are often a significant challenge to the optometrist and physician. This chapter considers the diagnostic features of Graves' ophthalmopathy and discusses the management of this important clinical syndrome.

Epidemiology

Noninfiltrative (Class 1) thyroid-related eye disease, the mildest form of ocular involvement, is the most frequent ocular manifestation of hyperthyroidism. This occurs in up to 50% of patients with toxic diffuse goiter and can begin at any age.[3] The more severe infiltrative (Classes 2 through 6) forms of ocular involvement, however, usually do not occur before adulthood. The incidence of ocular changes is inversely proportional to the severity of the manifestation; that is, most patients with ocular changes have relatively mild disease,

and very few patients develop the severe involvement characterized by significant corneal and optic nerve changes. Noninfiltrative disease occurs predominantly in females in a ratio of 4 to 6:1, with the most common age of onset during the second to third decade of life. Infiltrative disease, in contrast, is equally prevalent in male and female, but usually occurs at a later age.

Etiology

Although the precise etiopathogenesis of Graves' ophthalmopathy is not well understood, a basic knowledge of the pathology associated with the disease is essential for an understanding of the mechanisms of action of the various drugs and other therapeutic modalities used in managing this disorder. The ocular involvement associated with thyrotoxicosis is primarily an orbital disease. Although these orbital changes have been poorly understood, the most detailed report of the pathologic changes occurring in the orbital tissues and extraocular muscles of patients with Graves' disease has been that of Kroll and Kuwabara.[4] These investigators noted that the extraocular muscles may be grossly enlarged 2 to 5 times and that the orbital contents are under increased pressure. These changes are diffuse and progressive and histologically are represented by interstitial edema, increases in mucopolysaccharides, round cell infiltration (lymphocytes, plasma cells, macrophages, and mast cells), and degenerative changes within the muscle cells. This diffuse orbital infiltration involves all the connective tissues and extraocular muscles and is responsible for the proptosis and many of the other signs of Graves' ophthalmopathy.[5] Cant and Wilson[5] have hypothesized that almost all the secondary effects of thyroid-related orbital infiltration are circulatory and that the visual field loss and color vision dysfunction are typical of optic nerve involvement either by direct compression or by interference with circulation.

The role of the immune system in the pathophysiology of Graves' disease is presently well established.[6–11] A considerable amount of information has been obtained linking the human major histocompatibility complex (HLA) with Graves' disease.[9,12] For instance, there is an increased frequency of HLA-B8 in whites with this disorder. This is also true for the HLA-Dw3 that confers an even greater relative risk for Graves' disease than HLA-B8. On the other hand, Graves' disease in the Japanese has been found to be associated with HLA-B35, while in patients of Chinese origin HLA-Bw46 confers a greater risk.

In contrast to the systemic disorder, however, there is considerable disagreement regarding the association of HLA antigens and Graves' ophthalmopathy.[12] Although the immune system is clearly implicated, the immunologic basis and precise mechanism have not yet been defined to provide an explanation for the ocular disorder.[10,11,13,14] Kohn and Winand[15] have proposed a complex two-factor theory in which an IgG or exophthalmogenic immunoglobulin (EI) is postulated to be present in the serum of patients with Graves' ophthalmopathy. According to this theory, the EI sensitizes orbital tissues to the action of a fragment of thyrotropin (TSH) deprived of thyroid-stimulating activity but with exophthalmic properties, as demonstrated in fish. Kriss and associates[16] have provided some evidence that thyroglobulin (TG)-antithyroglobulin complexes bind to extraocular muscles and cause exophthalmos. These investigators base their argument on the hypothesis of lymphatic channels connecting the thyroid gland to the orbits, evidence that thyroglobulin-antihyroglobulin complexes bind specifically to extraocular muscle membranes, and that TG is present in extraocular muscles. Kidd and associates[6] have shown that an extraocular muscle antigen can induce in vitro secretion of the lymphokine, migration-inhibition factor (MIF), when using T-cell preparations from patients with Graves' ophthalmopathy. Consequently, T-cell-mediated immunity has also been implicated in the pathogenesis of the exophthalmos.

Doniach and Florin-Christensen[17] have offered a distinction between the way different tissues in the orbit are affected by these immune factors. These investigators suggest that the hypothesis of Kohn and Winand explains the edema of orbital fat, while that of Kriss and associates explains the changes of the extraocular muscles. To further complicate the issue, Solomon and associates[18] have provided evidence to support the concept that there are subclasses in so-called euthyroid Graves' ophthalmopathy, subclasses that cannot be explained entirely on the basis of the prevailing theories. More recently, circulating autoantibodies specific for eye muscle have been reported in 60% to 80% of patients with Graves' ophthalmopathy,[9,10] and antigenic differences between ocular and skeletal muscles have been found, which may explain the immunologic specificity of ocular muscle involvement in Graves' disease.[19] Furthermore, abnormal cell-mediated immunity appears to play an important role in the pathogenesis of Graves' ophthalmopathy.[9–11,20]

Diagnosis

The clinical diagnosis of Graves' ophthalmopathy can frequently be made without laboratory testing. Indeed, many patients will present with the classic signs of Graves' ophthalmopathy but will be found to be chemically and clinically euthyroid. In the patient who has a present or previous history of hyperthyroidism, the diagnosis is usually immediate. However, in those patients without such history, evidence of lid retraction is virtually pathognomonic. Vertical diplopia is particularly common, and intraocular pressure elevated more than 4 mm Hg on attempted upgaze signifies fibrosis of the inferior rectus muscle, an important diagnostic sign. The use of rose bengal solution may reveal superior limbic keratoconjunctivitis, which has been shown to have a possible association with hyperthyroidism.[21] These and other clinical findings, to be described, may serve to secure the clinical diagnosis. In 1 series of 52 patients[21] a diagnosis of Graves' ophthalmopathy based on the clinical findings alone was made in 42 of the patients with laboratory documentation of thyrotoxicosis.

Although Graves' disease and Hashimoto's thyroiditis account for the largest proportion of patients with bilateral proptosis, it can also be produced by neoplastic, vascular, and inflammatory processes as well as by infections, granulomatous processes, and other endocrine (Cushing's and acromegaly) diseases.[7,22] Thus, the diagnosis of Graves' ophthalmopathy can be made only by carefully excluding other possible causes of proptosis.[23,24]

Diagnosis of Thyrotoxicosis

In most cases the diagnosis of Graves' disease can be made on the basis of a careful clinical history and physical examination. The incidence of primary diagnostic symptoms and signs is listed in Table 27.1. In all cases, however, the laboratory confirmation of thyrotoxicosis is helpful in corroborating the diagnosis. Several laboratory tests are available for this purpose.[25–27] Figure 27.1 shows a suggested sequence of laboratory tests in the diagnosis of hyperthyroidism.

The concomitant determination of serum total thy-

TABLE 27.1
Incidence of Symptoms, Signs, and Laboratory Results

	Euthyroid Goiter (N = 321) (%)	Toxic Nodular Goiter (N = 108) (%)	Graves' Disease (N = 112) (%)
Symptoms			
1. Nervousness	66.5	83.0	90.5
2. Palpitations	60.0	78.3	83.6
3. Weight loss	48.1	84.0[a]	86.2[a]
4. Hyperhydrosis	46.5	68.0[b]	83.6[a]
5. Heat intolerance	38.4	65.1[b]	77.6[a]
6. Hair loss	38.4	67.0[b]	67.2[b]
7. Asthenia, fatigue, weakness	34.7	53.8[b]	57.7[b]
8. Dyspnea	24.7	55.7[a]	56.0[a]
9. Anorexia	22.8	35.8	42.2[b]
10. Amenorrhea	22.5	51.9[a]	38.8[b]
11. Diarrhea	22.5	47.2[a]	57.7[a]
12. Polyuria and polydipsia	17.5	44.3[a]	54.3[a]
13. Edema (pedal)	15.9	42.5[a]	45.7[a]
14. Eye symptoms	12.2	25.5[b]	36.2[a]
15. Emotional disturbance	9.0	15.1	23.2[b]
16. Increased appetite	5.3	12.3	32.7[a]
17. Increased bowel movements	1.5	5.7	14.6[a]
Signs			
1. Hyperreflexia	26.5	62.2[a]	62.0[a]
2. Tremor	24.4	64.1[a]	78.4[a]
3. Lymphocytosis (>40%)	23.4	26.4[b]	44.0[b]
4. Moderate tachycardia (95–110)	21.5	35.8[b]	27.5
5. Lid lag, stare, chemosis	13.7	30.2[b]	62.0[a]
6. Skin changes	12.8	52.8[a]	74.1[a]
7. Serum cholesterol (<150 mg/dl)	17.5	30.5	41.9[b]
8. Hyperkinesis	10.3	26.4[b]	38.8[a]
9. Wide pulse pressure	9.7	40.5[a]	25.0[b]
10. Marked tachycardia (>110)	8.1	49.0[a]	62.0[a]
11. Leukopenia	6.2	11.3	17.2[b]
12. Hepatosplenomegaly	4.0	17.0[b]	13.8[b]
13. Liver palms	3.4	17.0[b]	24.1[a]
14. Congestive heart failure	2.8	17.0[a]	7.7[b]
15. Onycholysis	0.9	5.7	6.0
16. Bruit	0.6	5.6	27.6[a]
17. Thyroid heart or atrial fibrillation	0.6	12.2[b]	10.3[b]
18. Exophthalmos	0.3	—	37.0[a]
19. Lagophthalmos	0.3	2.8	7.7[b]
20. Goiter	100.0	100.0	97.0

[a]Significantly different from euthyroid subjects ($P < 0.01$ by chi-square test).
[b]($P < 0.05$).
Adapted from Gaitan E, Wahner HW, Cuello C, et al. Endemic goiter in the Cauca Valley. II. Studies of thyroid pathophysiology. J Clin Endocrinol Metab 1969;29:675–683; Gaitan E. Thyroid Univ Case Reports 1980;1(5).

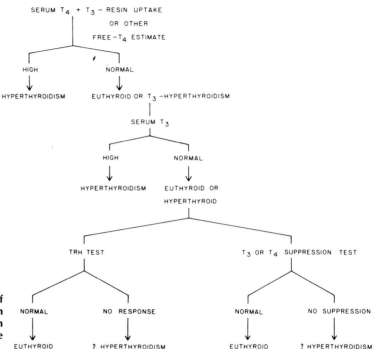

FIGURE 27.1 **Flowchart showing a suggested sequence of laboratory tests in the diagnosis of hyperthyroidism. (From Kaplan MM, Utiger RD. Diagnosis of hyperthyroidism. Clin Endocrinol Metab 1978;7:97–113, with permission of the authors and publisher.)**

roxine (T4) and triiodothyronine resin uptake (T3U) constitutes the best screening test for hyperthyroidism. In most laboratories T4 measured by radioimmunoassay (RIA) shows normal values ranging from 5 to 12 μg/dl. T3U is an indirect but simple in vitro technique reflecting the concentration and affinity of thyroid-binding globulin (TBG) such that T3U may be used to correct for changes in TBG. For this purpose the free T4 index (FTI) is used. To calculate this index, T4 is multiplied by the T3U, and the product is the FTI value, which correlates well in most instances with free T4 (FT4) concentrations. FTI values are high in hyperthyroidism. However, the FTI as calculated is subject to intraday and other variations in methodology so that often the result cannot be compared with that from other laboratories. To eliminate such variations, the FT4I was developed, where

$$FT4I = T4 \times \frac{T3U \text{ (patient)}}{T3U \text{ (lab standard)}}$$

Although a variety of methods to determine FT4 have been developed,[28] technical improvement is necessary before FT4 determinations can be routinely adopted in place of the combined measurements of T4 and T3U.

There are instances in which the FTI might be within normal limits in patients with Graves' ophthalmopathy, and the practitioner is confronted with the differential diagnosis between euthyroid Graves' ophthalmopathy and T3-toxicosis. In these instances measurement of total T3 by RIA will provide the diagnosis. T3-toxicosis is characterized by an elevated T3 level with normal T4 values. Since increased T3 concentrations can be found in conditions other than T3-toxicosis, it is mandatory to correlate the high T3 value with the clinical history and physical findings.

There are still other cases in which, in the absence of clear clinical manifestations and with normal values of T4, T3U, and T3 (RIA), the TRH test, which has replaced the Werner T3-suppression test, is necessary to document the autonomy of the thyroid gland. The TRH test involves the intravenous administration of TRH (Thypinone), 200 to 500 μg, and plasma concentrations of thyrotropin (TSH) are determined at the moment of injection and at 15-minute intervals thereafter for 60 to 90 minutes. For cost effectiveness, however, determinations at 0 and 30 minutes are usually sufficient. A prompt and significant increase (2 to 8 times) in TSH is observed in normal patients.[29] This functional test is of greatest value in the early diagnosis of hyperthyroidism, since administration of TRH to such patients fails to increase the plasma TSH concentration. The new sensitive TSH assays that can distinguish normal from subnormal serum TSH levels may become the front-line test in the diagnosis of hyperthyroidism.[30,31]

Both T3-suppression and TRH tests have been used to characterize various proposed subclasses of euthyroid Graves' ophthalmopathy,[18,141] in which the classic ocular changes of Graves' disease exist in patients who are clinically and chemically euthyroid, showing normal serum concentrations of T4, T3U, and T3 (RIA).[32,33] Some of these patients have an exaggerated increase in TSH following TRH administration and thus correspond with the early onset of hypothyroidism as seen in Hashimoto's thyroiditis. Other patients have no change in TSH after TRH administration, reflecting a very early stage of hyperthyroidism. Still others have an entirely normal response to TRH administration and to T3 suppression. The existence of ophthalmopathy identical to that seen in Graves' disease but with a normal pituitary-thyroid axis has permitted the speculation that Graves' ophthalmopathy might be closely associated with Graves' hyperthyroidism but may otherwise be a separate and distinct disorder.

Thyroid-stimulating immunoglobulins (TSI) have been found in almost all patients with Graves' disease and should provide additional information in categorizing those patients with euthyroid Graves' ophthalmopathy.[34–37] Two types of assays are used[36,37]: (1) assays for thyroid-stimulating antibody (TSAb) in which an increase in cyclic AMP in human thyroid in vitro indicates the presence of thyroid-stimulating immunoglobulin, and (2) the receptor-modulating assays in which TSH-binding inhibition (TBI) to the TSH receptor from human or porcine thyroid or guinea pig fat cell membranes is measured using ^{125}I-labelled TSH in the presence of serum or a solution of crude or purified IgG. Of these two assays, the TSAb is more sensitive and specific, so caution should be observed in the use of TBI data for clinical decision making.

A variety of assays to detect autoantibodies specific for ocular muscle have been developed,[9,10,20] which, along with measurement of TSAb or the thyroid microsomal autoantibody (TMAb), may assist in some instances in the diagnosis of Graves' ophthalmopathy. The measurement of TMAb, which is less expensive and more readily available, appears to have diagnostic significance similar to that of TSAb in euthyroid Graves' ophthalmopathy.[37]

In addition, determination of antibodies to thyroglobulin and to the thyroid microsomal antigen can be helpful in characterizing those patients with Hashimoto's thyroiditis and ophthalmopathy, in whom thyroid-stimulating antibodies are generally absent.[34]

Classification of Graves' Ophthalmopathy

In an attempt to achieve uniformity in terminology regarding the various ocular changes associated with thyroid disease, the American Thyroid Association adopted in 1968 an initial classification of the ocular changes of Graves' disease.[38] Various modifications to the original classification system have been proposed,[39,40] and one has been approved by the American Thyroid Association[39] (Tables 27.2 and 27.3). Each class usually, but not necessarily, includes the changes indicated in the preceding class. One should also note that the first letters of each definition form the mnemonic NO SPECS, the NO indicating the usually nonthreatening prognosis of Classes 0 and 1, and SPECS indicating the relatively serious nature of Classes 2 through 6.

CLASS 1 DISEASE

Class 1 disease, formerly termed *mild* or *noninfiltrative* disease, is characterized by upper lid retraction (Fig. 27.2) and occurs in over 90% of patients with hyperthyroidism.[5] This sign may initially occur unilaterally or bilaterally and is often asymmetric.[142] A helpful diagnostic sign often associated with lid retraction is the lid tug sign,[41] in which the retracted upper lid offers a sensation of increased resistance on attempted manual lid closure. The resistance to lid closure is noted by simply grasping the lashes of the upper lid and gently pulling down. The amount of resistance is compared with the contralateral lid in unilateral cases or with a control normal lid in cases of bilateral lid retraction. This test is particularly helpful in cases of questionable bilateral retraction or ambiguous unilateral retraction versus contralateral ptosis.

The most common cause of lid retraction is hyperthyroidism.[42] Thus, this sign is virtually pathognomonic of Graves' ophthalmopathy. There are three major hypotheses for the pathogenesis of thyroid-associated lid retraction[42–45]: (1) in the early stages there is exces-

TABLE 27.2
Abridged Classification of the Eye Changes of Graves' Disease

Class[a]	Definition
0	No physical signs or symptoms
1	Only signs, no symptoms (signs limited to upper eyelid retraction, stare, and eyelid lag)
2	Soft tissue involvement (symptoms and signs)
3	Proptosis
4	Extraocular muscle involvement
5	Corneal involvement
6	Sight loss (optic nerve involvement)

[a]Each class usually, but not necessarily, includes the involvements indicated in the preceding class.
From Werner SC. Modification of the classification of the eye changes of Graves' disease. Am J Ophthalmol 1977;83:725–727.

TABLE 27.3
Detailed Classification of the Eye Changes of Graves' Disease

Class	Grade	Suggestions for Grading
0		No physical signs or symptoms
1		Only signs
2		Soft tissue involvement with symptoms and signs
	o	Absent
	a	Minimal
	b	Moderate
	c	Marked
3		Proptosis 3 mm or more in excess of upper normal limit, with or without symptoms
	o	Absent
	a	3–4 mm increase over upper normal
	b	5–7 mm increase
	c	8 or more mm increase
4		Extraocular muscle involvement; usually with diplopia, other symptoms, and other signs
	o	Absent
	a	Limitation of motion at extremes of gaze
	b	Evident restriction of motion
	c	Fixation of a globe or globes
5		Corneal involvement primarily caused by lagophthalmos
	o	Absent
	a	Stippling of cornea
	b	Ulceration
	c	Clouding, necrosis, perforation
6		Sight loss caused by optic nerve involvement
	o	Absent
	a	Disc pallor or choking, or visual field defect; acuity 6/6 (20/20)–6/18 (20/60)
	b	Same; acuity 6/22 (20/70)–6/60 (20/200)
	c	Blindness (failure to perceive light), acuity less than 6/60 (20/200)

From Werner SC. Modification of the classification of the eye changes of Graves' disease. Am J Ophthalmol 1977;83(5):725–727.

sive stimulation of Mueller's muscle in the upper lid associated with the sympathicotonia of Graves' disease, resulting from the marked inhibition of liver mono-amine oxidase synthesis by high circulating thyroxine levels; (2) in long-standing Graves' disease, there may be overaction of the levator muscle, resulting from excessive stimulation of the superior rectus muscle acting against a fibrotic inferior rectus muscle; and (3) mechanical restriction or infiltration of the levator muscle.

Lid retraction can appear in the presence of chemical and clinical euthyroidism and is often unrelated to control of any existing thyroid dysfunction. Lid lag (Von Graefe's sign) often accompanies lid retraction (Fig. 27.3). Lid retraction disappears spontaneously after 15 years in about 60% of patients.[3]

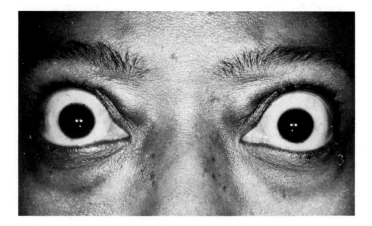

FIGURE 27.2 **Upper lid retraction characteristic of Class 1 Graves' ophthalmopathy.**

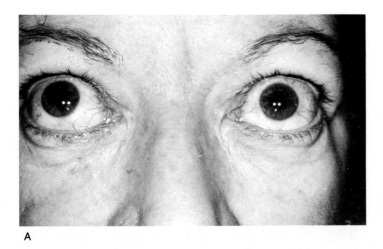

A

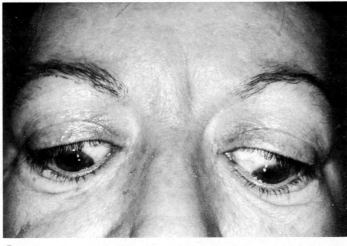

B

FIGURE 27.3 **Lid lag (Von Graefe's sign). Following extreme upgaze (A), the upper lids remain retracted and fail to assume their normal depressed position on downgaze (B).**

CLASS 2 DISEASE

Classes 2 through 6 disease, formerly termed *severe* or *infiltrative* disease, represent the more significant and vision-threatening changes associated with Graves' disease. The ocular manifestations of Class 2 disease include a variety of important clinical signs: swelling of the lids; prolapse of orbital fat, nasally in the upper lid and temporally in the lower lid; palpable lacrimal gland; injection of the conjunctival and episcleral vessels; and chemosis (Fig. 27.4). These changes result in symptoms relating to lacrimation, light sensitivity, and gritty or sandy foreign body sensation. These symptoms are frequently worse in the morning on awakening. Inflammation and hypertrophy of the insertions of the extraocular muscles (Fig. 27.5) are common and are of diagnostic value in those patients without proptosis.[21]

CLASS 3 DISEASE

The incidence of proptosis in patients with hyperthyroidism is high, with estimates ranging from 40% to 75%.[46] Two-thirds of patients with Graves' ophthalmopathy develop proptosis of 21 mm or more.[3] Although computed tomography (CT) and ultrasound evaluations reveal extraocular muscle involvement, the degree of proptosis does not necessarily parallel the severity of the orbital inflammatory process.[47] The proptosis may give rise to secondary lagophthalmos (Fig. 27.6). Like lid retraction, proptosis can begin unilaterally and should therefore be differentiated from the apparent proptosis simulated by unilateral lid retraction. This can be accomplished clinically by measurement using the Luedde or Hertel exophthalmometer,[48] with which the upper limits of normal are approximately 18 mm for Orientals, 20 mm for whites,

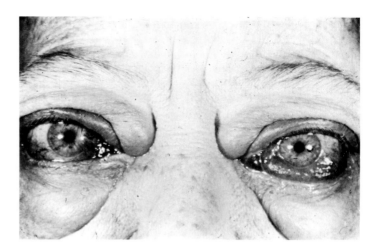

FIGURE 27.4 **Class 2 Graves' ophthalmopathy with upper and lower lid swelling, injection of conjunctival and episcleral vessels, and chemosis.**

and 23 mm for blacks[39,49] (Table 27.4). A difference between eyes of 2 mm or more should be considered abnormal and justification for further study.[50] Since hyperthyroidism is the most common cause of unilateral proptosis, the investigation of unilateral proptosis in patients without other signs of Graves' ophthalmopathy should include serum T4, T3U, and T3 (RIA).[21,51] If the results from these tests are normal, the TRH test should be performed.

CLASS 4 DISEASE

Approximately 14% of patients with thyrotoxicosis[52] and 33% of patients with Graves' ophthalmopathy[3] develop Class 4 involvement, in which the inflammatory changes result in loss of elasticity and fibrosis of the extraocular muscles. Most commonly the patient with Class 4 disease is a woman between age 40 and 60 years.[53] The patient is frequently chemically and clinically euthyroid and may present with extraocular muscle involvement as the only ocular change.[54–56]

Electromyography (EMG) and saccadic velocity studies have demonstrated that the mechanical restriction of the eye is caused by interstitial edema and fibrosis of the muscles rather than by myopathy.[57,58] The most common muscle to be involved is the inferior rectus, which is affected in 60% to 70% of cases (Fig. 27.7). Twenty-five percent of patients have a fibrotic medial rectus muscle, and only 10% or less demonstrate a fibrotic superior rectus muscle.[53] Differentiating a fibrotic muscle from paresis of its antagonist is essential and can be achieved by performing a forced duction test, as described in Chapter 15.

Since the inferior rectus muscle usually undergoes fibrosis early, attempted upgaze exerts traction on the globe, which elevates the intraocular pressure. This phenomenon occurs in approximately 20% of patients with Graves' disease[59] and indicates fibrosis of the

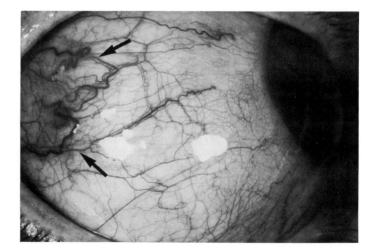

FIGURE 27.5 **Inflammation and early hypertrophy (arrows) of the insertion of the lateral rectus muscle in a patient with Class 2 Graves' ophthalmopathy. White spots in center are photographic artifacts.**

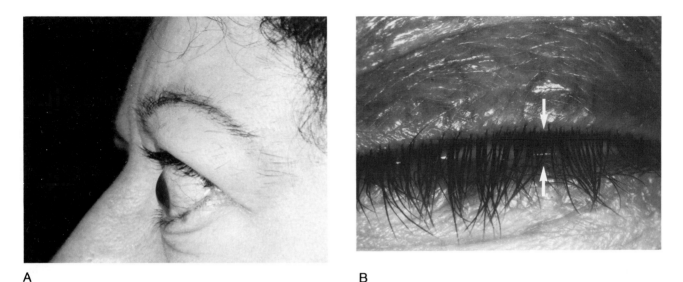

A   B

FIGURE 27.6   **White woman of 50 years with Class 3 Graves' ophthalmopathy.** *(A)* **Proptosis of 27 mm measured with the Hertel exophthalmometer.** *(B)* **Secondary lagophthalmos (arrows).**

inferior rectus muscle; more important, it should not mislead the clinician into pursuing a misdiagnosis of glaucoma.

CLASS 5 DISEASE

Class 5 involvement poses a significant threat to visual function because of exposure keratopathy secondary to lagophthalmos (Fig. 27.8). Corneal exposure may be particularly severe if there is significant upper lid retraction, proptosis, and an abolished Bell's reflex associated with fibrosis of the inferior rectus muscle and limitation of upgaze. Unless the patient is managed aggressively, secondary corneal ulceration can ensue with the potential risk of loss of the eye.

TABLE 27.4
Exophthalmometry Values in Healthy Black and White Adults

Race and Sex	Mean	Upper Limit of Normal
White male	16.5	21.7
White female	15.4	20.1
Black male	18.5	24.7
Black female	17.8	23.0

Adapted from Migliori ME, Gladstone GJ. Determination of the normal range of exophthalmometric values for black and white adults. Am J Ophthalmol 1984;98:438–442.

CLASS 6 DISEASE

Only a small number of patients with Graves' ophthalmopathy, perhaps 2% to 5%, develop optic nerve involvement.[46] Thyroid optic neuropathy may be evidenced by papilledema, papillitis, or retrobulbar neuritis and is usually characterized by a painless and gradual loss of visual acuity associated with central or paracentral scotomas. Thus, visual field examination is one of the best diagnostic tools for early optic neuropathy.[60] Occasionally, vision loss can occur precipitously over 1 or 2 weeks. Other features of optic nerve dysfunction frequently associated with the decreased visual acuity are color vision disturbances, afferent pupillary defects in patients with asymmetric involvement, and prolongation of the pupil cycle time.[46]

The precise pathogenesis of the optic neuropathy associated with Graves' disease has not been definitely established, but it is generally accepted that massively swollen extraocular muscles impinge on the optic nerve at the orbital apex, which interferes with blood supply to the nerve and results in the signs and symptoms of compressive optic neuropathy.[61–63] If prompt and aggressive treatment is not offered, optic atrophy often results.

Diagnostic Imaging of the Orbit

Orbital ultrasonographic examination[64] and CT scanning[65] are the most helpful noninvasive techniques for the diagnosis of Graves' ophthalmopathy. They are

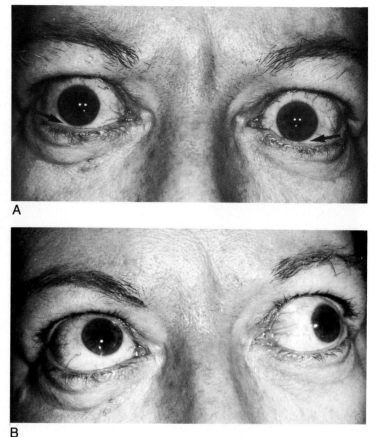

FIGURE 27.7   **Same patient as in Figure 27.6.** *(A)* **Note the asymmetry of visible sclera above each lower lid (arrows). By prism measurement this patient has an 8ᐃ left hypotropia in primary gaze.** *(B)* **Restriction of left inferior rectus on gaze up and left.**

particularly valuable when the patient is clinically and chemically euthyroid, since they may demonstrate evidence of enlarged extraocular muscles before clinical signs and symptoms arise. In general, the inflammatory and congestive orbital changes are most accurately defined using ultrasound rather than CT scanning, and detection of enlarged extraocular muscles occurs earlier with ultrasound.[64] Moreover, the use of ultrasound alone is often sufficient and more cost-effective than

is CT scanning in revealing enlarged extraocular muscles.[66] The diagnostic accuracy of ultrasound examination can be as high as 90%, with a diagnostic sensitivity of 70%.[67] This allows discovery of orbital involvement in the fellow eyes of about 50% of patients with unilateral ocular findings.[66]

CT scanning will confirm the diagnosis of Graves' ophthalmopathy in euthyroid patients and those with atypical or severe clinical manifestations, including

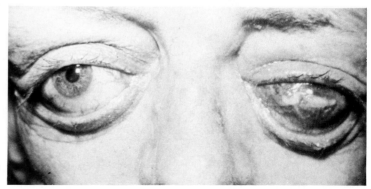

FIGURE 27.8   **Severe exposure keratopathy of the left eye of a patient with Class 5 Graves' ophthalmopathy.**

compressive optic neuropathy.[68] The extraocular muscle enlargement is seen to occupy the nontendonous (belly) portion of the muscles[66] (Fig. 27.9). However, when compared with ultrasound examination, the reduced diagnostic accuracy and diagnostic sensitivity of CT scanning make the former technique more reliable for detecting the orbital changes that define Graves' ophthalmopathy.[67] Zimmerman and associates[69] have shown that magnetic resonance imaging (MRI) of the orbit can reveal anatomic details superior to those from CT scanning.

Clinical Course of Graves' Ophthalmopathy

As stated previously, because of the sometimes ill-defined association with thyrotoxicosis, some investigators have questioned the relationship of the ocular changes to systemic hyperthyroidism. The ocular changes may appear before, during, or after the onset of thyrotoxicosis, but usually occur within 18 months before or after the diagnosis of hyperthyroidism.[70] Gamblin and associates[71] assert that ocular involvement, even if subclinical, is an inevitable complication of Graves' disease. All classes of ocular changes occur in euthyroid Graves' disease as well as in the euthyroid phase of hyperthyroidism. The course and duration of changes in Classes 2 through 6 are extremely unpredictable, with progression from Class 1 to Class 6 often being irregular. Progression from Class 1 through Class 6 occurs in about 5% of patients even after subtotal thyroidectomy or after radioactive iodine (RAI) therapy.[3] The onset is usually subacute, with one eye frequently being affected before its fellow. The natural history of the ocular disease from onset to spontaneous remission usually covers 6 months to 3 years (mean 2 years), after which the patient usually manifests a residual lid retraction, lid fullness, proptosis, and fibrotic changes of the extraocular muscles. Because of the tendency for Graves' ophthalmopathy to undergo spontaneous remission, medical or surgical treatment is intended to prevent permanent ocular damage rather than to arrest or retard progression of the disease process.

The clinical course of the ocular changes in hyperthyroidism seems to have two distinct phases,[72] rapid and plateau. The rapid phase lasts from several weeks to 6 months. During this time the ocular changes progress rapidly. During the plateau phase, the condition of the eyes either remains stationary or slowly moderates over several years before significant improvement occurs.

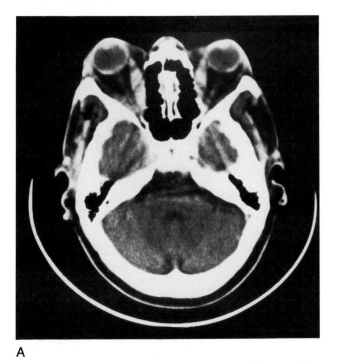

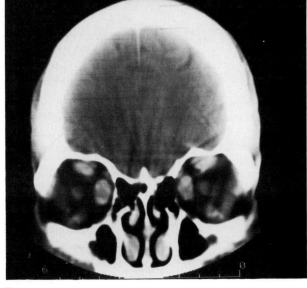

A   B

FIGURE 27.9 **CT scans of the orbit in a 63-year-old man with Graves' ophthalmopathy.** *(A)* **Proptosis and markedly enlarged extraocular muscles.** *(B)* **Coronal view showing extraocular muscle enlargement.**

Management

Since the natural history of Graves' ophthalmopathy is to undergo spontaneous remission, the effectiveness of various forms of treatment is sometimes difficult to evaluate. However, with the knowledge that some eyes are lost solely due to failure to provide treatment, appropriate therapeutic measures may serve to reduce the risk to visual function and provide the patient with symptomatic relief. In general, management of the ocular involvement includes treatment of the underlying hyperthyroidism, if present, and the provision of local treatment to protect the ocular tissues and preserve visual functions. Surgical intervention should be withheld until the ocular and thyroid disorders are stable. The presence of active Class 2 through Class 6 disease calls for prompt and aggressive treatment as soon as the diagnosis is confirmed. Regardless of the stage of ocular involvement, however, the following general principles of management[73] apply:

- Since most patients with Graves' ophthalmopathy go through a period of initial worsening followed by a plateau of variable length, and finally spontaneous improvement, patients should be monitored more closely if in the worsening phase. If spontaneous improvement is occurring, more vigorous forms of treatment such as surgery or high-dose steroids should be withheld.
- Many patients, if relieved of the fear of losing vision, are willing to accept surprising degrees of cosmetic change.
- The patient should be advised of the marked variations in the course of the ocular disease and its relatively imprecise association with thyrotoxicosis; this will serve to reassure the patient and maintain rapport with the practitioner if the condition should worsen in its later stages.

A major problem in devising effective treatment has been an inadequate understanding of the factors that cause the ocular disease. Despite this, the following recommendations are representative of the most effective treatment modalities currently available.

Management of the Thyrotoxicosis

As part of the treatment of Graves' ophthalmopathy, adequate control of the hyperthyroid state, if it exists, is essential.[74,75] The antithyroid drugs propylthiouracil (PTU) and methimazole (MMI), radioactive iodine (^{131}I), and surgery are the 3 major modalities used in the treatment of hyperthyroidism. In addition, β-adrenergic blocking agents such as propranolol are useful for the rapid control of sympathetic nervous system manifestations. There is general agreement that the hyperthyroid state and the ocular disease run their own courses. Although control of hypermetabolism is necessary, this control does not ensure that the ophthalmopathy will improve concomitantly with treatment of the hyperthyroidism. However, it is essential in the treatment of the thyrotoxicosis to bring the patient gradually to euthyroidism by avoiding abrupt and exaggerated changes in the thyroid state. The ocular changes may be more likely to progress following systemic treatment that causes rapid alteration in thyroid function.[2]

Most patients with Graves' disease will respond adequately to an initial dose of PTU, 300 to 450 mg, or MMI, 30 to 45 mg, daily in divided doses. Doses should be adjusted subsequently by clinical response and thyroid hormone determinations. Several management options exist once the patient's hyperthyroidism has been controlled with antithyroid drugs.[76] Some physicians reduce the dose of medication while others, to maintain a euthyroid state, provide thyroid hormone replacement without modifying the amount of antithyroid drug. Radioactive iodine (RAI) treatment is generally reserved for patients over 30 years of age. Most patients with Graves' disease will respond adequately to doses between 5 and 10 mCi of ^{131}I. Subtotal thyroidectomy is used in selected cases but should not be performed until the patient is under adequate control with antithyroid drugs. Patients developing hypothyroidism due to treatment should receive L-thyroxine, 0.1 to 0.2 mg daily. These patients should be monitored at regular intervals by careful clinical examination and serum T4 and, if necessary, TSH determinations.

The frequency and types of toxic reactions to PTU and MMI are similar but appear to be related to the doses employed. In about 5% of patients there are mild side effects, ranging from gastrointestinal complaints to mild skin reactions and pruritis, that can usually be controlled adequately with antihistamines without discontinuing the drug. The most severe and worrisome complication, however, is agranulocytosis, which occurs in about 0.2% of patients treated with these drugs. It always responds to discontinuation of the medication, but, in a few instances, concomitant administration of steroids may be indicated. Since this complication can be lethal if not quickly recognized, the patient should be advised to report to the physician whenever infection, sore throat, or general malaise occurs, in which case a complete blood count (CBC) should be obtained.

It is generally accepted that the outcome of Graves' ophthalmopathy after treatment of the hyperthyroidism with antithyroid drugs, radioactive iodine, or surgery is similar for the 3 groups. There is also clinical evidence that the development of severe ophthalmopathy does not seem to be related to the degree of hypothyroidism or hyperthyroidism, but that the careful, gradual control of thyroid function is important in minimizing the danger to these patients' eyes.

Local Management of the Ophthalmopathy

A variety of local measures can be used to provide the patient with symptomatic relief while protecting ocular tissues and preserving visual functions. These are discussed for each disease classification.

CLASS 1 DISEASE (LID RETRACTION)

The patient with Class 1 disease may have lagophthalmos ranging from very mild to very severe. The lid retraction and lagophthalmos accelerate tear film evaporation, thus increasing tear film osmolarity and causing ocular surface damage.[77] Any associated exposure keratopathy should be managed with mild ocular lubricating solutions or ointments. A variety of general measures may be helpful, such as the wearing of tinted lenses to shield the cosmetic appearance and to protect the eye from wind, dust, and other environmental factors. The eyelids can be taped shut at bedtime to protect the cornea. Likewise, a Saran Wrap shield can be constructed and taped over the eye, thus creating a moisture chamber during sleep. For moderate to severe cases of corneal exposure, applying a topical broad-spectrum antibacterial ointment (e.g., gentamicin or bacitracin–polymyxin B) at bedtime or continuously during the day will serve to prevent infection of the exposed corneal and conjunctival tissues.

In many instances, however, the patient's primary desire is to have an improved cosmetic appearance of the lid retraction. Since the relationship between the clinical signs of thyrotoxicosis and the effects of increased catecholamine activity has been apparent for many decades, various attempts have been made to control or alleviate the upper lid retraction by using adrenergic blocking agents such as guanethidine, reserpine, and thymoxamine. Because upper lid retraction may be mediated through sympathetic activity of Mueller's muscle, drugs with α-adrenergic blocking properties have been used topically and orally to manage this condition. However, these drugs do not affect the degree of proptosis, if present, because proptosis is associated with increased volume of the retrobulbar tissues and is not mediated through autonomic nervous system control. Topical bethanidine, an adrenergic blocking agent, has been used in 10% and 20% solutions to treat lid retraction.[78] When used in a dosage

of 2 or 3 drops daily, it effectively induces a pharmacologic Horner's syndrome with associated ptosis and miosis. Three or more weeks may be required to reach a maximum ptotic effect. No serious adverse ocular or systemic side effects have been observed. Propranolol, a β-adrenergic blocking agent, has been used both orally[53] and topically[79] to relieve lid retraction. For acute cases of lid retraction, propranolol, 10 mg 4 times daily, may be helpful. The topical use of 1% propranolol solution has produced variable results.[79] In addition, topical timolol has been used by some practitioners for lid retraction, but with variable results.[80]

Thymoxamine is a selective, competitive pure α-adrenergic blocking agent that is a theoretically ideal drug for the management of lid retraction. A substantial narrowing of the palpebral fissure occurs in about 75% of patients administered topical 0.5% thymoxamine.[43] The maximum reduction in palpebral fissure occurs within 30 minutes (Fig. 27.10). Unfortunately, however, topical instillation of this drug produces considerable transient ocular irritation, limiting its current usefulness for lid retraction. If this drug can be modified to reduce its ocular irritation, it may prove beneficial in the management of thyroid-related lid retraction.

The most commonly employed drug for the relief of lid retraction is orally or topically administered guanethidine. Guanethidine depletes sympathetic storage sites, initially causing release of norepinephrine that may lead to mydriasis and lid retraction but that eventually produces a chemical sympathectomy resembling postganglionic Horner's syndrome. Although guanethidine is somewhat unpredictable in the management of lid retraction, it seems to offer the best results with the fewest toxic effects when used in lower concentrations. Orally administered guanethidine, 15 mg daily, has been shown to lower the eyelid in some patients,[80] but most clinicians prefer the topical route of administration. When employed topically in a 10% concentration, this agent substantially reduces lid retraction (Fig. 27.11) but is associated with significant superficial punctate keratitis in about 50% of patients.[81] The 5% solution is equally effective but without the attendant side effects.[81] Unlike the effect associated with thymoxamine, the maximum effect on lid retraction requires several days (Fig. 27.12). Systemic side effects have not been noted in most studies, but 1 report of 2 patients with severe abdominal pains and diarrhea requiring emergency hospital admission should call for caution in the use of this drug.[82] The clinician should initiate therapy with 5% guanethidine,[a] 1 drop 3 times daily, until maximum improvement in the lid position is obtained, and then reduce the frequency of administration to daily instillation if this is adequate and, if possible, further reduce the instillation to alternate

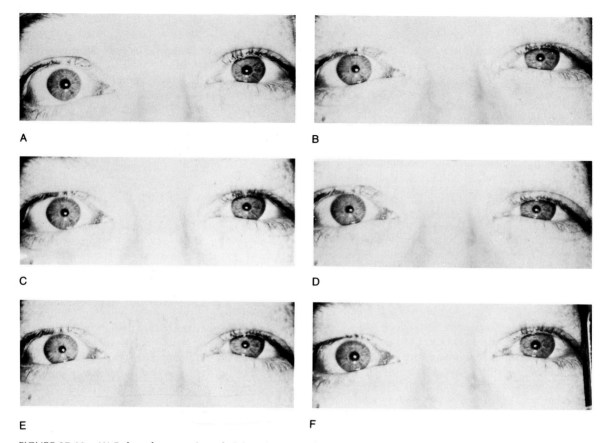

A

B

C

D

E

F

FIGURE 27.10   *(A)* **Before thymoxamine administration.** *(B)* **Fifteen minutes after thymoxamine administration.** *(C)* **Forty-five minutes after administration.** *(D)* **Two hours after administration.** *(E)* **Four hours after administration.** *(F)* **Five and one-half hours after administration. Miosis and reduction in palpebral fissure are evident at 15 minutes *(B)*. At 5½ hours *(F)*, pupils are redilating and fissures are wider than at 4 hours *(E)*. Note marked response in normal-appearing left fissure *(B)*. (From Dixon RS, Anderson RL, Hatt MU. The use of thymoxamine in eyelid retraction. Arch Ophthalmol 1979;97:2147–2150. Copyright 1979, American Medical Association.)**

days.[83] Table 27.5 lists the local side effects of guanethidine encountered in one series of patients.[84]

Several conditions may adversely affect the ability of guanethidine to lower the upper lid:[44] (1) if the patient is thyrotoxic, rather than euthyroid or hypothyroid[85]; (2) if the patient is concomitantly undergoing drug therapy with adrenergic agonists, either systemically or topically; and (3) if adhesions form between the levator and the superior rectus muscles in the later stages of the disease process.[80]

Surgery for Class 1 disease is usually not indicated because these patients are typically asymptomatic and because the lid retraction may resolve after treatment of the underlying thyrotoxicosis. Surgery, however, is a reasonable and necessary alternative for patients with severe lid retraction not responding to conservative measures. In some patients a small lateral tarsorrhaphy may be cosmetically justified,[86] and in other patients a scleral implant, levator tenotomy, levator recession,

resection of Mueller's muscle, or levator myotomy may be warranted.[87–89] In most cases surgery for lid retraction should not be considered until the ocular condition has been stable for at least 6 months to 1 year. If proptosis is present and is severe enough to require orbital decompression, this procedure should be done first, since the decompression itself may reduce the lid retraction.[90] The decision to lower the lids should then be postponed for several months. However, in emergencies in which corneal integrity is threatened, lid surgery could be contemplated together with the orbital decompression.[42]

CLASS 2 DISEASE (SOFT TISSUE INVOLVEMENT)

Many patients with mild Class 2 disease can be adequately managed with bland ocular lubricants. Elevating the head of the bed on 6 inch blocks during sleep with often minimize lid and periocular swelling on

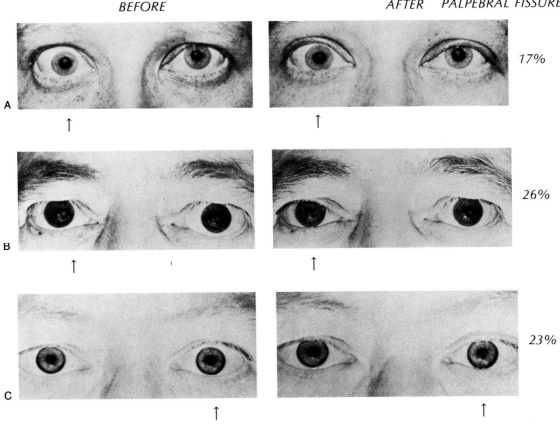

BEFORE   *AFTER*   *% DECREASE IN PALPEBRAL FISSURE*

17%

26%

23%

FIGURE 27.11   **Response of 3 patients to treatment with guanethidine 10% in 1 eye for 1 week. The average reduction in the palpebral fissure of the treated eye is about 20%. (From Sneddon JM, Turner P. Adrenergic blockade and the eye signs of thyrotoxicosis. Lancet 1966;2:525–527, with permission of the authors and publisher.)**

awakening.[2,3,53,82] The use of tinted lenses will afford relief from light sensitivity. Tinted lenses not only guard against irritation and light sensitivity, but they also have the advantage of masking the cosmetic problem. Occasionally, the use of orally administered diuretics is indicated. If the patient has unquestioned glaucoma concomitantly with Class 2 Graves' ophthalmopathy, the diuretic of choice, conveniently, is acetazolamide.[53] For patients with moderate to severe Class 2 disease, the use of systemically administered corticosteroids may be of immense benefit (Fig. 27.13). There is no doubt that the use of steroids in adequate dosages can decrease the severity of ocular complications, although they have minimal, if any, influence on the duration of the thyrotoxicosis.[82] In rare instances, surgical excision of pockets of fat from bulging upper and lower lids will be required, as will tightening of redundant skin of the lids by blepharoplasty.[88]

Locally administered steroids have been used with variable success. Although topically applied steroids are completely ineffective in alleviating the ocular signs or symptoms associated with Class 2 disease,[3] periocular steroids have been employed with some success.[3,53,73,82,91,92] Subconjunctival or retrobulbar injections of methylprednisolone are most commonly used, but sub-Tenon's injection of aqueous triamcinolone (Kenalog 40 mg/ml) can also be used.[53,82] The precise dosage of methylprednisolone must be guided by the individual patient, but 10 to 20 mg per injection (40 mg/ml) has been effective when repeated at varying intervals.[82] More concentrated preparations of methylprednisolone (Depo-Medrol 80 mg/ml) permit the injection of higher doses with smaller volumes,[82] which is particularly important when giving retrobulbar injections into an already tense orbit. Periocular injections may be repeated at monthly or longer intervals as required.

The results obtained from the use of periocular steroids can be quite dramatic. Most patients obtain

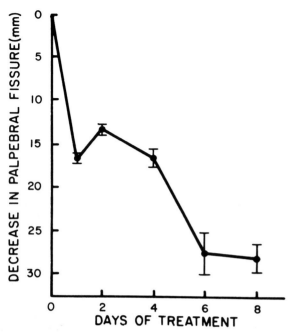

FIGURE 27.12 **The mean decrease in palpebral fissure of 1 eye compared with pretreatment values in 14 patients receiving guanethidine 10%, 2 drops twice daily. Each point represents the mean (±SEM). Measurements were obtained by projecting the clinical photographs to 8 times their original size. (From Sneddon JM, Turner P. Adrenergic blockade and the eye signs of thyrotoxicosis. Lancet 1966;2:525–527, with permission of the authors and publisher.)**

- The ocular tissues as well as most patients tolerate the injections very well.
- The injections are seldom needed more often than once every 2 weeks.
- A single injection often allows control of ocular signs and symptoms for 4 weeks.
- After periocular administration of steroids is begun, oral steroid therapy can often be discontinued or reduced.

Although periocular steroid administration is not without risk, associated side effects are virtually nonexistent, although one patient has developed steroid glaucoma.[91] Thus, it appears that subconjunctival or retrobulbar steroids can be an effective substitute in many cases for orally administered steroids. There are few complications, and local tolerance to the preparation and procedure is usually good.

CLASS 3 DISEASE (PROPTOSIS)

Since proptosis is a variable finding in Graves' ophthalmopathy, it is not a useful indication of the degree of orbital infiltration or of the response to treatment. Moreover, longstanding proptosis tends to be permanent, presumably because of the permanent changes in the tissues of the orbit, and is thus not often amenable to medical therapy.

As previously stated, Graves' ophthalmopathy may be more likely to progress following systemic treatment that causes rapid alteration in thyroid tissue and function.[2] Gwinup and associates,[93] however, have shown that proptosis progresses more slowly in patients treated with subtotal thyroidectomy and radioactive iodine in contrast to treatment with antithyroid drugs. The loss of thyroid tissue by these means may limit the progression of proptosis.

Proptosis as an isolated finding rarely requires treatment unless there is secondary exposure keratopathy or unless it represents a significant cosmetic problem.[45]

relief from the symptoms of ocular discomfort after the first injection.[91] If periocular steroids are to be used, treatment should not be delayed until after the ocular disease becomes severe but, rather, should be employed at an early stage to prevent complications. Periocular injections have the advantage of requiring only 10 to 15 mg of steroid monthly, whereas the equivalent effective oral dose of prednisone is at least 2000 mg.[91] Other advantages include[92]:

TABLE 27.5
Incidence of Side Effects of Guanethidine in 81 Patients

Side Effect	%	Side Effect	%
Miosis	100	Unilateral ptosis (both eyes treated)	5
Conjunctival congestion	100	Ptosis of contralateral eye (1 eye treated)	4
Microscopic only	10	Nasal congestion (bilateral)	2
Minimal (i.e., evident on naked eye examination)	74	Rhinorrhea (bilateral)	1
Cosmetic complaint	7	Burning on instillation	17
Discomfort (no corneal staining)	5	Itching on instillation	1
With superficial punctate keratitis	4	Exacerbation of viral keratoconjunctivitis	2
Conjunctival sensitivity	4	Effect on accommodation	0
Bilateral ptosis (both eyes treated)	1	Abnormal intraocular pressure	0

Modified from Cant JS, Lewis DRH. Unwanted pharmacological effects of local guanethidine in the treatment of dysthyroid upper lid retraction. Br J Ophthalmol 1969;53:239–245.

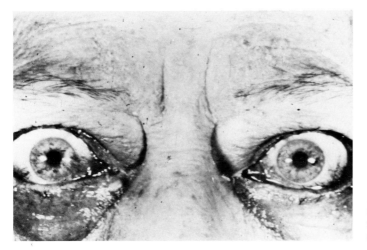

FIGURE 27.13 **Same patient as in Figure 27.4 following systemic steroid therapy. Note the marked improvement in lid swelling, conjunctival and episcleral injection, and chemosis.**

Such patients may benefit from a trial of systemic or periocular corticosteroids. A significant decrease in the severity of proptosis may be observed in some patients. In general, if regression of the proptosis occurs after the institution of steroid therapy, it will begin soon after the onset of therapy and reach a maximum in 2 or 3 months.[94]

Adrenergic blocking agents such as propranolol have been used but are generally ineffective in relieving proptosis, since this condition is associated with increased volume of the retrobulbar tissues rather than with sympathetic autonomic nervous system control of the eye.[95]

CLASS 4 DISEASE (EXTRAOCULAR MUSCLE INVOLVEMENT)

Many patients, perhaps up to 50%, may experience return of normal eye movements following medical control of the thyrotoxicosis.[52] For patients who do not experience improvement, the only pharmacologic interventions that have been shown to be effective for the specific changes associated with Class 4 disease are systemic prednisone[3,94,96] and local injections of botulinum toxin.[97-99]

In the early stages of Class 4 involvement, treatment with small doses of prednisone may be initiated when control of the hyperthyroidism or adequate therapy of hypothyroidism has not arrested the ocular activity. Improvement in motility usually occurs within 4 to 12 weeks.[45] Many patients experience enough subsequent improvement in ocular motility that severe Class 4 disease may be considered a relative but not absolute indication for steroid therapy.[94,100] However, conservative therapy is prudent in many cases and may include exercising the eyes to lessen the tendency for muscle fibrosis[53]; the use of Fresnel prisms, which serve a definite advantage in the management of unstable motility disorders; or simple monocular patching.

In patients with motility disorders with onset of less than 12 months, botulinum toxin can be injected directly into the affected muscle(s).[97,99] Following injection the toxin is rapidly bound to the muscle, where it inhibits liberation of the neurotransmitter, acetylcholine, into the neuromuscular junction.[98] Such "chemodenervation" can effectively, although temporarily, decrease or eliminate symptoms of diplopia.[97]

The drug is supplied in vials containing 50 ng of freeze-dried toxin, which is reconstituted with unpreserved saline before use. A typical dosage is 1.25 to 25 U (0.5 to 10 ng), and the usual maximum volume injected is 0.1 ml.[98] Injections may be repeated after 2 or 3 months if the motility disturbances persist.[99] Dramatic results are sometimes obtained with injections of botulinum toxin (Fig. 27.14), but the treatment is less effective for patients with long-standing deviations because of restrictions secondary to muscle fibrosis.[97] Side effects are minimal and include transient ptosis, involvement of adjacent muscles, and overcorrection.[97,98]

Many patients should be considered surgical candidates following the failure of steroid therapy, or other, more conservative therapeutic measures. Marked improvement can often be obtained in elevation of the globe following appropriate recession of the fibrotic inferior rectus muscle.[88,101,143] The recession of other extraocular muscles to correct existing heterotropias and associated diplopia should also be considered.[88,102] Surgery, however, should generally be postponed at least 6 to 12 months after stabilization of the metabolic and ocular conditions, since early surgical manipulation may acutely exacerbate the original disease process.[82,103] Significant complications from eye muscle surgery are rare but include an increase of the proptosis following release of the fibrotic ocular muscles.[104] For this reason, if the proptosis is more than 22 or 23 mm, serious consideration should be given to orbital decompression before muscle surgery even if there is no significant threat to vision.

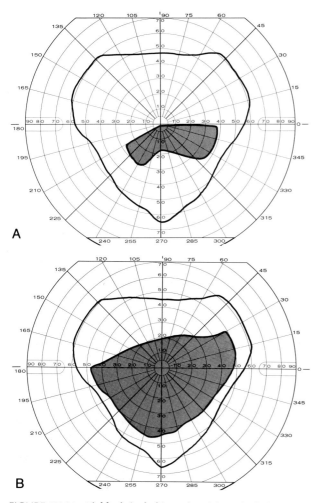

FIGURE 27.14   **Field of single binocular vision (shaded area) in patient with thyroid-related myopathy. (A) Before treatment with botulinum toxin. (B) One week following injection of botulinum toxin into left inferior rectus muscle. (Modified from Fells P, McCarry B. Diplopia in thyroid eye disease. Trans Ophthalmol Soc UK 1986;105:413–423.)**

CLASS 5 DISEASE (CORNEAL INVOLVEMENT)

Patients with Class 5 disease are at risk of serious ocular complications and loss of vision. In the milder forms of exposure keratopathy the administration of bland ocular lubricants at bedtime or continuously during the day may be of significant benefit in alleviating associated symptoms and preventing or delaying more serious ocular involvement. The topical application of broad-spectrum antibiotics (e.g., gentamicin) may be indicated for the prophylaxis of infection. Taping the lids shut at bedtime or employing a Saran Wrap shield may also prove beneficial. When frank corneal ulceration is imminent, systemic steroid therapy can prove useful.[105] In these cases high doses of steroid given for short periods (e.g., prednisone 120 to 140 mg daily for

7 days and gradually tapered) may bring about desired results. The use of systemic steroids sometimes obviates the need for surgery (orbital decompression) but generally involves long-term therapy with the possibility of adverse effects. Steroids are also useful for patients who cannot undergo orbital decompression because of contraindication to general anesthesia. In addition, the use of diuretics may be beneficial in some patients.

Orbital decompression should be considered for patients with severe Class 5 disease for whom steroids are ineffective or contraindicated, or for patients whose compliance may be poor or for whom follow-up may be difficult.

CLASS 6 DISEASE (OPTIC NERVE INVOLVEMENT)

Although as many as 70% of patients with optic neuropathy spontaneously improve without treatment,[106] the risk to vision is significant, and loss of vision may become permanent if the optic neuropathy is not quickly recognized and aggressively treated.[107] Therapy should ideally begin with correction of the thyroid imbalance.[76] Replacement thyroid hormone is mandatory for hypothyroid states. Some patients with optic neuropathy can be managed entirely by adjustment of the thyroid state, particularly if the clinician and patient are willing to wait several weeks for improvement to begin.

Systemic corticosteroids have been used for severe Class 6 disease since they first became available, but the early results were not satisfactory, probably because of the relatively small doses that were employed. Brown and associates[94] in 1963 were the first to show the often dramatic effects of large doses of prednisone in patients with Graves' ophthalmopathy, including documented optic nerve disease.

A gratifying response to steroid therapy may be observed in many patients with optic neuropathy (Fig. 27.15). Trobe and associates[108] reported a 48% success rate defined as 2 Snellen lines of improvement in visual acuity within 2 months of steroid treatment. A beneficial effect was usually noted within 72 hours of beginning therapy, and no further improvement was noted after 6 to 8 weeks. Fifty-two percent of eyes failed to respond to oral steroid therapy despite doses from 50 to 100 mg daily maintained for 2 to 6 months. Five eyes were subjected to repeated retrobulbar injections of triamcinolone (Kenalog) 60 mg but with no perceptible change in the clinical course. If a response to oral steroid is to occur at all, signs of improvement in visual function will usually be evident within 1 week and often earlier. There is no apparent justification for maintaining patients with optic neuropathy on prolonged high doses of systemic steroids in the absence of a reasonably rapid improvement in vision.

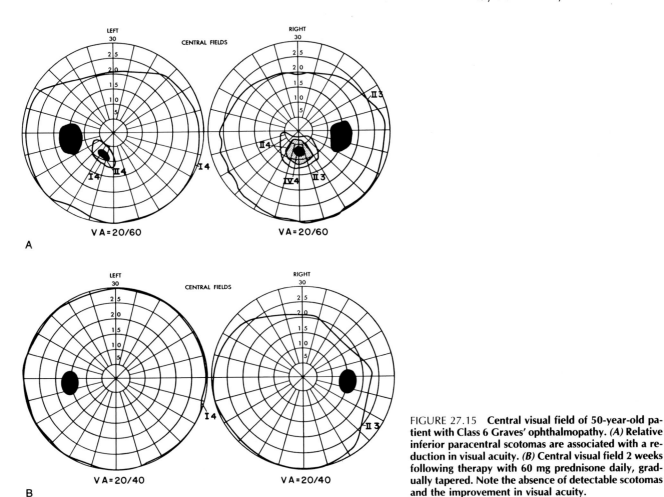

FIGURE 27.15   **Central visual field of 50-year-old patient with Class 6 Graves' ophthalmopathy.** *(A)* **Relative inferior paracentral scotomas are associated with a reduction in visual acuity.** *(B)* **Central visual field 2 weeks following therapy with 60 mg prednisone daily, gradually tapered. Note the absence of detectable scotomas and the improvement in visual acuity.**

Trobe and associates[108] have offered the following guidelines for the management of patients with optic neuropathy.

- Patients with minimal optic nerve dysfunction (visual acuity of 20/30 [6/9] or better) may be managed by observation alone. However, the tendency for rapid progression demands serial examinations of visual acuity and visual fields.
- Patients with progressive vision loss (with or without disc swelling), or with disc swelling and no visual defect should be treated. Oral steroids in large doses remain the primary therapeutic modality, but if a response has not occurred within 3 or 4 weeks, continued high doses are not likely to succeed.
- Prolonged steroid maintenance without improvement in visual function is not justified.

With failure of systemic steroids to control the optic nerve disease, low-dosage orbital irradiation (1600 to 2000 rad) may be considered or may be employed initially for patients with contraindications to steroids. With the failure of both oral steroids and orbital irradiation, orbital decompression must be considered the final management option.

Systemic Management of the Ophthalmopathy

As mentioned, the hyperthyroid state must be controlled before use of other therapeutic measures,[73,82] including diuretics, steroids, plasmapheresis, and immunosuppressive agents.

Diuretics are used occasionally in the treatment of Graves' ophthalmopathy, particularly when there is pronounced periorbital edema. These agents are thought to mobilize salt and water deposits retained locally by hydrophilic mucopolysaccharides. Diuretics might also be used in conjunction with other forms of treatment such as systemic steroids. As previously mentioned, the use of acetazolamide is a logical and convenient choice for patients who also have unquestioned glaucoma.[53]

Systemic steroids and plasmapheresis are effective only in ophthalmopathy that is recent or acute (less than 6 months) or that is rapidly advancing. These forms of treatment are ineffective in stable and chronic ophthalmopathy.

STEROIDS

Systemic steroids often effectively control the optic neuropathy and other inflammatory changes of the ophthalmopathy, although they must be used in high dosages at the expense of their known complications and side effects, including osteoporosis, hyperglycemia, hypertension, infection, gastric ulceration, cataract, Cushingoid features, and psychosis.[73,82,94,109,110] However, rapid progression of proptosis, ophthalmoplegia, and optic nerve involvement warrant such treatment. Development of visual field defects or decreased visual acuity are absolute indications for the use of steroids. In such instances systemic steroids often produce rapid and dramatic improvement of the ocular changes. Subjective improvement might occur within the first 24 hours, and extraocular muscle function and visual acuity might improve in a few days or weeks.[110] Treatment should be initiated with large doses of prednisone (50 to 100 mg daily). When improvement is apparent, the dosage should be reduced gradually. Whenever exacerbation occurs, the dosage must be increased until improvement is restored. Subsequently, the steroid should be tapered more gradually. In general, the longer the disease has existed before treatment, the longer the period of treatment required before recovery. Werner[109] has reported dramatic results with the use of very high doses of prednisone, 140 mg daily, in extreme emergencies such as severe corneal compromise or optic nerve involvement.

In general, if optic neuropathy is responsive to steroids, exacerbations will often occur if the drug is withdrawn within 2 to 4 weeks.[106,110] Therefore, steroids must be administered until the disease process undergoes spontaneous remission. Although this increases the potential risk of serious steroid-related complications, this risk is justified in many instances. Because of the risks inherent in systemic steroid therapy, the practitioner should educate the patient regarding the potential side effects of steroids and the need for regular and long-term medical supervision.

PLASMAPHERESIS

Plasmapheresis as a form of therapy for Graves' ophthalmopathy was first reported by Dandona and associates[111,112] in 1979. These investigators reported impressive results in a small group of patients. Although its cost-effectiveness has been questioned,[7,22,113] the procedure consists of 3 or 4 sessions of plasmapheresis, each of which involves removal of 2 or 3 liters of plasma. Lost plasma is replaced by human plasma or human albumin in 0.9% saline solution. Best results are obtained in patients with acute, recent, or rapidly advancing eye disease.[114] The treatment should be instituted concurrently with the administration of prednisone 80 mg for the first day, and then decreasing every second day to 60, 40, and 20 mg doses, which is then maintained for at least 3 weeks. The patient should also receive azathioprine 2.5 mg/kg body weight daily. Improvement in the ocular condition has been observed within 48 to 72 hours even before steroids and immunosuppressive drugs have been administered. The question still remains, however, whether the dramatic improvement in the ocular condition is due more to the administration of steroids and immunosuppressive agents than to the plasmapheresis itself. Dandona and associates[111,112] have observed that the levels of TSAb markedly decrease after the procedure, but this does not necessarily correlate with the ocular response. However, if steroids are not concomitantly administered, there is rebound in the production of these antibodies to values higher than those before treatment, with potential aggravation of the hyperthyroid state.

IMMUNOSUPPRESSIVE AGENTS

There is convincing evidence that Graves' disease is related to a defective immune system.[6,34,35] TSAb that correspond to immunoglobulins (IgG) are present in the serum of patients with Graves' disease. The long-acting thyroid stimulator (LATS) was the first immunoglobulin, class IgG, identified and the one that initiated the concept of the autoimmune origin of Graves' disease. Kidd and associates[6] have provided in vitro evidence indicating that abnormal T-lymphocyte suppressor function might be an essential component in the disturbance of the immune system. On the basis of these findings, it seemed justifiable to attempt immunosuppressive therapy in an effort to control the ocular changes. However, several therapeutic attempts using immunosuppressive drugs such as azathioprine have generally been unsuccessful in improving the ocular involvement.[2,105,115,116] Burrow and associates[116] administered azathioprine to 5 patients with the active eye changes of Graves' disease and noted objective evidence of immune suppression in each patient; despite this, however, there was no significant improvement in the ophthalmopathy. Several possible explanations exist for the failure of immunosuppressive therapy: (1) the orbital infiltration may occur and stabilize before therapy is begun, and (2) TSAb may not play a role in the etiology of the ocular changes, and suppression of TSAb production therefore has no effect on the ocular disease.

Bigos and associates[115] administered cyclophosphamide in the management of advanced Graves' ophthalmopathy with proptosis and diplopia. Withdrawal of steroid therapy was permitted in one patient, symptoms of diplopia completely resolved in 2 patients and improved in a third patient coincident with administration of the drug, and deteriorating visual acuity resolved in one patient. Although chemosis improved in the two affected patients, proptosis remained unchanged in all three patients. These authors concluded that cyclophosphamide deserves further study as a therapeutic agent in Graves' eye disease.

Cyclosporin A is a potent immunosuppressive agent with a high degree of specificity for T-cells.[117] Therapeutic results obtained with this drug have varied. Although use of cyclosporin was unsuccessful in small groups of patients reported by Howlett and associates[118] and Brabant and associates,[119] the drug improved ocular motility, visual acuity, proptosis, and muscle swelling in 2 patients reported by Weetman and associates[117] and in 9 patients reported by Utech and associates.[120] Concomitantly, thyroid antibodies fell and T-cell abnormalities returned toward normal.[117] The use of cyclosporin A and other immunosuppressive agents in the treatment of Graves' ophthalmopathy appears to be limited by their side effects and long-term carcinogenic properties.

The Role of Other Forms of Management

ORBITAL IRRADIATION

Attempts at orbital irradiation were begun about 50 years ago but involved relatively low-dose, low-energy, or poorly collimated beams. The results were generally unsatisfactory. In 1968 Donaldson[121] began an experimental program of supervoltage orbital radiotherapy for Graves' ophthalmopathy. The design was to treat the orbit laterally, targeting the muscle cone only, and sparing the lens, cornea, pituitary, and hypothalamus. The results have been favorable, and this approach seems to offer a reasonable alternative to steroid therapy and surgical decompression in some patients. Since the infiltration of lymphocytes may play a role in the pathogenesis of thyroid-related orbital disease, x-radiation may produce its beneficial effect by markedly reducing populations of these lymphocytes. Existing hyperthyroidism should be corrected if possible before irradiation. When systemic steroids are administered simultaneously, the dose should be kept constant during the period of irradiation and for several weeks thereafter.[106,122] Two thousand rads are usually deliv-

ered in 10 sessions. In the Kriss series[123] excellent or good results were obtained in 72% of patients monitored for a minimum of 1 year.

In general, orbital irradiation produces the most impressive results in patients with active and progressive ophthalmopathy rather than in patients with a more indolent disease course. The procedure is indicated for patients with[124,125]

- Rapidly progressive severe ophthalmopathy
- Troublesome soft tissue signs and symptoms
- Contraindications to use of steroids
- Side effects from or lack of disease control with steroids

Therapy may result in improved proptosis, lid retraction, visual acuity, and soft tissue signs,[125-127,144] but motility disorders respond less satisfactorily.[125,128,144] If treatment is administered early (within 6 to 24 months[127,129]), a positive response usually occurs within 6 weeks.[126] Acute and long-term complications are negligible,[125] but radiation retinopathy has been reported as a rare side effect, probably due to error in technique.[130]

ORBITAL DECOMPRESSION

When steroid therapy is unsatisfactory in improving the severe changes associated with Class 5 and 6 disease, surgical enlargement of the orbital volume should be considered. Dollinger[131] first reported orbital decompression for Graves' ophthalmopathy in 1911.[132-137,145] Since then, several surgical approaches for orbital decompression have been described (Fig. 27.16). In 1931 Naffziger introduced the concept of removal of the roof of the orbit by a neurosurgical transfrontal approach. Another approach, the Kronlein procedure, involves removing the lateral wall of the orbit with decompression into the temporal fossa. Both these procedures have the disadvantage of decompressing the orbit into an area of high tissue pressure. In addition, the Naffziger approach introduces the morbidity of an intracranial operation, and the Kronlein method is a lengthy procedure involving considerable bony resection. As an alternative approach, the procedure currently receiving widespread acceptance is the transantral approach described by Walsh and Ogura.[138] This procedure, or modifications thereof, involves removal of the medial wall and floor of the orbit, has the advantage of decompressing the orbital tissues into the maxillary antrum, a naturally dead space, and has relatively low morbidity.

Because of the inherent risks involved, orbital decompression should be considered only after more conservative therapeutic measures have been attempted. Most clinicians reserve the use of orbital decompres-

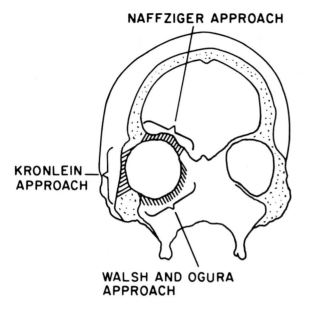

NAFFZIGER APPROACH

KRONLEIN APPROACH

WALSH AND OGURA APPROACH

FIGURE 27.16 **Surgical approaches to orbital decompression. The Naffziger approach involves removal of the roof of the orbit, the Kronlein approach involves removal of the lateral wall of the orbit, and the Walsh and Ogura procedure involves removal of the medial wall and floor of the orbit.**

TABLE 27.6
Medical and Surgical Management of Graves' Ophthalmopathy[a]

Class	Eye Signs	Medical Management	Surgical Management
0	None	Observation	
1	Lid retraction	Ocular lubricants	Scleral implant
		Tinted lenses	Levator tenotomy
		Topical adrenergic blocking agent (e.g., guanethidine)	Levator myotomy Levator recession
		Tape lids h.s.	Lateral tarsorrhaphy
		Saran shield h.s.	Recession of Mueller's muscle
2	Lid swelling, episcleral and conjunctival injection, chemosis, injection and hypertrophy of lateral recti insertions	Ocular lubricants Oral diuretic Elevate head during sleep Tinted lenses Systemic steroid Periocular steroid	Blepharoplasty
3	Proptosis	Ocular lubricants Tape lids h.s. Saran shield h.s. Systemic steroid Periocular steroid	Lateral tarsorrhaphy
4	Extraocular muscle fibrosis	Fresnel prisms Monocular patching Botulinum toxin Systemic steroid	Recession of fibrotic muscles
5	Exposure keratopathy	Ocular lubricants Topical antibiotic ointment Tape lids h.s. Saran shield h.s. Tinted lenses Systemic steroid Oral diuretic	Orbital decompression
6	Optic neuropathy	Systemic steroid Periocular steroid Orbital irradiation	Orbital decompression

[a]Any disorder of thyroid function should be simultaneously corrected. h.s., at bedtime.

sion for patients with severe corneal compromise associated with progressive proptosis and corneal exposure and for patients with optic neuropathy who have failed to respond to systemic steroids or for whom systemic steroids are contraindicated. In all cases, however, orbital decompression should not be considered until the thyroid state is stable.[104]

Orbital decompression allows the volume of the orbit to be expanded by as much as 2-fold,[139] often with significant improvement in visual acuity, visual field, disc edema, proptosis, lid closure, and corneal healing.[140] The degree of recession of proptosis can range from 2 to 12 mm.[135]

Although not without serious risks, this procedure, particularly the transantral approach, is remarkably free of significant complications in most patients. Up to 50% of patients with no ocular muscle imbalance before decompression will experience diplopia afterward.[73,104] However, the major complication of the transantral approach is infraorbital nerve anesthesia, which may last up to 18 months.[135] Other complications have included blindness, accentuation of the appearance of upper lid retraction associated with inferior displacement of the globe, substantial blood loss, nasolacrimal duct obstruction, ascending infection from the sinuses, and meningitis associated with cerebrospinal fluid leakage.[46,140] Chronic sinusitis with polyps is the main contraindication to transantral decompression.[135]

Fortunately, Graves' ophthalmopathy severe enough to warrant high-dosage steroids, orbital radiotherapy, or orbital decompression is estimated to occur in not more than 3% of patients with Graves' disease.[115] In the vast majority of cases, patients can be adequately managed with more conservative therapeutic measures. Table 27.6 summarizes the current therapeutic approaches to the patient with Graves' ophthalmopathy.

References

1. Graves RJ. Clinical lectures. Lond Med Surg J 1835;7:516.
2. Young LA. Dysthyroid ophthalmopathy: An update. J Natl Med Assoc 1979;71:855–860.
3. Werner SC, Fells P, Day RM, et al. Eye changes. In: Werner SC, Ingbar SH, ed. The thyroid: A fundamental and clinical text. Hagerstown, MD: Harper & Row, 1978; 4:655–683.
4. Kroll AJ, Kuwabara T. Dysthroid ocular myopathy. Anatomy, histology, and electron microscopy. Arch Ophthalmol 1966;76:244–257.
5. Cant JS, Wilson TM. The ocular and orbital circulations in dysthyroid ophthalmopathy. Trans Ophthalmol Soc UK 1974;94:416–429.
6. Kidd A, Okita N, Row VV, et al. Immunologic aspects of Graves' and Hashimoto's diseases. Metabolism 1980;29:80–99.
7. DeGroot LJ, Larsen PR, Refetoff S, Stanbury JB, eds. The thyroid and its diseases, ed. 5. New York: John Wiley & Sons, 1984;458–496.
8. Weetman AP, McGregor AM. Autoimmune thyroid disease: Developments in our understanding. Endocr Rev 1984;5:309–355.
9. Walfish PG, Wall JR, Volpe R, eds. Autoimmunity and the thyroid. New York: Academic Press, 1985.
10. Wall JR, Koroki T. Immunologic factors in thyroid disease. In: Kaplan MM, Larsen PR, eds. Symposium on thyroid disease. Philadelphia: W.B. Saunders Co, 1985;69:913–936.
11. Gorman CA. Extrathyroid manifestations of Graves' disease. In: Ingbar SH, Braverman LE, eds. Werner's the thyroid: A fundamental and clinical text, ed. 5. Philadelphia: J.B. Lippincott Co, 1986;1015–1038.
12. Farid NR, Bear JC. The human major histocompatibility complex and endocrine disease. Endocr Rev 1981;2:50–85.
13. Riddick FA Jr. Immunologic aspects of thyroid disease. Ophthalmology 1981;88:471–475.
14. Sergott RC, Felberg NT, Savino PJ, et al. The clinical immunology of Graves' ophthalmopathy. Ophthalmology 1981;88:484–487.
15. Kohn LD, Winand RJ. Experimental exophthalmos. Alterations of normal hormone-receptor interactions in the pathogenesis of a disease. Isr J Med Sci 1974;10:1348–1363.
16. Kriss JP, Konishi J, Herman M. Studies on the pathogenesis of Graves' ophthalmopathy (with some related observations regarding therapy). Recent Prog Horm Res 1975;31:533–566.
17. Doniach D, Florin-Christensen A. Autoimmunity in the pathogenesis of endocrine exophthalmos. Clin Endocrinol Metab 1975;4:341–350.
18. Solomon DH, Chopra IJ, Chopra U, et al. Identification of subgroups of euthyroid Graves' ophthalmopathy. N Engl J Med 1977;296:181–186.
19. Ahmann A, Baker JR Jr, Weetman AP, et al. Antibodies to porcine eye muscle in patients with Graves' ophthalmopathy: Identification of serum immunoglobulins directed against unique determinants by immunoblotting and enzyme-linked immunosorbent assay. J Clin Endocrinol Metab 1987;64:454–460.
20. Wang PW, Hiromatsu Y, Laryea E, et al. Immunologically mediated cytotoxicity against human eye muscle cells in Graves' ophthalmopathy. J Clin Endocrinol Metab 1986; 63:316–322.
21. Lawton NF. Dysthyroid eye disease: Medical investigations. Proc R Soc Med 1977;70:698–700.
22. Jacobson DH, Gorman CA. Diagnosis and management of endocrine ophthalmopathy. In: Kaplan MM, Larsen PR, eds. Symposium on thyroid disease. Philadelphia: W.B. Saunders Co, 1985;69:973–988.
23. Bullock JD, Bartley GB. Dynamic proptosis. Am J Ophthalmol 1986;102:104–110.
24. Hornblass A, Jakobiec FA, Reifler DM, et al. Orbital lymphoid tumors located predominantly within extraocular muscles. Ophthalmology 1987;94:688–697.
25. Kaplan MM, Utiger RD. Diagnosis of hyperthyroidism. Clin Endocrinol Metab 1978;7:97–113.

26. Chopra IJ. Laboratory aids in the diagnosis of hyperthyroidism. Thyroid Today 1978;1:1–6.

27. Surks MI. Assessment of thyroid function. Ophthalmology 1981;88:476–478.

28. Kaptein EM, MacIntyre SS, Weiner JM, et al. Free thyroxine estimates in nonthyroidal illness: Comparison of eight methods. J Clin Endocrinol Metab 1981;52:1073–1077.

29. Riddick FA Jr. Update on thyroid diseases. Ophthalmology 1981;88:467–470.

30. Spencer CA. Clinical utility of sensitive TSH assays. Thyroid Today 1986;9:1–8.

31. Klee GG, Hay ID. Assessment of sensitive thyrotropin assays for an expanded role in thyroid function testing: Proposed criteria for analytic performance and clinical utility. J Clin Endocrinol Metab 1987;64:461–471.

32. Peter SA. Euthyroid Graves' disease. Report of a case observed over a 12-year period. Am J Med 1986;80:1197–1198.

33. Rush JA, Older JJ. Graves' orbitopathy and the thyrotropin-releasing hormone (TRH) test. J Clin Neuro-ophthalmol 1981;1:219–224.

34. UCLA Conference. Autoimmune thyroid diseases—Graves' and Hasimoto's. Ann Intern Med 1978;88:379–391.

35. McKenzie JM, Zakarija M, Sato A. Humoral immunity in Graves' disease. Clin Endocrinol Metab 1978;7:31–45.

36. McKenzie JM. Thyroid-stimulating antibody (TSAb) in Graves' disease. Thyroid Today 1980;3:1–5.

37. McKenzie JM, Zakarija M. Hyperthyroidism: Autoimmune aspects. In: Van Middlesworth L, ed. The thyroid gland: A practical clinical treatise. Chicago: Year Book Medical Publishers, 1986;297–303.

38. Werner SC. Classification of the eye changes of Graves' disease. J Clin Endocrinol Metab 1969;29:982–984.

39. Werner SC. Modification of the classification of the eye changes of Graves' disease. Am J Ophthalmol 1977;83:725–727.

40. Van Dyk HJ. Orbital Graves' disease. A modification of the "NO-SPECS" classification. Ophthalmology 1981;88:479–483.

41. Laibovitz RA, Cain R. Lost lid signs in topical neuro-ophthalmic diagnosis. Tex Med 1977;73:68–69.

42. Meltzer MA. Surgery for lid retraction. Ann Ophthalmol 1978;10:102–106.

43. Dixon RS, Anderson RL, Hatt MU. The use of thymoxamine in eyelid retraction. Arch Ophthalmol 1979;97:2147–2150.

44. Gay AJ, Wolkstein MA. Topical guanethidine therapy for endocrine lid retraction. Arch Ophthalmol 1966;76:364–367.

45. Sergott RC, Glaser JS. Graves' ophthalmopathy. A clinical and immunologic review. Surv Ophthalmol 1981;26:1–21.

46. Linberg JV, Anderson RL. Transorbital decompression. Indications and results. Arch Ophthalmol 1981;99:113–119.

47. Frueh BR, Musch DC, Garber FW. Exophthalmometer readings in patients with Graves' eye disease. Ophthal Surg 1986;17:37–40.

48. Greenberg DA. Basic evaluation of exophthalmos. J Am Optom Assoc 1977;48:1431–1433.

49. DeJuan E, Hurley DP, Sapira JD. Racial differences in normal values of proptosis. Arch Intern Med 1980;140:1230–1231.

50. Migliori ME, Gladstone GJ. Determination of the normal range of exophthalmometric values for black and white adults. Am J Ophthalmol 1984;98:438–442.

51. Bar-Meir S, Pinkhas J, Golan A, et al. Malignant lymphoma presenting as unilateral exophthalmos and thyroid nodule. Haematologica 1975;60:85–87.

52. Schultz RO, Van Allen MW, Blodi FC. Endocrine ophthalmoplegia: With an electromyographic study of paretic extraocular muscles. Arch Ophthalmol 1960;63:217–225.

53. Smith JL. Recent advances in therapy of thyroid eye disease. In: Smith JL, ed. Neuro-ophthalmology. St. Louis: C.V. Mosby Co, 1972;6:1–10.

54. Newcomb R. Paralysis of elevation of one eye: A case report. Am J Optom Physiol Opt 1976;53:205–207.

55. Appen RE, Wendelborn D, Nolten WE. Diplopia in autoimmune thyroid disease. Arch Intern Med 1982;142:898–901.

56. Metz HS, Woolf PD, Patton ML. Endocrine ophthalmomyopathy in adolescence. J Pediatr Ophthalmol Strabismus 1982;19:58–60.

57. Metz HS. Saccadic velocity studies in patients with endocrine ocular disease. Am J Ophthalmol 1977;84:695–699.

58. Jensen SF. Endocrine ophthalmoplegia. Is it due to myopathy or to mechanical immobilization? Acta Ophthalmol 1971;49:679–684.

59. Stetz CA, Roman SH, Podos S, et al. Prevalence and clinical associations of intraocular pressure changes in Graves' disease. J Clin Endocrinol Metab 1985;61:183–187.

60. Gasser P, Flammer J. Optic neuropathy of Graves' disease. A report of a perimetric follow-up. Ophthalmologica 1986;192:22–27.

61. Frueh BR, Musch DC, Grill R, et al. Orbital compliance in Graves' eye disease. Ophthalmology 1985;92:657–665.

62. Feldon SE, Lee CP, Muramatsu SK, et al. Quantitative computed tomography of Graves' ophthalmopathy. Extraocular muscle and orbital fat in development of optic neuropathy. Arch Ophthalmol 1985;103:213–215.

63. Hufnagel TJ, Hickey WF, Cobbs WH, et al. Immunohistochemical and ultrastructural studies on the exenterated orbital tissues of a patient with Graves' disease. Ophthalmology 1984;91:1411–1419.

64. Dallow RL. Ultrasonography of the orbit. Int Ophthalmol Clin 1986;26:51–76.

65. Leib MC. Computed tomography of the orbit. Int Ophthalmol Clin 1986;26:103–121.

66. Char DH, Norman D. The use of computed tomography and ultrasonography in the evaluation of orbital masses. Surv Ophthalmol 1982;27:49–63.

67. Holt JE, O'Connor PS, Douglas JP, et al. Extraocular muscle size comparison using standardized A-scan echography and computerized tomography scan measurements. Ophthalmology 1985;92:1351–1355.

68. Trokel SL. Computed tomographic scanning of orbital inflammations. Int Ophthalmol Clin 1982;22:81–98.

69. Zimmerman RA, Bilaniuk LT, Yanoff M, et al. Orbital magnetic resonance imaging. Am J Ophthalmol 1985;100:312–317.

70. Gorman CA. Temporal relationship between onset of Graves' ophthalmopathy and diagnosis of thyrotoxicosis. Mayo Clin Proc 1983;58:515–519.

71. Gamblin GT, Harper DG, Galentine P, et al. Prevalence

of increased intraocular pressure in Graves' disease—evidence of frequent subclinical ophthalmopathy. N Engl J Med 1983;308:420–424.

72. Ali AS, Akavaram NR. Neuromuscular disorders in thyrotoxicosis. Am Fam Physician 1980;22:97–102.

73. Gorman CA. Management of the patient with Graves' ophthalmopathy. Thyroid Today 1977;1:1–6.

74. Braverman LE. Thyrotoxicosis. Therapeutic considerations. Clin Endocrinol Metab 1978;7:221–240.

75. McClung MR, Greer MA. Treatment of hyperthyroidism. Ann Rev Med 1980;31:385–404.

76. Knox DL. Optic nerve manifestations of systemic diseases. Trans Am Acad Ophthalmol Otolaryngol 1977;83:743–750.

77. Gilbard JP, Farris RL. Ocular surface drying and tear film osmolarity in thyroid eye disease. Acta Ophthalmol 1983;61:108–116.

78. Gay AJ, Salmon ML, Wolkstein MA. Topical sympatholytic therapy for pathologic lid retraction. Arch Ophthalmol 1967;77:341–344.

79. Sneddon JM, Turner P. Adrenergic blockade and the eye signs of thyrotoxicosis. Lancet 1966;2:525–527.

80. Hodes BL, Shoch DE. Thyroid ocular myopathy. Trans Am Ophthalmol Soc 1979;77:80–103.

81. Crombie AL, Lawson AAH. Long-term trial of local guanethidine in treatment of eye signs of thyroid dysfunction and idiopathic lid retraction. Br Med J 1967;4:592–595.

82. Kramar P. Management of eye changes of Graves' disease. Surv Ophthalmol 1974;18:369–382.

83. Cant JS, Lewis DRH, Harrison MT. Treatment of dysthyroid ophthalmopathy with local guanethidine. Br J Ophthalmol 1969;53:233–238.

84. Cant JS, Lewis DRH. Unwanted pharmacological effects of local guanethidine in the treatment of dysthyroid upper lid retraction. Br J Ophthalmol 1969;53:239–245.

85. Bowden AN, Rose FC. Dysthyroid eye disease. A trial of guanethidine eye drops. Br J Ophthalmol 1969;53:246–251.

86. Trevor-Roper PD. Diseases of the orbit. Int Ophthalmol Clin 1974;14:323–346.

87. Crawford JS, Easterbrook M. The use of bank sclera to correct lid retraction. Can J Ophthalmol 1976;11:304–308.

88. Schimek RA. Surgical management of ocular complications of Graves' disease. Arch Ophthalmol 1972;87:655–664.

89. Putterman AM, Fett DR. Müller's muscle in the treatment of upper eyelid retraction: A 12-year study. Ophthal Surg 1986;17:361–367.

90. Frueh BR, Musch DC, Garber FW. Lid retraction and levator aponeurosis defects in Graves' eye disease. Ophthal Surg 1986;17:216–220.

91. Garber MI. Methylprednisolone in the treatment of exophthalmos. Lancet 1966;1:958–960.

92. Gebertt S. Depot-methylprednisolone for subconjunctival and retrobulbar injections. Lancet 1961;2:344–345.

93. Gwinup G, Elias AN, Ascher MS. Effect on exophthalmos of various methods of treatment of Graves' disease. JAMA 1982;247:12135–2138.

94. Brown J, Coburn JW, Wigod RA, et al. Adrenal steroid therapy of severe infiltrative ophthalmopathy of Graves' disease. Am J Med 1963;34:786–795.

95. Grossman W, Robin NI, Johnson LW, et al. Effects of beta blockade on the peripheral manifestations of thyrotoxicosis. Ann Intern Med 1971;74:875–879.

96. Sisler HA, Jakobiec FA, Trokel SL. Ocular abnormalities and orbital changes of Graves' disease. In: Duane TD, Jaeger EA, eds. Clinical ophthalmology. Philadelphia: Harper & Row, 1987;2:1–30.

97. Dunn WJ, Arnold AC, O'Connor PS. Botulinum toxin for the treatment of dysthyroid ocular myopathy. Ophthalmology 1986;93:470–475.

98. Hoffman RO, Helveston EM. Botulinum in the treatment of adult motility disorders. Int Ophthalmol Clin 1986;26:241–250.

99. Fells P, McCarry B. Diplopia in thyroid eye disease. Trans Ophthalmol Soc UK 1986;105:413–423.

100. Frueh BR, Benger RS. Spontaneous reversal of vertical diplopia in Graves' eye disease. Trans Am Ophthalmol Soc 1985;83:387–396.

101. Miller JE, van Heuven W, Ward R. Surgical correction of hypotropias associated with thyroid dysfunction. Arch Ophthalmol 1965;74:509–515.

102. Long JC. Surgical management of the tropias of thyroid exophthalmos. Arch Ophthalmol 1966;75:634–638.

103. Apers RC, Bierlaagh JJM. Indications and results of eye muscle surgery in thyroid ophthalmopathy. Ophthalmologica 1976;173:171–179.

104. Dyer JA. Ocular muscle surgery in Graves' disease. Trans Am Ophthalmol Soc 1978;76:125–139.

105. Sachdev Y, Chatterji JC, Sharma RC. Heterogeneity of failure of visual acuity in Graves' disease. Postgrad Med J 1979;55:241–247.

106. Ravin JG, Sisson JC, Knapp WT. Orbital radiation for the ocular changes of Graves' disease. Am J Ophthalmol 1975;79:285–288.

107. Trobe JD. Optic nerve involvement in dysthyroidism. Ophthalmology 1981;88:488–492.

108. Trobe JD, Glaser JS, Laflamme P. Dysthyroid optic neuropathy. Clinical profile and rationale for management. Arch Ophthalmol 1978;96:1199–1209.

109. Werner SC. Management of the active severe eye changes of Graves' disease. Am Acad Ophthalmol Otolaryngol 1967;71:631–637.

110. Day RM, Carroll FD. Corticosteroids in the treatment of optic nerve involvement associated with thyroid dysfunction. Trans Am Ophthalmol Soc 1967;65:41–51.

111. Dandona P, Marshall NJ, Bidey SP, et al. Successful treatment of exophthalmos and pretibial myxoedema with plasmapheresis. Br Med J 1979;1:374–376.

112. Dandona P, Marshall NH, Bidey SP, et al. Treatment of acute malignant exophthalmos with plasma exchange. In: Stockigt JR, Nagataki S, eds. Thyroid research VIII. Canberra: Australian Academy of Science 1980;583–586.

113. McConahey WM. Ophthalmopathy. In: Van Middlesworth L, ed. The thyroid gland: A practical clinical treatise. Chicago: Year Book Medical Publishers, 1986:315–331.

114. Glinoer D, Etienne-Decerf J, Schrooyen M, et al. Beneficial effects of intensive plasma exchange followed by immunosuppressive therapy in severe Graves' ophthalmopathy. Acta Endocrinol 1986;111:30–38.

115. Bigos ST, Nisula BC, Daniels GH, et al. Cyclophosphamide in the management of advanced Graves' ophthalmopathy. A preliminary report. Ann Intern Med 1979;90:921–923.

116. Burrow GN, Mitchell MS, Howard RO, et al. Immunosup-

pressive therapy for the eye changes of Graves' disease. J Clin Endocrinol Metab 1970;31:307–311.

117. Weetman AP, Ludgate M, Mills PV, et al. Cyclosporin improves Graves' ophthalmopathy. Lancet 1983;2:486–489.

118. Howlett TA, Lawton NF, Fells P, et al. Deterioration of severe Graves' ophthalmopathy during cyclosporin treatment. Lancet 1984;2:1101.

119. Brabant G, Peter H, Becker H, et al. Cyclosporin in infiltrative eye disease. Lancet 1984;1:515–516.

120. Utech C, Wulle KG, Bieler EU, et al. Treatment of severe Graves' ophthalmopathy with cyclosporin A. Acta Endocrinol 1985;110:493–498.

121. Donaldson SS, Bagshaw MA, Kriss JP. Supervoltage orbital radiotherapy for Graves' ophthalmopathy. J Clin Endocrinol Metab 1973;37:276–285.

122. Leone CR. The management of ophthalmic Graves' disease. Ophthalmology 1984;91:770–779.

123. Kriss JP, McDougall IR, Donaldson SS. Supervoltage orbital radiotherapy for Graves' ophthalmopathy: Results of 141 consecutive cases. Proceedings of the 56th American Thyroid Association, San Diego, November 5–8, 1980; Abstr. p T8.

124. Glaser JS. Graves' ophthalmopathy. Arch Ophthalmol 1984;102:1448–1449.

125. Olivotto IA, Ludgate CM, Allen LH, et al. Supervoltage radiotherapy for Graves' ophthalmopathy: CCABC technique and results. Int J Radiat Oncol Biol Phys 1985;11:2085–2090.

126. Pinchera A, Bartalena L, Chiovato L, et al. Radiotherapy of Graves' ophthalmopathy. In: Gorman CA, Waller RR, Dyer JA, eds. The eye and orbit in thyroid disease. New York: Raven Press, 1984;301–316.

127. Hurbli T, Char DH, Harris J, et al. Radiation therapy for thyroid eye disease. Am J Ophthalmol 1985;99:633–637.

128. Brennan MW, Leone CR, Janaki L. Radiation therapy for Graves' disease. Am J Ophthalmol 1983;96:195–199.

129. van Ouwerkerk BM, Wijngaarde R, Hennemann G, et al. Radiotherapy of severe ophthalmic Graves' disease. J Endocrinol Invest 1985;8:241–247.

130. Kinyoun JL, Kalina RE, Brower SA, et al. Radiation retinopathy after orbital irradiation for Graves' ophthalmopathy. Arch Ophthalmol 1984;102:1473–1476.

131. Dollinger J. Die druchenllastung der augenhohle durch entfernung der ausseren orbitalwand bei hochgradigen exophthalmus und konsekotiver hornhauterkrantung. Dtsch Med Wochenschr 1911;37:1888–1890.

132. Shorr N, Seiff SR. The four stages of surgical rehabilitation of the patient with dysthyroid ophthalmopathy. Ophthalmology 1986;93:476–483.

133. McCord CD. Current trends in orbital decompression. Ophthalmology 1985;92:21–33.

134. Taylor W. Transantral orbital decompression in dysthyroid eye disease. Trans Ophthalmol Soc NZ 1974;26:51–53.

135. Fells P. Surgical management of dysthyroid eye disease: A review. Proc R Soc Med 1977;70:698–699.

136. Desanto LW. Surgical palliation of ophthalmopathy of Graves' disease: Transantral approach. Mayo Clin Proc 1972;47:989–992.

137. Riley FC. Surgical management of ophthalmopathy in Graves' disease: Transfrontal orbital decompression. Mayo Clin Proc 1972;47:986–988.

138. Walsh TE, Ogura JH. Transantral orbital decompression for malignant exophthalmos. Laryngoscope 1957;67:544–568.

139. Anderson RL, Linberg JV. Transorbital approach to decompression in Graves' disease. Arch Ophthalmol 1981;99:120–124.

140. Ogura JH. Surgical results of orbital decompression for malignant exophthalmos. J Laryngol Otol 1978;92:181–195.

141. Spector RH, Carlisle JA. Minimal thyroid ophthalmopathy. Neurology 1987;37:1803–1808.

142. Uldry PA, Regli F, Scazziga BR, et al. Palpebral asymmetry and hyperthyroidism. Two cases in connection with Graves' disease. J Neurol 1986;233:126–127.

143. Buckley EG, Meekins BB. Fadenoperation for the management of complicated incomitant vertical strabismus. Am J Ophthalmol 1988;105:304–312.

144. Palmer D, Greenberg P, Cornell P, et al. Radiation therapy for Graves' ophthalmopathy: A retrospective analysis. Int J Radiat Oncol Biol Phys 1987;13:1815–1820.

145. Wirtschafter JD, Chu AE. Lateral orbitotomy without removal of the lateral orbital rim. Arch Ophthalmol 1988;106:1463–1468.

CHAPTER 28

Pharmacologic Management of Strabismus

David M. Amos

The customary treatment of strabismus employs spectacle lenses, prisms, and orthoptics, with or without surgical intervention. These nonpharmacologic measures usually establish cosmetic alignment of the eyes and often allow functional binocular vision to be obtained. In some instances certain drugs can be used as the primary treatment modality. Although not commonly used, these agents may allow a cosmetic or functional cure when other management options are less effective. This chapter considers the clinical uses of anticholinesterase miotics for accommodative esotropia, and botulinum toxin for other forms of horizontal deviations.

Accommodative Esotropia

Etiology

Accommodative esotropia is a convergent concomitant strabismus associated with increased convergence innervation, usually accommodative in origin, often occurring in hyperopes.[1] If the fusional divergence amplitude is sufficient to allow fusion, it is termed *accommodative esophoria;* however, if fusion is not maintained, it is termed *accommodative esotropia.*

Accommodative esotropia is thought to have at least 2 etiologies. One etiology is the hyperopic patient's desire for clear vision. If the retinal image is allowed to remain blurred in hyperopia, the patient does not

accommodate, and the eyes remain orthophoric. If the patient clears the blurred image by accommodating, the resulting convergence can cause an accommodative esotropia. Although accommodative esotropia can become manifest from ages 6 months to 7 years, the average age of onset is 2.5 years.[2] At this age the child's developing intelligence begins to demand clarity of near objects, and the demand for clarity in hyperopia often dominates the accompanying diplopia and esodeviation.

Another etiology is a high accommodative convergence-to-accommodation (AC/A) ratio. Even if the patient is emmetropic, an abnormal relationship between accommodation and resulting accommodative-convergence can cause an esotropia at near. With a high AC/A ratio a small amount of accommodation triggers an excessive amount of convergence.

In some instances a patient may manifest both hyperopia and a high AC/A ratio. Although a high AC/A ratio without hyperopia usually results in an esodeviation at near only, an esodeviation resulting from hyperopia can cause the patient to have symptoms at both distance and near.

Accommodative esotropia is heritable, with siblings, parents, or relatives exhibiting the same disorder.[3]

Diagnosis

A cycloplegic refraction or retinoscopy should be performed on all children with suspected accommodative esotropia (see Chapter 17). It is essential to uncover as much hyperopia as possible to prescribe the appropriate spectacle correction. Atropine is usually the drug of choice for retinoscopy of children up to age 4 years with suspected accommodative esotropia.[4-7] The traditional dosage is 1 drop of 1% atropine solution instilled 3 times daily for 3 days before refraction. However, several instillations of 1% cyclopentolate or 1 drop of 2% cyclopentolate may produce a clinically effective cycloplegia approaching that of atropine. Patients with deeply pigmented irides may require 2 or 3 instillations of 1% cyclopentolate 5 minutes apart to obtain satisfactory cycloplegia. It should be emphasized that both atropine and cyclopentolate can cause ocular and systemic reactions including contact blepharodermatitis,[8,9] acute glaucoma,[10] hallucinations,[11] and severe anticholinergic effects.[12] Three instillations of 1% atropine solution 1 day before refraction of patients under 4 years of age is recommended and gives results comparable to the traditional atropine dosage regimen while minimizing the risk of side effects. This procedure requires a reliable parent to administer the drug at home.

Young children who are tense or anxious on examination may actually overcome a weak cycloplegic drug. The anxiety and accompanying blur caused by the drug will induce many children to forcefully attempt to accommodate to see clearly. This can diminish the full effect of the drug, resulting in no additional hyperopia and even less hyperopia or more myopia on retinoscopy. This psychogenic effect may be even more apparent in patients with existing functional accommodative problems. These factors must be considered in young children, and a strong, long-lasting cycloplegic such as atropine should be used if at all possible. In older patients with suspected accommodative esotropia, 1 drop of 1% cyclopentolate administered in the office usually allows adequate cycloplegia. If satisfactory cycloplegia is not achieved, additional drops of cyclopentolate can be instilled.

The clinical investigation of accommodative esotropia should also include an estimate of the AC/A ratio. This should be delayed for several days to allow the effect of the cycloplegic to subside. To determine the AC/A ratio, the patient should wear, in a trial frame, the plus lenses determined by the cycloplegic retinoscopy to correct the hyperopia. Fixation is alternated between distance (20 feet [6 m]) and near (13 inches [33 cm]) by using small interesting objects rather than a muscle light. Prism and alternate cover measurements should be made as the patient accommodates for each distance. A patient is considered to have a high AC/A ratio if the near esodeviation prism measurement is more than 10 prism diopters of the distance measurement.[3] A simple way of recognizing a high AC/A ratio is the finding of a relative esodeviation greater at near than at distance viewing. It is commonly found in esotropia that patients with lower amounts of hyperopia have the higher AC/A ratios. This is to be expected because a patient with a high AC/A ratio will have to accommodate less than a patient with a low AC/A ratio for both to have the same amount of esotropia.

Divergent fusional reserve should also be estimated by placing in the trial frame the least amount of hyperopic correction that permits fusion, and then performing the prism and alternate cover tests. The divergent fusional amplitude range is usually between 12 and 20 prism diopters. Patients with intermittent esotropia will usually have a much higher amount of divergent fusional reserve than patients who develop constant esotropia.

Management

Accommodative esotropia should be diagnosed and treated as early as possible to avoid a permanent strabismus or amblyopia and other complications of delayed treatment. Complications of long-standing esodeviations such as amblyopia, eccentric fixation, suppression, and anomalous retinal correspondence greatly influence the choice of treatment and invariably require a more sophisticated treatment plan. Three possible methods of therapy can be used, either singularly or in combination, to produce alignment: (1) spectacles for hyperopia, (2) anticholinesterase miotics, and (3) vision therapy-orthoptics. All these methods may be used to relieve the accommodative stress. Spectacle therapy and vision therapy-orthoptics will not be discussed in detail in this chapter.

SPECTACLE THERAPY

Spectacles provide the most conservative yet the most effective method of treatment for most patients with accommodative esotropia[13] (Table 28.1). Parks[3] recommends that the full correction determined by the cycloplegic refraction be prescribed for children under 4 years of age. If the full plus correction is not accepted

TABLE 28.1
Advantages of Glasses over Miotics

- No side effects
- Probably more effective for more patients
- Bifocals very effective for patients with high AC/A ratios
- More cosmetically acceptable to children now compared with years ago

by the patient, 1% atropine can be prescribed (1 drop 3 times daily for 1 day only) to assist with the plus lens acceptance. The cycloplegic refraction should be repeated several times during the first year of treatment, since it is not uncommon to reveal even more hyperopia, especially in patients under 4 years of age.[5]

After the young patient with esotropia and hyperopia has worn the full plus correction for several weeks or months, reexamination will probably reveal one of the following conditions: (1) orthophoria with near and distance fixation, (2) reduced amount of esotropia with near and distance fixation, or (3) orthophoria with distance fixation but a significant esodeviation with near fixation. This near esodeviation is thought to be caused by a high AC/A ratio.[14] To alleviate the near esodeviation, a plus lens addition over the full distance hyperopic correction has proved quite successful. This bifocal addition is determined by adding +0.50 to +1.00 D increments to the patient's spectacles until the least power is found that reduces the angle of strabismus sufficiently to permit stable fixation and fusion. The bifocal addition is usually between +1.00 D and +3.50 D. A flat top, executive style bifocal bisecting the pupils with the eyes in primary position is usually prescribed. However, some investigators[15,16] have shown that progressive addition lenses are also effective in the management of accommodative esotropia.

MIOTIC THERAPY

Since some children will not wear or tolerate spectacles or bifocals for a variety of reasons, anticholinesterase miotics have been used therapeutically as a "substitute" for spectacles.

History.   Miotics have been used in the treatment of convergent strabismus for over 100 years. In 1896 Javal[17] specifically mentioned the use of pilocarpine and physostigmine as substitutes for spectacles in several cases of convergent strabismus. In 1949 Abraham[18,19] first reported the effective use of isoflurophate in accommodative esotropia. It offered a great advantage over pilocarpine or physostigmine because of its effectiveness when used only once a day or less. In 1960 Miller[20] reported a similar effectiveness with the use of echothiophate iodide. Since then, there have been a myriad of studies published concerning the effectiveness and safety of anticholinesterase miotics in the treatment of accommodative esotropia.

Pharmacology.   The contraction of the ciliary muscle for accommodation is effected through the parasympathetic outflow of the third cranial nerve. The efferent arc consists of the preganglionic fiber from the central

nervous system (CNS) to the ciliary ganglion, and the postganglionic fiber from the ciliary ganglion to the effector cells in the ciliary muscle. The transmission of the nerve impulse is mediated by acetylcholine. Acetylcholine is hydrolyzed rapidly into choline and acetic acid by acetylcholinesterase (see Chapter 3). It is possible to simulate this parasympathetic effect by using either acetylcholine or another cholinergic drug, or by allowing acetylcholine to accumulate on the effector cells by preventing its inactivation by acetylcholinesterase. This latter action is accomplished by the use of anticholinesterase drugs.[21]

The classic theory that is held to explain their success is that these anticholinesterase drugs increase the accommodative output (ciliary muscle contraction) without increasing the usually associated neuronal input into the ciliary muscle. As a result, there is no increase in convergence associated with the drug-induced ciliary muscle contraction. This theory explains to some extent why these drugs often reduce the AC/A ratio (Figs. 28.1, 28.2). There are also reports of a more direct effect of cholinesterase inhibitors on the extraocular muscles. Bunke and Bito[22] have demonstrated that with prolonged use of cholinesterase inhibitors in rabbit eyes the extraocular muscles develop a hypersensitivity to the drugs, which causes direct stimulation of the muscle. This stimulation is relatively increased when the concentration of surrounding acetylcholine is low. When the level of acetylcholine is high, this stimulation becomes irrelevant, since there is increased stimulation at the respective neuromuscular junction due to the acetylcholine. These factors explain why such drugs have more of a stimulative effect on the lateral rectus muscles, which are normally less active in accommodative esotropia than are the medial rectus muscles.

The anticholinesterase miotics most commonly used in the treatment of accommodative esotropia, isoflurophate and echothiophate, "irreversibly" inactivate cholinesterases, so that more enzyme must be regenerated. Thus, their effects last several days.

Indications.   As previously noted, anticholinesterase miotics are useful for some children with accommodative esotropia who will not wear glasses for a variety of reasons. These include the usual childhood problems with broken or poorly adjusted frames, undesirable cosmesis, peer pressure, and insignificant improvement in visual acuity. Other possible advantages of miotics are[23] (1) to ensure a continuous therapeutic effect throughout the day, (2) to correct or diminish a near esotropia, (3) to replace glasses or bifocals, especially in accommodative esotropic patients with high AC/A ratios, and (4) to help wean older children (8 years and older) from their hyperopic glasses. Miotics do not

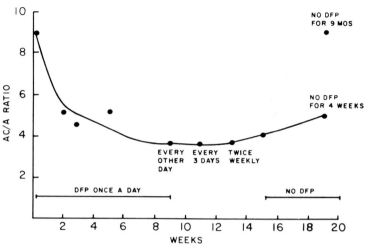

FIGURE 28.1   **Decrease in AC/A ratio during isofluro-phate therapy and subsequent return to previous values.** (Modified from Sloan LL, Sears ML, Jablonski MD. Convergence-accommodation relationships. Description of a simple clinical test and its application to the evaluation of isoflurophate (DFP) therapy. Arch Ophthalmol 1960;63:283–306. Copyright 1960, American Medical Association)

seem to be effective when used in conjunction with glasses, since the patient tends to peer over the lenses.[3]

There has been considerable debate regarding the true effectiveness of miotics as a permanent replacement for spectacles in hyperopic patients with accommodative esotropia. Hill and Stromberg[24] reported that echothiophate may be an effective substitute for bifocals, especially in patients with high AC/A ratios. Wheeler and Moore[25] reported approximately the same findings with isoflurophate. Bedrossian and Krewson[26] found that glasses and miotics were equally effective in 42% of cases and that glasses were more effective in 48%. Hiatt and associates[27] found an equal reduction in esodeviation in 48% of cases treated with echothiophate for 2 months compared with treatment using full hyperopic correction. However, 48% had a larger reduction in the esodeviation with glasses than with echo-

thiophate, while the miotic was more effective in only 4% of patients.

Goldstein[23] suggested the following guidelines for the use of miotics.

- Miotics should never be used unless some degree of binocularity can be achieved.
- Miotics tend to be less effective in the presence of amblyopia.
- Miotics are more useful in patients with high AC/A ratios.
- Miotics are more effective in reducing the near as compared to the distance deviation.

No studies have shown anticholinesterase miotics to be significantly *more* effective than glasses or bifocals in the treatment of accommodative esotropia.[28]

Dosage.   Since isoflurophate hydrolyzes in the presence of water, it must be dispensed in USP anhydrous peanut oil or as an ophthalmic ointment.[29] Currently it is commercially available only as an ointment in 0.025% concentration (Table 28.2). It should be instilled at bedtime to minimize blurring of vision.

In addition to its therapeutic use, isoflurophate may be employed as a diagnostic aid to determine if an accommodative component exists in very young children and in patients with relatively low hyperopic refractive errors. The ointment should be instilled nightly at bedtime for 2 weeks. An accommodative component is revealed if the esodeviation is reduced. This procedure is useful in supplementing standard evaluation techniques.

Echothiophate iodide is available in 0.03, 0.06, 0.125, and 0.25% solutions (see Table 28.2). The usual concentration for use in strabismus is 0.125%.[30] Echothio-

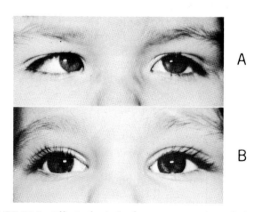

FIGURE 28.2   **Effect of miotic therapy on accommodative esotropia.** *(A)* Before therapy. *(B)* During anticholinesterase therapy. (From von Noorden GK. Atlas of strabismus, ed. 4. St Louis: C.V. Mosby Co, 1983, with permission of the author and publisher.)

TABLE 28.2
Anticholinesterase Miotics Used for Accommodative Esotropia

Generic Name	Trade Name	Dosage Form	Recommended Dosage
Diisopropylfluorophosphate (DFP, isoflurophate)	Floropryl	0.025% ointment	Instill at bedtime
Echothiophate iodide	Phospholine Iodide	0.03%–0.25% solution	Instill 0.125% solution at bedtime

phate is relatively stable in water, but refrigeration improves its stability. Instillation is once a day, preferably at bedtime. A 0.06% solution is sometimes used in older children in an effort to remove the glasses by expanding the fusional divergence amplitude through increased accommodation.

As with isoflurophate, echothiophate may be used diagnostically to confirm the presence of an accommodative component. The 0.125% solution should be instilled at bedtime for 2 to 3 weeks. If the esotropia is accommodative, a reduction of the deviation will be revealed.

Side Effects.   The most significant ocular side effects of the anticholinesterase miotics are the formation of iris cysts (see Fig. 3.42) and the development of anterior subcapsular lens opacities (see Fig. 3.43). Other ocular complications include retinal detachment,[31] angle-closure glaucoma,[32] iritis,[33] superficial punctate keratitis,[20] follicular conjunctivitis,[34] brow-ache, blurred distance vision, lid swelling, and fasciculation of eyelid muscles (see Chapter 3).[24]

The major systemic side effect of echothiophate is substantial reduction of plasma and erythrocyte cholinesterase, resulting in marked cholinergic overactivity.[35–46] Isoflurophate does not seem to depress cholinesterase levels, possibly due to rapid hydrolysis. Serious systemic toxicity is rare in children using anticholinesterase miotics for strabismus.[46] Nausea, abdominal discomfort, and diarrhea are the most frequently reported symptoms, but these problems are usually mild and of no serious consequence. If serious systemic toxicity is noted, atropine and pralidoxime chloride (Protopam) are effective antidotes. The use of these drugs in the management of anticholinesterase toxicity is discussed in Chapter 31.

Use of Botulinum Toxin

In the management of strabismus, if the more conservative modalities—prisms, spectacles, miotics, or orthoptics—fail to bring the eyes into alignment, the next step has often been surgical correction. During the last decade the injection of botulinum A neurotoxin[47,48] has been investigated as another means for treating strabismus.

Pharmacology

Botulinum A is a protein exotoxin produced by Clostridium botulinum, an anaerobic spore-forming bacterium. The toxin, in its nascent state, is composed of a neurotoxin and a larger hemagglutinin portion. The neurotoxin is composed of 2 polypeptide chains held together with interchain disulfide bonds.[49] Type A is the most potent of 8 immunologically distinct toxins produced by the species, which is the etiologic agent of botulism, a swift and often fatal food poisoning. The systemic disease, which often presents with cranial nerve palsies, is characterized by progressive functional disturbances of the peripheral nervous system leading to flaccid paralysis.[50]

The neurotoxin has been shown to act at the level of the neuromuscular junction to prevent the release of the neurotransmitter, acetylcholine. The neurotoxin binds to receptors on the surface of the nerve cell and enters through receptor-mediated endocytosis. Through a mechanism not entirely understood, the toxin interferes with transmitter release.[49] There is also evidence that the toxin alters the concentration of calcium ions at the neuronal junction, which, in turn, interferes with membrane excitability.[49,51] The result of this process is intracellular poisoning and complete paralysis of the cholinergic nerve fibers. The paralysis causes atrophy of the affected muscle(s) and functional loss that remains until a new motor end plate is formed.[52] Local, mild demyelination has been demonstrated histologically in muscles injected with the toxin.[51]

Clinical Procedures

In 1973, Scott demonstrated in primates that a dilute solution of botulinum A toxin (Oculinum) was capable of weakening extraocular muscles when it was injected directly into the muscles. In time human subjects were included in clinical trials, and the initial results were published in 1980.[47] Since then a number of strabismus specialists have experienced varying results using the technique in selected patients.

The method involves the injection, under local anesthesia, of 1.25 to 25 U (0.5 to 10 ng) of the toxin in a total volume of 0.1 ml saline into the muscle group to be weakened.[51] The injection is accomplished through a narrow-gauge needle guided by an electromyography signal. The needle is advanced between the conjunctiva and the orbital surface of the muscle and then into the middle third of the muscle itself, where the toxin is injected. This region is particularly rich in neuromuscular junctions, which then become binding sites for the toxin.[52]

The muscle weakens 24 to 36 hours following treatment. The initial result is paralysis of the injected muscle, often manifest as an opposite deviation in the treated eye; for example, an esotropic eye may become exotropic.[52] As the muscle recovers function, the eye gradually returns toward the pretreatment angle until it reaches a steady state, which, in some cases, represents a reduction in the angle of deviation (Fig. 28.3). The objective of this temporarily induced paresis in the treatment of strabismus is to allow the antagonist muscle to shorten and tighten, thereby improving the position of the eye when the paretic muscle recovers.[51,53] The response is a constant proportion of the pretreatment deviation and averages about 55% to 70% of the original deviation. Stabilization of alignment appears to depend on the patient's ability to fuse, since without fusion the eyes tend to drift back to the original deviation. The treatment can be repeated and the dose increased if necessary.

The rationale is slightly different when the toxin is used in the treatment of acute sixth nerve palsy. In this procedure the toxin is injected into the antagonist medial rectus muscle to bring about temporary reduction in the contracture of this muscle while awaiting functional recovery of the lateral rectus. Single binocular vision can then be preserved during the healing period in these patients.[51,54]

Early investigations suggest that the long-term results of botulinum injection are variable.[55] However, there are several advantages to botulinum treatment compared with the surgical alternative. The treatment is performed, usually within 5 to 10 minutes, on an outpatient basis using local anesthesia. This is preferred economically because not only is the procedure less expensive than surgery, it permits less time lost from employment.[53] Morbidity is less significant than that occurring with surgical treatment, and scar tissue is not formed.[56]

Patient Selection

Some variation exists in the criteria used by strabismologists in choosing the patient population best suited for this alternative therapy. Some investigators believe the procedure has merit in children, and Magoon and Scott[56] have published the results of a series of 82 children aged 13 years or younger treated for horizontal strabismus by toxin injection. Improvement was achieved in 81 of the children, although reinjection was necessary in 85% of the patients.[56] The advantage of using a local anesthetic is lost in children, since in much of this population general anesthesia is required. Low dose ketamine anesthesia has typically been used in this age group.[53] However, the procedure can be carried out successfully in children younger than 1 year and older than 6 years of age using only topical drop anesthesia and no sedation.[56]

Most investigators, however, reserve the therapy primarily for teenage and adult patients, often those who have undergone prior surgical attempts at correction.[53] Some clinicians actually restrict botulinum A injection to patients who represent a poor surgical risk. Included in that group are patients during the relatively acute phase of thyroid-related ophthalmopathy (see Chapter 27), patients with remaining free or restricted passive ductions after surgical procedures, patients with an intermittent deviation who reject surgery, and patients with acute and chronic muscle palsy. It has also been suggested that botulinum toxin can be used to "fine tune" the results of strabismus surgery. Nevertheless, for most clinicians, surgery remains the treatment of choice for primary strabismus, since it offers the advantage of cosmetically straight eyes after only one procedure in most cases.[55]

Complications

Pain, subconjunctival hemorrhage, expanded paralysis within the orbit, induced diplopia, and a prolonged period of ptosis have been reported.[51–53] Ptosis is a relatively common, but temporary, complication occurring to some extent in up to 53% of cases[57] and to a significant degree in 17% to 21% of cases.[51,57] The ptosis generally resolves within 8 weeks (see Fig. 28.3). Diplopia is brought on when the altered, usually overcorrected gaze takes the treated eye into an area where suppression does not occur.[51] This temporary complication can be managed with a patch.[52] In about 10% of cases, adjacent muscles will be affected by the toxin injection, with the levator being the most susceptible.[51] In some instances where the paralytic effect has expanded outside the injected muscle, surgical correction has been necessary.[52] The most serious complication associated with botulinum injection is inad-

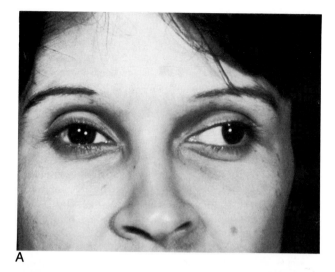

A

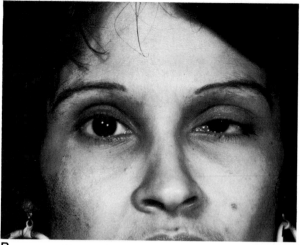

B

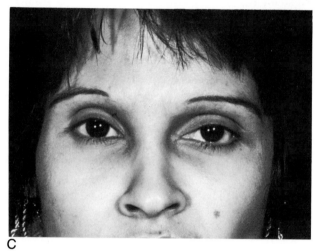

C

FIGURE 28.3   **Reduction of large angle exotropia using combination of surgery and botulinum toxin injection.** *(A)* **Preoperative left exotropia measured 100**△ **by Krimsky with 15**△ **left hypotropia. At surgery the left lateral rectus was injected with 10 units of botulinum toxin, followed by 10 mm recession of the left lateral rectus and 10 mm resection of the medial rectus.** *(B)* **One week postoperatively, deviation in primary gaze was 30**△ **left esotropia with no lateral rectus function. Note left ptosis.** *(C)* **Twelve weeks postoperatively, deviation was 3**△ **left exotropia with 10**△ **left hypotropia. Ptosis has resolved. (Courtesy Paul L. Owens, O.D., M.D.)**

vertent perforation of the globe. Five cases have been reported, with one patient suffering vitreous hemorrhage and subsequent decreased vision. Other rarely reported complications include retrobulbar hemorrhage, pupillary dilation, spatial disorientation, and rash.[51]

Perhaps the most important consideration in assessing the procedure at this time is its unknown long-term effectiveness. Additional patients with a range of indications must be treated to determine the ultimate role of this form of therapy.

References

1. Duke-Elder S, Wybar K, eds. System of ophthalmology. St Louis: C.V. Mosby Co, 1973;6:590–616.

2. Baker JD, Parks MM. Early-onset accommodative esotropia. Am J Ophthalmol 1980;90:11–18.

3. Parks MM, Wheeler MB. Concomitant esodeviations. In: Duane TD, Jaeger EA, eds. Clinical ophthalmology. Philadelphia: Harper & Row, 1987;vol. 1, Chap 12:1–14.

4. Chang FW. The pharmacology of cycloplegics. Am J Optom Physiol Opt 1978;55:219–222.

5. Amos DM. Cycloplegics for refraction. Am J Optom Physiol Opt 1978;55:223–226.

6. Bartlett JD. Administration of and adverse reactions to cycloplegic agents. Am J Optom Physiol Opt 1978;55:227–233.

7. Rosenbaum AL, Bateman JB, Bremer DL, et al. Cycloplegic refraction in esotropic children. Cyclopentolate versus atropine. Ophthalmology 1981;88:1031–1033.

8. Havener WH. Ocular pharmacology. 5th ed. St Louis: C.V. Mosby Co, 1983;379–398.

9. Michaels DD. Visual optics and refraction: A clinical approach. St Louis: C.V. Mosby Co, 1975:186–195.

10. Abraham SV. Mydriatic glaucoma—a statistical study. Arch Ophthalmol 1933;10:757–762.

11. Adcock EW. Cyclopentolate (Cyclogyl) toxicity in pediatric patients. J Pediatr 1971;79:127–129.

12. Gray LG. Avoiding adverse effects of cycloplegics in infants and children. J Am Optom Assoc 1979;50:465–470.

13. Wick B. Accommodative esotropia: Efficacy of therapy. J Am Optom Assoc 1987;58:562–566.

14. Von Noorden GK, Morris J, Edelman P. Efficacy of bifocals in the treatment of accommodative esotropia. Am J Ophthalmol 1978;85:830–834.

15. Jacob JL, Beaulieu Y, Brunet E. Progressive-addition lenses in the management of esotropia with a high accommodation-convergence ratio. Can J Ophthalmol 1980;15:166–169.

16. Smith JB. Progressive-addition lenses in the treatment of accommodative esotropia. Am J Ophthalmol 1985;99:56–62.

17. Javal E. Manuel du strabisme. Paris: Masson, 1896;45–87.

18. Abraham SV. The use of miotics in the treatment of convergent strabismus anisometropia: A preliminary report. Am J Ophthalmol 1949;32:233–240.

19. Abraham SV. The use of miotics in the treatment of nonparalytic convergent strabismus: A progress report. Am J Ophthalmol 1952;35:1191–1195.

20. Miller JE. A comparison of miotics in accommodative esotropia. Am J Ophthalmol 1960;49:1350–1355.

21. Taylor P. Anticholinesterase agents. In: Goodman L, Gilman A, eds. The pharmacological basis of therapeutics, ed. 6. New York: Macmillan, 1980;100–119.

22. Bunke A, Bito LZ. Gradual increase in the sensitivity of extraocular muscles to acetylcholine during topical treatment of rabbit eyes with isoflurophate. Am J Ophthalmol 1981;92:259–267.

23. Goldstein JH. The role of miotics in strabismus. Surv Ophthalmol 1968;13:31–46.

24. Hill K, Stromberg AE. Echothiophate iodide in the management of esotropia. Am J Ophthalmol 1962;53:488–494.

25. Wheeler MC, Moore S. DFP in the handling of esotropia. Am Orthop J 1964;14:178–188.

26. Bedrossian EH, Krewson WE. Isoflurophate versus glasses in evaluating the accommodative element in esotropia. Arch Ophthalmol 1966;76:186–188.

27. Hiatt RL, Ringer C, Cope-Troupe C. Miotics vs glasses in esodeviation. J Pediatr Ophthalmol 1979;16:213–217.

28. Hiatt RL. Management of accommodative esotropia. J Pediatr Ophthalmol Strabismus 1983;20:199–201.

29. Havener W. Ocular pharmacology. 5th ed. St Louis: C.V. Mosby Co, 1983;349–358.

30. Moss HM. Strabismus: Current use of therapeutic drugs. In: Srinivasan BD, ed. Ocular therapeutics. New York: Masson, 1980;111–114.

31. La Rocca V. Retinal detachment from diisopropyl fluorophosphate in an aphakic eye. NY State J Med 1952;52:1329–1330.

32. Butler WE. Acute glaucoma precipitated by DFP: Report of a case. Am J Ophthalmol 1952;35:1031–1033.

33. Becker B, Gage T. Demecarium bromide and echothiophate iodide in chronic glaucoma. Arch Ophthalmol 1960;63:102–107.

34. Knapp P. Use of miotics in esotropia. J Iowa State Med Soc 1956;46:581–585.

35. De Roeth A, Dettbarn WD, Rosenberg P, et al. Effect of phospholine iodide on blood cholinesterase levels of normal and glaucoma subjects. Am J Ophthalmol 1965;59:586–592.

36. Humphreys JA, Holmes JH. Systemic effects produced by echothiophate iodide in the treatment of glaucoma. Arch Ophthalmol 1963;69:737–743.

37. Klendshoj NC, Olmstead EP. Observation of dangerous side-effects of phospholine iodide in glaucoma therapy. Am J Ophthalmol 1963;56:247–250.

38. McGavi DM. Depressed levels of serum pseudocholinesterase with echothiophate iodide eyedrops. Lancet 1965;2:272–273.

39. Ripps H. Miotics in the treatment of accommodative strabismus. Trans Ophthalmol Soc UK 1963;88:199–210.

40. Klendshoj NC, Feldstein M. Cholinesterase of blood in relation to organic phosphate insecticides. NY State J Med 1953;53:2667–2669.

41. Leopold IH, Comroe JH. Effect of diisopropyl fluorophosphate ("DFP") on the normal eye. Arch Ophthalmol 1946;36:17–32.

42. Leopold IH. Ocular cholinesterase and cholinesterase inhibitors. Am J Ophthalmol 1961;51:885–919.

43. Humphreys JA, Holmes JH. Systemic effects produced by echothiophate iodide in treatment of glaucoma. Arch Ophthalmol 1963;69:737–734.

44. Ellis PP, Esterdahl M. Echothiophate iodide therapy in children. Effect upon blood cholinesterase levels. Arch Ophthalmol 1967;77:598–601.

45. Sampson CR, Hermann JS. Isoflurophate in esotropic children: Effects on serum cholinesterase. J Pediatr Ophthalmol 1970;7:44–45.

46. Apt L. Toxicity of strong miotics in children. In: Leopold IH, ed. Symposium on ocular therapy V. St Louis: C.V. Mosby Co, 1972; Chap. 2:30–35.

47. Scott AB. Botulinum toxin injection into extraocular muscles as an alternative to strabismus surgery. Ophthalmology 1980;87:1044–1049.

48. Scott AB. Botulinum toxin injection of eye muscles to correct strabismus. Trans Am Ophthalmol Soc 1981;79:735–770.

49. Simpson LL. Molecular pharmacology of botulinum toxin and tetanus toxin. Ann Rev Pharmacol Toxicol 1986;26:427–453.

50. Joklik WK, Willett HP, Amos DB, eds. Zinsser microbiology, ed. 18. Norwalk, CT: Appleton-Century-Crofts, 1984;711–717.

51. Hoffman RO, Helveston EM. Botulinum in the treatment of adult motility disorders. Int Ophthalmol Clin 1986;26:241–250.

52. Elston JS. The use of botulinum toxin A in the treatment of strabismus. Trans Ophthalmol Soc UK 1985;104:208–210.

53. Metz HS. Botulinum injections for strabismus. J Pediatr Ophthalmol Strabismus 1984;21:199–201.

54. Scott AB, Kraft SP. Botulinum toxin injection in the management of lateral rectus paresis. Ophthalmology 1985;92:676–683.

55. Helveston EM. Botulinum injections for strabismus. J Pediatr Ophthalmol Strabismus 1984;21:202–204.

56. Magoon E, Scott AB. Botulinum toxin chemodenervation in infants and children: An alternative to incisional strabismus surgery. J Pediatr 1987;110:719–722.

57. Burns CL, Gammon JA, Gemmill MC. Ptosis associated with botulinum toxin treatment of strabismus and blepharospasm. Ophthalmology 1986;93:1621–1627.

CHAPTER 29

The Glaucomas

J. Boyd Eskridge

Jimmy D. Bartlett

The term *glaukoma* was first used by Aristotle when referring to blue-eyed patients with "weakness of the eyes" in daylight.[1] It has been assumed that Aristotle was referring to blue-eyed patients with cataracts. Al-Tabari, an Arabian physician, is reported to be the first to associate the term *glaucoma* with an increased intraocular pressure (IOP).[2] In 1622, Banister, an English oculist, discussed the detection of glaucoma using finger palpation to evaluate hardness of the eyeball.[3] Over the years the term *glaucoma* came to be associated with an elevated IOP that produced damage to ocular structures. The emphasis in the theoretical considerations and in the clinical diagnosis was on elevated IOP.

In recent years, however, the emphasis has shifted from elevated IOP to impaired visual function.[4] An elevated IOP is a major risk factor for glaucoma, but the ability to predict the presence of impaired visual function from IOP alone is low. The essence of glaucoma is visual and ocular impairment manifested by optic disc changes, nerve fiber layer irregularities, visual field losses, and other factors that are associated with a disturbance of aqueous circulation and a constant or intermittent unphysiologic IOP.

Classification

The glaucomas can be divided into two broad classifications—primary and secondary. Primary glaucoma is associated with a direct known or unknown disturbance of the aqueous circulation. Secondary glaucoma de-velops because of another recognizable disease mechanism. The glaucomas can be further classified by the degree of the anterior chamber angle, with 20° usually considered to be the magnitude dividing narrow angle (less than 20°) from open angle (greater than 20°) (Fig. 29.1). Although this classification can generally be made clinically, the work of Douglas and associates[5] and Horie and associates[6] has suggested that the glaucomas may exist as a continuum from acute angle-closure to subacute angle-closure to chronic angle-closure to open-angle glaucoma. These investigators found that patients with acute angle-closure glaucoma had normal visual fields and normal optic discs, but patients with chronic angle-closure glaucoma had visual field and optic disc changes similar to those in open-angle glaucoma. This information suggests that although there are specific differences, the basic etiopathogenesis of primary angle-closure glaucoma and primary open-angle glaucoma is similar.

Congenital glaucoma is often classified separately. This form of glaucoma occurs in the young as the result of developmental or birth defects.

A clinical classification of the glaucomas is shown in Table 29.1.

Basic Etiology

As previously indicated, all glaucomas are associated with a disturbance of aqueous circulation and the resultant unphysiologic IOP.

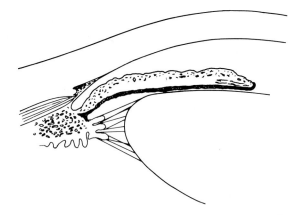

FIGURE 29.1 **An anterior chamber angle of about 20°. This is usually considered to be the degree that divides an open angle from a narrow angle.**

Characteristics of Aqueous

The aqueous humor is a secretion-diffusion clear fluid formed at the rate of about 2 to 3 µl/min. The total volume of aqueous in the eye is about 125 µl. The blood-aqueous barrier is highly permeable to water, so that if the blood osmotic pressure is high, water will be rapidly removed from the eye, resulting in reduction of IOP. This physiologic principle is used in the management of acute angle-closure glaucoma. Mannitol or oral glycerin may be administered, producing an increase in osmotic pressure of the blood, thereby increasing the removal of water from the eye and reducing a generally very high IOP.

Formation of Aqueous

Most of the aqueous is derived from blood plasma in the highly vascularized ciliary processes (see Chapter 7). Aqueous is formed from the blood by epithelial

TABLE 29.1
Clinical Classification of the Glaucomas

Congenital glaucoma
Primary glaucoma
  Angle closure
    Without pupillary block
    With pupillary block
  Open angle
    Chronic open angle
    Low tension
Secondary glaucoma
  Angle closure
  Open angle

cells in the ciliary processes (Fig. 29.2). Two enzymes are involved in the process of aqueous formation—adenosine triphosphatase and carbonic anhydrase. If these enzymes are inhibited, the rate of aqueous formation is decreased, reducing both the aqueous content in the eye and IOP. Ouabain inhibits adenosine triphosphatase, but it has too many side effects to be clinically useful. Acetazolamide and methazolamide inhibit carbonic anhydrase and are often used in the treatment of glaucoma.

Circulation of Aqueous

The capillary bed in the ciliary processes receives its blood supply from the large posterior ciliary arteries, the anterior ciliary arteries, and the major arterial circle in the iris. Aqueous is formed by epithelial cells in the ciliary processes and moves into the posterior chamber partly by active secretion (75%) and partly by ultrafiltration (25%). Aqueous flows from the posterior chamber to the anterior chamber through the pupil. Since the iris is in contact with the lens, a slight anatomic resistance to the flow of aqueous from the posterior to the anterior chamber is present. Aqueous

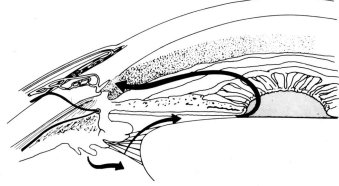

FIGURE 29.2 **Normal flow of aqueous humor. Aqueous is formed in the ciliary processes, moves out around the crystalline lens, through the pupil, and flows out of the anterior chamber through the trabecular meshwork into Schlemm's canal and then to the episcleral veins.**

leaves the anterior chamber by passing through pores in the trabecular meshwork and then through the endothelial cell lining into Schlemm's canal (see Fig. 29.2). From here 20 to 30 aqueous veins return the aqueous to the venous blood.

Aqueous is transferred through the endothelium into Schlemm's canal by endothelial vacuolization (Fig. 29.3). Johnstone and Grant[7] determined that this process of aqueous outflow was pressure regulated, since the number and size of the endothelial vacuoles changed as the IOP was raised and lowered. In the normal condition, the arterial blood pressure in the ciliary processes is high enough to maintain aqueous formation, and the intraocular pressure is high enough to maintain the flow of aqueous from the eye. The pressure in the aqueous veins is only about 10 mm Hg.[8]

It has been suggested that an active phagocytotic process occurs during the aqueous transfer, in which the endothelial cells of the trabecular meshwork engulf and digest the debris in the aqueous outflow, thereby providing a self-cleaning mechanism.[9] If this phagocytotic process is decreased due to reduced function of the endothelial cells, the outflow resistance would increase, resulting in decreased aqueous outflow and increased IOP. The efficiency of this process is reduced if the inflow of debris or undigestable particles is increased, as in pigmentary glaucoma. Steroids may also inhibit phagocytosis.[9] Reduced phagocytosis can occur in both open-angle and angle-closure glaucoma.

Aqueous humor also leaves the anterior chamber through a uveoscleral route. In this route, the aqueous leaves the anterior chamber near the base of the trabecular meshwork and passes into the supraciliary and the suprachoroidal spaces. From here, the fluid is absorbed by the choroidal and scleral circulation. In one study[10] in glaucomatous dogs, the uveoscleral outflow was significantly decreased or completely absent.

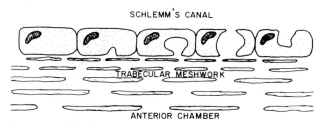

SCHLEMM'S CANAL

TRABECULAR MESHWORK

ANTERIOR CHAMBER

FIGURE 29.3 **Endothelial vacuoles. Aqueous flows through the trabecular meshwork and into Schlemm's canal by passing through the endothelium of Schlemm's canal. This is accomplished by a process of vacuolization. The endothelial cell indents, forms a vacuole, perforates to form a passage for the aqueous to flow into Schlemm's canal, and then repairs itself and repeats the process. During this process of endothelial vacuolization, a phagocytotic process is taking place.**

Any mechanism, process, activity, or condition, such as extracellular material, that decreases aqueous outflow can result in an unphysiologic increased IOP and glaucomatous visual impairment. Campbell and associates[11] have shown that in the early stages of glaucoma, the reduction in aqueous outflow probably occurs in certain areas or segments of the meshwork rather than throughout the entire trabecular meshwork.

Pathogenesis

Although changes in the eye that produce the unphysiologic IOP are located in the anterior segment, the ocular changes that produce the visual impairment in glaucoma occur in the posterior segment, in and around the optic nerve. The changes in the posterior segment can be due to a frank increase in IOP (mechanical theory), an imbalance between the IOP and the systemic blood pressure in the vessels supplying the anterior portion of the optic nerve (vasogenic theory), or both.

Although the vasogenic theory does not adequately explain all the clinical observations, there is still considerable evidence in its favor and general agreement that it is involved. Some recent reports,[12] however, have indicated that vascular insufficiency may not be the main mechanism of glaucomatous damage. Gallois,[13] as early as 1933, pointed out a relationship between a decrease in systemic blood pressure and the progression of visual field loss in glaucoma. Harrington[14] focused attention on the clinical relationship of blood pressure and visual field loss by presenting clinical evidence that arterial insufficiency and decreased blood flow in the anterior portion of the optic nerve are the primary factors producing visual field loss in glaucoma. He demonstrated that visual field losses occurred with IOPs that were formerly compatible with health and function when the systemic blood pressure was lowered medically for systemic hypertension. Hitchings and Spaeth[15] studied the blood supply to the optic nerve head using fluorescein angiography in patients with low tension and primary open-angle glaucoma matched for visual field loss. They found no difference in the circulation times between the 2 groups, suggesting that a decreased vascular supply to the optic nerve head can result from an unphysiologically high IOP or an unphysiologically low blood pressure in the vessels supplying the anterior portion of the optic nerve. Sebag and associates[16] have also shown that patients with arteritic anterior ischemic optic neuropathy have cupping of the optic disc that is similar to glaucomatous cupping.

Hayreh[17] proposed that the primary blood supply to the anterior portion of the optic nerve comes from the posterior ciliary arteries by way of peripapillary choroidal circulation and that the central retinal artery supplies only a thin superficial layer of tissue on the optic nerve head and possibly some tissue in the retrolaminar region (Fig. 29.4). The peripapillary choroidal circulation is more vulnerable to extracellular pressure than is the retinal circulation, so that with a given rise in IOP or a reduction in perfusion pressure in the posterior ciliary arteries, blood flow decreases in the peripapillary choroidal circulation and a vascular insufficiency develops in the anterior portion of the optic nerve. If this insufficiency continues beyond a critical period, ischemia of the optic nerve results, with corresponding optic disc cupping and visual field loss. High resolution fluorescein angiography of the optic nerve head has shown a significant correlation between fluorescein filling defects and visual field loss in glaucoma.[18,19] As cupping of the optic disc increases, the lamina cribrosa, which is flat in normal eyes, begins to bow backward and take on a concave shape. With this shape the optic nerve fibers passing through the fenestrated connective tissue sheets of the lamina cribrosa may be subjected to a shearing pressure, resulting in additional decreased function and visual field loss. Histologic evaluations of the optic nerve fibers of human glaucomatous eyes have shown that the main location

of optic nerve damage is in the area of the lamina cribrosa. The early nerve fiber injury usually occurs at the superior and inferior poles of the lamina. This suggests a correlation between structural changes in the lamina cribrosa and nerve fiber loss in glaucomatous optic nerves.[21]

Although ischemia of the optic nerve head is a significant factor in the pathogenesis of glaucoma, more than the posterior ciliary arteries and the peripapillary choroidal circulation are probably involved. Using a histologic approach to study the vascularity of the optic nerve, Anderson and Davis[22] and Lieberman and associates[23] determined that the retrolaminar area is profusely supplied with vessels from the pial sheath around the optic nerve and small branches from the central retinal artery. They also found that the lamina cribrosa does receive a blood supply from the short posterior ciliary arteries without passing through the peripapillary choroidal circulation and that the prelaminar area receives a blood supply directly from smaller short posterior ciliary branches as well as from branches from the choroidal circulation. These investigators do not deny some choroidal circulation at all areas but maintain that the major vascular supply to the anterior optic nerve does not come from the peripapillary choroidal circulation.

Anderson[24] has proposed an additional mechanism to account for some of the early changes that occur in the optic disc. He has shown that the glial tissue framework supporting the nerve fibers occupies almost the entire surface of the optic nerve head and about half the volume of the optic papilla. The capillaries feeding the optic nerve fibers are located in and supported by this glial tissue. He has proposed that the glial tissue is sensitive to pressure and that an increase in intraocular pressure results in damage and deterioration of the glial tissue from the mechanical stress. The loss of glial tissue support of the capillaries in a given area could expose the capillaries in that area to an unphysiologic extravascular pressure, resulting in localized closure of the capillaries and loss of blood supply to the adjacent nerve fibers. Visual field loss could result from the vascular insufficiency that follows the astroglial tissue breakdown. However, the more recent histologic studies of Quigley[12] have shown that there is very little loss of glial tissue from the optic nerve head in glaucoma, and thus the loss of glial tissue is probably not a factor in the neuropathy of optic nerve fibers or in cupping of the optic disc.

Another change in the optic nerve associated with an elevated IOP should be considered in the pathogenesis of glaucoma. The normal eye has a continuous rapid and slow flow of protein from the retinal ganglion cells through the optic nerve to the lateral geniculate nucleus. Levy[25] has shown that with even minor ele-

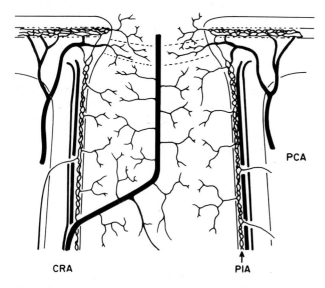

FIGURE 29.4 **Blood supply to the anterior segment of the optic nerve. The prelaminar and laminar portions of the optic nerve are primarily nourished by the posterior ciliary arteries (PCA) directly through their own branches and indirectly through branches from the peripapillary choroidal circulation. They probably also receive nourishment from branches of the pial (PIA) circulation. The postlaminar portion is probably nourished by branches from the central retinal artery (CRA) and the pial circulation.**

vations in IOP, the slow axonal flow of protein in the optic nerve is reduced. Anderson and Hendrickson[26] found a reduction in the rapid transport of protein in the optic nerve with moderately elevated IOP. Some of the blockage occurred in the retina, but most of it occurred in the region of the lamina cribrosa. One study[27] also reported blockage at the edge of the posterior scleral foramen. It is possible that if this blockage is present for a sufficient time, axonal damage could occur, resulting in visual field loss. Sakugawa and Chihara[27] have suggested that if the blockage is at the lamina, a paracentral scotoma will result, and if the blockage is at the scleral foramen, a peripheral nasal step will result. Reduction in the flow of protein in the optic nerve fibers is probably associated with mechanical pressure.

Other studies have indicated that the earliest changes in glaucomatous neuropathy are in the retina and not in the optic nerve. Nakatani and Suzuki[28] carefully evaluated the retinas of glaucoma patients and found excavations in the retinal surface that corresponded to the visual field defects. They concluded that the glaucomatous visual field defects resulted from degeneration of retinal ganglion cells and that the optic disc changes are secondary to this degeneration. The work of Anctil and Anderson,[29] showing a reduction in foveal threshold before any significant visual field loss or optic disc cupping occurs in early glaucomatous eyes, tends to support this.

Epidemiology

Prevalence

Glaucoma is currently the leading cause of legal blindness in the United States, and the incidence does not appear to be decreasing.[30] About 62,000 individuals are legally blind from glaucoma, and nearly 1 million have visual impairment due to glaucoma.[31] In a study[32] in England of patients 76 years of age and older, openangle glaucoma was found to be the third leading cause of sight reduction, with a prevalence of 6.6%.

In a study of people over the age of 60 years in Sweden,[33] the prevalence of glaucoma was found to be 0.86% for open-angle glaucoma, 0.06% for angleclosure glaucoma, 0.05% for congenital glaucoma, and 0.27% for secondary glaucoma. This suggests that about 80% of glaucoma is primary and about 20% is secondary.

The studies of Hollows and Graham[34] and of Bankes and associates[35] indicate that the prevalence of openangle glaucoma in the population over 40 years of age is 0.43% to 1.02%. These investigators found the prevalence of angle-closure glaucoma to be 0.09% to 0.21%. This suggests that open-angle glaucoma is about 5 times more prevalent than angle-closure glaucoma.

Risk Factors

Several risk factors have been identified whose presence increases the probability of primary glaucoma in any given patient (Table 29.2). Appreciation of these factors is important for the diagnosis and management of primary glaucoma.

AGE

The prevalence of primary glaucoma increases with age. Colenbrander[36] reported that the prevalence of glaucoma is about 0.25% at age 20 years and that it nearly doubles every 10 years. Although other studies[35,37,38] show somewhat different prevalence values, they do demonstrate a significant increase with age. David and associates[39] reported that the age group most frequently affected with angle-closure glaucoma is between 50 and 60 years of age. Every patient should be evaluated for glaucoma, but the older the patient, the more thorough should be the evaluation.

FAMILY HISTORY

Substantial evidence indicates a genetic basis for primary glaucoma. Becker and associates[40] studied the close relatives (parents, siblings, children) of patients with primary open-angle glaucoma and found that the average values for intraocular pressure and outflow facility were significantly different from those for a normal population. They also found a 5.5% prevalence of primary open-angle glaucoma in close relatives. Shin and associates[41] found a family history of glaucoma in 50% of the patients with primary open-angle glaucoma. Perkins[42] studied the children and siblings of patients with glaucoma and found a prevalence of 5.3% with open-angle glaucoma and 6% with angle-closure glaucoma. Paterson[43] studied the relatives of patients with angle-closure glaucoma and also found a prevalence of

TABLE 29.2
Risk Factors for Glaucoma

- Age
- Family history of glaucoma
- Race
- Ametropia
- Sex
- Mental set
- Systemic illness

primary angle-closure glaucoma of about 6%. These studies suggest that primary glaucoma is found from 5.5 to 13 times more often in close relatives of glaucoma patients and that the prevalence of a positive family history is 6 to 7 times greater on the maternal side than on the paternal side.

Although genetic factors are involved in primary glaucoma, the exact mode of inheritance is as yet unresolved. Studies have suggested that the inheritance patterns for angle-closure glaucoma could be multifactorial,[44] polygenic,[45] autosomal dominant,[46] and autosomal recessive.[47] Similarly, other studies have suggested several modes of inheritance for open-angle glaucoma—multifactorial,[48] autosomal dominant with variable penetrance,[49] and autosomal recessive.[50]

Infantile glaucoma occurs in 1 in 10,000 births and is bilateral in 75% of the infants. It appears to have an autosomal recessive transmittance with incomplete penetrance.[51,52]

Every patient should be questioned regarding a family history of glaucoma. Those indicating such a history have a much greater risk for glaucoma.

RACIAL INFLUENCE

Several reports have indicated that the prevalence of primary glaucoma varies in different racial groups. In their study of nearly 12,000 people, Packer and associates[53] found a prevalence of open-angle glaucoma of 1% in whites and 2.6% in blacks. In a comprehensive study of 15,000 patients by Turner,[54] the prevalence of open-angle glaucoma was 1% in whites and 3% in blacks. Wilensky and associates[55] found that the prevalence of open-angle glaucoma in blacks was 2.59 times the prevalence in whites and that it occurs at a younger age in blacks than in whites. They also suggested that glaucoma is a more severe disease in blacks, since blacks appear to be less responsive to glaucoma therapy. Martin and associates[56] also found a higher incidence of open-angle glaucoma in blacks, and that the age of diagnosis was younger, the mean cup/disc ratio was higher, the IOP at the time of diagnosis was higher, and the visual field loss at the time of diagnosis was greater in blacks than in whites.

The prevalence of angle-closure glaucoma has also been reported to vary with race. The prevalence of angle-closure glaucoma is 4 times greater than open-angle glaucoma among the Singaporean Chinese,[57] and is the most prevalent form of glaucoma among adults in the Philippines.[58] Alper and Laubach[59] reported that acute angle-closure glaucoma with its classic signs and symptoms is rare in American blacks but that chronic angle-closure glaucoma occurs with significant frequency. However, Luntz[60] reported that the prevalence and clinical features of angle-closure glaucoma are similar for blacks and for whites in South Africa.

The Eskimos in Greenland[61] and Canada[62] have the highest reported prevalence of angle-closure glaucoma. Drance[62] found the prevalence of primary angle-closure glaucoma in Canadian Eskimos over the age of 40 years to be 2.9%. The prevalence also increased substantially with age. Mann[63] has reported that glaucoma in all forms is rare in Orientals and in Indians of North and South America. The results of the study by Kass and associates[64] with Zuni Indians support this, but the results of Bettman[65] indicate that American Indians have a prevalence of open-angle glaucoma of 1.5%. Lowe[66] reported a low prevalence of angle-closure glaucoma in Italians and Greeks.

These studies suggest that blacks have a higher prevalence of open-angle glaucoma than do whites, that whites may have a higher prevalence of acute angle-closure glaucoma, that angle-closure glaucoma is rare in Italians and Greeks, and that glaucoma is rare in American Indians and Orientals.

AMETROPIA

Angle-closure glaucoma occurs more frequently in hyperopic eyes.[67] The influence of myopia in glaucoma is not as significant, but Perkins and Phelps[68] found a high incidence of open-angle glaucoma in patients with myopia.

ROLE OF SEX

Several studies[34,62,69] have suggested that the index of suspicion for open-angle glaucoma should be the same for males or females but that it should be higher in angle-closure glaucoma for females.

MENTAL SET

It has been shown[70,71] that people with low-stress jobs and relaxed personalities have a lower incidence of primary glaucoma, whereas people with chronic anxiety neuroses in high-stress environments have a higher incidence of glaucoma. Van Alphen and Stokvis[72] have also shown that the incidence of glaucoma increases in times of chronic societal stress and anxiety.

SYSTEMIC ILLNESS

Duke-Elder[73] has stated that "Glaucoma is a sick eye in a sick body." Numerous systemic diseases such as diabetes, hyperthyroidism, anemia, arthritis, hypertension, arteriosclerosis, and emphysema have been associated with glaucoma. The prevalence of glaucoma is greater in diabetic patients than in a nondiabetic matched control group, and high cup-disc (C/D) ratios occur with greater frequency in diabetic populations.[74] Becker and associates[75] found a significant correlation between thyroid disease and glaucoma. A high prevalence of arteriosclerosis and hypertension has been found in glaucoma patients and glaucoma suspects.[53] However, a recent study[76] has shown that although systolic blood pressure does increase with age, there is no statistical association between systolic blood pressure and glaucoma. Thus, hypertension itself is not a risk factor, but there may be an increased risk when patients with systemic hypertension and relatively high IOP receive systemic hypotensive therapy. This may cause a reduction in the blood perfusion pressure of the optic nerve head, with resulting ischemia and visual field loss.

Ocular Hypotensive Agents

Most drugs used to reduce IOP exert their ocular hypotensive effect by influencing the autonomic nervous system (Table 29.3). The specific mechanisms by which these drugs reduce IOP, as well as their recommended dosages, side effects, and contraindications, are considered in Chapters 3, 7, and 8.

Congenital Glaucoma

Etiology

The etiology of congenital glaucoma varies with the specific congenital abnormality. Some of the major causes and associated abnormalities are listed in Table 29.4. Congenital glaucoma is not solely due to genetic factors. In most cases, the condition results from an interaction between genetic predisposition and a combination of environmental causes.[77] In a recent study[78] of infantile glaucoma, glaucoma associated with congenital anomalies accounted for 46% of the patients,

TABLE 29.3
Commonly Employed Ocular Hypotensive Agents

Cholinergic agonists
  Pilocarpine
  Carbachol
  Echothiophate
Adrenergic agonists
  Epinephrine
  Dipivefrin
Adrenergic blockers
  Timolol
  Levobunolol
  Betaxolol
Carbonic anhydrase inhibitors
  Acetazolamide
  Methazolamide
  Dichlorphenamide
Hyperosmotic agents
  Glycerol (glycerin)

secondary infantile glaucoma was present in 31.8% of the patients, and primary congenital glaucoma occurred in 22.2% of the patients.

Diagnosis

Several conditions simulate congenital glaucoma and should be carefully considered in the differential diagnosis (Table 29.5). The diagnosis of congenital glaucoma is accomplished through careful patient history and examination.

PATIENT HISTORY

Some of the early indications of congenital glaucoma are lacrimation, epiphora, light sensitivity, and blepharospasm. Slight haziness or cloudiness of the cornea is also common. Buphthalmus may be present if the

TABLE 29.4
Congenital Glaucoma

Etiology	Associated Congenital Abnormality
Residual iris stump obstructing the trabecular meshwork	Aniridia
Anomalous attachment of iris tissue to the cornea, obstructing the trabecular meshwork	Anterior chamber cleavage syndrome
	Axenfeld's syndrome
	Reiger's anomaly
	Peters' anomaly
	Neurofibromatosis
Dislocated crystalline lens or microspherophakia, producing pupillary block	Marfan's syndrome
	Homocystinuria
	Marchesani's syndrome
Barkan's membrane (a thin translucent gelatinous-appearing membrane that covers the trabecular meshwork)	Infantile glaucoma
Improper development of the trabecular meshwork	Lowe's syndrome

TABLE 29.5
Conditions that Simulate Congenital Glaucoma

- Megalocornea
- Congenital corneal edema
- Rubella keratitis
- Corneal injury at birth producing tears in Descemet's membrane
- Corneal lipoidosis
- Mucopolysaccharidosis that produces corneal opacities

IOP has been elevated for some time. Infants should be closely observed for the presence of these signs.

Another indication is the presence of any abnormality known to cause congenital glaucoma such as aniridia, Reiger's anomaly, or Marfan's syndrome.

EXAMINATION

Using calipers for accuracy, the horizontal diameter of the cornea should be measured. Each corneal diameter should be approximately equal. The average in infants is 10.0 mm as compared with 11.8 mm in adults.[79] Corneal asymmetry exceeding 1.5 mm or a diameter over 12 mm in an infant suggests congenital glaucoma (Fig. 29.5).

Although the axial length is increased in congenital glaucoma, a study by Kiskis and associates[80] indicated that corneal diameter is a more sensitive and more reliable finding than axial length in the diagnosis of congenital glaucoma. The use of A-scan ultrasonography, however, can be helpful in the long-term follow-up of patients being treated for congenital glaucoma.[81] Axial length changes can be used to evaluate the effectiveness of therapy.

Each cornea should be evaluated with a penlight, loupe, or hand-held slit lamp. Haziness, cloudiness, or ruptures in Descemet's membrane suggest congenital glaucoma.

IOP should be measured with a Schiotz, Mackay-Marg, or hand-held applanation tonometer. IOP measurements in infants generally vary greatly, possibly due to lid pressure, anesthesia, or corneal curvatures. Grote,[82] using an applanation tonometer, determined an average normal intraocular pressure of 10.68 mm ± 6.0 mm Hg. Dominguez and associates[83] used the Mackay-Marg tonometer on 500 newborns and found an average normal IOP of 12.4 mm ± 2.58 mm Hg. This suggests that an IOP exceeding 18 mm Hg should create concern.

Gonioscopy should be performed using a 14 mm Koeppe lens. Abnormalities that would inhibit aqueous outflow, such as Barkan's membrane, pigment, or anomalous iris position, suggest congenital glaucoma.

The optic discs should be evaluated. Richardson[84] evaluated about 1000 eyes in normal newborns and reported cupping greater than 0.3 in only 2.7% and significant asymmetry in only 2.3%. Shaffer[85] reported much greater cupping (68% with greater than 0.3) and disc asymmetry (88%) in glaucomatous infants.

Management

Since the response of infantile (before 6 years of age) and juvenile (between 6 and 30 years of age) glaucoma to medical therapy is often poor, surgical treatment is usually necessary. Medical therapy, however, may be indicated as supplemental treatment, especially in children who have other significant congenital abnormalities that increase the risk of general anesthesia and in children who have a shortened life expectancy.[86] In addition, medical therapy may be useful for patients with other congenital ocular abnormalities for whom

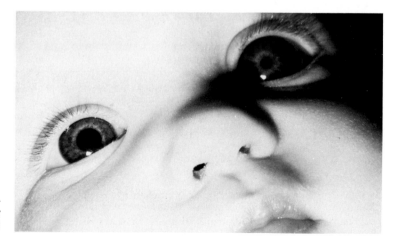

FIGURE 29.5 **An infant with congenital megalocornea. Note the enlarged lid aperture and relatively larger cornea in the left eye. (Courtesy Donald Bocken, O.D.)**

successful surgery is less likely and for patients whose IOP is reduced following surgery but who nevertheless have advanced optic disc cupping.

Goniotomy alone may control as many as 50% of uncomplicated cases of congenital glaucoma, and as many as 75% of these cases may be eventually controlled with combined surgical and medical therapy.[86] Combined surgical and medical therapy may allow about 50% of eyes with complicated congenital glaucoma to have acceptable IOP control.[86] However, once IOP has been normalized, it occasionally elevates even years later. Thus, it is essential to monitor these patients every 1 to 2 years.[87]

Despite aggressive management, congenital glaucoma still produces severe visual loss from a combination of corneal damage, optic nerve damage, and amblyopia. Delay in treatment results in rapid enlargement of the cornea with rupturing of Descemet's membrane, which produces corneal scarring and irregular astigmatism. The optic disc may undergo rapid cupping if elevated intraocular pressure is not controlled. Amblyopia can develop due to the resulting anisometropia.

The specific management of congenital glaucoma is determined from the etiology. The cause of glaucoma in patients with Marfan's syndrome is pupillary block secondary to malposition of the lens.[79] This complication is managed initially by pupillary dilation. Open-angle glaucoma can also develop that is usually of early onset and that is associated with congenital abnormalities of the anterior chamber angle. Management of such open-angle glaucoma is somewhat difficult because these eyes tend to be unresponsive to surgery. Thus, it is wise to attempt to control the IOP with medication.

In congenital rubella the glaucoma may be associated with a developmentally normal trabecular meshwork. Since these patients usually respond poorly to goniotomy, medical therapy is required during the acute phase.[79] Likewise, since surgery is hazardous and generally produces poor results in patients with aniridia, an attempt should be made initially to control the IOP pharmacologically.[79]

MEDICAL THERAPY

Some patients respond well to pharmacologic therapy initially, but long-term medical therapy is usually unsuccessful in adequately controlling IOP because of medication side effects and poor patient compliance. Short-term medical therapy may be used effectively before and between surgeries. Temporary treatment with miotics, adrenergic agonists, and carbonic anhydrase inhibitors is sometimes necessary and may be effective in some cases. Medications that have been used include topically administered pilocarpine, epi-

nephrine or dipivefrin, and β blockers, or orally administered acetazolamide (5 to 10 mg/kg body weight daily, not exceeding 250 mg every 6 hours), or both.[88] These medications usually produce no significant complications when used in recommended dosages. It should be noted, however, that topical β blockers have not yet been approved by the Food and Drug Administration (FDA) for use in children. This requires that patient (parental) informed consent be obtained (see Chapter 33) and that potential side effects be carefully explained before initiating β-blocker therapy.[89,90]

It is essential to discontinue echothiophate therapy at least 2 weeks before surgical procedures involving general anesthesia.[87] Because of drug-induced reduction of serum butyrocholinesterase levels, prolonged apnea may result if succinylcholine is administered to patients still influenced by the anticholinesterase medication.[87]

The dosage of oral acetazolamide used in infants and children should not be calculated by the child's age because there can be considerable variation in weight of children of the same age. Instead, dosages should be determined according to the child's weight. Clark's weight formula or Augsberger's rule by weight may be used. Clark's formula is widely employed for use in children 2 years of age or older:[87]

$$\text{pediatric dose} = \frac{\text{child's weight (kg or lb)} \times \text{adult dose}}{(70 \text{ kg or } 150 \text{ lb})}.$$

Augsberger's rule by weight is useful for children under 2 years of age and gives the percentage of the adult dose:[87]

$$\text{pediatric dose} = (\text{child's weight[kg]} \times 1.5) + 10.$$

SURGICAL AND LASER THERAPY

As previously mentioned, congenital glaucoma generally requires surgical intervention. Historically, goniotomy has been considered the safest and most effective treatment for control of infantile glaucoma.[87] This procedure is relatively simple and rapid and may be repeated several times without compromising integrity of the eye.[87] If this procedure fails, the intact external eye remains suitable for other procedures such as trabeculotomy or trabeculectomy. Although some surgeons still prefer goniotomy over trabeculotomy, trabeculotomy and trabeculectomy have become more popular in recent years, especially when corneal opacification precludes safe goniotomy or when goniotomy procedures have failed.[91–94]

In juvenile glaucoma the indications for surgery are similar to those for adult primary open-angle glaucoma. Patients with early onset glaucoma generally respond better to goniotomy, while those with late onset glaucoma usually respond better to trabeculotomy or trabeculectomy.[87,92]

Using the Nd:YAG laser to perform trabeculotomies, Melamed and associates[95] have reported successful lowering of IOP in a limited number of patients with juvenile open-angle glaucoma. This form of treatment might be considered before invasive goniotomy or filtering procedures.

TREATMENT OF AMBLYOPIA

Unless the treatment of infantile glaucoma is promptly and effectively instituted, anisometropia or strabismus can result, and amblyopia can develop. In the absence of significant organic lesions such as corneal irregularity, opacification of the media, or severe optic disc cupping, amblyopia therapy should be instituted in any child who demonstrates anisometropia and a fixation preference for one eye. The best sensory refractive correction as determined by retinoscopy should be prescribed, and amblyopia therapy should be employed in conjunction with medical or surgical management of the glaucoma. This will vastly improve the potential for useful vision following normalization of IOP.

Primary Angle-Closure Glaucoma

The etiology of angle-closure glaucoma is decreased aqueous outflow due to an anatomically restricted angle. The reduced aqueous outflow produces an unphysiologic excess of aqueous that increases the IOP. Tomlinson and Leighton[44] compared the ocular dimensions of patients with primary angle-closure glaucoma to those of matched normal control subjects and found that patients with primary angle-closure glaucoma have smaller corneal heights, smaller corneal diameters, and thicker crystalline lenses positioned more anteriorly than do normals. Thus, the anterior chamber depth is a useful diagnostic sign for identifying patients with primary angle-closure glaucoma and patients who are at risk for it.

Primary angle-closure glaucoma can be classified as acute, subacute, or chronic. There is a continuum from acute angle-closure glaucoma to chronic angle-closure glaucoma in symptoms and, to a lesser extent, in signs. Sudden, dramatic, severe, and persistent symptoms characterize acute angle closure, while mild and recurrent symptoms indicate subacute angle closure. Chronic angle-closure glaucoma has few or no symptoms.

Acute Angle-Closure Glaucoma

DIAGNOSIS

This condition is a true ocular emergency. There is a sudden (30 to 60 minutes) significant increase in IOP with dilation of vessels at the limbus, steamy cornea, an oval mid-dilated pupil that is unreactive to light, blurred vision, colored rings around point sources of light, significant ocular pain and discomfort, nausea, and often vomiting. The "attack" follows sudden obstruction of the trabecular meshwork. If the patient is not treated, loss of vision can occur within 24 hours, and blindness may follow in 2 or 3 days.[96]

The clinical examination consists of history, biomicroscopy, and when possible, gonioscopy and tonometry. If corneal edema is significant, the use of topical glycerin (75% to 100%) following topical anesthesia will often reduce the edema so that gonioscopy can be performed. In some cases use of glycerin as the gonioscopic bonding solution hastens the reduction of corneal edema by prolonging the drug contact with the cornea.

Because of the discomfort and accompanying signs, the diagnosis of acute angle-closure glaucoma is usually straightforward. The patient is more often an older person with a small globe and a significantly narrow anterior chamber angle. There is often a history of mild "attacks." The "attacks" are often associated with significant patient fatigue or follow a period of sudden emotional stress.

MANAGEMENT

Because the mechanism of acute angle closure relates to pupillary block and subsequent iris bombé, the initial treatment involves use of mild miotics to pull the iris away from the angle and reduce the intraocular pressure, followed by the use of laser iridotomy to eliminate the obstruction to aqueous flow from the posterior to the anterior chambers.[97]

As previously indicated, acute angle-closure glaucoma should be regarded as a true ocular emergency, and the immediate reduction of IOP is crucial to minimize vision loss. If laser intervention is not immediately available, the initial treatment is directed toward reducing the IOP medically.[98] This is usually achieved with the use of topically administered pilocarpine or β blocker, orally administered glycerin, or parenteral or oral acetazolamide (Fig. 29.6). Although any of these medications, when used alone, may be sufficient to relieve the angle closure attack, their combined use increases the chance of terminating the attack and shortening its duration.[403] Since the acute episode rarely resolves without medical treatment and may cause significant ocular damage, it is imperative to relieve the

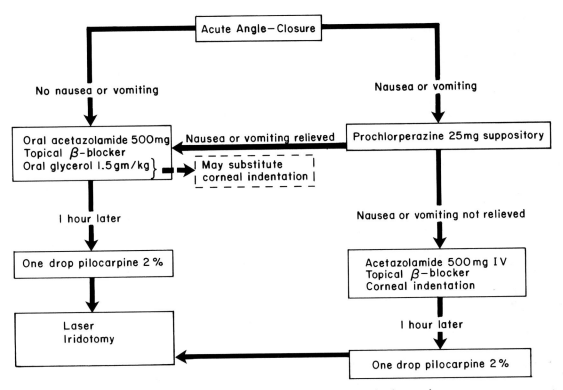

FIGURE 29.6   **Flowchart for the management of acute angle-closure glaucoma.**

attack promptly. Following medical reduction of IOP, a laser iridectomy or iridotomy is indicated.

The traditional recommendation for the use of pilocarpine involves the instillation of 1 or 2 drops of the 4% solution every minute for 5 minutes, every 5 minutes for 30 minutes, and then every 15 minutes for 90 minutes.[99] This dosage regimen, however, most probably represents an overdosage, and lower dosages are now recommended.[100] Less intense dosages should be used, such as 1 drop of the 2% solution every 10 minutes for a total of 3 or 4 doses,[101] or 1 drop of the 1% solution every 15 minutes for 1 hour.[102] It has been shown that the instillation of a single drop of 2% pilocarpine 3 or 4 hours after administration of intravenous acetazolamide 500 mg is sufficient to terminate an acute angle-closure attack.[103,104]

Pilocarpine concentrations exceeding 2% are contraindicated because these concentrations are no more effective than the 2% concentration and because such strong miotics cause further shallowing of the anterior chamber and can lead to intensified pupillary block, permanent peripheral synechiae, and permanent angle closure.[98,105,403] For these reasons anticholinesterase agents such as echothiophate are also contraindicated.

In the early stages of the attack, pilocarpine will often be completely ineffective in producing miosis because of ischemia of the iris sphincter caused by IOP exceeding 50 to 55 mm Hg.[105] Once the IOP has been reduced by drugs that decrease aqueous formation or withdraw intraocular water (acetazolamide, a β blocker, or glycerin), normal blood flow is reinstated to the iris sphincter, which then responds to the pilocarpine.[105] Thus, the instillation of pilocarpine should often be delayed for several hours until the IOP has been reduced to levels that permit normal activity of the iris sphincter.[103] When this regimen is followed, multiple doses of pilocarpine become unnecessary.[98] This eliminates the systemic side effects associated with the more traditional dosage recommendations, which administer approximately 40 to 80 mg of pilocarpine.[106] The symptoms of nausea, diaphoresis, and weakness frequently experienced by patients undergoing acute angle closure are often attributed to the glaucoma attacks themselves; however, these symptoms may also be associated with systemic pilocarpine toxicity.

In addition to the topical instillation of pilocarpine and a β blocker, the systemic administration of various drugs will hasten reduction of intraocular pressure. If the patient is not nauseated or vomiting, acetazolamide 500 mg and glycerin 1.5 g/kg body weight should be administered orally.[107] Glycerin is best tolerated if administered chilled, and the entire dose should be consumed within 5 minutes.[107] If the patient is vomiting, oral drug administration is impossible, and the patient should be given the acetazolamide intravenously. Alternatively, the topical administration of timolol may be substituted for acetazolamide. It has been shown that the use of topical 0.5% timolol, 2 drops within 1 hour, is effective in reducing the IOP to a level that permits pilocarpine to activate the iris sphincter and terminate the angle-closure attack.[104] Thus, the use of topical timolol may serve as a valuable alternative when systemic medication is contraindicated. Analgesic agents may be administered in cases of severe pain, and antiemetic agents, such as 25 mg prochlorperazine (Compazine) as a suppository, usually relieve nausea or vomiting.

As an alternative to the use of oral glycerin, a corneal indentation maneuver has been described by Anderson.[108] This procedure involves the use of a cotton-tipped applicator or Goldmann applanation prism to indent the cornea, thereby deepening the anterior chamber and allowing aqueous to escape from the anterior chamber. This maneuver serves the same purpose as do hyperosmotic agents—the removal of intraocular fluid leading to reduced IOP and relief of iris sphincter ischemia. Thus, the procedure may be used in lieu of hyperosmotic agents. Following gonioscopy for the initial diagnostic evaluation, the cornea is indented for about 30 seconds followed by release of indentation for another 30 seconds, and this process is continued for 15 to 20 minutes. The intermittent release of indentation reduces the risk of central retinal artery occlusion. The patient need not be positioned at the slit lamp, since the procedure can be performed with a hand-held device while the patient relaxes in the examination chair. This corneal indentation procedure appears to be safer, more rapid, more convenient, and less expensive than the use of glycerin. Although significant corneal damage does not occur, a soft contact lens can be placed over the cornea to minimize or prevent epithelial abrasions. It should be emphasized that this technique does not replace the need for pilocarpine, acetazolamide, or β blockers because these agents help to prevent the immediate recurrence of angle closure during the interval before surgery. In addition, since this procedure is ineffective in eyes with total peripheral anterior synechiae and rubeosis, hyperosmotic agents will be necessary in such eyes.[108]

The patient should be reevaluated periodically during the initial 2 or 3 hours of medical therapy. The desired response is a reduction of IOP, pupillary constriction, and deepening of the anterior chamber. After 2 or 3 hours of therapy usually 1 of 3 responses is observed:[97,107] (1) The eye may become stable following termination of the attack, as evidenced by opening of the anterior chamber and reduction of IOP to normal levels. If the IOP has been reduced to normal levels and gonioscopy reveals entirely open angles, the condition is temporarily relieved, but it may recur even with the use of miotic therapy. Thus, the patient should proceed to laser surgery within 1 or 2 days, since it is impossible to predict which patients will have recurrence of the acute angle-closure episode. (2) The intraocular pressure may decrease to normal or subnormal levels, but gonioscopy may reveal much or all of the angle to have remained closed. In such cases the low pressure is the result of a reduction of aqueous formation caused by the acetazolamide or β blocker or the hyperosmotic effect of the glycerin rather than a result of improvement in aqueous outflow. Such patients should proceed to laser surgery within 2 to 4 hours. (3) The eye may be totally unresponsive to medical therapy, as evidenced by persistence of a considerably elevated intraocular pressure, a mid-dilated pupil, and a closed angle. Laser surgery should be performed on such eyes within 2 to 4 hours.

Despite the success of pharmacologic therapy in lowering IOP and deepening the anterior chamber, surgical intervention is indicated to reduce the risk of a subsequent attack. Although surgical peripheral iridectomy has been the standard approach, laser iridotomy is now the treatment of choice.[109–113,402] Laser therapy has several advantages over surgical iridectomy, including simplicity, reduced cost, fewer complications, and the fact that it can be performed on an outpatient basis.[114,115] Although treatment with either argon or Nd:YAG laser can cause complications (Table 29.6), Nd:YAG laser iridotomy appears to be the preferred procedure in most patients because of its effectiveness and reduced complication rate.[109,111,116,402] When compared with traditional surgical procedures, laser therapy achieves comparable control of IOP and visual acuity[117] and is highly successful as well in pseudophakic pupillary-block angle closure.[118,119]

TABLE 29.6
Complications of Laser Iridotomy

- Iridotomy closure
- Corneal opacities/burns
- Microhyphema
- Reduced visual acuity
- Lenticular opacities
- Corectopia
- Hypopyon
- Transient elevation of IOP
- Posterior synechiae
- Iritis
- Retinal burns

IOP, intraocular pressure.

The laser iridotomy establishes a communication between the posterior and anterior chambers (Fig. 29.7), thus permitting aqueous to enter the anterior chamber. If the iridotomy remains patent, the laser procedure will generally protect the eye from future angle-closure attacks. For neglected cases of angle closure, in which the eye has been untreated for periods exceeding 48 hours and the IOP cannot be reduced with miotics or β blockers, iridotomy may succeed in completely normalizing the IOP.[120]

Pilocarpine 2% can be instilled 20 or 30 minutes before laser therapy if a miotic has not previously been administered. This produces a stretched and thinned iris, allowing easier iridotomy. It also avoids motion of the pupil during the procedure.[113,116] Postoperatively, IOP increases in 25% to 40% of eyes undergoing laser iridotomy and has a peak incidence between 1 and 3 hours after the procedure.[113] Although these pressure spikes are transient, resolving within several days, it is important to protect against large pressure increases, particularly in patients with severe glaucomatous damage. To this end, many practitioners use topical β blockers, oral carbonic anhydrase inhibitors, and topical steroids postoperatively as necessary.[113,114,116,121] The topical steroid can be tapered from a dosage frequency of every 6 hours on the day of laser therapy to discontinuation after 4 or 5 days. Alternatively, topical apraclonidine 1% (Iopidine, Alcon) can be administered 1 hour before laser surgery and immediately on completion of the procedure.[122–124] This new α2-adrenergic agonist became commercially available for ophthalmic use in 1988, and it lowers IOP probably by inhibiting aqueous formation.[401] As a consequence of its α-receptor stimulation, apraclonidine frequently causes conjunctival blanching and upper eyelid retraction lasting from 4 to 24 hours.[122,123a,400,401]

Angle-closure glaucoma eventually becomes bilateral in up to 70% of patients.[124] Thus, it is imperative that patients sustaining an acute angle-closure episode in one eye undergo prophylactic laser iridotomy in the fellow eye. The fact that optic nerve damage occurs within hours of the initial elevation in IOP emphasizes the need for such routine prophylactic iridotomy in fellow eyes.[125,126] This can be performed at the same time that the initial eye receives treatment.[126]

Subacute and Chronic Angle-Closure Glaucoma

DIAGNOSIS

Although these conditions are not true ocular emergencies, they do require prompt diagnosis and appropriate management to avoid a possible acute attack and gradual visual and ocular impairment. Although the symptoms are not as severe and are transient, they are similar to those in acute angle-closure glaucoma (Table 29.7). These symptoms are intermittent and have been reported to be present more often when the patient is hungry, tired, angry, worried, in a poorly ventilated room, or during periods of inactivity or following emotional stress.

The clinical examination consists of history, biomicroscopy, optic disc evaluation, tonometry, and visual fields.

Biomicroscopy should include an evaluation of the cornea, the anterior chamber angle, and the iris. The findings are similar to those in acute angle-closure

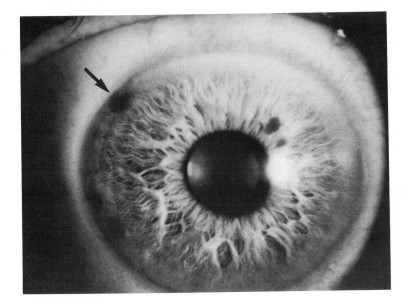

FIGURE 29.7   Nd: YAG laser iridotomy (arrow). (From Catania LJ, Lewis TL, eds. Primary care of glaucoma. Dresher, PA: Primary Eyecare, 1986.)

TABLE 29.7
**Symptoms of Subacute and Chronic
Angle-Closure Glaucoma**

- Red eye
- Blurred vision
- Colored rings around lights
- Tearing
- Ocular discomfort
- Headache located above the eyes

glaucoma but are not as severe. The angle in subacute angle closure is not closed for the entire 360°, but there should be evidence of some closure; otherwise open-angle glaucoma should be suspected.

There is a low incidence of narrow anterior chamber angles in the general population. Van Herick and associates[127] studied 2200 eyes and found that only 1% of angles were less than 20° and 0.6% were less than 10°. Therefore, when narrow angles are detected, careful evaluation is indicated (see Chapter 16).

The slit lamp should be used to estimate the depth of the anterior chamber angle, to evaluate the pupil margin, iris, lens, and anterior chamber for pigment and exfoliation debris, and to identify the presence of iris stromal atrophy, glaukomflecken, posterior synechiae, and neovascularization. If previous "glaucoma attacks" have occurred, patchy iris stromal atrophy, posterior synechiae, and glaukomflecken may be present.[128] Glaukomflecken appear as small gray-white areas just beneath the anterior capsule of the lens in the pupillary zone (Fig. 29.8). They are reported to be areas of necrotic lens epithelial tissue caused by the increased pressure. The presence of pigment on the corneal endothelium (Krukenberg spindle) or exfoliation debris on the anterior lens capsule suggests possible pigmentary dispersion or exfoliation syndrome, respectively. The presence of posterior synechiae or neovascularization suggests previous trauma, inflammation, ocular or systemic disease, and the possibility of secondary glaucoma.

The best way to evaluate the anterior chamber angle is with gonioscopy. Gonioscopy should be used to evaluate the anterior chamber for pigment, exfoliation debris, neovascularization, and posterior synechiae, but it is also used to evaluate depth of the anterior chamber angle. In assessing the angle, there are 3 things to consider.

- Shape or contour and position of the insertion of the iris. The iris normally inserts on the ciliary body. The closer the insertion is to the scleral spur, the greater the probability of a narrow angle. A flat iris is more often associated with an open angle. If the

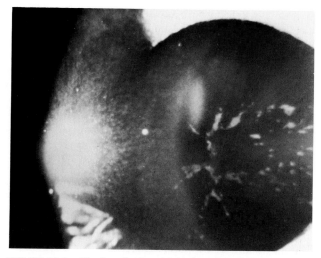

FIGURE 29.8   **Glaukomflecken. Note the white spots on the anterior surface of the crystalline lens. (Courtesy Anthony P. Cullen, O.D., Ph.D.)**

iris insertion is not visible, due to curvature of the iris, the probability of angle closure is increased.
- Amount of pigment or debris on the trabecular meshwork. The greater the amount of pigment or debris, the greater the possibility for decreased aqueous outflow. The amount of pigment present can be graded (Fig. 29.9). Pigment is usually greater in the inferior angle due to gravity. In angle-closure glaucoma, however, the anterior chamber angle is generally more narrow superiorly, and if there has been prolonged contact between the peripheral iris and the trabecular meshwork, more pigment may be found in the superior angle.[129] Pigment in the superior angle only may indicate angle-closure glaucoma.
- Assessment of the magnitude of the angle. The angle assessment is made by noting the amount of visible ciliary body and trabecular meshwork. The interpretation and classification of the angle according to Becker and Shaffer[130] is indicated in Table 16.5. A wide pigment-free anterior chamber angle is illustrated in Figure 29.10.

Although the anterior chamber angle has been assessed as being narrow or even dangerously narrow, further information is often needed. The clinical question is how to differentiate angles where closure is imminent from those where closure is not likely. Spaeth[131] has shown that asymptomatic narrow to closed angles are common in the elderly. This differentiation is thus often necessary but sometimes extremely difficult.

One procedure that can be used to indicate if very narrow or apparently closed angles are optically closed

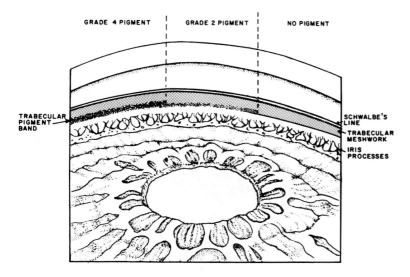

FIGURE 29.9 **Anterior chamber angle showing various pigment classifications.**

or closed due to peripheral anterior synechiae (PAS) is the Forbes test of indentation or pressure gonioscopy.[132] It is done during routine gonioscopy. If a very narrow or apparently closed angle is detected, the gonioscope can be gently pushed against the cornea. When this is done, the aqueous humor is displaced toward the iris, and causes the iris to move posteriorly (Fig. 29.11*B*). If the root of the iris fails to move away from the trabecular meshwork, PAS are probably present, and a diagnosis of angle-closure glaucoma is indicated (Fig. 29.11*C*). Even if the synechial closure is partial, therapy is still indicated.

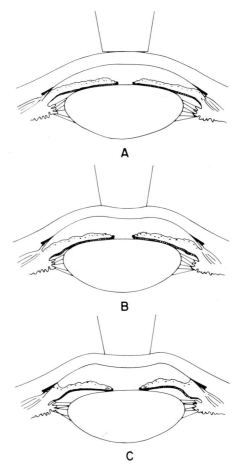

FIGURE 29.11 **The Forbes test. To differentiate angle closure from a very narrow angle *(A)*, the gonioscope is gently pressed against the cornea *(B)*. If a very narrow but open angle is present, the iris will move away, exposing the angle *(B)*, but if synechial angle closure is present, the central portion of the iris will move posteriorly, but the iris root will not move and expose the angle *(C)*.**

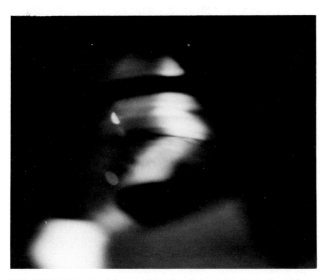

FIGURE 29.10 **A wide anterior chamber angle. Note the ciliary body and Schwalbe's line. Pigment classification is zero (0).**

PROVOCATIVE TESTS

The determination of which patients will develop angle-closure glaucoma is sometimes difficult. To assist in the clinical decision making, provocative tests have been developed. These procedures attempt to precipitate a mild acute attack of angle-closure glaucoma.

One way to precipitate an acute angle-closure attack is to dilate the pupil pharmacologically. Unfortunately, the results of such testing have not been of significant help. Since dilating the pupil artificially with drugs does not represent the normal physiologic situation, it does not determine which angles will close spontaneously.

Although it is highly desirable to have accurate provocative tests to identify those asymptomatic eyes with shallow anterior chambers and narrow angles that are at risk for angle-closure glaucoma, at present such testing is unsatisfactory. Currently, these provocative tests provide a relatively high percentage of false-negative results, and positive results indicating surgical intervention have not been shown to be totally valid.[133] It is generally considered that a carefully taken clinical history and examination of the eye, including gonioscopy, provide more accurate information regarding the need for surgical intervention than do provocative tests.[133]

One test, however, that appears to be helpful is the prone position test. Harris and Galin[134] have modified this test slightly by performing it in a dark room. After the IOP is measured, the patient is placed face down without pressure on the eyes in a dark room for 1 hour. Following this, the IOP is measured again. Patients who have an 8 mm Hg or more increase in IOP should be classified as significant angle-closure glaucoma suspects.

MANAGEMENT

Surgical intervention should be considered for all eyes with subacute angle-closure glaucoma. Although medical therapy may be initially successful in controlling the IOP, it is usually not satisfactory on a long-term basis because of the development of PAS. In the early stages before the development of PAS, a simple laser iridotomy usually prevents further angle-closure.[107] In the later stages of the disorder following the development of some PAS, the portion of the angle unaffected with peripheral synechiae will open with the iridotomy. In neglected cases, however, there is progression of the PAS caused by repeated attacks of angle closure, and the IOP gradually rises. If a carbonic anhydrase inhibitor or β blocker is administered at this stage, the IOP may be reduced to acceptable levels temporarily, but only at the expense of the formation of additional PAS and further elevation of IOP. Despite maximum medical therapy, the gradual synechial closure and as-

sociated elevated pressure require a filtering operation rather than a simple iridotomy.[107] Thus, it is mandatory that the laser iridotomy be performed early in the course of the subacute angle closure. As is the case in acute angle closure, eyes with subacute angle closure have fellow eyes that are similarly predisposed to closure. Prophylactic iridotomy should be performed in the fellow eyes if gonioscopy reveals a narrow angle predisposed to closure.

Some patients may have primary open-angle glaucoma in conjunction with subacute or chronic angle closure, the so-called combined mechanism glaucoma. If gonioscopy reveals a significant degree of angle closure while medical therapy is being employed for the primary open-angle component, laser iridotomy should be considered to eliminate the angle closure component.[107] Subsequent medical treatment of the residual open-angle glaucoma is often more successful following the surgical intervention.

Because of the lack of symptoms, chronic angle closure glaucoma can run a course of months or years with progressive closure of the angle and the development of PAS. As the closure progresses, the IOP slowly rises to a degree proportionate to the extent of angle closure.[107] The management generally follows the same principles as outlined for subacute angle closure. Surgical intervention is essential in all patients. Filtering operations are usually necessary because of the extent of angle compromise by the peripheral synechiae.

Primary Open-Angle Glaucoma

Etiology

The specific etiology of primary open-angle glaucoma is not well understood. Various studies[135,136] have indicated that the anterior chamber depth in both primary angle-closure and open-angle glaucoma is reduced from that in the normal, that the crystalline lens thickness is increased in both primary angle-closure and open-angle glaucoma compared with the normal, and that the flow of aqueous out of the eye is reduced in open-angle as well as in angle-closure glaucoma. Although the differences in angle size and the chamber depth from the normal in primary open-angle glaucoma are only about half as great as those in primary angle-closure glaucoma, the differences are significant and may be a factor in the etiology of primary open-angle glaucoma.

Another study[137] reported that there are more iris processes at all levels of insertion and more trabecular pigment, and that the insertion of the iris root is positioned more anteriorly in patients with primary open-angle glaucoma than in normal controls.

Collagen is modified in old age so that the trabeculae become limp and stick together, resulting in an increased resistance to aqueous outflow.[138] Weinstein and associates[139] have shown that there are enzyme defects in the trabecular meshwork of patients with primary open-angle glaucoma. In addition, it has been shown that the trabecular meshwork of eyes with primary open-angle glaucoma contains plasma cells and gamma globulin[140] and that positive antinuclear antibody reactions occur almost 6 times more often in patients with primary open-angle glaucoma than in the normal.[141] This suggests the presence of a connective tissue disorder or an altered immune function.

Other studies[142] have shown that there is an increase in the extracellular material containing acid mucopolysaccharide and glycoprotein in the endothelial lining of Schlemm's canal in primary open-angle glaucoma producing a partial blockage of Schlemm's canal. Rodrigues and associates[143] found that fibronectin, an extracellular glycoprotein, as well as collagen and laminin are present in the subendothelial regions of the trabecular meshwork in greater amounts in glaucomatous eyes compared with age-matched normal eyes. In addition, a quantitative and qualitative depletion of the endothelial vacuoles in the trabecular wall of Schlemm's canal has been found in enucleated eyes that have had primary open-angle glaucoma as well as those that have had angle-closure glaucoma.[144] One report[145] has shown that as the IOP increases, the number of endothelial vacuoles decreases.

These studies show that distinct cellular and morphologic changes occur in the anterior chamber in open-angle as well as in angle-closure glaucoma and suggest that the cause of increased IOP in primary open-angle glaucoma as well as in primary angle-closure glaucoma is an increased resistance to aqueous outflow. This information would also suggest that a more appropriate clinical classification of primary glaucoma should be based on the angular subtense of the anterior chamber angle, which can be clinically assessed, rather than on the supposed status of the aqueous outflow. Wide-angle glaucoma and narrow-angle glaucoma would therefore be more appropriate terms than open-angle and angle-closure glaucoma.

Open-angle glaucoma could theoretically occur due to an overproduction of aqueous humor—hypersecretion glaucoma. An increase in IOP would occur, however, only if the normal outflow capacity of the eye could not manage the increased production. Kolker and Hetherington[146] have concluded that true hypersecretion glaucoma is exceedingly rare.

This information strongly suggests that the cause of open-angle as well as of angle-closure glaucoma is reduced efficiency of aqueous outflow. Even though the general etiology is the same, the specific etiologies are different, and effective diagnosis and management require that the practitioner take these differences into account.

Diagnosis

The diagnosis of primary open-angle glaucoma is accomplished through an evaluation of patient characteristics (risk factors), symptoms, anterior segment, intraocular pressures, optic discs, and visual fields.

PATIENT CHARACTERISTICS

Epidemiologic studies suggest that the practitioner look more carefully for primary open-angle glaucoma in patients who are older, black, myopic, under stress, have relatives with glaucoma, or have diabetes, thyroid disease, or other chronic systemic disease.[147]

SYMPTOMS

Patients with primary open-angle glaucoma have essentially no symptoms associated with the glaucoma.

ANTERIOR SEGMENT

The anterior segment in primary open-angle glaucoma differs from that in the normal by having narrower anterior chambers, more iris processes, more trabecular pigment, and a more anterior insertion of the iris root. The presence of one more of these signs should indicate further evaluation for the presence of open-angle glaucoma.

Gonioscopic evaluation is necessary to differentiate open-angle from angle-closure glaucoma. It is also helpful in differentiating the type of open-angle glaucoma (e.g., pigmentary, exfoliation) from congenital angle abnormalities. Gonioscopic evaluation is therefore essential in the differential diagnosis of open-angle glaucoma.

The practitioner may find the presence of an afferent pupillary defect (positive Marcus Gunn pupil) in patients with asymmetric glaucoma.[148,149] In one study,[148] the afferent pupillary defect was detected before the onset of visual field loss. In patients who already had visual field losses, the depth of the pupillary defect quantified by neutral density filters correlated well with the visual field differences between the two eyes.[149] Thus, in any patient suspected of asymmetric glaucoma (asymmetric IOP or optic disc findings), the swinging flashlight test should be performed.

INTRAOCULAR PRESSURES

Although some patients develop glaucomatous visual field loss with IOPs of less than 20 mm Hg and others withstand IOPs exceeding 30 mm Hg without glaucomatous visual field loss,[150] 40% of new open-angle glaucoma patients have IOPs of less than 21 mm Hg,[151] indicating that the IOP level is not directly correlated with optic nerve damage. Tonometry, however, still provides valuable information for the diagnosis and management of glaucoma. Spaeth[152] has shown that in many cases there may be an improvement in visual field when the IOPs are lowered and an increasing loss of visual field when the IOPs are not lowered. To use the results of tonometry effectively, an accurate tonometric measurement must be obtained and the characteristics of IOP must be appreciated.

To obtain an accurate tonometric measurement, a reliable and accurate instrument is necessary (preferably Goldmann applanation), and an effective technique is vital, since a blink can increase the IOP by 10 mm Hg and a forced closure can increase the pressure by 75 to 100 mm Hg. The characteristics of IOP measurement are shown in Table 29.8.

Although tonometry does not provide a definitive diagnosis, it can provide significant diagnostic information, especially with high IOPs, change in IOP with time, and a difference in IOP between the two eyes.

Schappert-Kemmijser[154] correlated IOP and the incidence of glaucoma during a 5-year period and found that the higher the IOP, the greater the probability of developing glaucoma (Table 29.9). Pohjanpelto and Palva[155] related IOP to visual field loss and found that the frequency of visual field loss increased sharply at 34 mm Hg and that little visual field loss was present below 30 mm Hg. Patients with high IOP (exceeding 21 mm Hg) should be carefully evaluated for other signs of primary open-angle glaucoma.

Bengtsson[156] has shown that change in IOP with time in the nonglaucomatous population—from one examination to the next or with diurnal variations—is seldom greater than 5 mm Hg. He has also shown that if the IOP measurements are corrected for blood pressure, IOP does not change with age. Kitazawa and associates[157] measured the IOP every hour for 24 hours in normal patients, in those who were classified as ocular hypertensives, and in primary open-angle glaucoma patients. They found that the average diurnal variation in IOP was 6.4 mm in the normals, 8.4 mm in the ocular hypertensives, and 13.3 mm in the glaucoma patients. Thus, any patient who has a change in IOP during the day or over a period of time greater than 6 mm Hg should be more carefully evaluated for other signs of open-angle glaucoma.

The final factor to consider is a difference or asymmetry of pressure between the two eyes. Although primary open-angle glaucoma is a bilateral disease, the disorder generally appears in one eye before the other. In the normal population, the IOPs in the two eyes are generally symmetric.[158] A difference in IOP between the two eyes could therefore signal the presence of potential glaucomatous damage. Carel and associates[159] compared the IOPs in the two eyes of 13,000 nonglaucomatous patients over age 40 years. They found that the mean difference between the two eyes was 0.12 mm, that 78% had less than 3 mm difference, that 17% had a 3 mm to 4 mm difference, and that only 4.4% had a difference of 5 mm or more. They found a tendency for the difference in the IOP between the two eyes to increase with age and with an increase in the amount of the IOP. Thus, patients with IOP differences between the two eyes greater than 5 mm Hg should be carefully evaluated for other signs of primary open-angle glaucoma.

OPTIC DISCS

As previously indicated, optic disc changes do occur in subacute and chronic angle-closure glaucoma, but evaluation of the optic disc is of primary significance in open-angle glaucoma. The four aspects of optic disc evaluation are disc topography, disc hemorrhages, nerve fiber layer changes, and peripapillary changes.

TABLE 29.9
Intraocular Pressure and Incidence of Glaucoma

Intraocular Pressure	Percent Developing Glaucoma in 5 Years
Less than 25 mm Hg	3
25–30 mm Hg	26
Greater than 30 mm Hg	42

Adapted from Schappert-Kemmijser J. A five year follow-up of subjects with IOP of 22–30 mm Hg without anomalies of optic nerve and visual field typical for glaucoma at first investigation. Ophthalmologica 1971;162:289–295.

TABLE 29.8
Characteristics of Intraocular Pressure Measurement

- Average is approximately 16 mm ± 2.5 mm Hg
- Does not separate normal eyes from eyes with glaucoma
- Does not change with age if corrected for blood pressure
- No significant difference between the 2 eyes in nonglaucomatous patients
- Slightly higher average in females
- Slightly higher average in myopia[153]
- Diurnal variation of less than 5 mm Hg in the nonglaucomatous patient

Disc Topography. In evaluating disc topography, the factor of concern is the relationship between the optic disc and the optic cup. Six aspects must be evaluated: cup size, cup shape, cup position, cup depth, differences between the two eyes, and changes with time.

The size of the cup in relationship to the size of the disc, the C/D ratio, is the value used to specify cup size. It is the ratio of the horizontal and vertical dimensions of the cup to corresponding dimensions of the disc (Fig. 29.12). Both should be recorded. The vertical is sometimes more easily assessed because of less vessel interference, and it is more meaningful because glaucomatous tissue damage occurs more often near the vertical meridian.

Although there are great individual variations, cup size is hereditary, is slightly larger in myopes than hyperopes, is slightly larger in blacks than whites,[160] and changes very little with age. In the nonglaucomatous population, 32% have C/D ratios of 0.3 or greater, 7% have C/D ratios of 0.5 or greater, and only 1% have C/D ratios of 0.7 or greater.[161] Armaly[162] has also pointed out that the C/D ratio is 0.4 or greater in 61% of patients with glaucoma.

There is a general rough relationship between C/D ratio and IOP—the higher the IOP, the higher the C/D ratio. There is also a rough relationship between C/D ratio and visual field loss—the higher the C/D ratio, the greater the probability for visual field loss.

Two methods can be used to determine the size of the cup for calculating the C/D ratio. One method is to use the size of the cup determined by its color, and the other is to use the size of the cup determined by its 3-dimensional nature or contour.

The color of the disc is related more to glial tissue than to disc vascularity, and the change in color is

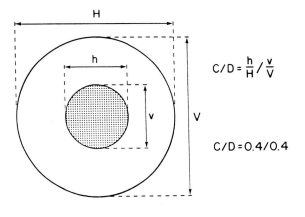

$$C/D = \frac{h}{H} / \frac{v}{V}$$

$$C/D = 0.4/0.4$$

CUP/DISC RATIO

FIGURE 29.12 **A diagrammatic representation illustrating the method to determine the cup-disc (C/D) ratio.**

reportedly due to degeneration of glial tissue and nerve fibers. This is not an absolute assessment, and errors in cup size can be made using color as the sole criterion.

Schwartz[163] has stressed the difference between C/D ratios determined by color and by contour and has pointed out that the contour C/D ratio changes before the color C/D ratio. Therefore, a difference in the C/D ratios using color and contour indicates possible glaucomatous damage (Fig. 29.13). Schwartz suggests that when using a direct ophthalmoscope, the C/D ratio by contour be determined by using the change in direction of the vessels as they leave the cup. This emphasizes the need for binocular stereoscopic evaluation of the disc with relatively high magnification in glaucoma suspects. This can be accomplished by using a

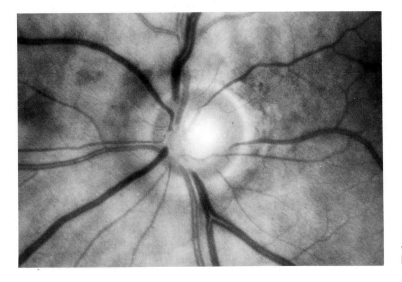

FIGURE 29.13 **An optic disc photograph illustrating the difference of the C/D ratio by color (0.6/0.6) and by contour (0.9/0.9).**

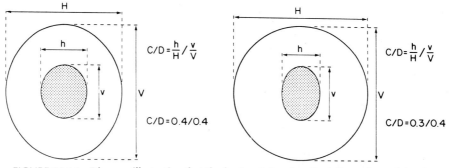

FIGURE 29.14 **Diagram illustrating that the horizontal and vertical dimensions of the disc as well as those of the cup must be considered to determine the proper C/D ratio.**

fundus contact lens, a Hruby lens, or by fundus biomicroscopy using a 90 D condensing lens. Any suspicious optic disc should be evaluated stereoscopically with relatively high magnification. The 90 D and fundus contact lenses also permit a better evaluation of the optic disc in patients with moderate to dense cataracts.

Cup shape is a useful indication of glaucomatous damage. When a cup is present, it is generally round. One of the early reliable disc signs of glaucoma is an oval C/D ratio (Fig. 29.14). Weisman and associates[164] have shown that whereas 30% of normals have a difference between the horizontal and vertical C/D ratios of 0.1, only 4% of normals have a difference of 0.2, while 60% of glaucomatous patients have differences of 0.1 or greater.

The optic cup is generally located in the center of the disc. Displacement of the cup is another indication of possible glaucomatous damage.[165] Gloster and Parry[166] showed that if the width of the neuroretinal rim is less than one-eighth of the disc diameter, a glaucomatous visual field loss is likely (Fig. 29.15).

Although considerable attention is given to the cup, the area, shape, and integrity of the neuroretinal rim are vital. A healthy, large, pink, evenly shaped neuroretinal rim suggests no visual field loss, whereas a small, unevenly colored, or unevenly shaped neuroretinal rim is often associated with a visual field loss. Airaksinen and associates[167,168] have shown that there is a reduction in area of the neuroretinal rim in early glaucoma and that this reduction is significantly correlated with visual field losses. There is a decrease in area of the neuroretinal rim before visual field loss develops in open-angle glaucoma.[169] Trobe and associates[170] have reported that *generalized* pallor of the neuroretinal rim appears to be associated more with nonglaucomatous optic atrophy, whereas *localized* pallor, focal obliteration, or "notching" of the neuroretinal rim is more indicative of glaucoma. "Notching" of the neuroretinal rim appears to be present more

frequently at the 12 or the 6 o'clock positions of the optic disc (Fig. 29.16). This is in the same areas where the early optic nerve fiber losses occur.[12]

Balaszi and associates[171] reported that the neuroretinal rim area of normal eyes, eyes with suspected glaucoma, and eyes with glaucomatous visual field loss differ significantly from each other. These investigators found that the neuroretinal rim area is more strongly correlated with visual field loss than is the C/D ratio. A method of recording the size, shape, and position of the optic cup in the optic disc is shown in Figure 29.17. Although photography is a better recording procedure, this method can be used to indicate changes in cup size, shape, and position and, more important, changes in area of the neuroretinal rim with time.

There are many variations in the depth and shape of the optic cupping due to the unique anatomy of each eye. If there is no cupping and glaucomatous damage begins, a cup will form centrally in a cone shape and increase in depth until it reaches the lamina

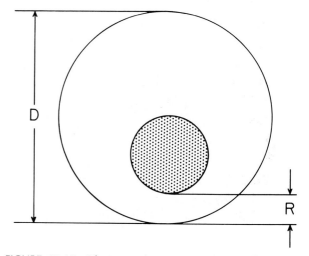

FIGURE 29.15 **Diagrammatic representation of the rim/disc (R/D) ratio.**

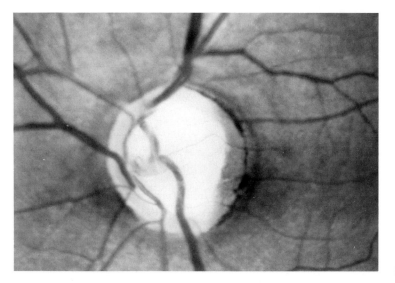

FIGURE 29.16 **Optic disc photograph illustrating an inferior "notching" of the neuroretinal rim.**

cribrosa, and then it will enlarge at the bottom. If a cup was already present, the cup will enlarge without significant deepening. Read and Spaeth[172] have called the appearance of the lamina the *laminar dot sign.* The depth and contour of the walls of the cup should be

recorded. A useful recording procedure is shown in Figure 29.18.

The evaluation of disc cupping can be a problem in patients with glaucoma and optic nerve head drusen.[173] The presence of drusen does not stop the cupping, but

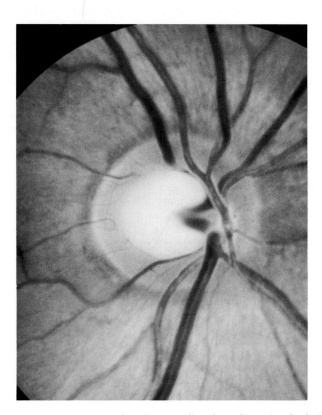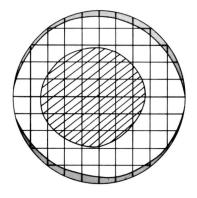

FIGURE 29.17 **Procedure for recording the 2-dimensional relationships of the optic cup to optic disc. Left, fundus photograph. Right, disc drawing.**

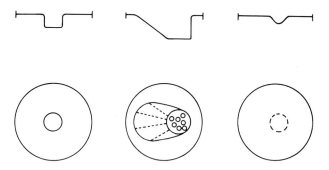

FIGURE 29.18 **Procedure for recording the 3-dimensional relationships of the optic cup to optic disc.**

it decreases it and makes it more difficult to evaluate. Drusen can also produce visual field loss, which can further create a problem of diagnosis, especially if the drusen is monocular.

Evaluation of the asymmetry of the C/D ratios between the two eyes is extremely helpful in detecting early glaucomatous damage. The C/D ratios are generally the same in each eye unless there is a high anisometropia or other abnormality.[174] Armaly[175] has shown that 99% of normals have an asymmetry of 0.2 or less and that 53% of the glaucomatous population can be detected by an asymmetry of the C/D ratios.

A change in the C/D ratio with time strongly suggests the presence of glaucoma.[176] This requires accurate recordkeeping. Ideally, the C/D ratio and disc architecture should be photographed stereoscopically on every glaucoma suspect so that any changes in the disc can be carefully monitored. Within a few years, computer analysis of stereophotographs of the disc will be more readily available and will provide valuable quantitative information for the monitoring of optic disc cupping.[177,178] Another procedure to evaluate disc architecture is photogrammetry.[19] Using stereophotographs, photogrammetry provides a 3-dimensional evaluation of the area of the surface opening, slopes of the cup walls, cup depth, and cup volume. This information can be used to thoroughly evaluate the cup and to monitor changes in the cup with time.[179]

A *reduction* in the C/D ratio with a reduction of IOP can and does occur, primarily in young people with early glaucoma, but it can also occur in the elderly.[179,180] Reversal of glaucomatous cupping has been reported in adults up to 62 years of age.[181] The reversal occurs more often in patients who are detected in the early stages of glaucoma and who have high IOP, moderate C/D ratios (not over 0.8), and little visual field loss. Reduction in the C/D ratio is probably due to a decrease in stretching of the sclera, a reduction in the posterior bowing of the lamina cribrosa, a proliferation of astroglial tissue, and a restoration of intracellular and extracellular fluid in the optic disc.

It is important to be able to correlate disc topography with visual field loss. If changes in the disc are associated with tissue changes and nerve damage, there should be a correlation between the type of disc change and the type of visual field loss. Several studies[166,182,184] have demonstrated that normal visual fields can be predicted with an accuracy of over 90%, and abnormal visual fields can be predicted with an accuracy of about 80%. Read and Spaeth[172] attempted to correlate the location of the visual field loss (Fig. 29.19). Although it is probably not completely reliable, it is a useful clinical tool.

Although visual field losses are generally associated with relatively large, deep, and decentered optic cups, a small, central, round cup does not exclude the presence of a glaucomatous visual field. Glaucomatous visual field loss can occur with normal-appearing discs.[185]

Studies have shown that patients with glaucoma have areas of absolute fluorescein filling defects in the optic disc as demonstrated by fluorescein angiography.[186,390,391] This further supports ischemia as one of the mechanisms of the pathogenesis of visual loss in glaucoma. One study[390] has shown that the absolute filling defects tend to be located in the outer third of the disc generally near the superior and inferior poles, and that their location corresponds with the location of the visual field defects. Another study[391] has shown that the number and size of the fluorescein filling defects in the optic disc increase with an increase in the visual field loss in glaucoma, showing a direct correlation between optic disc filling defects and visual field loss. This study also demonstrated that absolute fluorescein filling defects were present in the disc in some ocular hypertensive patients who had no visual field loss. This further suggests that damage to some optic nerve fibers occurs before visual field loss.

Disc Hemorrhages. Splinter hemorrhages near the disc margin are present in some patients with glaucoma. Shihab and associates[187] reported an incidence of 3% in open-angle glaucoma. Since they are small, vessel-like in appearance, and transient, they are difficult to detect. Disc hemorrhages are unilateral in about 80% of patients in whom they occur, and 88% of the hemorrhages are located on the temporal disc margin[187] (Fig. 29.20). They are present for about 3 to 5 weeks before they completely disappear. When they do absorb, they may do so without leaving a sign, or a pigmented spot or small whorl of vessels may be present. Disc hemorrhages have no associated visual symptoms and have no correlation with IOP.[188] These hemorrhages have been found more often in patients who have systemic hypertension, ischemic heart disease, and a positive glucose tolerance test.[189] They have also been associated with disc drusen, papilledema, and papillitis.[190]

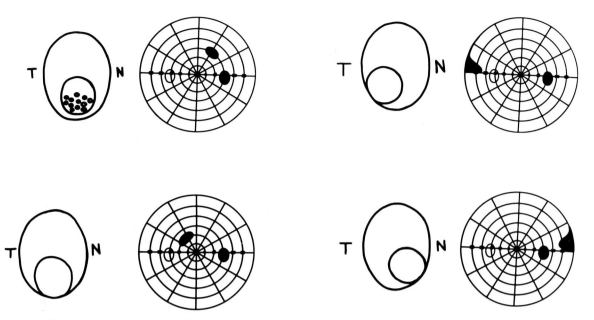

FIGURE 29.19 **Suggested correlation of the optic cup and disc relationship with visual field loss in glaucoma.**

A high correlation between disc hemorrhage location and the character of the visual field loss has been reported.[191] The cause of the disc hemorrhages is unknown, but they could be due to mechanical distortion of the lamina cribrosa, causing obliteration of the disc capillaries. Whatever the cause, the presence of disc hemorrhages suggests disc damage and a reduced prognosis.[187,191]

Nerve Fiber Layer Changes. Hoyt and associates[192] observed some subtle, thin, darkened slit-like gaps in the nerve fiber layer of patients with glaucoma and indicated that these nerve fiber layer changes may be the earliest objective evidence of glaucomatous tissue damage. The subtle slit-like changes appear as a lighter area among the arcuate bundles approaching the optic disc superiorly and inferiorly more often from the temporal retina (Fig. 29.21). They are usually found 1 to 3 disc diameters from the disc and are about 2 to 3 disc diameters long.[193] They give the nerve fiber layer a "raked" appearance. Slit-like or localized nerve fiber loss is more common in patients with ocular hypertension, and generalized reduction in nerve fibers or diffuse nerve fiber loss is more common in patients with glaucomatous visual field loss.[193–195] Other studies have reported a high correlation between nerve fiber layer changes and visual field loss,[392] and between nerve fiber layer changes and area of the neuroretinal rim,[393] further supporting nerve fiber layer changes as an important diagnostic sign in glaucoma. A correlation between nerve fiber layer changes and fluorescein angiographic defects has also been reported.[394] This suggests that photographs and fluorescein angiograms of the optic discs in glaucoma suspects may provide early objective evidence of glaucomatous damage. It has also been shown, however, that some patients with glaucomatous visual field loss do not have nerve fiber layer defects, and many patients with nerve fiber layer defects do not have glaucoma.[194,195]

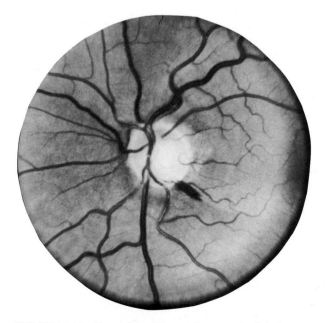

FIGURE 29.20 **Flame-shaped hemorrhage on the inferior temporal disc rim. (Courtesy John W. Potter, O.D.)**

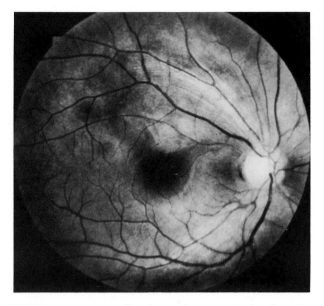

FIGURE 29.21 **Nerve fiber layer changes eminating from the optic disc and following the superior and inferior arcuate bundles.**

Nerve fiber layer changes can be seen with an ophthalmoscope, especially with red-free light, but they are best detected in black and white fundus photographs.[196] Computerized processing techniques have also been used to enhance visibility of the nerve fiber layer defects.[197] Nerve fiber layer defects are difficult to see in older patients due to the increase in opacification of the media and the decrease in number of optic nerve fibers with age.[38] They are more difficult to evaluate in black patients because the darker fundi increase visibility of the nerve fibers, which makes slight variations in the nerve fiber layer more apparent, resulting in detection of nerve fiber layer defects when none is actually present.[181] They are also more difficult to detect in patients with lightly pigmented fundi.[197] It is unfortunate that evaluation of the nerve fiber layer is more difficult in the elderly and blacks, because of the increased incidence of glaucoma in these populations. Although nerve fiber layer defects are not diagnostically definitive, their presence during a routine examination or in a glaucoma suspect should indicate the need for further evaluation for possible glaucomatous damage.

Peripapillary Changes. Changes in the tissue around the disc have been described in patients with glaucoma.[198] Some investigators have reported that a peripapillary halo (pale yellow ring adjacent to the disc with sharp borders and no pigment changes) might be a useful diagnostic sign for detection of glaucoma in the early stages. Later reports,[199] however, have not substantiated this but have indicated that peripapillary

atrophy (tissue change with irregular pigmentation) is often found in eyes with significant glaucoma of long duration. These changes should not be confused with peripapillary choroidal atrophy, a normal finding often observed in patients over 55 years of age.

VISUAL FIELDS

For many years, glaucoma was synonymous with visual field loss. In 1969, Armaly[200] suggested that a definitive diagnosis of glaucoma could not be made before the demonstration of a characteristic visual field loss. It is evident now that there is loss of optic nerve fibers and cupping of the optic disc before visual field loss can be detected. A histological study[20] of the optic nerve of patients with ocular hypertension found a diffuse loss of 40% of the optic nerve fibers in a patient who had a medium sized, vertically oval cup and a normal visual field. Increases in the C/D ratio often precede the detection of visual field defects.[201] However, the testing of visual fields is an essential part of the diagnostic evaluation of glaucoma and should be done on every patient suspected of having glaucoma. The results of visual field testing are also essential in determining the prognosis and effectiveness of medical and surgical therapy.

Although visual field testing is an essential part of the diagnostic evaluation for glaucoma, visual field testing is time-consuming, and the detection of glaucomatous visual field changes can be elusive. Sturmer[202] has shown that a relative scotoma, or early visual field loss, in glaucoma does not consist of a sharply bordered area with a definite loss of sensitivity, but instead is a region of increased scatter with poorly definable borders due to instability in the threshold. He suggested that these early sensitivity disturbances cannot be detected without extensive threshold perimetry. Not only is it difficult to detect early visual field sensitivity disturbances, but it has also been shown that it is difficult to detect progressive visual field losses in glaucoma using automated perimetry when only a few visual fields are available for evaluation.[207] Therefore, several visual fields should be taken on glaucoma suspects and on patients receiving glaucoma therapy using automated computerized perimetry that presents stimuli in a multi-flash (static) pattern.[203–206] The target size and intensity can be increased and decreased until the threshold has been determined in various areas of the visual field.

The earliest loss of optic nerve fibers in glaucoma usually occurs at the superior and inferior areas of the optic disc, indicating that the early visual field changes in glaucoma would be expected to be paracentral scotomas, nasal steps, and temporal wedges.[208] A recent study[395] has reported that quantitative testing of the central visual field is essential, quantitative testing of

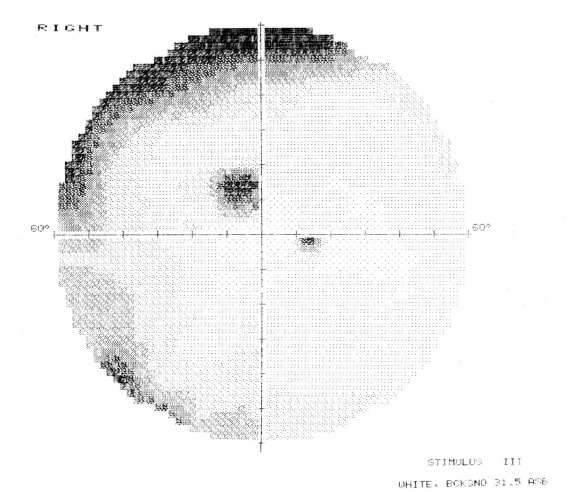

RIGHT

60°

60°

STIMULUS   III

WHITE, BCKGND 31.5 ASB

FIGURE 29.22 **Results of automated perimetry showing a nasal superior paracentral scotoma.**

the peripheral nasal field is valuable, and quantitative testing of the peripheral temporal field is less valuable for the detection of glaucoma.

Paracentral Scotomas.   Small paracentral scotomas located within the 20° meridian are the earliest visual field defects in glaucoma (Fig. 29.22). They are most often found in the superior nasal field.[209] These small scotomas are generally farther from the point of fixation on the temporal side and closer on the nasal side. Armaly[210] reported that they are the first and only visual field loss in about 70% of patients with glaucoma and are associated with a nasal step in another 18%. Therefore, paracentral scotomas are present in about 88% of all glaucomatous visual fields (Table 29.10). Bryars and associates[211] studied glaucomatous visual field losses for 5 years and concluded that 76% of all early visual field changes are paracentral scotomas between the 5° and the 20° meridian and appear about 4 times more often above than below the horizontal meridian.

Nasal Step.   A nasal step is a constriction of the visual field either above or below the horizontal meridian in the nasal field (Fig. 29.23). The nasal step may take on an acute-angle shape in the periphery, a right-angle shape in the mid-periphery, and an obtuse-angle shape near the point of fixation. It is present as the only visual field loss in 6% to 11% of glaucomatous patients (see Table 29.10).[210,212]

TABLE 29.10
Glaucomatous Visual Field Loss

Type of Visual Field Loss	Prevalence (%)
Paracentral scotoma	70
Nasal step	6–11
Paracentral scotoma and nasal step	18
Temporal step and concentric constriction	6

Adapted from Armaly MF. Selective perimetry for glaucomatous defects in ocular hypertension. Arch Ophthalmol 1972;87:518–524.

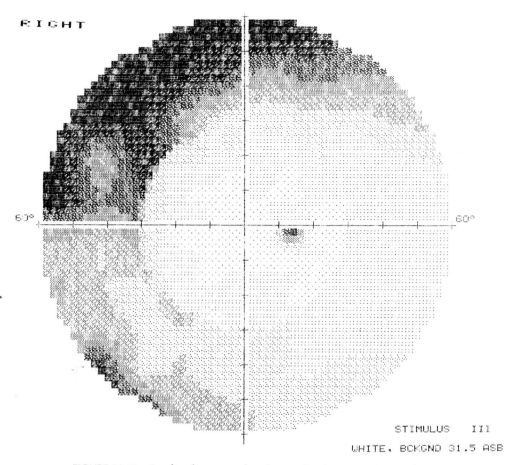

FIGURE 29.23   **Results of automated perimetry showing a superior nasal step.**

Temporal Wedge. A temporal wedge is a constriction of the visual field either above or below the horizontal meridian in the temporal field. It is a sector-shaped defect (Fig. 29.24) and can be the only manifestation of a glaucomatous visual field loss. Armaly[210] has reported that this occurs along with a generalized concentric constriction in about 6% of glaucomatous patients. In their study of glaucomatous visual field defects, Werner and Beraskow[213] found that isolated temporal visual field defects were present in 3% of eyes with open-angle glaucoma.

Bryars and associates[211] concluded that 91% of all early glaucomatous visual field defects will occur in a horizontal bow tie–shaped central area (Fig. 29.25). This is the area that must be thoroughly evaluated in patients with suspected glaucoma.[206,209,214,215]

To decrease the time involved and to increase the reliability of visual field evaluation, testing in certain areas of the visual field with certain target patterns has been developed.[204,206] This approach has been found to be both accurate and specific for glaucomatous visual field changes.[206]

Progression of visual field defects in glaucoma can occur even though treatment is provided.[216,217] Progression of the visual field loss can occur in two ways. In the first, there is gradual enlarging of the paracentral scotomas to form an arcuate scotoma along with a peripheral constriction[218] (Fig. 29.26). In the second, new paracentral scotomas and sector-shaped defects can occur separate from any previous defect, and then both gradually enlarge.

It is important to realize that visual field losses simulating glaucoma can be present with conditions such as cataract, pituitary tumor, drusen of the optic nerve head, sclerosis of the choroidal vessels, stenosis or sclerosis of the ciliary arteries, choroidal tumors, and ischemic optic neuropathy. If the optic disc topography does not correlate with the visual fields, the practitioner should search for other causes of the visual field loss.

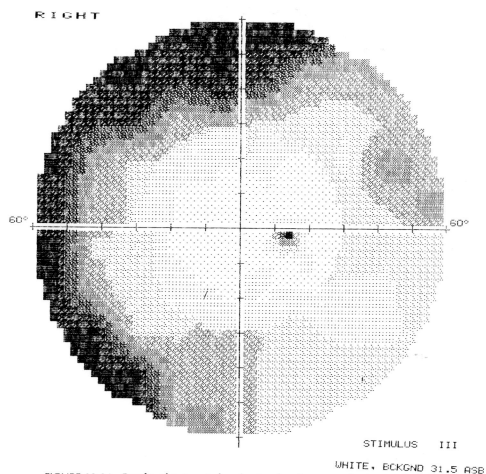

FIGURE 29.24 **Results of automated perimetry showing a superior temporal wedge.**

Visual field loss from glaucoma is generally permanent, but isolated paracentral scotomas occasionally disappear following therapy, and enlargement of a constricted visual field can occur with therapy. Visual field losses are more often reversible in young patients, patients with low C/D ratios and centered cups, and patients who have significant reductions in IOP with therapy.[219]

Visual fields are also a function of pupil size. There may be a considerable variation in size and shape of the visual field with changes in size of the pupil[220,221] (Fig. 29.27). Therefore, when considering the possibility of changes in the visual field, only those visual fields performed with approximately the same pupil size should be considered.

PROVOCATIVE TESTS

Many provocative tests have been developed to assist in the diagnosis of open-angle glaucoma. Unfortu-

nately, none of the tests contributes definitive information, so few of them are actually used.

PSYCHOPHYSICAL AND ELECTROPHYSIOLOGIC TESTING

Visual field defects in glaucoma are preceded by changes in the optic nerve fibers and retinal nerve fiber layer losses. To detect the earliest reliable clinical evidence of optic nerve damage, alternative methods of optic nerve evaluation are being investigated. These include the testing of color vision,[222,223] dark adaptation,[224] contrast sensitivity,[225,226] visually evoked potentials,[227] and the pattern electroretinogram.[228,229] Color contrast sensitivity[396] and the pattern electroretinogram[397] appear the most promising.

Management

The availability of a wide variety of ocular hypotensive agents often allows IOP to be adequately controlled,

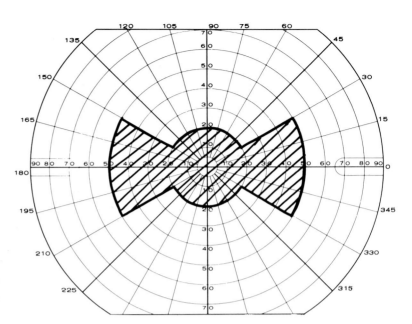

FIGURE 29.25 **Area of visual field where 91% of all early glaucomatous visual field changes occur, according to Bryars and associates.**[211]

thereby minimizing further optic disc damage and visual field loss.[231] The successful management of primary open-angle glaucoma requires careful attention to the patient's optic discs, visual fields, IOPs, and medication schedules. Failure of medical therapy to prevent further optic disc and visual field changes necessitates laser or surgical intervention.[232] The planning

of an appropriate treatment strategy helps ensure the success of medical therapy.

DETERMINING THE "TARGET PRESSURE"

The predominant objective in the treatment of primary open-angle glaucoma is to obtain a level of IOP that

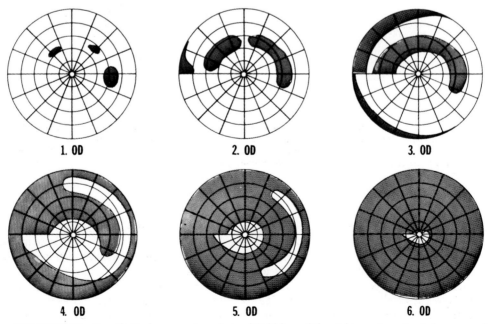

FIGURE 29.26 **Hypothetical progression of visual field loss of the right eye in untreated open-angle glaucoma.**

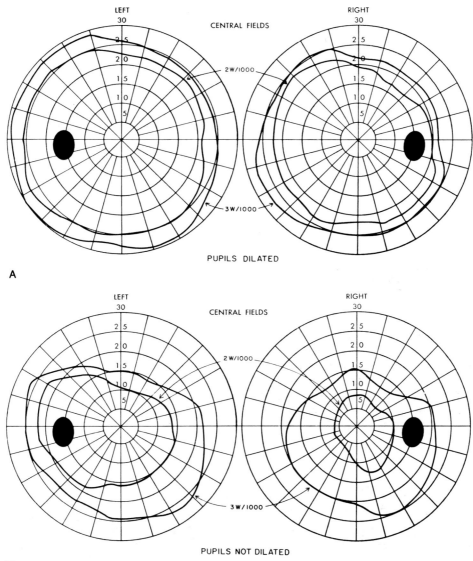

FIGURE 29.27   **Effect of pupil size on visual field. *(A)* Visual field plotted with dilated pupil. *(B)* The same visual field plotted with constricted pupil. This emphasizes the importance of recording pupil size when plotting visual fields and the need to keep pupil size approximately the same when evaluating visual field changes over time in a given patient.**

is compatible with preservation of optic nerve function and stability of the visual fields. In addition, the medical therapy must be compatible with the patient's lifestyle. Treatment that is inconvenient or that causes undesirable side effects encourages noncompliance, a significant factor in the failure of medical therapy. The most popular treatment strategies involve considering the initial status of the IOP, optic discs, and visual fields; and the use of uniocular therapeutic trials.

Initial Status of IOP, Optic Discs, and Visual Fields. The realization that eyes with ocular hypertension may withstand considerable elevation of IOP without damage to the optic disc and visual field has led to the development of a treatment strategy based on evaluation of the initial IOPs as well as initial status of the optic discs and visual fields. It is possible that a patient with an IOP of 28 mm Hg and no glaucomatous damage to the optic disc or visual field would require no treatment while, on the other hand, another patient with an IOP of 21 mm Hg and with significant glaucomatous damage would require aggressive medical therapy. Thus, this strategy entails an individualized approach to each patient based on evaluation of the initial IOP, optic discs, and visual fields.

By considering the initial pressure that produced the observed optic disc and visual field changes, the clinician is able to estimate the level of IOP reduction that should prevent further visual field loss. Examples of such an approach are illustrated in Table 29.11.

These examples are intended merely to illustrate the process. They should not be interpreted as necessarily defining specific management procedures for individual patients with IOPs, optic discs, and visual fields described. An extremely important principle that guides medical therapy is to reduce IOP to a greater extent in eyes with more advanced glaucomatous damage. That is, the greater the initial damage, the greater the IOP should be reduced to obtain adequate control and prevent further damage.[233]

The findings in each eye are particularly useful in

TABLE 29.11
Examples of Choosing Level of Intraocular Pressure that Controls the Glaucoma

	Patient A	Patient B
Initial IOP before treatment (mm Hg)	36	29
Initial discs		
Cupping (C/D ratio)	0.9	0.9
Pallor (% area of disc)	50	50
Initial visual field	Dense paracentral scotomas	Dense paracentral scotomas
"Target pressure"	Reduce IOP to mid 20s	Reduce IOP to low 20s

	Patient A	Patient B
Initial IOP before treatment (mm Hg)	36	29
Initial discs		
Cupping (C/D ratio)	0.95	0.95
Pallor (% area of disc)	70	70
Initial visual field	Dense arcuate scotoma	Dense arcuate scotoma
"Target pressure"	Reduce IOP to high teens	Reduce IOP to mid teens

	Patient A	Patient B	Patient C
Initial IOP before treatment (mm Hg)	29	24	24
Initial discs			
Cupping (C/D ratio)	0.9	0.9	0.9
Pallor (% area of disc)	50	50	70
Initial visual field	Dense arcuate scotoma	Dense arcuate scotoma	Loss of nasal quadrant
"Target pressure"	Reduce IOP to high teens	Reduce IOP to mid teens	Reduce IOP to low teens

	Patient A	Patient B
Initial IOP before treatment (mm Hg)	28	34
Initial discs		
Cupping (C/D ratio)	0.7	0.7
Pallor (% area of disc)	15	15
Initial visual field	No defect	No defect
"Target pressure"	None (Ocular hypertension)	Reduce IOP to high 20s

Adapted from Schwartz B. Primary open-angle glaucoma. In: Duane TD, Jaeger EA, eds. Clinical ophthalmology. Philadelphia: Harper & Row 1987; Chap. 52.

estimating the level of IOP at which control of the glaucoma should be obtained. Asymmetric findings, in particular, can be used to further define the decision to treat. This concept is illustrated in Table 29.12. Other factors may contribute to the decision regarding the level of IOP to be attained. Patients with central or branch vein occlusions may require lower IOP, as would those with low systemic blood pressure, cardiovascular disease, or diabetes.[234]

Since the changes in the optic discs and visual fields may have occurred at a pressure lower than that determined on the initial examination, the practitioner must not underestimate the pressure level at which no further damage is likely to occur. Once the decision is made about the desired IOP level that would be expected to control the glaucoma, the patient should be carefully monitored on treatment to determine the accuracy of this initial prediction. Serial examinations of IOPs, optic discs, and visual fields will verify the adequacy of the pressure reduction in controlling the glaucoma. Although these judgments are somewhat arbitrary in the beginning, the experienced clinician soon learns to predict such controlling IOP levels fairly accurately.

The Uniocular Therapeutic Trial. A uniocular therapeutic trial can be used to assess the therapeutic effectiveness of the medical regimen as well as to determine the patient's response to the intended drug therapy.

It has been shown that the IOP of patients with primary open-angle glaucoma can vary as much as 10 mm Hg or more within 1 hour.[235] Furthermore, the IOP of the 2 eyes varies synchronously, the difference in pressure between the 2 eyes remaining fairly constant for the full 24-hour period.[235] Thus, when evaluating the immediate effect of a drug on IOP, a comparison of the pressure before and after drug administration cannot be a reliable indicator of the drug effect, especially when the drug is administered to both eyes. With the exception of the use of timolol and other β blockers, which often have an effect in the untreated fellow eye,[236] the treatment of only 1 eye initially allows a more objective evaluation of the drug effect by using the fellow eye as a control.

A therapeutic trial of medication in only 1 eye allows evaluation of the effectiveness of the drug in reducing the pressure and allows assessment of the patient's response to the therapy.[237] The trial is performed by using the intended drug regimen in 1 eye only, preferably with simple and convenient dosage schedules and with low concentrations to prevent excessive side effects. The goal of the therapeutic trial is to obtain adequate reduction of IOP while minimizing undesirable side effects (Table 29.13).

An example of a uniocular therapeutic trial is a patient whose initial IOPs are OD 26 mm Hg and OS 35 mm Hg. If the topical medication administered initially only to the left eye resulted in tonometric readings of OD 23 mm Hg and OS 25 mm Hg without side effects, the trial would be considered successful and the medication could be increased if necessary as therapy is

TABLE 29.12
Example of Using Asymmetric Findings

	Normal Eye	Abnormal Eye	Maximal IOP Chosen for Control
Initial IOP before treatment (mm Hg)	27	33	
Initial discs			27
Cupping (C/D ratio)	0.4	0.6	
Pallor (% area of disc)	20	40	
Initial visual field	No defect	Paracentral scotoma	

	Normal Eye	Abnormal Eye	Maximal IOP Chosen for Control
Initial IOP before treatment (mm Hg)	27	33	
Initial discs			High teens
Cupping (C/D ratio)	0.6	0.6	
Pallor (% area of disc)	40	40	
Initial visual field	No defect	Paracentral scotoma	

Adapted from Schwartz B. Primary open-angle glaucoma. In: Duane TD, Jaeger EA, eds. Clinical ophthalmology. Philadelphia: Harper & Row 1987; Chap. 52.

TABLE 29.13
Uniocular Therapeutic Trial

Results	*Treatment Decision*
Adequate reduction of IOP without side effects	Continue medication or increase if necessary
Slight reduction of IOP without side effects	Increase medication
Adequate reduction of IOP, but with side effects	Decrease or change medication
Slight reduction of IOP with side effects	Change medication

instituted in both eyes. If, however, the resulting tonometric readings were OD 21 mm Hg and OS 28 mm Hg, it is clear that the medication is ineffective in adequately reducing the IOP—this would necessitate an alternative drug regimen.

TREATMENT METHODOLOGY

Since primary open-angle glaucoma is a bilateral disease, treatment should generally be instituted in both eyes even if the glaucomatous damage is evident in only one eye. This is often not the case, however, in many of the secondary glaucomas such as those associated with exfoliation or the pigmentary dispersion syndrome, in which unilateral treatment is justified.

It is generally unnecessary to advise patients to reduce fluid intake (including coffee or other stimulants) or to withhold treatment with topical or systemic over-the-counter medications. Although the pharmaceutic labelling of many systemic drugs—anticholinergic agents or drugs with anticholinergic side effects, and other drugs such as vasodilators and corticosteroids—often states that such medications are contraindicated in glaucoma, this advice fails to recognize that glaucoma is a multifaceted disease rather than a single disease entity. In patients with medically controlled primary open-angle glaucoma, there is no definite contraindication to the use of most systemic medications because the concentration of drug reaching the eye is usually too low to be of any significant influence. Although there have been reports of aggravation of existing open-angle glaucoma with the use of systemic steroids, these drugs can generally be safely used in such patients if the IOP is carefully monitored.[238] The concomitant use of some topical and systemic medications carries a greater risk in patients predisposed to angle-closure glaucoma (Table 29.14).[239]

In devising an effective treatment plan, the following guidelines should facilitate management of the patient by increasing the effectiveness of medical therapy, improving patient compliance, and reducing therapeutic failures.[234,240]

- Use the lowest concentration and dosage frequency compatible with acceptable control of IOP. This is determined by beginning with low concentrations of drug and increasing as necessary until the desired IOP is attained. Low initial doses cause fewer side effects and improve patient compliance with the prescribed therapy.
- IOP should ideally be determined just before a scheduled drug application to ensure that the desired effect is being reasonably maintained from one dose to the next.
- Observe the patient administer a drop of medication. Instruction regarding proper instillation technique may be required. If the patient has difficulty discerning when a drop of medication has been properly instilled, the drug can be refrigerated to improve the patient's sensitivity. In addition, the patient should be instructed to wait at least 5 minutes between drop instillations when multiple topical medications have been prescribed. Washing one medication out with another is a frequent cause of failure to obtain expected additive drug effects when topical medications are used in combination.
- When initially devising a medication schedule, the practitioner should attempt to integrate the therapy as smoothly as possible into the patient's daily routine. This is especially important in encouraging compliance with the use of every-6-hour medications (pilocarpine solutions). In such cases the patient can be instructed to use the medication on arising, before lunch, before dinner, and before retiring. For some employed patients, the use of 2 bottles of medication, 1 for home and 1 for work, may be beneficial.
- The practitioner should have regard for the patient's safety by keeping a total drug record that includes the name and address of the patient's primary physician as well as a complete list of all ophthalmic and systemic medications. In addition, the practitioner should remind the patient to inform his or her primary physician of the medications that have been prescribed for the glaucoma, or, alternatively, the patient may be encouraged to take the medications when other practitioners are visited. This is especially important when the glaucoma drug regimen includes a β blocker, anticholinesterase agent, epinephrine, or a carbonic anhydrase inhibitor.

TABLE 29.14
Estimate of Actual Risk Associated with Drugs "Contraindicated" in Glaucoma

Patient Group	High Risk (Avoid)	Slight Risk	Minimal Risk (in Usual Doses)

Patients with controlled open-angle glaucoma	None	Topical steroids
		  Dexamethasone
		  Prednisolone
		  Betamethasone
		Oral steroids
			Topical and oral
			  anticholinergics
			Antihistamines
			Tricyclic antidepressants
			Phenothiazines
			Benzodiazepines
			Vasodilators
			  Nitrites
			  Nitrates
			  Tolazoline
			  Hydralazine
			  Nylidrin
			  Nicotinic acid
			  Cyclandelate
			  Isoxuprine
			  Papaverine

Patients predisposed to angle-closure glaucoma	Topical anticholinergics
	  Atropine
	  Homatropine
	  Scopolamine
	  Cyclopentolate
	  Tropicamide
	Topical adrenergics
	  Naphazoline
	  Tetrahydrozoline
	  Epinephrine
	  Ephedrine
	  Phenylephrine
	  Hydroxyamphetamine
		Oral anticholinergics
		  Atropine
		  Scopolamine
		  Belladonna alkaloids
		Oral adrenergics
		  Pseudoephedrine
		  Phenylephrine
		  Phenylpropanolamine
		  Ephedrine
		  Methoxyphenamine
		Amphetamines
		Appetite suppressants
		Bronchodilators
		Central nervous system
		  stimulants
			Steroids
			Vasodilators
			Tricyclic antidepressants
			Phenothiazines
			Antihistamines

Modified from Durkee DP, Bryant BG. Drug therapy reviews: Drug therapy of glaucoma. Am J Hosp Pharm 1978;35:682–690.

Drug Schema.   The general approach to the medical management of primary open-angle glaucoma is shown in Figure 29.28. When beginning treatment, the choice of drug should generally be a β blocker. This approach usually allows a significant reduction of IOP without the ocular side effects of miotics. In addition, dosage frequency is only once or twice daily, which reduces the opportunity for noncompliance when compared with the more frequent instillation required of pilocarpine solutions. It must be stressed that the general recommendations given in Figure 29.28 must often be modified according to each patient's individual requirements. Some patients, for example, will have contraindications to specific drugs, and some medications will not be tolerated or will be ineffective. It is important to promptly modify therapy or discontinue any medications that are poorly tolerated or ineffective.

Once the patient has started initial drug therapy, 2 weeks is a useful follow-up time interval. This allows the patient to determine the ability to tolerate the medication and allows the practitioner to determine the clinical effectiveness of therapy. According to the results of this therapeutic trial, therapy can be increased, decreased, or otherwise modified to enhance the reduction of IOP while minimizing undesirable side effects. After the medication has been titrated to achieve the desired "target pressure," the patient should be monitored every 3 to 6 months according to the severity of the glaucomatous damage and the susceptibility of the patient to further optic disc and visual field changes. Specific procedures and guidelines for the long-term management of patients with primary open-angle glaucoma are discussed below.

Although single-medication therapy is preferred, patients often become tolerant of the initial drug or require additional medication as the glaucomatous damage progresses. In such cases additional medication may be added to the drug regimen, as shown in Figure 29.28. This step-wise approach reserves the more potent medications, such as the carbonic anhydrase in-

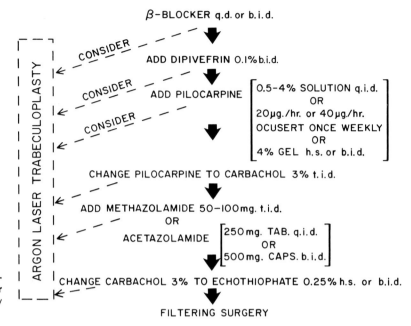

FIGURE 29.28 **Flowchart for the medical management of primary open-angle glaucoma. Argon laser trabeculoplasty is used as an adjunct to drug therapy (see text).**

hibitors and anticholinesterase agents, for patients with the more advanced and resistant forms of glaucoma. Patients with early or moderate degrees of glaucomatous damage are unlikely to require such medications.

SPECIFIC MANAGEMENT PLANS

Although the drug schema illustrated in Figure 29.28 can be used to treat most patients with primary open-angle glaucoma, the specific management plan will often vary according to the individual characteristics and requirements of each patient (Table 29.15). For example, miotic solutions may be used in elderly patients without cataracts, but the practitioner should be cautious in using carbonic anhydrase inhibitors because of drug-induced behavioral changes.

In patients with cataracts, miotic solutions are generally contraindicated because of their devastating effect on visual acuity and because of their acceleration of cataractous changes. A β blocker or dipivefrin is a reasonable drug of first choice for such patients, and, if needed, the carbonic anhydrase inhibitors may be added, followed finally by lower concentrations of pilocarpine.[234]

Miotic solutions should be avoided in young patients (under 40 years of age) because of drug-induced accommodative spasm and refractive changes. Instead, a β blocker or dipivefrin may be useful initial drugs that can be followed, if necessary, by a carbonic anhydrase inhibitor. Pilocarpine in the form of Ocusert or gel may be beneficial. The anticholinesterase agents are generally not tolerated by these patients.

All strong miotics, including carbachol and echothiophate, should be avoided in patients with a history of retinal detachment or in patients with high myopia. Dipivefrin or a β blocker is preferred as the initial drug, followed, if necessary, by lower concentrations of pilocarpine or a carbonic anhydrase inhibitor.

Epinephrine and dipivefrin should be avoided in aphakic or pseudophakic patients, since these drugs carry a risk of maculopathy. Instead, treatment should begin with low concentrations of pilocarpine or a β blocker and proceed, as needed, to a carbonic anhydrase inhibitor.[234] Since the anticholinesterase agents

TABLE 29.15
Contraindicated Drugs or Drug Classes

Situation	Contraindicated Drug or Drug Class
Elderly patients	Carbonic anhydrase inhibitors
Cataract	Miotic solutions
Young patients (<40 years of age)	Miotic solutions
History of retinal detachment	Strong miotics (e.g., anticholinesterase agents)
High myopia	Strong miotics (e.g., anticholinesterase agents)
Aphakia or pseudophakia	Epinephrine and dipivefrin
History of kidney disease	Acetazolamide
Chronic obstructive pulmonary disease	β blockers (β₁ blockers may be used with caution)
Congestive heart disease	β blockers

carry a greater risk of retinal detachment, they should be held in reserve until all other treatment modalities have been exhausted.

Patients with a history of kidney stones may be treated as shown in Figure 29.28. However, methazolamide should be the carbonic anhydrase inhibitor of choice because of its lower risk of kidney impairment.

PATIENT COMPLIANCE

The general factors contributing to noncompliance with medication schedules are discussed in Chapter 2. Primary open-angle glaucoma encompasses more of these factors than do most other ocular diseases because it is chronic, asymptomatic, sometimes requires complex therapeutic regimens often with associated side effects, and requires considerable time in patient education. It has been reported that patients take only about 75% of prescribed doses of pilocarpine drops, with 6% of patients taking less than one-fourth and 15% taking less than half of prescribed doses.[241] Unfortunately, there is no simple screening device that will help the practitioner identify the unreliable patient, or that will predict accurately at the time of initial diagnosis the potential for patient noncompliance.[242] In general, age, sex, education, visual ability, and ethnic background seem to have little influence on the potential for noncompliance.[243,244] The practitioner often assumes that the patient is properly complying with the prescribed treatment and interprets the progression of optic disc damage and visual field loss as indicating medication failure. This may be an inappropriate assumption, since the progression of glaucomatous damage may be related solely to patient failure to properly comply with the medical therapy.

Numerous factors contribute to noncompliance in patients with primary open-angle glaucoma (Table 29.16). The fact that primary open-angle glaucoma is a chronic disease that requires long-term management encourages at least occasional noncompliance with

TABLE 29.16
Factors Contributing to Noncompliance in Primary Open-Angle Glaucoma

- Use of multiple medications requiring frequent daily administration
- Medication expense
- Medication side effects
- Patient's understanding of the disease
- Asymptomatic disease (no noticeable effects of therapy)
- Requires long-term medication (chronic disease)
- Patient's ability to understand treatment procedure and to comply with drop instillation or oral medication

medication schedules. The asymptomatic nature of the disease, in which the beneficial effects of therapy are not readily appreciated or are associated with significant side effects, are other factors leading to noncompliance.

Factors related to the therapeutic regimen itself may promote poor compliance. These include the use of multiple medications requiring frequent administration, medication expense, and the frequency and severity of side effects. In general, the more a therapeutic regimen interferes with the patient's daily lifestyle, the less likely it is to be accepted and maintained.

Socioeconomic factors may also contribute to noncompliance. Medication expense, cost of office visits, and transportation may limit use of medications in some patients despite the willingness of the patient to accept and comply with the prescribed therapy. Patients should be encouraged to compare prices of medications at different pharmacies to obtain the most economical dosage regimen, and the practitioner can help reduce overall cost of therapy by prescribing generic equivalent drugs if available.[245]

Perhaps the most important factor is the patient's perception and understanding of the disease. Poor compliance occurs more frequently in patients who show little concern for their own health or well-being, who question the effectiveness of medical care or medications, or who do not understand the information or instructions provided by the practitioner or staff.[244]

Recognition of the patient's noncompliance is essential so that appropriate corrective measures can be instituted before further glaucomatous damage occurs. Noncompliance may be identified by instructing the patient to bring his or her medications to the office so that the amount used by the patient can be determined (Table 29.17). It is important to inspect the pupillary responses of patients taking miotics; normally reactive pupils that are not miotic are a strong indication of noncompliance. On the other hand, the practitioner should be alert to the occasional patient who instills the medication only on the day of examination. Despite acceptable IOPs, progression of glaucomatous damage to the optic disc and visual field is observed.[241] Once the clinician realizes the potential for such noncompliance, the assessment of visual fields and optic discs should take precedence over the measurement of IOP.

Methods for improving compliance are listed in Table 29.18.[246] Unfortunately, simple interventions rarely produce substantial, long-lasting improvement in compliance.[247] On the other hand, coercing or provoking fear may also be unsuccessful in improving compliance because the patient may fear the consequences of the glaucoma so much that he or she does not take the required medications, which only reinforce a feeling of vulnerability to the disease.[247]

TABLE 29.17
Approximate Longevity of Glaucoma Medications[a]

Medication	Bottle Size (ml)	Dosage Frequency		
		Once Daily	Twice Daily	Four Times Daily
β blocker, dipivefrin	10	100 days	50 days	
β blocker, pilocarpine, dipivefrin	15	150 days	75 days	38 days
Pilocarpine	30			75 days

[a]Assumes 20 drops/ml and good patient compliance for instillation into both eyes.

Perhaps the most effective method for improving compliance with medication schedules is by developing an attitude of concern and compassion and frequently communicating with the patient using understandable instructions for proper use of the medications. Brown and associates[248] found that 13% of glaucoma patients experienced in the use of topical eyedrops were unable to instill topical medications into both eyes successfully even after several attempts. In addition, counseling and education regarding the disease process and the importance of its treatment are vital.[249] This should be reinforced by the office assistant, technician, or nurse. On subsequent visits the practitioner or assistant should periodically reassess (by observation) the patient's ability to properly use the prescribed medication.[248,250] In addition, the patient should be asked to verbally recite the instructions for use of the medication. At each office visit the patient should be reminded about the importance of regular medication usage and should be reassured regarding minor medication side effects.

Another effective method for improving compliance is to devise an initial medication schedule that is easily integrated into the patient's daily lifestyle. This appears to be effective in reducing the number of missed doses and improving the regular dosage intervals. For example, the use of pilocarpine drops on awakening, before lunch, before dinner, and at bedtime avoids a rigid every-6-hour dosage schedule. On the other hand, patients who consistently administer their medication at unevenly spaced intervals may require such a rigid dosage schedule. It may be helpful for these patients to change from a q.i.d. dosage interval to a q.6.h. schedule to reduce diurnal variations of IOP. When appropriate, the use of a β blocker, requiring only once- or twice-a-day dosage instead of 4 times a day, will interfere less with the patient's normal lifestyle and often improves compliance.[249,251] In this regard, a compromise may be required by both the practitioner and the patient. A realistic drug schedule with which the patient is likely to comply may be far superior to a medically ideal regimen that requires substantial changes in the patient's lifestyle. A medication time-table card similar to the one shown in Table 29.19 can be used to reinforce medication schedules.[252] Another measure that may improve compliance in some patients is the dispensing of pilocarpine, dipivefrin, or levobunolol with C Cap Compliance Caps (Allergan) (Fig. 29.29). This dosing formulation allows the patient to keep track of the daily doses of medication and may help to minimize dosing confusion when multiple medications are prescribed.

Another method for improving compliance is to substitute a "new," equally effective medication for the older drug therapy. Novack and associates,[253] for example, have shown that patients may comply better with levobunolol as "new" therapy when they were previously uncontrolled with timolol. When 2 or more drugs are prescribed for use at different times, the patient must be able to identify the individual medications. He or she can be educated in this regard by identifying the pilocarpine as "the bottle with the green top" or the β blocker as "the bottle with the yellow top," and so on. When a particular medication may be expected to cause unfamiliar or uncomfortable side effects, these should be explained to the patient before beginning therapy. In those instances in which the side effects will decrease or disappear, the patient should be advised of this in advance.

If the problem of noncompliance is not properly addressed, it usually leads to progressive glaucomatous damage. In such cases laser therapy or filtering surgery become the only recourse.

TABLE 29.18
Methods for Improving Compliance

- Use of coercion or fear provocation
- Improve practitioner-patient communication
- Teach proper drop instillation
- Patient should recite instructions
- Devise medication schedule that is easily integrated into patient's lifestyle
- Some patients may require rigid dosage schedule
- Explain potential side effects in advance

TABLE 29.19
Glaucoma Medication Time-Table Card

Medication	Eye		Time				Comment
	R	L	AM	PM	PM	PM	
Timoptic 0.25%, 0.5%							
Betagan 0.5%							
Betoptic 0.5%							
Propine 0.1%							
Pilocarpine 1%, 2%, 4%							
Carbachol 3%							
Pholpholine Iodide 0.25%							
Neptazane tablets 25 mg, 50 mg							
Diamox tablets 250 mg							
Diamox capsules 500 mg							

Adapted from Kooner KS, Zimmerman TJ. A glaucoma medication timetable card. Ann Ophthalmol 1987;19:43–44.

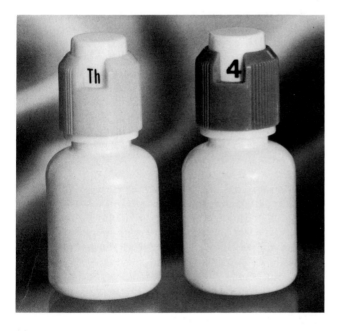

FIGURE 29.29 **Glaucoma medications with C Cap Compliance Caps (Allergan). When the medication cap is returned to the bottle after dispensing a drop of medication into the eye, the cap is turned to the next dosage indication. The number of instilled daily doses can thus be accounted for, and the device serves to remind the patient of the next indicated dosage.**

LONG-TERM MANAGEMENT

The long-term management of patients with primary open-angle glaucoma requires careful attention to a variety of parameters that serve to indicate the adequacy of IOP control. The most important factors to be carefully monitored are IOP, visual fields, and the optic discs. Depending on the extent of glaucomatous damage and rate of progression of the optic disc and visual field changes, it is generally useful to monitor patients every 3 to 6 months. IOP status should be determined at each visit, but visual fields and optic disc evaluations generally need be performed only every 6 months. Figure 29.30 shows a suggested long-term management plan for an every-3-month monitoring schedule. Regardless of the time interval chosen for the monitoring schedule, it is essential that evaluations of visual fields and optic discs be performed during the same office visit, or within a few weeks of each other, so that the optic disc changes can be accurately correlated with changes of the visual fields.

The large amount and variety of information collected on individual patients necessitates use of a control sheet such as the one illustrated in Table 29.20. Such a device facilitates the long-term monitoring of patients by consolidating the important diagnostic and therapeutic parameters into a form allowing rapid recognition of trends in the IOP or visual acuity.[254] A simple check mark may be used to indicate that visual field or optic disc evaluations were performed. The patient's chart must then be consulted to determine the actual status of the visual fields or optic discs. For simplicity, therapeutic drug regimens can be documented using easily identifiable abbreviations (Table 29.21).

Usage of Medications.   As previously discussed, the patient's improper use of medication is one of the most important factors in failure to control the glaucomatous damage. It is therefore vital to evaluate the patient's continued ability to properly use the prescribed medications. The practitioner should inquire about the frequency of medication use, the approximate percentage of missed doses, and convenience of the dosage schedule. Any medication side effects should be elicited, particularly those that might limit use of the medication. Because IOP status directly reflects duration of action of the various medications, it is essential to record in the patient's chart the time of the most recent dose of each medication.

Visual Acuity.   Stabilization of the IOP at a level that permits control of the glaucomatous optic disc changes should prevent any further loss of visual acuity. A gradual reduction in visual acuity may be associated with further visual field changes, indicating progression of optic disc damage. Corneal edema associated with corneal endothelial compromise may also reduce visual acuity. Other possible causes of visual acuity loss include the development or progression of cataract, the development of miotic cysts, retinal venous occlusive disease, and retinal detachment. A gradual or sudden reduction of visual acuity should be an indication for pupillary dilation and careful examination of the crystalline lens and retina.

Intraocular Pressure.   The IOP should be correlated with the most recent dose of medication. An apparent increase in pressure may be related solely to the interval between the last medication dose and the time of IOP measurement rather than to a true drug tolerance or exacerbation of the disease. Since diurnal variations have an important influence on IOP measurements, these influences should be taken into consideration when interpreting the IOP. The possibility of noncompliance should be considered when the IOPs are only occasionally elevated. Once the practitioner has determined that a true, consistent elevation in IOP has occurred, the medication or dosage schedules should be adjusted accordingly. When a sudden decrease in IOP occurs, uveitis or retinal detachment should be considered.

Visual Fields.   Since maintenance of the visual fields is a primary therapeutic objective in the treatment of glaucoma, periodic reevaluation of the visual field is one of the most important factors in the patient's long-term management. In comparing the visual field from one visit to the next, it is important to evaluate for consistent *trends* in visual field changes rather than changing medical therapy solely on the basis of a single

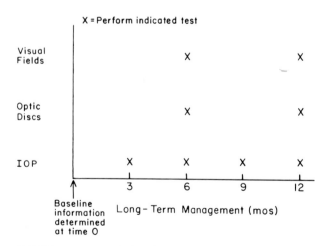

FIGURE 29.30   **Practical evaluation plan for long-term management of primary open-angle glaucoma.**

TABLE 29.20
Glaucoma Control Sheet

NAME: John A. Doe
DOB: 6/17/27
DIAGNOSIS: POAG OU
TARGET PRESSURE: Below 21

Date	IOP OD	IOP OS	Visual Fields	Optic Discs OD	Optic Discs OS	Gonio	Visual Acuity OD	Visual Acuity OS	Blood Pressure	Medication Schedule	Comments
2/10/86	31	28	√	√	√	√	20/25	20/25	140/88	$B_{1/2}$ OU BID	Emphysema
2/24/86	25	21					20/25	20/25	142/86	Add $P_{1/10}$ OU BID	
3/7/86	20	19					20/25	20/25	140/86		Good compliance
7/8/86	19	18					20/30	20/25			
11/10/86	20	18	√	√	√		20/25	20/30			
3/15/87	24	22					20/30	20/30			Missed last dosage
7/20/87	21	20	√	√	√		20/30	20/30			
11/13/87	22	22					20/30	20/30			
3/11/88	25	24	√	√	√	√	20/30	20/30	145/88	Add P_1 OU QID	
3/26/88	19	18					20/30	20/40			
8/3/88	21	21					20/40	20/30			
12/15/88	21	22	√	√	√		20/40	20/40			
4/3/89	23	22					20/40	20/40		Δ P_1 to P_2 OU QID	
4/20/89	18	18					20/40	20/40			
8/18/89	25	24	√	√	√	√	20/40	20/40			Patient to consider laser trabec

TABLE 29.21
Commonly Used Abbreviations for Glaucoma Medications

Medication	Trade Name	Concentration (%)	Abbreviation
Timolol	Timoptic	0.25, 0.50	$T_{1/4}$, $T_{1/2}$
Levobunolol	Betagan	0.50	$L_{1/2}$
Betaxolol	Betoptic	0.50	$B_{1/2}$
Dipivefrin	Propine	0.1	$P_{1/10}$
Epinephrine	Glaucon	1.0	E_1
Pilocarpine solution	Isoptocarpine	1.0, 2.0, 4.0	P_1, P_2, P_4
Pilocarpine gel	Pilopine H.S. Gel	4.0	P Gel
Carbachol	Isoptocarbachol	3.0	C_3
Acetazolamide[a]	Diamox	250[a], 500[a]	D_{250}, D_{500}
Methazolamide[a]	Neptazane	25[a], 50[a]	N_{25}, N_{50}
Echothiophate	Phospholine Iodide	0.25	$PI_{1/4}$

[a]The concentration for these medications is in milligrams (mg).

visual field evaluation. It is important, therefore, that the physical parameters of visual field testing—illumination, target size, pupil sizes, and procedure—be approximately the same for each visual field assessment. Pupillary dilation with 2.5% phenylephrine or a combination of 2.5% phenylephrine and 1% tropicamide is usually satisfactory for such evaluations. When Goldmann or static threshold perimetry is employed, the patient's vision should be optimally corrected. When evaluating the visual fields, it is important to realize that changes in the visual field may be due not only to progressive glaucoma, but may also be caused by many other disorders such as retinal venous occlusive disease, retinal detachment, cataracts, diabetic retinopathy, miotic cysts, or refractive error changes.[234]

Optic Discs. It is crucial to dilate the pupil for careful stereoscopic evaluation of the optic discs. The optic discs must be carefully reevaluated for changes in cupping, pallor, or the presence of neuroretinal rim compromise, which may indicate inadequate control of IOP.[234]

Systemic Disease. The patient's general health should be monitored. Patients who develop systemic hypertension or who have been given increases of antihypertensive medication should be monitored more carefully for optic disc and visual field changes. In some cases it may be appropriate to adjust the patient's medication schedule to allow for some additional reduction in IOP so that an optimum perfusion-pressure gradient is maintained. The development of diabetes, with associated small-vessel disease, may also indicate the need to further reduce IOP.[234]

FAILURE OF MEDICAL THERAPY

A variety of factors contribute to the failure of medical therapy to adequately prevent further glaucomatous optic disc and visual field changes:[234,255,256]

- The IOP measurement may not completely reflect the pressure control because of diurnal variations of pressure.[257]
- The practitioner may inaccurately estimate the level of IOP that is expected to reduce the risk of further progression. Such underestimation (i.e., selection of IOP that is too high) leads to further visual field loss even though lower pressures could have been obtained by adjusting the medical therapy.
- Drug tolerance may occur. This may lead to the use of maximum medical therapy, consisting of an anticholinesterase agent, dipivefrin, a β blocker, and a carbonic anhydrase inhibitor. If tolerance develops to this drug regimen, laser or filtering surgery is

usually required. In some cases, however, the practitioner may be able to change to a previously employed drug, with some occasional success in further reducing pressure.
- Medication side effects may necessitate discontinuation of certain drugs, leading in some cases to the need for laser therapy or filtering surgery.
- The development and treatment of other diseases can contribute to progressive optic disc damage. Patients may unknowingly be given topical or systemic anticholinergic drugs or steroids by other practitioners. These medications may prevent adequate reduction of IOP. The presence of diabetes or treatment of systemic hypertension may accelerate glaucomatous changes of the optic disc despite maximum medical glaucoma therapy.
- Noncompliance can significantly affect the success of medical therapy.

LASER SURGERY

Since the late 1970s argon laser trabeculoplasty (ALT) has been investigated as a means to lower IOP in patients uncontrolled with maximum tolerable medical therapy.[258–265] The technique is performed at the slit lamp following topical anesthesia. After placement of a mirrored contact lens on the cornea, the operator places 50 to 100 "burns" evenly spaced on the anterior portion of the trabecular meshwork. Most clinicians initially treat only 180° of the angle, reserving the balance of the angle for later treatment, if indicated.[264,266] The procedure produces an increase in aqueous outflow by opening the trabecular spaces due to the mechanical shrinkage of collagen at the burn sites.[266] Several investigators[267,268] have shown that laser trabeculoplasty induces mechanical, cellular, and biochemical changes within the trabecular meshwork, causing decreased outflow resistance.

When first introduced into clinical practice, ALT was reserved for use only in patients who remained uncontrolled with maximum tolerable medical therapy. Now, however, some authors[248,261,269] advocate its use as primary therapy, even before pharmacologic treatment is attempted. Although the indications for use of ALT are now more liberal than in the past, most clinicians favor an approach whereby the procedure is used when patients cannot tolerate simple drug regimens or when noncompliance, drug tolerance, or advancing disease preclude the success of pharmacologic therapy[258,262,404] (Table 29.22). Contraindications to ALT are listed in Table 29.23.

Although initial results of ALT can be impressive, the effectiveness of the procedure tends to decrease with time,[263,260,404] and most patients will continue to require medical therapy.[263,270] Pollack and associates[270] have shown that about 40% of eyes will require the

TABLE 29.22
Indications for Argon Laser Trabeculoplasty

- Medically uncontrolled primary open-angle glaucoma (POAG) before filtering surgery
- Failed filtering surgery in POAG where ALT not previously performed
- Unacceptable side effects from medical therapy
- Poor compliance with medical therapy
- Patient inability to instill topical medications

Adapted from Goldberg I. Argon laser trabeculoplasty and the open-angle glaucomas. Aust NZ J Ophthalmol 1985;13:243–248.

prelaser medical regimen, while only about 20% can discontinue all prior medical therapy. Many patients, however, can discontinue miotics or carbonic anhydrase inhibitors following ALT and can thus avoid annoying side effects from these medications. Although ALT can delay the need for filtering surgery,[271] the probability of treatment success after 4 years is only about 50%.[272,404]

Complications of ALT are listed in Table 29.24. Following the procedure topical steroids are routinely used to control ocular congestion and iritis.[260,266] Although some patients do not need steroids, a regimen consisting of 1% prednisolone acetate 4 times daily for 5 to 7 days is effective in reducing both the incidence and severity of anterior uveal reactions. A more serious postlaser complication is acute elevation of IOP, which can lead to optic disc damage and further visual field loss in susceptible patients. Since the incidence of IOP elevations of 10 mm Hg or greater is 20% to 40% following ALT,[273] it is important to minimize both the incidence and severity of these pressure responses to prevent iatrogenic glaucomatous damage. Such IOP elevations can often be prevented or controlled by giving 4% pilocarpine postoperatively and monitoring IOP for 2 or 3 hours before dismissing the patient to regular postoperative care.[274] Currently, however, apraclonidine 1% (Iopidine, Alcon), an α_2-adrenergic agonist, is commonly used 1 hour before laser treatment and immediately following ALT. This agent, which reduces IOP probably by inhibiting aqueous formation, is effective in reducing both the incidence and severity of acute postlaser IOP elevations.[122]

TABLE 29.23
Contraindications to Argon Laser Trabeculoplasty

- Corneal opacities
- Extensive peripheral anterior synechiae
- Patient inability to cooperate at slit lamp

From Goldberg I. Argon laser trabeculoplasty and the open-angle glaucomas. Aust NZ J Ophthalmol 1985;13:243–248.

TABLE 29.24
Complications of Argon Laser Trabeculoplasty[273]

- Transient blurred vision
- Iritis
- Microhyphema
- Acute elevation of IOP
- Peripheral anterior synechiae
- Corneal burns
- Corneal edema

FILTERING SURGERY AND OTHER TREATMENT MODALITIES

When argon laser trabeculoplasty and maximum tolerable medical therapy have failed to prevent further progression of optic disc damage and visual field loss, filtering surgery is indicated. Since the prognosis for retention of visual acuity and visual field is good following surgical intervention,[399] and since the risk of visual loss increases markedly in eyes with advanced glaucoma in which IOP exceeds 18 mm Hg, serious consideration should be given to a filtering procedure when the IOP is consistently over 22 mm Hg.[275]

Despite very definite risks, various filtering procedures may be used in an attempt to further reduce IOP. The most popular technique is trabeculectomy. This procedure involves providing a scleral filtration pathway to the subconjunctival space to allow the aqueous to escape. After a conjunctival flap is turned down over the cornea, a lamellar flap of sclera is created and the exposed trabeculum is excised. A peripheral iridectomy is performed, and the sclera and conjunctival flaps are replaced. This creates a filtering bleb at the site of aqueous drainage.

Various procedures may be carried out on the ciliary body in an attempt to functionally destroy this structure, thereby decreasing aqueous production. Such procedures are reserved for those cases that are resistant to control by standard filtering operations. Cyclocryotherapy uses transcleral freezing of the ciliary body at multiple locations.[276,277] This procedure has generally replaced cyclodiathermy and cyclodialysis because it is less invasive. Other procedures are currently being developed to more effectively manage patients with advanced glaucomatous damage. These techniques include transcleral Nd:YAG laser cyclocoagulation,[278,279] endolaser treatment of the ciliary body,[280] and therapeutic ultrasound.[281–283]

Low Tension Glaucoma

Diagnosis

Many clinicians believe that use of the term *low tension glaucoma* is inappropriate. Levene[284] has reviewed the literature and found 6 definitions of low tension glaucoma and about 15 classifications, an indication of the lack of consistency and understanding of this term.

From a practical clinical point of view, however, patients are found who have open anterior chamber angles, optic disc changes, typical glaucomatous visual field losses, but with normal or low IOPs (usually 21 mm Hg is considered to be the upper limit). These patients are said to have low tension glaucoma (LTG). The optic nerve appears to be abnormally vulnerable to an otherwise normal IOP. It has been shown that the level of IOP is a factor in producing the glaucomatous damage.[398] Patients with LTG and asymmetric IOPs were evaluated and in 86% of the patients, cupping of the optic disc and the amount of visual field loss were greater in the eye with the higher IOP. The incidence of LTG has been reported to be as low as 7%[129] and as high as 66%.[285] The most probable incidence is about 30%. The differential diagnosis includes the disorders listed in Table 29.25.

Gorin[286] contends that true LTG is rare and that most patients assumed to have the disorder have one of the following conditions.

- "Burned-out" open-angle glaucoma. These patients have had moderate open-angle glaucoma for many years that produced the damage. When they are examined in later years, the damage is evident and they have normal or low IOP because of aqueous hyposecretion due to ciliary body atrophy and advancing age. Even though the pressure is not high, damage may still be occurring. The appropriate treatment is usually surgery.
- Patients with high diurnal variations. Some patients with visual field loss and optic disc changes will have IOPs of 17 to 19 mm Hg at certain times of the day and 28 to 30 mm Hg at other times. These patients have primary open-angle glaucoma and should be treated as such. Variations in IOP can suggest the presence of LTG. A variation in IOP of 11 to 21 mm Hg, twice the normal range of diurnal variation, indicates the presence of LTG. One other IOP vari-

ation that may be helpful in the detection of LTG is the variation of pressure with postural changes. If IOP is measured with the patient sitting and then supine, the normal patient will have an average increase in pressure of about 3 mm Hg. Occasionally a difference of up to 6 mm Hg may be observed.[287] Hyams and associates[288] have reported that the IOP of patients with LTG is significantly higher in the supine position than in the sitting position. This testing procedure may thus be very helpful in the diagnosis of some patients with LTG.

- Patients with history of cardiovascular disease. Some patients with normal or low IOP, visual field loss, and optic disc changes may have histories of severe internal bleeding, low systemic blood pressure, myocardial infarction, or serious arrhythmia that produced a sudden and somewhat prolonged decrease in systemic blood pressure, resulting in ischemia of the optic nerve with glaucomatous disc changes and visual field losses.[289] This is more likely to occur in patients with myopia and preexisting large physiologic cupping. Generally no treatment is necessary if the cardiovascular problems have been properly treated.

An increased prevalence of optic disc hemorrhages in patients with LTG[290] indicates the presence of a possible ischemic factor in the pathogenesis of this disorder.

- Patients with hereditary optic atrophy. Such patients have low IOP, optic disc changes, and glaucoma-like visual field losses. A complete examination and thorough history, including a genetic evaluation, are necessary to determine the correct diagnosis. No medical or surgical treatment is effective.

Caprioli and Spaeth[291] compared the optic nerve head in LTG and high tension glaucoma and reported that the neuroretinal rim in LTG is significantly thinner than it is in high tension glaucoma. The greatest difference generally occurs in the inferior and inferotemporal areas. This suggests that the mechanism for optic nerve damage may differ in the two conditions. These investigators[292] also compared the visual fields in LTG and high tension glaucoma and have shown that the visual field losses in the two conditions differ. The scotomas in LTG are closer to fixation and are deeper than those in high tension glaucoma, also suggesting that the mechanism for damage of the optic nerve in the two conditions may differ. Another similar study[293] found the scotomas closer together, but with the scotomas in high tension glaucoma slightly closer to fixation.

Levene[284] has pointed out some of the clinical characteristics of LTG (Table 29.26). Patients with suspected LTG should be evaluated very carefully for

TABLE 29.25
Differential Diagnosis of Low Tension Glaucoma

- Congenital optic disc defects
- Optic atrophy
- Ischemic optic neuropathy
- Vascular disease
- Chronic angle-closure glaucoma
- Open-angle glaucoma
- Optic nerve tumors
- Optic nerve drusen

TABLE 29.26
Clinical Characteristics of Low Tension Glaucoma

Clinical Factor	Characteristic of Low Tension Glaucoma in Relationship to Primary Open-Angle Glaucoma
Age	More often found in older patients
Sex	Increased incidence and more progressive in females
Visual acuity	Reduced visual acuity reported by some patients
Optic disc changes	Disc cupping and visual field losses not well correlated. Cupping more significant in relationship to visual field loss
Splinter hemorrhages	More often present on the disc or disc margins
IOP	Usually a great diurnal variation
Visual fields	Early dense paracentral scotoma in the nasal field that extends to within 5° of the point of fixation. The field loss often has an altitudinal nature. Progression is often slower
Laterality	Monocular cases more frequent
Congruence	More noncongruent cases. Eye with the lowest IOP has greatest field loss

these clinical characteristics so that appropriate management decisions can be made.

Management

The significant risk factors that contribute to LTG must be diligently sought out and corrected if possible. These conditions include systemic vascular disease such as anemia, internal carotid occlusive disease, incipient cardiac failure, paroxysmal arrhythmias, and therapy of systemic hypertension.[256] It is not necessary to treat the group of patients with LTG who have had a preceding hemodynamic crisis because the likelihood of further progression of the glaucomatous damage is remote.

Patients with progressive optic nerve damage and visual field loss should be aggressively treated, but, unfortunately, medical therapy is only rarely effective in arresting the disease process.[284] In general, LTG progresses more slowly than does primary open-angle glaucoma, but females seem to have a more rapidly progressive disease than do males.[284] Thus, female patients should probably be treated more aggressively than males.

Despite the general lack of effectiveness of medical therapy, an attempt should be made to reduce the IOP as much as possible, even if the baseline value is not in the upper normal range.[284] The pretreatment baseline is probably an important factor—the higher the initial pressure, the more successful medical therapy will be in reducing the pressure. In approximately one-third of patients, medical therapy produces little or no reduction of IOP, while in perhaps two-thirds of patients a slight reduction, from 2 to 9 mm Hg, may occur.[284]

The ability of various medications to reduce the IOP depends on the type, concentration, and combi-

nation of drugs used. To achieve the lowest IOP possible, any combination of ocular hypotensive agents may be employed.[256] Echothiophate, however, should be avoided. In addition, since there is some evidence that patients with LTG have increased levels of cholesterol, it has been suggested that the oral administration of clofibrate (Atromid-S) may be beneficial.[294] There have been no controlled studies, however, to substantiate the effectiveness of this therapy.

Laser treatment (trabeculoplasty) or filtering surgery should be considered only after weighing the potential benefits and risks. Although not as effective in LTG as in patients with higher baseline IOPs,[295] ALT can further reduce the IOP to clinically acceptable levels that may slow the progression of optic disc damage and visual field loss.[296] Schwartz and associates[295] showed that ALT was clinically successful in 73% of patients with progressive LTG, and the procedure decreased the mean peak pressure during the diurnal curve, confirming the usefulness of laser therapy as an alternative to filtering surgery.

It is often difficult to determine the effectiveness of filtering surgery, since the natural course of visual field loss in LTG is more uncertain than in primary open-angle glaucoma. Thus, it may be less advisable to operate on the elderly patient with LTG who has a limited life expectancy than on the same patient with primary open-angle glaucoma. The spectrum of surgical results ranges from being completely ineffective to being occasionally successful.[284] In cases of LTG that are definitely progressive, surgery is likely to be more successful if the preoperative baseline IOP is in the upper normal range.[284] If filtering surgery is considered, it should be performed before visual field loss involves fixation. Abedin and associates[297] have reported successful management of progressive LTG by reducing the IOP to 10 mm Hg or less by filtering surgery.

Ocular Hypertension

Definition

Ocular hypertension is a controversial term. It was developed from a practical clinical perspective. A number of patients are found to have high IOPs (greater than 21 mm Hg), open anterior chamber angles, no suspicious optic disc changes, and no visual field losses. Such patients have been classified as having ocular hypertension. Other terms such as "preglaucoma," "early open-angle glaucoma," or "glaucoma suspect" have been proposed.[230] Although some patients with IOPs greater than 21 mm Hg will develop glaucoma, most will not, so that any classifying term using the word *glaucoma* seems inappropriate. Furthermore, use of any term that includes "glaucoma" frightens the patient and may carry legal and employment consequences. Regardless of the terminology, since a large number of such patients does exist, it is essential for the practitioner to understand the condition and to develop a methodology for managing these patients.

Epidemiology

The prevalence of ocular hypertension in patients over age 40 years has been reported to be 4% to 10%.[298] Cockburn[299] evaluated 1000 consecutive adult patients in a private optometric practice and classified 5.4% as having ocular hypertension.

The incidence of glaucoma in patients with ocular hypertension who have been monitored for several years is very low.[298] Cockburn[299] reviewed 21 studies that reported long-term follow-up evaluations of ocular hypertensive patients. Although different criteria for ocular hypertension were used, different lengths of follow-up time were involved, and although there were considerable variations in the findings, the evaluation probably yields useful information. The 21 studies included 2178 ocular hypertensive patients, and 10.6% were found to have progressed to true glaucoma.

Diagnosis

The diagnosis of ocular hypertension is relatively straightforward. Those patients with open anterior chamber angles, no suspicious optic disc change, and no visual field loss but with IOPs greater than 21 mm Hg are said to have ocular hypertension.

Management

The management of patients with ocular hypertension can be a challenging clinical problem. The problem is the detection of the 10% of ocular hypertensive patients who will develop glaucomatous damage. Although definitive predictive information is not yet available, the use of risk factor information is very helpful.

Levene[300] has classified the most significant risk factors according to their importance in contributing to early optic disc damage and visual field loss (Table 29.27). The decision to treat ocular hypertension may be based solely on the more important factors, sometimes in combination with the less important factors, but the decision is rarely based solely on the less important factors.

Although it is not now possible to predict which individual patients with ocular hypertension will eventually develop glaucomatous visual field loss, a management decision for each ocular hypertensive patient must be made—to treat or to monitor without treatment. The prevailing management guideline is to carefully weigh the benefits of "early" or "prophylactic" therapy against the risks of medication side effects,

TABLE 29.27
Risk Factors in Ocular Hypertension

More Important Factors	Less Important Factors
• Suspicious visual field	• Age and longevity
• Optic disc changes	• General vascular disease
• IOP elevation or asymmetry	• Unreliability in follow-up
• Useful vision in only 1 eye	• Poor cooperation in testing
• Family history of glaucoma	• Psychological considerations
• Idiopathic retinal vascular occlusion	• Myopia
	• Spontaneous ocular symptoms
	• Other tests of aqueous humor dynamics

Modified from Levene RZ. Indications for medical treatment of ocular hypertension and the initial use of pilocarpine. Surv Ophthalmol 1980;25:183–187.

noncompliance, and glaucomatous visual field loss. When all these factors are considered, it is reasonable to assume that about 5% of ocular hypertensive patients will be treated to reduce IOP.[300]

SELECTING PATIENTS FOR TREATMENT

It is generally accepted that the reduction of IOP in an eye with ocular hypertension decreases the risk of developing glaucomatous changes in that eye compared with similar eyes that are untreated.[301] Unfortunately, however, the development of such glaucomatous changes cannot be prevented in some eyes despite appropriate medical therapy.[302] Medical therapy is often expensive and inconvenient, and it may produce adverse psychological effects. The side effects of medication will also contribute to patient noncompliance in some patients. Thus, it is wise to carefully select patients for treatment based on the presence of substantial risk factors rather than to provide treatment for all patients with ocular hypertension.

The management decision should include an evaluation of systemic risk factors. Younger patients are likely to be treated more aggressively than are older patients because of their longer life expectancy.[334] Patients with one or more vascular diseases are more likely to be treated. These include diabetes, cerebrovascular disease, cardiac disease, and patients with systemic hypertension undergoing treatment. Levene,[300] however, believes that systemic vascular disease probably has only a weak association with glaucomatous visual field loss. Elderly patients (over 70 years of age) with IOPs greater than 26 mm Hg who also have systemic vascular disease should probably be treated because of the increased risk of retinal vein occlusion.[302,303] However, if such patients have IOPs lower than 26 mm Hg, there is probably no advantage in prescribing treatment. In addition, patient lifestyle as well as attitude toward and understanding of the condition will help to determine patient reliability in complying with the proposed management plan.

The management decision may be based primarily on the elevated IOP. This decision is justified if reliable visual fields cannot be obtained because of poor patient cooperation. Patients who have normal visual fields and optic discs, and IOPs greater than 30 mm Hg, should receive treatment regardless of the presence or absence of other significant risk factors. Most practitioners consider the risk of impending visual field loss to be substantial when the IOP exceeds 30 mm Hg, regardless of the absence of other risk factors.

The practitioner may decide to treat based primarily on the optic disc changes. It appears that the amount or degree of pallor of the optic disc (the color C/D ratio) is probably a better guideline than the amount of cupping (the contour C/D ratio), especially if the color C/D ratios are asymmetric between the two eyes.[234] Progression of optic disc changes is an important indication for treatment even if visual field loss is not apparent or is unreliable.

The management decision may be based primarily on visual field changes. If any consistent, reliable glaucomatous visual field change is present, it is essential that treatment be provided.

It has been reported that the use of medications in the treatment of ocular hypertension can improve compliance in patient follow-up by implying seriousness of the condition and by providing a daily reminder to the patient that an abnormal condition exists.[244] However, the institution of treatment for this reason alone cannot be advocated because of documented high noncompliance rates among the patients who are treated.[244] Instead, the decision to treat patients with ocular hypertension must be individualized by considering the major risk factors, with the potential for noncompliance being of secondary importance.

The existence of multiple risk factors increases the justification for medical therapy. Yablonski and associates[304] reported that patients with a mean IOP of 28 mm Hg or greater and a vertical contour C/D ratio of 0.6 or greater had a 100% incidence of glaucomatous visual field loss in 5 years. Under ideal situations it is probably more important to emphasize evaluation of the optic discs and visual fields rather than to rely on IOP, even though the only single risk factor that has been proved in prospective studies to be a valid predictor of glaucomatous visual field loss is the level of IOP.[302] However, when a dense cataract prevents adequate evaluation of the optic disc, or when the visual field evaluation is unreliable, the IOP assumes greater importance. The evaluation of multiple risk factors in the decision to treat ocular hypertension is summarized in Table 29.28.[300] This table illustrates 7 specific clinical situations, with an approximate ranking of the relative importance of 6 major risk factors from left to right. The importance of the optic disc is emphasized, since it is involved in 6 of the 7 clinical situations. One risk factor alone is sufficient to justify treatment in two cases—a definitely abnormal optic disc or an IOP repeatedly over 30 mm Hg. A combination of two risk factors is sufficient to justify treatment in the remaining situations.

MEDICAL THERAPY

Most practitioners favor the use of β blockers for the initial medical therapy of patients with ocular hypertension. These drugs do not produce the miosis and accommodative spasm characteristic of pilocarpine, and their long-term effectiveness and side effects have been

TABLE 29.28
The Decision to Treat Ocular Hypertension Based on 6 Risk Factors

	Visual Field	Optic Disc	Intraocular Pressure	Useful Vision in Only 1 Eye	Family History of Glaucoma	Retinal Vascular Occlusion
1	—	Abnormal	—	—	—	—
2	—	—	>30	—	—	—
3	Suspect	Suspect	—	—	—	—
4	—	Suspect	Progressive elevation or asymmetry	—	—	—
5	—	Suspect	—	+	—	—
6	—	Suspect	—	—	+	—
7	—	Suspect	—	—	—	+

Modified from Levene RZ. Indications for medical treatment of ocular hypertension and the initial use of pilocarpine. Surv Ophthalmol 1980;25:183–187.

established. If the β blocker causes undesirable side effects, dipivefrin or pilocarpine may be considered.[305,306] The more potent medications such as acetazolamide and echothiophate should be avoided because of their greater potentials for adverse effects. In addition, laser trabeculoplasty or filtering surgery is clearly without justification in patients with normal optic discs and visual fields.

In the treatment of patients with ocular hypertension, it must be emphasized that medical therapy is elective, not imperative.[307] The practitioner should respect the wishes of the patient who prefers treatment despite the absence of significant risk factors.[305,306] In many instances it is acceptable to provide medical therapy as long as it does not cause severe drug-related side effects and the patient has been informed about[308] (1) the individual risk factors present; (2) the insidious, painless nature of primary open-angle glaucoma; (3) the generally permanent nature of lost vision; (4) the treatable nature of primary open-angle glaucoma, especially in its early stages; (5) the low incidence of developing visual field changes; (6) the economic aspects of lifelong treatment.

MONITORING THE PATIENT WITHOUT MEDICAL THERAPY

Although most patients with ocular hypertension can be managed without medical therapy, these patients must be carefully monitored so that treatment can be instituted before glaucomatous damage occurs. Patients who appear to be least likely to develop such changes are those having normal visual fields and optic discs, IOPs between 21 and 30 mm Hg, and no other significant risk factors. Unfortunately, ocular hypertensive patients not receiving medical therapy do not return for follow-up examinations as often as do ocular hypertensives who are receiving medical therapy. Bigger[244] found that over a 12- to 20-month period, 37% of ocular hypertensive patients were lost to fol-

low-up evaluation. Noncompliance rates were highest in patients who were not prescribed medical therapy. The majority of noncompliant patients were lost to follow-up within 1 month following the initial diagnosis. Such high noncompliance rates can be decreased by careful patient education.

During the initial evaluation, complete baseline information should be obtained, including documentation of the appearance of the optic discs (preferably with stereophotography), visual fields, tonometry, gonioscopy, and evaluation for risk factors. According to the availability and reliability of the diagnostic information and clinical history, each patient's follow-up may be individualized according to the following general guidelines[307,309]: (1) reevaluate at yearly intervals if the IOP is 20 to 24 mm Hg; (2) reevaluate every 6 months if the IOP is 25 to 29 mm Hg; and (3) reevaluate every 3 or 4 months if the IOP is 30 mm Hg or higher if the decision is made to withhold treatment. Each follow-up visit should include evaluation of visual fields, IOPs, careful stereoscopic examination of the optic discs, and reevaluation of risk factors.

Secondary Angle-Closure Glaucoma: Neovascular Glaucoma

Secondary angle-closure glaucoma develops as a consequence of another recognizable disease process that produces a marked narrowing of the anterior chamber angle either by pulling the iris forward or by pushing the iris into the angle. The typical glaucomatous signs of angle-closure glaucoma are usually present. Although secondary angle-closure glaucoma can result from a variety of diseases, only neovascular glaucoma will be considered here.

Diagnosis

Neovascular glaucoma results from growth of new vessels on the iris—rubeosis iridis.[310] Its incidence is highest in patients with diabetic retinopathy or central retinal vein occlusion, but it also occurs in patients with other ocular disorders such as chronic retinal detachment, Coats' disease, retinopathy of prematurity (ROP), ocular neoplastic disorders, and endophthalmitis. It has also developed following helium irradiation for uveal melanoma,[311] and following Nd:YAG laser posterior capsulotomy in diabetic patients.[312]

The new vessels generally form near the pupillary margin and in small isolated areas on the iris. The small vessels then extend in an irregular pattern to cover the iris and the posterior corneal surface near the angle[313] (Fig. 29.31). A fibrovascular membrane develops along the new vessels, and, over time, it contracts and pulls the peripheral iris toward the cornea and physically restricts the aqueous outflow, producing glaucoma. The glaucoma can occur weeks to years following neovascularization of the iris.

One of the earliest diagnostic signs of neovascularization is leakage of fluorescein from the iris vessels into the anterior chamber. Another early sign is tiny dilated capillaries at the pupillary margin. These dilated capillaries can be mistaken for clumps of pigment. As the fibrovascular membrane develops in the pupillary area and contracts, it generally produces an ectropion uveae.

If angle-closure glaucoma does result, there will be significant neovascularization, a markedly narrow or closed angle, corneal edema and an extremely high IOP. Symptoms include ocular pain, conjunctival hyperemia, and blurred vision.

Management

Although neovascular glaucoma is one of the most difficult forms of glaucoma to manage successfully, recent advances have resulted in success rates up to 77%.[314] The most successful treatment occurs when the neovascular process is detected in its earliest phase, before the angle has become closed by peripheral anterior synechiae (PAS). Thus, it is imperative that all susceptible patients be evaluated periodically for the development of rubeosis at the pupillary margin and in the angle.[315] The use of anterior and posterior segment photocoagulation can maintain an open angle in up to 80% of eyes when they are treated before angle closure.[314] However, since progression from onset of neovascularization in the angle to a 360° closure of the angle may occur within weeks, treatment should be provided without delay.

It is practical to divide patients with neovascular glaucoma into those with useful vision and those without useful vision (Fig. 29.32). Patients with useful vision may be treated with panretinal photocoagulation (PRP), goniophotocoagulation (direct laser application to vessels in the angle), or both. PRP may result in regression of the anterior segment neovascularization,[316,317] while goniophotocoagulation may be successful in obliterating these vessels, thereby preventing angle closure. PRP generally requires several weeks to produce clinical regression of the neovascularization, whereas goniophotocoagulation usually results in immediate obliteration of the angle vessels.[314] In patients in whom media opacities preclude PRP, or in eyes that do not respond to photocoagulation therapy, panretinal cryotherapy may be effective.[318]

Once the angle has become closed by PAS, the

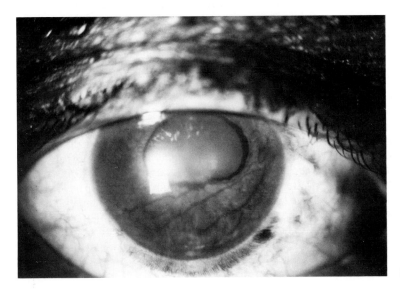

FIGURE 29.31 **Neovascularization of the inferior iris.**

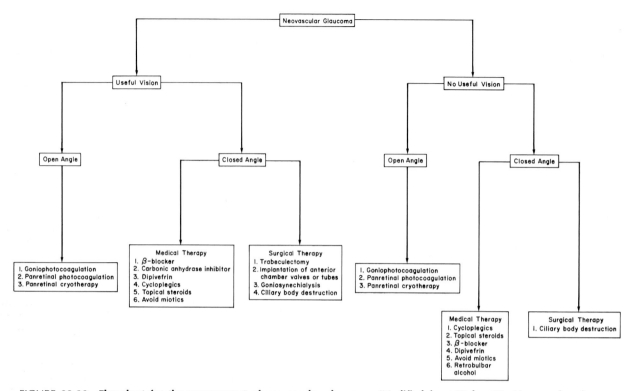

FIGURE 29.32   Flowchart for the management of neovascular glaucoma. (Modified from Weber PA. Neovascular glaucoma. Current management. Surv Ophthalmol 1981;26:149–153.)

prognosis diminishes considerably because laser therapy will be of no benefit in improving outflow facility. If the angle is closed 360° by PAS but there is potential for useful vision, a short clinical trial of medical therapy may be beneficial in some cases. A β blocker, dipivefrin, and carbonic anhydrase inhibitor may be helpful in controlling the IOP.[314] Since the angle is closed, pilocarpine and other miotics are of no benefit. Cycloplegics and topical steroids, however, can often reduce discomfort in these inflamed eyes.[319] Although such medical therapy is justified on a short-term basis, most eyes will prove to be resistant, and various nonmedical approaches will be required (see Fig. 29.32). Trabeculectomy, implantation of anterior chamber valves or tubes, goniosynechialysis, or ciliary body destruction can be attempted in an effort to control the IOP.[314,316,320–322]

If the angle is closed 360° by PAS and there is no potential for useful vision, the primary therapeutic goal is to provide comfort. This can be accomplished with the use of a β blocker or dipivefrin.[314] Carbonic anhydrase inhibitors may also be employed, but they should generally be avoided because of potential systemic side effects. Pilocarpine should also be avoided

because of its ineffectiveness in eyes with total PAS. In addition, pilocarpine causes increased vascular permeability, which leads to increased ocular inflammation and irritation. Additional comfort can be achieved in some eyes with the use of topical cycloplegics and steroids. When these efforts fail to provide an acceptable level of comfort, consideration may be given to cyclocryotherapy, laser therapy of the ciliary body, or retrobulbar alcohol injection.[314] Of these procedures, retrobulbar alcohol injection is the least expensive and the most convenient procedure to use.

Secondary Open-Angle Glaucoma

Secondary open-angle glaucoma develops as a consequence of another recognizable disease process that produces restricted aqueous outflow due to pretrabecular tissue growth, to "clogging" of the pores in the trabecular meshwork, or to an elevated pressure in the episcleral veins. The typical glaucomatous signs of elevated IOP, optic disc changes, or visual field losses are present. The pattern of visual field loss in patients with secondary open-angle glaucoma is similar to that in those with primary open-angle glaucoma, suggesting a similar pathogenic mechanism for the optic nerve damage.[323] Secondary open-angle glaucoma can be caused by many diseases. Some of the more well-known are discussed below.

Pigmentary Glaucoma

Pigmentary glaucoma is associated with the pigmentary dispersion syndrome, characterized by loss of pigment from the posterior surface of the iris and, probably, the ciliary body and by dispersion of this pigment into the anterior chamber. The pigment is moved by the aqueous flow and is deposited on the lens, iris, corneal endothelium, and trabecular meshwork. Because of the direction of aqueous flow, the pigment is often deposited on the corneal endothelium in the shape of a vertical line or spindle—Krukenberg's spindle (Fig. 29.33). It is logical that the circulating pigment could be deposited in the trabecular meshwork, decreasing aqueous outflow and producing a secondary glaucoma.

Pigmentary glaucoma is a rare disease and has a low prevalence even in patients with pigmentary dispersion syndrome. Becker and associates[324] studied 300 patients with and without glaucoma and reported that 10% of patients in each group demonstrated the pigmentary dispersion syndrome. These investigators concluded that pigmentary dispersion syndrome is not a high-risk factor for the development of glaucoma. Kupfer and associates[325] concluded that the occurrence of glaucoma in conjunction with pigmentary dispersion syndrome is probably coincidental. Wilensky and associates[326] stud-

ied patients with Krukenberg's spindle over a 5-year period and found the incidence of glaucoma to be very low, concluding that the presence of Krukenberg's spindle in patients with no visual field defect is not a particularly ominous sign.

There is other information to support the relatively benign nature of pigmentary dispersion syndrome. Although the syndrome occurs more often in myopic females, Lichter and Shaffer[327] have shown that pigmentary glaucoma occurs more often in myopic males. When glaucoma does occur in an eye with Krukenberg's spindle, the cause of glaucoma is frequently not the pigment, but a narrow angle. It has been suggested[327] that the cause of the glaucoma is a congenital deficiency of the mesodermal support tissue of the iris, or other functional angle defect, and that the pigment is simply a contributing factor or is secondary to the underlying etiology.

Even though patients with pigmentary dispersion syndrome do not have a high risk for the development of glaucoma, the risk is probably higher than normal. Thus, the patient with pigmentary dispersion syndrome should be thoroughly evaluated for glaucoma and then monitored at routine examination intervals.

Campbell[328] has proposed that the loss of pigment from the pigment epithelium of the iris occurs from mechanical rubbing of the iris against the anterior zonules during normal dilation and constriction of the pupil. Large globes, as in myopic males, would be more susceptible. The anterior chambers are significantly deeper and the crystalline lens significantly flatter in patients with pigmentary dispersion syndrome than in patients with other forms of open-angle glaucoma.[329,330] It has been suggested that blacks have less

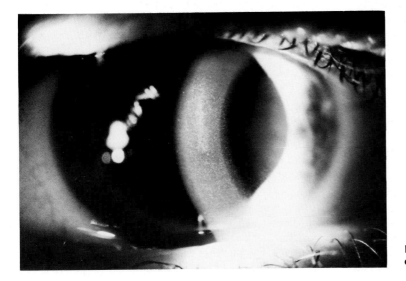

FIGURE 29.33 **Krukenberg's spindle on corneal endothelium.**

pigment dispersion because their iris pigment is more compact and secure. Some patients with pigmentary dispersion syndrome often have a shower of pigment into the angle following vigorous exercise.

Pigmentary glaucoma occurs more often in myopic males around age 35 years.[331] It has also been reported in patients who have had posterior chamber lens implants.[332–334] When it occurs in females, it is usually at an older age, around 50 years. It is a bilateral disease, occurring more often in whites than in blacks. The severity of pigmentary glaucoma decreases with age in some patients, probably due to a reduction in amount of available pigment or the continued phagocytosis of pigment particles by the trabecular endothelial cells and macrophages.[335] More often, however, the severity of pigmentary glaucoma increases with age, especially in patients with increasing iris transillumination, increasing corneal pigmentation, and increasing pigment on the anterior lens capsule.[336,337]

DIAGNOSIS

Evaluation of the patient with pigmentary dispersion syndrome should include gonioscopy, transillumination of the iris, tonometry, stereoscopic optic disc evaluation, and visual fields. The angle must be evaluated gonioscopically to verify the presence of significant pigment in the trabecular meshwork (Fig. 29.34). When the eye is transilluminated, wedge-shaped areas of iris depigmentation can be observed in the mid-periphery of the iris in patients with pigmentary loss.[338]

Epstein and associates[339] have shown that provocative testing with phenylephrine is not productive in identifying latent glaucoma in patients with pigmentary dispersion syndrome. In some patients the instillation of phenylephrine results in the dispersion of iris pigment granules into the aqueous. These investigators observed patients with pigmentary disperion syndrome after the administration of phenylephrine and found that less than one-third of the patients demonstrated a significant increase of pigment in the aqueous, and only 0.04% had an increase in IOP greater than 2 mm Hg. In fact, more patients demonstrated a reduction, rather than an increase, in IOP.

MANAGEMENT

Because of the sometimes wide fluctuations in IOP, pigmentary glaucoma may require treatment only during the acute elevations of pressure.[340] In general, however, it is treated medically, following the same guidelines as for primary open-angle glaucoma, since the major site of impairment is in the trabecular meshwork.[341]

Because most patients with pigmentary glaucoma are young, β blockers or dipivefrin are the initial drugs of choice.[342] Miotics are not generally used because affected patients are often young and the miotics produce spasm of accommodation with resulting blurred vision. Although many clinicians favor use of miotics based on the belief that they reduce iridozonular contact and consequently decrease further pigment liberation, there is no evidence to support such an approach, and, in fact, caution must be observed during miotic therapy because of the relatively high incidence of drug-induced retinal detachment.[336,342] Carbonic anhydrase inhibitors may be employed according to the usual guidelines governing these drugs. They may be effective on a short-term basis during acute elevations of IOP. It has been speculated that thymoxamine, an

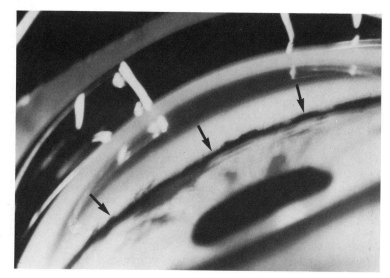

FIGURE 29.34 **Goniophotograph showing 4+ pigment (arrows) in the trabecular meshwork. Compare with Figure 29.10.** (Courtesy Leo P. Semes, O.D.)

α-adrenergic blocking agent, should be beneficial in these patients by constricting the pupil without affecting accommodation, thereby minimizing the iridozonular contact. This would tend to eliminate pigment release and accumulation in the trabecular meshwork.[340] Further studies are needed to substantiate the effectiveness of this treatment modality.

In some patients with pigmentary glaucoma, the pigment decreases in the trabecular meshwork with time (years) by presumably passing through the meshwork and out of the eye. Medical therapy can then be decreased or discontinued. Likewise, in pigmentary glaucoma associated with posterior chamber intraocular lenses (IOLs), the intensity of the glaucoma lessens with time as the pigment liberation from the localized area of IOL-iris contact decreases.[343,344] In the meantime, use of routine antiglaucoma medications is usually effective in controlling the pressure and preventing optic disc damage. Severe glaucoma not controlled medically may require repositioning of the IOL, laser trabeculoplasty, or trabeculectomy. Removal of the offending IOL is not generally advisable because of surgical complications.[343]

In patients for whom maximum-tolerated medical therapy does not allow adequate control of IOP, laser trabeculoplasty should be attempted.[341,342] This procedure, however, often has a high long-term failure rate.[345] Lunde[346] reported a 40% failure rate in eyes with pigmentary glaucoma and suggested that ALT is more beneficial for younger patients with a relatively recent onset of glaucoma.

The surgical management of pigmentary glaucoma follows the same general guidelines as for primary open-angle glaucoma. If medical and laser therapy are not effective, filtration procedures are used and are usually successful.[341,345]

Exfoliation Glaucoma

Exfoliation glaucoma is associated with the exfoliation syndrome. In 1917 Lindberg[347] first reported grayish flaky material at the pupillary margins, and Vogt[348] later associated the presence of the material with glaucoma resulting from decreased aqueous outflow due to exfoliated material in the trabecular meshwork. The flaky material was first considered to be desquamated debris from the crystalline lens capsule. Since further studies suggested that the material was not true exfoliation from the lens capsule, Dvorok-Theobald[349] proposed that the condition be called pseudoexfoliation syndrome. Recent studies, however, have indicated that the exfoliated material comes from multiple sources—lens epithelium, ciliary body epithelium, iris pigment epithelium, and endothelial cells in the tra-

becular meshwork—so the term *exfoliation glaucoma* is generally accepted. Sugar and associates[350] concluded that the exfoliation syndrome is probably a disease entity in which there is degeneration of the limiting basement membrane lining the anterior and posterior chambers.

The relationship between glaucoma and exfoliation syndrome is now well established. Some studies have shown the prevalence of glaucoma in patients with exfoliation syndrome to be as high as 89%.[351] Kozart and Yanoff[352] studied 100 patients with exfoliation syndrome and found that 7% had glaucoma. These investigators also reported that another 13% had ocular hypertension (IOP greater than 21 mm Hg) and that patients with bilateral exfoliation syndrome had a higher incidence of glaucoma. Other investigators have shown that the presence of exfoliation syndrome increases the risk of both ocular hypertension and glaucoma.[353,354]

Exfoliation syndrome is a disease entity that may exist without glaucoma, but it can intensify the condition in a patient with primary open-angle glaucoma, and it can be the primary cause of the glaucoma. Certainly glaucoma must be considered when exfoliation debris is detected.

The movement of the iris probably scrapes the exfoliated material off the anterior lens capsule, leaving a clear zone where the iris moves and depositing the material on the pupillary margins and on the lens surface in the pupillary area (Fig. 29.35). The flow of aqueous moves the debris to the iris, corneal endothelium, and trabecular meshwork, where it decreases aqueous outflow and produces a secondary glaucoma.

Exfoliation glaucoma develops slowly, and although

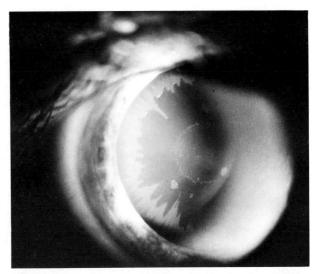

FIGURE 29.35 **Appearance of the crystalline lens in exfoliation syndrome.**

it is often observed in only one eye, it becomes bilateral in many patients.[353] The incidence increases with age and is much more prevalent after age 70 years. The incidence is probably higher in females, higher in people from Scandinavian countries, and much lower in people from central Europe and in American blacks. Familial occurrence of the exfoliation syndrome suggests an autosomal dominant mode of inheritance.[355] There is no apparent association with any systemic disease. It is found in patients with wide and with narrow anterior chamber angles but more often in patients with narrow angles.[356]

DIAGNOSIS

Exfoliation glaucoma is characterized by elevated IOP, optic disc or visual field changes, the presence of flaky, dandruff-like, white or light gray material on the pupillary margin, and a sugar-like frosting on the anterior lens capsule.[357] The material may be present on the iris and corneal endothelium, but it is difficult to see. There may also be slight depigmentation of the pupillary margin and some pigment granules on the corneal endothelium. There is generally heavy pigmentation of the trabecular meshwork, although less than that observed in pigmentary glaucoma. Since the diagnosis of exfoliation syndrome can be easily overlooked, the practitioner must not dismiss the subtle clinical signs that can reveal the disease (Table 29.29).

MANAGEMENT

The medical management of exfoliation glaucoma generally follows the same guidelines as for primary open-angle glaucoma.[358] However, medical therapy is usually not as satisfactory in exfoliation glaucoma as it is in primary open-angle glaucoma.[354,355,359] Pilocarpine can be employed, but the stronger miotics, such as the anticholinesterase agents, should be avoided because of the possibility of drug-induced cataract. Because many of these patients have nuclear sclerotic or posterior subcapsular cataracts, it is advantageous to avoid miosis by employing adrenergic agents such as topical

TABLE 29.29
Subtle Signs of Exfoliation Syndrome

- Pupillary ruff defects
- Iris sphincter transillumination
- Whorl-like particulate pigment deposition on iris sphincter
- Particulate pigment deposition on anterior iris surface and trabecular meshwork
- Exfoliation material on zonules and ciliary body

Adapted from Prince AM, Ritch R. Clinical signs of the pseudoexfoliation syndrome. Ophthalmology 1986;93:803–807.

dipivefrin or β blockers. ALT appears to be a useful adjunct to medical therapy, especially for patients who remain uncontrolled with maximum-tolerated drug therapy.[358] Sherwood and Svedbergh[360] found a 70% success rate with use of ALT in patients with exfoliation glaucoma, and 40% of patients were able to reduce or discontinue their drug therapy. It should be noted, however, that the long-term efficacy of ALT in these patients may be less satisfactory than in patients with primary open-angle glaucoma.[361]

Filtering surgery is indicated in cases that are unresponsive to medical or laser therapy. Although lens extraction may be temporarily beneficial, deposition of exfoliation material can continue following cataract extraction. Thus, it is probably unwise to depend solely on lens extraction as the primary therapeutic approach to exfoliation glaucoma.[359] Trabeculectomy appears to be an effective surgical procedure in most cases. Tarkkanen[355] reported that 85% of patients with exfoliation glaucoma were well controlled without medication 5 years following trabeculectomy, and 92% were controlled with concomitant medical therapy.

Steroid Glaucoma

Some patients receiving long-term topical steroid therapy, or in some cases systemic steroid therapy, respond with a marked increase in IOP.[362] In these patients, the steroid decreases the efficiency of the aqueous outflow mechanism in the trabecular meshwork or the endothelial vacuoles.

Before steroid therapy—especially topical—is instituted, baseline IOP should be recorded. During the course of therapy close observation of the patient is mandatory, monitoring the IOP every 2 to 4 weeks. Although the risk of steroid-induced glaucoma is greatest during the first 4 to 6 weeks of therapy, the patient may develop an acute elevation of pressure at any time, in some instances after several months of therapy.

Most cases of steroid-induced glaucoma respond promptly to discontinuation of the drug.[363] This is usually the only treatment required. In some cases of persistent elevation of IOP, treatment with ocular hypotensive medications may be necessary, following the principles outlined for treatment of primary open-angle glaucoma. Elevated IOP that is resistant to such medical management should be treated by laser trabeculoplasty or filtering procedures. However, it may be reasonable to monitor the patient carefully in cases in which there is no apparent optic nerve damage. Laser trabeculoplasty or filtering surgery should be reserved for patients with progressive optic nerve or visual field damage or for patients in whom such damage seems imminent.[363] Following filtering surgery, steroids can be employed as necessary to control inflammation and scarring without the risk for drug-induced elevation of IOP.[363]

If steroid therapy must be continued despite the presence of elevated IOP, a lower concentration of the drug should be employed or therapy may be continued by changing to medrysone or fluorometholone, both of which demonstrate less propensity to elevate IOP. If decreasing or changing steroid therapy does not reduce IOP, or if such changes in therapy are contraindicated, routine antiglaucoma therapy may be instituted.

Persistent elevation of IOP associated with the use of periocular steroids often responds to standard medical therapy. However, excision of the steroid material may be necessary if the pressure cannot be controlled medically.

Glaucoma Secondary to Uveitis

Uveitis can produce several changes in the anterior chamber that decrease aqueous outflow and elevate IOP. The reduction in aqueous outflow can be due to a decrease in size of the pores in the trabecular meshwork because the trabecular meshwork is swollen and edematous from the inflammation. It may also be caused by blockage of some of the trabecular meshwork pores by inflammatory debris (white blood cells and macrophages) and by an increased viscosity of aqueous due to protein leakage from blood vessels in the iris and ciliary body.

There may be a significant and rapid elevation in IOP with ocular discomfort and corneal edema. A complete glaucoma workup should be performed. Gonioscopy is necessary to differentiate the condition from angle-closure glaucoma and to assess the extent of peripheral anterior synechiae as well as the extent of compromise to the trabecular meshwork.

Management of glaucoma associated with active anterior uveitis is directed primarily toward the inflammation by employing cycloplegics, mydriatics, and steroids and is directed secondarily toward the elevated IOP by employing inhibitors of aqueous formation. If medical therapy fails to adequately control the IOP, surgical intervention may become necessary.

Posterior synechiae should be prevented or broken with the use of topical cycloplegic and mydriatic agents (Fig. 29.36). Use of a combination of 1% atropine twice daily and 2.5% or 10% phenylephrine 4 times daily is often effective in reducing patient discomfort associated with ciliary spasm, reducing intraocular inflammation associated with the uveitis, and preventing the development of posterior synechiae.

Topically applied steroids, along with the atropine,

will usually control the anterior segment inflammation. Since the anti-inflammatory effect is related to the frequency of instillation, a useful dosage regimen is 1 drop of 1% prednisolone acetate every 1 or 2 hours during the acute stage of inflammation. As the inflammatory process subsides, the dosage frequency may gradually be decreased. When persistent elevation of IOP is suspected to be associated with the steroid, changing the drug to medrysone or fluorometholone may be sufficient to reduce pressure while maintaining the steroid's desired anti-inflammatory effect. In some cases it is difficult to determine whether the elevated IOP is caused by the uveitis or the topical steroid.

If the uveitis does not respond adequately to the use of topical steroids, subconjunctival or systemic steroids can be employed. Subconjunctival steroid therapy is often effective with the use of dexamethasone phosphate 4 mg, prednisolone succinate 25 mg, triamcinolone acetonide 4 mg, or methylprednisolone acetate 20 mg.[102] The use of long-acting repository steroids should be avoided, since these may result in a delayed elevation of IOP. Systemic steroids become necessary when the topical or subconjunctival routes of administration have been ineffective. In such cases, prednisone, 80 to 100 mg daily, should be maintained until there is evidence of remission, at which time the daily dosage is decreased 5 mg every second or third day.[102]

Because the side effects of topical or systemic steroids are not insignificant, patients should be monitored carefully for the development of elevated IOP, posterior subcapsular cataracts, and other steroid-related effects. If the uveitis recurs after topical steroid therapy has been discontinued, the possibility of drug-induced inflammation should be considered, and the steroid therapy should be reinstituted and then tapered more slowly.

In addition to the control of the active anterior uveitis, treatment should be directed toward the elevated IOP by employing topical β blockers or dipivefrin.[102] Miotics should be avoided since they can increase the inflammation and lead to the formation of posterior synechiae. When topical antiglaucoma therapy is unsuccessful in adequately controlling the elevated pressure, systemic carbonic anhydrase inhibitors such as methazolamide may be employed. These agents are usually effective in treating glaucoma secondary to inflammatory diseases with obstruction of aqueous outflow.[102]

Elevated IOP that is unresponsive to medical therapy requires surgical intervention. Iridectomy is generally considered to be the procedure of choice, especially if pupillary block is a contributing factor.[102] ALT has been shown to be ineffective in cases of uveitic glaucoma and thus should not be attempted.[364]

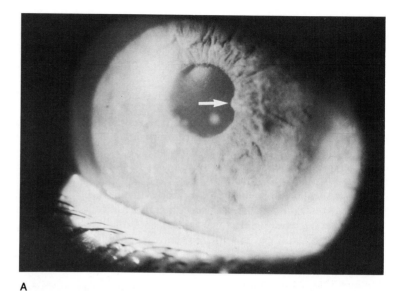

A

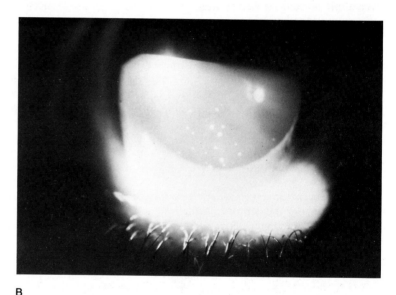

FIGURE 29.36 **Posterior synechiae.** *(A)* **Posterior synechiae (arrow) at the nasal pupillary margin before dilation.** *(B)* **The same eye after dilation. Small white spots are keratic precipitates on corneal endothelium.**

B

Glaucoma Secondary to Cyclitis (Posner-Schlossman Syndrome)

Patients who have recurrent attacks of mild cyclitis can develop glaucoma, since cyclitis can produce an increase in IOP. The increase in IOP is usually rapid. This condition is called glaucomatocyclitic crisis, or the Posner-Schlossman syndrome.[365] It is generally unilateral and occurs in patients between the ages of 20 and 50 years, who report a history of recurrent attacks of unilateral blurred vision. There is usually only slight discomfort associated with the attack, and the attack may last from a few hours to several weeks. The patient

may report that the eye with the blurred vision had a larger pupil during the attack, and the patient can even present with a larger pupil in the affected eye. These patients usually have open anterior chamber angles and do not have any posterior or anterior synechiae, ciliary injection, or numerous cells in the anterior chamber.[366] However, mild conjunctival injection is common. If the patient is not treated for the cyclitis, keratic precipitates can develop on the corneal endothelium, more cells can be present in the aqueous, and the visual acuity can be reduced. These patients generally have normal optic discs and no visual field loss. The increase in IOP is probably due to numerous mononuclear cells in the trabecular meshwork interspaces[367] and to increased aqueous formation.[368]

Since a glaucomatocyclic crisis is a self-limited glaucoma, it will usually subside spontaneously within a few days regardless of treatment. Medical therapy, however, is usually effective in controlling the acute elevations of IOP. The use of a topical β blocker, dipivefrin, or a systemic carbonic anhydrase inhibitor will usually reduce the IOP to normal. Because of the inflammatory process, miotics should be avoided. In addition to this antiglaucoma therapy, topical steroids may be effective in controlling the inflammation, but the patient should be monitored carefully for the development of steroid-induced elevations of IOP.

Prolonged medical therapy with antiglaucoma agents and steroids should be avoided, since such treatment does not prevent recurrences and is unnecessary between attacks. In addition, prolonged steroid therapy increases the risk of cataract, elevated IOP, and other undesirable steroid-related side effects.

Surgical procedures are generally ineffective in preventing recurrent attacks and, indeed, are contraindicated because of the risks they impose in this self-limiting condition.[369] Varma and associates,[370] however, have reported one patient who had no documented recurrent episodes of glaucomatocyclitis crisis during a 12-year period following a trabeculectomy for glaucomatous damage to the optic nerve.

Angle-Recession Glaucoma

Blunt trauma to the eye can result in damage to the anterior chamber angle, reduction in aqueous outflow, and secondary glaucoma. The trauma produces a tear in the ciliary muscle, usually between the circular and longitudinal muscles, creating a recession of the anterior chamber angle[371] (Fig. 29.37). Direct damage to the trabecular meshwork can also occur. In some patients, glaucoma can develop immediately following the trauma or may not occur until months or years later.[374]

Studies have indicated that the incidence of late-onset glaucoma following blunt trauma varies from 2% to 10%.[371,372] The incidence is higher if the angle recession involves 270° or more of the angle,[371] if the patient is older, and if there is familial predisposition for the development of primary open-angle glaucoma. The glaucoma is generally unilateral.

The immediate elevation of IOP may be due to trabecular damage or to the presence of prostaglandins that are released in the anterior chamber. The elevated IOP often lasts for hours, days or weeks. It is generally self-limiting.

Some patients, months to years later, have a gradual increase in IOP and develop glaucoma. These patients generally have a marked angle recession. The elevation of pressure is due to a reduction of aqueous outflow believed to be caused by the resultant scarring of the trabecular meshwork or by the gradual growth of a membrane over the trabecular meshwork.[373]

Patients who have sustained blunt trauma to the eye should be evaluated for possible angle-recession glaucoma by performing gonioscopy, tonometry, stereoscopic optic disc evaluation, and visual fields. In the absence of glaucoma, these patients should be routinely evaluated on an annual basis.[374]

Eyes with angle-recession glaucoma are treated following the same guidelines that apply to the management of primary open-angle glaucoma. It should be

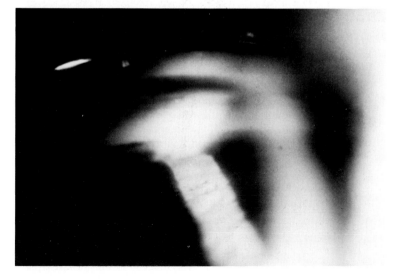

FIGURE 29.37 **Goniophotograph of angle recession. Note that the light beam on the iris appears to be depressed into the angle, exposing a wider than normal band of ciliary body.**

realized, however, that miotics may be ineffective because of the interruption of the normal ciliary muscle-scleral spur relationship induced by the initial traumatic episode.[375] Rarely, a paradoxical elevation of IOP occurs in response to pilocarpine.[376] Paradoxically, the use of atropine in such cases may reduce the pressure and be of therapeutic value by forestalling the need for carbonic anhydrase inhibitors or surgical therapy.[376] Robin and Pollack[364] have shown poor responses to ALT in patients with angle-recession glaucoma.

Glaucoma Secondary to Hyphema

Blunt, nonpenetrating trauma to the eye may cause hyphema, vitreous hemorrhage, iridodialysis, cyclodialysis, or recession of the anterior angle. Blood in the anterior chamber (hyphema) can compromise aqueous outflow and produce glaucoma. Following a total hyphema where the entire anterior chamber is filled with blood ("8-ball" hyphema), the trabecular meshwork is overloaded with blood cells and blood clots, and aqueous outflow decreases, resulting in elevated IOP. On the other hand, hyphemas that occupy less than half the anterior chamber will usually resolve spontaneously within 7 days without complications.[377] However, recession of the angle occurs in about 70% of eyes with hyphema, with the potential risk for acute or late-onset glaucoma.[377]

One of the most important considerations in the patient with hyphema is that of secondary hemorrhage, or rebleeding. This occurs during the first 5 days in about 25% of cases and substantially reduces the prognosis.[378,379] Secondary hemorrhage is associated with a higher incidence of elevated IOP than is the initial hyphema, the incidence of the former being about 50%.[380,381] Any hyphema, however, regardless of its size, can cause elevated IOP, but hyphemas filling at least half the anterior chamber are more likely to produce pressure increases.[382] About one-third of eyes with hyphema will develop an IOP exceeding 24 mm Hg during the acute episode.[379]

The treatment of hyphema has been controversial and has included miotics, cycloplegics, steroids, bed rest, unilateral or bilateral patching, hospitalization, and sedation.[382] There is little difference in outcome, however, between patients treated with bilateral patching, bed rest, and sedation and those who remain ambulatory wearing a patch and shield over the injured eye.[379,383] As a practical matter, elevation of the head of the bed to 30° to 45° seems to facilitate the settling of blood in the anterior chamber, allowing more rapid improvement in vision and an earlier view of the fundus.[382] Since many patients have an associated anterior

uveitis, treatment with cycloplegics and steroids improves comfort and places the iris at rest during the healing process. Hospitalization is not mandatory for small hyphemas, but it allows for daily monitoring of the resolution of the hyphema and of its effects on IOP.[382] Since patients with sickle cell trait are more susceptible to complications from hyphema,[384] black patients presenting with hyphema should be screened for hemoglobin abnormalities.

Although not effective in cases of total hyphema, topical β blockers can be used to reduce elevated IOP. Miotics are generally contraindicated, since they increase vasodilatation and can aggravate any existing uveitis. In addition, one of the most effective drug groups for treatment of elevated IOP is the carbonic anhydrase inhibitors. One should be cautious, however, with the use of acetazolamide, since this drug can increase the ascorbate concentration of the aqueous and lower the pH, producing sickling of erythrocytes in the anterior chamber. This can possibly cause the hyphema to resolve more slowly and lead to additional complications. Methazolamide is a better choice, especially in patients with sickle cell disease.[383] If necessary, hyperosmotic agents (oral glycerol or intravenous mannitol) can also be used.

Since the risk of complications increases with recurrent episodes, it is important to minimize the risk of secondary hemorrhage. Aminocaproic acid (Amicar), an antifibrinolytic agent, has been shown to reduce the incidence of secondary hyphema in adults.[385-388] It is given in an oral dosage of 100 mg/kg body weight every 4 hours for 5 days.[a] Side effects of nausea, vomiting, and systemic hypotension can often be minimized without diminishing efficacy by reducing the dosage to 50 mg/kg body weight.[387] Aminocaproic acid should not be used for hyphemas larger than 75% because it may cause blood clotting in the anterior chamber.[382] The rate of secondary hemorrhage during aminocaproic acid use has been reported to be reduced from about 25% to 7%.[386-388]

Surgical intervention is necessary for cases of total hyphema that are unresponsive to medical therapy. Such treatment, however, should be delayed for at least 7 days, since early surgical intervention is often accompanied by rebleeding and because a significant number of cases will spontaneously resolve during that time.[389] Surgical procedures that have been employed include paracentesis, irrigation with balanced salt solution or fibrinolytic agents, aspiration with an emulsification or vitrectomy unit, or draining the anterior chamber through a trabeculectomy incision.[389]

---

[a]Not approved by the FDA for ophthalmic use.

It should be noted that the ultimate visual outcome is determined more often by damage to the retina or optic nerve by the initial traumatic episode than by the elevation of IOP.

References

1. Mailer CM. Glaucoma: An argument that began with Aristotle. Arch Ophthalmol 1966;76:623–636.
2. Duke-Elder S. System of ophthalmology. St. Louis: C.V. Mosby Co, 1969;3:381.
3. Banister R. A treatise of one hundred and thirteen diseases of the eyes and eye-liddes. London, 1622.
4. Leopold IH. Glaucoma masque. Am J Ophthalmol 1967;63:174–178.
5. Douglas GR, Drance SM, Schulzer M. The visual field and nerve head in angle-closure glaucoma. Arch Ophthalmol 1975;93:409–411.
6. Horie T, Kitazawa Y, Nose H. Visual field changes in primary angle closure glaucoma. Jpn J Ophthalmol 1975;19:108–115.
7. Johnstone MA, Grant WM. Pressure-dependent changes in structures of the aqueous outflow system of human and monkeys' eyes. Am J Ophthalmol 1973;75:365–383.
8. Wollensak J, Mildner I. Pressure in Schlemm's canal and the anterior chamber of the normal as well as the glaucomatous eye of man. Trans Am Acad Ophthalmol Otolaryngol 1975;79:340–341.
9. Bill A. The drainage of aqueous humor. Invest Ophthalmol 1975;14:1–3.
10. Barrie KP, Gum GG, Samuelson DA, et al. Morphologic studies of uveoscleral outflow in normotensive and glaucomatous beagles with fluorescein-labeled dextran. Am J Vet Res 1985;46:89–97.
11. Campbell DG, Boys-Smith JW, Woods WD. Variations of pigmentation and segmentation of pigmentation in primary open-angle glaucoma. Invest Ophthalmol Vis Sci 1984;25(Suppl):122.
12. Quigley HA. The pathogenesis of optic nerve damage in glaucoma. Trans New Orleans Acad Ophthalmol. St. Louis: C.V. Mosby Co, 1985, 111–128.
13. Gallois J. Glaucoma chronique et abaissement de la tension arterielle generale. Bull Soc Ophthalmol 1933;45:110–112.
14. Harrington DO. The pathogenesis of the glaucoma field. Clinical evidence that circulatory insufficiency in the optic nerve is the primary cause of visual field loss in glaucoma. Am J Ophthalmol 1959;47:177–185.
15. Hitchings RA, Spaeth GL. Fluorescein angiography in chronic simple and low-tension glaucoma. Br J Ophthalmol 1977;61:126–132.
16. Sebag J, Thomas JV, Epstein DL, et al. Optic disc cupping in arteritic anterior ischemic optic neuropathy resembles glaucomatous cupping. Ophthalmology 1986;93:357–361.
17. Hayreh SS. Pathogenesis of cupping of the optic disc. Br J Ophthalmol 1974;58:863–876.
18. Nanba K, Schwartz B. Fluorescein angiographic defects of the optic disc in glaucomatous visual field loss. Doc Ophthalmol Proc Ser 1983;35:67–73.
19. Schwartz B. Changes in optic disc in ocular hypertension and glaucoma. Jpn J Ophthalmol 1986;30:143–153.
20. Quigley HA, Addicks EN, Green WR. Optic nerve damage in human glaucoma. III. Quantitative correlation of nerve fiber loss and visual field defect in glaucoma, ischemic neuropathy, papilledema, toxic neuropathy. Arch Ophthalmol 1982;100:135–146.
21. Quigley HA, Hohman RM, Addicks EM, et al. Morphologic changes in the lamina cribrosa correlated with neural loss in open-angle glaucoma. Am J Ophthalmol 1983;95:673–691.
22. Anderson DR, Davis EB. Retina and optic nerve after posterior ciliary artery occlusion. Arch Ophthalmol 1974;92:422–426.
23. Leiberman MF, Maumenee AE, Green WR. Histologic studies of the vasculature of the anterior optic nerve. Am J Ophthalmol 1976;82:405–423.
24. Anderson DR. Pathogenesis of glaucomatous cupping: A new hypothesis. In: Symposium on glaucoma. St. Louis: C.V. Mosby Co, 1975; Chap. 6.
25. Levy SN. The effects of elevated intraocular pressure on slow axonal protein flow. Invest Ophthalmol 1974;13:691–696.
26. Anderson DR, Hendrickson A. Effect of intraocular pressure on rapid axoplasmic transport in monkey optic nerve. Invest Ophthalmol 1974;13:771–783.
27. Sakugawa M, Chihara E. Blockage at two points of axonal transport in glaucomatous eye. Arch Clin Exp Ophthalmol 1985;223:214–218.
28. Nakatani H, Suzuki N. Correlation between the stereographic shape of the ocular fundus and the visual field in glaucomatous eyes. Doc Ophthalmol Proc Ser 1983;35:51–58.
29. Anctil JL, Anderson DR. Early foveal involvement and generalized depression of the visual field in glaucoma. Arch Ophthalmol 1984;102:363–370.
30. Report of the Glaucoma Panel: Vision Research, a National Plan. Bethesda, MD, National Institutes of Health, 1983; vol. 2, part 4:1–10.
31. Vision problems in the US, Data analysis. New York: National Society to Prevent Blindness, 1980.
32. Gibson JM, Rosenthal AR, Lavery J. A study of the prevalence of eye disease in the elderly in an English community. Trans Ophthalmol Soc UK 1985;104:196–203 (Pt. 2).
33. Bengtsson B. The prevalence of glaucoma. Br J Ophthalmol 1981;65:46–49.
34. Hollows FC, Graham PA. Intra-ocular pressure, glaucoma, and glaucoma suspects in a defined population. Br J Ophthalmol 1966;50:570–586.
35. Bankes JLK, Perkins ES, Tsolakis S, et al. Bedford glaucoma survey. Br Med J 1968;1:791–796.
36. Colenbrander MC. The early diagnosis of glaucoma. Ophthalmologica 1971;162:276–281.
37. Hyans SW, Keroub C, Pokotilo E. The computer in clinical research. Prevalence of glaucoma. Doc Ophthalmol 1977;43:17–21.
38. Kini MM, Leibowitz HM, Colton T, et al. Prevalence of senile cataract, diabetic retinopathy, senile macular degeneration, and open-angle glaucoma in the Framingham Eye Study. Am J Ophthalmol 1978;85:28–34.

39. David R, Tessler Z, Yassur Y. Epidemiology of acute angle-closure glaucoma: Incidence and seasonal variations. Ophthalmologica 1985;191:4–7.

40. Becker B, Kolker AE, Roth FD. Glaucoma family study. Am J Ophthalmol 1960;50:557–567.

41. Shin DH, Becker B, Kolker AE. Family history in primary open-angle glaucoma. Arch Ophthalmol 1977;95:598–600.

42. Perkins ES. Family studies in glaucoma. Br J Ophthalmol 1974;58:529–535.

43. Paterson G. Studies on siblings of patients with both angle-closure and chronic simple glaucoma. Trans Ophthalmol Soc UK 1961;81:561–576.

44. Tomlinson A, Leighton DA. Ocular dimensions in the heredity of angle-closure glaucoma. Br J Ophthalmol 1973;57:475–486.

45. Lowe RF. Aetiology of the anatomical basis for primary angle-closure glaucoma. Br J Ophthalmol 1970;54:161–169.

46. Lowe RF. Primary angle-closure glaucoma. Br J Ophthalmol 1964;48:191–195.

47. Biro I. Notes upon the question of hereditary glaucoma. Ophthalmologica 1951;122:228–238.

48. Armaly MF, Monstavicius BF, Sayegh RE. Ocular pressure and aqueous outflow facility in siblings. Arch Ophthalmol 1968;80:354–360.

49. Francois J. Genetics and primary open-angle glaucoma. Am J Ophthalmol 1966;61:652–665.

50. Waardenburg PJ. Genetics and opthalmology. Springfield, IL: Charles C Thomas, 1961.

51. Pollack IP. Diagnosis of the glaucomas. In: Symposium on glaucoma. St Louis: C.V. Mosby Co, 1967; Chap. 2.

52. Luntz MH. Congenital, infantile, and juvenile glaucoma. Ophthalmology 1979;86:793–802.

53. Packer H, Deutsch AR, Lewis PM, et al. Study of the frequency and distribution of glaucoma. JAMA 1959; 171:1090–1093.

54. Turner CC. Open-angle glaucoma—a survey of racial incidence. Am J Optom Physiol Opt 1967;44:56–57.

55. Wilensky JT, Gandhi N, Pan T. Racial influences in open-angle glaucoma. Ann Ophthalmol 1978;10:1398–1402.

56. Martin MJ, Sommer A, Gold EB, et al. Race and primary open-angle glaucoma. Am J Ophthalmol 1985;99:383–387.

57. Lim ASM. Primary angle-closure glaucoma in Singapore. Aust J Ophthalmol 1979;7:23–30.

58. Genio CA, Gavino BC. Glaucoma profile in the Phillipines General Hospital. Philipp J Ophthalmol 1983;15:1–2.

59. Alper MG, Laubach JL. Primary angle-closure glaucoma in the American Negro. Arch Ophthalmol 1963;79:663–668.

60. Luntz MH. Primary angle-closure glaucoma in urbanized South African caucasoid and negro communities. Br J Ophthalmol 1973;57:445–456.

61. Alsbirk PH. Anterior chamber depth and primary angle-closure glaucoma. Acta Ophthalmol 1975;53:89–104.

62. Drance SM. Angle-closure glaucoma among Canadian Eskimos. Can J Ophthalmol 1973;8:252–260.

63. Mann I. Culture, race, climate and eye disease. Springfield, IL: Charles C Thomas, 1966;539.

64. Kass MA, Zimmerman TJ, Alton E, et al. Intraocular pressure and glaucoma in the Zuni Indians. Arch Ophthalmol 1978;96:2212–2213.

65. Bettman JW. Eye disease among American Indians of the Southwest. Arch Ophthalmol 1972;88:263–268.

66. Lowe RF. Comparative incidence of angle-closure glaucoma among different national groups in Victoria, Australia. Br J Ophthalmol 1963;47:721–727.

67. Sugar HS. The mechanical factors in the etiology of acute glaucoma. Am J Ophthalmol 1941;24:851–873.

68. Perkins ES, Phelps CD. Open-angle glaucoma, ocular hypertension, low-tension glaucoma, and refraction. Arch Ophthalmol 1982;100:1464–1467.

69. Alsbirk PH. Primary angle-closure glaucoma. Acta Ophthalmol 1976; Suppl 127:5–31.

70. Tassman IS. The role of stress in ocular disease. Trans Am Acad Ophthalmol Otolaryngol 1957;61:179–193.

71. Weinstein P. Nervism in ophthalmology. Ophthalmologica 1954;127:164–178.

72. Van Alphen GW, Stokvis B. Psychosomatic aspects of intraocular pressure. Nederl Tijdschr Geneesk 1951;95:2246–2256.

73. Duke-Elder S. Textbook of ophthalmology. St. Louis: C.V. Mosby Co, 1942;3:3336.

74. Becker B. Diabetes mellitus and primary open-angle glaucoma. Am J Ophthalmol 1971;71:1–16.

75. Becker B, Kolker AE, Ballin N. Thyroid function and glaucoma. Am J Ophthalmol 1966;61:997–999.

76. Schulzer M, Drance SM. Intraocular pressure, systemic blood pressure, and age: A correlational study. Br J Ophthalmol 1987;71:245–250.

77. Bardelli AM, Hadjistilianou T, Frezzotti R. Etiology of congenital glaucoma. Genetic and extragenetic factors. Ophthalmic Paediatr Genet 1985;6:265–270.

78. Barsoum-Homsy M, Chevrette L. Incidence and prognosis of childhood glaucoma. A study of 63 cases. Ophthalmology 1986;93:1323–1327.

79. Hetherington J. Congenital glaucoma. In: Duane TD, Jaeger EA, eds. Clinical ophthalmology. Philadelphia: Harper & Row, 1979; Chap. 51.

80. Kiskis AA, Markowitz SN, Morin JD. Corneal diameter and axial length in congenital glaucoma. Can J Ophthalmol 1985;20:93–97.

81. Krieglstein GK. Congenital glaucoma—diagnosis and management. Trans Ophthalmol Soc UK 1986;105:549–554.

82. Grote P. Augeninnendruckmessungen bei kleinkindern ohne glaukom in halothanmaskennarkose. Ophthalmologica 1975;171:202–206.

83. Dominguez A, Alvarez MG, Banos MS. Electronic tonometry in the newborn. Adv Ophthalmol 1975;29:88–125.

84. Richardson KT. Optic cup symmetry in normal newborn infants. Invest Ophthalmol 1968;7:137–140.

85. Shaffer RN. New concepts in infants glaucoma. Can J Ophthalmol 1967;2:243–248.

86. Morgan KS, Black B, Ellis FD, et al. Treatment of congenital glaucoma. Am J Ophthalmol 1981;92:799–803.

87. Feman SS, Reinecke RD, eds. Handbook of pediatric ophthalmology. New York: Grune & Stratton, 1978;85–86.

88. deLuise VP, Anderson DR. Primary infantile glaucoma (congenital glaucoma). Surv Ophthalmol 1983;28:1–19.

89. Boger WP. Timolol in childhood glaucoma. Surv Ophthalmol 1983;28:259–261.

90. Haskins HO, Hetherington J, Magee SD, et al. Clinical experience with timolol in childhood glaucoma. Arch Ophthalmol 1985;203:1163–1165.

91. Luntz MH. The advantages of trabeculotomy over goniotomy. J Pediatr Ophthalmol Strabismus 1984;21:150–153.

92. Haskins HD, Shaffer RN, Hetherington J. Goniotomy vs trabeculotomy. J Pediatr Ophthalmol Strabismus 1984;21:153–158.

93. Anderson DR. Trabeculotomy compared to goniotomy for glaucoma in children. Ophthalmology 1983;90:805–806.

94. Cibis GW. Congenital glaucoma. J Am Optom Assoc 1987;58:728–733.

95. Melamed S, Latina MA, Epstein DL. Neodymium:YAG laser trabeculopuncture in juvenile open-angle glaucoma. Ophthalmology 1987;94:163–170.

96. David R, Tessler Z, Yassur Y. Long-term outcome of primary acute angle-closure glaucoma. Br J Ophthalmol 1985;69:261–262.

97. Chandler PA. Narrow-angle glaucoma. Arch Ophthalmol 1952;47:695–716.

98. Kramer P, Ritch R. The treatment of acute angle-closure glaucoma revisited. Ann Ophthalmol 1984;16:1101–1103.

99. Hillman JS. Management of acute glaucoma with pilocarpine-soaked hydrophilic lens. Br J Ophthalmol 1974;58:674–679.

100. Ritch R. Argon laser treatment for medically unresponsive attacks of angle-closure glaucoma. Am J Ophthalmol 1982;94:197–204.

101. Greco JJ, Kelman CD. Systemic pilocarpine toxicity in the treatment of angle-closure glaucoma. Ann Ophthalmol 1973;5:57–59.

102. Krupin T. Glaucoma associated with uveitis. In: Ritch R, Shields MB, eds. The secondary glaucomas. St. Louis: C.V. Mosby Co, 1982;290–306.

103. Ganias F, Mapstone R. Miotics in closed-angle glaucoma. Br J Ophthalmol 1975;59:205–206.

104. Airaksinen PJ, Saari KM, Tiainen TJ, et al. Management of acute closed-angle glaucoma with miotics and timolol. Br J Ophthalmol 1979;63:822–825.

105. Zimmerman TJ. Pilocarpine. Ophthalmology 1981;88:85–88.

106. Hillman JS, Marsters JB, Broad A. Pilocarpine delivery by hydrophilic lens in the management of acute glaucoma. Trans Ophthalmol Soc UK 1975;95:79–84.

107. Simons RJ, Dallow RL. Primary angle-closure glaucoma. In: Duane TD, Jaeger EA, eds. Clinical ophthalmology. Philadelphia: Harper & Row, 1982; Chap. 53.

108. Anderson DR. Corneal indentation to relieve acute angle-closure glaucoma. Am J Ophthalmol 1979;88:1091–1093.

109. Robin AL, Pollack IP. Q-switched neodymium-YAG laser iridotomy in patients in whom the argon laser fails. Arch Ophthalmol 1986;104:531–535.

110. Rivera AH, Brown RH, Anderson DR. Laser iridotomy vs surgical iridectomy. Have the indications changed? Arch Ophthalmol 1985;103:1350–1354.

111. Moster MR, Schwartz LW, Spaeth Gal, et al. Laser iridectomy. A controlled study comparing argon and neodymium:YAG. Ophthalmology 1986;93:20–24.

112. Wise JB. Low-energy liner-incision neodymium:YAG laser

113. Drake MV. Neodymium:YAG laser iridotomy. Surv Ophthalmol 1987;32:171–177.

114. Cashwell LF. Laser iridotomy for management of angle-closure glaucoma. South Med J 1985;78:288–291.

115. Cohen JS, Bibler L, Tucker D. Hypopyon following laser iridotomy. Ophthalmic Surg 1984;15:604–606.

116. Haut J, Gaven I, Moulin F, et al. Study of the first hundred phakic eyes treated by peripheral iridotomy using the N.D. Yag laser. Int Ophthalmol 1986;9:227–235.

117. Yamamoto T, Shirato S, Kitazawa Y. Treatment of primary angle-closure glaucoma by argon laser iridotomy: A long-term follow-up. Jpn J Ophthalmol 1985;29:1–12.

118. Willis DA, Stewart RH, Kimbrough RL. Pupillary block associated with posterior chamber lenses. Ophthalmic Surg 1985;16:108–109.

119. Cinotti DJ, Reiter DJ, Maltzman BA, et al. Neodymium:YAG laser therapy for pseudophakic pupillary block. J Cataract Refract Surg 1986;12:174–179.

120. Gieser DK, Wilensky JT. Laser iridectomy in the management of chronic angle-closure glaucoma. Am J Ophthalmol 1984;98:446–450.

121. Pollack IP. Current concepts in laser iridotomy. Int Ophthalmol Clin 1984;24:153–180.

122. Brown RH, Stewart RH, Lynch MG, et al. ALO 2145 reduces the intraocular pressure elevation after anterior segment laser surgery. Ophthalmology 1988;95:378–384.

123. Robin AL, Pollack IP, deFaller JM. Effects of topical ALO 2145 (p-aminoclonidine hydrochloride) on the acute intra-ocular pressure rise after argon laser iridotomy. Arch Ophthalmol 1987;105:1208–1211.

123a. Robin AL. Short-term effects of unilateral 1% apraclonidine therapy. Arch Ophthalmol 1988;106:912–915.

124. Robin AL, Pollack IP, House B, Enger C. Effects of ALO 2145 on intraocular pressure following argon laser trabeculoplasty. Arch Ophthalmol 1987;105:646–650.

125. Hillman JS. Acute closed-angle glaucoma. An investigation into the effect of delay in treatment. Br J Ophthalmol 1979;63:817–821.

126. Ingram RM, Ennis JR. Acute glaucoma: Results of treatment by bilateral simultaneous iridectomy, now without admission to hospital. Br J Ophthalmol 1983;67:367–371.

127. Van Herick W, Shaffer RN, Schwartz A. Estimation of width of angle of anterior chamber. Am J Ophthalmol 1969;68:626–630.

128. Wilensky JT. Current concepts in primary angle-closure glaucoma. Ann Ophthalmol 1977;9:963–972.

129. Desjardins D, Parrish RK. Inversion of anterior chamber pigment as a possible prognostic sign in narrow angles. Am J Ophthalmol 1985;100:480–481.

130. Becker B, Shaffer RN. Diagnosis and therapy of glaucoma. St Louis: C.V. Mosby Co, 1961.

131. Spaeth GL. Classification and management of patients with narrow or closed angles. Ophthalmic Surg 1978;9:39–44.

132. Forbes M. Gonioscopy with corneal indentation. A method for distinguishing between a positional closure and synechial closure. Arch Ophthalmol 1966;76:488–492.

133. Lowe RF. Primary angle-closure glaucoma. Br J Ophthalmol 1967;51:727–731.

134. Harris LS, Galin MA. Prone provocative testing for narrow-angle glaucoma. Arch Ophthalmol 1972;87:493–496.

135. Tomlinson A, Leighton DA. Ocular dimensions and the heredity of open-angle glaucoma. Br J Ophthalmol 1974;58:68–74.

136. Walker MW. Ocular hypertension. Trans Ophthalmol Soc UK 1974;94:525–534.

137. Kimura R, Levene RZ. Gonioscopic differences between primary open-angle glaucoma and normal subjects over 40 years of age. Am J Ophthalmol 1975;80:56–61.

138. Verhoeff FH. The pathogenesis of glaucoma. Arch Ophthalmol 1925;54:20–37.

139. Weinstein BI, Munnangi P, Gordon GG, et al. Defects in cortisol-metabolizing enzymes in primary open-angle glaucoma. Invest Ophthalmol Vis Sci 1985;26:890–893.

140. Becker B, Unger HH, Coleman SL, et al. Plasma cells and gamma-globulin in trabecular meshwork of eyes with primary open-angle glaucoma. Arch Ophthalmol 1963;70:38–41.

141. Waltman SR, Yarian D. Antinuclear antibodies in open-angle glaucoma. Invest Ophthalmol 1974;13:695–697.

142. Segawa K. Ultrastructural changes of the trabecular tissue in primary open-angle glaucoma. Jpn J Ophthalmol 1975;19:317–338.

143. Rodrigues MM, Katz SI, Foidart JM, Spaeth GL. Collagen, factor VIII antigen, and immunoglobulins in the human aqueous drainage channels. Ophthalmology 1980;87:337–342.

144. Alvardo J, Murphy C, Juster R. Trabecular meshwork cellularity in primary open-angle glaucoma and nonglaucomatous normals. Ophthalmology 1984;91:564–579.

145. Tripathi RC. Aqueous outflow pathway in normal and glaucomatous eyes. Br J Ophthalmol 1972;56:157–174.

146. Kolker AE, Hetherington LJ. Becker-Shaffer's diagnosis and therapy of the glaucomas, ed. 3. St Louis: C.V. Mosby Co, 1970;249.

147. Johnson DH, Brubaker RF. Glaucoma: An overview. Mayo Clinic Proc 1986;61:59–67.

148. Kohn AN, Moss AP, Podos SM. Relative afferent pupillary defects in glaucoma without characteristic field loss. Arch Ophthalmol 1979;97:294–296.

149. Brown RH, Zilis JD, Lynch MG, et al. The afferent pupillary defect in asymmetric glaucoma. Arch Ophthalmol 1987;105:1540–1543.

150. Armaly MF. The visual field defect and ocular pressure level in open-angle glaucoma. Invest Ophthalmol 1969;8:105–124.

151. Cameron D, Finlay ET, Jackson CRS. Tonometry and tonography in the diagnosis of chronic simple glaucoma. Br J Ophthalmol 1971;55:738–741.

152. Spaeth GL. The effect of change in intraocular pressure on the natural history of glaucoma: Lowering intraocular pressure in glaucoma can result in improvement of visual fields. Trans Ophthalmol Soc UK 1985;104:256–264 (Pt. 3).

153. David R, Zangwill LM, Tessler Z, et al. The correlation between intraocular pressure and refractive status. Arch Ophthalmol 1985;103:1812–1815.

154. Schappert-Kemmijser J. A five year follow-up of subjects with IOP of 22-30 mm Hg without anomalies of optic nerve and visual field typical for glaucoma at first investigation. Ophthalmologica 1971;162:289–295.

155. Pohjanpelto PEJ, Palva J. Ocular hypertension and glaucomatous optic nerve damage. Acta Ophthalmol 1974;52:194–200.

156. Bengtsson B. Some factors affecting the distribution of intraocular pressure in a population. Acta Ophthalmol 1972;50:33–46.

157. Kitazawa Y, Horie T. Diurnal variation of intraocular pressure and its significance in the medical treatment of primary open-angle glaucoma. In: Krieglstein GK, Leydhecker W, eds. Glaucoma update. New York: Springer-Verlag, 1979;169–176.

158. Drance SM. The significance of the diurnal tension variations in normal and glaucomatous eyes. Arch Ophthalmol 1960;64:494–501.

159. Carel RS, Korczyn AD, Rock M. Ocular tension: Comparison between the two eyes. Ophthalmologica 1985;190:98–101.

160. Beck RW, Messner DK, Musch DC, et al. Is there a racial difference in physiologic cup size? Ophthalmology 1985;92:873–876.

161. Armaly MF. The optic cup in the normal eye. Am J Ophthalmol 1969;68:401–407.

162. Armaly MF. Cup/disc ratio in early open-angle glaucoma. Doc Ophthalmol 1969;26:526–533.

163. Schwartz B. Cupping and pallor of the optic disc. Arch Ophthalmol 1973;89:272–277.

164. Weisman RL, Asseff CF, Phelps CD, et al. Vertical elongation of the optic cup in glaucoma. Trans Am Acad Ophthalmol Otolaryngol 1973;77:157–161.

165. Kirsch RE, Anderson DR. Clinical recognition of glaucomatous cupping. Am J Ophthalmol 1973;75:442–454.

166. Gloster J, Parry DG. Use of phonographs for measuring cupping in the optic disc. Br J Ophthalmol 1974;58:850–862.

167. Airaksinen PJ, Drance SM, Douglas GR, et al. Neuroretinal rim areas and visual field indices in glaucoma. Am J Ophthalmol 1985;99:107–110.

168. Airaksinen PJ, Drance SM, Schulzer M. Neuroretinal rim area in early glaucoma. Am J Ophthalmol 1985;99:1–4.

169. Caprioli J, Miller JM, Sears M. Quantitative evaluation of the optic nerve head in patients with unilateral visual field loss from primary open-angle glaucoma. Ophthalmology 1987;94:1484–1487.

170. Trobe JD, Glaser JS, Cassady J, et al. Non-glaucomatous excavation of the optic disc. Arch Ophthalmol 1980;98:1046–1050.

171. Balaszi AG, Drance SM, Schulzer M, et al. Neuroretinal rim area in suspected glaucoma and early chronic open-angle glaucoma. Arch Ophthalmol 1984;102:1011–1014.

172. Read RM, Spaeth GL. The practical clinical appraisal of the optic disc in glaucoma. Trans Am Acad Ophthalmol Otolaryngol 1974;78:255–274.

173. Samples JR, van Buskirk M, Shults WT, Van Dyk HJ. Optic nerve head drusen and glaucoma. Arch Ophthalmol 1985;103:1678–1680.

174. Fishman RS. Optic disc asymmetry. Arch Ophthalmol 1970;84:590–594.

175. Armaly MJ. Genetic determination of cup/disc ratio of the optic nerve. Arch Ophthalmol 1967;78:35–43.

176. Odberg T, Riise D. Early diagnosis of glaucoma. The value of successive stereophotography of the optic disc. Acta Ophthalmol 1985;63:257–263.

177. Algazi VR, Keltner JL, Johnson CA. Computer analysis of the optic cup in glaucoma. Invest Ophthalmol Vis Sci 1985;26:1759–1770.

178. Caprioli J, Klingbeil U, Sears M, et al. Reproducibility of optic disc measurements with computerized analysis of stereoscopic video images. Arch Ophthalmol 1986;104:1035–1039.

179. Schwartz B, Takamoto T, Nagin P. Measurements of reversibility of optic disc cupping and pallor in ocular hypertension and glaucoma. Ophthalmology 1985;92:1396–1407.

180. Greenidge KC, Spaeth GL, Traverso CE. Change in appearance of the optic disc associated with lowering of intraocular pressure. Ophthalmology 1985;92:897–903.

181. Pederson JE, Herschler JH. Reversal of glaucomatous cupping in adults. Arch Ophthalmol 1982;100:426–431.

182. Hoskins HD, Gelber EC. Optic disk topography and visual field defects in patients with increased intraocular pressure. Am J Ophthalmol 1975;80:284–290.

183. Douglas GR, Drance SM, Schulzer M. A correlation of fields and discs in open-angle glaucoma. Can J Ophthalmol 1974;9:391–398.

184. Hitchings RA, Spaeth GL. The optic disc in glaucoma. II. Correlation of the appearance of the optic disc with the visual field. Br J Ophthalmol 1977;61:107–113.

185. Motolko M, Drane SM. Features of the optic disc in preglaucomatous eyes. Arch Ophthalmol 1981;99:1992–1994.

186. Nagin P, Schwartz B, Reynolds G. Measurement of fluorescein angiograms of the optic disc and retina using computerized image analysis. Opthalmology 1985;92:547–552.

187. Shihab ZM, Lee PF, Hay P. The significance of disc hemorrhage in open-angle glaucoma. Ophthalmology 1982;89:211–213.

188. Heijl A. Frequent disc photography and computerized perimetry in eyes with optic disc hemorrhage. A pilot study. Acta Ophthalmol 1986;64:274–281.

189. Poinoosawmy D, Gloster J, Nagasubramanian S, et al. Association between optic disc hemorrhages in glaucoma and abnormal glucose tolerance. Br J Ophthalmol 1986;70:599–602.

190. Cockburn DM. Clinical significance of hemorrhages in the optic disc. Am J Optom Physiol Opt 1987;64:450–457.

191. Bengtsson B, Holmin C, Krakau CET. Disc hemorrhage and glaucoma. Acta Ophthalmol 1981;59:1–14.

192. Hoyt WF, Frisen L, Newman NM. Fundoscopy of the nerve fiber layer defects in glaucoma. Invest Ophthalmol 1973;12:814–829.

193. Quigley HA, Miller NR, George T. Clinical evaluation of nerve fiber layer atrophy as an indicator of glaucomatous optic nerve damage. Arch Ophthalmol 1980;98:1564–1571.

194. Sommer A, Miller N, Quigley H, et al. Assessment of the nerve fiber layer as a predictor of glaucoma. Invest Ophthalmol Vis Sci 1985;26:122–128.

195. Airaksinen PJ, Drance SM, Douglas GR, et al. Diffuse and localized nerve fiber layer loss in glaucoma. Am J Ophthalmol 1984;98:566–571.

196. Fulk GW, Van Veen HG. How to photograph and evaluate the retinal nerve fiber layer. J Am Optom Assoc 1986;57:760–763.

197. Peli E, Hedges TR, Schwartz B. Computerized enhancement of retinal nerve fiber layer. Acta Ophthalmol 1986;64:113–122.

198. Primrose J. Early signs of the glaucomatous disc. Br J Ophthalmol 1971;55:820–825.

199. Wilensky JT, Kolker AE. Peripapillary changes in glaucoma. Am J Ophthalmol 1976;81:341–345.

200. Armaly MF. Ocular pressure and visual fields. Arch Ophthalmol 1969;81:25–40.

201. Pederson JE, Anderson DR. The mode of progressive disc cupping in ocular hypertension and glaucoma. Arch Ophthalmol 1980;98:490–495.

202. Sturmer J. What do glaucomatous visual fields really look like in fine-grid computerized profile perimetry? Dev Ophthalmol 1985;12:1–47.

203. Wilensky JT, Mermelstein JR, Siegel HC. The use of different-sized stimuli in automated perimetry. Am J Ophthalmol 1986;101:710–713.

204. Postaire JG, Hache JC, Diaf M. Fully automated screening procedure for early detection of visual field defects. J Biomed Eng 1986;8:156–161.

205. Brussell EM, White CW, Fauber J, et al. Multi-flash campimetry as an indicator of visual field loss in glaucoma. Am J Optom Physiol Opt 1986;63:32–40.

206. Duggan C, Sommer A, Auer C, et al. Automated differential threshold perimetry for detecting glaucomatous visual field loss. Am J Ophthalmol 1985;100:420–423.

207. Werner EB, Bishop KI, Koelle J, et al. A comparison of experienced clinical observers and statistical tests in detection of progressive visual field loss in glaucoma using automated perimetry. Arch Ophthalmol 1988;106:619–623.

208. Quigley HA, Addicks EM, Green WR, et al. Optic nerve damage in glaucoma. II. The site of injury and the susceptibility to damage. Arch Opthalmol 1981;99:635–649.

209. Heijl A, Lundquist L. The frequency distribution of earliest glaucomatous visual field defects documented by automatic perimetry. Acta Ophthalmol 1984;62:658–664.

210. Armaly MF. Selective perimetry for glaucomatous defects in ocular hypertension. Arch Ophthalmol 1972;87:518–524.

211. Bryars JH, Cowan EC, Linton D. The earliest visual field changes in glaucoma simplex. Trans Ophthalmol Soc UK 1974;94:1050–1052.

212. Caprioli J, Spaeth GL. Static threshold examination of the peripheral nasal visual field in glaucoma. Arch Ophthalmol 1985;103:1150–1154.

213. Werner EB, Beraskow J. Temporal visual field defects in glaucoma. Can J Ophthalmol 1980;15:13–14.

214. Weber J, Dobek K. What is the most suitable grid for computer perimetry in glaucoma patients. Ophthalmologica 1986;192:88–96.

215. Henson DB, Chauhan B. Informational content of visual field location in glaucoma. Doc Ophthalmol 1985;59:341–352.

216. Hart WM, Becker B. The onset and evolution of glaucomatous visual field defects. Ophthalmology 1982;89:268–279.

217. Mikelberg FS, Schulzer M, Drance SM, Lau W. The rate

of progression of scotomas in glaucoma. Am J Ophthalmol 1986;101:1–6.

218. Hart WM, Becker B. The onset and evolution of glaucomatous visual field defects. Ophthalmology 1982;89:268–279.

219. Forbes M. Influence of miotics on visual fields in glaucoma. Invest Ophthalmol 1966;5:139–145.

220. Schwartz B. Management of ocular hypertension. Surv Ophthalmol 1980;25:208–221.

221. McCluskey DJ, Douglas JP, O'Connor PS, et al. The effect of pilocarpine on the visual field in normals. Ophthalmology 1986;93:843–846.

222. Hamill TR, Post RB, Johnson CA, et al. Correlations of color vision deficits and observable changes in the optic disc in a population of ocular hypertensives. Arch Ophthalmol 1984;102:1637–1939.

223. Gundvy K, Arden GB, Perry S, et al. Color vision defects in ocular hypertension and glaucoma. Arch Ophthalmol 1988;106:929–935.

224. Goldthwaite D, Lakowski R, Drance SM. A study of dark adaptation in ocular hypertensives. Can J Ophthalmol 1976;11:55–60.

225. Motolko MA, Phelps CD. Contrast sensitivity in asymmetric glaucoma. International Ophthalmol 1984;7:45–50.

226. Lundh B. Centeral and peripheral contrast sensitivity for static and dynamic sinusoidal grating in glaucoma. Acta Ophthalmol 1985;63:487–492.

227. Towle VL, Moskowitz A, Sokol S, et al. The VEP in glaucoma and ocular hypertension. Invest Ophthalmol Vis Sci 1983;24:175–183.

228. Weinstern GW, Arden GB, Hitchings RA, et al. The pattern electroretinograph (PERG) in ocular hypertension and glaucoma. Arch Ophthalmol 1988;106:923–928.

229. Drum B, Johnson MA, Quigley HA, et al. Pattern ERG and optic nerve histology in monkeys with laser-induced glaucoma. Invest Ophthalmol Vis Sci 1986;27(Suppl):40.

230. Eskridge JB. Ocular hypertension or early undetected glaucoma? J Am Optom Assoc 1987;58:747–769.

231. Sears ML. Clinical and scientific basis for the management of open-angle glaucoma. Arch Ophthalmol 1986;104:191–195.

232. Quigley HA. A reevaluation of glaucoma management. Int Ophthalmol Clin 1984;24:1–11.

233. Grant WM, Burke JF. Why do some people go blind from glaucoma? Ophthalmology 1982;89:991–998.

234. Schwartz B. Primary open-angle glaucoma. In: Duane TD, Jaeger EA, eds. Clinical ophthalmology. Philadelphia: Harper & Row 1982; Chap. 52.

235. Kitazawa Y, Horie T. Diurnal variation of intraocular pressure in primary open-angle glaucoma. Am J Ophthalmol 1975;79:557–566.

236. Kwitko GM, Shin DH, Ahn BH, et al. Bilateral effects of long-term monocular timolol therapy. Am J Ophthalmol 1987;104:591–594.

237. Smith J, Wandel T. Rationale for the one-eye therapeutic trial. Ann Ophthalmol 1986;18:8.

238. Durkee DP, Bryant BG. Drug therapy reviews: Drug therapy of glaucoma. Am J Hosp Pharm 1978;35:682–690.

239. Soll DB, Saxon AM. Drugs and glaucoma. Am Fam Physician 1986;34:181–185.

240. Olander K, Zimmerman TJ. Practical aspects of controlling

glaucoma medically or how to make your glaucoma medicines work for you. Ann Ophthalmol 1980;12:717–718.

241. Kass MA, Meltzer DW, Gordon M, et al. Compliance with topical pilocarpine treatment. Am J Ophthalmol 1986;101:515–523.

242. Kass MA, Gordon M, Meltzer DW. Can ophthalmologists correctly identify patients defaulting from pilocarpine therapy? Am J Ophthalmol 1986;101:524–530.

243. Granström P-A, Norell S. Visual ability and drug regimen—relation to compliance with glaucoma therapy. Acta Ophthalmol 1983;61:206–219.

244. Bigger JF. A comparison of patient compliance in treated vs untreated ocular hypertension. Trans Am Acad Ophthalmol Otolaryngol 1976;81:277–285.

245. Kooner KS, Zimmerman TJ. The cost of antiglaucoma medications. Ann Ophthalmol 1987;19:327–328.

246. Zimmerman TJ, Zalta AH. Facilitating patient compliance in glaucoma therapy. Surv Ophthalmol 1983;28:252–257.

247. Ashburn FS, Goldberg I, Kass MA. Compliance with ocular therapy. Surv Ophthalmol 1980;24:237–248.

248. Brown MM, Brown GC, Spaeth GL. Improper topical self-administration of ocular medication among patients with glaucoma. Can J Ophthalmol 1984;19:2–5.

249. MacKean JM, Elkington AR. Compliance with treatment of patients with chronic open-angle glaucoma. Br J Ophthalmol 1983;67:46–49.

250. Zimmerman TJ, Ziegler LP. Successful topical medication: Methodology as well as diligence. Ann Ophthalmol 1984;16:109.

251. Kass MA, Gordon M, Morley RE, et al. Compliance with topical timolol treatment. Am J Ophthalmol 1987;103:188–193.

252. Kooner KS, Zimmerman TJ. A glaucoma medication timetable card. Ann Ophthalmol 1987;19:43–44.

253. Novack GO, David R, Lee PF, et al. Effect of changing medication regimens in glaucoma patients. Ophthalmologica 1988;196:23.

254. Kowal DJ, Fingeret M. A glaucoma control chart. J Am Optom Assoc 1987;58:734–737.

255. Sugar HS. Pitfalls in the medical treatment of simple glaucoma. Ann Ophthalmol 1979;11:1041–1050.

256. Drance SM. Medical control of open-angle glaucoma. Can J Ophthalmol 1978;13:123–127.

257. Wilensky JT, Gieser DK, Mori MT, et al. Self-tonometry to manage patients with glaucoma and apparently controlled intraocular pressure. Arch Ophthalmol 1987;105:1072–1075.

258. Remis LL, Epstein DL. Treatment of glaucoma. Ann Rev Med 1984;35:195–205.

259. Tuulonen A, Airaksinen PJ, Kuulasmaa K. Factors influencing the outcome of laser trabeculoplasty. Am J Ophthalmol 1985;99:388–391.

260. Grinich NP, Van Buskirk EM, Samples JR. Three-year efficacy of argon laser trabeculoplasty. Ophthalmology 1987;94:858–861.

261. Migdal C, Hitchings R. Primary therapy for chronic simple glaucoma. The role of argon laser trabeculoplasty. Trans Ophthalmol Soc UK 1984;104:62–66.

262. Watson PG, Allen ED, Graham CM, et al. Argon laser trabeculoplasty or trabeculectomy. A prospective randomised block study. Trans Ophthalmol Soc UK 1984;104:55–61.

263. Schwartz AL, Love DC, Schwartz MA. Long-term follow-up of argon laser trabeculoplasty for uncontrolled open-angle glaucoma. Arch Ophthalmol 1985;103:1482–1484.

264. Goldberg I. Argon laser trabeculoplasty and the open-angle glaucomas. Aust NZ J Ophthalmol 1985;13:243–248.

265. Krupin T, Patkin R, Kurata FK, et al. Argon laser trabeculoplasty in black and white patients with primary open-angle glaucoma. Ophthalmology 1986;93:811–816.

266. Thomas JV, Simmons RJ, Belcher CD, et al. Laser trabeculoplasty: Technique, indications, results, and complications. Int Ophthalmol Clin 1984;24:97–120.

267. Van Buskirk EM, Pond V, Rosenquist RC, et al. Argon laser trabeculoplasty. Studies of mechanism of action. Ophthalmology 1984;91:1005–1010.

268. Bylsma SS, Samples JR, Acott TS, et al. Trabecular cell division after argon laser trabeculoplasty. Arch Ophthalmol 1988;106:544–547.

269. Tuulonen A, Niva A-K, Alanko HI. A controlled five-year follow-up study of laser trabeculoplasty as primary therapy for open-angle glaucoma. Am J Ophthalmol 1987;104:334–338.

270. Pollack IP, Robin AL, Sax H. The effect of argon laser trabeculoplasty on the medical control of primary open-angle glaucoma. Ophthalmology 1983;90:785–789.

271. Gilbert CM, Brown RH, Lynch MG. The effect of argon laser trabeculoplasty on the rate of filtering surgery. Ophthalmology 1986;93:362–365.

272. Shingleton BJ, Richter CU, Bellows AR, et al. Long-term efficacy of argon laser trabeculoplasty. Ophthalmology 1987;94:1513–1518.

273. Hoskins HD, Hetherington J, Minckler DS, et al. Complications of laser trabeculoplasty. Ophthalmology 1983;90:796–799.

274. Ofner S, Samples JR, Van Buskirk EM. Pilocarpine and the increase in intraocular pressure after trabeculoplasty. Am J Ophthalmol 1984;97:647–649.

275. Kolker AE. Visual prognosis in advanced glaucoma: A comparison of medical and surgical therapy for retention of vision in 101 eyes with advanced glaucoma. Trans Am Ophthalmol Soc 1977;75:539–555.

276. Caprioli J, Strang SL, Spaeth GL, et al. Cyclocryotherapy in the treatment of advanced glaucoma. Ophthalmology 1985;92:947–954.

277. Brindler G, Shields MB. Value and limitations of cyclocryotherapy. Arch Clin Exp Ophthalmol 1986;224:545–548.

278. Klapper RM, Wandel T, Donnenfeld E, et al. Transscleral neodymium:YAG thermal cyclophotocoagulation in refractory glaucoma. A preliminary report. Ophthalmology 1988;95:719–722.

279. Devenyi RG, Trope GE, Hunter WH, et al. Neodymium:YAG transscleral cyclocoagulation in human eyes. Ophthalmology 1987;94:1519–1522.

280. Patel A, Thompson JT, Michels RG, et al. Endolaser treatment of the ciliary body for uncontrolled glaucoma. Ophthalmology 1986;93:825–830.

281. Margo CE. Therapeutic ultrasound. Light and electron microscopic findings in an eye treated for glaucoma. Arch Ophthalmol 1986;104:735–738.

282. Coleman DJ, Lizzi FL, Driller J, et al. Therapeutic ultrasound in the treatment of glaucoma. II. Clinical applications. Ophthalmology 1985;92:347–353.

283. Burgess SEP, Silverman RH, Coleman DJ, et al. Treatment of glaucoma with high-intensity focused ultrasound. Ophthalmology 1986;93:831–838.

284. Levene RZ. Low tension glaucoma: A critical review and new material. Surv Ophthalmol 1980;24:621–664.

285. Shiose Y. Prevalence and clinical aspects of low tension glaucoma. In: Henkind P, ed. Acta XXIV International Congress of Ophthalmology. Philadelphia: JB Lippincott Co, 1983.

286. Gorin G. Clinical glaucoma. New York: Marcel Dekker, 1977.

287. Galin MA, McIvor JW, Magruder GB. Influence of position in intraocular pressure. Am J Ophthalmol 1963;55:720–723.

288. Hyams SW, Frankel A, Keroub C, et al. Postural changes in intraocular pressure with particular reference to low tension glaucoma. Glaucoma 1984;6:178–181.

289. Demailly P, Cambien F, Plouin PF, et al. Do patients with low tension glaucoma have particular cardiovascular characteristics? Ophthalmologica 1984;188:65–75.

290. Kitazawa Y, Shirato S, Yamamoto T. Optic disc hemorrhages in low tension glaucoma. Ophthalmology 1986;93:853–857.

291. Caprioli J, Spaeth GL. Comparison of the optic nerve head in high- and low-tension glaucoma. Arch Ophthalmol 1985;103:1145–1149.

292. Caprioli J, Spaeth GL. Comparison of visual field defects in the low-tension glaucomas with those in the high-tension glaucomas. Am J Ophthalmol 1984;97:730–737.

293. King D, Drance SM, Douglas G, et al. Comparison of visual field defects in normal-tension glaucoma and high-tension glaucoma. Am J Ophthalmol 1986;101:204–207.

294. Gloster J. Atromid and glaucoma. Trans Ophthalmol Soc UK 1974;94:567–569.

295. Schwartz AL, Perman KI, Whitten M. Argon laser trabeculoplasty in progressive low-tension glaucoma. Ann Ophthalmol 1984;16:560–566.

296. Sharpe ED, Simmons RJ. Argon laser trabeculoplasty as a means of decreasing intraocular pressure from "normal" levels in glaucomatous eyes. Am J Ophthalmol 1985;99:704–707.

297. Abedin S, Simmons RJ, Grant WM. Progressive low-tension glaucoma. Ophthalmology 1982;89:1–6.

298. Kass MA, Hart WM, Gordon M, et al. Risk factors favoring the development of glaucomatous visual field loss in ocular hypertension. Surv Ophthalmol 1980;25:155–162.

299. Cockburn DM. The prevalence of ocular hypertension in patients of an optometrist and the incidence of glaucoma occurring during long-term follow-up of ocular hyptertensives. Am J Optom Physiol Opt 1982;59:330–337.

300. Levene R. Indications for medical treatment of ocular hypertension and the initial use of pilocarpine. Surv Ophthalmol 1980;25:183–187.

301. Shin DH, Kolker AE, Kass MA, et al. Long-term epinephrine therapy of ocular hypertension. Arch Ophthalmol 1976;94:2059–2060.

302. David R, Livingston DG, Luntz MH. Ocular hypertension—a long-term follow-up of treated and untreated patients. Br J Ophthalmol 1977;61:668–674.

303. Luntz MH, Schenker HI. Retinal vascular accidents in glaucoma and ocular hypertension. Surv Ophthalmol 1980;25:163–167.

304. Yablonski ME, Zimmerman TJ, Kass MA, et al. Prognostic significance of optic disc cupping in ocular hypertensive patients. Am J Ophthalmol 1980;89:585–592.

305. Shuster J, Kass MA. When to treat ocular hypertension. Ann Ophthalmol 1983;15:301–302.

306. Kass MA. When to treat ocular hypertension. Surv Ophthalmol 1983;28:229–232.

307. Phelps CD. The no treatment approach to ocular hypertension. Surv Ophthalmol 1980;25:175–182.

308. Johnson TD, Zimmerman TJ. Glaucoma? High-pressure decisions. Ann Ophthalmol 1986;18:207–209.

309. Phelps CD. Ocular hypertension: To treat or not to treat? Arch Ophthalmol 1977;95:588–589.

310. Feibel RM, Bigger JF. Rubeosis iridis and neovascular glaucoma. Am J Ophthalmol 1972;74:862–867.

311. Kim MK, Char DH, Castro JL, et al. Neovascular glaucoma after helium ion irradiation for uveal melanoma. Ophthalmology 1986;93:189–193.

312. Weinreb RN, Wasserstrom JP, Parker W. Neovascular glaucoma following neodymium-YAG laser posterior capsulotomy. Arch Ophthalmol 1986;104:730–731.

313. Gartner S, Henkind P. Neovascularization of the iris (rubeosis iridis). Surv Ophthalmol 1978;22:291–312.

314. Weber PA. Neovascular glaucoma. Current management. Surv Ophthalmol 1981;26:149–153.

315. Rodgin SG. Neovascular glaucoma associated with uveitis. J Am Optom Assoc 1987;58:499–503.

316. Flanagan DW, Blach RK. Place of panretinal photocoagulation and trabeculectomy in the management of neovascular glaucoma. Br J Ophthalmol 1983;67:526–528.

317. Clearkin LG. Recent experience in the management of neovascular glaucoma by pan-retinal photocoagulation and trabeculectomy. Eye 1987;1:397–400.

318. Brodell LP, Olk RJ, Arribas NP, et al. Neovascular glaucoma: A retrospective analysis of treatment with peripheral panretinal cryotherapy. Ophthalmic Surg 1987;18:200–206.

319. Pavan PR, Folk JC. Anterior neovascularization. Int Ophthalmol Clin 1984;24:61–70.

320. Campbell DG, Vela A. Modern goniosynechialysis for the treatment of synechial angle-closure glaucoma. Ophthalmology 1984;91:1052–1060.

321. Krupin T, Kaufman P, Mandell AI, et al. Long-term results of valve implants in filtering surgery for eyes with neovascular glaucoma. Am J Ophthalmol 1983;95:775–782.

322. Schocket SS, Nirankari VS, Lakhanpal V, et al. Anterior chamber tube shunt to an encircling band in the treatment of neovascular glaucoma and other refractory glaucomas. A long-term study. Ophthalmology 1985;92:553–562.

323. Lewis RA, Phelps CD. A comparison of visual field loss in primary open-angle glaucoma and the secondary glaucomas. Ophthalmologica 1984;189:41–48.

324. Becker B, Shin DH, Cooper DG, et al. The pigment dispersion syndrome. Am J Ophthalmol 1977;83:161–166.

325. Kupfer C, Kuwabara T, Kaiser-Kupfer M. The histopathology of pigmentary dispersion syndrome with glaucoma. Am J Ophthalmol 1975;80:857–862.

326. Wilensky JT, Buerk KM, Podos SM. Krukenberg's spindles. Am J Ophthalmol 1975;79:220–225.

327. Lichter PR, Shaffer RN. Diagnostic and prognostic signs in pigmentary glaucoma. Trans Am Acad Ophthalmol Otolaryngol 1970;74:984–998.

328. Campbell DG. Pigmentary dispersion and glaucoma: A new theory. Arch Ophthalmol 1979;97:1667–1672.

329. Strasser G, Hauff W. Pigmentary dispersion syndrome. A biometric study. Acta Ophthalmol 1985;63:721–722.

330. Caprioli J, Spaeth GL, Wilson RP. Anterior chamber depth in open-angle glaucoma. Br J Ophthalmol 1986;70:831–836.

331. Scheie HG, Cameron JD. Pigment dispersion syndrome; a clinical study. Br J Ophthalmol 1981;65:264–269.

332. Samples JR, Bellows AR, Rosenquist RC, et al. Pupillary block with posterior chamber intraocular lenses. Arch Ophthalmol 1987;105:335–337.

333. Smith JP. Pigmentary open-angle glaucoma secondary to posterior chamber intraocular lens implantation and erosion of the iris pigment epithelium. J Am Intraocul Implant Soc 1985;11:174–176.

334. Caplan MB, Brown RH, Love LL. Pseudophakic pigmentary glaucoma. Am J Ophthalmol 1988;105:320–321.

335. Epstein DL, Freddo TF, Anderson PJ, et al. Experimental obstruction to aqueous outflow by pigment particles in living monkeys. Invest Ophthalmol Vis Sci 1986;27:387–395.

336. Migliazzo CV, Shaffer RN, Nykin R, et al. Long-term analysis of pigmentary dispersion syndrome and pigmentary glaucoma. Ophthalmology 1986;93:1528–1536.

337. Richter CU, Richardson TM, Grant WM. Pigmentary dispersion syndrome and pigmentary glaucoma. A prospective study of the natural history. Arch Ophthalmol 1986;104:211–215.

338. Fine BS, Yanoff M, Scheie HG. Pigmentary glaucoma: A histological study. Trans Am Acad Ophthalmol Otolaryngol 1974;78:314–325.

339. Epstein DL, Boger WP, Grant WM. Phenylephrine provocative testing in the pigmentary dispersion syndrome. Am J Ophthalmol 1978;85:43–50.

340. Richardson TM. Pigmentary glaucoma. In: Ritch R, Shields MB, eds. The secondary glaucomas. St Louis: C.V. Mosby Co, 1982;84–98.

341. Sugar S. Pigmentary glaucoma and the glaucoma associated with the exfoliation-pseudoexfoliation syndrome: Update. Ophthalmology 1984;91:307–310.

342. Ritch R. Pigmentary glaucoma: A self-limited entity? Ann Ophthalmol 1983;15:115–116.

343. Samples JR, Van Buskirk EM. Pigmentary glaucoma associated with posterior chamber intraocular lenses. Am J Ophthalmol 1985;100:385–388.

344. Woodhams JT, Lester JC. Pigmentary dispersion glaucoma secondary to posterior chamber intra-ocular lenses. Ann Ophthalmol 1984;16:852–854.

345. Gillies WE. Pigmentary glaucoma: A clinical review of anterior segment pigment dispersal syndrome. Aust NZ J Ophthalmol 1985;13:325–328.

346. Lunde MW. Argon laser trabeculoplasty in pigmentary dispersion syndrome with glaucoma. Am J Ophthalmol 1983;96:721–725.

347. Lindberg JG. Klinska undersokningar over depigmentering av pupillarrandeh och genomlysbarket av aris. Helsingfors 1917.

348. Vogt A. Ein neues spaltlampenbild obschilferung der linsenvorderkapsel als wahrscheinliche ursache von seilem

chronischen glaukom. Schweiz Med Wochenschr 1926; 56:413–415.

349. Dvorak-Theobald G. Pseudoexfoliation of the lens capsule. Am J Ophthalmol 1954;37:1–12.

350. Sugar HS, Harding C, Barsky D. The exfoliation syndrome. Ann Ophthalmol 1976;8:1165–1181.

351. Horven I. Exfoliation of the superficial layer of the lens capsule. Br J Ophthalmol 1937;21:626–637.

352. Kozart DM, Yanoff M. Intraocular pressure status in 100 consecutive patients with exfoliation syndrome. Ophthalmology 1982;89:214–218.

353. Henry JC, Krupin T, Schmitt M, et al. Long-term follow-up of pseudoexfoliation and the development of elevated intraocular pressure. Ophthalmology 1987;94:545–552.

354. Brooks AMV, Gillies WE. The presentation and prognosis of glaucoma in pseudoexfoliation of the lens capsule. Ophthalmology 1988;95:271–276.

355. Tarkkanen AH. Exfoliation syndrome. Trans Ophthalmol Soc UK 1986;105:233–236.

356. Wishart PK, Spaeth GL, Poryzees EM. Anterior chamber angle in the exfoliation syndrome. Br J Ophthalmol 1985;69:103–107.

357. Roth M, Epstein DL. Exfoliation syndrome. Am J Ophthalmol 1980;89:477–481.

358. Ritch R, Podos S. Laser trabeculoplasty in the exfoliation syndrome. Bull NY Acad Med 1983;59:339–344.

359. Layden WE. Exfoliation syndrome. In: Ritch R, Shields MB, eds. The secondary glaucomas. St Louis: C.V. Mosby Co, 1982;99–120.

360. Sherwood MB, Svedbergh B. Argon laser trabeculoplasty in exfoliation syndrome. Br J Ophthalmol 1985;69:886–890.

361. Higginbotham EJ, Richardson TM. Response of exfoliation glaucoma to laser trabeculoplasty. Br J Ophthalmol 1986;70:837–839.

362. Goldman H. Cortisone glaucoma. Arch Ophthalmol 1961; 68:621–626.

363. Hodapp EA, Kass MA. Corticosteroid-induced glaucoma. In: Ritch R, Shields MB, eds. The secondary glaucomas. St Louis: C.V. Mosby Co, 1982;258–265.

364. Robin AL, Pollack IP. Argon laser trabeculoplasty in secondary forms of open-angle glaucoma. Arch Ophthalmol 1983;101:382–384.

365. Posner A, Schlossman A. Syndrome of unilateral recurrent attacks of glaucoma with cyclitic symptoms. Arch Ophthalmol 1948;39:517–535.

366. Naveh-Floman N, Spierer A, Blumenthal M, et al. Protein glaucoma as a possible mechanism in a case of glaucomatocyclitic crisis and periphlebitis. Metab Pediatr Syst Ophthalmol 1983;7:85–88.

367. Harstad HK, Ringvold A. Glaucomatocyclitic crises (Posner-Schlossman syndrome). A case report. Acta Ophthalmol 1986;64:146–151.

368. Spivey BE, Armaly MF. Tonographic findings in glaucomatocyclitic crises. Am J Ophthalmol 1963;55:47–51.

369. de Roetth A. Glaucomatocyclitic crisis. Am J Ophthalmol 1970;69:370–371.

370. Varma R, Katz LJ, Spaeth GL. Surgical treatment of acute glaucomatocyclitic crisis in a patient with primary open-angle glaucoma. Am J Ophthalmol 1988;105:99–100.

371. Herschler J. Trabecular damage due to blunt anterior seg-ment injury and its relationship to traumatic glaucoma. Trans Am Acad Ophthalmol Otolaryngol 1977;83:239–248.

372. Tonjum AM. Intraocular pressure and facility of outflow late after ocular contusion. Acta Ophthalmol 1968;46:886–908.

373. Kaufman JH, Tolpin DW. Glaucoma after traumatic angle recession: A ten year prospective study. Am J Ophthalmol 1974;78:648–654.

374. Pilger IS, Khwarg SG. Angle recession glaucoma: Review and two case reports. Ann Ophthalmol 1985;17:197–199.

375. Layden WE. Cataracts and glaucoma. In: Duane TD, Jaeger EA, eds. Clinical ophthalmology. Philadelphia: Harper & Row, 1979; Chap. 55.

376. Bleiman BS, Schwartz AL. Paradoxical intraocular pressure response to pilocarpine. A proposed mechanism and treatment. Arch Ophthalmol 1979;97:1305–1306.

377. Morin JD. Secondary glaucoma. In: Duane TD, Jaeger EA, eds. Clinical ophthalmology. Philadelphia: Harper & Row 1979; Chap. 54.

378. Motolko MA, Phelps CD. The secondary glaucomas. In: Duane TD, Jaeger EA, eds. Clinical ophthalmology. Hagerstown, MD: Harper & Row, vol. 3, Chap. 54; 1987:1–23.

379. Read JE, Goldberg MF. Traumatic hyphema: Comparison of medical treatment. Trans Am Acad Ophthalmol Otolaryngol 1974;78:794–815.

380. Darr JL, Passmore JW. Management of traumatic hyphema: A review of 109 cases. Am J Ophthalmol 1967;63:134–136.

381. Thygeson P, Beard C. Observations of traumatic hyphema. Am J Ophthalmol 1952;35:977–985.

382. Jones WL. Posttraumatic glaucoma. J Am Optom Assoc 1987;58:708–715.

383. Rakusin W. Traumatic hyphema. Am J Ophthalmol 1972; 74:284–292.

384. Goldberg MF. Sickled erythrocytes, hyphema, and secondary glaucoma. Ophthalmic Surg 1979;10:17–31.

385. Crouch ER, Frenkel M. Aminocaproic acid in the treatment of traumatic hyphema. Am J Ophthalmol 1976;81:355–360.

386. McGetrick J, Jampol L, Goldberg MF, et al. Aminocaproic acid decreases secondary hemorrhage after traumatic hyphema. Arch Ophthalmol 1983;101:1031–1033.

387. Palmer DJ, Goldberg M, Frenkel M, et al. A comparison of two dose regimens of epsilon aminocaproic acid in the prevention and management of secondary traumatic hyphemas. Ophthalmology 1986;93:102–108.

388. Kutner B, Fourman S, Brein K, et al. Aminocaproic acid reduces the risk of secondary hemorrhage in patients with traumatic hyphema. Arch Ophthalmol 1987;105:206–208.

389. Herschler J, Cobo M. Trauma and elevated intraocular pressure. In: Ritch R, Shields MB, eds. The secondary glaucomas. St Louis: C.V. Mosby Co, 1982;307–319.

390. Fishbein SL, Schwartz B. Optic disc in glaucoma. Arch Ophthalmol 1977;95:1975–1979.

391. Schwartz B, Rieser JC, Fishbein SL. Fluorescein angiographic defects of the optic disc in glaucoma. Arch Ophthalmol 1977;95:1961–1974.

392. Airaksinen PJ, Drance SM, Douglas GR, et al. Visual field and retinal nerve fiber layer comparisons in glaucoma. Arch Ophthalmol 1985;103:205–207.

393. Airaksinen PJ, Drance SM. Neuroretinal rim area and ret-

inal nerve fiber layer in glaucoma. Arch Ophthalmol 1985;103:203–204.

394. Nanba K, Schwartz B. Nerve fiber layer and optic disc fluorescein defects in glaucoma and ocular hypertension. Ophthalmology 1988;95:1227–1233.

395. Seamone C, LeBlanc R, Rubillowiez M, et al. The value of indices in the central and peripheral visual fields for the detection of glaucoma. Am J Ophthalmol 1988;106:180–185.

396. Gunduz K, Arden GB, Perry S, et al. Color vision defects in ocular hypertension and glaucoma. Arch Ophthalmol 1988;106:929–935.

397. Weinstein GW, Arden GB, Hitchings RA, et al. The pattern electroretinogram (PERG) in ocular hypertension and glaucoma. Arch Ophthalmol 1988;106:923–928.

398. Cartwright MJ, Anderson DR. Correlation of asymmetric damage with asymmetric intraocular pressure in normal-tension glaucoma (low-tension glaucoma). Arch Ophthalmol 1988;106:898–900.

399. Lamping KA, Bellows AR, Hutchinson BT, et al. Long-term evaluation of initial filtration surgery. Ophthalmology 1986;93:91–101.

400. Jampel HD, Robin AL, Quigley HA, et al. Apraclonidine. A one-week dose-response study. Arch Ophthalmol 1988; 106:1069–1073.

401. Gharagozloo NZ, Relf SJ, Brubaker RF. Aqueous flow is reduced by the alpha-adrenergic agonist, apraclonidine hydrochloride (ALO 2145). Ophthalmology 1988;95:1217–1220.

402. Priore LVD, Robin AL, Pollack IP. Neodymium:YAG and argon laser iridotomy. Long-term follow-up in a prospective, randomized clinical trial. Ophthalmology 1988;95:1207–1211.

403. Kooner KS, Zimmerman TJ. Management of acute elevated intraocular pressure: Part II. Treatment. Ann Ophthalmol 1988;20:87–88.

404. Fink AI, Jordan AJ, Lao PN, et al. Therapeutic limitations of argon laser trabeculoplasty. Br J Ophthalmol 1988;72:263–269.

PART IV

Toxicology

The remedy often times proves worse than the disease.

—William Penn

CHAPTER 30

Ocular Effects of Systemic Drugs

Jimmy D. Bartlett
Siret D. Jaanus

During the past several decades the effects of systemic drug therapy on ocular function have received considerable attention. Monographs have been devoted to this subject,[1,2] and mechanisms have been devised whereby clinical observations can be reported and possible causal connections between systemic drug use and ocular effects can be established.[3,4] The aim is to promote awareness and aid in the early recognition of possible ocular reactions.

The eye, because of its rich blood supply and relatively small mass, exhibits an unusually high susceptibility to toxic substances. Drug molecules present in systemic circulation can reach the ocular structures by way of the uveal or retinal vasculature. Once in the eye, the systemic drugs can be deposited in several anatomic sites acting as drug depots, such as the cornea, lens, and retina. In addition, many ocular functions, including pupil size, accommodation, intraocular pressure, and lid position, are controlled by what appears to be a delicate balance of interactions between the cholinergic and adrenergic nervous systems. Thus, many systemically administered drugs can cause adverse ocular effects, and nearly all ocular structures are vulnerable. Moreover, multiple drug therapy as well as predisposing factors in individual patients add to the complexity of the problem.[5,6]

With our present state of knowledge, few ocular drug reactions are predictable or avoidable, since the patient's welfare usually depends on continued use of the drug. Nevertheless, adverse reactions can be reduced or prevented by understanding the major factors that lead to ocular side effects as well as by knowing which systemic drugs cause adverse ocular effects.

This chapter considers determinant aspects of adverse drug reactions and presents the most common drugs that can affect the eye. Clinically important drug effects are related to the anatomic ocular structures or functions involved, rather than to specific drug classes.

Determinants of Adverse Drug Reactions

Amount of Drug Administered

Nearly every drug, if administered in excessive dosage, may produce toxic effects. Toxic levels of drugs can result from high daily doses, following prolonged administration, or when drug detoxification or excretion mechanisms occur more slowly than normal.[5] The effect of excessive drug intake has been observed with several drugs and is particularly well documented with chloroquine.[7,8] When it is used as a malaria suppressant, ocular complications are rare. In control of rheumatoid arthritis and systemic lupus erythematosus, however, relatively larger dosages of chloroquine are administered and ocular complications involving the retina have been observed. Since the visual loss occurring with chloroquine is often irreversible,[9] regular ocular examinations of patients taking chloroquine or other quinoline derivatives are necessary.

Nature of Drug

The inherent pharmacologic properties of a drug determine its pharmacokinetic effects in the body, including its absorption, metabolism, and excretion. The ease with which a drug passes into the general circulation and its ability to penetrate the blood-brain, blood-aqueous, or blood-retinal barrier determine its ability to affect ocular tissue and function.

It has been suggested that the binding of drugs to melanin can lead to ocular toxicity.[6] The free, radical nature of melanin, present in ocular structures such as the uveal tract and retinal pigment epithelium, has been proposed to contribute to the binding ability of certain drugs, including phenothiazines and chloroquine. Drugs can also bind to ocular structures other than melanin. Digitalis has been observed to accumulate in the retina and ciliary body.[10] Other drugs are thought to produce ocular reactions by their effects on the general circulation, such as subconjunctival or retinal hemorrhages caused by use of anticoagulants such as heparin or aspirin.[11]

Route of Administration

All routes of drug administration can affect ocular function. Most adverse ocular reactions have been associated with oral or parenteral administration. However, topical application to the skin, particularly if abraded or burned, can result in sufficient systemic absorption to lead to ocular side effects. Dermatologic use of antibiotics has resulted in ocular hypersensitivity reactions.[8]

Pathophysiologic Variables

The presence of systemic disease can often alter the way an individual detoxifies or excretes a drug. Liver and kidney disease, in particular, can markedly influence drug response by allowing the drug to accumulate to toxic levels.[8] The rate of excretion of digoxin, for example, is markedly reduced in patients with renal impairment.[5] These patients could be more prone to ocular effects of this drug, such as the frequently observed alterations in color vision.[1]

The presence of systemic disease can also make it difficult in some instances to determine whether the ocular effect is the result of the disease process itself or a toxic manifestation of the drug used in therapy. For example, ocular effects occurring in hypertensive patients could be associated with the disease process or be due to drugs used for control of blood pressure, such as clonidine, which has been implicated in macular depigmentation with reduced vision.[1]

Age and Sex

Adverse drug reactions are more likely to occur in the very young and the elderly. Deficiencies in liver and kidney function can result in marked delay of drug detoxification and elimination. Lower dosages of drugs are generally indicated at these two extremes of life.

In general, more adverse systemic drug reactions are reported in women than in men. It is not clear whether this also applies to toxic ocular effects. A possible sex hormone–linked response to certain drugs may exist in humans.[5]

Multiple Drug Therapy

In general, the incidence of adverse drug reactions increases with the number of drugs administered. Interactions can occur when a drug is added to or withdrawn from a therapeutic regimen.

Many different sites or mechanisms can be involved. For example, one drug can alter the absorption, distribution, metabolism, or excretion of other drugs. In addition, a drug may alter the sensitivity of certain tissues to other drugs or act at the same cellular site or on the same physiologic system. Other factors such as chemical incompatibility between drugs can lead to inactivation and loss of pharmacologic activity.[5]

History of Allergy to Drugs

Adverse reactions to drugs are generally more likely to occur in patients with a history of previous reactions. For a drug to cause an allergic reaction, it must combine with an endogenous protein and form an antigenic complex. Subsequent exposure of the patient to the drug or an agent similar to it results in an antigen-antibody interaction that provokes the allergic response. Such reactions are not usually dose related, and relatively small quantities of drugs that act as allergens can provoke a reaction.[5]

Allergic reactions are not infrequent and, more often than not, are unpredictable and sometimes difficult to manage. The skin is most commonly involved. Reactions can range from a mild rash to exfoliative dermatitis and erythema multiforme. Ocular structures most commonly affected are the eyelids and the conjunctiva.

Numerous systemic drugs have been implicated, including the penicillins and sulfonamides, which can cause swelling of the lids and conjunctiva as part of a generalized urticaria or localized angioneurotic edema. Other drugs implicated in ocular allergic reactions are antidepressants, antipsychotics, antihypertensives, antirheumatics, sedatives, and hypnotics.[1]

Individual Idiosyncrasy

Idiosyncrasy refers to an unexpected reaction that can occur in some patients following administration of ordinary doses of a drug. These qualitatively abnormal responses have been attributed to heritable characteristics that result in altered handling of, or abnormal tissue responsiveness to, drugs.[5,12]

In ocular therapeutics the autosomal dominant inheritance of a glaucomatous response to topical ocular steroid therapy has been well documented. One-third of the general population responds to a 4- to 6-week challenge of topical ocular dexamethasone or betamethasone with a significant rise in intraocular pressure.[13,14] Patients with open-angle glaucoma, diabetes mellitus, or myopia greater than 5 D also have a greater incidence of increased intraocular pressure response to steroids. Genetic influences have also been implicated in the development of posterior subcapsular cataracts in patients receiving high-dose systemic steroid therapy.[15] At present the role of genetics in toxic drug reactions remains an enigma.

It has been proposed that alterations in enzymatic mechanisms could be responsible for some observed toxicities. Thus, the drug itself or metabolites formed in the liver or other organs of the body could enter the eye. It is also likely that metabolites can be formed locally in the eye, since a number of enzymes capable of metabolizing drugs have been isolated from various ocular tissues such as the corneal epithelium, iris, ciliary body, and retinal pigment epithelium.[6]

Diagnosis of Adverse Reactions

An adverse ocular drug reaction can be a challenging diagnosis, since cause and effect are often difficult to establish. A rewarding approach is a detailed drug history that includes over-the-counter (OTC) drugs as well as prescription agents. A temporal relationship between drug use and ocular signs or symptoms is an important clue. Another, equally important factor is the practitioner's familiarity with the possible ocular effects of any drugs the patient is taking. This will allow prompt recognition and management.

Ocular Manifestations of Systemic Drug Therapy

When used in normal dosage amounts, most drugs have a relatively low incidence of drug-induced ocular complications.[16] Many drugs, however, may often cause side effects, and others can affect ocular tissues or visual functions when taken in excessive quantities or when abused. The following sections consider the most important drugs that have the potential to affect the eye.

Drugs Affecting the Cornea and Lens

Perhaps because of its avascularity, the cornea is less frequently affected by systemic drugs than are other anterior segment structures such as the iris and ciliary body. Sporadic reports have implicated isotretinoin[17] and phenytoin[18] as causes of anterior subcapsular or posterior subcapsular cataract. Aside from such isolated case reports, however, a variety of ocular toxicities are well recognized, and the drugs responsible for these side effects are listed in Tables 30.1 and 30.2.

Chloroquine and Hydroxychloroquine

Chloroquine and hydroxychloroquine are usually reserved for the treatment of rheumatoid arthritis, discoid and systemic lupus erythematosus, and other collagen diseases. These quinoline drugs have been used for such purposes since the early 1950s. In 1958

TABLE 30.1
Drugs that Can Affect the Cornea

Drug	Side Effect
Chloroquine and hydroxychloroquine	Whorl-like epithelial opacities
Chlorpromazine	Pigmentation of endothelium and Descemet's membrane
Indomethacin	Stromal opacities or whorl-like epithelial opacities
Gold salts	Minute stromal gold deposits
Amiodarone	Whorl-like epithelial opacities

TABLE 30.2
Drugs that Can Affect the Lens

Drug	Side Effect
Chlorpromazine	Anterior subcapsular stellate-shaped cataract
8-Methoxypsoralen	Cataract
Gold salts	Anterior capsular or subcapsular gold deposits
Corticosteroids	Posterior subcapsular cataract
Amiodarone	Anterior subcapsular opacities

Hobbs and Calnan[19] were first to report corneal changes associated with these drugs.

CLINICAL SIGNS AND SYMPTOMS

The pattern of chloroquine keratopathy can be divided into 3 stages:[7] In the early stages diffuse punctate deposits appear in the corneal epithelium. Later the deposits aggregate into curved lines that converge and coalesce just below the central cornea. Finally, green-yellow pigmented lines appear in the center of the cornea as a whorl-like opacity.

Less than half of affected patients with corneal changes have visual symptoms,[20] but the most common complaints relate to halos around lights, glare, and photophobia. Visual acuity usually remains unchanged.[20,21] On discontinuation of drug therapy, both subjective symptoms and objective corneal signs invariably disappear.[22–24]

Keratopathy occurs in 30% to 75% of patients treated with either chloroquine or hydroxychloroquine,[20,21,25] but the corneal changes are much less frequently found in patients treated with hydroxychloroquine.[20,21,23] Although Calkins[26] reported the corneal findings to be related to total (cumulative) drug dosage or duration of therapy, more recent studies[25,27] have found no correlation between the severity of keratopathy and the dosage or duration of drug therapy. Corneal deposits can be observed as early as 2 to 6 weeks after beginning therapy,[20,26] and there is no relationship between the development of corneal deposits and the occurrence of retinopathy.[27] About half of patients treated with chloroquine exhibit decreased or absent corneal sensitivity unrelated to the development of corneal opacities.[21]

In recent years hydroxychloroquine has become the preferred quinoline drug for the treatment of collagen diseases because of fewer side effects, and its ocular toxicity is considerably less than that of chloroquine.[24,28,29] Tobin and associates[28] monitored 99 patients treated with hydroxychloroquine during a 7-year period. All patients received the drug for at least 1 year, and most patients received a daily dosage of 400 mg. No keratopathy was observed in any patient. At higher dosage levels, however, a higher incidence of keratopathy has been reported.[29] In a group of patients receiving an average daily dosage of 800 mg of hydroxychloroquine, 6% developed keratopathy within 6 months of therapy, while the incidence increased to 32% during the second 6 months. Corneal changes were present in all patients after 4 years of hydroxychloroquine therapy. Shearer and Dubois[29] have reported a rapid rise in the incidence of keratopathy when the total drug dosage exceeds 150 g. On reducing or discontinuing drug dosage, the corneal opacities decreased or disappeared during an average of 8 months.

MECHANISM

The origin of the corneal opacities is somewhat obscure but appears to represent reversible binding of the drug to intracellular nucleoproteins.[21] The changes are limited to the corneal epithelium, which the drug may reach by deposition in the tear film or by the limbal vasculature.[30]

Individual susceptibility probably plays an important role in the development of chloroquine keratopathy, since at lower dosages (e.g., 250 mg of chloroquine or 200 mg of hydroxychloroquine daily), there appears to be no relationship between the occurrence of keratopathy and total dosage or duration of therapy.[25] Patients receiving chloroquine doses exceeding 750 mg daily or hydroxychloroquine doses exceeding 800 mg daily appear to develop keratopathy earlier in the course of treatment.[26,29]

MANAGEMENT

Patients taking chloroquine or hydroxychloroquine should receive careful baseline and periodic slit-lamp examinations. Early identification of the corneal changes is facilitated by using retroillumination.[26] The practitioner should be careful to distinguish early chloroquine keratopathy from the normal development of Hudson-Stahli lines, which it can resemble. Fabry's keratopathy is another important condition in the differential diagnosis. The verticillate corneal findings are quite similar to those induced by chloroquine, but the systemic implications in Fabry's disease warrant consultation with an internist.

Since the condition is relatively benign and only rarely results in debilitating visual symptoms, the development of chloroquine keratopathy does not contraindicate continued use of the medication.[20,23] If, however, symptoms of glare, halos, or reduced vision bother the patient, drug therapy can be decreased or changed. This, however, must be done only in consultation with the prescribing physician.

Chlorpromazine

Chlorpromazine is a phenothiazine derivative used in the treatment of various psychiatric disorders.[31] Often high, prolonged dosages are required, and these have led to well-documented changes in the cornea and lens. In 1964 Greiner and Berry[32] reported the first cases of chlorpromazine-induced corneal and lens changes, and it is now generally accepted that chlorpromazine is the only phenothiazine to cause such ocular changes.[20]

CLINICAL SIGNS AND SYMPTOMS

Both corneal and lens changes are associated with chlorpromazine therapy.[33–37] Thaler and associates[33] have divided the lenticular pigmentation into 5 stages. The earliest sign of lenticular toxicity is fine, dot-like opacities on the anterior lens surface. At this stage the pigmentary deposits are small and tend to assume a disciform distribution within the pupillary area. Grade II lenticular changes consist of dot-like opacities that are more opaque and denser than in grade I. The pigmentary granules may begin to assume a stellate pattern. As the condition progresses, grade III changes are characterized by larger granules of pigment with an anterior subcapsular stellate pattern that is easily recognized. At this stage the opacity can range from white to yellow to tan. The stellate pattern has a dense central area with radiating branches (Fig. 30.1). A readily visible stellate pattern with 3 to 9 star points characterizes grade IV lenticular pigmentation. The lens changes at this stage can be recognized with a penlight, and diagnosis does not necessarily require slit-lamp examination. Grade V lenticular changes are characterized by a central, lightly pigmented, pearl-like, opaque mass surrounded by smaller clumps of pigment.

Corneal pigmentary changes almost invariably occur only in patients who have concomitant lens opacities in the higher grades.[33,34,36] There is often little or no corneal involvement with lens grades I and II, but grades III and higher have detectable corneal pigmen-

tation ranging from light to heavy.[33] The pigmentation is white, yellow-white, brown, or black and occurs at the level of the endothelium and Descemet's membrane primarily in the interpalpebral fissure area (Fig. 30.2). In severe cases it can affect the deep stroma.[34]

The most prevalent ocular side effect associated with chlorpromazine therapy is anterior capsular and subcapsular lens pigmentation, followed by corneal endothelial pigmentary changes. Alexander and associates[31] found 67% of a group of patients to have the former, while 45% exhibited the latter. Both conditions, however, only rarely reduce visual acuity, and patients may occasionally report glare, halos around lights, or hazy vision.

Both the corneal and lenticular pigmentary changes usually progress to a point beyond which no further changes are observed.[37] On reduction or discontinuation of drug therapy, the pigmentary deposits are generally irreversible.[34,36,37] This is not surprising because the deposits associated with chlorpromazine therapy are located in avascular tissues. In rare instances the lenticular pigmentation can begin after chlorpromazine therapy is discontinued.[35]

The ocular changes associated with chlorpromazine are dose related. Lenticular pigmentation is rarely evident when the total dosage is less than 500 g, and the prevalence of pigmentary changes increases with total

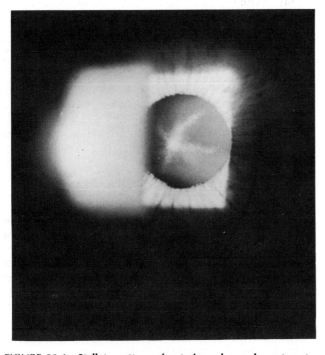

FIGURE 30.1 **Stellate pattern of anterior subcapsular cataract associated with chlorpromazine administration. (Courtesy Jerome Thaler, O.D.)**

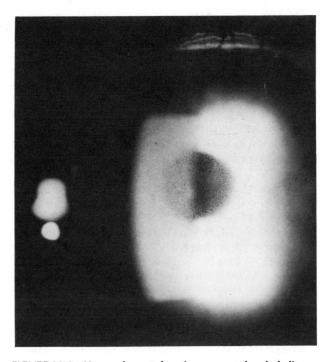

FIGURE 30.2 **Heavy pigment deposits on corneal endothelium, caused by chlorpromazine administration. (Courtesy Jerome Thaler, O.D.)**

dosages between 1000 and 2000 g, until 90% of patients demonstrate pigmentation when the total dosage exceeds 2500 g.[31,33] Since some psychiatric conditions may require daily dosages exceeding 800 mg, lenticular pigmentation can appear in as early as 14 to 20 months of therapy.[33] Dosages consisting of 2000 mg daily have been reported to cause lenticular changes in as early as 6 months of therapy.[36]

Corneal toxicity has been reported to occur within 6 months of therapy in 12% of patients receiving 2000 mg of chlorpromazine daily but in only 1% of patients receiving 300 mg of chlorpromazine daily.[36]

MECHANISM

The precise nature of the pigmentary granules in the cornea and lens is unknown. A popular hypothesis, however, is that the pigmentary changes are a result of drug interaction with ultraviolet light as it passes through the cornea and lens, causing exposed proteins to denature, opacify, and accumulate in the anterior subcapsular region of the lens as well as in corneal stroma.[38] This would explain why the keratopathy is localized to the interpalpebral fissure area.

MANAGEMENT

Patients receiving high-dosage or long-term, low-dosage chlorpromazine therapy should be monitored annually by careful slit-lamp examination. Since lens pigmentation is the most frequent ocular change observed, slit-lamp examination of the lens with the pupil dilated is the most direct method for detecting early chlorpromazine toxicity.

It may be possible to delay ocular pigmentary changes by avoiding long-term, high-dosage therapy or by employing intervals of treatment with nonphenothiazine drugs such as haloperidol (Haldol).[34,36] The use of spectacle lenses, presumably to reduce the amount of ultraviolet light entering the eye, has been found to be unsuccessful in reducing the prevalence of ocular toxicity.[31]

If corneal and lens changes occur but visual acuity is not affected and the patient is asymptomatic, the drug dosage can generally be continued without modification. If the patient becomes symptomatic, however, the dosage should be reduced or therapy should be changed to a different drug. The use of d-penicillamine has been unsuccessful in reversing the ocular pigmentary changes associated with long-term chlorpromazine therapy.[34]

Nonsteroidal Anti-Inflammatory Agents

Nonsteroidal anti-inflammatory agents (NSAIAs) are commonly used for their analgesic, anti-inflammatory, and antipyretic actions in the treatment of arthritis, musculoskeletal disorders, dysmenorrhea, and acute gout. Although these drugs are widely used and are often employed for prolonged periods, ocular side effects occur very rarely.[39]

CLINICAL SIGNS AND SYMPTOMS

The prevalence of corneal toxicity associated with indomethacin therapy has been reported to be 11% to 16%.[40,41] The corneal lesions appear either as fine stromal, speckled opacities or have a whorl-like distribution resembling that seen in chloroquine keratopathy. These corneal changes diminish or disappear within 6 months of discontinuing indomethacin therapy.[40,41] Although no definite relationship has been established between dosage of drug and corneal changes,[41] Palimeris and associates[40] found corneal opacities in patients who had taken indomethacin for 12 to 18 months, with the daily dosage ranging from 75 to 200 mg and the total dosage ranging from 20 to 70 g.

Symptoms associated with the corneal opacities can include mild light sensitivity or even frank photophobia. Corneal sensitivity, however, is normal.[40]

Szmyd and Perry[42] have observed whorl-like corneal opacities in a 76-year-old woman who had used naproxen for 2 months. There was complete regression of the corneal changes when the medication was discontinued.

MECHANISM

Controlled, prospective clinical trials are needed to further establish and clarify the association between NSAIAs and corneal opacities. The mechanism of such ocular changes is unknown.

MANAGEMENT

Since the corneal opacities associated with NSAIAs are benign and represent no significant threat to vision, patients taking these drugs can be monitored annually for evidence of corneal changes. Patients who develop evidence of keratotoxicity should be reassured regarding the benign nature of these changes, and the prescribing physician should be notified. The benign nature of the corneal opacities does not necessitate reduction or discontinuation of drug therapy except in circumstances in which severe corneal toxicity causes visual symptoms that are annoying or incapacitating.

Photosensitizing Drugs

Photosensitizing drugs are compounds that absorb optical radiation (ultraviolet [UV] and visible) and undergo a photochemical reaction, resulting in chemical modifications in nearby molecules of the tissue.[43] The psoralen compounds are photosensitizing drugs and are widely used by dermatologists to treat psoriasis and vitiligo. This treatment is commonly referred to as PUVA therapy and involves the administration of 8-methoxypsoralen (8-MOP) or related compounds, followed by exposure to UV radiation (320 to 400 nm) for short periods.[43] The most common photosensitizing reactions involve the skin and eye. Cataract formation is now well documented in patients undergoing PUVA therapy,[43] but the association between allopurinol therapy and cataracts has been disputed.[44]

MECHANISM

The eye and the skin are the only tissues of the body that are particularly susceptible to damage from non-ionizing wavelengths of optical radiation (280 to 1400 nm).[43] The crystalline lens can absorb varying amounts of UV radiation and thus photobind susceptible drugs present in that tissue. Most ocular damage from photosensitizing drugs occurs on exposure to UV radiation.[43] Because the adult crystalline lens effectively filters most UV radiation, there is minimal risk of photobinding susceptible drugs in the retina. UV radiation, however, can penetrate to the retina in aphakic and pseudophakic individuals and in young eyes, thus causing potential photosensitizing damage to the retina.[43]

MANAGEMENT

If the eye is protected from UV radiation during PUVA therapy, free 8-MOP can be found in the lens for only 24 hours.[43] Thus, to prevent permanent photobinding of this drug, dermatologists usually provide UV-filtering lenses to patients undergoing PUVA therapy. The patient should wear the lenses for at least 24 hours beginning when the drug is first taken. These filters must be worn both indoors as well as outdoors, since there is sufficient UV radiation in ordinary fluorescent lighting to photobind the 8-MOP.[43] These measures are generally effective in preventing cataracts associated with PUVA therapy.

Gold Salts

Both parenteral and oral gold salts are used in the treatment of rheumatoid arthritis. After prolonged administration, gold can be deposited in various tissues of the body, a condition known as chrysiasis. Ocular chrysiasis was reported as early as 1937 by Bonnet[45] and can involve the conjunctiva, cornea, and lens. In 1987 Weidle[46] first reported ocular chrysiasis in a patient using oral gold.

CLINICAL SIGNS AND SYMPTOMS

Corneal chrysiasis consists of numerous, minute gold particles appearing as yellowish-brown to violet and red particles distributed irregularly in the stroma.[47,48] The deposition of gold generally spares the peripheral 1 to 3 mm as well as superior one-fourth to one-half of cornea,[47] and the deposits tend to localize to the posterior one-third of the stroma.[47,49] There is typically no involvement of the epithelium, Descemet's membrane, or endothelium.[47] Figure 30.3 shows the general distribution of gold deposits in a typical case of corneal chrysiasis.

Corneal chrysiasis is a common finding in patients receiving long-term maintenance gold therapy for rheumatoid arthritis. McCormick and associates[47] found gold deposits in 97% of patients receiving continuous gold therapy consisting of a cumulative dosage of at least 1000 mg. Gottlieb and Major[48] reported corneal chrysiasis in 45% of patients who had received a mean cumulative dosage greater than 7 g during a mean 6-year period. Although no correlation exists between the density of corneal deposits and the cumulative dosage, there is a positive correlation between the duration of gold therapy and the density of corneal deposits.[47]

Lenticular chrysiasis appears as fine, dust-like, yellowish, glistening deposits in the anterior capsule or in the anterior suture lines.[48] Oral auranofin is deposited in the anterior subcapsular region[46] (Figure 30.4).

Various studies[47,48] have established the prevalence of lenticular chrysiasis from parenteral gold to be from 36% to 55%. Although there is no correlation between the dosage of gold and the presence of lenticular deposits,[48] the deposition of gold deposits in the lens generally requires at least 3 years of parenteral chrysotherapy.[47] The lowest cumulative dosage to produce such lenticular deposits is about 2500 mg.[47] Weidle[46] reported lenticular chrysiasis in a 72-year-old woman who had received 960 mg of oral auranofin during a 5-month period.

There is no significant correlation between corneal

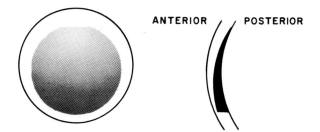

FIGURE 30.3 **General distribution of gold deposits in corneal chrysiasis. The deposits spare the peripheral and superior cornea and are more dense inferiorly. (Modified from McCormick SA, DiBartolomeo AG, Raju VK, et al. Ocular chrysiasis. Ophthalmology 1985;92:1432–1435.)**

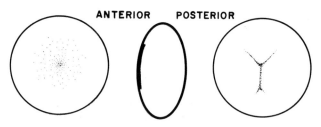

ANTERIOR   POSTERIOR

FIGURE 30.4   Lenticular chrysiasis. Gold deposits can diffusely involve the anterior capsule and concentrate within the axial region, or can involve the anterior suture line. (Modified from McCormick SA, DiBartolomeo AG, Raju VK, et al. Ocular chrysiasis. Ophthalmology 1985;92:1432–1435.)

chrysiasis and lenticular chrysiasis, and there is no evidence that gold therapy leads to cataract formation.[48] Deposits of gold in the cornea or lens do not cause visual disturbances or other symptoms.[47,48]

MECHANISM

The available evidence suggests that gold is deposited in the cornea and lens by circulation in the aqueous fluid in the anterior chamber.[47]

MANAGEMENT

Since ocular chrysiasis does not lead to visual impairment, inflammation, or corneal endothelial changes, gold therapy does not need to be reduced or discontinued.[46,47] This benign process requires only routine follow-up. The deposits often disappear within 3 to 6 months following cessation of therapy, but they may occasionally be found years after chrysotherapy has been discontinued.

Corticosteroids

Because of the potential for systemic side effects, use of steroids is limited to conditions for which less conservative therapy is inadequate. Steroids are sometimes used in the treatment of collagen diseases such as rheumatoid arthritis and systemic lupus, and they are used in the treatment of sarcoidosis. The association between steroid use and cataracts has been well known for several decades. However, direct interpretation of published reports of patients with steroid-induced cataracts is often subject to error because of variations in duration of treatment and in the steroid dosages employed.

In 1960 Black and associates[50] were the first to suggest that systemic steroid therapy could lead to posterior subcapsular (PSC) cataracts. They had observed PSC cataracts in 39% of a group of patients with rheumatoid arthritis who had undergone prolonged systemic steroid therapy. Although several au-

thors subsequently refuted the relationship between systemic steroids and PSC cataracts,[51–53] it is now widely accepted that under certain circumstances systemic steroid therapy can induce cataract formation.

CLINICAL SIGNS AND SYMPTOMS

Systemic steroids can produce PSC cataracts that are clinically indistinguishable from complicated cataract and cataracts caused by exposure to ionizing radiation.[50] They often cannot be distinguished from age-related PSC cataracts except that the latter frequently have other associated findings such as anterior capsular or subcapsular vacuoles, cortical opacities, or nuclear sclerosis. Even if the steroid dosage is reduced or discontinued, the cataract usually remains unchanged and will neither progress in size nor become smaller or less dense.[54,55] On rare occasions, however, the size of the opacity may decrease following reduction of steroid therapy. It has been suggested that spontaneous regression of steroid-induced PSC cataract might occur in cases associated with relatively low doses of steroid or when the duration of treatment is less than 2 years.[54] In other cases progressive changes may occasionally occur when the steroid dosage is reduced or discontinued.[54]

Several of the early studies on the relationship between systemic steroids and cataracts suggested that the dosage or duration of treatment was significantly correlated with the development of cataract.[55–57] Furst and associates,[55] however, proposed that it is possible for patients to develop steroid-induced cataract even when taking very low doses of steroid. In 1961 Oglesby and associates[56] provided data to suggest that no patient taking steroids for less than 1 year would develop PSC cataracts, whereas 48% of patients treated for 1 year or longer would develop lens opacities. Patients receiving less than 10 mg of prednisone daily, regardless of duration, or patients treated for less than 1 year, regardless of steroid dosage, would be unlikely to develop PSC cataracts. On the other hand, patients who receive at least 15 mg of prednisone daily for more than 1 year were very likely to develop PSC cataracts.[56] The relationship of dosage and duration of therapy was further defined by Crews,[58] who suggested that steroids could cause cataracts with short-term therapy only if the dosage was extremely high.

More recently the relationship between PSC cataract and daily dosage or duration of prednisone therapy has been called into question.[59,60] Because of considerable variation in the numbers of patients studied, dosage and duration of treatment, criteria for diagnosis, route of drug administration, and the underlying disease process itself, attention has focused on the possibility that PSC cataract formation may be related more to factors of individual susceptibility than to drug-related factors of dosage or duration of therapy.[15,61,62] Skalka and Prchal[62] found no statistically significant correlation between PSC opacities and total steroid dosage, weekly dosage, duration of therapy, or patient age. There may also be special susceptibility among various ethnic groups. Hispanics are apparently more predisposed to steroid-induced PSC cataracts than are either whites or blacks.[63,64]

It has been suggested that children are more susceptible than adults to develop steroid-induced cataracts,[54] developing them at a lower dosage and in a shorter time.[54,55] This can be attributed to the relatively massive doses of steroids in relation to body weight sometimes prescribed in children.[15]

Visual impairment is rare in patients with steroid-induced PSC cataracts.[15,54,57] Astle and Ellis[59] reported that 88% of a group of patients with steroid-induced cataracts had visual acuity of 20/40 or better in each eye. Although severe visual reduction is uncommon, patients may report light sensitivity, frank photophobia, reading difficulty, or glare.

MECHANISM

Although the precise mechanism whereby steroids lead to cataract formation is unknown, Urban and Cotlier[15] have proposed that steroids gain entry to the fiber cells of the crystalline lens and then react with specific amino groups of the lens crystallins. This alteration frees protein sulfhydral groups to form disulfide bonds, which subsequently lead to protein aggregation and ultimately to complexes that refract light. Other mechanisms have also been proposed.[65–67]

MANAGEMENT

Patients taking systemic steroids should have careful slit-lamp examinations performed through a dilated pupil every 6 months. Since it is possible for patients to develop cataracts even when taking very low doses of steroid,[68] every patient, regardless of dosage or duration of treatment, should be carefully evaluated for the presence of drug-induced cataract. When drug-induced cataracts are discovered, the prescribing practitioner should be notified so that the dosage can be reduced, if possible, to the minimum that will control the disease process. Alternatively, alternate-day therapy can be considered,[62] or a NSAIA may be selected. Episodes of renal transplant rejection can often be equally well controlled by lower doses of steroid, and these reduced dosages may help to prevent cataracts following transplantation.[60] If cataract extraction becomes necessary, the procedure generally carries an excellent prognosis.

Amiodarone

Amiodarone, a benzofurane derivative, has been used for several decades to treat a variety of cardiac abnormalities.[69,70] The drug is highly effective in the treatment of both atrial and ventricular arrhythmias and Wolff-Parkinson-White syndrome.[71] Almost since its first introduction into clinical practice, however, amiodarone has been observed to cause keratopathy early in the course of treatment.

CLINICAL SIGNS AND SYMPTOMS

Onset of keratopathy may be as early as 6 days following initiation of drug therapy,[72] but it more commonly appears after 1 to 3 months of treatment.[73] Virtually all patients will demonstrate corneal changes after 3 months of therapy.[72,74] The corneal deposits are bilateral but are often asymmetric, and they are easily observed with the slit lamp. The development of keratopathy can be divided into several stages.[72,73,75]

1. A faint horizontal line, similar to a Hudson-Stahli line, appears in the interpalpebral fissure at the junction of the middle and lower third of the cornea. It consists of golden-brown microdeposits in the epithelium just anterior to Bowman's layer.

2. Transition to grade II occurs by 6 months, during which the deposits become aligned in a more linear pattern and extend toward the limbus. The grade II pattern does not necessarily proceed to grade III.

3. The deposits increase in number and density, and the lines extend superiorly to produce a whorl-like pattern into the visual axis.

4. Irregular, round clumps of deposits characterize grade IV keratopathy. The development of each stage of keratopathy is shown in Figure 30.5, and a clinical representation of amiodarone keratopathy is shown in Figure 30.6.

On discontinuation of drug therapy, the keratopathy gradually resolves within 6 to 18 months.[73]

The severity of the keratopathy appears to be significantly correlated with total drug dosage as well as duration of treatment.[70,75,76] It is possible, however, for patients taking lower doses of amiodarone to demonstrate marked keratopathy while other patients taking high doses of drug show only mild corneal changes.[75] In general, patients taking low dosages of drug (100 to 200 mg daily) retain clear corneas or demonstrate only mild keratopathy regardless of duration of treatment or cumulative dosage. Patients taking higher dosages (400 to 1400 mg daily) demonstrate more advanced keratopathy depending on the duration of treatment.[70] Once the keratopathy becomes fully developed, it remains relatively stationary until the drug dosage is reduced or discontinued.[75]

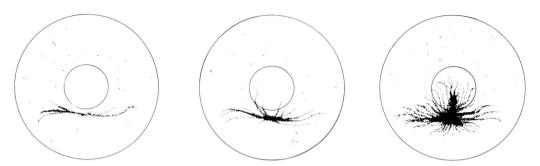

FIGURE 30.5 **Stages of amiodarone keratopathy. Left, grade I; Center, grade II; Right, grade III. (Modified from Klingele TG, Alves LE, Rose EP. Amiodarone keratopathy. Ann Ophthalmol 1984;16:1172–1176.)**

Amiodarone-induced lens opacities have also been reported.[73,75,77] Fine anterior subcapsular lens deposits occur in about 50% of patients taking amiodarone in moderate to high doses (600 to 800 mg daily)[77] after 6 to 18 months of treatment. The deposits first appear small, golden-brown or white-yellow punctate opacities located just below the anterior lens capsule. They are loosely packed and cover an area greater than 2 mm within the pupillary aperture.[77] Unlike the lenticular deposits associated with chlorpromazine therapy, which develop before corneal changes, the lens opacities associated with amiodarone develop in the presence of marked keratopathy.

Amiodarone-induced lens deposits can be differentiated from the axial punctate opacities (epicapsular stars) found physiologically in about 10% of individuals over 40 years of age. The latter have a brown or metallic pigmentation and often penetrate several millimeters into the anterior cortex from their anterior subcapsular location.[73] The lenticular opacities related to amiodarone, however, are less darkly pigmented and are limited to the superficial anterior subcapsular area. Once drug therapy is discontinued, it is unknown whether the lens opacities resolve.

Symptoms associated with amiodarone-induced corneal and lens changes are minimal or absent.[73–75] Lenticular opacities generally cause no visual symptoms, but moderate to severe keratopathy can lead to complaints of blurred vision, glare, halos around lights, or light sensitivity. Visual acuity is usually normal but may be slightly decreased if the keratopathy is severe.

MECHANISM

Amiodarone belongs to a group of drugs having the physical and chemical properties of cationic amphiphilia.[78] Amphiphilic drugs bind to polar lipids and accumulate within lysosomes. Several investigators[71,75,79] have

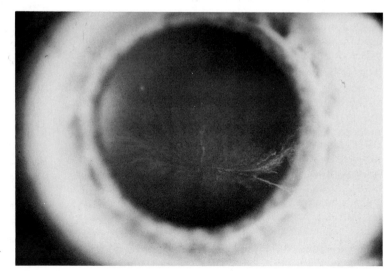

FIGURE 30.6 **Clinical photograph of grade III amiodarone keratopathy. (Courtesy Jerry Pederson, O.D.)**

performed electron microscopy on ocular tissues of patients who had taken amiodarone, and these studies have consistently revealed intracytoplasmic membrane-bound lamellar bodies similar to myelin. These changes have been noted not only in the corneal epithelium, the conjunctiva, and the lens, but have also been found in the corneal endothelium, the iris, ciliary body, choroid, and retina.[71,75] The presence of such complex lipid deposits within these tissues has led recent investigators to conclude that amiodarone keratopathy is probably a drug-induced lipid storage disease.[71,75,79] The whorl-like pattern of the keratopathy may result from an effect at the limbus on the epithelial cells that are migrating centripetally.[80]

MANAGEMENT

Because the corneal and lenticular changes associated with amiodarone therapy are benign, special follow-up of affected patients is not required unless the opacities have induced visual symptoms. In the rare cases in which visual symptoms are annoying or incapacitating, reduction or discontinuation of drug dosage usually resolves the corneal findings. It is unusual for ocular side effects to necessitate discontinuation of drug therapy,[73] but occasionally treatment must be discontinued because of drug intolerance or other side effects such as diarrhea, vomiting, pulmonary fibrosis, or liver damage.[75]

Since the early stages of amiodarone keratopathy can mimic a Hudson-Stahli line, a careful drug history relative to amiodarone use should be carefully elicited. More advanced stages of amiodarone keratopathy may resemble the corneal changes of Fabry's disease or chloroquine toxicity. Because of the systemic implications of Fabry's disease, patients with no history of amiodarone or chloroquine use should be evaluated by an internist.

Donor corneas affected by amiodarone can be safely used in penetrating keratoplasty without removing the affected epithelium. The keratopathy has been reported to quickly resolve following the operation.[81]

Oral Contraceptives

Although ocular side effects have been widely reported with oral contraceptive use, most of these effects have been based primarily on isolated, anecdotal case reports. Animal studies as well as prospective clinical trials in humans have failed to document any significant relationship between use of oral contraceptives and ocular side effects.[82] Although various authors have speculated that oral contraceptives may influence contact lens wear, sometimes leading to contact lens in-

tolerance, there is no evidence to suggest that such a relationship exists.[83,84]

Anderson and Martin,[85] in an uncontrolled study, found that a significant number of women taking oral contraceptives experienced steepening of corneal curvature. The etiology of contact lens intolerance during use of oral contraceptives could potentially include changes in corneal curvature, corneal edema due to hypoxia,[86] or changes in the quality of the precorneal tear film such as excessive mucus formation or a reduction of the aqueous component of the tears.[84] None of these changes, however, has been definitely implicated, and the practitioner is cautioned to investigate other potential causes for any observed objective signs or subjective symptoms. The contact lens parameters, solutions, lens hygiene, wearing schedules, and other factors should be taken into consideration before recommendations are made regarding oral contraceptive use.

Although small anterior and posterior subcapsular opacities have been reported in patients using oral contraceptives,[87] most authorities believe there is no relationship between oral contraceptive use and cataract formation.[82]

Drugs Affecting the Conjunctiva and Lids

Drug effects on the conjunctiva and lids can be irritative, allergic, or involve pigmentary inclusions (Table 30.3).

Isotretinoin

An analog of vitamin A, isotretinoin (Accutane), or 13-*cis*-retinoic acid, is used for control of severe recalcitrant cystic acne and other keratinizing dermatoses.[88] Oral administration of 1 or 2 mg/kg body weight daily temporarily suppresses sebaceous gland activity, changes

TABLE 30.3
Drugs that Can Affect the Conjunctiva and Lids

Drug	Side Effect
Isotretinoin	Blepharoconjunctivitis, dry eye, contact lens intolerance
Chlorpromazine	Slate-blue discoloration of conjunctiva and dermis of lids
Sulfonamides	Lid edema, conjunctivitis, chemosis
Gold salts	Gold deposits in conjunctiva
Tetracycline	Pigmented conjunctival inclusion cysts

surface lipid composition of the skin and inhibits keratinization. The therapeutic effect is resolution of lesions and, in most patients, prolonged remission of the disease.

CLINICAL SIGNS AND SYMPTOMS

Both systemic and ocular side effects have been reported with use of this drug. Dryness of the face and mucous membranes is frequently observed. Other systemic effects include hair loss, colitis, and skeletal hyperostosis.[88]

Ocular complications include blepharoconjunctivitis, dry eye symptoms, contact lens intolerance, and subepithelial corneal opacities. In 1979 Blackman and associates[89] first reported blepharoconjunctivitis in association with isotretinoin therapy. Milson and associates[90] later observed a dose-dependent relationship between isotretinoin therapy and blepharoconjunctivitis. Dosages of 2 mg/kg body weight daily of isotretinoin resulted in blepharoconjunctivitis in 43% of patients, whereas dosages of 1 mg/kg body weight daily showed a 20% incidence of blepharoconjunctivitis. A retrospective study[110] of 237 patients showed the most common ocular side effect was blepharoconjunctivitis, occurring in 37% of patients.

MANAGEMENT

Since as many as half the patients who develop blepharoconjunctivitis have symptoms before the start of therapy, the drug may aggravate preexisting conditions.[89] Decreasing the dosage or discontinuing the drug will usually alleviate the side effect, although a few months may be required in some patients before significant relief is obtained.

Chlorpromazine

Discoloration of the conjunctiva, sclera, and exposed skin have been reported with administration of phenothiazine derivatives.[91-94] The skin of the face and lids can be equally pigmented, while the palpebral folds contain an area of nonpigmented skin deep within the creases.[91] The discoloration is usually slate-blue. Melanin-like granules have been observed in the superficial dermis of the skin.[91,92] The oculo-skin syndrome is usually associated with pigmentary deposits in the exposed interpalpebral area of the bulbar conjunctiva, especially near the limbus.[91-94] The palpebral conjunctiva does not appear to be involved. Patients exposed to dosages of chlorpromazine ranging from 500 to 3000 mg daily for 1 to 6 years may develop discoloration of the exposed skin, lids, and bulbar conjunctiva.[93,94]

There have been sporadic reports of allergic conjunctivitis and edema of the lids associated with phenothiazine use.[95]

Sulfonamides

Ocular complications are rare with systemic use of this class of anti-infective drugs. Lid edema, conjunctivitis, chemosis, and scleral reactions have been reported with high-dose administration of sulfanilamide.[96] The observed reactions appear to be analogous to systemic hypersensitivity reactions such as urticaria and edema seen in some patients who are allergic to sulfonamides.

Gold Compounds

Chrysiasis, or gold deposition in various tissues of the body, can also occur in the conjunctiva following gold injection for rheumatoid arthritis. In 1956 Roberts and Wolter[49] observed during a biomicroscopic examination the presence of irregular, brownish deposits in the cornea and superficial layers of the conjunctiva. On biopsy of the conjunctiva, the particles proved to be metallic gold. No deposits were found in the skin of the lid. Inflammation or foreign body reaction was not present. The patient had received a total of 4555 mg of sodium thiomalate (Myochrysine) and 2188 mg of aurothioglucose (Solganal) over a 9-year period.

A more recent investigation[47] of 34 patients with rheumatoid arthritis who had received intramuscular injections of either Myochrysine or Solganal failed to show deposits in the conjunctiva under slit-lamp examination although deposits were present in the cornea and lens (see above). The total dosage range of gold administered was 2250 to 10,410 mg. No tissue biopsies were performed on these patients.

Conjunctivitis and eyelid exfoliative dermatitis have also been observed. Discontinuation of therapy usually eliminates these side effects.[8]

Tetracyclines

Tetracycline and its derivative, minocycline, are used for control of acne vulgaris. Conjunctival deposits similar to those seen in epinephrine-treated glaucoma patients have been observed in patients treated orally with these compounds.[97,98] Dosages ranged from 250 to 1500 mg daily of tetracycline and at least 100 mg daily of minocycline.

The deposits appear as dark-brown to black granules in the palpebral conjunctiva, located nasally and temporally in the upper tarsus and temporally in the lower tarsus.[97] The granules vary in size and are located in conjunctival cysts, surrounded by minute, gray-white, noncrystalline soft spots. Under UV light microscopy the brown pigment concentrations give a yellow fluorescence characteristic of tetracycline.[98]

Along with pigment, calcium is also present in the cysts. It has been hypothesized that either tetracycline or its metabolites form an insoluble chelation complex that results in the pigmentation.[98] Considering the large number of patients who have received these drugs for prolonged periods for acne, it is interesting that conjunctival pigmentation has not been reported more frequently.

Amiodarone

Although chronic administration of this antiarrhythmic agent has produced no visible biomicroscopic changes in the conjunctiva, electron microscopic studies of human autopsy material have indicated that some ultrastructural changes may occur during therapy.[75,99] Intracytoplasmic membrane-bound deposits similar to myelin have been demonstrated in the cytoplasm of nearly all ocular structures, including the conjunctival epithelium.[99] It has been suggested that these findings represent a drug-induced lipidosis.[75,99] Amiodarone has also been reported to concentrate within a chalazion that developed in a patient who had been taking the drug for 2 years for ventricular arrhythmias.[100]

Miscellaneous Drugs

A variety of other systemic drugs have been implicated to cause irritative or allergic reactions in the conjunctiva or lids.[2,8,95] Barbiturates have rarely been reported to cause conjunctival hyperemia and chemosis. Dermatitis, lid swelling, and ptosis have also been related to chronic barbiturate use. The reaction can persist for months after the drug is discontinued.[101]

Salicylates may cause allergic conjunctivitis, which may be associated with urticaria of the lids.[95] Chloroquine has been reported to cause ptosis, and phenytoin may cause chronic conjunctivitis.[8] Drugs of abuse such as marijuana may lead to conjunctival injection, sometimes with eyelid edema.[1,2]

Drugs Affecting the Lacrimal System

Human lacrimal fluid consists of a combination of secretions from the lacrimal gland, meibomian glands,

and the goblet cells of the conjunctiva. Aqueous tear secretion from the lacrimal gland is controlled by the autonomic nervous system. The lacrimal gland is innervated by cholinergic fibers from the seventh cranial nerve as well as by adrenergic fibers from the pericarotid plexus.[102] Chemically the tears are 98.2% water and 1.8% solids. Thus, drugs that directly or indirectly affect the autonomic nervous system may cause hypersecretion or, more commonly, dry eye.

Several classes of drugs can affect aqueous tear secretion, influence tear constituents, or appear in the tears following systemic administration.[103] Patients complaining of watery or dry eyes, eye infections, or uncomfortable contact lens wear could be exhibiting symptoms relating to actions on the tears of a variety of prescription as well as OTC drugs.[104]

Drugs reported to affect aqueous tear secretion are listed in Table 30.4. Among the agents that frequently reduce tear secretion are the anticholinergics and antihistamines. Both these classes of drugs are also present in numerous OTC products such as sedatives, sleep aids, cold preparations, antidiarrheals, and nasal decongestants.

TABLE 30.4
Drugs that Can Affect Aqueous Tear Secretion

Drug Class	Example
Agents decreasing aqueous tears	
Anticholinergics	Atropine
	Scopolamine
Antihistamines	Chlorpheniramine
	Diphenhydramine
Vitamin A analogs	Isotretinoin
β-adrenergic blockers	Practolol
	Propranolol
	Timolol
Phenothiazines	Chlorpromazine
	Thioridazine
Antianxiety agents	Chlordiazepoxide
	Diazepam
Tricyclic antidepressants	Amitriptyline
	Doxepin
Agents increasing aqueous tears	
Adrenergic agonists	Ephedrine
Antihypertensives	Reserpine
	Hydralazine
Cholinergic agonists	Neostigmine

Drugs that Decrease Aqueous Tears and Tear Film Constituents

ANTICHOLINERGICS

Dryness of mucous membranes is a common side effect of anticholinergic drug use, since atropine and related drugs inhibit glandular secretion in a dose-dependent manner.

In one study,[105] oral administration of atropine caused tear secretion to fall from 15 μl/min to 3 μl/min. A similar dose of atropine given subcutaneously gave a nearly 50% reduction in lacrimal secretion.[106] Scopolamine, 1 to 2 mg orally, reduced tear secretion from 5 μl/min to 0.8 μl/min.[105]

ANTIHISTAMINES

This class of drugs consists of agents that block two types of histamine receptors, H_1 or H_2. Agents blocking H_1 receptor types are commonly used for symptoms associated with colds, hay fever and other allergies, to prevent motion sickness, and for control of Parkinson's disease. The H_2 receptor antagonists are clinically useful for gastric ulcer therapy.

In addition to their receptor-blocking effects, H_1 antihistamines have varying degrees of atropine-like actions, including the ability to alter tear film integrity.[103,106,107] Both aqueous and mucin production have been reported to decrease with antihistamine use.[105] Koeffler and Lemp[108] administered 4 mg daily of chlorpheniramine maleate to a 20-year-old age group of volunteers. Tear secretion was measured by use of the standard Schirmer's test. A significant reduction in tear flow was observed on the days when chlorpheniramine was taken. The difference between the mean values of Schirmer strip wetting for days on which antihistamines were taken and nondrug days was highly significant.

Systemic use of antihistamines can aggravate an existing condition of keratitis sicca.[109] Use of 200 mg daily of diphenhydramine (Benadryl) has resulted in reoccurrence of filamentary keratitis in a female arthritic patient. When the medication was discontinued, the symptoms disappeared. This suggests that patients with a compromised tear film may aggravate this condition by use of antihistamines or other agents that can affect ocular surface wetting.

ISOTRETINOIN

Dry eye symptoms have been reported as one of the side effects of systemic isotretinoin therapy for acne. The prevalance has been estimated to be as high as 20%, with about 8% of patients experiencing contact lens intolerance.[110]

Isotretinoin has been observed to decrease tear breakup time.[110,111] It is possible that lipid secretion by the meibomian glands may be decreased, reducing the lipid layer and thereby increasing the evaporation rate of the aqueous tear film.[110]

Analysis of lacrimal gland fluid of rabbits and human tears of subjects treated with isotretinoin has shown the presence of this vitamin derivative in tears. Thus, the actual presence of isotretinoin in tear fluid could decrease stability of the lipid layer of the tear film, which would enhance the formation of dry spots. This effect could be responsible, in turn, for the dry eye symptoms, contact lens intolerance, and conjunctival irritation accompanying isotretinoin therapy.[112] Use of artificial tear preparations may help to alleviate the associated discomfort.

BETA-ADRENERGIC BLOCKING AGENTS

Drugs classified as β-adrenergic blocking agents have become the mainstay in the treatment of systemic hypertension, ischemic heart disease, cardiac arrhythmias, and migraine headache. Use of these drugs is not without systemic and ocular side effects (see Chapter 3).

Reduced tear secretion is a reported side effect of oral β-blocking drugs. Although most of the reported cases deal with practolol,[113] other β blockers such as propranolol and timolol have also been implicated in dry eye syndrome.[114,115] Ocular side effects of practolol have been described as an oculomucocutaneous syndrome in which patients suffer from symptomatic lesions of the outer eye.[113] A reduction of lysozyme and an absence of IgA may also occur.[115] The ocular side effects of practolol can be so serious that this drug is no longer marketed for clinical use.

Atenolol, metoprolol, oxyprenolol and pindolol have all been implicated in patients with dry eye symptoms and in reduction of tear lysozyme.[115,116] Metoprolol has also been associated with conjunctival injection and keratoconjunctivitis sicca.[115]

ORAL CONTRACEPTIVES

Although oral contraceptives have been implicated to cause reduced tear production and problems associated with contact lens wear, the literature is devoid of well-documented studies showing a definite cause-and-effect relationship.[117-119]

MISCELLANEOUS AGENTS

Other drugs with possible anticholinergic actions, such as phenothiazines, antianxiety agents, and tricyclic antidepressants, have been associated with dry eye syndromes.[1] Diuretics such as hydrochlorothiazide can also reduce tear production.[120]

Drugs that Increase Aqueous Tears and Tear Film Constituents

Several studies indicate that systemic administration of certain cholinergic, adrenergic, and antihypertensive agents stimulates lacrimation. Subcutaneous pilocarpine can increase tear production in normal eyes.[105] Neostigmine, given subcutaneously or intramuscularly, will also induce lacrimation.[121] Among the adrenergic agonists, ephedrine has been reported to increase tear production.[1,2] Several antihypertensive agents can increase tear production. Reserpine, hydralazine, and diazoxide at therapeutic dosages can induce lacrimation in humans.[2] Chronic use of marijuana has been reported to increase tear secretion.[122] Tear samples have shown the presence of small amounts (2.1%) of Δ^9-tetrahydrocannabinol. Other authors,[123] however, have reported a reduction in tear secretion following marijuana use, along with a subjective feeling of dryness.

Several investigators have studied the effects of systemic agents on tear protein and other constituents.[106,115] Atropine increases tear protein and lysozyme, but since tear secretion is reduced, production of protein and lysozyme per unit time remains unchanged.[106] In the same study the adrenergic stimulator, ephedrine, increased tear lysozyme production threefold per unit time.

Among the β-adrenergic antagonists, timolol and propranolol increase tear lysozyme, whereas practolol decreases its concentration, particularly in patients with the oculomucocutaneous syndrome of decreased tear secretion, conjunctival keratinization, scarring, and shrinkage.[115]

Drug penetration into tears has been reported with certain antimicrobial agents and aspirin. Sulfonamides, tetracyclines, erythromycin, and rifampin have been assayed in tears of human subjects.[124] Ampicillin and penicillin penetrate into the tears very poorly, and important bioactive concentrations are most likely not obtained.[124] In contrast, erythromycin levels in tears have been found to be higher than the serum concentration, implying active transport of this antibiotic into tears following systemic administration.[124] Following its oral administration, 36% to 88% of the daily erythromycin dosage is present in tears. Aspirin and isotretinoin also appear to penetrate into human tears following high-dose oral administration.[110,112]

An observation worth noting is that the tears can become discolored after the use of systemic rifampin.[125] The tears usually become orange but may also be light pink or red. Contact lenses may also stain, and it has therefore been suggested that lens wear may need to be discontinued during rifampin therapy in patients who secrete this drug in tears.[126]

Drugs Affecting the Pupil

Pupil size and function can be affected by both peripheral autonomic action as well as by centrally initiated impulses. The iris is an excellent indicator of autonomic activity because of the delicate balance between adrenergic and cholinergic innervation to the iris dilator and iris sphincter muscles, respectively. By acting directly on these muscles both adrenergic and cholinergic agents can influence pupil size and activity.

Drugs Causing Mydriasis

Anticholinergics, central nervous system stimulants and depressants, antihistamines, and phenothiazines can all cause mydriasis (Table 30.5).

ANTICHOLINERGICS

Drugs with anticholinergic effects such as atropine or related compounds can cause significant mydriasis. Systemic administration of 2 mg or more of atropine can result in pupillary dilation and cycloplegia.[127]

Scopolamine, a semisynthetic derivative of atropine, is marketed as a transdermal delivery system (Transderm Scōp) to prevent motion sickness. The device, which is placed behind the ear, consists of a 2.5 cm² disk containing 1.5 mg of scopolamine in a polymeric gel. Approximately 0.5 mg of drug is released into systemic circulation over a 3-day period.[128] Both mydriasis and reduced pupillary light response can occur when this device is used for 3 or more days.[129] Direct contamination of the eye by rubbing with fingers following application of the patch to the skin or during wear has been suggested as the cause for the observed pupillary dilation.[128]

CENTRAL NERVOUS SYSTEM STIMULANTS

This class of drugs includes agents such as the amphetamines (Dexedrine), methylphenidate (Ritalin), and

TABLE 30.5
Drugs that Can Cause Mydriasis

Anticholinergics
CNS stimulants
   Amphetamines
   Methylphenidate
   Cocaine
CNS depressants
   Barbiturates
   Antianxiety agents
Antihistamines
Phenothiazines

cocaine. Their mechanism of action is to augment actions of the adrenergic nervous system. Amphetamines are used to elevate mood, suppress appetite, and control hyperkinetic disorders in children.

High-dose, chronic use of amphetamines has been observed to cause mydriasis and decreased pupillary light response. The dilation can be to such an extent that the drug abuser seems to have unusually bright and shiny eyes.[130] In patients with potentially narrow angles, the mydriasis can precipitate an attack of acute or subacute angle-closure glaucoma.

CENTRAL NERVOUS SYSTEM DEPRESSANTS

These drugs include the barbiturates, such as phenobarbital, and the antianxiety drugs, including diazepam (Valium), chlordiazepoxide (Librium), oxazepam (Serax), flurazepam (Dalmane), and lorazepam (Ativan). These agents act by potentiating the neural inhibition mediated by the GABA system.

Barbiturates have little effect on the pupils, although in acute or chronic poisoning a sluggish pupillary light reaction is common.[2] The benzodiazepines including diazepam (Valium) can occasionally cause mydriasis, presumably because of their anticholinergic side effects.

MISCELLANEOUS DRUGS

Other drugs with potential to cause mydriasis include the antihistamines and antipsychotic agents.[1] Both these classes of drugs have anticholinergic properties.

Pupillary dilation has also been observed on exposure to certain plants. The dried pods of the jimson weed *(Datura stramonium)* are often used for floral arrangements during the winter. Children have been known to consume the "berries," which contain significant concentrations of belladonna alkaloids. Systemic side effects are those typical of anticholinergic drugs and include bilaterally dilated pupils.[131]

Drugs Causing Miosis

Opiates such as heroin, morphine, and codeine, and anticholinesterase agents can cause miosis.

OPIATES

Heroin, morphine, and codeine characteristically constrict the pupil. Moreover, the pupillary light response is enhanced.[132] This appears to be due to action on the central nervous system, possibly on the visceral nucleus of the oculomotor nuclear complex.[133]

ANTICHOLINESTERASE AGENTS

Systemic absorption of agents that inhibit the cholinesterase enzymes can result in miosis. Such substances are present in most insecticides and many toxic nerve gases. Toxic episodes involving the pupil have occurred in workers in fields being dusted with insecticides from an airplane.[134] The miotic pupils of affected patients may not return to normal until 30 to 45 days after exposure to the toxic agent.[309]

Drugs Affecting Extraocular Muscles

The effects of systemic drugs on extraocular muscles remain obscure. Drugs affecting the autonomic nervous system, central vestibular system, or causing extrapyramidal effects have been associated with ocular manifestations such as nystagmus, diplopia, extraocular muscle palsy, and oculogyric crisis.[135] Table 30.6 lists drugs that can affect extraocular muscles.

Various classes of drugs have been implicated in patients with nystagmus, including salicylates, phenytoin (Dilantin), antihistamines, gold, and barbiturates.[135] Diplopia has been associated with many drugs that affect central nervous system activity. Included are the phenothiazines, anti-anxiety agents, and antidepressants.[135]

Alcohol is well documented to affect eye movement.[136–138] Both smooth pursuits and saccades are impaired when blood ethanol concentrations reach the range of 60 to 100 mg/dl. Bittencourt and associates[137] have reported a direct linear relationship between blood alcohol concentration and a reduction in smooth-pursuit velocity. Their results indicate that at a blood ethanol concentration of 80 mg/dl, the capacity of the eyes to track objects moving across the visual fields is impaired by 25%.

TABLE 30.6
Drugs that Can Affect Extraocular Muscles

Drug	Side Effect
Salicylates	Nystagmus
Phenytoin	Nystagmus
Antihistamines	Nystagmus
Gold salts	Nystagmus
Barbiturates	Nystagmus
Phenothiazines	Diplopia
Anti-anxiety agents	Diplopia
Antidepressants	Diplopia
Alcohol	Impairment of version movements

The fact that alcohol can affect eye movement ability has been employed to devise a test known as the alcohol gaze nystagmus test. This procedure was developed to augment the traditional field evaluation of suspected drunk drivers by law enforcement officials. The test involves the observation of ocular version movements, end-point nystagmus, and angle of lateral deviation at which the nystagmoid movements begin. When properly administered and evaluated, the test can help to correctly identify about 80% of drivers with blood alcohol levels of 0.10% or higher.[139,140]

Drugs Causing Myopia

Numerous reports have described patients with acute onset of myopia following use of various oral medications or drugs applied as vaginal suppositories or creams. In most cases the amount of drug-induced myopia has been slight, but in some cases myopia exceeding 5 D has occurred.[141] Commonly prescribed drugs that are widely recognized to cause myopia include sulfonamides, diuretics, and carbonic anhydrase inhibitors. In most instances the myopia is acute in onset following administration of the drug and subsides within days or weeks following withdrawal of the medication.

Clinical Signs and Symptoms

Among the drugs most commonly implicated are the sulfonamides.[141–144] Mattsson[144] described two cases of transient myopia associated with oral sulfonamides in which there was reduced accommodation, shallow anterior chamber angles, and moderate mydriasis. In one case there was chemosis. In 1986 Hook and associates[142] described a 23-year-old woman who had 4 D of increased myopia in one eye and 3 D increase in the fellow eye following the use of oral sulfonamides. Vaginal absorption of sulfonamides can also lead to myopia. Chirls and Norris[143] reported a patient with 1.0 to 1.5 D of myopia following use of a vaginal sulfonamide suppository, and Maddalena[141] described a patient with 7 D of induced myopia following use of a sulfonamide vaginal cream. This case was complicated by retinal edema, narrowing of the anterior chamber angle, and acute angle-closure glaucoma.

Diuretic agents can also cause myopia.[145–149] Beasley[145] reported transient myopia associated with perimacular edema apparently caused from the use of 100 mg of hydrochlorothiazide. The drug induced approximately 3 D of myopia, which resolved within 3 days. Carbonic anhydrase inhibitors are also known to cause myopia.[146,147,149] Muirhead and Scheie[149] described a case of transient myopia associated with acetazolamide, in which there was also narrowing of the anterior chamber angle, suggesting increased volume (edema) of the ocular contents behind the iris, or diminished volume of the anterior chamber.

Drug-induced myopia has also been reported with prochlorperazine (Compazine) therapy[150] and with use of aspirin.[151]

Mechanism

In general, transient myopia results from edema of the ciliary body, lenticular edema, or accommodative spasm.[142] Topically administered cholinergic agonists are well known to cause myopia by stimulating accommodation, but systemically administered cholinergic agents are only infrequently implicated as a cause of myopia. Most drugs that cause myopia do so by producing ciliary body edema, resulting in relaxation of the zonules, which causes thickening and anterior movement of the lens.[142]

Drug-induced myopia associated with sulfonamides has been documented by ultrasonographic A-scan measurements and refractions to be due to edema of the ciliary body.[142,152] The ciliary body edema, occasionally associated with retinal edema, has led to the speculation that sulfonamide-induced myopia may be related to a hypersensitivity reaction.[141,144]

Since carbonic anhydrase inhibitors (CAI) are sulfonamide derivatives, the mechanism for CAI-induced myopia would be expected to be similar to that associated with sulfonamides. Indeed, Galin and associates[147] have speculated that myopia resulting from use of acetazolamide is due to a hypersensitivity reaction resulting in ciliary body edema. The instillation of cycloplegics has had little influence on the refractive error, suggesting that the mechanism is unrelated to ciliary spasm.[146]

Management

Patients with well-documented acute myopia should be carefully evaluated to eliminate other causes of the refractive change. Intumescence of the lens associated with nuclear sclerosis is a common cause of increasing myopia related to this type of lens change is often associated with somewhat reduced best-corrected visual acuity. After eliminating these other factors, the patient's drug therapy may be investigated as a cause of the myopia by reducing or discontinuing the drug under suspicion. This should be done only in consultation with the patient's physician. By reducing or discontinuing the offending agent, the refractive error change should subside within several days or several weeks.

Drugs Causing Cycloplegia

Some drugs administered systemically are well known to have mild anticholinergic properties or side effects, including antianxiety agents, antihistamines, and tricyclic antidepressants. Agents with strong anticholinergic effects include atropine and scopolamine. Although these drugs can dilate the pupil and can cause dry eye symptoms due to the peripheral effects on the parasympathetic nervous system, the cycloplegic effects are less commonly encountered in clinical practice. Sulfadiazine[153] and disopyramide[154] have been reported to cause paralysis of accommodation, but the most common drugs associated with clinical cycloplegia are chloroquine and the phenothiazines.

Chloroquine

CLINICAL SIGNS AND SYMPTOMS

Accommodative insufficiency, with associated reading difficulty, is a common side effect of long-term chloroquine therapy.[20,21,155–157] This usually begins within several weeks after treatment is started, and the effect appears to be dose related.[21,155,157] As many as 40% of patients taking 500 to 750 mg daily will have impaired accommodation.[158] The accommodative insufficiency is often rapid in onset but is reversible on reduction or discontinuation of drug therapy.[21,155]

MECHANISM

The precise mechanism underlying the cycloplegic effect of chloroquine is unknown. However, the fact that the accommodative insufficiency is rapid in both onset and reversibility suggests that the effect is not related to melanin binding.[21] The changes in amplitude of accommodation might also be explained by a drug effect on the central nervous system.[155]

MANAGEMENT

Because the cycloplegic effects of chloroquine are transient and are related to drug dosage, symptoms of accommodative insufficiency can be managed by prescribing appropriate reading lenses during long-term drug therapy, or, in consultation with the patient's physician, drug dosages may be reduced or discontinued. The cycloplegic effects of chloroquine will often abate when the dosage is reduced, and accommodation will completely return to pretreatment levels after drug therapy is discontinued.[155]

Phenothiazines

Transient disturbances of accommodation often occur in patients taking chlorpromazine and other phenothiazines.[159,160] These effects are most likely due to the anticholinergic properties of the medication[159] and are most pronounced when benztropine (Cogentin) is administered along with the phenothiazine.[161,162] The visual symptoms may also be ascribed to reduced tearing and drying of the cornea, causing blurred vision. In patients with narrow anterior chamber angles, acute or subacute angle-closure glaucoma secondary to dilated pupils could also contribute to symptoms of blurred vision.[159]

Drugs Affecting Intraocular Pressure

A variety of drugs can affect intraocular pressure (Table 30.7). Drugs capable of dilating the pupil can cause acute or subacute angle-closure glaucoma if the anterior chamber is narrow. Steroids are widely known to elevate intraocular pressure in the presence of open angles. Other drugs, such as β-adrenergic blocking agents, can reduce intraocular pressure.

Clinical Signs and Symptoms

Since patients with extremely narrow anterior chamber angles are at risk for the development of angle-closure glaucoma, drugs that can potentially dilate the pupil may induce acute or subacute angle-closure glaucoma. This includes any medication with anticholinergic or strong adrenergic agonist properties.[154] Hiatt and associates[163] have shown, however, that the risk of elevating intraocular pressure with systemically administered anticholinergic agents is small, even in patients with narrow angles.

Of greater importance is the influence of systemically administered steroids on intraocular pressure. In addition to their systemic effects, steroids administered

TABLE 30.7
Drugs that Can Affect Intraocular Pressure

Drugs Causing Elevated IOP (with open angle)	Drugs Potentially Causing Angle-Closure Glaucoma	Drugs Causing Decreased IOP
Corticosteroids	Anticholinergics Antihistamines Phenothiazines Tricyclic antidepressants	β-adrenergic blockers Ethyl alcohol Cardiac glycosides

IOP, intraocular pressure.

orally can elevate intraocular pressure, although the prevalence of elevated pressure is less than that occurring with topical steroids.[164,165] This is probably due to the lower concentration of steroid within the anterior chamber when steroids are administered systemically.[165] Nevertheless, systemic steroids can elevate pressure enough to cause glaucomatous damage to the optic disc and visual field.[166]

The long-term administration of systemic steroids typically produces a relatively small increase in pressure,[59,167] and the elevated pressure is self-limiting as the drug therapy is reduced or discontinued. In one study[168] about 34% of the patients receiving systemic steroids had ocular pressures of 20 mm Hg or higher, while only 6% of the control group had similar pressure elevations.

As with topically applied steroids, the degree of response to systemic steroids is not related to dosage or duration of treatment but is due, rather, to factors of individual susceptibility or responsiveness to the effects of steroids.[168–171] In patients who are steroid responders, pressure elevations with systemic steroids average about 60% of those produced by topically applied steroids.[172] Thus, patients with glaucoma would be expected to be particularly sensitive to the pressure-elevating effects of systemic steroids.

Systemically administered β-adrenergic blocking agents are well known to reduce intraocular pressure.[173–175] This occurs both in patients with normal pressure as well as in those with glaucoma.[173,174] The ocular hypotensive effects of systemic β blockers are discussed in detail in Chapter 7.

Ethyl alcohol is widely consumed in the form of beer, whiskey, and other alcoholic beverages. Normal individuals demonstrate only a minimal reduction of pressure following consumption of 50 ml of 43% ethyl alcohol in the form of whiskey.[176] Patients with open-angle glaucoma, however, have a much greater reduction of pressure lasting for 3 to 5 hours. These effects are discussed further in Chapter 8.

Mechanism

As previously discussed, drugs that dilate the pupil can acutely elevate intraocular pressure in eyes predisposed to angle-closure glaucoma. The pathogenesis of steroid-induced pressure elevation is less well understood. As with topically applied steroids, steroids administered systemically may reduce aqueous outflow facility in susceptible patients,[172] but there is substantial evidence that systemically administered steroids may also increase aqueous formation, leading to elevated pressure.[53,168,169,172,177] Diotallevi and Bocci[177] have shown that systemically administered steroids can increase aqueous production without elevating intraocular pressure, implying a concomitant increase of aqueous outflow. Compared with topical steroids, systemic steroids may evoke different changes in the ocular fluid dynamics because of the distinctly different route of administration.[168] Patients receiving long-term systemic steroids may accumulate excessive amounts of mucopolysaccharide in the trabecular meshwork, obstructing aqueous outflow by hydrating the trabeculum.[178]

Management

Patients who sustain acute or subacute angle-closure glaucoma should be managed following the guidelines given in Chapter 29. It is imperative, of course, that the offending drug be immediately withdrawn.

Ocular hypertension or open-angle glaucoma associated with systemic steroid therapy should be managed according to the guidelines given in Chapter 29. Reducing steroid dosage, if possible, almost always reduces pressure. If continuation of steroid therapy is deemed necessary, the ocular pressure can often be controlled with topical antiglaucoma therapy despite continuation of systemic steroids.[164]

Because propranolol and other systemic β blockers are widely used for treatment of systemic hypertension,

TABLE 30.8
Drugs that Can Affect Retinal Function

Drug	Side Effect
Chloroquine and hydroxychloroquine	Retinal pigmentary changes, visual field defects, color vision loss
Thioridazine	Retinal pigmentary changes, disturbances of dark adaptation, color vision loss, visual field defects
Quinine	Impairment of dark adaptation, visual field defects, vascular attenuation
Talc	Intra-arteriolar talc particles, retinal nonperfusion, neovascularization
Cardiac glycosides	Color vision disturbances, entoptic phenomena
Nonsteroidal anti-inflammatory agents	
Salicylates	Retinal hemorrhage
Indomethacin	Pigmentary changes, color vision loss, visual field defects
Antineoplastic agents	
Tamoxifen	Refractile opacities in posterior pole
Carmustine	Retinal vascular disease
Isotretinoin	Impairment of dark adaptation

angina, or cardiac arrhythmias, the possibility of drug-induced lowering of intraocular pressure should always be considered. This can potentially mask primary open-angle glaucoma or falsely lead to a diagnosis of low tension glaucoma. On the other hand, once the diagnosis of glaucoma is made, systemic β blockers can be of value in the treatment of the glaucoma if the systemic agents are needed for other purposes.[174]

Since ethyl alcohol is widely used socially and can temporarily lower intraocular pressure, it is possible that the ocular hypotensive effect could contribute to errors in evaluation, diagnosis, or management of glaucoma during a clinical examination. The practitioner, therefore, should consider this effect in patients who have recently consumed alcohol.[176]

Drugs Affecting the Retina

Numerous drugs have been associated with retinal toxicity (Table 30.8). These include medications obtained by prescription as well as drugs available over the counter. Phenylpropanolamine, an adrenergic agonist available over the counter and used as an anorectic, has been reported to cause central retinal vein occlusion associated with systemic hypertension.[179] This emphasizes the importance of a careful drug history.

Drugs can be retinotoxic through a variety of mechanisms (Table 30.9). Depending on the specific drug, its dosage, and duration of treatment, these retinotoxic effects are often reversible if recognized early.[180]

The following sections discuss the systemic drugs that are well known to be toxic to the retina.

Chloroquine and Hydroxychloroquine

Both chloroquine and hydroxychloroquine have been widely used for the treatment of rheumatoid arthritis, discoid and systemic lupus erythematosus, and other collagen diseases since the early 1950s. Presently hydroxychloroquine (Plaquenil) is used almost exclusively as the quinoline agent of choice for the treatment of rheumatic diseases.[181] Cambiaggi[182] first described chloroquine retinopathy, although he believed the lesions to be associated with the patient's systemic lupus. In 1959 Hobbs and associates[183] confirmed these findings and appropriately related them to the chloroquine treatment. Since that time numerous cases of chloroquine-related retinopathy have been reported, and the mechanism underlying these drug-induced changes has been largely confirmed.

CLINICAL SIGNS AND SYMPTOMS

The first visible evidence of chloroquine retinopathy is a fine pigmentary mottling within the macular area

TABLE 30.9
Mechanisms of Retinal Drug Toxicity

- Overdosage
- Idiosyncrasy
- Side effects
- Secondary
- Hypersensitivity
- Photosensitization

Modified from Crews SJ. Some aspects of retinal drug toxicity. Ophthalmologica 1969;158:232–244.

with or without loss of the foveal reflex.[184,185] Even before visible ophthalmoscopic changes are detectable, however, a "premaculopathy" state can exist in which the drug interferes with metabolism of the macular tissues, causing subtle relative visual field defects in patients with ophthalmoscopically normal maculas.[156,157] As the macular pigmentary changes progress, a classic pattern develops consisting of a granular hyperpigmentation surrounded by a zone of depigmentation, which in turn is surrounded by another ring of pigment. Although this clinical picture can vary in intensity, it is pathognomonic of chloroquine retinopathy and is referred to as a "bull's eye" lesion[21,184–189] (Fig. 30.7).

Variations of retinal pigment epithelial (RPE) disturbances can occur and are commonly observed as a well-circumscribed area of RPE atrophy in the macular area, which resembles a macular hole[21,184] (Fig. 30.8). In moderate to advanced cases of retinal toxicity, the arterioles may become attenuated, and the optic disc can become pale.[21,186,187] Occasionally there may be signs of macular edema.[21,187] There usually is a high degree of bilateral symmetry between eyes, but occasionally the toxicity can affect one eye more than the other.

Fluorescein angiography demonstrates dramatic fluorescence of the macular area in patients with chloroquine maculopathy. Atrophy of the RPE allows the underlying choroidal fluorescence to become visible during the early, pre-arterial phase of the angiogram.[21,190]

Some patients with chloroquine retinopathy may have retinal changes resembling retinitis pigmentosa.[21,188,191–194] There is peripheral RPE hyperplasia, but, in contrast to retinitis pigmentosa, the pigment does not tend to accumulate around the retinal veins.[194] These peripheral lesions can occur with or without simultaneous macular involvement[21] (Fig. 30.9). Other changes include attenuated retinal vessels, optic atrophy, peripheral visual field loss, and a subnormal electroretinogram (ERG). The fact that the dark-adaptation threshold is normal or only minimally abnormal further differentiates this condition from retinitis pigmentosa.[192]

Although the visual fields may be normal even in the presence of definite macular pigmentary changes,[27] visual field loss generally correlates well with the degree of retinal damage. The typical visual field defects in chloroquine retinopathy consist of central, paracentral, or pericentral scotomas.[22,194,195] The paracentral scotomas may become confluent and form a complete ring scotoma.

In the early stages of retinopathy electrodiagnostic studies are usually of little value in detecting early chloroquine toxicity.[21,185] Both the ERG and electrooculogram (EOG) can be normal or abnormal. Advanced cases of chloroquine retinopathy, however, are generally characterized by markedly abnormal or even extinguished ERGs.[192,194] This is especially true in cases involving the retinal periphery.

Although it is possible for patients with chloroquine

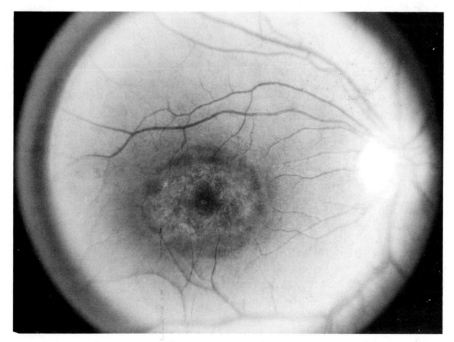

FIGURE 30.7   **Characteristic bull's eye maculopathy associated with chloroquine toxicity.**

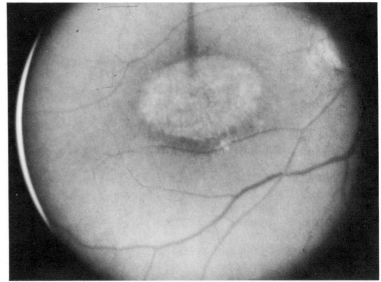

FIGURE 30.8 **Retinal pigment epithelial atrophy in macular area as a consequence of chloroquine therapy.**

maculopathy to be asymptomatic,[27] extensive macular damage will often lead to symptoms of decreased visual acuity, metamorphopsia, and visual field disturbances.[21,156,186] Pericentral ring scotomas can cause reading difficulty.[196] Although color vision is normal in the early stages of chloroquine toxicity, more extensive macular damage can lead to severe impairment of color vision. Dark adaptation is typically normal, an impor-

tant feature distinguishing the peripheral retinal changes from those seen in retinitis pigmentosa.[21]

Risk factors for the development of chloroquine retinopathy include daily dosage, duration of treatment, serum drug levels, and patient age. The incidence of retinopathy increases with patient age, and in older patients retinal toxicity appears to be correlated with total drug dosage.[27,197,198] Ehrenfeld and

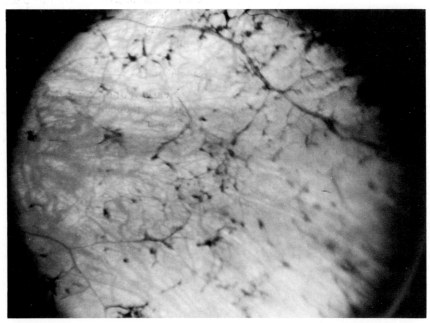

FIGURE 30.9 **Peripheral retinal pigment epithelial hyperplasia characteristic of pseudoretinitis pigmentosa in 42-year-old male with chloroquine toxicity.**

associates[197] contend that daily dosage is the most critical risk factor. Most cases of chloroquine retinopathy occur in patients taking 500 mg daily,[a] but dosages as low as 250 mg daily can also be retinotoxic.[20,21,188] No adult cases of retinopathy have been associated with dosages less than 250 mg daily.[21] Retinopathy can develop when the total cumulative dosage is as little as 100 g (the equivalent of 250 mg daily for 1 year), but the risk increases significantly when the total dosage exceeds 300 g.[20] Marks and Power[27] found retinopathy in 10% of patients receiving a total dosage of less than 200 g, while 50% of patients receiving more than 600 g developed retinopathy. The duration of therapy required to produce chloroquine retinopathy can be as little as 6 months, but most patients require 2 to 4 years of therapy before retinal changes develop.[20,186,199]

Chloroquine retinopathy tends to remain stable once therapy is discontinued.[188] Some patients, however, may demonstrate regression of macular changes if the retinal involvement is mild and if visual acuity is normal.[185,188] Although some patients with the classic "bull's eye" maculopathy may have reversible macular changes,[27] patients with moderately advanced retinopathy may show progression after drug therapy is discontinued.[188] Progressive impairment of visual acuity can occur for up to 5 years following discontinuation of chloroquine therapy.[200]

Occasionally retinopathy does not develop until chloroquine therapy is discontinued. Such delayed-onset chloroquine retinopathy can occur from 1 to 10 years following discontinuation of drug therapy.[187,196,197]

The risk of retinopathy associated with hydroxychloroquine appears to be considerably less than that associated with chloroquine.[181,198] Tobin and associates[28] reported retinal toxicity in only 4 of 99 patients receiving hydroxychloroquine in a daily dosage of 400 mg for at least 1 year. No patient, however, sustained significant vision loss, and the abnormalities were reversible after the medication was discontinued. In some cases the macular changes may be reversible without recurrence even if the medication is reinstituted.[181] As little as 73 g of hydroxychloroquine taken over 6 months has been reported to cause retinopathy,[181] and the incidence of retinopathy may be as high as 29% if the cumulative dosage exceeds 800 g.[189] Several investigators,[28,201] however, have discounted the role of cumulative dosage and believe that the risk of maculopathy associated with hydroxychloroquine therapy is more closely related to daily dosage. Johnson and Vine[201] found no evidence of retinopathy in 9 patients treated with massive total dosages of hydroxychloroquine ranging from 1054 to 3923 g. These authors suggest that patients who take prudent daily dosages of hydroxychloroquine (400 mg daily or 6.5 mg/kg body weight daily, whichever is less) are at little risk of developing retinopathy even when therapy is prolonged.

MECHANISM

Although the precise mechanism by which chloroquine and hydroxychloroquine cause retinal toxicity is unknown, it is widely recognized that these drugs bind tenaciously to melanin within the eye.[202,203] Moreover, histopathologic analysis has revealed that the pigmented tissues of the eye will continue to hold the drug for prolonged periods after drug therapy is discontinued.[202] This can lead to degenerative changes of the RPE. Rosenthal and associates,[202] however, have shown that chloroquine also accumulates in the retina itself, suggesting that the neurosensory retina may also be able to bind the drug. Investigations in monkeys have shown that chloroquine initially causes degenerative effects in the ganglion cells, followed by disruption of the photoreceptors and finally the RPE and choroid.[202] Ramsay and Fine[204] have confirmed in humans that the initial pathologic change occurs in the ganglion cells and that the changes within the RPE and photoreceptors occur late in the disease process. The destructive process within the RPE leads to migration of pigment-laden cells from the RPE to the outer nuclear and outer plexiform layers.[21,205] There is frequently sparing of the foveal cones, which explains the ophthalmoscopic appearance seen in cases of bull's eye maculopathy.[203] Attenuation of the retinal arterioles is thought to be secondary to the extensive retinal damage.[203]

MANAGEMENT

Since early retinopathy is frequently reversible if drug dosage is reduced or discontinued, patients taking chloroquine or hydroxychloroquine should be monitored very carefully. Patients should receive baseline examinations before starting therapy and should be examined periodically for evidence of retinal changes. Baseline examinations of the fundus are especially important, since chloroquine and hydroxychloroquine maculopathy can resemble age-related macular disease. Once treatment has started, it is prudent to monitor patients every 6 months,[28,181] especially if the patient is over 65 years of age.[197] Elderly patients should be monitored more carefully, since chloroquine and hydroxychloroquine are detoxified and eliminated from the body by the liver and kidney, respectively, which might be impaired in the elderly.[24]

Fundus and visual field evaluations are among the most important clinical procedures to be performed.

---

[a]For comparison purposes, 500 mg of chloroquine phosphate is equivalent to 400 mg of hydroxychloroquine sulfate.

Careful ophthalmoscopic examination of the fundus, including retinal periphery, is one of the most sensitive indicators of early maculopathy.[189,206] Subtle macular changes can often be detected using slit lamp biomicroscopy. Visual field assessment using static threshold techniques are of value in detecting the early stages of visual field loss associated with chloroquine retinopathy.[195]

The indecisive quality of the ERG and EOG in cases of early maculopathy preclude their use in the detection of early chloroquine retinopathy. Likewise, fluorescein angiography has been shown to be less sensitive than routine ophthalmoscopy or color photography in the detection of early chloroquine retinopathy.[184] Thus, fluorescein angiography is generally not required to establish the diagnosis. However, in patients with preexisting macular disease, fluorescein angiography may help differentiate underlying macular disease from that induced by drug toxicity.

Since the clinical signs and symptoms of toxic retinopathy may not appear until after drug therapy is discontinued, it is important to monitor patients for several years after drug therapy has been stopped. This is more important for patients who have received at least 300 g of chloroquine or the equivalent of hydroxychloroquine.[196,197]

Thioridazine

Chlorpromazine and thioridazine, both phenothiazine derivatives, are commonly used for their antipsychotic effects. Although pigmentary changes of the retina have occasionally been reported in association with chlorpromazine therapy,[160] it is now generally recognized that only thioridazine produces retinal toxicity. Pigmentary retinopathy associated with thioridazine therapy was first reported in 1959 by Kinross-Wright.[207]

CLINICAL SIGNS AND SYMPTOMS

Blurred vision associated with thioridazine therapy is often due to the anticholinergic effects of the medication. More important, however, thioridazine can cause significant retinal toxicity, leading to reduced visual acuity, changes in color vision, and disturbances of dark adaptation. These symptoms typically occur 30 to 90 days after treatment is begun.[159,208] Visual field changes consist of concentric contraction or irregular paracentral or ring scotomas.[208] The fundus appearance is often normal during the early stages of symptoms, but within several weeks or months a pigmentary retinopathy develops characterized by fine clumps of pigment developing first in the periphery and progressing toward the posterior pole (Fig. 30.10).[159,209] In milder cases the pigment remains fine and peppery, but in more severe cases the pigment can form plaque-like lesions with multiple confluent areas of hypopigmentation and choroidal atrophy.[208] Retinal edema can also occur,[159] but the optic disc and retinal vasculature are usually normal.[209]

The ERG and EOG are often normal during the early stages of toxicity, but as the RPE becomes diffusely abnormal, the EOG becomes attenuated.[210] The

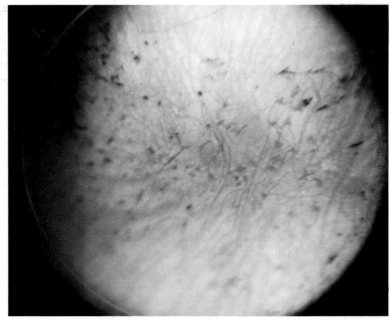

FIGURE 30.10 **Retinal pigment epithelial hyperplasia and atrophy in 33-year-old man with thioridazine retinopathy.**

amplitude of the oscillatory potential of the ERG decreases in proportion to the daily dosage of thioridazine, but the a- and b-waves as well as the latencies are normal.[211]

It is now recognized that the primary clinical factor associated with thioridazine retinopathy is the daily drug dosage.[209] Before the dose-related retinal toxicity was recognized, dosages exceeding 1600 mg daily were commonly used.[208] Few cases of pigmentary retinopathy have been reported, however, with daily dosages of less than 800 mg. Thus, thioridazine therapy appears to be safe with regard to retinal toxicity as long as daily dosages of less than 800 mg are employed.[35,209,212]

Although it is possible for thioridazine retinopathy to resolve despite continued drug therapy, this usually occurs only in patients taking low dosages.[159] If significant resolution is to occur, drug therapy must generally be reduced or discontinued. Depending on the severity of toxicity, retinal function can return to normal, but the pigmentary changes are often permanent. In severe cases there may be permanent impairment of visual acuity, visual field, and dark adaptation.[35,209] The pigmentary retinopathy may even progress after the drug therapy has been discontinued, and some cases of progressive retinopathy can have a late onset, occurring from 4 to 10 years following discontinuation of thioridazine.[209,210]

MECHANISM

Thioridazine and other phenothiazines bind to melanin in the uveal tract, especially the choroid.[209,213] Drug uptake by the choroid occurs even in patients whose serum levels of thioridazine are in the nontoxic range.[214] It has been proposed that such drug binding is retinotoxic by damaging the choriocapillaris, thus leading to changes in the RPE.[208,209] It is also possible that thioridazine may alter retinal enzyme kinetics, inhibiting the oxidation of retinol. Alterations in the enzyme systems of Mueller cells and photoreceptors may lead to atrophy and disorganization of the rods and cones as one of the initial degenerative changes, followed later by loss of the RPE and choriocapillaris.[208]

MANAGEMENT

Since the danger of retinal toxicity with thioridazine is significantly correlated with daily dosage, patients should generally be placed on dosages of less than 800 mg daily.[208,209] Patients should receive careful fundus examinations during the first 2 to 4 months of therapy and every 6 months thereafter.[209] Electrodiagnostic tests such as ERG and EOG are generally of no value in detecting early retinopathy.[215] If symptoms or objective signs of retinal toxicity are observed, the medication must be promptly discontinued to improve the chances of resolution. This must be done only in consultation with the patient's physician. Since the pigmentary retinopathy may be progressive even after thioridazine has been discontinued, patients should receive follow-up examinations on an annual basis.

Quinine

Historically quinine has been employed for the treatment of malaria, but it is now used primarily for the management of leg cramps, myotonia congenita, and eyelid myokymia.[216] Quinine toxicity has been recognized for 150 years, and overdosage of quinine is still encountered in patients who attempt abortion or suicide. Accidental ingestion of quinine can also lead to serious side effects. Among the various features of quinine toxicity, acute vision loss is one of the most significant and dangerous.

CLINICAL SIGNS AND SYMPTOMS

Mild toxic reactions are characterized by slight reduction of visual acuity, "flickering" of vision, tinnitus, weakness, or confusion. In more severe cases symptoms consist of sudden complete loss of vision, dizziness, and even deafness. Coma with circulatory collapse characterize the most severe form of quinine toxicity.[216] Patients presenting with acute quinine overdose frequently have no light perception in both eyes, and pupils are often dilated and nonreactive to light.[217–219] Patients may complain of impairment of night vision, but color vision is usually normal.[219] The visual fields usually demonstrate concentric contraction, and improvement of the visual fields following the acute episode may require days or months, but the field loss may show no recovery and become permanent.[216,217]

Ophthalmoscopic examination of the fundus soon after acute quinine overdose may reveal a normal fundus,[219,220] but constriction of the arterioles, optic disc pallor, venous dilatation, or retinal edema can also be observed. Several authors,[216,221] have reported normal ERG findings in the early stages of quinine toxicity, but as visual acuity improves, the ERG becomes distinctly abnormal. Yospaiboon and associates[217] have shown, in contrast, that the ERG is initially abnormal and gradually improves as visual function recovers. The EOG is initially abnormal but improves as visual function returns.[216,221]

The visual prognosis for patients with acute quinine toxicity is guarded. Visual acuity can improve from no light perception to 20/20 within days[219] to several weeks.[216,220] Sometimes vision does not improve to normal for several months.[217] As vision recovers there is progressive constriction of the retinal vessels, and the optic disc becomes pale.[216,219] Although central vision often returns to normal levels, the visual fields can remain constricted.[216,218,220] Any impairment of night vision and color vision can be permanent.[216,218]

The maximum daily dosage of quinine should generally not exceed 2 g, and quinine toxicity is common in dosages over 4 g. The lethal oral dose in adults is about 8 g.[219] Toxic reactions to relatively small doses of quinine are probably idiosyncratic in nature but can result in a clinical picture similar to that caused by higher doses.

MECHANISM

Several decades ago the concept of vascular spasm was widely held as the primary mechanism for the retinal damage associated with quinine toxicity.[222] This prompted treatment regimens aimed at promoting vascular dilatation in efforts to improve retinal circulation. However, our current understanding of the pathogenesis of quinine retinal toxicity is largely derived from various electrodiagnostic studies that have demonstrated that quinine probably has a direct toxic effect on the photoreceptors and ganglion cells.[217,219,220,310] Moreover, fluorescein angiographic studies have shown no significant circulatory disturbances.[217] Damage to the RPE is indicated by the abnormal EOG, the increased visibility of the choroid in the late stages of toxicity, and the increased background fluorescence seen on angiography.[219,221] Visual evoked potential (VEP) findings confirm the conduction abnormality in the nerve fiber layer associated with the secondary optic atrophy.[216]

MANAGEMENT

Several decades ago, when the concept of vascular spasm was accepted as the cause of retinal damage in quinine toxicity, attempts at retinal vasodilatation were made to improve retinal circulation. Stellate ganglion block was commonly used for this purpose.[222-224] Efforts were also made to accelerate removal of quinine from the body with techniques such as hemodialysis, peritoneal dialysis, plasmapheresis, and forced diuresis.[225,226] More recent investigations, however, have shown that these procedures have no rational basis and are without proven benefit.[219,220,310] Since central vision tends to recover spontaneously even without treatment,[219] patients with acute quinine toxicity should be managed by immediate gastric emptying, administration of activated charcoal, and other supportive measures. It is important to emphasize preventive measures such as patient education and dispensing of quinine in child-resistant containers, and efforts should be made to reformulate quinine tablets to enhance their bitter taste.[220]

Following the acute episode, patients should be monitored carefully for improvement in visual acuity, visual fields, and fundus appearance.

Talc

Tablets of medication intended for oral use contain inert filler materials such as talc (magnesium silicate), corn starch, cotton fibers, and other refractile and nonrefractile substances.[227] Chronic drug abusers are known to prepare a suspension of medication for injection by dissolving the crushed tablet of cocaine, heroin, methylphenidate, or other narcotic in water. They then boil the solution and filter it through a crude cigarette or cotton filter before injecting the solution intravenously, subcutaneously, or intramuscularly.[228] The talc particles eventually embolize to the retinal circulation and produce a characteristic form of retinopathy. Talc retinopathy was first reported in 1972 by AtLee,[229] and since then numerous cases have been described.

CLINICAL SIGNS AND SYMPTOMS

Fundus examination reveals multiple, tiny, yellow-white, glistening particles scattered throughout the posterior pole, but they are more numerous in the capillary bed and small arterioles of the perimacular area[229-231] (Fig. 30.11). In addition to these characteristic lesions, some patients can have macular edema, venous engorgement, punctate and flame-shaped hemorrhages, as well as arterial occlusion.[229,232] Foreign body granulomas of the retina have also been described.[227]

Retinal neovascularization as a consequence of talc injection was first reported in 1979 by Kresca and associates.[233] These lesions appear in the retinal periphery as neovascular tufts in the shape of seafans at the junction of the perfused and nonperfused retina. This is a potentially serious complication of talc injection because it can lead to retinal detachment, massive vitreal hemorrhage, and optic disc neovascularization.[228,234]

Most patients have no significant visual symptoms, and visual acuity is normal.[234] Some patients, however, may report blurring of vision, blind spots in the visual fields, and occasionally can have severe reduction of visual acuity.[228,232,234] Neither the extent of drug abuse nor the degree of filtration of the prepared suspension appears to be correlated with visual symptoms.[228]

The extent and concentration of talc particles observed in the posterior pole appear to correlate with the duration of drug abuse as well as with the cumulative number of tablets injected.[228,229] Often the drug abuser injects from 10 to 40 tablets daily, and some abusers inject as many as 100 tablets daily for several years.[229,235] Talc retinopathy is usually not found in drug abusers who have injected less than 9000 tablets, but it is consistently found in most patients who have injected more than 12,000 tablets.[235,236]

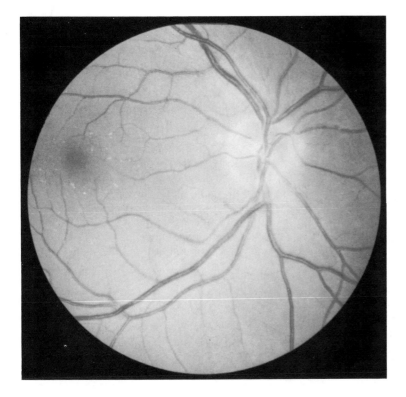

FIGURE 30.11 **Talc retinopathy characterized by numerous yellow-white intra-arteriolar particles scattered throughout perimacular area.**

MECHANISM

As the talc, corn starch, and other insoluble tablet fillers embolize to the lungs, they become trapped within the pulmonary tissues and eventually cause pulmonary hypertension. This leads to the development of collateral vessels that allow part of the venous return to bypass the lungs and enter the left side of the heart, where the particles are further embolized to the eye and other organs of the body.[228,230] The presence of talc particles in the eye indicates that substantial foreign body damage has occurred in the lungs.[229]

The talc particles are more numerous in the perimacular region than in other areas of the retina probably because of the rich blood supply and greater blood flow in that area.[237] The particles lodge in the walls of the precapillary arterioles and capillaries, producing focal occlusion of these vessels in the retina and choroid.[238] The occlusions are caused primarily by the cellular reaction to the emboli.[239]

The neovascular lesions of talc retinopathy are thought to be associated with peripheral arteriolar nonperfusion, which leads to retinal ischemia and secondary neovascularization. Such a pathogenesis is quite similar to that seen in sickle cell retinopathy and is confirmed by the predominantly superotemporal location of the neovascular proliferation.[228,233,234]

MANAGEMENT

Because of the implications involved in the diagnosis, the practitioner must rule out other conditions that may have a similar clinical appearance. The differential diagnosis includes Gunn's dots, multiple cholesterol emboli, drusen, and Stargardt's disease.

Once the diagnosis has been established, appropriate drug abuse counseling should be given to prevent further risk of severe pulmonary or ocular complications. Consideration should also be given to pulmonary consultation, since patients with eye findings usually have acute or chronic impairment of pulmonary function.[235] The patient should be monitored carefully for the development of progressive ocular lesions, especially of the neovascular type. Proliferative retinopathy can be treated with the use of argon laser photocoagulation, and vitreal hemorrhage may require vitrectomy.[228]

Cardiac Glycosides

Digitoxin and digoxin, both digitalis derivatives, have been widely used in the treatment of congestive heart disease and certain cardiac arrhythmias. Visual symptoms associated with digitalis have been recognized

TABLE 30.10
Visual Symptoms in Digitalis Intoxication[241,243]

- Dyschromatopsia
- Flickering or flashes of light
- Colored spots surrounded by coronas
- Snowy vision
- Disturbances of visual acuity
- Dimming of vision
- Glare sensitivity

since 1785 when Withering[240] recorded the effects from large doses of foxglove. Since that time many patients have incurred symptoms of dimness of vision, flickering or flashing scotomas, and significant disturbances of color vision.

CLINICAL SIGNS AND SYMPTOMS

The most common symptoms reported by patients are changes in color vision and impaired vision.[241] These symptoms can take many forms and include the visual phenomena listed in Table 30.10. They often precede cardiac abnormalities as the earliest symptoms of digitoxin intoxication.[242] A common symptom is snowy vision, wherein objects of regard appear to be covered with frost or snow, and this observation is intensified in brightly illuminated environments.[241,243] Elevated dark-adaptation thresholds have been reported, which gradually return to normal within 2 to 3 weeks after digitalis is discontinued.[244] There is also evidence that digoxin may contribute to rhegmatogenous retinal detachment by decreasing the normal adhesion of the retina to the retinal pigment epithelium.[245]

Complaints of color vision disturbances are common with both digoxin and digitoxin, but color vision impairment can often be detected even in patients without symptoms.[246] Both the incidence and severity of color vision impairment tend to correlate with the plasma glycoside level.[246,247] Figure 30.12 shows the results of color vision testing in patients receiving therapeutic doses and toxic serum levels of digoxin. About 80% of patients with digoxin intoxication will demonstrate generalized color vision deficiencies,[246] but detectable color vision impairment occurs even at therapeutic drug levels (Fig. 30.13). In contrast, patients treated with digitoxin in therapeutic concentrations usually show no significant color vision abnormality.[247] Haustein and associates[247] showed that at toxic plasma concentrations, nearly all digoxin-treated patients, but only about half of digitoxin-treated patients, will demonstrate impaired color vision. Thus, at therapeutic concentrations digoxin tends to impair color vision more than does digitoxin. This difference may be related to plasma protein binding or to different distributions in the retina.[247] Digoxin can also interact with quinidine, raising the digoxin level approximately twofold.[243]

The prevalence of digitalis intoxication is from 16% to 20%,[248] and the incidence of visual complaints among intoxicated patients may be as high as 10% to 25%.[241] Color vision disturbances, in particular, are especially common and have a higher incidence than any other

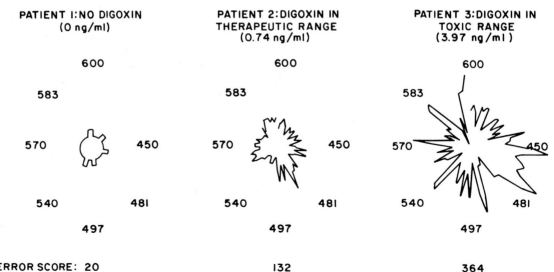

FIGURE 30.12   **Farnsworth Munsell 100-hue test results in 3 patients with differing digoxin serum levels (0.0, 0.74, 3.97 ng/ml, respectively). Total error scores were 20, 132, and 364, respectively. (Modified from Rietbrock N, Alken RG. Color vision deficiencies: A common sign of intoxication in chronically digoxin-treated patients. J Cardiovasc Pharmacol 1980;2:93–99.)**

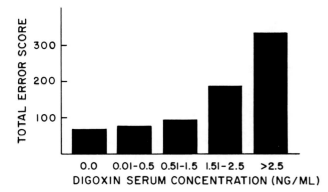

FIGURE 30.13 **Mean total error scores on Farnsworth Munsell 100-hue test according to digoxin serum concentration ranges. (Modified from Rietbrock N, Alken RG. Color vision deficiencies: A common sign of intoxication in chronically digoxin-treated patients. J Cardiovasc Pharmacol 1980;2:93–99.)**

single sign of digitalis toxicity.[246] These color vision disturbances may occur before, simultaneously with, or after the onset of cardiac toxicity.

The onset of visual symptoms following drug administration may be as soon as 1 day but is often within 2 weeks of initial therapy. Occasionally ocular toxicity is not shown until after several years of treatment.[241] Once digitalis therapy is discontinued, however, visual symptoms quickly subside, usually within several weeks.

MECHANISM

Early reports suggested that the cause of the visual symptoms in patients with digitalis toxicity was retrobulbar neuritis or disturbances in the visual cortex.[249] Gibson and associates,[250] however, were among the first investigators to propose that the retina, rather than the optic nerve, was the site of digitalis toxicity. Binnion and Frazer[251] have demonstrated in dogs that the highest concentrations of digoxin are found in the choroid and retina, and ERG studies as well as dark adaptometry have confirmed cone dysfunction in patients with digitalis intoxication.[243,244]

The precise mechanism whereby digoxin produces a toxic effect may involve inhibition of Na^+-K^+-activated ATPase, an enzyme that plays a vital role in maintaining normal cone receptor function. This would explain the drug-induced interference with both dark adaptation and color vision.[243,244]

MANAGEMENT

Patients taking cardiac glycosides should be monitored carefully for visual symptoms, including color vision changes, flashing or flickering lights, and other entoptic phenomena Color vision evaluation, especially during

the first several weeks of therapy, can be especially helpful in detecting signs of early intoxication. Although the Panel D-15 test can be useful for this purpose, the Farnsworth Munsell 100-hue test has been shown to be particularly sensitive for detecting digitalis-induced color vision deficiencies.[246,248] Periodic color vision testing should be performed as long as the patient continues taking the medication, and detectable changes in color vision should warrant consultation with the prescribing physician with regard to potential digitalis intoxication.

Nonsteroidal Anti-Inflammatory Agents

NSAIAs are commonly used for their analgesic, anti-inflammatory, and antipyretic actions in the treatment of arthritis, musculoskeletal disorders, dysmenorrhea, and acute gout. Although these drugs are widely used and are often employed for prolonged periods, retinal toxicity is rare.[39]

CLINICAL SIGNS AND SYMPTOMS

Salicylates are well known to have anticoagulant properties, and in high dosages or prolonged use these drugs can cause retinal hemorrhage.[252]

Most of the reported cases of retinopathy associated with NSAIAs have involved indomethacin therapy. Although there have been no prospective, controlled clinical trials investigating the relationship between indomethacin and retinopathy, there is evidence that the drug can induce pigmentary changes of the macula and other areas of the retina.[39–41,253,308] The lesions usually consist of discrete pigment scattering of the RPE perifoveally as well as fine areas of depigmentation around the macula. In some cases the pigmentary changes can be more marked in the periphery of the retina.[39] Depending on the amount of retinal involvement, the ERG and EOG can be normal or abnormal.[39–41] Likewise, the amount of retinopathy will dictate whether changes occur in visual acuity, dark adaptation, and visual fields. Acquired color vision deficiencies of the blue-yellow type have been reported.[40,253]

No definite relationship has been established between the dosage of indomethacin and retinal toxicity. When drug therapy is discontinued, however, most of the functional disturbances associated with the retinopathy will usually improve, although the pigmentary changes of the retina are generally irreversible.[39–41,253] Significant improvement of color vision, visual acuity, dark adaptation, and visual fields may require at least 6 to 12 months following discontinuation of drug therapy.

MECHANISM

Most investigators have speculated that indomethacin may have a direct or indirect effect on the retinal pigment epithelium, but the precise mechanism has not been clarified.[39-41] The localization of the retinotoxic effect to the RPE is supported by changes observed in the ERG and EOG in patients with indomethacin retinopathy.[39]

MANAGEMENT

Patients taking high or prolonged doses of salicylates or indomethacin should be monitored carefully for evidence of retinal hemorrhage or pigmentary changes, especially in the macular area. Evaluation of color vision may be helpful in identifying patients with early retinotoxic effects associated with indomethacin.[253] Consideration should also be given to other functional disturbances, and these can be monitored by performing serial visual acuity, visual fields, and studies of dark adaptation. Once retinal toxicity is documented, the prognosis for improved retinal function is good provided indomethacin therapy is decreased or discontinued. Drug therapy, however, should be changed only on the advice of the prescribing physician.

Antineoplastic Agents

TAMOXIFEN

Tamoxifen citrate (Nolvadex), an orally administered nonsteroidal antiestrogen, is one of the most effective antitumor agents for the palliative treatment of metastatic breast carcinoma in postmenopausal women.[254] This drug has been in clinical use since 1970 without serious side effects in most patients. It is used both alone and in combination with other agents, and the recommended oral dosage is 10 mg twice daily, increasing to 20 mg twice daily if no response is obtained within 1 month.[255]

Clinical Signs and Symptoms.   Tamoxifen retinopathy has been documented in a number of patients, and the retinal findings include white or yellow refractile opacities in the macular and perimacular area, with or without macular edema (Fig. 30.14).[256,257] Although the lesions are usually more numerous in the macular area, they can also extend to the ora serrata.[257] The lesions occur at all levels of the sensory retina, and many appear superficial to the retinal vessels. Subjectively the patient may experience reduced visual acuity associated with the macular lesions, and the visual fields can show abnormalities such as constrictions and central scotomas.

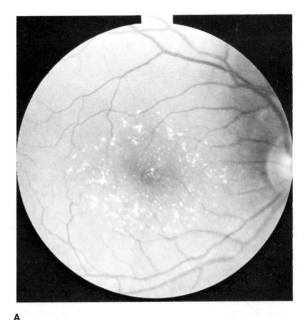

A

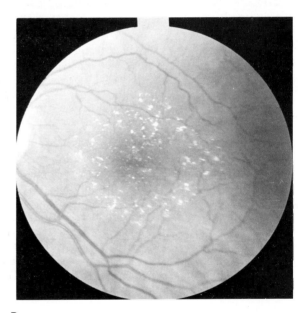

B

FIGURE 30.14   **Macular edema with yellow-white crystalline deposition in 66-year-old woman administered 120 mg of tamoxifen twice daily for 2 years.** *(A)* **Right eye, visual acuity 20/180 (6/54).** *(B)* **Left eye, visual acuity 20/60 (6/18).**

At normal dosage levels tamoxifen rarely causes retinal toxicity,[255] but when taken in high dosages (e.g., 90 to 120 mg twice daily) the toxic effects can be observed within 17 to 27 months as the total cumulative dosage exceeds 90 g.[254,256,257] In rare cases, however, tamoxifen can be retinotoxic in low dosages. Griffiths[258] has reported a patient with tamoxifen retinopathy who had received less than 8 g of drug.

Once tamoxifen therapy is discontinued, the number and size of retinal lesions generally remain unchanged, and the degenerative changes are irreversible.[254]

Mechanism.   Kaiser-Kupfer and associates[254] provided the first clinicopathologic correlation of tamoxifen retinopathy. These investigators have shown that high-dosage tamoxifen therapy causes widespread axonal degeneration, primarily in the paramacular area. The yellow-white lesions seen on fundus examination appear to represent products of the axonal degeneration. They are 3 to 10 μm in diameter in the macular area, from 30 to 35 μm in diameter in the paramacular area, and are confined to the nerve fiber and inner plexiform layers.

Management.   Since tamoxifen retinopathy can occur at relatively low total doses of drug, it is important to obtain a baseline examination before therapy is begun. This should include best-corrected visual acuity, visual fields, Amsler grid evaluation, and fundus photography. It is important to monitor the patient carefully during therapy, since macular compromise can result in irreversible loss of vision. Annual examinations are sufficient if normal drug dosages are administered. Patients receiving higher than normal doses, however, should be monitored every 6 months.

CARMUSTINE

Carmustine (BCNU) is a commonly used chemotherapeutic agent for the treatment of various malignant neoplasms, including metastatic malignant melanoma, malignant gliomas of the central nervous system, metastatic breast cancer, and leukemia.[259] It has been administered by infusion into the internal carotid artery as a method of increasing bioavailability of the drug to brain tumors within the supply of this vessel. This has led to ocular toxicity in some patients.[260]

Clinical Signs and Symptoms.   Retinal toxicity usually begins within 2 to 14 weeks following intra-arterial infusion of BCNU.[259] Approximately 65% of patients develop retinal complications (Table 30.11).[261] It is common to have loss of vision from the retinopathy, and visual acuity can be reduced to 20/60 to light perception or even no light perception.[259,261] A definite relationship between dosage of BCNU and retinopathy has not been established, but retinal complications can be avoided using intracarotid administration by passing the infusion catheter beyond the origin of the ophthalmic artery.[262]

TABLE 30.11
Retinal Complications of Carmustine

- Retinal infarction
- Retinal periarteritis
- Retinal periphlebitis
- Changes of retinal pigment epithelium
- Branch retinal artery occlusion
- Nerve fiber layer hemorrhages
- Macular edema

Mechanism.   The retinal toxicity resulting from intracarotid BCNU is probably related to the increased flow of drug into the ophthalmic artery. The precise mechanism whereby BCNU causes retinal toxicity is unknown, but several investigators have suggested that the drug may be toxic to the retinal and choroidal vasculature, causing segmental intraretinal vasculitis with or without vascular obstruction. This process would lead to nerve fiber layer infarcts and retinal hemorrhage.[259,261]

Management.   As previously mentioned, the retinotoxic effects of intracarotid BCNU can be largely minimized or avoided by employing an infusion catheter that is advanced beyond the origin of the ophthalmic artery.[262] If retinal complications develop, the risk/benefit ratio must be considered regarding the advisability of continued therapy.

Oral Contraceptives

Since the early 1960s, when oral contraceptives became a popular means of birth control, there have been numerous reports of ocular as well as systemic side effects associated with this medication. Although the relationship between the use of oral contraceptives and systemic thromboembolic disease is now well established,[82,263] the reports linking oral contraceptives with ocular side effects have been based solely on isolated case reports and uncontrolled retrospective studies. Most case reports of ocular side effects involve drug therapy from 48 hours to several years, and complications have been observed for up to 5 months following discontinuation of oral contraceptive use.[82] Controlled, prospective studies, however, have consistently failed to document any significant relationship between use of oral contraceptives and ocular side effects.[82,264–267] Nevertheless, there is circumstantial evidence that retinal vascular disease may be associated with oral contraceptives because patients have been reported with retinal lesions that disappeared when the drug was discontinued, promptly reappearing when the drug was resumed, and then regressing when treatment was again discontinued.[268,269] Furthermore, the retinal vascular disturbances occur at an unusually young age when vascular damage associated with arteriosclerosis is quite rare. Thus, the practitioner should be aware of the most common retinal vascular lesions that have been linked with oral contraceptive therapy.

CLINICAL SIGNS AND SYMPTOMS

The most common retinal findings reportedly associated with oral contraceptive use are retinal vascular occlusions. These may present as typical branch or central retinal vein occlusion,[270] branch or central retinal artery occlusion,[271] or they may involve atypical presentations such as tortuosity of the perimacular venules[272] or combined central retinal artery and vein occlusion.[273]

Acquired color vision deficiencies have also been reported. Marre and associates[274] found acquired tritanomaly in 28% of women using oral contraceptives when tested with the Panel D-15 test.

Other retinotoxic effects reportedly associated with oral contraceptives are listed in Table 30.12.

MECHANISM

The mechanism underlying retinal vascular complications associated with oral contraceptives is unknown. Schenker and associates[275] have shown that oral contraceptives may cause changes in the retinal microvasculature. Fluorescein angiography was used to demonstrate narrowing of the capillary arterioles and postcapillary venules. Women who complained of headache while taking oral contraceptives demonstrated dilatation of perimacular vessels several weeks after the drug was discontinued. Retinal vascular occlusive episodes might also occur as a consequence of marked intimal proliferation, or as a result of contraceptive-enhanced platelet adhesiveness. Fibrinogen and clotting factors may also be increased.[82,273]

MANAGEMENT

The risk of retinal vascular disease associated with oral contraceptive use in women of child-bearing age is generally considered to be minimal. However, certain predisposing factors may increase the risk of retinal vascular episodes. Women with any of the conditions listed in Table 30.13 may be at increased risk for vascular complications associated with oral contraceptives.[82,86,268,276] These patients should therefore be monitored more carefully for evidence of retinal disease. If the patient develops retinal vascular complications that are suspected to be associated with the oral contraceptive, consideration can be given to changing the mode of contraception. This should be done only in consultation with the patient's physician.

Isotretinoin

Isotretinoin, or 13-*cis*-retinoic acid, is widely used for the treatment of cystic acne. Although this drug more commonly affects the external tissues of the eye, there is evidence to suggest that this agent may also have a retinotoxic effect.

CLINICAL SIGNS AND SYMPTOMS

Impairment of dark adaptation with or without excessive glare sensitivity has been reported with isotretinoin therapy in dosages of 1 mg/kg body weight daily.[277] These complaints may be associated with an abnormal ERG or abnormal EOG. Once therapy is discontinued, both the abnormal dark adaptation and abnormal ERG usually resolve within several months.

MECHANISM

Although the precise mechanism explaining isotretinoin's effect on dark adaptation is unclear, it has been suggested that the drug could become incorporated into the rod photoreceptor elements during the process of outer disc shedding and renewal.[43] Weleber and

TABLE 30.12
Reported Retinotoxic Effects of Oral Contraceptives[86,268]

- Central retinal vein occlusion
- Branch retinal vein occlusion
- Central retinal artery occlusion
- Branch retinal artery occlusion
- Perivasculitis
- Impending occlusion of central retinal vein
- Attenuation of retinal arteries
- Macular hemorrhage
- Retinal edema

TABLE 30.13
Risk Factors for Vascular Complications Associated with Oral Contraceptives

- Migraine headache
- Phlebitis
- Inclination to varicosity
- Systemic hypertension
- Hyperlipidemia or hypercholesterolemia
- Diabetes
- Cigarette smoking
- Obesity

TABLE 30.14
Drugs that Can Affect the Optic Nerve

Drug	Side Effect
Ethambutol	Retrobulbar neuritis
Chloramphenicol	Optic neuritis, retrobulbar neuritis
Isoniazid	Optic neuritis
Oral contraceptives	Pseudotumor cerebri, optic neuritis
Tamoxifen	Optic neuritis
Corticosteroids	Pseudotumor cerebri
Tetracycline	Pseudotumor cerebri
Amiodarone	Papillitis

associates[277] have hypothesized that isotretinoin may compete for normal retinol binding sites on cell surfaces or transport molecules, accounting for the reduced retinal sensitivity.

MANAGEMENT

Patients taking isotretinoin should be monitored for changes in night vision. A history of night vision impairment should suggest more definitive evaluation procedures such as visual fields, dark adaptometry, and electroretinography. If retinal function is documented to be abnormal, the drug should be withdrawn in consultation with the patient's physician. Once drug therapy has been discontinued, retinal function should be monitored for improvement.

Drugs Affecting the Optic Nerve

Drug toxicity must always be considered in the differential diagnosis of optic neuropathy. A careful history should attempt to uncover any prescribed or self-administered drugs that may have been taken in the past or present. There has been speculation that maternal drug use during pregnancy may lead to optic nerve hypoplasia. Drugs reported to cause this condition include phenytoin,[278] quinine,[279] and alcohol.[280] Other drugs known or reported to cause significant optic nerve disease are listed in Table 30.14.

Ethambutol

Introduced in 1961 for the treatment of tuberculosis, ethambutol has supplanted paraaminosalicyclic acid for the initial and retreatment of tuberculosis.[281] Severe toxic side effects were initially reported, but these were linked to use of the racemic mixture of the drug. Consequently, the dextro isomer was selected as the most therapeutically useful and has been found to have a lower incidence of ocular toxicity than the racemic form.[282] Ocular side effects usually occur in the form of retrobulbar neuritis.

CLINICAL SIGNS AND SYMPTOMS

Ethambutol is well recognized to cause ocular symptoms of reduced visual acuity, changes in color vision, and visual field loss.[283] Signs of ocular toxicity can appear as early as several weeks following initial therapy, but the onset of ocular complications usually occurs several months after therapy is begun.[284–286] Although various forms of optic neuritis have been described,[287] the primary ocular manifestation of ethambutol toxicity is retrobulbar neuritis. This commonly occurs in several forms (Table 30.15).[285,288–290] The most common form involves loss of visual acuity associated with a central or paracentral scotoma along with color vision disturbances. This type is caused by compromise of the central optic nerve fibers. Less commonly ethambutol can affect the peripheral optic nerve fibers, causing defects in the peripheral visual field. Finally, in rare cases ethambutol can cause visible retinal manifestations, including hyperemia and swelling of the optic disc, flame-shaped hemorrhages on the optic disc and in the retina, and macular edema. After several weeks these signs can be followed by primary optic atrophy.[287,291]

TABLE 30.15
Characteristics of Ethambutol Optic Neuropathy

	Central (Axial)	Peripheral
Toxic dosage	Low	High
Visual acuity	Reduced	Normal
Visual field	Central scotoma	Peripheral contraction
Color vision	Red-green deficiency	Normal

Modified from Garrett CR. Optic neuritis in a patient on ethambutol and isoniazid evaluated by visual evoked potentials: Case report. Military Med 1985;150:43–46.

Color vision deficiencies are probably the most sensitive indicator of early ethambutol optic neuropathy.[186,292] When the patient is examined with sensitive tests such as the Farnsworth Munsell 100-hue or desaturated Panel D-15, both red-green or blue-yellow defects may be observed in early stages of toxicity.[253,292] These changes in color vision can occur even before visual acuity and visual fields are affected.

Once changes have occurred in visual acuity, visual field, or color vision, these functional changes may continue to deteriorate even after ethambutol has been discontinued.[291] More often, however, there is recovery of pretreatment visual acuity and visual field several months or years following discontinuation of drug treatment.[283,286] The degree of recovery depends largely on the extent to which ethambutol has compromised optic nerve function, and if the ocular toxicity is not recognized early, the drug can cause permanent loss of vision.[291,293]

There is considerable evidence that ocular toxicity associated with ethambutol therapy is dose-related.[282,293] It is now recognized that ethambutol rarely induces ocular changes at a dosage of 15 to 20 mg/kg body weight daily,[286] and this has led to the current recommendation that ethambutol dosages should not generally exceed 15 mg/kg body weight daily. Some practitioners employ the drug in dosages of 25 mg/kg daily for a period not exceeding 2 months, followed by a maintenance dose of 15 mg/kg daily, and this has been shown to cause virtually no ocular complications.[284,289]

MECHANISM

Although the mechanism by which ethambutol causes retrobulbar neuritis is largely unknown, van Dijk and Spekreijse[294] have suggested that ethambutol may affect the amacrine and bipolar cells of the retina, since color vision can be affected without altering visual acuity. This concept deserves further study before definitive conclusions can be reached.

MANAGEMENT

It is important for patients beginning treatment with ethambutol to have baseline examination and frequent monitoring of visual acuity, visual fields, color vision, and fundus appearance. Since it is rare for ocular toxicity to occur with dosages as low as 15 mg/kg daily, patients taking such doses can be monitored every 3 to 6 months.[292] Patients with renal insufficiency, however, have impaired ability to excrete the drug and therefore may be at greater risk for developing ocular changes.[287,291] These patients should be monitored monthly.[295]

Evaluations of color vision and visual fields are usually more sensitive indicators of early optic neuropathy than is visual acuity testing.[290] Use of the desaturated Panel D-15 test or the Farnsworth Munsell 100-hue test is effective for detecting subtle color vision changes associated with early ethambutol toxicity.[286,292] Visual field studies using static threshold techniques will aid in detecting early visual field abnormalities.[296] Several authors have recommended use of VEPs for the routine monitoring of patients taking ethambutol.[288,293] This procedure has been shown to be effective for detecting subclinical optic nerve disease that can precede changes in visual acuity and color vision.

Nair and associates[281] have suggested that symptoms of peripheral neuropathy may indicate early ethambutol toxicity and should serve as a warning sign of impending optic neuropathy. Thus, the ethambutol dosage in patients encountering peripheral neuropathy should be reduced to prevent the development of ocular toxicity. Ethambutol therapy must be discontinued in patients who develop reduced visual acuity, color vision deficiency, or visual field defects characteristic of optic neuropathy.[285,290] If discontinuation of drug therapy alone does not result in improvement of visual function, consideration can be given to treatment with hydroxycobalamin. Guerra and Casu[297] have reported recovery of visual acuity in 4 patients treated with hydroxycobalamin several months after the discontinuation of ethambutol had failed to improve the visual acuity. Although the mechanism of action of hydroxycobalamin in the treatment of ethambutol-induced optic neuropathy is elusive, this vitamin may act by neutralizing the chelating action of ethambutol on the optic nerve. Further clinical trials are needed to clarify the role of hydroxycobalamin.

Chloramphenicol

Chloramphenicol is used for the treatment of typhoid fever, bacterial meningitis, and certain anaerobic infections. However, because of the risk of serious systemic toxicity, including blood dyscrasias and death, use of the drug is generally limited to conditions for which other, less toxic, agents are ineffective. Optic neuropathy as a consequence of chloramphenicol therapy is well known, especially when the drug is used to treat cystic fibrosis in children.

CLINICAL SIGNS AND SYMPTOMS

Chloramphenicol causes both optic neuritis and retrobulbar neuritis.[298] Characteristic of most cases is severe, bilateral reduction of visual acuity accompanied by dense central scotomas.[298–300] Visual acuity can range from 20/100 to 5/400.[301] Although there may be no fundus changes, the optic discs are usually edematous and hyperemic, the retinal veins are engorged and tortuous, and hemorrhages are often seen in the parapapillary area.[165,301] Optic atrophy is a late sign.[201] Peripheral neuritis characterized by numbness and cramps of the feet often precedes the visual complaints by 1 to 2 weeks and may therefore serve as an early warning sign of impending ocular toxicity.[298]

Visual impairment associated with chloramphenicol therapy usually recovers after the drug is discontinued, but pretreatment visual acuity is often not regained and visual field defects may persist.[165,298,302] Some patients may tolerate further prolonged treatment with chloramphenicol without recurrent optic neuritis, and on occasion patients can demonstrate improvement of visual function despite continued therapy.[165]

Most cases of optic neuritis associated with chloramphenicol therapy have occurred in children with cystic fibrosis who were treated with large daily dosages of drug, 1 to 6 g daily. Although visual symptoms can occur as early as 10 days after beginning therapy, ocular toxicity commonly occurs after several months or years of treatment.[299,303] Harley and associates[299] have reported a dosage-dependent relationship between chloramphenicol therapy and optic neuritis. The incidence of optic neuritis varied from 5% of patients treated with a daily dosage of 10 to 25 mg/kg body weight to 38% of patients treated with a daily dosage exceeding 50 mg/kg body weight. There was no vision loss among patients treated for less than 3 months, but the incidence of optic neuritis increased to 16% in patients treated longer than 12 months.

MECHANISM

The precise mechanism by which chloramphenicol produces optic neuritis is unknown, but VEP abnormalities have confirmed optic nerve involvement in patients taking chloramphenicol.[304] Although not substantiated, several authors have proposed that chloramphenicol may induce optic neuropathy by causing a vitamin deficiency.[305] Genetic factors may be involved, and it has also been hypothesized that chloramphenicol may be metabolized to degradation products that are potentially toxic to the optic nerve.[165]

Histopathologic studies have found bilateral optic atrophy with primary involvement of the papillomacular bundle, loss of the retinal ganglion cells, and gliosis of the nerve fiber layer.[299] The presence of peripheral visual field defects in some patients is evidence that there is also involvement of the peripheral portion of the visual pathway.[300]

MANAGEMENT

Patients who are to receive long-term chloramphenicol therapy should receive a comprehensive baseline examination consisting of visual acuity, visual fields, color vision, and fundus examination. The risk of optic neuropathy is minimized if the daily dosage of drug is limited to 25 mg/kg body weight or less for a period not exceeding 3 months.[299] Patients or their parents should be encouraged to be alert to the development of peripheral neuritis, which might indicate impending loss of vision. Once signs or symptoms of optic neuropathy are detected, drug therapy should be promptly discontinued, in consultation with the prescribing physician. Because the outcome of vitamin therapy is uncertain, the case for megadose vitamins is not compelling.[298]

Prevention of Adverse Reactions

Health care practitioners must protect their patients' well-being by detecting signs and symptoms of drug toxicities so that appropriate action can be taken to prevent or minimize serious ocular consequences. The detection process begins with the initial patient interview, during which a detailed drug history may reveal use of medications with potential ocular side effects.[306] A careful history is especially important in elderly patients, who typically use more medications than do younger individuals.[307] Although most patients over age 60 years regularly take several medications, many patients are unable to identify the drugs they take.[306] This emphasizes the importance of patient education regarding prescribed and self-administered medications.

The practitioner should record on the patient's chart both prescribed and self-administered medications, including drug dosage, duration of therapy, and any adverse reactions noted by the patient. If documented ocular side effects are discovered in the examination, it is wise to advise the prescribing practitioner so that appropriate remedial action can be taken. If no side effects are found, but the patient is using high-risk medications such as steroids, the patient should be monitored closely so that any significant adverse reaction can be detected before serious consequences develop.

References

1. Fraunfelder FT. Drug induced ocular side effects and drug interactions. Philadelphia; Lea & Febiger, 1982.

2. Grant WM. Toxicology of the eye, ed. 2. Springfield, IL: Charles C Thomas, 1974.

3. Fraunfelder FT, Meyer SM. The national registry of drug-induced ocular side effects. J Toxicol Cut Ocular Toxicol 1982;1:65–70.

4. Applebaum M, Jaanus SD. A study of utilization of diagnostic pharmaceutical agents and the incidence of adverse effects. Am J Optom Physiol Opt 1983;60:384–388.

5. McQueen EG. Pharmacological basis of adverse drug reactions. In: Avery GS, ed. Drug treatment. New York: Adis Press, 1980; Chap. 7.

6. Koneru PB, Lien EJ, Koda RT. Oculotoxicities of systemically administered drugs. J Ocul Pharmacol 1986;2:385–404.

7. Hobbs HE, Eadie SP, Somerville F. Ocular lesions after treatment with chloroquine. Br J Ophthalmol 1961;45:284–298.

8. Willetts GS. Ocular side effects of drugs. Br J Ophthalmol 1969;53:252–255.

9. Leopold IH. Ocular complications of drugs. JAMA 1968;205:285–287.

10. Lufkin MW, Harrison CE, Henderson JW, et al. Ocular distribution of digoxin-H[3] in the cat. Am J Ophthalmol 1967;64:1134–1140.

11. Yamamoto GK. Ocular drug toxicity. In: Langston-Pavan D. Manual of ocular diagnosis and therapy. Boston: Little, Brown, 1980; Chap. 15.

12. Abel A, Leopold IH. Ocular diseases. In: Avery GS, ed. Drug treatment. New York: Adis Press, 1980; Chap. 12.

13. Armaly MF. Statistical attributes of the steroid hypertensive response in the clinically normal eye. I. The demonstration of three levels of response. Invest Ophthalmol 1965;4:187–197.

14. Becker B. Intraocular response to topical corticosteroids. Invest Ophthalmol 1965;4:198–205.

15. Urban RC, Cotlier E. Corticosteroid-induced cataracts. Surv Ophthalmol 1986;31:102–110.

16. Davidson SI. Reports of ocular adverse reactions. Trans Ophthalmol Soc UK 1973;93:495–510.

17. Herman DC, Dyer JA. Anterior subcapsular cataracts as a possible adverse ocular reaction to isotretinoin. Am J Ophthalmol 1987;103:236–237.

18. Bar S, Feller N, Savir H. Presenile cataracts in phenytoin-treated epileptic patients. Arch Ophthalmol 1983;101:422–425.

19. Hobbs HE, Calnan CD. The ocular complications of chloroquine therapy. Lancet 1958;1:1207–1209.

20. Bernstein NH. Some iatrogenic ocular diseases from systemically administered drugs. Int Ophthalmol Clin 1970;10:553–619.

21. Bernstein HN. Chloroquine ocular toxicity. Surv Ophthalmol 1967;12:415–447.

22. Goldhammer Y, Smith JL. Bitemporal hemianopia in chloroquine retinopathy. Neurology 1974;24:1135–1138.

23. Petrohelos MA. Chloroquine-induced ocular toxicity. Ann Ophthalmol 1974;6:615–618.

24. Mantyjarvi M. Hydroxychloroquine treatment and the eye. Scand J Rheumatol 1985;14:171–174.

25. Cullen AP, Chou BR. Keratopathy with low dose chloroquine therapy. J Am Optom Assoc 1986;57:368–372.

26. Calkins LL. Corneal epithelial changes occurring during chloroquine (Aralen) therapy. Arch Ophthalmol 1958;60:981–988.

27. Marks JS, Power BJ. Is chloroquine obsolete in treatment of rheumatic disease? Lancet 1979;1:371–373.

28. Tobin DR, Krohel GB, Rynes RI. Hydroxychloroquine. Seven-year experience. Arch Ophthalmol 1982;100:81–83.

29. Shearer RV, Dubois EL. Ocular changes induced by long-term hydroxychloroquine (Plaquenil) therapy. Am J Ophthalmol 1967;64:245–252.

30. Beebe WE, Abbott RL, Fung WE. Hydroxychloroquine crystals in the tear film of a patient with rheumatoid arthritis. Am J Ophthalmol 1986;101:377–378.

31. Alexander LJ, Bowerman L, Thompson LR. The prevalence of the ocular side effects of chlorpromazine in the Tuscaloosa Veterans Administration patient population. J Am Optom Assoc 1985;56:872–876.

32. Greiner AC, Berry K. Skin pigmentation and corneal and lens opacities with prolonged chlorpromazine therapy. Can Med Assoc J 1964;90:663–665.

33. Thaler JS, Curinga R, Kiracofe G. Relation of graded ocular anterior chamber pigmentation to phenothiazine intake in schizophrenics—quantification procedures. Am J Optom Physiol Opt 1985;62:600–604.

34. Mathalone MBR. Ocular effects of phenothiazine derivatives and reversibility. Dis Nerv Syst 1968;29:29–35.

35. Siddall JR. Ocular complications related to phenothiazines. Dis Nerv Syst 1968;29:10–13.

36. Prien RF, DeLong SL, Cole JO, et al. Ocular changes occurring with prolonged high dose chlorpromazine therapy. Arch Gen Psychiat 1970;23:464–468.

37. Rasmussen K, Kirk L, Faurbye A. Deposits in the lens and cornea of the eye during long-term chlorpromazine medication. Acta Psychiat Scand 1976;53:1–6.

38. Deluise VP, Flynn JT. Asymmetric anterior segment changes induced by chlorpromazine. Ann Ophthalmol 1981;13:953–955.

39. Henkes HE, van Lith GHM, Canta LR. Indomethacin retinopathy. Am J Ophthalmol 1972;73:846–856.

40. Palimeris G, Koliopoulos J, Velissaropoulos P. Ocular side effects of indomethacin. Ophthalmologica 1972;164:339–353.

41. Burns CA. Indomethacin, reduced retinal sensitivity, and corneal deposits. Am J Ophthalmol 1968;66:825–835.

42. Szmyd L, Perry HD. Keratopathy associated with the use of naproxen. Am J Ophthalmol 1985;99:598.

43. Lerman S. Photosensitizing drugs and their possible role in enhancing ocular toxicity. Ophthalmology 1986;93:304–313.

44. Jick H, Brandt DE. Allopurinol and cataracts. Am J Ophthalmol 1984;98:355–358.

45. Bonnet P. Sur une forme particulière de granulations miliaires de l'iris. Bull Soc Ophthalmol Paris 1937;49:413–416.

46. Weidle EG. Lenticular chrysiasis in oral chrysotherapy. Am J Ophthalmol 1987;103:240–241.

47. McCormick SA, DiBartolomeo G, Raju VK, et al. Ocular chrysiasis. Ophthalmology 1985;92:1432–1435.

48. Gottlieb NL, Major JC. Ocular chrysiasis correlated with gold concentrations in the crystalline lens during chrysotherapy. Arth Rheumat 1978;21:704–708.

49. Roberts WH, Wolter JR. Ocular chrysiasis. Arch Ophthalmol 1956;56:48–52.

50. Black RL, Oglesby RB, von Sallmann L, et al. Posterior subcapsular cataracts induced by corticosteroids in patients with rheumatoid arthritis. JAMA 1960;174:166–171.

51. Toogood JH, Dyson C, Thompson CA, et al. Posterior subcapsular cataracts as a complication of adrenocortical steroid therapy. Can Med Assoc J 1962;86:52–56.

52. Havre DC. Cataracts in children on long-term corticosteroid therapy. Arch Ophthalmol 1965;78:818–821.

53. Lindholm B, Linnér E, Tengroth B. Effects of long-term systemic steroids on cataract formation and on aqueous humour dynamics. Acta Ophthalmol 1965;43:120–127.

54. Kobayashi Y, Akaishi K, Nishio T, et al. Posterior subcapsular cataract in nephrotic children receiving steriod therapy. Am J Dis Child 1974;128:671–673.

55. Fürst C, Smiley WK, Ansell BM. Steroid cataract. Ann Rheum Dis 1966;25:364–368.

56. Oglesby RB, Black RL, von Sallmann L, et al. Cataracts in patients with rheumatic diseases treated with corticosteroids. Further observations. Arch Ophthalmol 1961;66:625–630.

57. Giles CL, Mason GL, Duff IF, et al. The association of cataract formation and systemic corticosteroid therapy. JAMA 1962;182:719–722.

58. Crews SJ. Posterior subcapsular lens opacities in patients on long-term corticosteroid therapy. Br Med J 1963;1:1644–1647.

59. Astle JN, Ellis PP. Ocular complications in renal transplant patients. Ann Ophthalmol 1974;6:1269–1274.

60. Pavlin CR, de Veber GA, Cook GT, et al. Ocular complications in renal transplant recipients. Can Med Assoc J 1977;117:360–362.

61. Kristensen P. Posterior subcapsular cataract (PSC) and systemic steroid therapy. Acta Ophthalmol 1968;46:1025–1032.

62. Skalka HW, Prchal JT. Effect of corticosteroids on cataract formation. Arch Ophthalmol 1980;98:1773–1777.

63. Loredo A, Rodriguez RS, Murillo L. Cataracts after short-term corticosteroid treatment. N Engl J Med 1972;286:160.

64. Rooklin AR, Lampert SI, Jaeger EA, et al. Posterior subcapsular cataracts in steroid-requiring asthmatic children. J Allergy Clin Immunol 1979;63:383–386.

65. Harris JE, Gruber L. The electrolyte and water balance of the lens. Exp Eye Res 1962;1:372–384.

66. Mayman CI, Miller D, Tijerina ML. In vitro production of steroid cataract in bovine lens: II. Measurement of sodium-potassium adenosine triphosphatase activity. Acta Ophthalmol 1979;57:1107–1116.

67. Bucala R, Fishman J, Cerami A. Formation of covalent adducts between cortisol and 16 α-hydroxyestrone and protein: Possible role in the pathogenesis of cortisol toxicity and systemic lupus erythematosus. Proc Natl Acad Sci USA 1982;79:3320–3324.

68. Bluming AZ, Zeegen P. Cataracts induced by intermittent Decadron used as an antiemetic. J Clin Oncol 1986;4:221–223.

69. Ward DE, Butrous G, Camm J. Clinical uses of amiodarone—a potent antiarrhythmic drug. Intern Med Special 1985;6:44–55.

70. Kaplan LJ, Cappaert WE. Amiodarone keratopathy. Correlation to dosage and duration. Arch Ophthalmol 1982;100:601–602.

71. Chew E, Ghosh M, McCulloch C. Amiodarone-induced cornea verticillata. Can J Ophthalmol 1982;17:96–99.

72. Orlando RG, Dangel ME, Schaal SF. Clinical experience and grading of amiodarone keratopathy. Ophthalmology 1984;91:1184–1187.

73. Dolan BJ, Flach AJ, Peterson JS. Amiodarone keratopathy and lens opacities. J Am Optom Assoc 1985;56:468–470.

74. Ingram DV, Jaggarao NSV, Chamberlain DA. Ocular changes resulting from therapy with amiodarone. Br J Ophthalmol 1982;66:676–679.

75. Ghosh M, McCulloch C. Amiodarone-induced ultrastructural changes in human eyes. Can J Ophthalmol 1984;19:178–186.

76. Nielsen CE, Andreasen F, Bjerregaard P. Amiodarone-induced cornea verticillata. Acta Ophthalmol 1983;61:474–480.

77. Flach AJ, Dolan BJ, Sudduth B, et al. Amiodarone-induced lens opacities. Arch Ophthalmol 1983;101:1554–1556.

78. Gittinger JW, Asdourian GK. Papillopathy caused by amiodarone. Arch Ophthalmol 1987;105:349–351.

79. D'Amico DJ, Kenyon KR, Ruskin JN. Amiodarone keratopathy. Drug-induced lipid storage disease. Arch Ophthalmol 1981;99:257–261.

80. Bron AJ. Vortex patterns of the corneal epithelium. Trans Ophthalmol Soc UK 1973;43:455–472.

81. Garrett SN, Waterhouse WJ, Parmley VC. Amiodarone keratopathy in the donor cornea. Am J Ophthalmol 1988;105:425–427.

82. Wood JR. Ocular complications of oral contraceptives. Ophthal Sem 1977;2:371–402.

83. Koetting RA. The influence of oral contraceptives on contact lens wear. Am J Optom Arch Am Acad Optom 1966;43:268–274.

84. Ruben M. Contact lenses and oral contraceptives. Br Med J 1966;1:1110.

85. Anderson RD, Martin PL. Oral contraceptives and eye changes. Pac Coast Oto-Ophthalmol Soc 1969;50:137–146.

86. Radnot M, Follmann P. Ocular side effects of oral contraceptives. Ann Clin Res 1973;5:197–204.

87. Varga M. Recent experiences on the ophthalmologic complications of oral contraceptives. Ann Ophthalmol 1976;8:925–934.

88. Dickens CH. Retinoids. A review. J Am Acad Dermatol 1984;11:541–552.

89. Blackman MJ, Peck GL, Olsen TG, et al. Blepharoconjunctivitis: A side effect of 13- cis-retinoic acid therapy for dermatologic disease. Ophthalmology 1979;86:753–758.

90. Milson J, Jones DH, King K. Ophthalmological effects of 13- cis-retinoic acid therapy for acne vulgaris. Br J Dermatol 1982;107:491–495.

91. Hays GB, Lyle CB, Wheeler CE. Slate gray color in patients receiving chlorpromazine. Arch Dermatol 1964;90:471–476.

92. Cairns RH, Capoore HS, Gregory JDR. Oculocutaneous changes after years of high doses of chlorpromazine. Lancet 1965;1:239–241.

93. Siddal JR. The ocular toxic findings with prolonged and high dosage chlorpromazine intake. Arch Opthalmol 1965;74:460–464.

94. McClanahan WS, Harris JE, Knobloch WH, et al. Ocular

manifestations of chronic phenothiazine derivative administration. Arch Ophthalmol 1966;75:319–325.

95. Editorial. Iatrogenic symptoms in ophthalmology. Br Med J 1969;2:199–200.

96. Alvaro ME. Effects other than antiinfections of sulfonamide compounds on eye. Arch Ophthalmol 1943;29:615–632.

97. Brothers DM, Hidayat AA. Conjunctival pigmentation associated with tetracycline medication. Ophthalmology 1981; 88:1212–1215.

98. Messmer E, Font RL, Sheldon G, et al. Pigmented conjunctival cysts following tetracycline/minocycline therapy. Ophthalmology 1983;90:1462–1468.

99. D'Amico DS, Kenyon RR. Drug-induced lipidoses in the cornea and conjunctiva. Int Ophthalmol 1981;4:67–76.

100. Reifler DM, Verdier DD, Davy CL, et al. Multiple chalazia and rosacea in a patient treated with amiodarone. Am J Ophthalmol 1987;103:594–595.

101. Ruth JH. Luminal poisoning with conjunctival residue. Am J Ophthalmol 1926;9:533–534.

102. Fraunfelder FT, Meyer MS. Ocular toxicology. In: Duane TD, Jaeger EA, eds. Clinical ophthalmology. Hagerstown, MD: Harper & Row, 1987; vol. 5, Chap. 37.

103. Crandall DC, Leopold IH. The influence of systemic drugs on tear constituents. Ophthalmology 1979;86:115–125.

104. Farber AS. Ocular side effect of antihistamine-decongestant combinations. Am J Ophthalmol 1982;94:565.

105. Balik J. Effect of atropine and pilocarpine on the secretion of chloride ion into the tears. Cesk Oftalmol 1958;14:28–33.

106. Erickson OF. Drug influences on lacrimal lysozyme production. Stanford Med Bull 1960;18:34–39.

107. Miller D. Role of the tear film in contact lens wear. Int Ophthalmol Clin 1973;13:247–262.

108. Koeffler BH, Lemp MA. The effect of an antihistamine (chlorpheniramine maleate) on tear production in humans. Am J Ophthalmol 1980;12:217–219.

109. Seedor JA, Lamberts D, Bermann RB, et al. Filamentary keratitis associated with diphenhydramine hydrochloride (Benadryl). Am J Ophthalmol 1986;101:376–377.

110. Fraunfelder FT, Baico JM, Meyer SM. Adverse ocular reactions possibly associated with isotretinoin. Am J Ophthalmol 1985;100:534–537.

111. Ensink BW, Van Voorst Vader PC. Ophthalmological side effects of 13- cis-retinoic therapy. Br J Dermatol 1983; 108:637–641.

112. Ubels JL, MacRae SM. Vitamin A is present as retinol in tears of humans and rabbits. Curr Eye Res 1984;3:815–817.

113. Felix FH, Ive FA, Dahl MGC. Cutaneous and ocular reactions with practolol administration. Oculomucocutaneous syndrome. Br Med J 1975;1:595–598.

114. Scott D. Another beta blocker causing eye problems. Br Med J 1977;2:1221.

115. Mackie IA, Seal DV, Pescod JM. Beta-adrenergic receptor blocking drugs: Tear lysozyme and immunological screening for adverse reactions. Br J Ophthalmol 1977;61:354–359.

116. Almog Y, Monselise M, Almog CH, et al. The effect of oral treatment with beta blockers on tear secretion. Metab Ped Syst Ophthalmol 1983;6:343–345.

117. Chizek DJ, Franceschetti AT. Oral contraceptives: Their side effects and ophthalmological manifestations. Surv Ophthalmol 1969;14:90–101.

118. Verbeck B. Augenbefunde und stoffwechselverhalten bei einnahme von ovulation-schemmern. Klin Monatsbl Augenheilkd 1973;162:612–615.

119. Frankel SH, Ellis PP. Effect of oral contraceptives on tear production. Ann Ophthalmol 1978;10:1585–1588.

120. Berman MT, Newman BL, Johnson NC. The effect of a diuretic (hydrochlorothiazide) on tear production in humans. Am J Ophthalmol 1985;99:473–475.

121. De Haas EBH. Lacrimal gland response to parasympathomimetics after parasympathetic denervation. Arch Ophthalmol 1960;64:34–43.

122. Dawson WW, Jimenez-Antillon CF, Perez JM, et al. Marijuana and vision—after 10 years use in Costa Rica. Invest Ophthalmol Vis Sci 1977;16:689–699.

123. Shapiro D. The ocular manifestations of cannabinols. Ophthalmologia 1974;168:366–369.

124. Melon J, Reginster M. Passage into normal salivary, lacrimal and nasal secretions of ampicillin and erythromycin administered intramuscularly. Acta Otorhinolaryngol Belg 1976;30:643–651.

125. Fraunfelder FT. Orange tears. Am J Ophthalmol 1980;89:752.

126. Lyons RW. Orange contact-lenses from rifampin. N Engl J Med 1979;300:372.

127. Leopold IH, Comroe JH. Effect of intramuscular administration of morphine, atropine, scopolamine and neostigmine on the human eye. Arch Ophthalmol 1948;40:285–290.

128. Verdier DD, Kennerdell JS. Fixed dilated pupil resulting from transdermal scopolamine. Am J Ophthalmol 1982;93:803–804.

129. McCrary JA, Webb NR. Anisocoria from scopolamine patches. JAMA 1982;248:353–355.

130. Burns RP, Steele AS. Ocular change in drug abusers. In: Leopold IH. Symposium on ocular therapy. St Louis: C.V. Mosby Co, 1973; vol. 6;6–10.

131. Goldey JA, Dick DA, Porter WL. Cornpicker's pupil: A clinical note regarding mydriasis from jimson weed dust (Stramonium). Ohio State Med J 1966;62:921.

132. Upholt JP, Qunby GE, Batchelor GS, et al. Visual effects accompanying TEPP induced miosis. Arch Ophthalmol 1956;56:128–134.

133. Lee HK, Wang SC. Mechanism of morphine induced miosis in the dog. Am J Ophthalmol 1982;14:436–438.

134. Crews SJ. Toxic effects on the eye and visual apparatus resulting from the systemic absorption of recently induced chemical agents. Trans Ophthalmol Soc UK 1962;82:387–406.

135. Leebeck MJ. Effect of drugs on ocular muscles. Int Ophthalmol Clin 1971;11:35–62.

136. Wilkinson IMS, Kime R, Purnell M. Alcohol and human eye movement. Brain 1974;97:785–792.

137. Bittencourt P, Wade P, Richens A, et al. Blood alcohol and eye movements. Lancet 1980;16:981.

138. Wilson G, Mitchell R. The effect of alcohol on the visual and ocular motor systems. Aust J Ophthalmol 1983;11:315–319.

139. Halperin E, Yolton RL. Is the driver drunk? Oculomotor sobriety testing. J Am Optom Assoc 1986;57:654–657.

140. Tiffany DV. Optometric expert testimony. Foundation for the horizontal gaze nystagmus test. J Am Optom Assoc 1986;57:705–708.

141. Maddalena MA. Transient myopia associated with acute

glaucoma and retinal edema. Arch Ophthalmol 1968;80:186–188.

142. Hook SR, Holladay JT, Prager TC, et al. Transient myopia induced by sulfonamides. Am J Ophthalmol 1986;101:495–496.

143. Chirls IA, Norris JW. Transient myopia associated with vaginal sulfanilamide suppositories. Am J Ophthalmol 1984;98:120–121.

144. Mattsson R. Transient myopia following the use of sulphonamides. Acta Ophthalmol 1952;30:385–398.

145. Beasley FJ. Transient myopia and retinal edema during hydrochlorothiazide (Hydrodiuril) therapy. Arch Ophthalmol 1961;65:212–213.

146. Beasley FJ. Transient myopia and retinal edema during ethoxzolamide (Cardrase) therapy. Arch Ophthalmol 1962;68:490–491.

147. Galin MA, Baras I, Zweifach P. Diamox-induced myopia. Am J Ophthalmol 1962;54:237–240.

148. Michaelson JJ. Transient myopia due to Hygroton. Am J Ophthalmol 1962;54:1146–1147.

149. Muirhead JF, Scheie HG. Transient myopia after acetazolamide. Arch Ophthalmol 1960;63:315–318.

150. Yasuna E. Acute myopia associated with prochlorperazine (Compazine) therapy. Am J Ophthalmol 1962;54:793–796.

151. Sandford-Smith JH. Transient myopia after aspirin. Br J Ophthalmol 1974;58:698–700.

152. Bovino JA, Marcus DF. The mechanism of transient myopia induced by sulfonamide therapy. Am J Ophthalmol 1982;94:99.

153. Laval J. Paresis of accommodation following sulfadiazine therapy. Am J Ophthalmol 1943;26:303.

154. Frucht J, Freimann I, Merin S. Ocular side effects of disopyramide. Br J Ophthalmol 1984;68:890–891.

155. Rubin ML, Thomas WC. Diplopia and loss of accommodation due to chloroquine. Arth Rheumat 1970;13:75–82.

156. Percival SPB, Behrman J. Ophthalmological safety of chloroquine. Br J Ophthalmol 1969;53:101–109.

157. Percival SPB, Meanock I. Chloroquine: Opthalmological safety, and clinical assessment in rheumatoid arthritis. Br Med J 1968;3:579–584.

158. Howell R. Treatment of discoid lupus erythematosus. St John's Hosp Dermat Soc 1957;39:48.

159. Kjaer GCD. Retinopathy associated with phenothiazine administration. Dis Nerv Syst 1968;29:316–319.

160. Alkemade PPH. Phenothiazine-retinopathy. Ophthalmologica 1968;155:70–76.

161. Thaler JS. The effect of multiple psychotropic drugs on the accommodation of prepresbyopes. Am J Optom Physiol Opt 1979;56:259–261.

162. Thaler JS. Effects of benztropine mesylate (Cogentin) on accommodation in normal volunteers. Am J Optom Physiol Opt 1982;59:918–919.

163. Hiatt RL, Fuller IB, Smith L, et al. Systemically administered anticholinergic drugs and intraocular pressure. Arch Ophthalmol 1970;84:735–740.

164. Wilson DM, Martin JHS, Niall JF. Raised intraocular tension in renal transplant recipients. Med J Aust 1973:482–484.

165. Lieberman TW. Ocular effects of prolonged systemic drug administration (corticosteroids, chloramphenicol, and anovultory agents). Dis Nerv Syst 1968;29:44–50.

166. Covell LL. Glaucoma induced by systemic steroid therapy. Am J Ophthalmol 1958;45:108–109.

167. Bernstein HN, Schwartz B. Effects of long-term systemic steroids on ocular pressure and tonographic values. Arch Ophthalmol 1962;68:742–743.

168. Godel V, Feiler-Ofry V, Stein R. Systemic steroids and ocular fluid dynamics. I. Analysis of the sample as a whole. Influence of dosage and duration of therapy. Acta Ophthalmol 1972;50:655–663.

169. Godel V, Feiler-Ofry V, Stein R. Systemic steroids and ocular fluid dynamics. II. Systemic versus topical steroids. Acta Ophthalmol 1972;50:664–676.

170. Godel V, Feiler-Ofry V, Stein R. The genetic nature of the hypertensive ocular response to long-term systemic steroids. Ann Ophthalmol 1970;1:462–467.

171. Schwartz B. The response of ocular pressure to corticosteroids. Int Ophthalmol Clin 1966;6:929–989.

172. Feiler-Ofry V, Godel V, Stein R. Systemic steroids and ocular fluid dynamics. III. The genetic nature of the ocular response and its different levels. Acta Ophthalmol 1972;50:699–706.

173. Smith SE, Smith SA, Reynolds F, et al. Ocular and cardiovascular effects of local and systemic pindolol. Br J Ophthalmol 1979;63:63–66.

174. Borthne A. The treatment of glaucoma with propranolol (Inderal). A clinical trial. Acta Ophthalmol 1976;54:291–300.

175. Rennie IG, Smerdon DL. The effect of a once-daily oral dose of nadolol on intraocular pressure in normal volunteers. Am J Ophthalmol 1985;100:445–447.

176. Peczon JD, Grant M. Glaucoma, alcohol, and intraocular pressure. Arch Ophthalmol 1965;73:495–501.

177. Diotallevi M, Bocci N. Effect of systemically administered corticosteroids on intraocular pressure and fluid dynamics. Acta Ophthalmol 1965;43:524–527.

178. Spaeth GL, Rodrigues MM, Weinreb S. Steroid-induced glaucoma. A. Persistent elevation of intraocular pressure. B. Histopathological aspects. Trans Am Ophthalmol Soc 1977;75:353–381.

179. Gilmer G, Swartz M, Teske M, et al. Over-the-counter phenylpropanolamine: A possible cause of central retinal vein occulsion. Arch Ophthalmol 1986;104:642.

180. Cerasoli JR. Effects of drugs on the retina. Int Ophthalmol Clin 1971;42:121–135.

181. Rynes RI, Krohel G, Falbo A, et al. Ophthalmologic safety of long-term hydroxychloroquine treatment. Arth Rheumat 1979;22:832–836.

182. Cambiaggi A. Unusual ocular lesions in a case of systemic lupus erythematosus. AMA Arch Ophthalmol 1957;57:451–453.

183. Hobbs HE, Sorbsy A, Freedman A. Retinopathy following chloroquine therapy. Lancet 1959;2:478–480.

184. Cruess AF, Schachat AP, Nicholl J, et al. Chloroquine retinopathy. Is fluorescein angiography necessary? Ophthalmology 1985;92:1127–1129.

185. Henkind P, Carr RE, Siegel IM. Early chloroquine retinopathy: Clinical and functional findings. Arch Ophthalmol 1964;71:157–165.

186. Carlberg O. Three cases of chloroquine retinopathy. A follow-up investigation. Acta Ophthalmol 1966;44:367–374.

187. Martin LJ, Bergen RL, Dobrow HR. Delayed onset chlor-

oquine retinopathy: Case report. Ann Ophthalmol 1978; 10:723–726.

188. Brinkley JR, Dubois EL, Ryan SJ. Long-term course of chloroquine retinopathy after cessation of medication. Am J Ophthalmol 1979;88:1–11.

189. Mills PV, Beck M, Power BJ. Assessment of the retinal toxicity of hydroxychloroquine. Trans Ophthalmol Soc UK 1981;101:109–113.

190. Kearns TP, Hollenhorst RW. Chloroquine retinopathy: Evaluation by fluorescein fundus angiography. Trans Am Ophthalmol Soc 1966;64:217–231.

191. Lowes M. Peripheral visual field restriction in chloroquine retinopathy. Report of a case. Acta Ophthalmol 1976;54:819–826.

192. Krill AE, Potts AM, Johanson CE. Chloroquine retinopathy. Investigation of discrepancy between dark adaptation and electroretinographic findings in advanced stages. Am J Ophthalmol 1971;71:530–543.

193. Kolb H. Electro-oculogram findings in patients treated with antimalarial drugs. Br J Ophthalmol 1965;49:573–589.

194. Nylander U. Ocular damage in chloroquine therapy. Acta Ophthalmol 1966;44:335–348.

195. Hart WM, Burde RM, Johnston GP, et al. Static perimetry in chloroquine retinopathy. Perifoveal patterns of visual field depression. Arch Ophthalmol 1984;102:377–380.

196. Burns RP. Delayed onset of chloroquine retinopathy. N Engl J Med 1966;275:693–696.

197. Ehrenfeld M, Nesher R, Merin S. Delayed-onset chloroquine retinopathy. Br J Ophthalmol 1986;70:281–283.

198. Finbloom DS, Silver K, Newsome DA, et al. Comparison of hydroxychloroquine and chloroquine use and the development of retinal toxicity. J Rheumatol 1985;12:692–694.

199. Voipio H. Incidence of chloroquine retinopathy. Acta Ophthalmol 1966;44:349–354.

200. Ogawa S, Kurumatani N, Shibaike N, et al. Progression of retinopathy long after cessation of chloroquine therapy. Lancet 1979;1:1408.

201. Johnson MW, Vine AK. Hydroxychloroquine therapy in massive total doses without retinal toxicity. Am J Ophthalmol 1987;104:139–144.

202. Rosenthal AR, Kolb H, Bergsma D, et al. Chloroquine retinopathy in the Rhesus monkey. Invest Ophthalmol Vis Sci 1978;17:1158–1175.

203. Bernstein HN, Ginsberg J. The pathology of chloroquine retinopathy. Arch Ophthalmol 1964;71:238–245.

204. Ramsey MS, Fine BS. Chloroquine toxicity in the human eye. Histopathologic observations by electron microscopy. Am J Ophthalmol 1972;73:229–235.

205. Wetterholm DH, Winter FC. Histopathology of chloroquine retinal toxicity. Arch Ophthalmol 1964;71:116–121.

206. Fleck BW, Bell AL, Mitchell JD, et al. Screening for antimalarial maculopathy in rheumatology clinics. Br Med J 1985;291:782–784.

207. Kinross-Wright VJ. Newer phenothiazine drugs in treatment of nervous disorders. JAMA 1959;170:1283–1288.

208. Miller FS, Bunt-Milam AH, Kalina RE. Clinical-ultrastructural study of thioridazine retinopathy. Ophthalmology 1982;89:1478–1488.

209. Davidorf FH. Thioridazine pigmentary retinopathy. Arch Ophthalmol 1973;90:251–255.

210. Meredith TA, Aaberg TM, Willerson D. Progressive chorioretinopathy after receiving thioridazine. Arch Ophthalmol 1978;96:1172–1176.

211. Miyata M, Imai H, Ishikawa S, et al. Change in human electroretinography associated with thioridazine administration. Ophthalmologica 1980;181:175–180.

212. Cameron ME, Lawrence JM, Olrich JG. Thioridazine (Melleril) retinopathy. Br J Ophthalmol 1972;56:131–134.

213. Potts AM. The concentration of phenothiazines in the eye of experimental animals. Invest Ophthalmol Vis Sci 1962; 1:522–530.

214. Kimbrough BO, Campbell RJ. Thioridazine levels in the human eye. Arch Ophthalmol 1981;99:2188–2189.

215. Henkes HE. Electro-oculography as a diagnostic aid in phenothiazin retinopathy. Trans Ophthalmol Soc UK 1967;87:285–287.

216. Gangitano JL, Keltner JL. Abnormalities of the pupil and visual-evoked potential in quinine amblyopia. Am J Ophthalmol 1980;89:425–430.

217. Yospaiboon Y, Lawtiantong T, Chotibutr S. Clinical observations of ocular quinine intoxication. Jpn J Ophthalmol 1984;28:409–415.

218. Dickinson P, Sabto J, West RH. Management of quinine toxicity. Aust J Ophthalmol 1983;11:265–269.

219. Brinton GS, Norton EWD, Zahn JR, et al. Ocular quinine toxicity. Am J Ophthalmol 1980;90:403–410.

220. Dyson EH, Proudfoot AT, Bateman DN. Quinine amblyopia: Is current management appropriate? Clin Toxicol 1985–86;23:571–578.

221. Behrman J, Mushin A. Electrodiagnostic findings in quinine amblyopia. Br J Ophthalmol 1968;52:925–928.

222. Stuart P. Quinine blindness: The value of stellate ganglion block. Br J Anaesth 1963;35:728–730.

223. Bankes JLK, Hayward JA, Jones MBS. Quinine amblyopia treated with stellate ganglion block. Br Med J 1972;4:85–86.

224. Vainio-Mattila B, Zewi M. Quinine amblyopia and the electroretinogram (ERG). Acta Ophthalmol 1954;32:451–461.

225. Sabto J, Pierce RM, West RH, et al. Hemodialysis, peritoneal dialysis, plasmapheresis, and forced diuresis for the treatment of quinine overdose. Clin Nephrol 1981;16:264–268.

226. Floyd M, Hill AVL, Ormston BJ, et al. Quinine amblyopia treated by hemodialysis. Clin Nephrol 1974;2:44–46.

227. Michelson JB, Whitcher JP, Wilson S, et al. Possible foreign body granuloma of the retina associated with intravenous cocaine addiction. Am J Ophthalmol 1979;87:278–280.

228. Tse DT, Ober RR. Talc retinopathy. Am J Ophthalmol 1980;90:624–640.

229. AtLee WE. Talc and cornstarch emboli in eyes of drug abusers. JAMA 1972;219:49–51.

230. Lederer CM, Sabates FN. Ocular findings in the intravenous drug abuser. Ann Ophthalmol 1982;14:436–438.

231. Carman CR. Talc retinopathy. J Am Optom Assoc 1985;56:129–130.

232. Lee J, Sapira JD. Retinal and cerebral microembolization of talc in a drug abuser. Am J Med Sci 1973;265:75–77.

233. Kresca LJ, Goldberg MF, Jampol LM. Talc emboli and retinal neovascularization in a drug abuser. Am J Ophthalmol 1979;87:334–339.

234. Bluth LL, Hanscom TA. Retinal detachment and vitreous hemorrhage due to talc emboli. JAMA 1981;246:980–981.

235. Paré JAP, Fraser RG, Hogg JC, et al. Pulmonary "mainline" granulomatosis: Talcosis of intravenous methadone abuse. Medicine 1979;58:229–239.

236. Murphy SB, Jackson B, Paré JAP. Talc retinopathy. Can J Ophthalmol 1978;13:152–156.

237. Jampol LM, Setogawa T, Rednam KRV, et al. Talc retinopathy in primates. A model of ischemic retinopathy. I. Clinical studies. Arch Ophthalmol 1981;99:1273–1280.

238. Kaga N, Tso MOM, Jampol LM, et al. Talc retinopathy in primates: A model of ischemic retinopathy. II. A histopathologic study. Arch Ophthalmol 1982;100:1644–1648.

239. Kaga N, Tso MOM, Jampol LM. Talc retinopathy in primates: A model of ischemic retinopathy. III. An electron microscopic study. Arch Ophthalmol 1982;100:1649–1657.

240. Withering W. An account of the foxglove and some of its medical uses: With practical remarks on dropsy and other diseases. London: Broomsleigh Press, 1785.

241. Robertson DM, Hollenhorst RW, Callahan JA. Ocular manifestations of digitalis toxicity. Discussion and report of three cases of central scotomas. Arch Ophthalmol 1966;76:640–645.

242. Sykowski P. Digitoxin intoxication. Resulting in retrobulbar optic neuritis. Am J Ophthalmol 1949;32:572–574.

243. Weleber RG, Shults WT. Digoxin retinal toxicity. Clinical and electrophysiologic evaluation of a cone dysfunction syndrome. Arch Ophthalmol 1981;99:1568–1572.

244. Robertson DM, Hollenhorst RW, Callahan JA. Receptor function in digitalis therapy. Arch Ophthalmol 1966;76:852–857.

245. Frambach DA, Matthews JD, Weiter JJ, et al. Digoxin in the subretinal spaces of humans with rhegmatogenous retinal detachments. Am J Ophthalmol 1985;100:490–491.

246. Rietbrock N, Alken RG. Color vision deficiencies: A common sign of intoxication in chronically digoxin-treated patients. J Cardiovasc Pharmacol 1980;2:93–99.

247. Haustein K-O, Oltmanns G, Rietbrock N, et al. Differences in color vision impairment caused by digoxin, digitoxin, or pengitoxin. J Cardiovasc Pharmacol 1982;4:536–541.

248. Chuman MA, LeSage J. Color vision deficiencies in two cases of digoxin toxicity. Am J Ophthalmol 1985;100:682–685.

249. Wagener HP, Smith HL, Nickeson RW. Retrobulbar neuritis and complete heart block caused by digitalis poisioning. Report of a case. Arch Ophthalmol 1946;36:478–483.

250. Gibson HC, Smith DM, Alpern M. II₅ specificity in digitoxin toxicity. A case report. Arch Ophthalmol 1965;74:154–158.

251. Binnion PF, Frazer G. [³H] digoxin in the optic tract in digoxin intoxication. J Cardiovasc Pharmacol 1980;2:699–706.

252. Mortada A, Abboud I. Retinal hemorrhages after prolonged use of salicylates. Br J Ophthalmol 1973;57:199–200.

253. Koliopoulos J, Palimeris G. On acquired colour vision disturbances during treatment with ethambutol and indomethacin. Mod Probl Ophthalmol 1972;11:178–184.

254. Kaiser-Kupfer MI, Kupfer C, Rodriques MM. Tamoxifen retinopathy. A clinicopathologic report. Ophthalmology 1981;88:89–93.

255. Beck M, Mills PV. Ocular assessment of patients treated with tamoxifen. Cancer Treat Rep 1979;63:1833–1834.

256. Kaiser-Kupfer MI, Lippman ME. Tamoxifen retinopathy. Cancer Treat Rep 1978;62:315–320.

257. McKeown CA, Swartz M, Blom J, et al. Tamoxifen retinopathy. Br J Ophthalmol 1981;65:177–179.

258. Griffiths MFP. Tamoxifen retinopathy at low dosage. Am J Ophthalmol 1987;104:185–186.

259. Shingleton BJ, Bienfang DC, Albert DM, et al. Ocular toxicity associated with high-dose carmustine. Arch Ophthalmol 1982;100:1766–1772.

260. Grimson BS, Mahaley MS, Dubey HD, et al. Ophthalmic and central nervous system complications following intracarotid BCNU (carmustine). J Clin Neuro-ophthalmol 1981;1:261–264.

261. Miller DF, Bay JW, Lederman RJ, et al. Ocular and orbital toxicity following intracarotid injection of BCNU (carmustine) and cisplatinum for malignant gliomas. Ophthalmology 1985;92:402–406.

262. Chrousos GA, Oldfield EH, Doppman JL, et al. Prevention of ocular toxicity of carmustine (BCNU) with supraophthalmic intracarotid infusion. Ophthalmology 1986;93:1471–1475.

263. Kaplan NM. Clinical complications of oral contraceptives. Adv Intern Med 1975;20:197.

264. Connell EB, Kelman CD. Ophthalmologic findings with oral contraceptives. Obstet Gynecol 1968;31:456–460.

265. Drill VA, Rao KS, McConnell RG, et al. Ocular effects of oral contraceptives. I. Studies in the dog. Fertil Steril 1975;26:908–913.

266. Faust JM, Tyler ET. Ophthalmologic findings in patients using oral contraception. Fertil Steril 1966;17:1–6.

267. Andelman MB, Zackler J, Slutsky HL, et al. Family planning and public health. Int J Fertil 1968;13:405–414.

268. Smith MS, Kreiger A. Visual loss associated with oral contraceptives. Am J Ophthalmol 1970;69:874–876.

269. Goren SB. Retinal edema secondary to oral contraceptives. Am J Ophthalmol 1967;64:447–449.

270. Ruskiewicz JP. Birth control linked to vein occlusion. Rev Optom 1983;120:58–60.

271. McGrand JC, Cory CC. Ophthalmic disease and the pill. Br Med J 1969;2:187.

272. Gombos GM, Moreno DA, Bedrossian PB. Retinal vascular occlusion induced by oral contraceptives. Ann Ophthalmol 1975;7:215–217.

273. Stowe GC, Zakov ZN, Albert DM. Central retinal vascular occlusion associated with oral contraceptives. Am J Ophthalmol 1978;86:798–801.

274. Marre M, Neubauer O, Nemetz U. Colour vision and the "pill." Mod Probl Ophthalmol 1974;13:345–348.

275. Schenker JG, Ivry M, Oliver M. The effect of oral contraceptives on microcirculation. Obstet Gynecol 1972;39:909–916.

276. Salmon ML, Winkelman JZ, Gay AJ. Neuro-ophthalmic sequelae in users of oral contraceptives. JAMA 1968;206:85–91.

277. Weleber RG, Denman ST, Hanifin JM, et al. Abnormal retinal function associated with isotretinoin therapy for acne. Arch Ophthalmol 1986;104:831–837.

278. Hoyt CS, Billson FA. Maternal anticonvulsants and optic nerve hypoplasia. Br J Ophthalmol 1978;62:3–6.

279. McKinna AJ. Quinine induced hypoplasia of the optic nerves. Can J Ophthalmol 1966;1:261–265.

280. Strömland K. Ocular abnormalities in the fetal alcohol syndrome. Acta Ophthalmol (Suppl) 1985;171:1–50.

281. Nair VS, LeBrun M, Kass I. Peripheral neuropathy associated with ethambutol. Chest 1980;77:98–100.

282. Roberts SM. A review of the papers on the ocular toxicity of ethambutol hydrochloride Myambutol an anti-tuberculosis drug. Am J Optom Physiol Opt 1974;51:987–992.

283. Carr RE, Henkind P. Ocular manifestations of ethambutol. Toxic amblyopia after administration of an experimental antituberculosis drug. Arch Ophthalmol 1962;67:50–55.

284. Addington WW. The side effects and interactions of antituberculosis drugs. Chest 1979 (Supp); 76:782–784.

285. Karmon G, Savir H, Zevin D, et al. Bilateral optic neuropathy due to combined ethambutol and isoniazid treatment. Ann Ophthalmol 1979;11:1013–1017.

286. Trusiewicz D. Farnsworth 100-Hue test in the diagnosis of ethambutol-induced damage to optic nerve. Ophthalmologica 1975;171:425–431.

287. Kuming BS, Braude L. Anterior optic neuritis caused by ethambutol toxicity. S Afr Med J 1979;55:4.

288. Garrett CR. Optic neuritis in a patient on ethambutol and isoniazid evaluated by visual evoked potentials: Case report. Military Med 1985;150:43–46.

289. Barron GJ, Tepper L, Iovine G. Ocular toxicity from ethambutol. Am J Ophthalmol 1974;77:256–260.

290. Citron KM, Thomas GO. Ocular toxicity from ethambutol. Thorax 1986;41:737–739.

291. Brontë-Stewart J, Pettigrew AR, Foulds WS. Toxic optic neuropathy and its experimental production. Trans Ophthalmol Soc UK 1976;96:355–358.

292. Polak BCP, Leys M, van Lith GHM. Blue-yellow colour vision changes as early symptoms of ethambutol oculotoxicity. Ophthalmologica 1985;191:223–226.

293. Yiannikas C, Walsh JC, McLeod JG. Visual evoked potentials in the detection of subclinical optic toxic effects secondary to ethambutol. Arch Neurol 1983;40:645–648.

294. van Dijk BW, Spekreijse H. Ethambutol changes the color coding of carp retinal ganglion cells reversibly. Invest Ophthalmol Vis Sci 1983;24:128–133.

295. Yoshikawa TT, Nagami PH. Adverse drug reactions in TB therapy: Risks and recommendations. Geriatrics 1982;37:61–67.

296. Friedmann AI. Visual field examination in the toxic and nutritional optic neuropathies. Trans Ophthalmol Soc UK 1970;40:795–808.

297. Guerra R, Casu L. Hydroxycobalamin for ethambutol-induced optic neuropathy. Lancet 1981;2:1176.

298. Huang NN, Harley RD, Promadhattavedi V, et al. Visual disturbances in cystic fibrosis following chloramphenicol administration. J Pediatr 1966;68:32–44.

299. Harley RD, Huang NN, Macri CH, et al. Optic neuritis and optic atrophy following chloramphenicol in cystic fibrosis patients. Trans Am Acad Ophthalmol Otolaryngol 1970;74:1011–1031.

300. Godel V, Nemet P, Lazar M. Chloramphenicol optic neuropathy. Arch Ophthalmol 1980;98:1417–1421.

301. Leibold JE. Drugs having a toxic effect on the optic nerve. Int Ophthalmol Clin 1971;11:137–157.

302. Lasky MA, Pincus MH, Katlan NR. Bilateral optic neuritis following chloramphenicol therapy. JAMA 1953;151:1403–1404.

303. Walker GF. Blindness during streptomycin and chloramphenicol therapy. Br J Ophthalmol 1961;45:555–559.

304. Spaide RF, Diamond G, D'Amico RA, et al. Ocular findings in cystic fibrosis. Am J Ophthalmol 1987;103:204–210.

305. Keith CG. Optic atrophy induced by chloramphenicol. Br J Ophthalmol 1964;48:567–570.

306. Wilcox TK, Bartlett JD. Systemic drug profiles in adult optometric outpatients. J Am Optom Assoc 1988;59:122–126.

307. Ostrom JR, Hammarlund ER, Christensen DB, et al. Medication usage in an elderly population. Med Care 1985;23:157–164.

308. Graham CM, Blach RK. Indomethacin retinopathy: Case report and review. Br J Ophthalmol 1988;72:434–438.

309. Rengstorff RH. Accidental exposure to sarin: Vision effects. Arch Toxicol 1985;56:201–203.

310. Bacon P, Spalton DJ, Smith SE. Blindness from quinine toxicity. Br J Ophthalmol 1988;72:219–224.

CHAPTER 31

Systemic Effects of Ocular Drugs

Robert D. Newcomb
Marlon L. Priest

Many topically administered drugs are widely used in the evaluation and treatment of ocular disorders. Side effects of these agents can be divided into:

1. Ocular or visual
2. Systemic
   a. Allergic
   b. Toxic

The ocular-visual effects are discussed in Part II of this book. Allergic manifestations can be limited to the eye or may present as a more generalized allergic phenomenon (e.g., urticaria or anaphylaxis). Although a potential risk with most pharmacologic agents, life-threatening allergic systemic reactions to topically administered ocular drugs are exceedingly rare. The diagnosis and management of such life-threatening reactions will be considered in this chapter.

Toxic systemic side effects are frequently predictable from knowledge of the pharmacologic properties of the agents involved. However, Yolton and associates[1] reported no side effects specifically requiring urgent or emergency medical intervention in a series of over 15,000 applications of diagnostic pharmaceutical agents covering much of the spectrum of the various classes of drugs presented below. The safety of such agents seems unequivocally established, although isolated reports of serious reactions occasionally appear in the medical literature.

Awareness of these potential side effects is necessary for clinicians using drugs in the delivery of primary health care services. One would suspect that primary care physicians and other health care practitioners who have no special interest in ocular diseases are, for the most part, uninformed about the potentially serious side effects from these drugs. How often does the drug history obtained by the primary physician include phrases such as "eyedrops for glaucoma" as a generic term imputed to have some descriptive value when, in fact, the phrase refers to a pharmacologically diverse group of drugs, each having specific pharmacologic characteristics and differing potentials for systemic toxicity? These side effects may be caused by systemic absorption and action of the drug itself, by interaction with other drugs, or by increased susceptibility due to local ocular disorders or preexisting systemic illness. In addition, individual hypersensitivities or idiosyncratic responses can never be predicted with certainty.

The following sections will address the potential systemic side effects of 6 groups of topically administered drugs selected on the basis of their prevalence of use in clinical practice or their potential for adverse systemic side effects.

- Anticholinergic agents
- Cholinergic agonists
- Adrenergic agonists
- Adrenergic blocking agents
- Anti-infective agents
- Local anesthetics

Epidemiologic Methodology

The epidemiology of systemic side effects associated with the topical administration of ophthalmic drugs is an important but elusive area of clinical research. It is important because of the potentially serious consequences of unwanted or unexpected systemic manifestations, and elusive because of the very rare occurrences of these unwanted or unexpected side effects.

To investigate this subject from a scientific rather than anecdotal basis, one must first conceptualize the epidemiologic approach to research as well as appreciate the nuances of standardized clinical trials. With this background, one is then prepared to consider the importance of clinical research protocols in the area of ocular pharmacology and toxicology.

The science of epidemiology evolved from a need to study the causes of epidemics logically and systematically, with the goal of ultimately preventing their occurrence. Epidemiologic research is now used to identify risk factors that cause a person (or group of persons) to become affected with a certain disease while another person (or group of persons) is somehow protected against it. The science of epidemiology is based on the premise that disease[a] does not occur in a random fashion but generally has predictable and sequential events that must occur before its clinical onset. Thus, modern epidemiology is more precisely defined as "the study of the distribution and determinants of disease frequency in man."[2] Epidemiologists today are concerned with the frequency of diseases (measured by incidence and prevalence rates), antecedent events, and personal characteristics such as age, sex, and race, which must be present for a disease to occur in persons exposed to common risk factors. The corollary to this approach is that individuals who are not exposed to certain antecedent events or do not have certain personal characteristics are not "at risk" for a certain disease.

Confounding Variables

When one attempts to study the epidemiology of systemic side effects associated with the topical administration of ophthalmic drugs, one must be very careful to limit the scope of investigation to consistent and verifiable systemic side effects in individuals exposed to the same risk factor or factors.

The first problem encountered in studying side effects is the realization that the same drug, in the same concentration and dosage, administered in the same manner by the same clinician, can cause systemic side effects in one person and no side effects in another. This may be due to individual hypersensitivity (allergy), potentiation by other drugs (synergism), underlying general medical conditions that either increase or decrease a drug's intended action (as in the use of mydriatics in an eye that has a corneal abrasion), psychological states (anxiety reaction), or a completely random occurrence with no known etiology (idiosyncratic reaction).[3]

In addition to the logical analysis of these etiologic factors, a systemic side effect must be qualified and quantified clinically. For example, was the side effect a rash? A headache? Fainting? Nausea and vomiting? Hyperventilation? Hypertension or hypotension? Hallucination? Death? It should be obvious that the type and frequency of systemic side effects should be qualified and quantified as much as possible to minimize and hopefully eliminate factors known as confounding variables. These are individual attributes frequently found in combination with others, and they make identification of a single causative factor difficult.

The Research Protocol

From an epidemiologic perspective, any investigation of systemic side effects caused by the topical administration of ophthalmic drugs must have a sufficient study population in which a statistically significant number of people experienced a similar systemic side effect associated with a standardized drug concentration, dosage, and uniform instillation technique. If there were a significant variation in the endpoint (type and severity of systemic side effect) or the precursor (drug concentration, dosage, or instillation technique), then it would be impossible to employ the concept of "relative risk" to evaluate accurately the suspected relationship between drug use and systemic side effects.

Relative Risk

Relative Risk (RR) is defined as the "ratio of the rate of the disease among those exposed, to the rate of disease among those not exposed."[4] Mathematically, this relationship is expressed as

$$RR = \frac{\text{Exposed}}{\text{Not Exposed}}$$

where the numerator is the rate of morbidity (or mortality) from a specific disease in a group of individuals exposed to a given risk factor, and the denominator is

---

[a]In this context the word "disease" is used in its broadest sense, meaning any abnormal health condition regardless of its infectious, degenerative, traumatic, or genetic etiology.

the rate of morbidity (or mortality) from the same disease in a group of individuals not exposed to the same risk factor. An RR equal to 1.0 indicates that exposure to the factor under study had no influence upon the rate of disease. An RR less than 1.0 indicates the likelihood of a factor protecting against the disease (i.e., reducing the rate of disease in the exposed group compared to the rate of disease in the nonexposed group). An RR greater than 1.0 indicates the likelihood of a factor being a precursor for the disease (i.e., increasing the rate of disease in the exposed group compared with the rate of disease in the nonexposed group). By employing various biostatistical tests, the RR can be evaluated for statistical significance, and this is important to permit the epidemiologist to determine whether differences in the rates between exposed and nonexposed groups are real and not due to chance.

The Investigation of Systemic Side Effects

There is little reliable information in the medical literature that proves that certain systemic side effects are definitely caused by the topical administration of ophthalmic drugs. Very few published reports have well-defined endpoints (side effects) and risk factors (age, sex, race, known allergies, general medical condition, drug concentration, drug dosage, instillation techniques, etc.). Most reports of side effects associated with topically applied ophthalmic drugs fall into the category of "anecdotes," which simply means that the author *believed* that a cause-and-effect relationship existed between the instillation of the drug and the observation of a systemic side effect. All clinicians should know that this type of contribution to the medical literature is only minimally useful in determining cause-and-effect relationships because of the variety of unknown and potentially confounding variables that may apply. Although anecdotal evidence provides interesting reading and may become a catalyst for large-scale clinical trials, it clearly cannot be considered to delineate a cause-and-effect relationship.

Given the fact that topically applied ophthalmic drugs are used or prescribed only by licensed health care professionals or their ancillary personnel and that these drugs are almost always used in small doses and low concentrations, they are among the safest of pharmacologic agents. However, to provide an overview of the frequency and types of systemic side effects reported to be associated with the use of topically applied ophthalmic drugs, 6 general classes of agents are analyzed in an attempt to determine the prevalence and seriousness of these side effects. This analysis is not exhaustive, but it does provide an epidemiologic approach to the investigation of systemic side effects purported to be caused by topically applied ophthalmic drugs. The method of investigation and the appreciation of the RR concept is stressed.

Anticholinergic Agents

Anticholinergic agents are used for their cycloplegic effect in the course of refraction, for routine dilation of the pupil, and in the treatment of anterior uveitis. Before the newer synthetic drugs became available, atropine and homatropine were the mainstays of cycloplegic refraction. However, since the newer drugs more nearly meet the ideal specifications for clinical cycloplegia, their use now predominates.

Toxic effects associated with these agents reflect their anticholinergic activity, which is manifest either within the central nervous system (CNS) or peripherally. "Hot as a hare, red as a beet, dry as a bone, blind as a bat, and mad as a hatter" is a mnemonic that reflects these signs and symptoms. Tables 3.23 and 3.24 list the clinical signs and symptoms of anticholinergic toxicity. Drug toxicities reportedly associated with specific anticholinergic agents are discussed in the following section.

Systemic Side Effects

TROPICAMIDE

Reports in the literature of adverse reactions to tropicamide are conspicuous by their rarity.[5] Tropicamide "syncope" has been reported as a complication of the drug, although review of the reported cases raises significant questions as to the mechanism of signs and symptoms observed. In both cases the syncopal episodes resolved spontaneously without specific medical treatment.[6,7] The benign course with spontaneous resolution argues against "anaphylactic shock" as a pathophysiologic mechanism underlying the one episode described as such.[7] Hopkins and Lyle[5] point out that children have been known to faint during testing of visual acuity, without administration of any ocular drug.

SCOPOLAMINE

Toxic reactions in which indications of CNS toxicity predominate have been described in association with the ocular administration of scopolamine. Hallucinations and ataxia have been noted.[8] These reactions have been transient, and no deaths have been reported.

HOMATROPINE

Little literature on adverse effects of homatropine has been published.[5] Four cases of ataxia, hallucinations, and speech difficulty have been reported in children, all of whom probably received dosages in excess of those recommended.

ATROPINE

The development of systemic toxicity associated with the ocular use of atropine appears well established. Gray[9] reported 6 deaths appearing in the literature from 1833 to 1979, all involving the ocular administration of atropine. All deaths involved children less than 3 years of age who received dosages exceeding recommended levels and who often had underlying systemic illnesses. A causal relationship between the drug and subsequent death has not always been clearly established.

CYCLOPENTOLATE

Reports of systemic toxicity related to the use of cyclopentolate abound in the literature.[10–16] Several reports describe unusual psychotic reactions in which ataxia, restlessness, hallucinations, and tachycardia were observed. Two cases of grand mal seizures have been reported.[16] An 82-year-old man with "chronic compensated dementia" is reported to have undergone permanent mental deterioration after administration of 0.2% cyclopentolate.[10] However, the permanent nature of his disability was felt to be caused by factors other than cyclopentolate toxicity. It is important to recognize that a large number of the cases of reported toxicity with this agent involved use of the 2% solution. The clinical use of concentrations of 1% or less seems clearly associated with much less frequent toxic manifestations.[5]

Epidemiology

In 1938 Hughes[17] reported a girl of 9½ years with suspected belladonna poisoning (increased temperature, pulse rate, and respirations; sore throat; dizziness; dry mouth and dry skin; urinary retention; disorientation; and muscular cramps in her hands and feet) following the instillation of 1% atropine ointment. The ointment had been prescribed for instillation in each eye, twice a day, for 3 days before a scheduled examination for a symptom of "suspected eyestrain." There was no lid edema, and no ocular findings were reported other than fixed and widely dilated pupils. The patient completely recovered with appropriate treatment.

Twelve years later Heath[18] reported the death of a boy, aged 2 years and 9 months, secondary to 1% atropine ointment. According to the report, the child did not feel well after his mother had given him the first 2 applications on 1 day, but a third dose was given on the following day despite his symptoms, and the child died at the hospital within 48 hours.

In 1961 Hoefnagel[19] reported 5 cases of toxic effects in children following the instillation of either 0.5% atropine or 2% homatropine eyedrops for cycloplegia before scheduled eye examinations. A brief summary of the 5 cases follows.

CASE 1

A 5-year-old girl who was born prematurely received a total of 14 drops of 0.5% atropine during a 3-day period. Following this medication, she was reported to have dry skin and dry mucous membranes, visual hallucinations, excessive talking, and an ataxic gait. She had increased temperature, pulse, and respiration rate but normal blood pressure. The symptoms completely subsided after 12 hours with conservative medical management.

CASE 2

A 9-year-old boy experienced ataxia, marked hyperactivity, and constant conversation with imaginary animals and people after receiving 6 drops of 2% homatropine in each eye within 1 hour. After 6 hours of observation in the hospital, the toxic side effects resolved.

CASE 3

An 11-year-old girl who had reported "feeling dizzy" after the first few doses of 2% homatropine eyedrops continued to receive the full dosage recommended by her practitioner: 1 drop in each eye every 10 minutes for 30 minutes. According to the report, "the fifth and sixth doses had to be given with the child lying down, because she was too ataxic to sit or stand." She displayed some of the classic signs and symptoms of toxicity as described in the cases cited above, but she was oriented after 12 hours and normal after 24 hours without medical intervention other than a precautionary hospital admission for observation.

CASE 4

A 12-year-old boy was admitted to the hospital because of ataxia and hyperkinetic behavior following the instillation of a total of 10 drops of 2% homatropine within a short period. After 12 hours of observation, the ataxia and restlessness had subsided without complications.

CASE 5

An 11-year-old boy was admitted to the hospital because of ataxia, combative behavior, and hallucinations. These signs and symptoms were believed to be caused by the instillation of 6 drops of 2% homatropine in each eye within 1 hour. Although he reported dizziness and "a funny feeling in his mouth" after the first dose, subsequent drops were administered by his mother as originally directed by the practitioner. Within 24 hours after admission to the hospital, the ataxia had disappeared. The tachycardia (pulse rate had been 120 on admission) persisted for about 3 days, and moderately severe hallucinatory experiences lasted for about 5 days after admission.

Despite the fact that systemic side effects caused by the use of topical ophthalmic atropine and other less potent anticholinergic drugs are potentially harmful, the incidence and prevalence of these side effects has not been calculated. This deficiency in the ophthalmic literature is due to at least 3 factors.

1. Since the total number of patients actually receiving the various types and amounts of ophthalmic anticholinergic drugs has not been documented, the "population at risk"[20] for these relatively rare systemic side effects has never been quantified. Without having at least an estimate of this population at risk, the denominator of the relative risk formula is unknown, and therefore no reliable relative risk computation is possible. However, it appears that the advantages of using these drugs by competent clinicians far outweigh their potential disadvantages. This viewpoint is supported by Norden.[21]

2. Except for age, few epidemiologic variables (risk factors) have been consistently found. Hoefnagel[19] suggested some variables, including blonde children (although 3 of the 5 cases he reported were black), Down's syndrome (also shown to be a risk factor by Berg and associates[22] and Harris and Goodman[23]), children with spastic paralyses, and environmental factors such as high temperature and relative humidity (4 of the 5 cases he reported were admitted to the hospital in either July or August).

3. For most diagnostic purposes strong anticholinergic drugs such as 1% atropine ointment, 0.5% atropine drops, and 2% homatropine drops have been replaced by less potent ones such as 0.5% and 1% tropicamide and 0.5% and 1% cyclopentolate. With these latter drugs the clinician can achieve adequate mydriasis for peripheral fundus examination and accommodative paralysis for cycloplegic refraction, and these drugs are much less likely to cause serious systemic side effects.

Precautions

The practitioner should follow an in-office protocol for the use of these drugs as proposed by Gray.[9]

- Avoid overdosage. Two human studies strongly indicate that cyclopentolate toxicity is dose related rather than related to individual idiosyncrasy.[13,24]
- Select the least toxic drug available that will produce the desired cycloplegia.
- Be prepared for adverse systemic side effects, and recognize toxic reactions quickly.
- Be aware of the few biologic variables that have been suggested as risk factors for systemic side effects.
- Avoid high environmental temperatures and relative humidities when anticholinergic drugs are used.

Hoefnagel[19] commented that the systemic effects of eyedrops occur more from the drug reaching the nasal mucosa and ultimately the intestinal tract through nasolacrimal duct drainage rather than through the conjunctival membranes. For this reason, he advised that light pressure be exerted briefly on the lower puncta and canaliculi (see Fig. 2.5) to prevent nasolacrimal duct drainage after the instillation of potentially toxic eyedrops. This recommendation has also been made by Praeger and Miller,[11] Adcock,[12] and Beitel,[25] and is a good rule to follow, especially in patients who have an increased susceptibility to anticholinergic toxicity.

Management

Toxicity from this class of agents is self-limiting in the vast majority of cases. Discontinuation of the drug and observation of the patient until symptoms subside, without pharmacologic intervention, is the approach of choice. Patients who develop behavioral aberrations that make them a threat to themselves or others should perhaps be considered for hospitalization. Hoefnagel,[19] in a discussion of toxicity from atropine and homatropine, suggests that all but the mildest cases should be hospitalized. He points out that cholinergic drugs such as pilocarpine and methacholine do not counteract CNS symptoms and are therefore of little use. Thus, therapy is largely symptomatic and should focus on:

- Protecting the patient from injury to self or others
- Controlling high body temperature
- Reducing sensory stimuli.

Physostigmine, cholinergic because of its inhibitory effect on cholinesterase, may be useful in doses of 1 or 2 mg intravenously or intramuscularly every 30 to 60 minutes as necessary to control major CNS or cardiac manifestations. However, the self-limited nature of these manifestations dictates that considerable restraint be exercised in its use. It should be noted that potentially life-threatening cardiac dysrhythmias and grand mal seizures can occur with parenteral administration of physostigmine.

Cholinergic Agonists

Systemic Side Effects

Cholinergic drugs are commonly used to reduce intraocular pressure in glaucoma. Table 3.16 shows the clinical signs and symptoms of systemic toxicity from cholinergic agonists. Such toxic manifestations appear to be rare, are almost always associated with drug overdoses, and are usually self-limited. Abdominal cramps and diarrhea may develop,[26] which has mistakenly led, on occasion, to laparotomy. A case has been reported[27] of cardiac arrest in a 72-year-old woman following 0.125% echothiophate eyedrops 3 times daily. The cardiac arrest was attributed to a reduction in blood cholinesterase.

One report[28] described a 75-year-old white man who received 30 drops of 2% pilocarpine over about 1 hour. The patient experienced profuse sweating and complained of nausea, followed by marked diaphoresis, retching, salivation, and tremor of his arms, legs, and thoracic muscles. His blood pressure fell from 170/89 to 110/60, and his pulse fell from 84 and regular to 70 and irregular. With timely medical intervention, the patient recovered fully within 7 hours.

Another report[29] described a 67-year-old white man who received 2 drops of 3% pilocarpine in each eye every 5 minutes for 75 minutes. The patient experienced profuse diaphoresis, systemic hypotension, tremors in his extremities, generalized weakness, and diarrhea. With supportive treatment, the patient fully recovered.

In both of the above cases, the ophthalmologist treating the patient was attempting to counteract attacks of angle-closure glaucoma.

Since blood cholinesterase levels are reduced after the use of echothiophate eyedrops,[30] the use of succinylcholine during general anesthesia as a muscle relaxant can cause protracted apnea and is dangerous within 6 weeks of discontinuation of anticholinesterase miotics.

Epidemiology

The frequency with which systemic side effects occur secondary to pilocarpine drops has never been documented. Risk factors associated with these adverse reactions have also not been determined. Basic research protocols, which include the age, race, sex, general medical condition, and the concentrations and dosages of drugs of both affected (i.e., cases) and nonaffected (i.e., controls) patients must be developed and performed.

Ellis[31] reported the prevalence of systemic side effects from the use of topical echothiophate to be from 0% to 37.5%. Patients frequently do not associate symptoms such as diarrhea and increased sweating with the use of eyedrops, and they should be asked whether they have encountered specific symptoms that might be attributed to these drugs.

On the basis of clinical experience and the relative paucity of reported side effects, one can only conclude that, since pilocarpine and, to a lesser extent, the anticholinesterase agents such as echothiophate are commonly used in the treatment of glaucoma, the benefits far exceed the potentially serious and rare side effects.

Precautions

The prudent clinician should use these drugs only when indicated and then only in their recommended concentrations, dosages, and routes of administration. Since bronchospasm can occur with use of these agents, a history of asthma contraindicates their use. The use of succinylcholine during general anesthesia as a muscle relaxant is contraindicated within 6 weeks of discontinuation of anticholinesterase miotics.

Management

Toxic manifestations that pose no threat to life are treated by reducing or discontinuing the offending agent. Severe toxic manifestations such as respiratory distress or serious cardiac disturbances may be treated with atropine, 1 to 4 mg intravenously, repeated every 30 to 60 minutes until evidence of atropinization (dry mouth, tachycardia, etc.) develops. Pralidoxime (2-PAM), a cholinesterase reactivator, may be used in a dosage of 1 or 2 g intravenously, slowly, but should not be used as a substitute for atropine in circumstances where drug therapy is required. If experience with systemic toxicity from organophosphate cholinesterase inhibitors can be applied, 2-PAM should perhaps be reserved for those patients with measurably depressed levels of plasma cholinesterase. Attention must be directed to maintaining adequate intravascular volume, and appropriate measures for ventilatory support should be instituted if necessary.

Adrenergic Agonists

Systemic Side Effects

Mydriatics such as hydroxyamphetamine and phenylephrine are commonly used adrenergic agonists. Semes and Bartlett[32] reported no cases of adverse reactions related to the use of hydroxyamphetamine. Phenylephrine, however, has been the subject of a number of reports pertaining to systemic toxicity.[33–39] Major toxic effects from the 10% concentration include acute hypertension and some propensity for the development of cardiac arrythmias following its topical administration. There are conflicting reports concerning the risk of systemic hypertension, but major systemic effects with concentrations less than 10% appear to be exceedingly rare. Additional systemic side effects of adrenergic agonists include paleness, faintness, trembling, excessive perspiration, and occipital headache. The clinical signs and symptoms of adrenergic toxicity are summarized in Table 3.8.

Epidemiology

In 1956 McReynolds and associates[33] concluded that adrenergic drugs have a wide margin of safety and that serious toxic effects are very rare. However, the same authors[33] went on to report a case of subarachnoid hemorrhage in a 35-year-old white man following the use of a cotton wick soaked with 10% phenylephrine. The pledget was placed in the lower cul-de-sac of 1 eye in an attempt to break posterior synechiae that had formed secondary to uveitis. The patient's blood pressure increased from 118/68 to 230/130, which required hospitalization for a month before complete recovery.

In 1936 Heath[34] suggested a cause-and-effect relationship between topically applied phenylephrine powder and elevated blood pressure in dogs, and in 1958 Drill[35] reported the possibility of cerebral vascular accidents in humans associated with increased arterial pressure following overdoses of adrenergic agents. But case reports describing these phenomena were rare, and sound epidemiologic research protocols to investigate these alleged associations were nonexistent. This

was especially true when the drugs were used topically in their recommended concentrations and dosages for ophthalmic diagnostic and therapeutic purposes. Although minor and transient toxic effects such as anxiety, tremor, headache, and palpitation were occasionally observed with these drugs, life-threatening effects were very poorly documented.

In 1966 Lansche[36] described 2 patients with marked hypertension secondary to topically applied 2% epinephrine and 10% phenylephrine ophthalmic drops. In each case, the drugs were applied to an anesthetized eye having either conjunctival hyperemia or a damaged corneal epithelium. Lansche[36] concluded that these conditions allowed a relatively large amount of the drug to be absorbed into the patient's systemic circulation. This hypothesis had been previously proposed by Beckman[37] in 1958.

Three additional cases of severe hypertension following the use of 10% phenylephrine ophthalmic drops were reported by Solosko and Smith[38] in 1972, and Wilensky and Woodward[39] added another case report in 1973. The latter authors concluded that it was not possible to say whether the rise in blood pressure represented a drug overdose or an individual idiosyncratic reaction unrelated to dosage.

Since 1975 several investigators have reported the results of their controlled studies to evaluate the relationship between topically applied ophthalmic adrenergic agents and systemic hypertension in adults.[40–43] An abbreviated discussion of their protocols and conclusions is presented below.

Samantary and Thomas,[40] in 1975, studied the systemic side effects of 10% phenylephrine eyedrops in 30 hypertensive and 30 normotensive patients matched for age and sex. They found elevated blood pressure in both groups after a total of 6 drops was administered to each subject. According to their report, systolic and diastolic blood pressure rose by about 10 to 40 mm Hg and 10 to 30 mm Hg, respectively, and this rise was accompanied by reduced heart rate. However, they did not observe palpitation, sweating, trembling, or fainting in any subjects. These investigators did not report the duration of the apparent drug-induced hypertension, and did not measure blood pressure in a matched control group of subjects who did not receive any eyedrop to ascertain the reliability and validity of their measurements.

In 1979 Sud and Grewal[41] repeated the Samantary and Thomas study using 50 hypertensive and 100 normotensive patients. They found elevated blood pressure and reduced pulse rate in 18% of the hypertensive subjects and in 21% of the normotensive subjects. The range of increases in systolic blood pressure was from 4 to 24 mm Hg in the hypertensive group and from 2 to 20 mm Hg in the normotensive group. The range of increases in diastolic blood pressure was from 4 to 20 mm Hg in the hypertensive group and from 2 to 20 mm Hg in the normotensive group. Paradoxically, blood pressure fell and pulse rate rose in 8% of the hypertensive group and in 10% of the normotensive group. These investigators[41] concluded that it was unclear whether the increase in blood pressure and decrease in pulse rate was due to overdose, individual idiosyncrasy unrelated to dosage, or other factors. Like Samantary and Thomas,[40] Sud and Grewal[41] did not measure blood pressure in a matched control group of subjects who received saline eyedrops as placebo to ascertain the reliability and validity of their measurements.

Kim and associates[42] in 1978 retrospectively studied 298 ocular surgery patients according to 3 constructed groupings. Group 1 included patients who had no history of insulin-dependent diabetes or prior treatment with adrenergic blocking drugs such as reserpine and guanethidine ($N = 230$). Group 2 included patients who were insulin-dependent diabetics ($N = 41$), and group 3 included patients who were taking reserpine or guanethidine ($N = 27$). The 3 groups were further subdivided into those patients who underwent ocular surgery preceded by topical administration of 10% phenylephrine eyedrops ($N = 202$) and those who did not ($N = 96$). The results of their study revealed no statistically significant change in preoperative and postoperative blood pressure measurements in the 176 patients who did receive preoperative 10% phenylephrine eyedrops but were neither insulin-dependent diabetics nor taking reserpine or guanethidine. However, after the administration of 10% phenylephrine eyedrops, both the systolic and the diastolic blood pressure measurements increased significantly in those groups of patients who were either insulin-dependent diabetics or taking adrenergic blocking drugs ($N = 12$). Thus, this research appears to indicate that insulin-dependent diabetes and severe hypertension are both risk factors for potentially harmful systemic side effects following the administration of topical 10% phenylephrine eyedrops. However, a similar statement cannot be made about the potential systemic side effects of 2.5% phenylephrine eyedrops, since this dosage formulation was not included in the study protocol.

Another controlled investigation was conducted by Brown and associates[43] in 1980. These investigators performed a double-blind study to determine the systemic hypertensive effects of topically administered 10% phenylephrine eyedrops compared to a control group of patients who received topically administered 1% tropicamide eyedrops. Using a standardized instillation technique, the investigators administered to both groups a total of 3 drops in the lower cul-de-sac of each eye within 4 minutes. The results of this study indicated no statistically significant difference between the experimental (10% phenylephrine) and control (1% tropicamide) groups with respect to drug effect on either blood pressure or pulse rate. The investigators concluded that idiosyncratic responses to very small amounts of drug (10% phenylephrine) may account for some of the increases in blood pressure in patients described in the literature. The incidence of severe hypertensive response to topically administered 10% phenylephrine is most probably very low.

In summary, one cannot conclude that a cause-and-effect relationship exists between the topical ocular administration of 10% phenylephrine and an increase in systemic blood pressure. However, the prudent clinician should be aware of very rare but potentially serious side effects when using this class of drugs. Fraunfelder and Scafidi[44] have proposed guidelines for the clinical use of 10% phenylephrine to minimize the possibility of potentially serious systemic side effects, but Leopold[45] has stated that even when a practitioner is familiar with the side effects and risks of using a drug for a specific ocular purpose, it cannot always be predicted whether side effects will occur.

Precautions

Subgroups of patients that appear to be at increased risk for systemic side effects include those with insulin-dependent diabetes, cardiac disease, hypertension, thyrotoxicosis, aneurysms, and advanced arteriosclerosis as well as the very young or very old.[44] Robertson[46] reported a significant pressor response to 2.5% phenylephrine in patients with idiopathic orthostatic hypotension and suggested that the drug be avoided in these patients.

Other precautions should include[44]: (1) avoid the 10% solution in infants and the elderly; (2) avoid irrigation, administration by conjunctival pledget, or subconjunctival injection of 10% phenylephrine; (3) avoid the drug in patients taking monoamine oxidase (MAO) inhibitors (for up to 3 weeks after their discontinuation) or tricyclic antidepressants; and (4) recognize that use of phenylephrine in the atropinized patient may cause an exaggerated pressor response and tachycardia.

Management

The paleness, faintness, trembling, excessive perspiration, or occipital headache will generally subside rapidly with rest and recumbency. Parenteral hydralazine (Apresoline) is recommended to treat major elevations of blood pressure. Dosage is 20 to 40 mg intravenously or intramuscularly, repeated as necessary. It should be emphasized, however, that specific antihypertensive therapy is usually not required and should be reserved for those patients with major CNS or cardiac symptoms or other evidence of significant target organ damage from acute elevation of blood pressure.

Adrenergic Blocking Agents

Systemic Side Effects and Epidemiology

There are currently 3 β-adrenergic blocking agents available in the United States for the topical treatment of open-angle glaucoma: timolol maleate (Timoptic), levobunolol (Betagan), and betaxolol (Betoptic). Because of their importance in treating a major cause of blindness in the United States, each will be discussed separately.

TIMOLOL

Timolol maleate is a nonselective β-adrenergic blocking agent. Although initially hailed as an effective new drug with relatively few side effects, the ophthalmic and medical literature since the introduction of timolol has shown this agent to have numerous undesirable ocular and systemic side effects. A variety of systemic side effects have been reported, including CNS (disorientation, depression, fatigue), cardiovascular (bradycardia, arrhythmias, syncope), pulmonary (dyspnea, wheezing), and gastrointestinal (nausea, vomiting, diarrhea, and abdominal pain) effects[47] (see Table 3.11).

McMahon and associates[48] in 1979 reported a study of 165 known glaucoma patients who were treated during a period of 14 months with timolol according to a rigid protocol approved by the Food and Drug Administration (FDA). These investigators found a 23.0% prevalence rate of adverse reactions from the drug, and 15 patients (9.1%) had side effects requiring discontinuation of the drug. The most common side effects involved the CNS (39.5%), eyes (25.6%), cardiovascular system (18.6%), respiratory system (7.0%), and other organs (9.3%).

In 1980, Wilson and associates[49] reported a 15.9% prevalence rate of systemic and ocular side effects associated with the use of timolol in 489 patients. These side effects included blurred vision, burning of the eyes, superficial punctate keratitis, cardiovascular involvement, headaches, visual hallucinations, dizziness, and drowsiness.

Also in 1980, Van Buskirk[47] reported 547 cases of adverse reactions to timolol that were recorded by the

National Registry of Drug-Induced Ocular Side Effects from October 1, 1978, to September 1, 1979. Of these cases, 46.0% were systemic side effects, 41.8% were ocular side effects (both external eye diseases and visual disturbances), and 12.2% were a failure to achieve the desired therapeutic response. According to this survey, the most commonly reported adverse systemic reactions were CNS effects (31.5%), cardiac abnormalities (27.9%), respiratory symptoms (14.7%), and dermatologic complications (6.0%). Since the number of patients throughout the United States who actually received timolol for the treatment of glaucoma during the 11-month study period is unknown, one is unable to calculate the true incidence and prevalence of adverse reactions. It is assumed that all 547 patients in the Van Buskirk study were receiving the drug in accordance with the standard prescribing practices recommended by the FDA. Moreover, since the influence of confounding variables was not specifically addressed by the author, one cannot dismiss the possibility of their contribution to reported adverse drug reactions.

In 1986 Nelson and associates[50] published a report of adverse respiratory and cardiovascular events attributed to timolol over an 8-year period. They concluded that ophthalmic timolol is contraindicated in patients with bronchial asthma, a history of bronchial asthma, severe chronic obstructive pulmonary disease, sinus bradycardia, second or third degree heart block, overt cardiac failure, or cardiogenic shock. In their study of 450 case reports of serious respiratory and cardiovascular events and 32 cases of death, they found 47.1% had respiratory and 51.2% had cardiovascular events linked to the topical use of timolol.

LEVOBUNOLOL

Levobunolol is a nonselective β-adrenergic blocking agent. Since its pharmacologic action is similar to that of timolol, all the precautions recommended for timolol should also be observed before prescribing levobunolol. Adverse reactions are rare, but may include CNS disorders such as headache, transient ataxia, dizziness, and lethargy as well as dermatologic disorders such as urticaria and pruritis.[51]

In 1983, Partamian and associates[52] established that levobunolol was an effective drug for lowering intraocular pressure in a group of 48 ocular hypertensive patients, and they reported no side effects, either ocular or systemic, attributed to the drug. In a study of 141 patients who had either ocular hypertension or primary open-angle glaucoma, Berson and associates[53] found that levobunolol was as effective and as safe as timolol for long-term control of intraocular pressure. These authors also reported that both drugs produce clinically insignificant decreases in systemic blood pressure but significant decreases in mean pulse rate (5 to 10 beats/min).[53] They recommend that neither drug be used in patients with abnormally low pulse rates. Similar findings were reported in 1985 by Cinotti and associates[54] and Silverstone and associates.[55]

BETAXOLOL

Betaxolol is a cardioselective (β_1) adrenergic blocking agent. In 1982, Berrospi and Leibowitz[56] reported a study of 12 patients who had used betaxolol to reduce intraocular pressure. The authors concluded that the drug was safe and effective for this purpose and suggested that it might be preferable over timolol because betaxolol has little effect on the β_2 receptors associated with the relaxation of bronchiolar and peripheral vascular smooth muscles and thus offers the potential advantage of fewer asthmatic toxic side effects.[56]

Berry and associates[57] in 1984 studied 46 patients with primary open-angle glaucoma and concluded that both betaxolol and timolol were comparable in both side effects and their ability to lower intraocular pressure. Since betaxolol is a selective β_1-adrenergic antagonist, it might be advantageous for patients in whom β_2 blockade could be harmful.[57]

In 1985, Dunn and associates[58] reported a study of 24 patients with known reactive obstructive airway disease (ROAD). The patients were given a timolol challenge, and 58.3% developed bronchospasm, but when 8 patients who had experienced bronchospasm were given either betaxolol or a placebo, there were no significant differences in the forced expiratory volumes (FEVs) observed between the 2 groups.[58]

Allen and associates[59] in 1986 compared the effects of timolol and betaxolol in a prospective 6-month double-blind randomized trial of 38 patients with primary open-angle glaucoma. The found betaxolol to be an effective drug for reducing intraocular pressure, but not as effective as timolol. In their study, there were no adverse ocular side effects and only minimal cardiovascular changes.[59] However, in 1986, Harris and associates[60] and Orlando[61] described cases in which respiratory difficulties and clinical depression were cited as possible side effects of betaxolol. In 1987, Ball[62] reported a case that implicated betaxolol as the agent exacerbating a patient's previously well-compensated congestive heart failure.

There have been no large-scale epidemiologic studies conducted to investigate the types and true incidences of side effects associated with betaxolol.

Precautions

As with all pharmaceutical agents, the prudent clinician must evaluate the beneficial effects of β-adrenergic blocking agents in light of their potential for adverse reactions. Until further data are available to accurately calculate the relative risks of the drugs and to identify the numerous nondrug confounding variables, β-adrenergic blocking agents should be avoided or used with caution in patients with asthma or a history of asthma, chronic obstructive pulmonary disease, and congestive heart failure. Cardiac arrhythmias may be particularly likely in patients who have hypokalemia related to concomitant therapy with carbonic anhydrase inhibitors. Since their long-term effects are not known, these drugs should also be used with caution in young patients.

Management

Side effects generally respond to discontinuation of the drug. Cardiac arrhythmias or respiratory symptoms may require treatment following the usual guidelines for the management of such disorders.

Anti-Infective Agents

Most topically applied ophthalmic anti-infective drugs can be used without fear of serious side effects, but two agents deserve special consideration. The first is chloramphenicol, a broad-spectrum antibiotic, and the second is the sulfonamides.

Chloramphenicol

Chloramphenicol is effective against a wide range of gram-positive and gram-negative bacteria, rickettsias, and viruses and is available in both solution and ointment form as topical ophthalmic preparations.

SYSTEMIC SIDE EFFECTS

Chloramphenicol should not be used to treat minor infections, either topically or systemically, because of its well-established potential for serious side effects such as bone marrow depression and aplastic anemia.[63–66]

In 1965, Rosenthal and Blackman[63] reported the first case of bone marrow hypoplasia following the use of topical ocular chloramphenicol. This case, however, could hardly be considered typical, since the patient had used 0.5% chloramphenicol eyedrops almost daily for 23 consecutive months, without medical supervision, for chronically red eyes. The patient also had a

5-year-old niece who had died of aplastic anemia following ingestion of chloramphenicol 2 years previously, indicating the possibility of a genetic predisposition to toxic side effects.

Since then, 3 other cases of serious adverse reactions have been reported, including 2 deaths.[64,66] According to 1 source,[66] the prevalence of bone marrow toxicity following the use of topical chloramphenicol is theoretically 1 in 30,000 to 50,000 cases, but a large-scale study to document the risk-benefit ratio has never been undertaken.

PRECAUTIONS

Systemic use of chloramphenicol is beneficial in patients who have intraocular infections because of its broad antimicrobial spectrum and its ability to penetrate the blood-aqueous barrier. However, topical ocular chloramphenicol should not be used to treat minor ocular infections, nor should it be used for serious infections in which less toxic antibacterial drugs are equally effective. Although the RR of adverse reactions occurring as a result of appropriate topical chloramphenicol usage is obviously extremely small, Fraunfelder and associates[66] have proposed the following guidelines for the use of this drug: (1) Its use is contraindicated in patients who have a personal or family history of drug-related hematopoietic failure, and (2) long-term ocular therapy of 40 days or more is seldom indicated.

MANAGEMENT

A patient receiving chloramphenicol therapy should have his or her white blood count monitored, and the drug should be discontinued at the first sign of an allergic or toxic reaction. The patient who experiences an adverse reaction may need aggressive medical intervention to counteract leukopenia or other acute hematologic deficits.

Sulfonamides

In 1938, Domagk, a German researcher, received the Nobel Prize in Medicine for his discovery of the chemotherapeutic value of sulfonamide drugs to combat bacterial infections in mice. The considerable medical and public health importance of this discovery and the subsequent widespread use of these drugs resulted in the sharp decline in morbidity and mortality figures for the treatable infectious diseases.[67] Although systemic sulfonamides are commonly used to treat urinary tract infections, topical ocular sulfonamides such as sodium sulfacetamide and sulfasoxazole are used to exert a bacteriostatic effect against a wide range of nonpurulent gram-positive and gram-negative bacteria.

SYSTEMIC SIDE EFFECTS

Adverse reactions to systemic sulfonamides occur in about 5% of all treated patients, and these reactions are highly variable.[67] The drugs can cause allergic disorders, renal and hepatic complications, blood dyscrasias, and transient myopia.

In 1922, Stevens and Johnson[68] published a report of a new clinical syndrome that was later named for them. The Stevens-Johnson syndrome, also known as erythema multiforme, is a potentially serious mucocutaneous disease consisting of a generalized maculopapular rash, severe stomatitis, and purulent conjunctivitis that may progress to symblepharon, corneal ulcers or perforations, and even panophthalmitis. It also can affect the respiratory, gastrointestinal, genitourinary, and central nervous systems, and death occurs in approximately 25% of all cases.[67] One of the first reports of this disease's being linked to the use of sulfonamides appeared in 1966.[69] Carroll and associates[69] studied 116 cases of Stevens-Johnson syndrome that the FDA had collected worldwide and concluded that adverse effects of sulfonamides could pose a serious public health hazard. Following that report, a warning was placed in the package insert and a letter was sent to all U.S. physicians to alert them to this hazard.

Similar reports of the Stevens-Johnson syndrome occurring in patients using a topical ophthalmic sulfonamide have been published,[70,79] and these cases have led to an increased awareness among optometrists and ophthalmologists of the potentially serious side effects that can result from the topical ocular use of sodium sulfacetamide.

PRECAUTIONS

The use of sulfonamides should be avoided in any patient who has a history of a hypersensitivity reaction to previously administered sulfonamides, regardless of the route of administration. In addition, the development of a rash or dry mucous membranes in a patient who is using any of the sulfonamide agents is an indication to discontinue the drug immediately.

MANAGEMENT

Patients who experience adverse reactions to sulfonamides should be given supportive care after discontinuing the drug, including artificial tears and ocular lubricants to treat dry eyes and antibiotics for secondary ocular infection.

Local Anesthetics

Systemic Side Effects

Although life-threatening allergic reactions are possible, serious systemic reactions to commonly used local anesthetic are rare.[71-75] Cases of convulsions and arrhythmias have been reported with overdosage of injectable agents.

Epidemiology

Serious systemic side effects from topically applied ocular anesthetics are exceedingly rare, but relatively mild ocular side effects are not uncommon. According to Lyle and Page,[71] in at least 98% of the cases in which a severe systemic reaction from a local anesthetic has occurred, it was due to an overdose of the drug. Adriani and Campbell[72] and Havener[73] support the concept that excessive amounts of topically applied ocular anesthetics can be absorbed by mucous membranes in sufficient quantity to potentially produce severe systemic reactions. However, there has been only one report of a severe systemic reaction to a topically applied ocular anesthetic. Cohn and Jocson[74] reported a case of grand mal seizures occurring in a 28-year-old patient following the administration of a benoxinate-sodium fluorescein solution. These authors acknowledged that the anesthetic component, benoxinate, may not necessarily have been implicated, since the combination solution also contains sodium fluorescein, polyvinylpyrrolidone as a vehicle, and chlorobutanol as a preservative. Appropriate testing for a possible immune mechanism could not be performed. Because of the speed and severity of the reaction, the authors preferred to characterize the reaction as idiosyncrasy rather than as an immune response. Except for this case, there have been no other reports of severe systemic toxic or allergic reactions to commonly used topically applied ocular anesthetics.[71,75]

In a prospective study of 6 schools and colleges of optometry, Yolton and associates[1] reported a 0% ocular side effect rate for 0.4% benoxinate and a 0.5% ocular side effect rate for 0.5% proparacaine when used in the recommended dosages before tonometry. There were no systemic side effects reported from either drug in the study population of 1942 optometry clinic patients representing all age groups.

Except for mild, local, self-limiting corneal and conjunctival side effects occurring in less than 1% of patients, anesthetic eyedrops, when used in the proper concentration, dosage, and route of administration, are among the safest classes of drugs used by ophthalmic practitioners.

Precautions

Multiple instillations of topical anesthetics should be avoided, particularly in patients with marked conjunctival hyperemia, liver disease, or kidney disease, since these can result in enhanced systemic absorption and reduced rates of metabolism and excretion.[76] In patients with a history of hypersensitivity to a specific anesthetic agent, it is advisable to use a drug from a different chemical family (see Chapter 4). Topical anesthetics should be used conservatively in patients with glaucoma or accommodative esotropia who are being treated with anticholinesterase drugs.[77] Anticholinesterase agents inhibit the action of plasma cholinesterase and thus delay metabolism of the ester anesthetics.

Management

CNS stimulation resulting from systemic absorption of local anesthetics is usually short-lived. Since 1 minimum lethal dose of a local anesthetic is destroyed in the plasma or liver in 20 to 60 minutes, recovery from local anesthetic poisoning is rapid.[78] Generalized seizures, reflecting the most dramatic extreme of cortical stimulatory effects, should be expected to be self-limited. Therefore, the major therapeutic objective should be protection of the patient from self-injury during the course of convulsions.

Supplemental oxygen should be available. Moore and Bridenburgh[76] report that in most cases oxygen alone prevents convulsions or corrects them. If the convulsions are short and the period between them is long enough to allow adequate oxygenation of the patient during the apneic phase of a convulsive episode, specific drug therapy may not be necessary.

Sustained convulsive activity may require the administration of specific drugs by qualified medical personnel. Diazepam (Valium), barbiturates, and succinylcholine have all been suggested as appropriate agents for parenteral administration in this setting. However, it must be emphasized that seizures related to local anesthetic agents are expected to be self-limited. The critical management consideration, therefore, is preventing self-injury to the patient by appropriate physical restraint. Tongue biting may be prevented by the use of an oral airway or padded tongue blade. However, unduly vigorous efforts to insert such devices may result in broken teeth, airway obstruction, or bitten fingers (the practitioner's). If placement cannot be accomplished rapidly and easily, attempts should be abandoned and reinstituted during the relaxation phase that inevitably follows the burst of convulsive activity.

Systemic Emergencies

Anaphylaxis

Anaphylaxis is an immediate hypersensitivity reaction usually mediated by IgE antibodies.[80] The reaction of the antigen with IgE-sensitized mast cells and basophils results in degranulation. Increased vascular permeability, vasodilatation, and bronchial smooth muscle constriction result from the actions of histamine and other biologically active substances.[81–85] The presenting symptoms are as varied as the distribution of the IgE-sensitized cells. Anaphylactic reactions may occur to agents administered by a number of routes. Although rare, acute allergic reactions following transmucosal absorption of agents are well recognized. Clinicians who use topically administered drugs in the diagnosis and management of ocular disease should be prepared to recognize and treat acute allergic reactions when they are encountered.

DIAGNOSIS

The manifestations of an acute IgE-mediated allergic reaction can range from bothersome but non-life-threatening cutaneous reactions to sudden vascular collapse followed rapidly by death. Although cutaneous reactions such as urticaria or hives are very annoying to the patient, they do not pose a threat to life. The clinician should view any cutaneous reaction, until proved otherwise, as a premonitory sign of full-blown life-threatening anaphylaxis. The majority of patients who experience cutaneous manifestations before a life-threatening episode of anaphylaxis describe a "deep diffuse burning pain."

Anaphylaxis produces airway obstruction in 2 forms. The most localized and often rapidly fatal is upper airway obstruction secondary to laryngeal edema. Stridor reflecting upper airway obstruction is manifest by a sensation of tightness in the throat, hoarseness, difficulty speaking, or dyspnea. Rarely, upper airway obstruction progresses so rapidly that sudden collapse from hypoxemia is the first sign.

Lower airway obstruction reflects the effect of the released mediators on the bronchial smooth muscles. Pure lower airway obstruction without other manifestations of anaphylaxis may be indistinguishable from asthma except for the historical component of a temporally related drug exposure. More diffuse wheezing reflecting distal airway obstruction aids in distinguishing lower from the more rapidly fatal upper airway obstruction. Patients with both upper and lower airway obstruction are anxious, tachypnea, and tachycardiac and describe a sensation of air hunger.

Vasodilatation and diffuse increased vascular permeability produce a relative hypovolemia. Manifestations may range from mild hypotension and tachycardia to circulatory collapse. Progressive alteration in sensorium associated with worsening hypotension is from a state of anxiety to confusion to lethargy and finally unresponsiveness. In anaphylaxis a varying combination of hypoxemia and hypotension is responsible for the inconsistent correlation of blood pressure and changes in sensorium.

MANAGEMENT

Prompt treatment is lifesaving. Patients with cutaneous manifestations without alterations in breathing or hemodynamics within 20 to 30 minutes of the onset of the reaction will probably not have progressive symptoms. This is not to say these patients can simply be observed in the office or discharged home. Evaluation of the patient with an allergic reaction should follow the "ABC"'s rule (see Evaluation of the Emergent Patient): Assessing the airway (A) followed by breathing (B), then circulation (C), and finally disability (D), which represents the central nervous system. The "ABCs" are to prevent "D," death and disability.

All patients with systemic allergic reactions who complain of chest tightness, throat tightness, dizziness, or difficulty breathing should be immediately transferred to an acute care facility. Notification of the Emergency Medical System (EMS) is crucial. Statutory limitations imposed upon the practitioner may govern additional treatment. If permissible, however, more aggressive therapy should be instituted.

First, supplemental oxygen should be administered. However, the critical pharmacologic intervention in acute anaphylaxis with signs and symptoms of hypotension or respiratory compromise is the administration of epinephrine. Patients without significant hypotension or alteration in sensorium should receive 0.3 to 0.5 ml of aqueous epinephrine 1:1000 subcutaneously or intramuscularly (0.01 ml/kg body weight in children).[85,86] Intravenous epinephrine in a dose of 3 to 5 ml of a 1:10,000 solution is preferred in the patient with hypotension. If a blood pressure is unavailable, patients with altered sensorium can be assumed to have both hypotension and hypoxemia. Titration of the epinephrine intravenously utilizing 1 ml increments of a 1:10,000 solution at 5 minute intervals is safest. In addition, if tolerated the patient should be placed in the supine position with the legs raised to aid in the treatment of hypotension.

Antihistamines and glucocorticoids, although widely used, should be regarded as ancillary measures in these critically ill patients. There is evidence that progression from cutaneous manifestations to full-blown anaphylaxis can be prevented in some patients if treated quickly with antihistamines. Patients with only lower airway obstruction may respond to a pulmonary β_2-receptor stimulant such as aerosolized isoproterenol or metaproterenol in addition to intramuscular diphenhydramine.[87] In animal studies, pretreatment with both H_1 and H_2 blockers prevents nearly all manifestations of anaphylaxis.[81,88]

Although epinephrine by the subcutaneous route will give prompt relief of cutaneous manifestations, it has been associated with the development of cardiac dysrhythmias and myocardial ischemia related to coronary spasm, tachycardia, hypertension, or varying combinations. Therefore, the administration of epinephrine should not be taken lightly. In addition, rapid metabolism limits its usefulness in the treatment of pruritus and hives (urticaria) in the office setting. A variety of antihistamines will provide relief for such cutaneous symptoms.

Drug administration to all patients should be monitored closely, but patients with a history suggestive of an allergic diathesis, i.e., previous asthma, hay fever, or urticaria, are at even greater risk for the development of severe reactions to drugs administered topically to the eyes. It is generally agreed, however, that if no systemic reaction has occurred within 20 to 30 minutes of administration of the drug, the likelihood is small of the subsequent appearance of life-threatening manifestations of immediate hypersensitivity.

Chest Pain

The patient who develops chest pain in the practitioner's office represents a medical emergency. Approximately 1 million deaths each year are related to coronary artery disease.[89] The majority of these patients die within 1 hour of the onset of pain. As high as 25% of patients dying from coronary artery disease suffer the sudden death syndrome as the first manifestation of their disease.[90]

When myocardial oxygen demand exceeds supply, ischemic chest pain or dysrhythmias follow. A mismatch in the myocardial oxygen supply and demand can result from blood pressure and heart rate changes produced by the systemic effects of topical ocular β blockers, phenylephrine, allergic reactions, or even the stress of an office visit. Any patient with risk factors for coronary artery disease who develops chest or epigastric pain lasting for more than 2 minutes should be considered for further evaluation.[90] The office evaluation or therapy should be terminated immediately and the patient referred to the nearest emergency facility. Patients with nausea, vomiting, radiation of the pain, or associated diaphoresis should be transported by emergency medical service (EMS) personnel.

Evaluation of the Emergent Patient

A plan for rapid sequential evaluation of the patient with a suspected medical threat to life is constructed with a prior understanding of the requirements for oxygen delivery and carbon dioxide removal to preserve useful life. A mnemonic for evaluation is the "ABCs" of life.

Oxygen must first transverse the upper airway, "A," which extends from the orifice of the nose and mouth to just distal to the larynx. Breathing, "B," is the flow of oxygen to the lung's aveolar capillary membrane where erythrocytes passively exchange oxygen and carbon dioxide. Circulation, "C," is the delivery of oxygen absorbed across the aveolar capillary membrane to distant tissues by the flowing erythrocytes. The brain, with the highest oxygen demand and lowest tolerance to anoxia, is the time-limiting organ.

Although the final diagnosis of cardiopulmonary arrest is usually not difficult, the practitioner is often presented with an unresponsive patient. True unresponsiveness must be determined by the practitioner, since cardiopulmonary resuscitation (CPR) is not without complications. A simple, "Are you all right?" or "Can you hear me?" followed in the unresponding patient by shaking the upper torso while repeating the verbal stimulus will awaken most sleeping patients. Rubbing the sternum, a painful stimulus, accompanied by repeating the verbal stimulus may be required in a small minority of patients. Metabolic, structural, and toxic causes of altered sensorium are myriad and may require evaluation and treatment in an emergency facility, since the office practitioner is usually not equipped to provide definitive care for such problems.[91] The initial question that must be answered in any unresponsive patient is, "Does this patient require cardiopulmonary resuscitation?" Immediate transfer to an acute care facility is indicated for any patient requiring a painful stimulus for arousal. Any patient with altered sensorium or who requires a painful stimulus to arouse should be monitored closely until EMS personnel arrive.

Cardiopulmonary Arrest

Any patient with absent spontaneous respirations and pulses has sustained a cardiopulmonary arrest. It represents the ultimate medical emergency. Cardiopulmonary arrest requires that the practitioner rapidly recognize and immediately institute appropriate therapy to minimize the chances of death and disability. The most common event leading to a cardiopulmonary arrest is a cardiac dysrhythmia resulting in oxygen delivery below metabolic demands of the brain and heart. The rhythmn disturbances most likely to result in cardiopulmonary arrest are ventricular fibrillation, ventricular tachycardia, and asystole. In the practitioner's office setting there are three common presentations of cardiopulmonary arrest.[92] Most commonly the rhythm disturbance abruptly interrupts oxygen delivery to the brain, causing a generalized seizure followed by a lack of breathing. Second, the patient may provide some warning by suddenly complaining of chest tightness, shortness of breath, or a smothering sensation. The warning is followed rapidly by a lack of respiratory effort, unresponsiveness, pallor, cyanosis, and a mottled appearance. Finally, the patient may quietly become limp and unresponsive. In either of these three situations, the "ABCs" must be rapidly evaluated and therapy instituted in a predetermined sequence to reestablish oxygen delivery.

Simultaneous notification of EMS services must be accomplished if the arrest occurs outside the hospital setting. All health care personnel including ancillary staff should be aware of the mechanism for activating EMS service. Telephone numbers for contacting these services should be properly displayed for reference in an emergency. The universal emergency number 911, in areas where it has been implemented, provides instant access to police, fire, and EMS. The caller should provide (1) the exact address, (2) the telephone number from which the call is being made, (3) what has happened, and (4) the number of victims. In addition, it is important for the caller to give the emergency dispatcher the opportunity to ask necessary questions. Ideally, personnel functioning within the prehospital EMS phase will be able to respond to such commonly occurring problems as hypoglycemia, analgesic overdose, stroke, and cardiopulmonary arrest.

The awake patient who suddenly develops crushing chest tightness associated with a presyncope feeling presents a special situation. The patient may well be suffering from ventricular tachycardia or ventricular fibrillation. In some of these patients, blood pressure and thus consciousness can be maintained for a short time by initiating a cough that increases peripheral vascular tone. Repeated coughing maintained cerebral perfusion until definitive therapy could be instituted in a small number of hospitalized patients. In addition, 10% of patients with ventricular dysrhythmia will cardiovert to a normal sinus with a vigorous cough. Thus, patients presenting with chest tightness associated with a near syncope feeling should be directed to cough. This may prevent a full cardiopulmonary arrest.[93–95]

Although the following discussion outlines the current approach to basic cardiopulmonary resuscitation, it must be understood that proficiency in the techniques requires training that incorporates "hands-on" experience (with mannequins) and periodic recertification to maintain skills (Fig. 31.1).

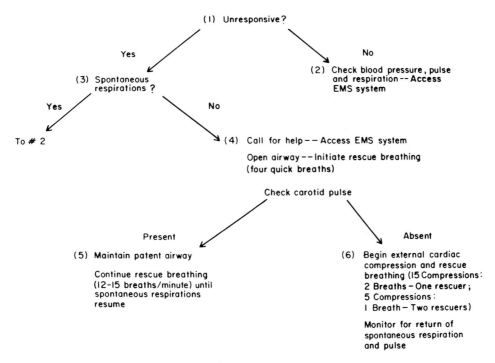

FIGURE 31.1   **Flowchart for basic cardiopulmonary resuscitation (CPR).**

Once patient unresponsiveness is established, the first measure is to open the airway, "A." The patient should be positioned supine on a hard flat surface so that the airway can be opened and cardiopulmonary resuscitation performed if indicated. In the unconscious patient, relaxation of the pharyngeal muscles may allow the tongue to fall back into the airway, resulting in mechanical obstruction. Simple manuevers such as the head-tilt-neck-lift, head-tilt-chin-lift, or jaw thrust will relieve the obstruction. In some cases restoration of airway patency may be all that is required to prevent deterioration of the patient's condition to complete cardiopulmonary arrest. Breathing, "B," can be ascertained by placing a hand or ear next to the patient's nose to detect air movement. If there is no air movement, breathing is inadequate. Four quick breaths should be delivered, and the chest wall should be observed for movement with each breath to reevaluate "A." Patients who have potential cervical spine injuries, although not likely to be encountered in the practitioner's office setting, pose a special problem. Maneuvers that depend on hyperextension of the neck in these patients should be avoided in favor of jaw thrust, which maintains the neck in the neutral position. The rescuer thereby minimizes the likelihood of a potential devastating spinal cord injury in the patient with a neck injury. The possibility of airway obstruction by vomitus, denture, or other foreign bodies must be kept in mind, and appropriate maneuvers should be undertaken to clear the airway. The lack of movement of the chest wall during rescue breathing means the airway has not been established. Prompt reevaluation and institution of additional manuevers to restore patency must be performed before proceeding.

Breathing, "B," must be instituted immediately if the patient is not breathing once appropriate measures to open the airway have been performed. Mouth-to-mouth breathing using exhaled air is the technique of choice. Concentrations of oxygen approaching 18% to 20% can be delivered by this method.[96] Pocket masks (Fig. 31.2), now available with a 1-way valve preventing the regurgitation of stomach contents or air into the rescuers mouth, are inexpensive and useful adjuncts to ventilation that can be used to overcome both aesthetic and health objections. These should be readily available to prevent delay in instituting CPR. A good seal over the face can be established, and with a simple oxygen delivery system it is possible to substantially increase the concentration of oxygen delivered to the patient. Observing movement of the chest wall confirms a patent airway and effective breathing, which together deliver oxygen to the aveolar capillary membrane for exchange.

The carotid pulse should be checked to assess circulation, "C," following the 4 quick breaths. The res-

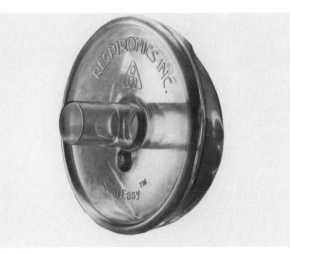

FIGURE 31.2   **Pocket mask, which aids ventilation procedures in CPR. (Courtesy Respironics, Inc., Monroeville, PA)**

cuer should attempt to palpate a spontaneous carotid pulse (femoral pulse is an acceptable alternative in the infant). If there is no palpable carotid pulse, a single firm precordial thump should be delivered. The thump will generate approximately 25 joules of energy and successfully cardiovert up to 25% of patients with ventricular fibrillation to a rhythmn-producing cardiac output and thus a palpable carotid pulse. External cardiac compression should be initiated when no spontaneous pulse is present following the precordial thump. The heart serves as a passive conduit with blood flow resulting from the intrathoracic pressure changes produced during external chest compressions. When properly applied, external cardiac compressions can generate a cardiac output approaching 30% of normal.[96–98] When promptly and efficiently applied, external cardiac compressions support perfusion and oxygenation to vital organs until spontaneous circulation is reestablished.

The time-critical nature of CPR must be recognized. Irreversible brain death occurs within 4 to 6 minutes from the cessation of cerebral perfusion. Variables such as body age, body temperature, certain drugs, and coexistent disease may modify tolerance of the brain to ischemia. However, the overriding consideration for the practitioner confronted with the unresponsive patient remains the prompt institution of measures for the support of breathing and circulation.

Adjunctive measures including mechanical devices and drugs (Table 31.1) are used in keeping with statutory limitations imposed on the practitioner, availability of EMS resources, and the interest and commitment of the practitioner.[96,99,100] Commercially available kits (Fig. 31.3) can be useful in an office setting where

TABLE 31.1
Basic Emergency Equipment and Drugs

Item	Description
Airway	Oral, resuscitation mask, Ambu bag
Oxygen	With appropriate delivery tubing
Blood pressure cuff	
Drugs	Epinephrine 1:1000 injectable
	Diphenhydramine injectable
	Isoproterenol or metaproterenol inhaler
	Hydrocortisone sodium succinate injectable

immediate access to equipment is essential. It must be reemphasized, however, that the critical element in the overall approach is the trained rescuer and that basic CPR requires essentially no adjunctive equipment. Nevertheless, current concerns for disease transmission dictate the availability of a 1-way valved pocket mask to prevent delays in instituting CPR.[101]

The institution of basic cardiopulmonary resuscitation is designed as an emergency measure before EMS personnel have arrived. What, then, is the responsibility of the practitioner in health care settings where cardiopulmonary arrest might reasonably be expected to occur on an infrequent basis? He or she should (1) obtain and maintain cardiopulmonary certification, (2) provide cardiopulmonary resuscitation training for all office personnel, (3) maintain proficiency in the recognition and treatment of cardiopulmonary arrest by periodic training, and (4) educate office personnel about available EMS resources and how to activate these resources in an emergency.

Summary

The basic descriptive epidemiologic information that would permit determination of the incidences, prevalences, and risk factors of systemic side effects caused by topically administered ocular drugs is not available in the ophthalmic or medical literature. This information is needed by all eyecare practitioners, and its absence can only indicate that other areas of clinical research have been judged to have a higher priority.

Perhaps the extremely rare occurrences of serious systemic side effects secondary to the topical use of ocular drugs is another reason for this lack of information. A third reason could be the previous lack of a national, coordinated effort to collect and analyze reports of alleged systemic side effects associated with ophthalmic drugs.

There now exists a center that serves as a clearinghouse for this type of information.[a] The National Registry of Drug-Induced Ocular Side Effects was established in 1976 to coordinate research efforts in this area, and all eyecare practitioners are encouraged to report to the National Registry any adverse reactions suspected to be associated with an ocular drug. It is hoped that protocols will be developed to determine the number of patients in various age, sex, and racial categories who are actually exposed to specific ocular drugs. This will allow calculation of the relative risk values for a number of antecedent events and personal characteristics. After these data are properly collected and statistically analyzed, the true incidence, prevalence, and risk factors of adverse drug reactions will begin to be determined. Only after this information is compiled and made available to all clinicians will we be able to prevent, to the maximum extent possible, unwanted or unexpected complications associated with ocular drugs.

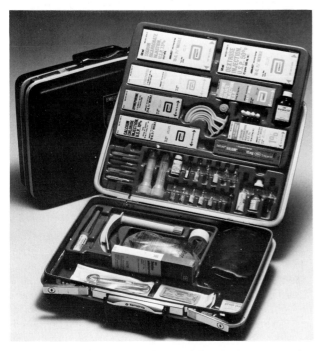

FIGURE 31.3 **Commercially available emergency drug kit. (Courtesy Banyan International Corporation, Abilene, TX)**

[a]National Registry of Drug-Induced Ocular Side Effects, Department of Ophthalmology, The Oregon Health Sciences University, 3181 S. W. Sam Jackson Park Road, Portland, Oregon 97201.

References

1. Yolton DP, Kandel JS, Yolton RL. Diagnostic pharmaceutical agents: Side effects encountered in a study of 15,000 applications. J Am Optom Assoc 1980;51:113–118.
2. MacMahon B, Pugh TF. Epidemiology: Principles and methods. Boston: Little, Brown, 1970;1.
3. Ross EM, Gilman AG. Pharmacodynamics: Mechanisms of drug action and the relationship between drug concentration and effect. In: Gilman AG, Goodman LS, Rall TW, Murad F, eds. Goodman and Gilman's The pharmacological basis of therapeutics. New York: Macmillan, 1985;7:35–48.
4. MacMahon B, Pugh TF. Epidemiology: Principles and methods. Boston: Little, Brown, 1970;232.
5. Hopkins GA, Lyle WM. Potential systemic side effects of six common ophthalmic drugs. J Am Optom Assoc 1977; 48:1241–1245.
6. Schmidt I. Two patients with unusual reaction to drugs used in optometric practice. Am J Optom Physiol Opt 1970; 47:312–315.
7. Wahl JW. Systemic reactions to tropicamide. Arch Ophthalmol 1969;82:320–321.
8. Freund M, Merin S. Toxic effects of scopolamine eye drops. Am J Ophthalmol 1970;70:637–639.
9. Gray LG. Avoiding adverse effects of cycloplegics in infants and children. J Am Optom Assoc 1979;50:465–470.
10. Carpenter WT. Precipitous mental deterioration following cycloplegia with 0.2% cyclopentolate HCl. Arch Ophthalmol 1967;78:445–447.
11. Praeger DL, Miller SN. Toxic effects of cyclopentolate (Cyclogyl). Am J Ophthalmol 1964;58:1060–1061.
12. Adcock EW. Cyclopentolate (Cyclogyl) toxicity in pediatric patients. J Pediatr 1971;79:127–129.
13. Simcoe CW. Cyclopentolate (Cyclogyl) toxicity: Report of a case. Arch Ophthalmol 1962;67:406–408.
14. Awan KJ. Adverse systemic reactions of topical cyclopentolate hydrochloride. Ann Ophthalmol 1976;8:695–698.
15. Awan KJ. Systemic toxicity of cyclopentolate hydrochloride in adults following topical ocular instillation. Ann Ophthalmol 1976;8:803–806.
16. Kennerdell JS, Wucher FP. Cyclopentolate associated with two cases of grand mal seizure. Arch Ophthalmol 1972; 87:634–635.
17. Hughes CA. Poisoning from use of atropine ointment 1%. Trans Ophthalmol Soc UK 1938;58:444–446.
18. Heath WE. Death from atropine poisoning. Br Med J 1950;2:608.
19. Hoefnagel D. Toxic effects of atropine and homatropine eyedrops in children. N Engl J Med 1961;264:168–171.
20. Werner SB, Austin DF. Epidemiology for the health sciences. Springfield, IL: Charles C Thomas, 1976;62.
21. Norden LC. Adverse reactions to topical ocular autonomic agents. J Am Optom Assoc 1978;49:75–80.
22. Berg JM, Brandon MWG, Kirman BH. Atropine in mongolism. Lancet 1959;441–442.
23. Harris WS, Goodman RM. Hyper-reactivity to atropine in Down's syndrome. N Engl J Med 1968;279:407–410.
24. Binkhorst RD, Weinstein GW, Baretz RM, et al. Psychotic reaction induced by cyclopentolate (Cyclogyl): Results of pilot study and a double-blind study. Am J Ophthalmol 1963;55:1243–1245.
25. Beitel RJ. Cycloplegic refraction. In: Duane TD, Jaeger EA, eds. Clinical ophthalmology. Philadelphia: Harper & Row, 1987;1, Chap. 41:1–4.
26. Markman HD, Rosenberg P, Dettbarn W. Eye drops and diarrhea. Diarrhea as the first symptom of echothiophate iodide toxicity. N Engl J Med 1964;271:197–198.
27. Hiscox PE, McCulloch C. Cardiac arrest occurring in a patient on echothiophate iodide therapy. Am J Ophthalmol 1965;60:425–427.
28. Epstein E, Kaufman I. Systemic pilocarpine toxicity from overdosage. Am J Ophthalmol 1965;
29. Greco JJ, Kelman CD. Systemic pilocarpine toxicity in the treatment of angle closure glaucoma. Ann Ophthalmol 1973;5:57–59.
30. DeRoetth A, Dettbarn WD, Rosenberg P, et al. Effect of phospholine iodide on blood cholinesterase levels of normal and glaucoma subjects. Am J Ophthalmol 1965;59: 586–592.
31. Ellis PP. Ocular therapeutics and pharmacology. St. Louis: C.V. Mosby Co, 1981;6:58.
32. Semes LP, Bartlett JD. Mydriatic effectiveness of hydroxyamphetamine. J Am Optom Assoc 1982;53:899–904.
33. McReynolds WU, Havener WH, Henderson JW. Hazards of the use of sympathomimetic drugs in ophthalmology. Arch Ophthalmol 1956;56:176–179.
34. Heath P. Neosynephrin hydrochloride: Some uses and effects in ophthalmology. Arch Ophthalmol 1936;16:839–846.
35. Drill VA, ed. Pharmacology in medicine. New York: McGraw-Hill, 1958;12.
36. Lansche RK. Systemic reactions to topical epinephrine and phenylephrine. Am J Ophthalmol 1966;61:95–98.
37. Beckman H. Drugs: Their nature, action, and use. Philadelphia: W.B. Saunders Co, 1958;345.
38. Solosko D, Smith RB. Hypertension following 10% phenylephrine ophthalmic. Anesthesiology 1972;36:187–189.
39. Wilensky JT, Woodward HJ. Acute systemic hypertension after conjunctival instillation of phenylephrine hydrochloride. Am J Ophthalmol 1973;76:156–157.
40. Samantary S, Thomas A. Systemic effects of topical phenylephrine. Ind J Ophthalmol 1975;23:16–17.
41. Sud RN, Grewal SS. Phenylephrine—systemic effects from its topical use. Ind J Ophthalmol 1979;26:33–37.
42. Kim JM, Stevenson CE, Mathewson HS. Hypertensive reactions to phenylephrine eyedrops in patients with sympathetic denervation. Am J Ophthalmol 1978;85:862–867.
43. Brown MM, Brown GC, Spaeth GL. Lack of side effects from topically administered 10% phenylepherine eyedrops. Arch Ophthalmol 1980;98:487–489.
44. Fraunfelder FT, Scafidi AF. Possible adverse effects from topical ocular 10% phenylephrine. Am J Ophthalmol 1978;85:447–453.
45. Leopold IH. The phenylephrine saga—a drug dilemma. Am J Ophthalmol 1978;85:572–574.
46. Robertson D. Contraindication to the use of ocular phenylephrine in idiopathic orthostatic hypotension. Am J Ophthalmol 1979;87:819–822.
47. Van Buskirk EM. Adverse reactions from timolol administration. Ophthalmology 1980;87:447–450.
48. McMahon CD, Shaffer RN, Hoskins HD, et al. Adverse effects experienced by patients taking timolol. Am J Ophthalmol 1979;88:736–738.

49. Wilson RP, et al. The place of timolol in the practice of ophthalmology. Ophthalmology 1980;87:451–454.

50. Nelson WL, Fraunfelder FT, Sills JM, et al. Adverse respiratory and cardiovascular events attributed to timolol ophthalmic solution, 1978–1985. Am J Ophthalmol 1986; 102:606–611.

51. American Society of Hospital Pharmacists. AHFS Drug Information 87. Bethesda, MD: American Society of Hospital Pharmacists. 1987;1491–1494.

52. Partamian LG, Kass MA, Gordon M. A dose-response study of the effect of levobunolol on ocular hypertension. Am J Ophthalmol 1983;95:229–232.

53. Berson FG, Cohen HB, Foerster RJ, et al. Levobunolol compared with timolol for the long-term control of elevated intraocular pressure. Arch Ophthalmol 1985;103: 379–382.

54. Cinotti A, Cinotti D, Grant W, et al. Levobunolol vs timolol for open-angle glaucoma and ocular hypertension. Am J Ophthalmol 1985;99:11–17.

55. Silverstone DE, Arkfeld D, Cowan G, et al. Long-term diurnal control of intraocular pressure with levobunolol and with timolol. Glaucoma 1985;7:138–140.

56. Berrospi AR, Leibowitz HM. Betaxolol: A new β-adrenergic blocking agent for treatment of glaucoma. Arch Ophthalmol 1982;100:943–946.

57. Berry DP, Van Buskirk EM, Shields MD. Betaxolol and timolol: A comparison of efficacy and side effects. Arch Ophthalmol 1984;102:42–45.

58. Dunn TL, Gerber MJ, Shen AS, et al. Timolol-induced bronchospasm: Utility of betaxolol as an alternative ocular hypotensive agent in patients with asthma. Clin Res 1985; 33:20A.

59. Allen RC, Hertzmark E, Walker AM, et al. A double-masked comparison of betaxolol vs timolol in the treatment of open-angle glaucoma. Am J Ophthalmol 1986;101:535–541.

60. Harris LS, Greenstein SH, Bloom AF. Respiratory difficulties with betaxolol (letter). Am J Ophthalmol 1986; 102:274.

61. Orlando RG. Clinical depression associated with betaxolol (letter). Am J Ophthalmol 1986;102:275.

62. Ball S. Congestive heart failure from betaxolol. Arch Ophthalmol 105:320,1987.

63. Rosenthal RL, Blackman A. Bone-marrow hypoplasia following use of chloramphenicol eye drops. JAMA 1965; 191:148.

64. Carpenter G. Chloramphenicol eye drops and marrow aplasia. Lancet 1975;2:326–327.

65. Abrams SM, Degnan TJ, Vinciguerra V. Marrow aplasia following topical application of chloramphenicol eye ointment. Arch Intern Med 140:576,1980.

66. Fraunfelder FT, Bagby GC, Kelly DJ. Fatal aplastic anemia following topical administration of ophthalmic chloramphenicol. Am J Ophthalmol 1982;93:356–360.

67. Mandell GL, Sande MA. Antimicrobial agents. Sulfonamides, trimethoprim-sulfamethox-azole, and agents for urinary tract infections. In: Gilman AG, Goodman LS, Rall TW, Murad F, eds. Goodman and Gilman's The pharmacological basis of therapeutics, ed. 7. New York: Macmillan, 1985;1095–1114.

68. Stevens AM, Johnson FC. New eruptive fever associated with stomatitis and ophthalmia. Am J Dis Child 1922;24:526–533.

69. Carroll OM, Bryan PA, Robinson RJ. Stevens-Johnson syndrome associated with long-acting sulfonamides. JAMA 1966;195:179–181.

70. Gottschalk AR, Stone OJ. Stevens-Johnson syndrome from ophthalmic sulfonamide. Arch Dermatol 1976;112:513–514.

71. Lyle WM, Page C. Possible adverse effects from local anesthetics and the treatment of these reactions. Am J Optom Physiol Opt 1975;52:736–744.

72. Adriani J, Campbell D. Fatalities following topical application of local anesthetics to mucous membranes. JAMA 1956;162:1527–1530.

73. Havener WH. Ocular pharmacology. St Louis: C.V. Mosby Co, 1974;3:67.

74. Cohn HC, Jocson VL. A unique case of grand mal seizures after Fluress. Ann Ophthalmol 1981;13:1379–1380.

75. Norden LC. Adverse reactions to topical ocular anesthetics. J Am Optom Assoc 1976;47:730–733.

76. Moore DC, Bridenburgh LD. Oxygen: The antidote for systemic toxic reactions from local anesthetic drugs. JAMA 1960;174:842–847.

77. Leopold IH. Advances in anesthesia in ophthalmic surgery. Ophthalmic Surg 1974;5:13–23.

78. Bryant JA. Local and topical anesthetics in ophthalmology. Surv Ophthalmol 1969;13:263–283.

79. Genvert GI, Cohen EJ, Donnenfeld ED, et al. Erythema multiforme after use of topical sulfacetamide. Am J Ophthalmol 1985;99:465–468.

80. Austen KF. Systemic anaphylaxis in the human being. N Engl J Med 1974;291:661–664.

81. Bristow MR, Ginsburg R, Harrison DC. Histamine and the human heart: The other receptor system. Am J Cardiol 1982;49:249–251.

82. Criep LH, Woehler TR. The heart in human anaphylaxis. Ann Allergy 1971;29:399–408.

83. Elenbaas RM. Anaphylactic shock. Crit Care 1980;2:77–84.

84. Hanashiro PK, Weil MH. Anaphylactic shock in man: Report of two cases with detailed hemodynamic and metabolic studies. Arch Intern Med 1967;119:129–139.

85. Lucke WC, Thomas H. Anaphylaxis: Pathophysiology, clinical presentations and treatment. J Emerg Med 1983;1:83–95.

86. Lockey RF, Bukantz SC. Allergic emergencies. Med Clin North Am 1974;58:147–156.

87. Ricker JG, Cacace LG. Double blind comparison of metaproterenol and isoetharine-phenylephrine solutions in intermittent positive pressure: Breathing in bronchospastic conditions. Chest 1980;78:723–725.

88. Kaliner M. Four immunologic mechanisms for release of chemical mediators of anaphylaxis from human lung tissue. Can Med Assoc J 1974;110:431–435.

89. American Heart Association. Heart attack: Signals and actions for survival. Dallas: 1976.

90. Feinleib M, Simon AB, Gillum RF, et al. Prodromal symptoms and signs of sudden death. Circulation 1975;52 (Suppl 3):155–159.

91. Weil LT. Coma. In: Rosen P, Baker FJ II, Brean BG, et al (eds). Emergency medicine: Concepts and practice. St. Louis: C.V. Mosby Co, 1983;166–176.

92. Baker, FJ II, Stauss R, Walter JJ. Cardiac arrest. In: Rosen P, Baker FJ II, et al (eds). Emergency medicine: Concepts and clinical practice. St. Louis: C.V. Mosby Co, 1988;83–141.

93. Caldwell G, Millar G, Quinn E, et al. Simple mechanical methods for cardioversion: Defense of the precordial thump and cough version. Br Med J 1985;291:627–630.

94. Criley JM, Neimann JT, Rosborough JP, et al. The heart is a conduit in CPR. Crit Care Med 1981;9:373–374.

95. Criley JM, Ung S, Neimann JT. What is the role of newer methods of cardiopulmonary resuscitation? Cardiovasc Clin 1983;13:297–307.

96. American Heart Association. Standards and guidelines for cardiopulmonary resuscitation (CPR) and emergency cardiac care (ECC). JAMA 1986;255:2905–2984.

97. Taylor GJ, Rubin R, Ticker M, et al. External cardiac compression. A randomized comparison of mechanical and manual techniques. JAMA 1978;240:644–646.

98. McDonald J. Systolic and mean arterial pressures during manual and mechanical CPR in humans. Ann Emerg Med 1982;11:292–295.

99. Goldberg A. Current concepts, cardiopulmonary arrest. N Engl J Med 1974;290:5.

100. Harris LC, Kirimli B, Safar P. Augmentation of artificial circulation during cardiopulmonary resuscitation. Anesthesiology 1967;28:730–734.

101. Centers for Disease Control. Recommendations for preventing transmission of infection with HIV during invasive procedures. MMWR 1986;35:221–223.

PART V

Legal Aspects of Drug Utilization

Ignorance of the law excuses no man; not that all men know the law, but cause 'tis an excuse every man will plead, and no man can tell how to confute him.
—John Selden (1892)

CHAPTER 32

Legal Basis for Drug Use in Optometry

John G. Classé

The use of drugs while rendering professional services has not traditionally been a clinical component of optometry. The reason lies in the historical basis for the licensure of optometrists. The clinical practice of optometry began as an extension of the science of optics, in a lineage that can be traced back for centuries.[1] This development occurred quite independently of medicine, which eschewed refractive services in favor of the use of drugs and surgery to treat disorders of the eye. In America, the two callings continued to evolve separately, although the clinical distinction between them lessened when physicians began practicing refraction as a "medical" function. The situation was further complicated by the emergence of two types of opticians: dispensing opticians, who performed no refractive services and whose sole function was to dispense ophthalmic materials on a physician's prescription; and refracting opticians (the forerunners of optometrists), who performed refractions, detected disease, and dispensed their own ophthalmic materials. In performing these services the refracting opticians were in direct competition with physicians who offered eyecare.[a] By the late 1800s physicians began to regard these services as "infringing" on the practice of medicine. The reason was the licensure laws passed by the states to regulate medicine.

The practice of medicine was largely unregulated during the first half of the 19th century, and legitimate physicians despaired over their inability to prevent quackery and to stem the proliferation of cult practitioners and unsound practices.[2] Their major problem was the lack of regulatory standards for medical schools, which produced graduates of widely varying levels of knowledge, skill, and experience. A solution was found in licensure: medical school graduates would be required to pass an examination and receive a license before they would be legally entitled to practice their profession within a state. Beginning in the 1870s the "modern" medical practice acts were passed to achieve this end, and they succeeded in elevating both the competence and the esteem of physicians nationwide.[2] However, out of necessity the laws incorporated a definition of medicine that was sufficiently broad to regulate any form of medical practice, including refraction. Refracting opticians, themselves unlicensed, found that their historical right to practice their calling was subservient to the legal right of the states to prevent them from doing so (under the guise of illegally practicing medicine). It was a situation ripe for conflict between the refracting opticians and their physician rivals, the ophthalmologists.

---

[a]Physicians were themselves divided into different camps: ophthalmologists were physicians who had undergone a residency in medical and surgical management of the eye and had restricted their practice to the eye; oculists were physicians who had learned eyecare through experience (without the benefit of formal training) and who specialized in treatment of the eye; and general practitioners were physicians who treated eye problems (including refractive errors) as part of the general practice of medicine but without having undergone any specialized training for this purpose.

Legislative Authorization

The "legalization" of optometry began with the efforts of Charles Prentice of New York City, whose Optical Society for the State of New York drafted the first bill intended to regulate the practice of "optometry."[3] Introduced in the New York legislature in 1897, the law required licensure of any individual—whether optician or physician—seeking to practice refraction and related services. Regulation was to be achieved through a 4-member Board of Optometry. Prentice and his colleagues, realizing that compromise was necessary to have the bill passed, agreed to an all-physician board. Despite this concession, physicians killed the bill, thereby ending the best opportunity they were to have to end the licensure of optometrists.[4]

But Prentice's idea caught the imagination of refracting opticians across the country, and in 1901 the state of Minnesota enacted the first optometry practice act.[1] This law recognized the practice of optometry, provided for examination and licensure, and established an all-optician board for regulatory purposes. In states throughout the nation similar laws were introduced, but to secure their passage the legislatures had to be convinced that the practice of optometry was not an aspect of medicine. Prentice and others devised strategies to impress this point on legislators, inventing slogans such as "A lens is not a pill" and "A lens treats light" to illustrate the difference between the two professions. A widely discussed lawsuit, brought at the urging of Albert Fitch of Philadelphia,[5] resulted in a ruling that optometry was not a branch of medicine and thus could not be regulated by physicians.[6] The distinction was further emphasized by the actual bills being introduced in the legislatures, which expressly or implicitly prohibited the use of drugs and surgery because these were "medical" functions. This strategy was a successful one; by 1924 all states and the District of Columbia had passed optometry laws. But the result was a drugless profession.

Judicial Regulation

By the late 1960s, almost 50 years after licensure had been won in the last jurisdiction, optometrists found the restrictive nature of these laws to be incompatible with their newly assumed role as health care providers. The ophthalmoscope was routinely used to detect abnormalities; the tonometer and the contact lens required physical contact with the eye; participation in Medicare, Medicaid, and other health insurance plans obligated the optometrist to make "medical" diag-

noses. As a result optometry became recognized as an aspect of health care, first as an entry point into the system, then as a primary care profession. Clinicians were frustrated because they were prevented from employing improved ophthalmic equipment and instrumentation due to statutory prohibitions against use of the pharmaceutical agents necessary to utilize these advances. Thus began a movement that has not yet run its course, the effort to amend the original optometry practice acts to permit optometrists to use pharmaceutical agents.

The first state law expressly authorizing the use of pharmaceutical agents was enacted in 1971 by the Rhode Island legislature after 3 years of effort. This law, which allowed Rhode Island optometrists to use drugs for diagnostic purposes, was the beginning of a new era in optometry. It was also the cause of a lawsuit, testing the right of state legislatures to enact such laws.[7]

Although the right to enact laws is strictly a legislative function, it is the duty of the courts, when presented with a case or controversy, to examine laws to ensure that they are not in conflict with the constitution. Therefore, although a law may be duly enacted, it will be void if the courts rule it is unconstitutional. Such was the purpose of the Rhode Island case.

The lawsuit was brought by the Rhode Island Ophthalmological Society and maintained that the legislature had endangered the public health by permitting optometrists to use these drugs. The ophthalmologists argued that the law was an unconstitutional exercise of legislative power and that it would cause them economic injury. Both the trial court and the Rhode Island Supreme Court rejected the ophthalmologists' arguments, and the law has not been subjected to further challenge.[8]

A similar fate awaited the first law authorizing optometric use of drugs for therapeutic purposes, passed by the West Virginia legislature in 1976. The law was immediately subjected to legal attack by an ophthalmologist, who argued that it was an unconstitutional application of the legislature's responsibility to protect the public from injury.[8,9] But again the courts ruled against the ophthalmologists, observing that the scope of optometric services was a legislative matter and that if the legislature conferred on optometrists the authority to use drugs for therapeutic purposes, such an exercise of legislative power was constitutional.

Further changes in the scope of optometry practice acts may bring additional lawsuits. However, it should be noted that no power ever granted to optometrists by the legislatures has been ruled unconstitutional by the courts, and it seems reasonable to assume that subsequent amendments of state optometry laws permitting an expanded scope of practice will meet a similar judicial response if challenged.

Administrative Regulation

Although the right to use ophthalmic drugs may be authorized by the jurisdiction's optometry statutes, various legal requirements may have to be satisfied to exercise this right. Two common requirements are certification and registration.

Certification

To employ pharmaceutical agents, an optometrist must have been granted this right at licensure[b] or must be certified by the board of optometry as qualified to exercise it. Certification—a process of education and examination—is necessary to ensure that pharmaceutical agents are employed only by qualified practitioners. Optometrists who have satisfied the educational requirements and have passed the examination are given a certificate, which usually must be displayed with the optometrist's license. Certification confers legal standing on a practitioner to use the permitted pharmaceutical agents within the bounds of state law. However, if an optometrist acts outside the scope of certification, such an action may subject the practitioner to discipline by the board of optometry. Similarly, if an optometrist uses drugs in the course of patient care, without first obtaining the necessary certification, the optometrist may be disciplined by the board, even though the state law authorizes use of the drug by optometrists. Certification is a legal prerequisite to drug use in these circumstances, and failure to satisfy certification requirements violates the optometry practice act.

Registration

Although an optometrist has complied with licensure and certification requirements, certain federal regulations must be observed if the optometrist wishes to use controlled substances. The dispensing of central nervous system drugs with significant potential for abuse is regulated by federal law[10,11]; enforcement is the responsibility of the Drug Enforcement Administration

(DEA). If a state optometry practice act (or board ruling) authorizes the use of controlled substances, the optometrist must register with the DEA and obtain a registration number before employing them clinically (see Chapter 2). The DEA number must also be written on any prescription for controlled substances given to a patient. Failure to observe these requirements violates federal law.

An additional administrative matter concerns the dispensing of drugs to patients by optometrists. Although state pharmacy acts regulate the sale of pharmaceutical products to consumers, a direct sale by a licensed health care practitioner to a patient is usually excluded from the provisions of these laws. Therefore, optometrists may dispense pharmaceutical agents to patients directly. If controlled substances are among the drugs provided to patients, the optometrist must be certain to comply with all record-keeping requirements (see Chapter 2).

Delegations of Authority

Under certain circumstances an optometrist may be authorized to use, in conjunction with a physician, otherwise prohibited pharmaceutical agents. These circumstances most commonly arise in multidisciplinary settings and in practices in which optometrists and physicians work together. The physician and the optometrist comanage the patient's care through a delegation of responsibility to the optometrist, who actually examines the patient and initiates the treatment. The authority for the optometrist to utilize pharmaceutical agents that would otherwise be outside the scope of licensure is obtained through the use of standing orders that are specifically written for the optometrist and that carefully delineate the conditions for which treatment may be undertaken. The mode of treatment (specific drugs, dosages, and patient follow-up) are also specified in the document. The optometrist, while following the orders, is acting as an agent of the physician under the physician's license, and is primarily responsible for the patient's well-being. However, the optometrist must confer with the physician within a reasonable period concerning the patient's care, and the physician should authenticate the record by signing it after determining that the care is satisfactory. These formalities are necessary to ensure that a legal delegation has been achieved.[c]

---

[b]A license confers the licensee all rights that may be exercised in the jurisdiction. Therefore, an optometrist who qualifies for licensure within a state receives a license that enables him or her to employ all the techniques and methods available to optometrists within that state. For example, if the state allows the use of therapeutic pharmaceutical agents by optometrists, successful passage of the licensing examination confers on the optometrist the right to use these agents. An optometrist who is already licensed at the time the definition is changed will have to be certified before he or she can employ this new right. Thus, certification inevitably occurs after licensure.

---

[c]There are at present no precedent-setting cases concerning the use of standing orders by optometrists. There have been two noteworthy legal disputes, one concerning the use of standing orders by optometrists at a multidisciplinary clinic in New York, and the other

Should the optometrist be negligent—while acting within the scope of the orders—both the physician and the optometrist will share legal responsibility for any injury the patient suffers.[12] If the optometrist acts outside the limits of the delegated authority, or in contravention to them, the optometrist is liable for any negligence. For this reason the physician must have great confidence in the optometrist's knowledge and skill before issuing a set of orders.

Without a delegation of authority such as has been described above, an optometrist who uses a pharmaceutical agent that is outside the scope of licensure commits an act for which discipline may be imposed by the appropriate state regulatory agency.[d] Even an averral that the circumstances constituted an "emergency" cannot provide legal justification for such an act, for Good Samaritan statutes generally do not provide legal immunity for in-office procedures even if the condition threatens vision.[e] Optometrists must understand the proscriptions of their optometry laws with regard to the use of pharmaceutical agents and must observe these limitations. Only through the use of a legal delegation of authority may an optometrist act outside these limits, and then only within specified bounds. Legal and insurance counsel should be consulted before initiating such a relationship.

The right to use drugs carries with it additional legal obligations, which are intended to protect patients from the risk of injury. These obligations include the doctrine of informed consent, which obliges the optometrist to inform the patient of the side effects and risks of drug use in some circumstances; the duty to conform to the standard of care, the breach of which constitutes negligence and subjects the optometrist to an action for damages if the patient has suffered any physical injury; and product liability law, under which an optometrist can be drawn into the legal dispute created by a drug that is unreasonably dangerous and injures the patient. These matters are discussed in Chapters 33 through 35.

References

1. Hirsch M, Wick R. The optometric profession. Philadelphia: Chilton, 1968.
2. Shyrock RH. Medical licensing in America, 1650–1965. Baltimore: Johns Hopkins University Press, 1967.
3. Prentice C. Legalized optometry and memoirs. Seattle: Casperin Fletcher Press, 1926;128–133.
4. Stevens R. American medicine and the public interest. New Haven: Yale University Press, 1977;103–109.
5. Fitch A. My fifty years in optometry. Philadelphia: Press of the Pennsylvania State College of Optometry, 1955;7–8.
6. *Martin v. Baldi,* 249 Pa 253, 94 A 1091 (1915).
7. *Rhode Island Ophthalmological Society v. Cannon,* 317 A2d 124 (1974).
8. Classé J. The right to practice primary care. J Am Optom Assoc 1986;57:549–553.
9. *Esposito v. Shapero,* C.A. 76-1214, West Virginia Circuit Court, Cabell County, December 16, 1976, *cert. denied* June 6, 1977.
10. Comprehensive Drug Abuse Prevention and Control Act of 1970. In: Physician's manual: An informational outline of the Controlled Substances Act of 1970. Washington, DC: U.S. Department of Justice, 1978.
11. Bartlett JD, Wood JW. Optometry and the Drug Enforcement Administration. J Am Optom Assoc 1981;52:495–498.
12. Holder A. Medical malpractice law. New York: John Wiley & Sons,1975;200–204.

---

involving the use of those orders by a clinic of the Pennsylvania College of Optometry, but these cases have not been adjudicated by an appellate court. However, the use of delegated orders for optometrists has been upheld as constitutional by the Texas Attorney General where they are part of the medical practice act. The use of standing orders is a standard aspect of medical practice, and the adoption of procedures similar to those employed in medical settings (such as hospitals) lessens the likelihood that a legal tribunal would rule the orders invalid.

[d]An optometrist who commits an act that is outside the scope of licensure is subject to discipline by the state board of optometry. Disciplinary measures that the board may use include reprimand, suspending licensure, and revoking licensure. Boards may also seek injunctions against continuation of the prohibited activity or may enter into consent agreements in which the defendant optometrist agrees not to continue the proscribed conduct.

[e]Good Samaritan statutes in most states do not include optometrists as a covered party. Furthermore, in most states these statutes do not cover in-office treatment of routine ocular urgencies or emergencies. See Classé J. Clinicolegal aspects of practice: Liability for ocular urgencies and emergencies. South J Optom 1986;4:51–58.

CHAPTER 33

Informed Consent

John G. Classé

The relationship between doctor and patient establishes several legal duties that the practitioner must observe. One of these is the affirmative duty of disclosure, which obliges the practitioner to communicate warnings, findings, and other pertinent information to the patient. The reason for this obligation lies in the legal status that doctors occupy as *fiduciaries,* who are persons occupying a special position of trust and confidence with those they serve.[1] The function of this duty of disclosure is to enable the less knowledgeable patient to understand the treatment recommended by the doctor. It has long been a precept of American law that no treatment may be undertaken without the consent of the patient, a philosophy succinctly stated by Judge Benjamin Cardozo[2]: "Any human being of adult years and sound mind has a right to determine what shall be done with his own body; and a surgeon who performs an operation without his patient's consent commits an assault, for which he is liable for damages."

Cardozo's opinion concerned a case in which surgery was performed without the patient's consent, but the principle he expressed can be applied to any procedure that contains some risk of harm to the patient. Treatment may not be instituted without the patient's consent, and this consent cannot be legally secured without the patient's being informed of the hazards, the possible complications, and both the expected and the unexpected results of treatment. Additionally, the practitioner must not make any misrepresentations, either by misstating known facts or by withholding pertinent information. This requirement forms the basis for the doctrine of informed consent.

Requirements for informed consent can arise in many areas of optometry: in the diagnosis of disease,[3] in contact lens practice,[4] when recommending binocular vision therapy,[5] or when ophthalmic pharmaceutical agents are employed.[6] The latter category is the one on which this chapter focuses. Optometrists must understand their legal obligation to discuss the risks of pharmaceutical use and must comply with the doctrine of informed consent when doing so. This legal duty has 2 aspects: (1) recognizing when the duty arises, and (2) determining the amount of information that must be divulged.

Disclosure Requirements

Generally speaking, an optometrist must disclose to the patient information sufficient to engender an informed consent. But the legal test of how much information must be divulged to satisfy this duty varies among states. In fact, conflicting opinions have been expressed by the courts and have proved to be a source of consternation for health care practitioners.[7] Even so, these opinions must be understood and complied with, since informed consent issues arise routinely in clinical practice.

Two standards may be applied to determine if the practitioner has met disclosure requirements: a "professional community" standard and a "reasonable patient" standard.

The "Professional Community" Standard

The first court decisions applied the same legal test to informed consent cases as was applied to negligence cases: the practitioner was held to the standard of the reasonable person.[8] Liability would be imposed if the practitioner were found to have breached the duty to do that which a reasonable practitioner would have done under the same or similar circumstances. In determining the standard of care expected of the practitioner, the courts allowed other practitioners to testify concerning the warnings or disclosures that were necessary. Hence, the standard was a profession-set one, based on expert testimony and determined by the conduct of other practitioners (Table 33.1). If the defendant practitioner divulged that amount of information deemed to be reasonable by other practitioners, then he or she had not breached the duty. However, this standard was soon rivaled by another which today is found in a minority of jurisdictions.

The "Reasonable Patient" Standard

This rival standard is based on what a reasonable patient must know rather than on what a reasonable practitioner must divulge.[9] Evidence is offered to establish what a prudent person in the patient's position would have done if suitably informed of all significant risks. The patient no longer must obtain expert testimony, since the issue concerns what the patient needs to know rather than what the practitioner is reasonably expected to divulge. This standard has become the subject of much discussion in the medical profession, although studies of professional liability claims have shown that physicians are rarely subjected to informed consent claims.[10] Jurisdictions that have adopted the objective standard are listed in Table 33.2.

Since in some states the courts have not been required to adjudicate the issue, the standard expected of practitioners cannot be determined.[a] But in most jurisdictions the courts have ruled on this issue, so health care practitioners—including optometrists—are required to observe these disclosure requirements. The other major issue posed by this doctrine is its application to drug use.

The Duty to Disclose Risks of Proposed Treatment

There are certain circumstances under which the practitioner may be under a duty to warn the patient of

---

[a]Those states in which the courts have not determined the applicable standard are Connecticut, Indiana, Maine, Nevada, South Carolina, South Dakota, and West Virginia. For a discussion of informed consent requirements, see Rosoff AJ. Informed consent: A guide for health care practitioners. Rockville, MD: Aspen, 1981.

TABLE 33.1
States Applying the "Professional Community" Standard

Alabama	Missouri
Arizona	Montana
Arkansas	Nebraska
Colorado	New Hampshire
Delaware	New Jersey
Florida	New York
Georgia	North Carolina
Hawaii	North Dakota
Idaho	Oregon
Illinois	Tennessee
Indiana	Texas
Kansas	Utah
Massachusetts	Vermont
Michigan	Virginia
Mississippi	Wyoming

Adapted from Rosoff AJ. Informed consent: A guide for health care practitioners. Rockville, MD: Aspen, 1981.

the risks of ophthalmic drug use, both for drugs used diagnostically and for those used therapeutically. Of the 2 classes, the greater obligation arises when therapeutic agents are employed. There may also be occasions when a patient should be warned of the potential risks of refusing to allow a drug to be administered.

Diagnostic Agents

The common diagnostic drugs used by optometrists are anesthetics, mydriatics, cycloplegics, and dyes. Routine use of these drugs creates a risk of injury only in very unusual circumstances. Therefore, informed consent is rarely a legal issue when they are employed.

The use of a topical anesthetic carries a small risk that a patient will experience a toxic response resulting in the disruption or desquamation of the corneal epithelium. Because this is an idiosyncratic response and cannot be predicted, it does not create the kind of risk for which informed consent is necessary. Even if an allergic or toxic reaction does occur, the effect is tran-

TABLE 33.2
States Applying the "Reasonable Patient" Standard

Alaska	Ohio
California	Oklahoma
District of Columbia	Pennsylvania
Kentucky	Rhode Island
Louisiana	Washington
Minnesota	Wisconsin
New Mexico	

Adapted from Rosoff AJ. Informed consent: A guide for health care practitioners. Rockville, MD: Aspen, 1981.

sient and limited and thus should not prevent a prudent patient from having the drug administered.

Dilation of the pupil is a diagnostic procedure with potentially serious side effects (i.e., angle-closure or pupillary-block glaucoma), and this risk may need to be communicated to patients for whom it is significant. However, studies have estimated that only 2% to 6% of the general population have angles that will close,[11] and of the age population most at risk—those over 30 years of age—the chance of precipitating an angle-closure glaucoma is 1 in 45,000.[12] These statistics indicate that for the great majority of patients the risk is minimal or nonexistent. Thus, for routine dilation the clinician has no duty to discuss the potential complications of mydriasis. But for that small percentage of the population with anterior chamber angles narrow enough to be closed by dilation, the decision to dilate should be made jointly with the patient after the patient has been informed of the benefits of dilation and of the risks and implications of angle closure. The determination of whether to employ dilation should be made in light of the need for it (e.g., if ophthalmoscopy of the retinal periphery is deemed necessary) and after the risk of angle closure has been reasonably determined (e.g., through the use of gonioscopy). The patient's decision to allow pupil dilation should be documented in the patient record.[13]

Cycloplegia is reserved for a limited number of conditions (e.g., patients suspected to have latent hyperopia or accommodative esotropia). Hyperopic patients may have shallow anterior chamber angles that require assessment before instillation of the cycloplegic. Because this technique is most often needed for young patients, careful attention must be given to the concentration and dosage of the cycloplegic employed, so that the risk of toxic effects can be minimized. Assuming that the angle is open and that the appropriate drug is selected for use, the risk of angle closure is no different than in patients undergoing routine mydriasis. Consequently, the clinician does not have to obtain an informed consent. If risk factors are present and clinical complications are a consideration, the practitioner should discuss these factors with the patient (or, if a child, with the parent or guardian) and obtain the necessary consent to administer the drug. One additional circumstance requiring communication is whenever atropine is to be administered to an infant before performing a cycloplegic examination. The use of atropine is probably justified clinically only in patients 4 years of age or younger with suspected accommodative esotropia[6] and should be used conservatively in terms of concentration and dosage. The signs and symptoms of atropine toxicity should be explained to parents in these cases to minimize the risk of an overlooked toxic drug reaction.

Although sodium fluorescein and rose bengal are routinely administered topically to the eye as indicator dyes, sodium fluorescein can also be administered orally in the evaluation of retinal and choroidal lesions. Such oral fluorography (or angioscopy) has been documented to be safe and effective for some clinical conditions,[14] but the oral administration of sodium fluorescein is not yet approved by the Food and Drug Administration (FDA). In these circumstances it is permissible for the practitioner to use the oral route of administration, but informed consent should be obtained (see Chapter 2). An example of such a consent form is shown in Table 33.3.

The preceding circumstances are not the only ones in which risks may have to be communicated to the patient. Occasionally, a patient will refuse to allow a drug to be administered for diagnostic purposes. The usual circumstances involve mydriatics for dilation and topical anesthetics for tonometry.[15] As previously discussed, the patient has the right to refuse any test, and the clinician cannot obtain a lawful consent by coercion or legally perform the test against the patient's will. In such a case the practitioner is obliged to ensure that the patient understands the potential ramifications of refusal. For example, an elderly patient with visual field loss and optic nerve atrophy should be warned of the need for tonometry; a patient with reduced visual acuity who complains of floaters and flashes has an

TABLE 33.3
Informed Consent for Oral Fluorography

I, _____, hereby consent to photography of my eyes or associated areas for the documentation and/or diagnosis of certain retinal conditions or diseases that may be present.

I also understand that the photographs may be used to document my ocular status as well as for future use in publications, video tapes, or other educational presentations that may or may not benefit me.

I understand that the medication, sodium fluorescein, is not yet approved by the Food and Drug Administration for oral use, although it has been documented to be effective in revealing certain abnormalities of the retina when taken orally. I also understand that no side effects have been reported from the use of oral fluorescein with the occasional exception of slight discoloration of the skin or urine lasting up to 24 hours. *Possible* side effects include nausea, vomiting, and allergic reactions such as hives or anaphylactic shock (breathing, heart, and blood pressure problems).

Signed: _____
Witness: _____
Dated: _____

Used with permission from the School of Optometry, University of Alabama at Birmingham.

obvious need for ophthalmoscopy under conditions of dilation. The practitioner must weigh the need for the test in light of the clinical situation and should advise the patient accordingly. Refusals should always be documented in the patient record. Some practitioners employ forms that are signed by the patient and retained in the patient record, and these are a satisfactory means of documenting the patient's decision. A patient's refusal that goes against the practitioner's advice should not go undocumented.[13]

Therapeutic Agents

The duty to inform the patient of potential toxic effects of drug therapy is greatest when therapeutic agents are prescribed.[6] The reason for this is due, in part, to the clinician's lack of control over drug administration. Whereas the use of drugs for diagnostic purposes is carefully controlled by the practitioner and is usually an in-office procedure, the prescribing of therapeutic agents results in extended drug use that is entirely within the patient's control. Abuse of therapeutic agents has been documented in the ophthalmologic patient population,[16] and optometrists should be aware of this potential problem, especially when using therapeutic drugs—such as steroids and antiglaucoma medications—with possible adverse effects.

Patients should be warned of the side effects of extended use of therapeutic agents and should be required to consult the clinician if additional prescription renewals are desired. As with diagnostic agents, the need to communicate with the patient depends on the clinician's assessment of the risk. If a drug is used for only a brief time, the risk is far less than if an extended period of treatment is anticipated. Likewise, greater dosages create larger risks and greater necessity for disclosure. Optometrists must be familiar with the allergic and toxic effects of the therapeutic drugs they prescribe and should inform patients of potential risks in the appropriate circumstances. Some examples of agents and their known complications are listed in Table 2.2

Of the commonly employed therapeutic drugs, the greatest risks are encountered when the clinician prescribes topical steroids (for extended periods), systemic steroids, miotic antiglaucoma agents, and carbonic anhydrase inhibitors.[16] Optometrists should be aware of the toxic effects that attend the use of these drugs and should warn patients accordingly. Disclosures should be documented in the patient record.

The doctrine of informed consent may also be applied to situations in which the optometrist fails to disclose alternatives to therapy. This issue can occasionally arise when the optometrist uses drugs for therapy.

Alternatives to Therapy

Disclosure requirements obligate clinicians not only to warn of the risks of treatment but also to describe alternatives to therapy.[17] This duty may arise in various ways when drug use is contemplated. For example, if echothiophate therapy is recommended for the treatment of accommodative esotropia in a young child, alternative treatment—such as lens therapy—should be discussed as well. Another example involves glaucoma suspects. The patient with elevated intraocular pressure and no optic disc damage or visual field loss should be appraised of the alternatives: receive medical therapy or be monitored by the optometrist until disc damage or measurable field loss occurs. In these and analogous situations the clinician should avoid choosing the mode of treatment for the patient and should ensure that the course of therapy is obtained with the patient's consent.

In clinical situations in which there are alternatives to treatment, the optometrist should note in the patient record that the alternatives were discussed and that the treatment chosen was obtained with full patient consent.

One other application of the doctrine of informed consent may influence the clinical practice of optometry, and that is the duty to disclose abnormalities.

Disclosure of Abnormalities

Not infrequently, diagnostic drug use will disclose an ambiguous or suspicious finding. In this instance the clinician must explain these results so that the patient can determine if he or she wishes to undergo further testing.[17] An example case will illustrate how informed consent can be applied to such a situation.[3]

A 58-year-old woman complaining of poor focus and of gaps in her vision was examined by an ophthalmologist. He attributed the cause of her complaints to her contact lenses, but during the course of the examination he performed Schiotz tonometry and obtained readings of 23.8 mm Hg in each eye. Despite this result, he did not perform a dilated fundus examination or a visual field assessment, and he did not discuss the potential significance of the intraocular pressure findings with the patient. During the next 2 years the patient was seen a dozen times, but it was not until the end of this period that she was diagnosed as having open-angle glaucoma. Despite medical and surgical therapy, her visual acuity decreased to 20/200 and she suffered a profound visual field loss. She sued the ophthalmologist, alleging that he was negligent in failing to diagnose the disease and in failing to warn her of the elevated intraocular pressures. The physician won at trial but she appealed, and the state supreme court reversed the decision of the trial court, ruling that under the doctrine of informed consent the ophthalmologist was under a duty to inform her of any abnormal findings and to advise her of any diagnostic procedures that could be undertaken to determine the significance of the findings.

An optometrist is under a similar duty to discuss the results of diagnostic tests with patients and to advise the patient of the availability of further testing to rule out the presence of disease.[3] Ambiguous or suspicious findings should be resolved, and if the patient does not return for recall appointments or does not wish to undergo further evaluation, these facts should be documented in the patient record.

Although the doctrine of informed consent is an important legal consideration when ophthalmic drugs are employed, the most likely source of a professional liability claim against an optometrist is negligence. How such a claim may arise in clinical practice is discussed in Chapter 34.

References

1. Black's Law Dictionary, Rev. ed.4. St. Paul, MN: West, 1968.
2. *Schloendorff v. Society of New York Hospital,* 211 NY 125, 105 NE 92(1914).
3. Thal LS. *Gates v. Jensen:* Another precedent for glaucoma testing. J Am Optom Assoc, 1981;52:349–353.
4. Harris MG, Dister RE. Informed consent in contact lens practice. J Am Optom Assoc 1987;58:230–236.
5. Luttjohann L. Informed consent and release of patient records. Kansas Optom J 1984;51:6–7.
6. Classé J. Liability for use of ophthalmic pharmaceutical agents. South J Optom 1984;2:43–49.
7. Kraushar MF, Steinberg JA. Informed consent: Surrender or salvation? Arch Ophthalmol 1986;104:352–355.
8. *Natanson v. Cline,* 187 Kan 186, 354 P2d 670 (1960).
9. *Woods v. Brumlop,* 1 NM2d 221, 377 P2d 520 (1962); *Canterbury v. Spence,* 464 F2d 772 (D.C. Cir., 1972); and *Cobbs v. Grant,* 8 Cal3d 229, 502 P2d 1 (1972).
10. Curran WJ. Malpractice claims: New data and new trends. N Engl J Med 1979;300:26.
11. Cockburn DM. Prevalence and significance of narrow anterior chamber angles in optometric practice. Am J Optom Physiol Opt 1981;58:171–175.
12. Keller JT. The risk of angle closure from the use of mydriatics. J Am Optom Assoc 1975;46:19–21.
13. Classé J. Record-keeping and documentation in clinical practice. South J Optom 1987;5:11–25.
14. Potter JW, Bartlett JD, Alexander LJ, et al. Oral fluorography. J Am Optom Assoc 1985;56:784–792.
15. Alexander LJ, Scholles J. Clinical and legal aspects of pupillary dilation. J Am Optom Assoc 1987;58:432–437.
16. Bettman JW. A review of 412 claims in ophthalmology. Int Ophthalmol Clin 1980;20:131–142.
17. Classé J. Optometrist's duty to detect glaucoma. South J Optom 1984;2:6–10.

CHAPTER 34

Negligence

John G. Classé

The most significant legal issue facing optometrists who use ophthalmic drugs is negligence. As various reports have demonstrated,[1-3] large liability claims against optometrists typically allege misdiagnosis, and the need for topical anesthesia and mydriasis is common to these claims. In the majority of instances the misdiagnosis is due to failure to use the appropriate pharmaceutical agent rather than toxic or allergic drug reactions.[3] Consequently, it may be argued that the likelihood of a negligence claim is highest when an optometrist fails to use an ophthalmic drug that, when used appropriately, would permit a proper diagnosis. Claims most commonly allege failure to diagnose open-angle glaucoma,[4] intraocular tumor,[5] or retinal detachment.[6]

Misdiagnosis is also an important aspect of claims involving the use of therapeutic ophthalmic agents. Although the toxic effects of these drugs have been the most common cause of liability claims against ophthalmologists,[7] failure to make the correct diagnosis, followed by institution of the inappropriate therapeutic regimen, has become the major concern of optometrists.[8] Because of the restricted nature of most optometry practice acts, which usually limit therapy to the anterior segment of the eye, claims against optometrists most frequently allege mismanagement of corneal problems.

Although negligence represents the most important legal complication of clinical practice, the exposure of optometrists to malpractice claims remains at a relatively low level, far below that of physicians.[3,9,10] Within the optometric profession there is presently little difference between diagnostic and therapeutic drug use with regard to the risk of malpractice, since professional liability insurance premiums do not vary on this basis.[3] However, as optometry laws continue to be amended to enable optometrists to serve as primary providers of eyecare, this increased clinical responsibility will inevitably result in increased litigation. Because the use of pharmaceutical agents will be an integral part of these responsibilities, optometrists must be familiar with the concept of negligence and must understand how negligence may arise in clinical practice.

Proof of Negligence

The law holds every individual to a reasonable standard of conduct, and failure to exercise reasonable care will create liability if it results in harm to others. Accordingly, negligence may be defined as "the omission to do something which a reasonable man, guided by those ordinary considerations which ordinarily regulate human affairs, would do, or the doing of something which a reasonable and prudent man would not do."[11]

In terms of an optometrist's conduct, there is an obligation to adhere to a reasonable standard of care when rendering services to patients. This standard may be summarized by the question, "What would a reasonable optometrist do under the same or similar circumstances"? From this question it is apparent that the defendant optometrist's conduct is to be compared with the conduct expected of a hypothetical "reasonable optometrist."[12] If the defendant optometrist's conduct fails to measure up to the conduct expected of this reasonable practitioner, there is a breach of the standard of care.

However, proof of negligence entails more than a demonstration that the defendant breached the standard of care. There are, in fact, 4 elements to this tort,[a] and to state a cause of action in a court of law the plaintiff-patient must offer evidence in support of each.[12] In a malpractice case, these 4 elements are as follows:

1. A duty on the part of the practitioner to adhere to a reasonable standard of care to minimize the risk of injury to the patient
2. Breach of this standard of care by the practitioner
3. Actual, physical injury suffered by the patient
4. A proximate relationship between the patient's injury and the practitioner's actions (or failure to act)

Duty

The duty to adhere to a reasonable standard of care is established by the doctor-patient relationship. Proof of the duty is rarely a problem for the plaintiff-patient, since in the great majority of cases the patient will be examined by the optometrist in an office or under circumstances that make the relationship apparent. The lack of formal surroundings, or even failure of the optometrist to charge for services, will not defeat the duty if a doctor-patient relationship has been formed. Once the optometrist has created the relationship, he or she is legally obligated to adhere to the standard of care expected of a reasonable optometrist acting under the same or similar circumstances. Since proof of this standard can be offered only by an individual actually familiar with it, expert testimony will be required.

Breach of the Standard of Care

An expert witness is not limited to reporting the perceptions of his or her senses but may testify concerning an otherwise prohibited matter: an opinion. To do so, an expert first must be qualified, which is a process intended to convince the trial judge that the witness is competent to testify about the matter at issue, in this instance the standard of care expected of an optometrist. Traditionally, only practitioners of the same "school" have been considered competent to testify about the standard of care expected of a defendant practitioner.[13] However, the growing liberality of rules

of evidence and the lessening distinction clinically between optometrists and ophthalmologists have combined to change this traditional pattern, so that ophthalmologists are frequently deemed competent to testify concerning the standard of care expected of an optometrist. This development has led to the imposition of a medical standard of care for optometrists in cases involving misdiagnosis of ocular disease.[14]

The likelihood of testimony by physicians—and the imposition of a medical standard of care—is greatest in cases involving ophthalmic drugs because of the use of these agents to diagnose or treat disease. Of course, expert testimony on behalf of the defendant optometrist may allege that he or she acted in conformance with the standard of care. It is then left to the jury to determine liability. This element of proof is usually the most difficult for a plaintiff to establish and is frequently the most contentious aspect of a malpractice trial.

Injury

Assessment of the patient's injury is also a matter requiring an expert's opinion, and either an optometrist or an ophthalmologist may provide this testimony. Visual impairment is usually evaluated as loss of visual acuity, visual field, or ocular motility or a combination.[15] Other ocular disturbances that result in loss of functions such as color vision, accommodation, and binocular vision may also be evaluated, as may deformities or disfigurements of the orbit or face.[15] Optometrists who testify concerning the degree of injury suffered by a patient should be familiar with the accepted standards used in legal proceedings by physicians.[b]

Proximate Cause

The fourth element of negligence is proximate cause, sometimes referred to as legal cause, which serves to tie together the negligent act (or failure to act) and the resulting injury.[12] For example, failure to employ a mydriatic for an ophthalmoscopic examination may be the proximate cause of a clinician's failure to detect an intraocular disease. Expert testimony is necessary to link together what the practitioner did (or did not do) and the injury.

---

[a]A tort is a "breach of duty (other than a contractual or quasi-contractual duty) which gives rise to an action for damages." (Prosser WL. Law of torts, ed. 4. St. Paul, MN: West, 1971;1.) This rather unsatisfactory definition leaves one with more of an indication of what a tort is not: it is not a crime, it is not based on contract, and it does not result in loss of liberty. It is a civil action, brought for the purpose of receiving monetary compensation for damages, and is based on a breach of duty.

---

[b]The assessment of visual impairment is described in *Guides to the Evaluation of Permanent Impairment,* ed. 2. Chicago: American Medical Association, 1984; 141–151. *The Physician's Desk Reference for Ophthalmology* contains a reprint of this information.

The plaintiff-patient must prove each of these 4 elements by a preponderance of the evidence to state a case.[c] As the preceding discussion has demonstrated, expert testimony is crucial to the presentation of this evidence, and it is equally important to the defendant optometrist, since he or she seeks to refute the plaintiff's allegations. The focus of a malpractice case is usually the standard of care, which has particular requirements when applied to the use of ophthalmic drugs.

Standard of Care

An optometrist is expected to display that degree of skill and learning that is commonly possessed by members of the profession in good standing and to exercise what is referred to as "due care."[d] This obligation has broad implications whenever an optometrist employs ophthalmic drugs, since the standard of care requires that the optometrist[8]:

1. Understand the allergic and toxic side effects of all drugs administered or prescribed
2. Take an adequate history to determine if there has been any previous allergic or toxic response to a drug, especially an ophthalmic agent
3. Select the appropriate drug for the patient's needs or condition
4. Warn the patient of side effects of drug use that may create a risk of injury
5. Monitor the patient while he or she is under the influence of the diagnostic or therapeutic agent so that complications can be managed in a timely manner

To conform to these due care requirements, an optometrist is expected to act as a reasonable practitioner would by observing the following clinical and legal guidelines.

Knowledge

Practitioners are under a legal duty to keep abreast of new developments, especially information that will af-

fect patient care, such as reports of drug toxicity.[16] Therefore, a practitioner not only must understand the properties of any drugs that are employed for patient care, but also must remain knowledgeable concerning more efficacious drugs or warnings of adverse effects. Failure to stay abreast of these developments has resulted in successful claims against physicians[17] and could also serve as a cause of action against optometrists.[8]

History

The standard of care requires that an adequate drug history be taken, including:

- The patient's history of past drug use
- Drugs currently being taken
- Any allergic or toxic reactions to drugs, past or present
- History of ophthalmic drug use, including a determination of whether anesthesia and mydriasis have been employed at a previous examination

Failure to take an adequate history, if it results in an allergic or toxic response to a drug, may render the practitioner liable for this otherwise preventable injury.[18]

Use of the Appropriate Agent

Adherence to the standard of care is necessary to minimize the risk of injury to the patient. An optometrist is obligated to choose the pharmaceutical agent that fulfills this requirement and, in so doing, is expected to exercise that degree of skill and learning that is commonly possessed by like practitioners. The drug that is most appropriate for the patient's condition and its most appropriate route of administration must be determined to minimize the risk of adverse effects. If an optometrist uses an inappropriate agent—such as proparacaine when a patient has previously experienced a toxic response to the drug—thereby precipitating an otherwise preventable injury, the optometrist has failed to meet this duty and is legally responsible for the resulting pain, discomfort, and reduced acuity. The same would be true if an optometrist attempted to treat an iritis with a systemic steroid without first establishing that a topical route of administration was inadequate or inappropriate.[7] In each instance the optometrist's conduct must measure up to that of a reasonable optometrist or liability will result.

---

[c]To state a case, the plaintiff must present evidence in support of each of the 4 elements of negligence, and this evidence must be more believable than that presented by the defendant. Otherwise, the plaintiff's case will be dismissed.

[d]Due care may be defined as "that care which an ordinarily prudent person would have exercised under the circumstances." (Black's Law Dictionary, rev. ed. 4. St. Paul, MN: West, 1968.)

Warnings

Because of the doctrine of informed consent, under some circumstances an optometrist must discuss the risks and possible side effects of drug use with the patient. For example, if a patient were to undergo prolonged treatment with a topical steroid, the optometrist would be obligated to warn the patient of potential side effects, including glaucoma, ocular infection, and cataract. Although the amount of information that must be communicated to the patient varies among states due to different state requirements (see Chapter 33), the circumstances under which warnings are necessary generally do not vary. For example, only patients with anterior chamber angles that are susceptible to closure must be warned of that potential side effect before instillation of a mydriatic, but all patients should be warned of the potential photophobia, discomfort, and blur caused by pupillary dilation. Warnings are an essential aspect of drug use and should not be overlooked or ignored.

Management of Side Effects

If a patient experiences a drug-related allergic or toxic effect, the clinician must meet reasonable standards of detection and management. A post-dilation telephone call from a patient complaining of severe headache and blurred vision may require an examination rather than a brusque, "Take an aspirin and call me in the morning." Likewise, a patient who is being treated with topical steroids must be recalled with sufficient regularity to detect adverse effects before they have significantly affected the patient's vision.

For each of these due care requirements, an optometrist must satisfy reasonable standards of conduct, and because the use of ophthalmic drugs is essentially a medical act, ophthalmologists may be competent to state the standard of care expected of optometrists under these circumstances.[8]

Another aspect of the standard of care involves optometrists who decide, for personal or professional reasons, not to employ pharmaceutical agents. No optometrist is under a legal duty to use these agents, but individuals who choose not to use ophthalmic drugs face some formidable standard of care issues, particularly with regard to the use of drugs for diagnostic purposes. If a patient seeks an optometrist's care, and if during the course of the examination a reasonable optometrist would have recognized that the use of an ophthalmic drug was needed to make the appropriate diagnosis of the patient's condition, then a legal duty arises either to use the ophthalmic agent or to refer the patient to another practitioner for the necessary

examination. The most common drugs that create this situation are mydriatics.

A hypothetical example illustrates how the standard of care can be applied to a practitioner who does not use drugs for diagnostic purposes. If a patient has received a blow to the eye from a fist, ball, or other blunt object, the optometrist must rule out the possibility of a retinal tear.[19] To perform a reasonable examination—one that will conform to the expected standard of care—dilation of the pupil is necessary.[20] In fact, it may be argued that examination of the retinal periphery with a binocular indirect ophthalmoscope is required under these circumstances.[6] If the optometrist does not dilate the pupil, any ophthalmic examination will be below the standard of care. The only recourse available to the optometrist is to refer the patient to another clinician so that the patient can receive the appropriate evaluation. The optometrist who chooses not to employ drugs is subject to the same standard as those who do; in this case, a reasonable practitioner would realize that a dilated fundus examination is necessary to rule out the presence of retinal disease. An optometrist who does not measure up to this standard is liable for any injury the patient suffers due to failure to receive a timely diagnosis.

Misdiagnosis

Misdiagnosis of open-angle glaucoma, intraocular tumors, and retinal detachment is the leading cause of large malpractice claims against optometrists.[3] In the great majority of cases, failure to make the appropriate diagnosis is linked to failure to perform a key diagnostic test (e.g., tonometry, or ophthalmoscopy through a dilated pupil). Therefore, failure to use an ophthalmic agent is the most likely legal problem that a clinician will encounter. Example cases illustrate how claims of misdiagnosis can arise when encountering these 3 important disorders.

Open-Angle Glaucoma

The standard of care for the detection of open-angle glaucoma has been established by a series of cases involving ophthalmologists.[21-23] The leading case[21] involved a 22-year-old woman who was fitted for contact lenses and examined intermittently over the course of 10 years, but it was not until the end of this period that the ophthalmologists discovered she had open-angle glaucoma and a visual field reduced to less than 10 degrees. She sued the ophthalmologists for negligence, and at trial tonometry became the key issue.

She alleged that the physicians had a duty to perform the test while she was a contact lens patient; they defended on the basis that tonometry was not a routine test for patients under 40 years of age.

Although the ophthalmologists won the trial, the case was reversed on appeal, a decision that evoked a storm of commentary.[24] Ironically, the court's opinion proved to be a legal dead end, but the intense publicity surrounding the case succeeded in changing the standard of care in both ophthalmology and optometry.[25]

Cases brought today against optometrists for failure to diagnose open-angle glaucoma almost uniformly allege failure to perform tonometry. Just as uniformly, defendant optometrists resort to procedural defenses that seek to avoid this issue.[26-28] The result has been a standard of care that requires routine use of tonometry, regardless of patient age. For this reason, topical anesthesia is an important procedure. Dilation of the pupil for ophthalmoscopy, visual field assessment, and other appropriate tests for glaucoma may be necessary as well.[4]

Intraocular Tumors

The detection of intraocular tumors presents one of the most difficult diagnostic dilemmas encountered by optometrists. To make the diagnosis, a dilated fundus examination is needed, but a patient with a "silent" tumor may not evince symptoms that would lead a reasonable practitioner to determine that dilation is required. A practitioner is not legally obligated to discover all that may be wrong with a patient but merely to perform an examination that is in keeping with the standard of care.[29] Therefore, failure to detect a "silent" tumor—because dilation is not demanded by the patient's complaint or history—may not be construed as negligence. A different result may be obtained, however, if the patient is symptomatic.

This principle is illustrated by the following case.[30] An optometrist who was employed by a multidisciplinary clinic examined a middle-aged woman who complained of reduced vision. He found her best-corrected visual acuity to be 20/25 and 20/40, which he attributed to cataracts. Although refraction, tonometry, and ophthalmoscopy were performed, the optometrist did not dilate the patient's pupils. He discussed his findings with the patient and dismissed her, but 2 months later she realized that the vision in one eye was markedly reduced. She returned to the clinic, where the diagnosis of retinal detachment secondary to a von Hippel–Lindau tumor was made. Despite surgery the patient was left with a permanent loss of acuity. She sued the optometrist, alleging that he was negligent for failing to make the diagnosis in a timely manner. Although the optom-

etrist prevailed at the trial, she was awarded damages on appeal, with the court stating that, "the evidence is overwhelming that the (plaintiff's) eye should have been dilated" and that the optometrist should be held to "the same rules relating to the duty of care and liability as ophthalmologists."[31]

The rationale for the court's opinion was that the diagnosis of cataract (a "disease") required dilation of the pupil and that had dilation been performed at the time of the optometrist's examination, the possibility of a tumor-caused retinal detachment could have been ruled out. In finding the optometrist liable, the court imposed a medical standard of care.[14] Therefore, a dilated fundus examination should be employed whenever best-corrected visual acuity is reduced, and coexisting disease should be considered a possibility until an examination determines otherwise. Optometrists may be held responsible for the diagnosis of intraocular tumors—even those as rare as malignant melanoma—in symptomatic patients.[5]

Retinal Detachment

The necessity for dilation of the pupil is probably most evident in cases where retinal detachment is, or should be, suspected. Many patients are at risk for retinal detachment, and it can be argued that dilation is necessary whenever a patient is found to have any of the following[6,20]:

- Significant myopia
- Aphakia
- Glaucoma
- Lattice degeneration
- Blunt trauma to the eye
- Any of the proliferative retinopathies (e.g., sickle cell, diabetes, branch retinal vein occlusion)

Another important precursor of retinal detachment is acute onset, symptomatic, posterior vitreous detachment (PVD). It has been reported that 8% to 15% of patients with an acute, symptomatic PVD have a retinal tear.[32,33] If a patient complains of spots, specks, floaters, or other entoptic phenomena that indicate the possibility of PVD, the optometrist must conduct a dilated fundus examination to rule out the presence of a tear. Although failure to detect the detachment may not be below the standard of care, failure to examine the patient under conditions of dilation may be so construed.[7]

Symptoms of reduced visual acuity also require careful assessment of the interior of the eye. In a case involving a diabetic patient,[34] the patient complained of blurred vision and the defendant optometrist performed a refraction and prescribed spectacles that he assured the patient would relieve her symptoms. Because of the patient's history of diabetes and the complaint of reduced acuity, the standard of care required a dilated fundus examination. The optometrist did not perform this evaluation, however, and after dispensing spectacles to the patient did not undertake any further treatment. Six months later the patient consulted an ophthalmologist, who found that the patient had proliferative retinopathy due to diabetes that had caused a retinal detachment in one eye and unmanageable complications in the other. A lawsuit was instituted against the optometrist for negligence in failing to make the diagnosis and to refer the patient for treatment. Diabetic patients constitute an important and challenging clinical problem for optometrists because of the number of afflicted individuals, the frequency of ocular complications, and the long-term management that is required.[35,36]

Although other causes of misdiagnosis have been alleged against optometrists,[37–40] these 3 types of claims are the most frequent and represent the most significant clinical and legal challenges to diagnostic skill. Failure to diagnose these conditions poses the greatest risk of litigation for optometrists.

Complications of Diagnostic Drug Use

Optometrists must be familiar with the allergic and toxic effects of any ophthalmic drugs used for diagnostic purposes and must be prepared to manage these complications when they occur. This obligation is frequently encountered when using the common diagnostic agents: anesthetics, mydriatics, and cycloplegics.

Anesthetics

Topical anesthesia is necessary for applanation tonometry, gonioscopy, and the use of fundus contact lenses. Proparacaine and benoxinate are the agents most commonly employed. Because use of these agents may cause an allergic or toxic response, the optometrist should determine if the patient has experienced a previous reaction before applying the drug. If the optometrist has observed such a reaction while the patient was under his or her care, this fact should be noted conspicuously in the patient record to prevent a second episode. Of course, the optometrist may choose an alternative drug in this event, since proparacaine and benoxinate are structurally dissimilar and an allergic reaction to one drug does not mean that the patient will also be allergic to the other (see Chapter 4).

If the patient experiences an adverse reaction, the worst result—desquamation of the corneal epithelium—is transient and the discomfort is not severe.[41] Most episodes resolve within 24 to 48 hours, and there is no permanent effect on vision. Thus, there is little opportunity for negligence or for substantial damages.

Injury may be permanent, however, if a topical anesthetic is applied copiously to a compromised cornea.[42] Anesthetics should never be dispensed to patients for use at home, and if other practitioners have dispensed anesthetics to a patient for use on an "as needed" basis, these patients should be counselled concerning this ill-advised use of topical anesthesia.

Mydriatics

These drugs constitute the most important class of diagnostic agents because of their use for dilating the pupil for ophthalmoscopy. A history must be taken to ensure that the patient has not experienced angle closure after dilation by a previous examiner, and the anterior chamber angle should be examined to determine the risk of precipitating an angle-closure attack. It has been estimated that only 2% to 6% of the population has angles that are sufficiently narrow to close[43] and that, of those most at risk (i.e., persons over 30 years of age), the chances of causing angle closure are 1 in 45,000.[44] For the general population, this risk is even more remote, estimated at 1 in 180,000.[44]

Therefore, for 94% to 98% of the population—those whose angles cannot be closed—there is no requirement under the doctrine of informed consent to warn them of this risk. Only those rare individuals whose histories or angles indicate a risk must be informed of the possibility of angle closure, so that their consent can be obtained before performing the procedure. The clinician should document that the warning was given and that the patient's consent was received.

A clinical and legal issue of some importance is posed by the necessity for dilation.[20] If there is litigation, the use of expert testimony will be required to determine if, in a specific instance, dilation was needed to conform to the standard of care. If a reasonable practitioner would have realized that a dilated fundus examination was necessary under the circumstances, then the patient must receive that evaluation or be referred to another practitioner so that it can be performed. There are numerous circumstances under which the obligation for dilation seems to arise (see Chapter 16). Failure to recognize the necessity for dilation is a leading cause of malpractice claims against optometrists.[1–3]

Because patients who have undergone mydriasis typically experience photophobia, discomfort, and loss of accommodation (if tropicamide is employed), the optometrist should be certain to safeguard them from injury while they are in the office and on the premises. Elderly[45] and handicapped[46] patients are particularly susceptible to injury from falls or similar mishaps and may successfully claim damages if it can be shown that the optometrist did not take reasonable steps to protect them. The optometrist's staff should be prepared to assist patients who are on the premises.

Because patients whose pupils have been dilated usually leave the premises with their vision impaired, the optometrist's obligation is extended to include a warning of the effects of mydriasis on such tasks as driving a motor vehicle, operating machinery, or other foreseeable activities for which there is a risk of injury.[47] If it is known in advance that patients will undergo a dilated fundus examination, they should be advised when making the appointment so that appropriate arrangements for transportation can be made. If the risk of injury to the patient is deemed significant, a reschedule examination may be arranged (e.g., at the same time ophthalmic materials are to be dispensed) so that the patient can make provisions for transportation. In all cases it is wise to ensure that the patient has sunglasses to protect against glare or to provide the patient with disposable mydriatic sunglasses designed for this purpose (see Chapter 16).

Failure to warn the patient not only subjects the optometrist to claims for injuries suffered by the patient but also can widen liability to include third parties who may be injured by the patient (e.g., in an automobile accident).[48,49] Optometrists should routinely document the warnings given to patients rather than relying on the patient's memory after the fact.[c]

Another important matter that should be documented is a patient's refusal to undergo dilation of the pupil. The optometrist is obligated to explain the importance of a dilated fundus examination to the patient in terms that will engender understanding. If, despite this warning, the patient refuses to undergo the procedure, an entry should be made in the patient's record, or the patient can be asked to sign a form, signifying that he or she has rejected the optometrist's advice and understands the significance of the refusal. In rare cases, the matter may be of such importance that a certified letter, return receipt requested, should be sent to the patient, with a copy retained in the patient's record. By whatever means selected, optometrists should not overlook the necessity for documentation in these cases.

Cycloplegics

The two cycloplegic drugs most frequently employed are cyclopentolate and atropine. Because of their potential side effects, a careful history and assessment of the anterior chamber angle must be made before their use. Selection of the appropriate agent is also important (see Chapter 17). If there is a risk of angle closure, this risk must be communicated to the patient, and an informed consent should be obtained before the drug is administered.

If atropine is used, the clinician must be aware of the signs and symptoms of atropine toxicity. A similar concern exists when 2% cyclopentolate is used in infants or children.[50] If the patient experiences side effects, the optometrist should be prepared to manage them, either through direct intervention or referral to another practitioner (see Chapter 31).

As with mydriatics, the patient may be affected by photophobia and loss of accommodation. Therefore, patients must be monitored while in the office and on the premises and must be warned of the drug's effects while operating a vehicle or performing other tasks that pose a risk of injury to the patient or others. Documentation of this warning should be included in the patient record.

Interestingly, failure to employ cycloplegia for the purpose of prescribing spectacles for a young patient with latent hyperopia has resulted in a claim of negligence against an optometrist.[51] However, the toxicity of these agents, if they are used inappropriately, and their effects on vision, if no warning is given or no protection is provided, pose the greatest legal risks.

Although the toxic and allergic side effects of diagnostic pharmaceutical agents can be the cause of a malpractice claim, the side effects of therapeutic drugs are a much more likely source of litigation.

---

[c]The ability of patients to recall warnings is highly suspect, because several studies have revealed that patients, in fact, remember very little. See Robinson G, Merav A. Informed consent: Recall by patients tested postoperatively. Ann Thorac Surg 1976;22:209–212; Priluck IA, Robertson DM, Buettner H. What patients recall of the preoperative discussion after retinal detachment surgery. Am J Ophthalmol 1979;87:620–623; and Morgan LW, Schwab IR. Informed consent in senile cataract extraction. Arch Ophthalmol 1986;104:42–45.

Complications of Therapeutic Drug Use

The complications of therapeutic drug use are a leading cause of malpractice claims against ophthalmologists[7] and potentially pose a significant malpractice risk for optometrists.[3] Because drug use occurs outside the practitioner's office and may involve an extended time, there is greater opportunity for complications to arise, particularly those related to drug toxicity. If patient follow-up is not timely, the complications may go undetected, thus compounding the injury. Worst of all, if the practitioner fails to make the correct diagnosis, the treatment not only fails to remedy the patient's problem but also delays institution of the correct therapy. For these reasons optometrists who employ therapeutic agents face malpractice risks that differ from those encountered by optometrists who use diagnostic agents.

Negligence claims against ophthalmologists involving the use of therapeutic agents can be grouped into 3 categories: (1) misuse of steroids, (2) complications of glaucoma therapy, and (3) misdiagnosis, followed by institution of an inappropriate therapeutic regimen.[7,8] Each of these legal problems has important legal implications for optometrists.

Misuse of Steroids

The leading cause of drug-related claims against ophthalmologists is misuse of steroids, particularly those topically applied.[7] The usual situation is one in which the patient uses the drug for prolonged therapy, resulting in cataracts, open-angle glaucoma, or both.[52] Two legal issues are present in these cases. The first involves the practitioner's obligation to warn the patient of side effects as required by the doctrine of informed consent (see Chapter 33). Failure to satisfy this duty can result in a successful liability claim against the practitioner.[53] The prudent practitioner will also ensure that this warning is documented in the patient record.

The second issue concerns the patient's ability to obtain prescription refills, which is often a complex web of entanglements between the prescribing practitioner, the practitioner's staff, the patient, and the pharmacist filling the prescription. To reduce the opportunity for misunderstanding or mistake, the prescription should specify the drug quantity and the number of refills and should include a statement that these orders may not be changed.[7] Practitioners should always retain a copy of the prescription given to the patient (see Chapter 2).

Systemic steroids are also the cause of numerous negligence claims. These drugs have side effects that can result in serious injury, even death, and consequently must be used conservatively. Systemically administered drugs—with their risk of systemic complications—should not be used if a topical route of administration will suffice, and practitioners must be prepared to justify the selection of a systemic route of administration when complications result and a topical route of administration

was not employed first.[7,8] Whenever systemic steroids are prescribed, the practitioner must warn the patient of side effects, monitor the patient adequately so that preventable injuries can be detected, and document the care rendered.

Glaucoma Therapy

Legal claims arising from glaucoma therapy must be divided into two categories: (1) retinal detachments following initiation of miotic therapy, and (2) complications resulting from use of carbonic anhydrase inhibitors.

The use of miotics in myopic patients has been the cause of negligence claims when therapy has resulted in retinal detachment.[54] Patients who are at risk for detachment should be treated with nonmiotic agents initially, and to comply with the doctrine of informed consent, use of miotics should be preceded by a discussion with the patient of the risks and benefits. Patients should be examined carefully to rule out the presence of risk factors (e.g., lattice degeneration) that may increase the likelihood of a retinal detachment.

Carbonic anhydrase inhibitors such as acetazolamide have well-known side effects (e.g., renal calculi) that require an assessment of the benefits and risks before initiating therapy. If the practitioner cannot demonstrate that topically applied drugs would be inadequate to control the patient's glaucoma, the choice of a carbonic anhydrase inhibitor may be difficult to justify.[7,8] The risks of a systemic route of administration obligate the practitioner to discuss potential complications and to obtain an informed consent from the patient. Because of the prolonged nature of glaucoma therapy, the patient must be examined periodically, both to assess the effectiveness of treatment and to rule out the presence of drug-related complications. The prudent practitioner will note even negative findings in the record to document that a proper examination was performed.

Misdiagnosis

Unlike claims of misdiagnosis involving diagnostic agents (which usually concern intraocular disorders), allegations involving therapeutic agents usually concern the cornea and the anterior segment. Optometrists who undertake to treat diseases of the cornea and the external adnexa may be held to a medical standard of care and must be prepared to justify the treatment rendered accordingly. This area of therapeutic drug use is probably the one in which optometrists are most vulnerable to legal claims.

Litigation can arise out of misdiagnosis of corneal complications due to herpes simplex,[55] *Pseudomonas*,[56] fungal infections,[7] and corneal abrasions occurring in the contact lens population, particularly among patients fitted with extended wear lenses.[57] Optometrists must be certain to conform to the standard of care in making diagnoses, scheduling patient follow-up visits, and arranging consultations and referrals. Because complications can rapidly lead to permanent injuries and loss of visual acuity, optometrists must be vigilant when diagnosing and managing corneal and external disease. The treatment rendered should be documented with the same meticulous concern.

Documentation

The patient record is a vital aspect of any litigation in which the optometrist has been charged with negligence. A properly maintained record may offer an irrefutable defense; an inadequate record may make the optometrist's position indefensible. Recordkeeping is an important task that should not be neglected.[58–60] Although there are no legally established requirements for organizing or maintaining records, because of the episodic nature of much of the care rendered by optometrists (particularly when using therapeutic pharmaceutical agents), the problem-oriented record system is preferable.[61] Optometrists should record the patient's drug history, the drugs used for diagnosis or treatment, any appropriate warnings, and the outcome of the case if there are complications (Table 34.1).

For clinical and legal reasons, optometrists should be certain to document recalls and referrals in the following manner.

TABLE 34.1
Documentation of Drug Use

1. All drugs the patient is taking, including any drugs taken for prolonged periods that may have adverse effects on the eyes or vision
2. Previous allergic or toxic responses to any drugs, including ophthalmic drugs
3. Drugs employed by the optometrist for diagnostic or therapeutic purposes, including concentration and dosage; if therapeutic drugs are prescribed, a copy of the prescription should be retained
4. Allergic or toxic responses to any drugs administered, which should be conspicuously noted
5. Warnings concerning the risks of drug use that are communicated to the patient
6. Treatment or disposition of the patient if an adverse effect is experienced
7. Recalls and referrals or consultations

Recalls

If a patient requires follow-up care, a recall appointment will be necessary. Recalls should be scheduled for a specific date and time before the patient leaves the office, even if the date of the appointment is weeks or months away. The optometrist should note on the patient's record the reason for the recall and should be certain that the recall examination addresses the problem for which the patient is required to return. To minimize "no-show" appointments, it is best to contact the patient before the scheduled date to confirm the day and time of the appointment. In some instances a "no-show" patient may need to be contacted to determine why he or she failed to keep the appointment.[f]

Referrals

The preferable means of making a referral is to choose the practitioner and arrange the appointment before the patient has left the office. This information should be noted in the patient's record, along with any other pertinent data relative to the referral. If a referral letter is written, a copy of the letter should also be retained in the record. Because of the importance of documenting referrals,[62] clinicians should establish a "fail-safe" system of review that ensures the appropriate entries have been made. The omission of this information, if litigation should ensue, unalterably weakens an optometrist's defense.[62]

Consultations with other practitioners should be similarly scheduled and documented. Recordkeeping is a responsibility of clinical practice that cannot be emphasized too greatly.

References

1. Bowers SA. Precedent-setting professional liability claims involving optometrists. J Am Optom Assoc 1986;57:397–401.
2. Scholles J. A review of professional liability claims in optometry. J Am Optom Assoc 1986;57:764–766.
3. Classé, JG. Malpractice and optometry: A personal commentary. South J Optom 1987;5:26–31.
4. Classé JG. Optometrist's duty to test for glaucoma. South J Optom 1984;2:6–10.

[f]Although a practitioner is under no legal duty to contact patients who fail to keep appointments, there are circumstances under which follow-up may be wise. For example, a patient who is undergoing treatment with therapeutic agents and who is in need of further evaluation faces a much higher risk than a daily wear contact lens patient who fails to keep a 6-month recall appointment. Follow-up in the former case may prevent an injury—and a lawsuit.

5. Classé JG. Optometrist's duty to detect ocular tumors. South J Optom 1985;3:26–32.

6. Classé JG. Optometrist's duty to detect retinal detachment. South J Optom 1985;3:7–13.

7. Bettman JW. A review of 412 claims in ophthalmology. Int Ophthalmol Clin 1980;20:131–142.

8. Classé JG. Liability for use of ophthalmic pharmaceutical agents. South J Optom 1984;2:43–49.

9. National Association of Insurance Commissioners. Malpractice Claims, vol. 2, no. 2. Madison, WI: National Association of Insurance Commissioners, 1980.

10. Elmstrom G. Malpractice: What can O.D.s expect?. Opt J Rev Optom 1977;114:42–45.

11. *Black's Law Dictionary,* rev. ed. 4. St. Paul, MN: West, 1968.

12. Prosser WL. Law of torts, ed. 4. St. Paul, MN: West, 1971;139–235.

13. Prosser WL. Law of torts, ed. 4. St. Paul, MN: West, 1971;162–163.

14. Classé J. Liability and the primary care optometrist. J Am Optom Assoc 1986;57:926–929.

15. Guides to the evaluation of permanent impairment, ed 2. Chicago: American Medical Association, 1984;141–151.

16. *Reed v. Church,* 8 S.E. 2d 285 (Va. 1940).

17. *Trogun v. Fruchtman,* 209 N.W. 2d 297 (Wis. 1973).

18. *Yorston v. Pennell,* 153 A. 2d 255 (Pa. 1959).

19. Cox MS, Schepens CL, Freeman HM. Retinal detachment due to ocular contusion. Arch Ophthalmol 1966;76:678–685.

20. Alexander LJ, Scholles J. Clinical and legal aspects of pupillary dilation. J Am Optom Assoc 1987;58:432–437.

21. *Helling v. Carey,* 83 Wash. 2d 514, 519 P. 2d 981 (Wash. 1974).

22. *Gates v. Jensen,* 92 Wash. 2d 246, 595 P. 2d 919 (Wash. 1979).

23. *Harris v. Groth,* 99 Wash. 2d 438, 663 P. 2d 113 (Wash. 1983).

24. Wechsler S, Classé JG. *Helling v. Carey:* Caveat medicus (let the doctor beware). J Am Optom Assoc 1977;48:1526–1529.

25. Classé JG. *Helling* revisited: How the "tale" wagged the dog. J Am Optom Assoc 1987;58:343–345.

26. *McMahon v. Glixman,* 393 N.E. 2d 875 (Mass. 1979).

27. *Collins v. American Optometric Association,* 693 F. 2d 636 (7th Cir. 1982).

28. *Holmes v. Iwasa,* 104 Ida. 179, 657 P. 2d 476 (Idaho 1983).

29. Semes L, Gold A. Clinical and legal considerations in the diagnosis and management of ocular tumors. J Am Optom Assoc 1987;58:134–139.

30. *Fairchild v. Brian,* 354 So. 2d 675 (La. App. 1977).

31. 354 So. 2d at 679.

32. Linder B. Acute posterior vitreous detachment and its retinal complications. Acta Ophthalmol 1966;87:30–38.

33. Tasman WS. Posterior vitreous detachment and peripheral breaks. Trans Am Acad Ophthalmol Otolaryngol 1968;72:217–224.

34. *Whitt v. Columbus Cooperative Enterprises,* 64 Ohio St. 355, 415 N.E. 2d 985 (Ohio 1980).

35. Alexander LJ. Vision care for the patient with diabetes (editorial). J Am Optom Assoc 1987;58:872–873.

36. Lipson LG, ed. Diabetes mellitus in the elderly. Am J Med 1986;80:1–56.

37. *Steele v. United States,* 463 F. Supp 321 (D.C. Alaska 1978).

38. *Tempchin v. Sampson,* 262 Md. 156, 277 A. 2d 67 (Md. 1971).

39. *Kime v. Aetna,* 66 Ohio App. 277, 33 N.E. 2d 1008 (Ohio App. 1940).

40. *Wills v. Klingenbeck,* 455 So. 2d 806 (Ala. 1984).

41. Norden LC. Adverse reactions to topical ocular anesthetics. J Am Optom Assoc 1976;47:730–733.

42. Burns RP, Forster RK, Laibson P, Gibson IK. Chronic toxicity of local anesthetics on the cornea. In: Leopold IH, Burns RP, eds. Symposium on ocular therapy. New York: John Wiley & Sons, 1977;10:31–44.

43. Cockburn DM. Prevalence and significance of narrow anterior chamber angles in optometric practice. Am J Optom Physiol Opt 1981;58:171–175.

44. Keller JT. The risk of angle closure from the use of mydriatics. J Am Optom Assoc 1975;46:19–21.

45. *Graham v. Whitaker,* 321 S.E. 2d 40 (S.C. 1984).

46. *Truxillo v. Gentilly Medical Building, Inc.,* 225 So. 2d 488 (La. 1969).

47. *Welke v. Kuzilla,* 144 Mich. App. 245, 375 N.W. 2d 403 (Mich. App. 1985).

48. Gold AR. Failure to warn. J Am Optom Assoc 1986;57:317–319.

49. Classé JG. Optometrist's duty to warn of vision impairment. South J Optom 1986;4:66–69.

50. Gray LG. Avoiding adverse effects of cycloplegics in infants and children. J Am Optom Assoc 1979;50:465–470.

51. *Kahn v. Shaw,* 65 Ga. App. 563, 16 S.E. 2d 99 (Ga. App. 1941).

52. *Lorentzon v. Rowell,* 321 S.E. 2d 341 (Ga. App. 1984).

53. *Ortiz v. Allergan Pharmaceuticals,* 489 S.W. 2d 135 (Tex. Civ. App. 1972).

54. *Fykes v. Chatow,* docket no. 976896, Superior Court, Los Angeles County, Cal., 1974; reported in The Citation, 1975;30:120.

55. Classé JG, Harris MG. Liability and extended wear contact lenses. J Am Optom Assoc 1987;58:848–854.

56. Classé JG. Optometrist's liability for contact lenses. South J Optom 1986;4:52–57.

57. *Beaman v. Schwartz,* 738 S.W. 2d 632 (Tenn. App. 1986).

58. Scholles J. Documentation and record-keeping in clinical practice. J Am Optom Assoc 1986;57:141–143.

59. Miller PJ. Documentation as a defense to legal claims. J Am Optom Assoc 1986;57:144–145.

60. Classé JG. Record-keeping and documentation in clinical practice. South J Optom 1987;5:11–25.

61. Scope of practice: Patient care and management manual. St. Louis: American Optometric Association, 1986.

62. Gerber P. How to blow your own malpractice defense. Optom Man 1981;17:19–25.

CHAPTER 35

Product Liability

John G. Classé

Drug-related product liability claims involving clinicians are rare. Because drugs are customarily sold to patients by pharmacists, on the prescription of a duly licensed practitioner, if the patient suffers an injury because the drug is "defective," it is the manufacturer or seller of the drug who is held liable. However, clinicians may become defendants because the drug was inappropriately or improperly prescribed or because there was insufficient follow-up of the patient's condition while the patient was taking the drug (see Chapter 34). Clinicians may also be charged with failing to comply with the doctrine of informed consent by inadequately warning the patient of drug-related side effects (see Chapter 33). Therefore, optometrists—as clinicians who prescribe and dispense drugs—should be familiar with the requirements of product liability law, since the adverse effects of a drug may precipitate a legal dispute among the patient, the pharmacist, and the drug manufacturer, to which the optometrist is a party.

An example case[1] can be used to illustrate a typical product liability claim. A patient who was severely allergic to a variety of substances was treated by a physician who prescribed an extensive course of therapy, including steroids taken topically, orally, and by injection. After more than 20 years of treatment, the patient developed osteoporosis and bilateral cataracts, which were removed surgically. He subsequently sued the manufacturer of the steroids, alleging that the drug was a defective product because the package inserts did not warn specifically enough of its dangerous side effects. He also sued the physician for negligence, alleging that the physician had failed to warn him of the risks associated with the use of steroids and had inadequately monitored the effects of treatment.

Because drug-related side effects may provide the motivation for a lawsuit, optometrists should be familiar with the ophthalmic drugs that have been the subject of product liability claims. This chapter will describe these ophthalmic drugs, the theory of product liability, and how together they may be applied to the practice of optometry.

Basis for Product Liability

Product liability law is an attempt to reduce the economic impact of product-caused injuries on consumers. The underlying theory is that the designer, manufacturer, or seller of a product is better able to absorb the economic loss—through the purchase of liability insurance, which becomes part of the cost of the product—than is the injured consumer, who suffers lost time from work and the cost of medical and hospital bills as well as the possibility of impairment. Product liability claims allow the consumer to recover these costs and to receive compensation for both temporary and permanent injuries.

If a product is being used for its customary and intended purpose, without having undergone substantial change in the condition in which it was sold, and the product injures a consumer as a result of defective design or manufacture, then the designer, manufacturer, or seller bears the legal responsibility for the consumer's injury as a matter of law.[2] This rule applies even though the designer, manufacturer, or seller has exercised all possible care in the preparation and sale of the product. The distinction between product liability law and negligence is made most apparent by the "strict liability" of the former: The standard of care is no longer the legal measure; rather, it is the "defective" character of the product that establishes the defendant's liability.

Proof that a drug is "defective" requires evidence that it is unreasonably dangerous for the purpose sold or, alternatively, that it does not meet the expectations of an ordinary consumer as to its safety. Injury caused by the side effects of a drug, however, will not create an action for which damages may be awarded if the manufacturer has adequately warned of the known side effects. In a representative case,[3] a patient who received chloroquine over an 8-year period for the treatment of systemic lupus erythematosus developed retinopathy and ultimately became almost totally blind. She sued the drug manufacturer for failure to warn, and the company defended the claim by producing evidence that warnings had been issued after investigators had established a scientific basis for attributing the retinal changes to the drug. These warnings were not issued, however, until years after the publication of the first case reports that linked the drug to ocular side effects. The trial court found in favor of the manufacturer, but the decision was reversed on appeal, with the court holding that the manufacturer failed to issue a timely warning. A similar conclusion has been reached in other cases.[4,5]

The manufacturer's duty to warn extends to the prescriber of the drug and not to the patient.[6] For example, a patient who had taken thioridazine (Mellaril) for a psychiatric disorder experienced a pigmentary retinopathy so severe that she became legally blind.[7] She sued the manufacturer, alleging that the warning of drug side effects was inadequate. The manufacturer's defense was that the risk of pigmentary retinopathy was well known, that this risk had been communicated to physicians for more than 20 years, and that the warning (supplied on the package insert) was sufficient. The jury found in favor of the manufacturer and the patient appealed, but the appellate court upheld the decision, noting that the drug manufacturer's duty was to provide an adequate warning to the physician and not to her.[7]

Because the clinician must communicate the warning to the patient (required by the doctrine of informed consent), optometrists are legally obligated to understand the side effects of any drugs that are prescribed.[8] Optometrists must stay abreast of reports in the literature and warnings from drug manufacturers and must explain these risks to patients before initiating treatment.[9]

The duty to warn also extends to the side effects of drugs administered systemically. A series of cases has delineated the obligation to warn patients of drugs that will impair operation of a motor vehicle and has resulted in the imposition of liability against practitioners for failing to fulfill this obligation, including cases in which the patient injures a third party.[10,11] For example, a bus driver who was given a prescription for the antihistamine tripelennamine (Pyribenzamine) by a physician became groggy and drowsy after taking a tablet before work and "blacked out or went to sleep" while driving, causing his bus to strike a telephone pole and injure a passenger.[12] In the resulting lawsuit, the passenger alleged that the physician was negligent in failing to warn the driver of the effects of the drug. Although the claim was dismissed by the trial court, it was upheld on appeal. The appellate court ruled that even if a jury found the driver to be negligent, the physician could also be held liable if the jury found he had failed to warn of the side effects of the drug.[12]

A common source of information concerning the risks of drug use is the package insert that accompanies the drug. The package insert also describes the recommended dosage and treatment regimen for the drug. Optometrists should be familiar with this information and should be prepared to justify any deviation from these recommendations.[13] The risk of side effects and the benefit to be obtained must be discussed with the patient before an informed consent that meets legal requirements can be secured. Because the treatment of eye disease raises the possibility that a court will impose a medical standard of care on a defendant optometrist,[14] deviation from a recommended treatment regimen described in the package insert should be undertaken only with clear clinical justification.

Another aspect of this obligation concerns the management of adverse reactions. Practitioners are fiduciaries and owe the patient a duty of affirmative disclosure, which means that not only misleading statements but also silence may constitute a breach of the practitioner's obligation.[15] An example case[16] will illustrate this principle. A patient who complained of chronic eyelid problems that caused numerous hordeola was treated by an ophthalmologist with Inflamase 1/8%. The treatment was successful, but 2 years after therapy began a pharmacist mistakenly refilled the prescription with Inflamase 1%, which caused blurred vision and pain due to disruption of the corneal epithelium. Afterwards the ophthalmologist avoided the patient's inquiries about the effects of the medication on his vision. Ultimately the patient sued the drug manufacturer, alleging that the product was defective, and the ophthalmologist, claiming that he was negligent and that his conduct constituted fraud. Although the trial court found that the statute of limitations barred the claim, on appeal the decision was reversed, with the appellate court ruling that the ophthalmologist's conduct in avoiding the patient's questions could not be used as a basis on which to defeat the patient's claim as a matter of law.[16]

The nexus among drug side effects, the duty to warn, and the torts of product liability and negligence makes it necessary for clinicians to recognize those drugs that have been the cause of legal claims in order to take the steps necessary to minimize the risk of injury—and litigation.

Ophthalmic Drugs and Liability Claims

The ophthalmic drugs that have been the most frequent causes of product liability and negligence claims are (1) acetazolamide, (2) echothiophate iodide, (3) hydrocortisone, (4) neomycin sulfate with dexamethasone sodium phosphate, (5) prednisolone acetate with phenylephrine hydrochloride, and (6) tropicamide. Cases will be used to illustrate the basis for legal claims involving these drugs.

Acetazolamide

This carbonic anhydrase inhibitor is used in the treatment of glaucoma (see Chapters 7 and 29). A known side effect of prolonged use is the formation of kidney stones.

A glaucoma patient who had been using Diamox for many years was hospitalized twice within 2 years for kidney stones.[17] After the second hospitalization another drug was substituted for the acetazolamide, and the patient's intraocular pressure was well controlled without further complications. The patient then sued the physician who had prescribed the Diamox, alleging that he was negligent, and this claim was eventually settled for an undisclosed sum. She also sued the drug manufacturer, alleging that there was a failure to warn users of the drug of its potential side effects. However, the manufacturer was held not to be liable, the court finding that the manufacturer had satisfied the legal duty to warn the physician and that there was no legal duty to warn the patient.[17]

Echothiophate Iodide

This strong miotic is used in the treatment of open-angle glaucoma when the disease does not respond to more conventional forms of therapy (see Chapters 3 and 29). A suspected side effect of treatment is retinal detachment, particularly in "at risk" patients, such as those with high myopia.[18]

A patient who had received glaucoma therapy for 8 years was changed to Phospholine Iodide.[19] Three weeks later he began seeing "spots" before his eyes, and 4 days later he suffered an acute loss of vision. Because the physicians he consulted were unable to see him immediately, there was a week's delay before the diagnosis of retinal detachment was made. Surgery was not successful, and the patient filed suit against the manufacturer of the drug and the physicians who had prescribed it. Although the drug manufacturer denied that there was a causal relationship between the use of echothiophate and the detachment, the patient's product liability claim was settled before trial. After a jury trial a substantial judgment was awarded to the patient for the negligence claim.[19]

Hydrocortisone

This anti-inflammatory agent is found in a number of ophthalmic drugs and is a well-documented cause of open-angle glaucoma when used for an extended time.

A 10-year-old boy was given Cortisporin by an ophthalmologist to treat a rash that affected the patient's eyelids.[20] The child's mother administered the drug for 15 months before it was discovered that he had bilateral open-angle glaucoma that caused loss of vision in one eye and severe visual impairment in the other. A lawsuit was filed against the prescribing physician and the pharmacy that had supplied the drug, and the case was settled before trial for a substantial amount.[20]

Neomycin Sulfate with Dexamethasone Sodium Phosphate

This antibiotic-steroid combination is applied topically for numerous ocular disorders. Known side effects of prolonged use are cataracts and open-angle glaucoma.

A pediatrician prescribed NeoDecadron for a young girl who had conjunctivitis, and the child's mother used the ointment intermittently for 2 years, during which time the prescription was refilled 6 times.[21] By the end of this period the child had developed bilateral open-angle glaucoma that caused loss of vision. During the time the child was receiving treatment the physician did not monitor her intraocular pressure. A sizable judgment was awarded the child by the trial court.[21]

Prednisolone Acetate with Phenylephrine Hydrochloride

This steroid-vasoconstrictor combination is applied topically to treat various ocular inflammations. Long-term use of the drug is known to cause open-angle glaucoma.

An ophthalmologist prescribed Prednefrin 1/8% solution for conjunctivitis, and 1 month later the patient's pharmacist called the physician to ask if he could refill the prescription in 2 bottles (the patient requested 1 for work and 1 for home).[22] The ophthalmologist gave his permission but offered no advice concerning future refills. The pharmacist continued to refill the prescription over 5 months, and at an examination 1 year later the patient was found to have elevated intraocular pressure. Eventually the patient was diagnosed as having open-angle glaucoma and cataracts, and she filed suit against the ophthalmologist, the pharmacist, and the drug manufacturer. During the trial the patient settled her claims against the ophthalmologist and the pharmacist, but the jury found in favor of the drug manufacturer, holding that the patient had misused the drug.[22]

Tropicamide

This mydriatic and cycloplegic agent is used to dilate the pupils. It causes photophobia and loss of accommodation.

An elderly patient who was to be examined by an ophthalmologist received drops of Mydriacyl from a nurse and then was seated in the waiting room without being informed of the drug's effects.[23] When she was called for examination, her blurred vision caused her to fall as she attempted to get up from the chair and cross the room. Despite her complaints of pain, the physician continued the examination, and after she insisted she could not walk to leave the office, an ambulance was called and she was taken to the hospital. She was found to have fractured her hip and spent considerable time recovering. She sued the ophthalmologist for negligence, and the trial court awarded her both compensatory and punitive damages.[23]

Documentation

Documentation of patient care is essential to the defense of legal claims. If pharmaceutical agents are used, the clinician should ensure that the patient record includes an adequate history, a description of the drugs used, any warnings communicated to the patient, and an explanation of the treatment rendered if the patient experiences allergic or toxic side effects (see Chapter 34).

If this information is recorded, the clinician will be able to substantiate the treatment rendered, and as long as that treatment has been in compliance with the standard of care, the clinician will defeat an action for damages. Inadequate documentation, however, may produce the opposite result.[24,25] Clinicians should take the time to maintain accurate, thorough, contemporaneous records that reflect the care and attention given to each patient.

References

1. *Hill v. Squibb and Sons,* 592 P. 2d 1383 (Mont. 1979).
2. Section 402A of the Restatement of Torts, 2nd. (may not be applicable in all jurisdictions).
3. *Basko v. Sterling Drug, Inc.,* 416 F. 2d 417 (D.C. Conn. 1969).
4. *Krug v. Sterling Drug, Inc.,* 416 S.W. 2d 143 (Mo. 1967).
5. *Kershaw v. Sterling Drug, Inc.,* 415 F. 2d 1005 (5th Cir. 1969).
6. Dixon MG. Drug product liability. New York: Matthew Bender,1974; §9.01–9.09.
7. *Hatfield v. Sandoz-Wander, Inc.,* 464 N.E. 2d 1105 (Ill. App. 1984).
8. Dixon MG. Drug product liability. New York: Matthew Bender, 1974: §7.01–7.26.
9. Classé JG. Liability for use of ophthalmic pharmaceutical agents. South J Optom 1984;2:43–49.
10. Gold AR. Failure to warn. J Am Optom Assoc 1986;57:317–319.
11. Classé JG. Optometrist's duty to warn of vision impairment. South J Optom 1986;4:66–69.
12. *Kaiser v. Suburban Transportation System,* 65 Wash. 2d 461, 398 P. 2d 14, *modified* 401 P. 2d 350 (Wash. 1965).
13. Bettman JW. A review of 412 claims in ophthalmology. Int Ophthalmol Clin 1980; 20:131–142.
14. *Fairchild v. Brian,* 354 So. 2d 675 (La App. 1977).
15. Holder AR: Medical malpractice law. New York: John Wiley & Sons, 1975;225.
16. *Lorentzon v. Rowell,* 321 S.E. 2d 341 (Ga. App. 1984).
17. *Bacardi v. Holzman,* 182 N.J. Super. 422, 442 A. 2d 617 (N.J. 1981).
18. Bettman JW. A review of 412 claims in ophthalmology. Int Ophthalmol Clin 1980;20:136–137.
19. *Fykes v. Chatow,* docket no. 976896, Superior Court, Los Angeles County, Cal., 1974. Reported in The Citation 1975;30:120.
20. *Kong v. Clay-Grant Pharmacy,* docket no. 619350, Superior Court, San Francisco County, Cal., 1972. Reported in The Citation 1973;26:122.
21. *Aetna Casualty and Surety Co. of Illinois v. Medical Protective Co. of Ft. Wayne, Indiana,* 575 F. Supp. 901 (Ill. D.C. 1983).

22. *Ortiz v. Allergan Pharmaceuticals,* 489 S.W. 2d 135 (Tex. Civ. App. 1972).
23. *Graham v. Whitaker,* 321 S.E. 2d 40 (S.C. 1984).
24. Scholles J. Documentation and record keeping in clinical practice. J Am Optom Assoc 1986;57:141–143.

25. Classé JG. Record keeping and documentation in clinical practice. South J Optom 1987;5:11–25.

Index